Core Psychiatry

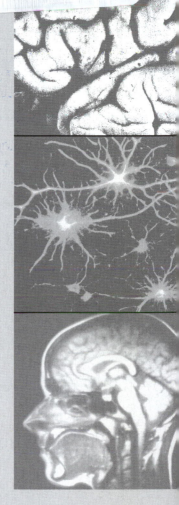

This book is dedicated to our families

Commissioning Editor: Michael Parkinson
Project Development Manager: Lynn Watt
Project Manager: Nancy Arnott
Designer: Erik Bigland

Core Psychiatry

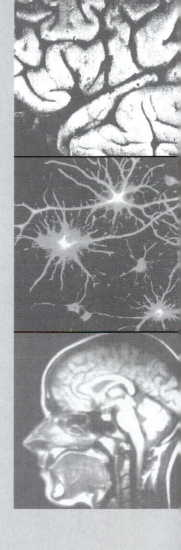

Pádraig Wright LRCP&SI LM MB BCh BAO(NUI) MRCPsych MD
Senior Lecturer (Honorary), Department of Psychological Medicine,
Institute of Psychiatry, London

Julian Stern BA MB ChB FRCPsych
Consultant Psychiatrist in Psychotherapy,
St Mark's Hospital, Harrow

Michael Phelan BSc MB BS MRCPsych
Consultant Psychiatrist, Department of psychiatry,
Charing Cross Hospital, London

SECOND EDITION

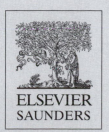

ELSEVIER
SAUNDERS

EDINBURGH LONDON NEW YORK OXFORD PHILADELPHIA ST LOUIS SYDNEY TORONTO 2005

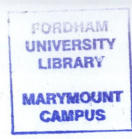
**ELSEVIER
SAUNDERS**

List publication years of previous editions:
First edition 2000
Second edition 2005

ISBN 0 7020 2718 9

British Library Cataloguing in Publication Data
A catalogue record for this book is available from the British
Library

Library of Congress Cataloging in Publication Data
A catalog record for this book is available from the Library of
Congress

Note
Medical knowledge is constantly changing. Standard safety
precautions must be followed, but as new research and clinical
experience broaden our knowledge, changes in treatment and
drug therapy may become necessary or appropriate. Readers are
advised to check the most current product information provided
by the manufacturer of each drug to be administered to verify the
recommended dose, the method and duration of administration,
and contraindications. It is the responsibility of the practitioner,
relying on experience and knowledge of the patient, to determine
dosages and the best treatment for each individual patient.
Neither the Publisher nor the author/editor/contributor (delete as
appropriate) assumes any liability for any injury and/or damage
to persons or property arising from this publication.
The Publisher

 ELSEVIER your source for books,
journals and multimedia
in the health sciences

www.elsevierhealth.com

The
Publisher's
policy is to use
**paper manufactured
from sustainable forests**

Typeset by IMH(Cartrif), Loanhead, Scotland
Printed in Spain

PREFACE TO SECOND EDITION

Our intention in producing the first edition of *Core Psychiatry* was to provide a single volume postgraduate textbook for candidates sitting the examinations for Membership of the Royal College of Psychiatrists. We have tried to remain faithful to this intention while preparing this second edition. Thankfully however, we have been thwarted in this intention by the current pace of discovery and development in psychiatry. This is such that every chapter (including the chapter on Clinical Neuroanatomy) has required considerable revision and the book has grown overall by five chapters.

Like the first edition of *Core Psychiatry*, this second edition is divided into three parts. The first two sections describe the sciences that underpin the practice of psychiatry (*The foundations of psychiatry*) and the clinical syndromes and their treatment, along with the health care settings, with which psychiatrists must be familiar (*Clinical psychiatry*). The final section (*Diagnosis, investigation and treatment*) provides a description of the clinical evaluation and investigation of patients and of current psychotherapeutic, psychopharmacological and other treatments. Again like the first edition, the authors contributing to this second edition are or have been associated with the Maudsley Hospital and Institute of Psychiatry or with other leading London teaching hospitals.

It is our hope that this second edition of *Core Psychiatry* will prove a useful addition to the bookshelves (and better still the desktops and briefcases) of all students of psychiatry, be they trainee or consultant psychiatrists, clinical psychologists, psychiatric nurses or senior medical students.

PREFACE TO FIRST EDITION

This book originated from a highly successful revision course for candidates sitting the Parts I and II examinations for Membership of the Royal College of Psychiatrists that two of us (JS, MP) have organized twice yearly in London since 1994 and from the suggestion by one of us (PW) that the knowledge and expertise of the lecturers on this revision course should be collected in a single volume.

Core Psychiatry is divided into three parts. Part I (The Foundations of Psychiatry) describes the historical development of psychiatry and the basic sciences with which all psychiatrists must be familiar, including the rapidly expanding field of psychiatric genetics, and discusses the skills required when reviewing scientific publications. Part II (Clinical Psychiatry) describes the major psychiatric syndromes and disorders, including the sequelae of childhood sexual abuse, and provides a detailed discussion of community psychiatry. Finally, Part III (Diagnosis, Investigation and Treatment) describes how patients should be interviewed and examined and how a diagnosis should be made, provides accounts of contemporary psychotherapeutic, psychopharmacological and other treatments, and discusses contemporary investigational techniques.

All of the authors contributing to *Core Psychiatry* are, or have been, associated with the world-renowned Maudsley Hospital/Institute of Psychiatry or with other London teaching hospitals and most now hold senior clinical or academic appointments in the UK, Ireland or Iceland. They have assumed little previous knowledge of psychiatry and have attempted to provide both introductory and in-depth coverage of their topics.

Thus while *Core Psychiatry* is primarily intended as a postgraduate textbook for candidates sitting the Parts I and II examinations for Membership of the Royal College of Psychiatrists and other similar examinations, it is also a suitable text for postgraduate medical and psychology students, for senior undergraduate medical students and for nursing students. *Core Psychiatry* will also serve as an excellent single volume reference for newly appointed consultant psychiatrists and for other specialists such as neurologists and general practitioners.

PW   2000
JS
MP

CONTRIBUTORS

Sadgun Bhandari MB BS MRCPsych
Consultant Psychiatrist
East Ham Memorial Hospital
London, UK

Kamaldeep Bhui MB BS MRCPsych
Professor of Social & Epidemiological Psychiatry
Queen Mary's School of Medicine & Dentistry
London, UK

Peter Byrne MB MRCPsych
Senior Lecturer and Honorary Consultant Psychiatrist
Mascalls Park Hospital
Brentwood, UK

David Castle MB MRCPsych PhD
Professor of Psychiatry
University of Melbourne
Victoria
Australia

Anthony Cleare BSc MB BS MRCPsych PhD
Senior Lecturer in Affective Disorders and Consultant
Psychiatrist
Section of Neurobiology of Mood Disorders
Institute of Psychiatry and Maudsley Hospital
Weston Education Centre
London, UK

John Cookson D Phil FRCP FRCPsych
Consultant Psychiatrist
The Royal London Hospital (St Clements)
London, UK

John Cooney MD MRCPI MRCPsych MD
Consultant Psychiatry
St Patrick's Hospital
Dublin
Ireland

Aiden Corvin MRCPsych
Lecturer in Psychiatry
Trinity College Dublin
Neuropsychiatric Genetics Group
Institute of Molecular Medicine
St James' Hospital
Dublin, Ireland

Michael Crawford MD
Professor of Medicine
Associate Chief of Cardiology for Clinical Programs
Division of Cardiology
University of California
San Francisco
USA

Martin Feakins MRCPsych
Consultant Psychiatrist
North Essex Mental Health Partnership NHS Trust
Colchester

Michael Gill MD MRCPsych FTCD
Associate Professor of Psychiatry
Trinity Centre for Health Sciences
St James' Hospital
Ireland

Nick Goddard BSc MB BS MRCPsych
Consultant/Senior Lecturer Child and Adolescent
Psychiatry
Lewisham Child and Family Psychiatry Centre
London, UK

Sarah Helps BSc D Clin Psy C Psychol
Clinical Psychologist
South London and Maudsley NHS Trust
London, UK

Claire Henderson MPH MRCPsych
Training Fellow in Health Services Research
Section of Community Psychiatry (PriSM)
Institute of Psychiatry
London

Matthew Hotopf MRCPsych MSc PhD
Clinical Senior Lecturer in Psychological Medicine
Department of Psychological Medicine
Weston Education Centre
London, UK

Louise Howard BSc MPhil MRCP MRCPsych
Research Fellow and Honorary Lecturer
Department of Psychiatry
Institute of Psychiatry
London, UK

Assen Jablensky MD DMSc FRCPsych FRANZCP
Professor of Psychiatry
School of Psychiatry and Clinical Neurosciences
The University of Western Australia
Australia

Mark Jones MB BS MRCPsych FRSA
Consultant Psychiatrist
Directorate of Mental Healthcare for Older People
Goodmayes Hospital
Goodmayes, UK

Anne Lingford-Hughes MA PhD BM BCh MRCPsych
Senior Lecturer in Biological Psychiatry and Addiction
Division of Psychiatry
University of Bristol
Bristol, UK

James Lucey MD FRCPI MRCPsych PhD
Senior Lecturer in Psychiatry
St Patrick's Hospital
Dublin
Ireland

Paul Mackin MB MRCPsych
Academic Specialist Registrar
School of Neurology, Neurobiology and Psychiatry
Royal Victoria Infirmary
Newcastle upon Tyne, UK

Sarah Majid MB BChir MRCPsych
Special Registrar in Adult Mental Illness
Maudsley Hospital
London, UK

Carine Minne MB BCh BAO DRCOG MRCPsych
Consultant Psychiatrist in Forensic Psychotherapy
Broadmoor Hospital and Portman NHS Clinic
London, UK

Joanna Moncrieff
Senior Lecturer/Honorary Consultant Psychiatrist
Mascalls Park Hospital
Brentwood, UK

Stirling Moorey BSc MB BS FRCPsych
Consultant Psychiatrist in Cognitive Behaviour Therapy
Bethlem and Maudsley NHS Trust
London, UK

Jean O'Hara MB MRCPsych
Consultant Psychiatrist in Learning Disability
South London and the Maudsley NHS Trust and the Estia Centre
Guy's Hospital
London, UK

Oyedeji Oyebode MB BS Dip Criminol M Phil MRCPsych
Clinical Director
Consultant and Honorary Senior Lecturer in Forensic Psychiatry
Forensic Mental Health Services
Springfield University Hospital
London, UK

Lisa Page BSc MBBS MRCPsych
Clinical Research Fellow and Honorary Specialist Registrar
Academic Department of Psychological Medicine
Weston Education Centre
London, UK

David Perahia BSc MB MRCPsych
Clinical Neurosciences
Eli Lilly
Europe

Michael Phelan BSc MB BS MRCPsych
Consultant Psychiatrist
Department of Psychiatry
Charing Cross Hospital
London, UK

Martin Prince MD MSc MRCPsych
Professor of Epidemiology
Institute of Psychiatry and
London School of Hygiene and Tropical Medicine
London, UK

Ajit Shah MB ChB MRCPsych
Consultant in Psychiatry of Old Age
West London Mental Healthcare Trust
Southall, UK

Thordur Sigmundsson MD MRCPsych
Consultant Psychiatrist
Department of Psychiatry
The University Hospital (Landspitalinn)
Reykjavik
Iceland

Shubuladè Smith MB BS MRCPsych
Department of Medicine
Maudsley Hospital
London, UK

Shankarnarayan Srinath BSc MB MRCPsych
Consultant Psychotherapist
Young People's Service
Psychological Treatment Services
Addenbrooke's NHS Trust
Cambridge

Julian Stern BA MB ChB FRCPsych
Consultant Psychiatrist in Psychotherapy
St Mark's Hospital
North West London NHS Trust
Harrow, UK

Sue Stuart-Smith BA MBBS MRCPsych
Consultant Psychotherapist
St Albans and Dacorum
Hertfordshire Partnership Trust
UK

Elizabeth Tovey MA MBBS BSc(Hons)
Senior House Officer
West London Mental Healthcare Trust
Southall, UK

Janet Treasure PhD FRCP FRCPsych
Consultant Psychiatrist
Eating Disorders Unit
Institute of Psychiatry
London, UK

Séan Whyte MA BM BCh MRCPsych
Specialist Registrar in Psychiatry
Chelsea and Westminster Hospital
London, UK

Adam Winstock MBBS BSc MSc MRCP MRCPsych FAChAM
Area Clinical Director Drug Health Services
South Western Sydney Area Health Service
Sydney
Australia

Pádraig Wright LRCP&SI LM MB BCh BAO(NUI) MRCPsych MD
Honorary Senior Lecturer
Division of Psychological Medicine
Institute of Psychiatry
London, UK

Eli Lilly
Clinical Neurosciences
Europe

Allan Young MB BCh MRCPsych PhD
Professor of Psychiatry
School of Neurology, Neurobiology and Psychiatry
Royal Victoria Infirmary
Newcastle upon Tyne, UK

CONTENTS

PART 1
The foundations of psychiatry

Part 2
Clinical psychiatry

Part 3
Diagnosis, investigation and treatment

The foundations of psychiatry

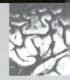

A brief history of psychiatry

John Cookson

INTRODUCTION

Many lessons can be learned about the treatment of mental illness from the earlier history of psychiatry. Furthermore, it is useful to consider the use of modern drug treatment and contemporary psychological therapy in the light of the effects of their predecessors. Edward Shorter's *A History of Psychiatry* (1997) and Roy Porter's *The Greatest Benefit to Mankind* (1997) provide excellent comprehensive accounts by professional historians of much that is discussed in this chapter, which summarizes the history of psychiatry over the last 7000 years.

ANCIENT AND CLASSICAL TIMES

Neolithic skulls dating from 5000 BC show evidence of trephination, the oldest known form of surgery, which was carried out in ancient times on living patients to release evil spirits or to relieve skull fractures, headaches, convulsions or insanity. The procedure must often have been fatal, but some skulls show bony callus formation, indicative of survival. We know little of what other desperate remedies were attempted by stone-age man, as herbal medicine began its evolution. Archaeological evidence of the use of psychotropic substances in Mexico dates from 8500 BC, with the mescal bean and peyote cactus; samples of peyote containing mescaline from a cave in Texas have been carbon-dated to 5700 years ago (Bruhn et al. 2002).

Medicine developed in Mesopotamia and Egypt almost simultaneously and descriptions of epilepsy, dementia and psychotic disorders in the form of spiritual possession are available from both cultures, as indeed they are from the Old Testament of the Bible. Treatment at the time appears to have involved the use of drugs (derived from plants, minerals and animal parts), diets, magical spells and incantations.

Hippocrates (460–377 BC) is regarded as the father of medicine and was among the first to challenge the view that disease was punishment sent from the gods. He especially ridiculed the idea that epilepsy was a 'sacred disease'. Hippocratic texts propounded the notion of four 'humors', of which black bile was associated with melancholia. This broad explanatory scheme (elaborated by Galen, a Greek of the first century AD) survived to some extent until the 19th century and probably impeded scientific advance.

Mania, melancholia and paranoia were prominent categories in Greek medicine. The writings of Aretaeus (from Cappodocia in Turkey in about 150 AD) certainly contain descriptions resembling modern depression and mania. However, it is very difficult to relate ancient accounts of mental illness (or even those from 100 years ago!) to their counterparts in modern diagnostic systems.

THE MIDDLE AGES

Mentally ill people were the responsibility of their family or community and were often excluded from general society. Mental illness was widely regarded as a spiritual affliction associated with witchcraft or possession by the Devil. This led to the burning of mentally ill people as witches during the Inquisition, to religious institutions becoming responsible for caring for mad people, and to the use of exorcism as a treatment. Thus Bethlem Hospital in London was founded in 1247 to care for the insane and was run by a religious order. 'Shock' was also used in various forms.

THE RENAISSANCE AND THE REFORMATION

The French philosopher and antipsychiatrist, Foucault (1926–1984), has written of the alienation and plight of the insane in these periods, although the historical basis for his statements seems slender (Foucault 1961).

During the Renaissance, at least in literature and painting, the mentally ill were treated with curiosity and fear or even romanticized, but were still excluded from general society and displaced or left to wander.

In the 17th century, mental illness began to rank as a problem of the cities. Places of confinement were developed which grouped the poor and the unemployed with criminals and the mentally ill. Workhouses were first established during the Elizabethan era, more from concern about the disruptive social effects of vagrancy than to administer charitable welfare. Houses of correction (bridewells) existed in England from 1575 for the punishment of vagabonds and relief of the poor. The Poor Law of 1601 made local parishes responsible for electing overseers to provide relief for the sick and work for the able-bodied poor in workhouses. An Act of 1670 gave an increasing sense of a duty of assistance, coupled with the view that work was the cure for idleness and poverty.

In France a decree of 1656 created establishments (*Hôpital General*), to which the poor 'in whatever state they may be' could be assigned. One such was the Salpetrière (previously an arsenal) in Paris. In 1676, an edict of the King required that a *Hôpital General* be established in each city of France. They were not medical establishments, and the Church was excluded from their administration. Within such places, when the insane became dangerous, their rages were dealt with by mechanical restraint, iron chains, cuffs and bars, leading Foucault to conclude that they were treated as animals, or wild beasts.

THE ASYLUM AND MORAL THERAPY

The history of 'psychiatry' began with the custodial asylum – an institution to confine raging individuals who were dangerous or a nuisance. The discovery that the institution itself could have a therapeutic function led to the birth of psychiatry as a medical speciality. This notion can be traced to clinicians such as William Battie (St Luke's, 1751), Chiarugi (Florence, 1785) and Pinel (Paris, 1795), and lay people such as William Tuke (1796), a Quaker tea merchant who founded the Retreat in York. Such a development was in keeping with the style of thinking of the Age of Enlightenment (that ended after the French revolution in 1789), with its religious scepticism and its quest for understanding. Pinel (at the Salpetrière for women and the Bicetre for men), in particular, anticipated several trends, abolishing the use of restraining chains and recognizing a group of 'curable lunatics' (mainly with melancholia or mania without delusions), for whom a more humanitarian approach in an 'institution morale' seemed to be therapeutic.

The term 'psychiatry' was first used in 1808 by Reil, a professor of medicine in Germany, to describe the evolving discipline, although its practitioners were known as alienists (those who treated mental alienation) until the 20th century.

During the 18th century, there had been a growing trade in lunacy throughout Europe. In Britain, for example, the insane were confined to private madhouses, to which physicians had limited access and input. In 1788, King George III suffered a bout of mental illness for which eventually he received attention from Francis Willis, a 'mad-doctor' renowned for his piercing stare. The constitutional implications were considerable, and parliament subsequently instituted a committee to enquire into this and into the care of the mentally ill in general.

The therapeutic asylums, which sprang up in the 19th century, had in common a routine of work and activity, and an approach by the staff encompassed in the term 'moral therapy' and variously described as 'a mildness of manner and expression, an attention to their narrative and seeming acquiescence in its truth' (Haslam, Bedlam, 1809), 'the soothing voice of friendship' (Burrows, London, 1828) and 'encouraging esteem . . . conducive to a salutary habit of self-restraint' (Samuel Tuke, York, 1813). Uplifting architecture, as well as access to sunlight and the opportunity to work in the open air, were also valued.

Many of these institutions had charismatic directors and employed attendants who could be trusted not to beat the patients. Reil (1803) described the qualities of a good psychiatrist as having 'perspicacity, a talent for observation, intelligence, good-will, persistence, patience, experience, an imposing physique and a countenance that commands respect'. These are recognizable ingredients contributing to a placebo effect, and most of the physical treatments at their disposal were largely that: purgatives, enemas, blood letting (advocated for example for mania by Benjamin Rush, the founding father of American medicine, 1812) and emetics, aimed to 'draw out' nervous irritants ('catharsis').

During the 19th century the confining of patients to an asylum passed from an unusual procedure born of grave necessity, to society's first response when dealing with psychotic illness. Therapeutic asylums were built on a vast scale as politicians responded to the claims of the early enthusiasts. Unfortunately, while the doctors had no effective treatments, the asylums were destined to accumulate more and more incurable patients, leaving the staff overwhelmed, demoralized, and with insufficient time or conviction to sustain their 'moral' approach. The situation was exacerbated by an increase in the numbers of mentally ill people, especially through neurosyphilis and alcoholism, and by the increasing reluctance of families in industrialized society to tolerate their mentally ill relatives.

In 1894 the American neurologist Silas Weir Mitchell told asylum physicians that they had lost contact with the rest of medicine, and that their treatments were 'a sham'. In Britain, apart from the Maudsley Hospital, which opened in 1923 for teaching and research and for the treatment of recently ill patients, asylum psychiatry remained virtually divorced from the rest of medicine until the 1930s.

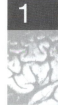

ACADEMIC PSYCHIATRY

During the 19th century many developments occurred in academic centres in Germany where the new techniques of neuroanatomy (Wernicke), histology (Meynert) and pathology (Alzheimer) were brought to bear. Griesinger wrote an influential textbook (1861) and strove to link psychiatry with general medicine, being of the view that 'psychological diseases are diseases of the brain'. The old humoral theories began to be replaced with new ideas about the connection between mental illness and brain function, and the pursuit of these links was successful for neurosyphilis, cretinism and dementia. By 1900 German academic centres had set a model for psychiatry to be taught alongside medicine.

But despite these developments, the scene was set for a period of therapeutic nihilism, and the rise of the new ideology of psychoanalysis. By the turn of the century, many leading clinicians believed that psychiatric illness was largely incurable, and therefore dedicated themselves to research rather than patient care. Kraepelin (1896) had concluded that mental illness should be defined by its prognosis rather than its cause, and that brain sciences were as yet too nascent to provide an understanding of mental illness. This nullified the premise that enthusiasm for research is a hallmark of better clinical care and failed to recognize that better treatments can be developed without a knowledge of aetiology provided one retains confidence that the illness has a biological basis. Wernicke did attempt to link psychiatric symptoms to brain regions and while successful for aphasia and the speech areas (1874), this approach led to a confusing attempt at classification which Karl Jaspers (1913) later described as 'brain mythology'. Furthermore, the attitude of many clinicians was affected by the doctrine of 'degeneracy' promulgated by Morel (1857) and the early sexologist Krafft-Ebing (1879), according to which severe mental illness represents the action of hereditary processes progressing over generations, constituting a threat to society. In France the excessive emphasis by Charcot (1825–1893) on 'hysteria' shows us, in retrospect, that illness behaviour may produce the very symptoms that the doctor is keen to treat, through the mechanism of suggestibility.

In the first half of the 20th century, American psychiatry became dominated by the ideas of Adolf Meyer (Johns Hopkins University) who elevated history-taking, investigations and note-keeping above treatment. Furthermore, academic psychiatrists began to devote more attention to the less severe mental conditions encountered outside the asylum.

A notable voice retaining enthusiasm for developing better treatments was that of Thomas Clouston in Edinburgh, whose textbook (1896) described clearly the shortcomings of available physical treatments and the hope for better.

NERVOUS ILLNESS. REST CURES AND PSYCHOANALYSIS

By 1900 the public was so frightened of psychiatry that care had often to be delivered under the guise of 'nervous illness', and accurate diagnostic terms had to be avoided. The less severely ill and the better-off sought help in less stigmatizing nerve clinics or 'hydros' (spas offering spring mineral water, showers and baths in pleasant resorts). In 1869 George Beard (New York) invented the term 'neurasthenia' to encompass many non-psychotic or psychosomatic disorders attributed to exhaustion of nerves. In 1875 Weir Mitchell – despite his subsequent debunking of 'sham' treatments – devised a 'rest cure' consisting of seclusion, enforced bedrest, a diet of milk products, electrical treatments and massage. It transpired that the essence of the cure was in fact the physician's authority and the patient's submission to it. Its effectiveness in some cases illustrated the importance of the one-to-one relationship between doctor and patient. This method remained in widespread use by neurologists and psychiatrists until the 1940s.

The introduction of psychoanalysis – with its concepts of transference and countertransference – made doctors more aware of the active nature of the therapeutic relationship. It also helped them to understand the content, though not the form, of mental symptoms, while its depth made psychiatrists rather than neurologists the appropriate specialists to deal with nervous illness. However, its initial promise of hope for the treatment of psychosis and other diagnostic groups proved unjustified, and concepts such as that of the schizophrenogenic mother (Frieda Fromm-Reichmann, 1935) were dogmatic and misleading.

PLANT ALKALOIDS AND THE FIRST DRUGS

Dioscordes (57 AD), Nero's surgeon, compiled a list –'materia medica'– of medicines including almost 500 derived from plants. Paracelsus (b.1493, Switzerland) is regarded as the grandfather of pharmacology; he taught that each drug (or plant) should be used alone, that chemistry was the science to produce medicines, and that it is only the dose that makes a thing a poison.

Plants with medicinal uses affecting the mind include the poppy (opium, morphine) (mentioned in the Ebers papyrus of about 1550 BC Egypt), hellebore (veratrum), rauwolfia serpentina (reserpine), the Solanacea henbane (hyoscine), belladonna (atropine), St John's wort (hypericum alkaloids) and cannabis. Kava root from South Pacific islands has at least fifteen chemical ingredients and effects including relaxation and sedation. Gingko biloba may help dementia. In their natural forms the medicines derived from plants lacked purity and varied in strength. They were consequently dangerous to administer, with a significant risk of overdose. Chemical techniques of the 19th century enabled the active alkaloid ingredients to be extracted, purified and identified.

Opium had long been used, and morphine was isolated in 1806 and used both orally and by subcutaneous injection as a sedative (after the introduction of the hypodermic syringe by the Scots physician Alexander Wood in 1855), until it was realized how addictive it was. Henbane and later hyoscine (isolated in 1880) were used to calm agitated and manic patients, as was atropine. Rauwolfia serpentina was used in India more than 2000 years ago for *Oonmaad* (insanity). Reserpine was isolated from it in 1953, and synthesized and introduced as an antipsychotic in 1954; it provided insights into the role of dopamine, noradrenaline and serotonin (5HT) in the brain, and the mechanisms of antidepressant drug actions. Veratrum was the source of modern calcium antagonists, some of which may have psychotropic properties. St John's wort has been confirmed recently to have mild antidepressant activity, and its ingredients share biochemical properties with modern monoamine reuptake inhibitors and serotonin agonists.

Heroin (diacetyl morphine) was synthesized in Bayer laboratories towards the end of the 19th century and was initially promoted as a cough remedy. Its name arose because it was said to make factory workers feel 'heroic'. At about that time chemists at Bayer were creating aspirin by acetylating salicylic acid, the active ingredient of myrtle, meadowsweet and willow bark; a drug was thus made that was more stable and less bitter. Such was the success of Bayer in making vast sums from healing common ailments that at the Treaty of Versailles the Allies expropriated the Bayer trademark – and with it aspirin – as part of First World War reparations. Only in the 1970s did Vane discover that aspirin blocked prostaglandin production, work for which he received a Nobel prize, and which led to further uses for aspirin, including stroke prophylaxis.

The French physiologist Claude Bernard (1856) had predicted that certain drugs (such as curare from South American arrow poison) could be used as 'physiological scalpels' to dissect the workings of neurotransmission. This proved prophetic with regard to biochemical theories of depression and schizophrenia, which arose from knowledge of the mechanism of action of antidepressants and antipsychotics, and anticipated the search for drugs with selective actions at particular receptors.

SEDATIVES. ANTICONVULSANTS AND BROMIDES

The synthesis by chemists, particularly in Germany, of sedative drugs in the 19th century, represents the beginning of the modern pharmaceutical industry. Chloral (1832) was synthesized by von Liebig (the founder of organic chemistry), found to be a sedative (1869), and produced by the pharmaceuticals division formed by Bayer (1888). It became widely used in psychiatry, although prone to abuse and addiction, and was the occasional cause of sudden death.

Paraldehyde was introduced into medicine in 1882 and used as an anticonvulsant and sedative, being regarded as relatively safe, albeit unpleasant treatment.

Bromide salts were produced by French chemists in the 19th century and found to be sedative, and in 1857 Locock (London) reported the use of potassium bromide for epilepsy and hysteria. Bromides became popular and remained in use as cheap alternatives to chloral for sedation until the 1940s. In higher doses they produce bromism, a toxic confusional state. McLeod (1899) used high doses of bromides to induce long periods of deep sleep in patients with mania, with reportedly good results.

Barbituric acid was first synthesized in 1864 but its first useful hypnotic and anticonvulsant derivative, diethyl barbituric acid (Veronal), was only produced much later, in 1904. Sedatives were used to assist catharsis or abreaction in victims of 'shell shock' in the first World War.

Many other barbiturates followed, including pheno-barbitone. These drugs induced sleep and relieved agitation, and paved the way for deep sleep therapy, or prolonged narcosis, in which patients were induced to sleep for 16 hours a day for several days, with drowsy intervals to eat and drink. Although widely used, and much appreciated by hospital personnel, the long-term efficacy of this treatment was never proven in a controlled trial. Prolonged narcosis also carried a significant risk of respiratory and cardiovascular depression, pneumonia and death. The subsequent use of benzodiazepines for prolonged sedation was safer. The first benzodiazepine, chlordiazepoxide, was introduced in 1961, and diazepam, which became the most commonly prescribed drug in the world, followed soon after. The risk of dependence on therapeutic doses of benzodiazepines was not widely recognized until 1981.

MALARIA, INSULIN COMA AND ECT

Wagner-Jauregg, an Austrian, had noted in 1883 that a psychotic patient was cured when she developed a streptococcal fever with erysipelas. In 1887 he proposed fever treatment with malaria for psychosis. In 1917 he returned to the subject, treating advanced neurosyphilis patients successfully by injecting blood infected with malaria, which induced a series of fevers that were later terminated by the use of quinine. In 1927 he was awarded a Nobel prize for this. Subsequently, penicillin, discovered by Fleming in 1929 and available clinically from 1944, virtually put an end to neurosyphilis in the developed world. These discoveries provided the first evidence to psychiatrists that a mental illness could be cured, and suggested that heroic methods might be justified.

Insulin was isolated by Banting and Best in 1922. Sakel thought that insulin-induced hypoglycaemic coma could relieve opiate withdrawal problems, and suggested its use in schizophrenia, claiming success in 1934. Insulin units were set up in many hospitals; in some centres coma was induced with increasing doses of insulin until convulsions occurred. By 1944 insulin coma therapy was the main physical treatment recommended for acute schizophrenia, for instance by Sargant and Slater in London. However, in 1953 Bourne, a junior psychiatrist, challenged its efficacy; several academic psychiatrists wrote in its defence, but the controlled trial that followed, comparing insulin coma and barbiturate-induced sleep, failed to demonstrate any advantage of insulin coma therapy (Ackner 1957). This dangerous treatment gradually fell into disuse and the antipsychotic drugs took its place.

Camphor was used to induce convulsions and claimed to effectively treat melancholia in the 18th century (although the convulsions could result in fractured bones). Convulsions induced by the chemical metrazol (Cardiazol), were proposed by von Meduna (1934) to relieve schizophrenia. However, the procedure itself was extremely unpleasant and a more controlled means of inducing convulsions was subsequently devised by Cerletti and Bini (Rome, 1938), using brief electrical currents applied through electrodes on the temples. Electroconvulsive therapy (ECT) was found to alleviate schizophrenia temporarily. The treatment was introduced at St Bartholomew's Hospital in London by Strauss in 1940; Felix Post (1978) has described its dramatic impact on the practice of psychiatry at the Bethlem Hospital in relation to depressive psychosis during the 1940s. The subsequent introduction of anaesthetics and muscular relaxants reduced many of the dangers associated with ECT, and its efficacy was established scientifically in double-blind controlled trials in the 1980s.

DIAGNOSTIC PRECISION

Accurate diagnosis becomes more important when treatments are discovered that are effective in specific conditions. The description of schizophrenia has developed from Kraepelin (1899), through Eugen Bleuler (1911) and Kurt Schneider (1959). The notion of bipolar disorder has developed from Falret's (1794–1870) circular insanity, through Baillarger's (1809–1890) 'folie a double forme' to Kraepelin's manic-depressive insanity (1899), and thence to the refinement by Leonard (1957) into 'bipolar' and 'unipolar' forms.

There is a tendency to overdiagnose conditions for which a new treatment has been discovered, as occurred in the USA with bipolar disorder after the introduction of lithium. When Baldessarini (1970) compared the frequency of affective illness to schizophrenia in patients discharged from hospital before and after the introduction of lithium, a reciprocal pattern was noted, with increasingly frequent diagnosis of bipolar illness and decreasing frequency of schizophrenia. Stoll et al. (1993) confirmed this finding in the discharge diagnoses of six psychiatric hospitals from the early 1970s. In the UK, the situation was different. There, affective illness was often diagnosed in patients whom US colleagues regarded as having schizophrenia. This resulted from differences in definition, with a broader concept of schizophrenia in the USA, as shown by the US–UK diagnostic project (Cooper et al. 1972). Subsequently the general acceptance of criteria-based diagnostic systems, particularly the DSM-III in 1982, introduced greater diagnostic reliability. However, the definition of bipolar mood disorder was broadened to include patients with mood-incongruent psychotic features, who would previously have been regarded as having schizoaffective disorder or schizophrenia. Thus the availability of lithium and the wider use of standard diagnostic systems have led patients to receive a diagnosis of bipolar disorder who might previously have been diagnosed with schizophrenia, at least in the USA.

PSYCHOTHERAPIES

Sigmund Freud (1856–1939), a Viennese neurologist who studied with Charcot in 1885, abandoned hypnosis in favour of free association and the interpretation of dreams, as a means of attaining 'catharsis' and understanding symptoms. The other ingredients of his 'models', which changed over the years, included the role of the unconscious, infantile sexuality, repression (developed from Pierre Janet) and other 'defence mechanisms' (later listed systematically by his daughter Anna Freud), identification with the lost 'object' in mourning, and the ambivalence of feelings. He also described the dangers and the therapeutic potential of 'transference' – the feelings directed towards the doctor by a patient re-enacting experiences from earlier influential relationships. Many of his ideas were too general to be amenable to experimental testing and possible refutation, and he was criticized for this by Jaspers. Other analysts who provided insights into the development of mental symptoms included Melanie Klein ('the paranoid-schizoid position') and Donald Winnicott, who worked in London (1935) and mainly with children. Since the 1960s, however, the application of psychoanalysis for the treatment of severe mental illness has been progressively eroded. Other forms of psychotherapy have been developed, mainly for non-psychotic conditions, with firmer foundations in terms of evidence of efficacy and practicability. These include cognitive therapies (after Beck), behavioural therapies (after Skinner and Wolpe) and more time-limited and focused forms such as interpersonal psychotherapy (see Chapters 36 and 37). In childhood disorders and in schizophrenia the techniques of family therapy retain value. Some of the ideas arising from psychoanalysis are now ubiquitous and some are part of the armamentarium of everyday clinical practice. They are not only treatments, they also help to make sense of complex behaviour.

THE SLOW EMERGENCE OF DRUG TREATMENT

By the end of the 19th century, drugs were available to calm manic or agitated patients, including chloral, paraldehyde, bromides and hyoscine. There were no specific drugs known for treating depression or paranoid psychoses. Fifty years later, the first edition of Sargant & Slater's book (1946) on physical treatments in psychiatry referred still to the Weir Mitchell method, but recommended ECT for melancholia and mania, insulin coma for schizophrenia, and malaria treatment for neurosyphilis. For chemical sedation, paraldehyde and barbiturates were used, while bromides were regarded as relatively ineffective and unsafe. The authors stated 'most people would rather have their relatives dead than linger on for years, depressed or demented in a mental hospital'. By the time of the second edition in 1948 the authors say 'apathy has given way to enthusiasm in mental hospitals', as facilities for ECT, deep insulin treatment and leucotomy (first proposed by Egas Moniz in Lisbon in 1935) became more accessible. The fourth edition in 1963 described the advent of many new drugs, which had allowed a 'therapeutic community approach and open doors' in hospitals, 'and with these drugs, community care becomes possible'.

The discovery by Bradford Hill of the experimental design known as the randomized controlled trial was such a potentially powerful one that it was guarded as part of the British war effort. Its importance continues to be appreciated as evidence-based medicine gathers momentum, for example through the efforts of the Cochrane Collaboration.

LITHIUM AND MOOD STABILIZERS

John Cade in Australia (1948) was studying the effects caused by injecting the urine of manic patients into guinea pigs when he noticed the calming effect of lithium (as its uric acid salt). He decided to inject lithium into psychotic patients and discovered the antimanic effect of lithium in patients with mania. It remained to Mogens Schou (1954), an academic pharmacologist in Aarhus, Denmark, to confirm this effect in a controlled trial. The prophylactic efficacy of lithium in manic-depressive illness was established by 1968. Thus from about 1950 psychiatrists stopped giving their patients the sedative large-anion bromide, and began to administer the small-cation lithium, on a surer scientific footing.

The anticonvulsant carbamazepine was first recognized as useful in bipolar patients by Okuma et al. (1973). Post & Ballenger (1980) subsequently surmised that certain anticonvulsants might be useful by preventing the 'kindling' of electrical excitability in limbic areas of the brain. A seminal report by Bowden et al. (1994) proved the efficacy of another anticonvulsant, valproate, in mania. This report stimulated much-needed research into the treatment of bipolar disorder, which is only recently coming to fruition with the publication of controlled trials of atypical antipsychotics in mania and in the longer-term management of bipolar disorder. Although lithium is still viewed as the 'gold standard' for the prevention of mania, the role of anticonvulsants and of atypical antipsychotics in the prophylaxis of bipolar disorder is becoming clearer.

ANTIHISTAMINES. CHLORPROMAZINE AND THE ANTIPSYCHOTICS

More than a quarter of a century elapsed between the description of the actions of histamine by Dale and Laidlaw (1910) and the discovery of the first clinically useful antihistamine in 1942. By the late 1940s, drug manufacturers were in a frenzy to synthesize new antihistamines. These drugs, although sedative, were not otherwise advantageous in schizophrenia, but they were to pave the way for the first drug that was.

Chlorpromazine was synthesized in France as a variant of the antihistamine, promethazine. Following Laborit's description of its effects in anaesthesia (1951), the psychiatrists Delay and Deniker (1952) reported its effects in psychosis, calming patients without deep sedation and relieving psychotic symptoms in only a few weeks. The use of the drug spread rapidly, beginning a psycho-pharmacological revolution. Many other phenothiazines were synthesized. In 1958 the creative genius of Paul Janssen, the Belgian clinician and chemist, led to the introduction of haloperidol, a butyrophenone with antipsychotic properties. This was synthesized as a variant of the pethidine molecule and had been observed to block the activating effects of amphetamines in animals. Amphetamines were associated with psychotic reactions in racing cyclists, who were taking them to enhance their performance, and this led Janssen to study the effects of haloperidol in schizophrenia and mania. The occurrence of neurological (parkinsonian) side-effects indicated that drugs such as chlorpromazine and haloperidol affected neurons, and the name 'neuroleptic' (seizes neurons) was used to describe them. The term 'antipsychotic' is now preferred. Later, newer drugs would be developed that would be relatively free from these side-effects (the 'atypical antipsychotics' or 'New Generation Antipsychotics').

The antipsychotic drugs enabled many patients to be discharged from hospital and many others to avoid hospitalization, and the number of inpatients with schizophrenia declined by 80% between 1955 and 1988. This continued a slight downward trend that had occurred in the 1940s when alternatives to inpatient care, such as day hospitals and group therapy, were established by proponents of social and community psychiatry.

The first depot injectable forms of antipsychotic medication, fluphenazine enanthate (Moditen) and decanoate (Modecate) were introduced in 1968 and stimulated the development of community psychiatric nursing services, in which nurses largely administered injections initially, and subsequently became the primary professional contacts for psychotic patients outside hospital.

A more recent breakthrough was the proof in a controlled trial by Kane et al. (1987) that clozapine may be effective in schizophrenia that had been resistant to all other types of antipsychotic therapy. Clozapine had been studied for almost 30 years and had many side-effects (including agranulocytosis) that restricted its usefulness, but the confirmation of its value in treatment-resistant schizo-phrenic patients stimulated a search for better drugs. Among those discovered were risperidone, developed because it was known to share with clozapine the ability to potently block the effects of both dopamine and serotonin. Olanzapine and quetiapine were developed because of their structural similarity to clozapine, and are also potent dopamine and serotonin receptor antagonists. Other atypical antipsychotics are ziprasidone, sertindole, zotepine, amisulpride and aripiprazole. The latter represents a further pharmacological development as the drug is a 'partial agonist' at dopamine receptors and is hypothesized to 'stabilize' dopamine systems by avoiding excessive blockade and by providing a degree of stimulation of dopamine receptors in the absence of dopamine. It is now widely accepted that the new generation of antipsychotics represent advance in terms of avoiding neurological side-effects and, with some drugs, avoiding endocrinological side-effects from hyperprolactinaemia.

IMIPRAMINE AND THE ANTIDEPRESSANTS

Imipramine, the first antidepressant, like the first antipsychotics, was also synthesized as an antihistamine, and was tried clinically at first in patients with schizophrenia. Its activating effects led Ronald Kuhn to give it to depressed patients, and in 1958 he reported its dramatic effects in some depressed patients, thus heralding the 'tricyclic' antidepressants era.

Another group of antidepressants, the monoamine oxidase inhibitors, evolved from antituberculous therapy. Iproniazid – in contrast to isoniazid – was devoid of antibiotic effects but improved the mood of the patients with tuberculosis. Iproniazid (introduced in 1957) was at first called a 'psychic energizer', and only later an antidepressant.

The discovery that both tricyclic and monoamine oxidase inhibitor classes of antidepressants acted to enhance noradrenaline and 5HT transmission led to strategies for developing drugs aimed specifically at those neuro-transmitters. The first of the selective serotonin reuptake inhibitors (SSRIs) was zimelidine, developed under the guidance of Arvid Carlsson and launched by Astra (Sweden) in 1981 but soon withdrawn because of an association with flu-like symptoms and Guillain-Barré syndrome. A more successful SSRI, fluoxetine (Prozac), was approved in 1987. This drug caught the public imagination perhaps more than any other psychotropic drug. It has been taken by more than 30 million people, books have been written about it (mostly praising but some vilifying it) and its huge financial success acted as a spur to pharmaceutical companies to develop better psychotropic medications. The adverse effects of SSRIs attracted public attention more recently when there was concern about the possible initial exacerbation of anxiety in some patients, and about the unpleasant effects of abrupt discontinuation of certain of this class of drugs, particularly paroxetine.

DRUGS AND BIOLOGICAL PSYCHIATRY

Many of the theories of biological psychiatry have been developed from knowledge of the mechanisms of action of psychotropic drugs. Thus the discovery that reserpine, which can cause depression as a side-effect, depletes neurones of 5HT (and noradrenaline and dopamine) contributed to the monoamine hypothesis of affective disorders. Similarly, the discovery by Carlsson and Linquist (1963) that antipsychotics worked largely by blocking dopamine receptors became one of the cornerstones of the dopamine hypothesis of schizophrenia. (In 2000 Arvid Carlsson shared the Nobel prize for medicine). In this manner, the development of an effective treatment could generate an explosion of interest in a previously poorly studied area, as well as funds for further investigations. Thus the surprising finding that the SSRI fluvoxamine is effective in panic disorder (Den Boer 1988) – and also in obsessive-compulsive disorder – focused attention on the role of 5HT in anxiety, and stimulated research in these areas.

DRUG DEPENDENCE

Drug misuse and dependence is an important accompaniment of drug discovery. Problems were recognized with opium, chloral and barbiturates but assumed greater significance with heroin. The report of the

Rolleston Committee (1926) led to the British System of treating opiate addicts, with maintenance substitutes. The ideas were revised in the reports of Russell Brain (1960 and 1965), with more emphasis on strategies of reduction. Methadone was introduced as an oral substitute in 1965 (Dole and Nyswander). In 1989, however, the Advisory Council on the Misuse of Drugs stated that 'the spread of HIV is a greater danger to individual and public health than drug misuse.' This changed prescribing practice back towards maintenance rather than reduction strategies, under the justification of 'harm minimization.' Recently the management of substance misuse (particularly cannabis and cocaine) among people with mental illness ('dual diagnosis') has become recognized as a priority. New approaches to treatment of substance dependence are being required and drugs that may reduce craving (acamprosate), or reduce the reinforcing effects of alcohol (naltrexone) and stimulants are being developed. The opiate partial agonist buprenorphine has to some extent displaced methadone as a substitute for heroin.

ANTIPSYCHIATRY

It may be no coincidence that following a decade of genuine innovation and progress in treatment in the 1950s, the following decade became known as the era of antipsychiatry. It was also a time of liberal thinking, student socialism, experimentation with mind-altering drugs and the beginning of the widespread abuse of illicit addictive drugs, which later expanded in epidemic proportions. Abuse of the new psychopharmacological agents by prescribers was also seen in the almost indiscriminate use of benzodiazepines in general practice, and in the use of inappropriately high doses of antipsychotic drugs in hospitalized patients who seemed resistant to treatment.

The success of psychiatry, which had led to open-door policies and the rundown of psychiatric beds, left the mental hospitals even more vulnerable to criticism. Indeed they were blamed for causing some of the very diseases that patients suffered, such as institutionalization or the deficits of chronic schizophrenia. The influential 'three hospitals' study, by Wing & Brown appeared in 1961. This seemed to show that patients deteriorated more in a hospital where they were given less individual attention, had fewer personal possessions and were generally treated less well than they would be in a family – the antithesis of moral therapy. This finding in a non-randomized study was often misinterpreted. The terms 'institutionalism' and 'institutionalization' were misapplied as descriptions of, and as an explanation for, the social impoverishment of chronic schizophrenia, even though the same phenomenon could be seen in patients who had little exposure to psychiatric wards, let alone spent years in a mental hospital.

The asylum in its 20th-century incarnation was rightfully criticized by Goffman (1961) as a total institution that could degrade its inmates. At the same time, however, attacks – regarded by many as sinister and unwarranted – were made upon the very concept of mental illness, and upon the claims of doctors to be able to treat it. Those articulating these ideas included Szasz and Scheff in the USA, R.D. Laing in the UK, and Foucault in France. Gradually their claims were exposed and discredited by thoughtful argument, based on well-conducted studies of the epidemiology, genetics and psychopharmacological responses of the major mental disorders. Vestiges of these philosophies are still occasionally encountered, however, usually among those who became acquainted with sociology during the 1960s, but also understandably in those with bad personal experiences of psychiatric services.

INTEGRATING TREATMENT APPROACHES

Accompanying the clinical and financial success of modern drug treatments, there has been a tendency to polarize treatment approaches into the 'organic' or 'biological' and the 'psychological'. The polarization can also be extended to the doctors who favour one or other approach. Such a division may be valid for focusing research interests, but is unhelpful for clinicians. Doctors should avoid becoming identified as solely organic; it may give a sense of knowledge and authority, but it undermines the basis of the doctor–patient relationship, which has been important for as long as psychiatry, and indeed medicine, has existed. The expanding knowledge base of psychopharmacology places an additional strain upon the therapeutic relationship, which is one that entails a degree of trust. The doctor is expected to be knowledgeable about the treatments being used. Patients may easily acquire detailed information, which can seem to expose gaps in their doctor's knowledge rather than supporting a constructive dialogue. There is also a growing expectation about what the doctor should tell the patient about his/her illness and treatment; again, trust in the doctor can be eroded if the patient feels that he or she has not been given accurate or sufficient information.

The pharmaceutical industry recognizes the value of promoting drugs directly to the public, and uses various means of 'health awareness' to achieve this. Such campaigns became so prevalent that in 1997 the US Food and Drugs Administration made direct-to-consumer advertising of prescription drugs legal. Doctors now have an important role in helping patients to make decisions based on information they may have received from a variety of sources.

REGULATORY AUTHORITIES

Disasters with drugs, such as that associated with thalidomide and foetal malformations in 1961, have led to legislation to regulate the marketing of medicines, for instance the Medicines Act of 1968 in the UK. These agencies, the Food and Drug Administration (FDA) in the USA and the European Medicines Evaluation Agency (EMEA), now set standards for the approval of new drugs and dictate much of the research that is done.

CONCLUSIONS

At the start of the 21st century the physical treatments available in psychiatry include an increasing number of highly 'crafted' molecules with selective actions on neurochemical systems. They also include three older treatments that are relatively crude in their mechanism of action: two drugs, lithium and clozapine, which have extensive biological actions and side-effects, and ECT. Although relatively crude, these treatments are still used because they are of proven efficacy. As our understanding of the mechanisms of action of drugs develops, so too does the possibility of developing more sophisticated treatments, with greater efficacy and with fewer side-effects. Psychopharmacology is particularly fascinating because it spans the spectrum of knowledge and understanding from molecules to the mind of the patient.

Experimental techniques play a crucial role in advancing scientific knowledge. The new techniques of structural and functional imaging combined with isotope-labelled drugs with known sites of action, provide powerful tools with which to explore the brain in health and disease and to expand our understanding of treatments. Together with the new science of molecular genetics, they offer hope that the era of effective treatments in psychiatry will advance much further, and will do so rapidly.

FURTHER READING

Bourne H (1953). The insulin myth. *Lancet* 2: 964–969.

Healy D (1996, 1998) *The Psychopharmacologists I and II: Interviews by David Healy*. London: Altman.

Healy D (1998) *The Antidepressant Era*. London: Harvard University Press.

REFERENCES

Baldessarini RJ (1970) Frequency of diagnoses of schizophrenia versus affective disorders from 1944 to 1968. *American Journal of Psychiatry* **127**: 757–63.

Bruhn JG, De Smeet PAGM, El-Seedi HR and Beck O (2002). Mescaline use for 5700 years. *Lancet* **359**: 1866.

Foucault M (1961) *Madness and Civilisation*, English translation. Routledge, Cambridge University Press.

Goffman E (1961) *Asylums. Essays on the Social Situation of Patients and other Inmates*. New York: Anchor Books.

Mitchell PB, Hadzi-Pavlovic D and Manji HK (eds) (1999) Fifty years of treatments for bipolar disorder: A celebration of John Cade's discovery. *Australia and New Zealand Journal of Psychiatry*, **33**(suppl): S1–S122.

Porter R (1997) *The Greatest Benefit to Mankind: A Medical History of Humanity from Antiquity to the Present*. London: Harper Collins.

Post F (1978) Then and now. *British Journal of Psychiatry* **133**: 83–6.

Sargent W & Slater E (1946) *An Introduction to Physical Methods of Treatment in Psychiatry*. Edinburgh: Churchill Livingstone.

Shepherd M (1990). The 'neuroleptics' and the Oedipus effect. *Journal of Psychopharmacology*, **4**: 131–135. Part of a special issue on the History of Psychopharmacology, including papers by Carlsson and Kuhn. Discusses the early impact of phenothiazines, and the term 'neuroleptic'.

Shorter E (1997) *A History of Psychiatry: From the Age of the Asylum to the Era of Prozac*. New York: Wiley.

Stoll AL, Tohen M, Baldessarini RJ et al. (1993) Shifts in diagnostic frequencies of schizophrenia and major affective disorders at six North American psychiatric hospitals, 1972–1988. *American Journal of Psychiatry* **150**: 1668–73.

Wing JK & Brown GW (1961) Social treatment of chronic schizophrenia. *Journal of Mental Science* 847–61.

THE HISTORY OF PSYCHOTROPIC AGENTS

1831	Atropine isolated
1857	Bromides synthesized
1869	Chloral as sedative
1880	Hyoscine isolated
1882	Paraldehyde
1903	Barbiturates (Veronal)
1917	Malaria for neurosyphilis
1930	Insulin coma for schizophrenia
1935	Amphetamine (narcolepsy)
1938	Phenytoin introduced; ECT
1942	Antihistamines
1948	Lithium in mania (Cade)
1952	Chlorpromazine (Delay & Deniker)
1954	Lithium (Schou)
1957	Iproniazid, psychic energizer – MAOIs
1958	Haloperidol (Janssen)
	Imipramine (Kuhn): TCAs, MARIs
1961	Chlordiazepoxide: benzodiazepines
1967	Depot antipsychotic injections: Modecate
1968	Lithium prophylaxis
1973	Carbamazepine in mania
1982	Zimelidine: SSRIs
1987	Clozapine (Kane et al.)
	Fluoxetine (Prozac) approved
1988	SSRIs in panic disorder
1994	Valproate in mania (Bowden et al.)
	Atypical antipsychotics: risperidone, olanzapine
1999	Atypical antipsychotics for bipolar disorder

Clinical neuroanatomy

Anne Lingford-Hughes

INTRODUCTION

The ultimate biological substrate for all human behaviour, physiological and pathological, is the human brain. Elucidating the function of the different parts of the brain has until relatively recently relied on studying patients with neurological lesions. Recently, neuroimaging (see elsewhere in this volume) has revolutionized our ability to characterize what functions different parts of the brain perform in both health and disease. The development and structure of the human central nervous system (CNS), and its role in health and disease, are discussed in this chapter.

BRAIN DEVELOPMENT

The cranial end of the neural tube develops into three vesicles after four weeks of gestation. The forebrain develops from the prosencephalon, the midbrain from the mesencephalon and the hindbrain from the rhombencephalon. The prosencephalon divides into the telencephalon and the diencephalon. The cerebral hemispheres, the rhinencephalon (or 'nosebrain', i.e. olfactory mucosa, tracts and bulbs) and corpus striatum develop from the telencephalon. The rhombencephalon divides into the metencephalon and myelencephalon, from which the cerebellum and spinal cord are formed.

CELLULAR CONSTITUENTS AND CONNECTIVE TISSUES OF THE BRAIN
(Box 2.1)

The neuron

A neuron consists of a body (soma) that contains the nucleus and an axon which conducts impulses from the body to the synapse. The axon is surrounded by a myelin sheath, which is generated by oligodendrocytes. Dendrites are projections from any part of the neuron. Receptors for neurotransmitters and drugs can be located on the body, dendrites or synaptic terminals of a neuron.

Neuroglia

The predominant neuroglia present in the brain are astrocytes. These are multipolar and provide structural, metabolic and phagocytic support to neurons. They occur in both white and grey matter. Processes from astrocytes terminate as 'end feet' on capillaries to form part of the blood–brain barrier and also as pial attachments to form part of the pia–glial membrane. Oligodendrocytes are smaller than astrocytes and form myelin sheaths. Microglia are the smallest form of neuroglia and proliferate in response to injury. They increase in size as they phagocytose degraded matter. There are three different types of the last type of neuroglia, the ependyma. They line cavities of brain and spinal cord and maintain cerebrospinal fluid (CSF) flow. Ependymocytes line the ventricles and central canal of the spinal cord, tanycytes line the floor of the third ventricle over the hypothalamic median eminence and choroidal epithelial cells cover the surface of choroidal plexus.

Box 2.1   Cellular constituents and connective tissue of the brain
Neuron

Neuroglia
    astrocytes
    oligodendrocytes
    microglia
    ependyma: tanycytes, ependymocytes, choroidal epithelium

Connective tissue
    dura mater
    arachnoid
    pia mater

Connective tissue

The connective tissue layers covering the brain and spinal cord are called the meninges, and comprise the dura, arachnoid and pia mater. The dura mater lines the skull and is the thickest membrane. The tentorium cerebelli is a fold of this membrane between the cerebellum and occipital lobe. Adjacent to the dura mater is the arachnoid, which is a thin membrane. The pia mater lies on the brain and spinal cord itself and between this and the arachnoid is the subarachnoid space, containing CSF.

CEREBRAL CORTEX

The lobes and surface markings of the cerebral cortex

The right and left cerebral hemispheres are separated by the longitudinal or sagittal fissure. Each hemisphere is further demarcated by the central sulcus or fissure of Rolando and the lateral sulcus or Sylvian fissure (Fig. 2.1). The frontal lobe lies anterior to the central sulcus and the parietal lobe posteriorly. The posterior border of the parietal lobe is more difficult to demarcate. Inferior to the lateral sulcus lies the temporal lobe. The occipital lobe lies posterior to the parietal and temporal lobes.

The surface of the cerebral hemisphere is very convoluted, thus increasing its surface area. The fissures are deepest, dividing the hemispheres, with sulci defining smaller areas or gyri.

The neocortex, which includes the frontal lobes, has six layers. The phylogenetically older paleocortex, rhinencephalon and archicortex or limbic lobe, have only three layers.

Cellular constituents of the cortex

The cerebral cortex is stratified into six layers (Box 2.2). The most common cells are stellate, which are present in all layers except layer I, and pyramidal cells. Starting at the surface, layer I contains glial cells and dendrites from neurons of deeper layers, and the horizontal cells of Cajal. Layers II and III comprise small pyramidal cells, whose axons project out of and within the hemispheres. Stellate and fusiform cells lie in layer IV and provide local connections and receive ascending fibres. Layer V consists of large pyramidal cells.

Intra- and interhemispheric white matter tracts

There are a number of short and long association tracts that provide intrahemispheric communication within the cerebral cortex. The cingulum is an example of a long association tract. Commissural fibres provide communication between homologous regions of the hemispheres. The largest such interhemispheric fibre bundle is the corpus callosum. Other commissures include the anterior commissure, which connects homologous cortical areas, and the fornix, which is the efferent projection from the hippocampus.

The internal capsule is a projection tract that contains many fibres carrying information between cortical and subcortical regions and the spinal column. It descends lateral to the head of the caudate nucleus and medial to the lentiform nucleus and thalamus. The corona radiata is where the internal capsule fans out superiorly. It is divided into several parts: the anterior limb contains frontopontine and corticothalamic fibres; the genu contains corticobulbar fibres; the posterior limb contains corticospinal and parieto-occipito-temporopontine fibres; and the retrolenti-form/sublentiform part includes the auditory and optic radiations. The internal capsule becomes the crus cerebri in the midbrain.

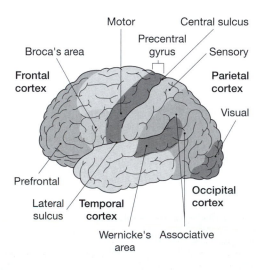

Motor   Central sulcus

Precentral gyrus

Broca's area   Sensory

Frontal cortex   Parietal cortex

Visual

Prefrontal

Occipital cortex

Lateral sulcus / Temporal cortex

Wernicke's   Associative area

Figure 2.1 Lateral view of left hemisphere.

Box 2.2	Layers of the cerebral cortex
Surface	
Layer I	Molecular or plexiform layer
Layer II	External granular layer
Layer III	External pyramidal layer
Layer IV	Internal granular layer
Layer V	Internal pyramidal layer
Layer VI	Multiform or polymorphic layer
Deep	

THE LOBES OF THE CEREBRAL CORTEX AND THEIR FUNCTION

Cerebral dominance

The general rule is that the hemisphere contralateral to the dominant hand is the dominant hemisphere and mediates language and speech functions. Thus in right-handed people, the left hemisphere is dominant. This is not necessarily so, however, and in approximately 10% of right-handed people the right hemisphere is dominant. In left-handed people, only about 20% are right hemisphere-dominant as expected, with 64% left hemisphere-dominant and 16% showing bilateral dominance.

Although not an absolute maxim, apraxia generally results from dysfunction in the dominant hemisphere and agnosia from dysfunction in the non-dominant hemisphere. These terms are more fully described after discussing signs and symptoms associated with dysfunction in specific lobes of the cerebral cortex.

Frontal lobe

The frontal lobe includes the prefrontal cortex, motor and supplementary motor cortices, Broca's area and frontal eye fields. Damage to the frontal lobes generally results in changes in personality, often profound, but in the presence of few other symptoms or signs. Consequently, changes or lesions in the frontal lobe can be 'silent' for a considerable length of time.

Functions of the frontal lobe

The prefrontal cortex (PFC) is divided into the medial and lateral surface and the latter into the ventrolateral, dorsolateral and anterior prefrontal regions. The PFC mediates executive functions of the brain such as focusing attention on relevant information and processes, and inhibiting irrelevant ones, switching focused attention between tasks, planning a sequence to achieve a goal, updating working memory to make sure a plan is 'on-task' as well as coding this information. Tests of frontal lobe function therefore generally include tasks that require attention, switching attention, planning and manipulation of information such as learning new rules, e.g. Wisconsin Card Sort Test.

The prefrontal cortex is also involved in encoding and retrieval of memories. The dorsolateral prefrontal cortex is particularly involved in working memory, i.e. short-lasting memory associated with active maintenance and rehearsal of information to achieve a goal in behaviour, speech or reasoning. The prefrontal cortex is also part of the mesolimbic or mesocorticolimbic system and receives dopaminergic projections from the ventral tegmental area in the brainstem. It is hypothesized that hypofunction in this pathway contributes to the negative features of schizophrenia.

The anterior cingulate cortex is part of the limbic system and is strongly implicated in attention and emotional processing. For example, its activity increases in response to emotionally significant stimuli. Its ventral subdivision appears to be the 'affective' component and impaired function here is strongly implicated in depression. The orbitofrontal cortex (OFC) is also part of the limbic system and is involved in processing the reward value of stimuli and in suppressing motor responses. It therefore plays a key role in decision-making and appropriate responsiveness. OFC dysfunction has been reported in some disorders of impulse control such as obsessive-compulsive disorder and addiction. Patients with OFC dysfunction can show inability to appreciate and avoid possible negative future consequences of their actions.

Personality changes

Damage to the prefrontal cortex results in changes in personality which broadly fit into categories of disturbed mood, poor judgement, and impaired social awareness and motivation (Box 2.3).

The changes seen in mood tend to be those of euphoria rather than depression, but all changes have an 'empty' feeling to them. Childishness may be a feature, including making jokes and performing pranks (*Witzelsucht*). Lack of drive and motivation coupled to an inability to plan, impaired judgement and poor social awareness often results in profound disability. Other features include perseveration, both of speech and movements, pallilalia or repetition of phrases and sentences, and decreased verbal fluency.

Motor changes

The primary motor cortex lies in the posterior part of the frontal lobe. The body is represented somatotopically and inverted with areas such as the face taking up more area than the lower limb. If this area is damaged, contralateral hemiparesis will be present. The signs can be subtle but the

Box 2.3 Personality changes associated with frontal lobe dysfunction	
Disinhibition	Reduced social awareness and control
Loss of finer feelings	Sexual indiscretions
Errors of judgement	Decreased abstracting ability
Irritability	Elevated mood (fatuous, childish)
Lack of concern for others	Lack of drive
Catastrophic response	Inability to adapt to the unexpected
Impaired initiation	Impaired concentration and attention

grasp reflex is invariably elicited. If the frontal lobe superior to the eye is damaged 'forced utilization' may be seen. Here, when objects are placed in front of the subject, an object will be picked up and used appropriately, even when the subject is told not to do so. Urinary incontinence can also be a sign of frontal lobe dysfunction.

Other changes

If the lesion is in the posterior part of the dominant frontal lobe, apraxia of the face, motor aphasia and motor agraphia may also be present. A lesion of Broca's area, which is in the motor area in the posterior frontal cortex, will result in problems with verbal expression. This is revealed by poor articulation and sparse speech. This is known as expressive or Broca's aphasia.

Clinical examination

The appearance and behaviour of the subject will provide many clues to frontal lobe dysfunction. The following bedside tests are sensitive to frontal lobe dysfunction: verbal fluency; ability to interpret proverbs (abstract thinking); and movements requiring coordinated series of actions.

Temporal lobe

Damage to the temporal lobe can result in amnesia, personality disturbances and visual field and sensory deficits, depending on the location of the lesion. Typically, lesions involving the dominant lobe result in more symptoms and signs. Components of the temporal lobe, such as the hippocampus and amygdala, play important roles within the limbic system and are more fully described below.

Sensation

The temporal lobe is the final destination for different sensory modalities including auditory, vestibular, gustatory and olfactory senses.

Memory and amnesia

The medial temporal lobe, including the hippocampus, plays a crucial role in mediating declarative memory, i.e. memory of personal events (episodic memory) and factual knowledge (semantic memory). The hippocampus serves as a final common pathway for other structures in the medial temporal cortex, such as the amygdala, parahippocampal and entorhinal cortices. Profound amnesia results from bilateral medial temporal lobe lesions. Causes of such lesions include infections, tumours, epilepsy and bilateral occlusion of the posterior cerebral artery. Subjects with such lesions will have preserved performance at tasks requiring intact immediate memory (e.g. digit span). Both retrograde and anterograde memory, i.e. memory of events before and after the lesion respectively, will be impaired. Retrograde amnesia may not be as severe as the anterograde amnesia and

memory for remote events may be well preserved. Semantic memory remains intact. More specific lesions of the hippocampal formation, if they occur bilaterally, will also result in global amnesia. The deficit resulting from unilateral lesions of the temporal cortex involving the hippocampus will depend on whether the dominant or the non-dominant lobe is affected. Problems with learning new verbal material results from dysfunction of the dominant lobe, with impaired learning of new nonverbal information (e.g. music) resulting from lesions of the non-dominant lobe.

Personality changes

Personality changes include depersonalization, emotional instability, aggression and antisocial behaviour. Psychosis may also be present, as can be seen in temporal lobe epilepsy.

Visual field deficit

Lesions deep within the temporal lobe which involve the optic radiation result in a contralateral homonymous upper quadrant visual field defect.

Other changes

If lesions are in the dominant lobe, sensory or receptive aphasia will be present. Lesions in the posterior part of the temporal lobe will also result in alexia and agraphia. Hemisomatognosia, prosopagnosia and visuospatial problems may be present after damage to either hemisphere, but more commonly occur with nondominant hemisphere dysfunction.

Lesions within Wernicke's auditory association area in the dominant superior temporal cortex, result in problems of reduced verbal comprehension and reading and writing abilities. Despite their speech being fluent, reduced comprehension means that the speech may be nonsensical or so-called jargon aphasia. This is also referred to as Wernicke's or receptive aphasia.

Kluver–Bucy syndrome

This syndrome results from bilateral ablation of temporal lobes and destruction of the uncus, amygdala and hippocampus. In monkeys, an increase in oral and sexual behaviours, placidity and a loss of fear or anger with apathy and pet-like compliance is seen. A similar syndrome is seen in humans in association with a number of disorders such as Pick's disease, Alzheimer's dementia, arteriosclerosis, cerebral tumours and herpes simplex encephalitis. The syndrome is also associated with visual agnosia and sometimes prosopagnosia and hypermetamorphosis (patients touch everything).

Parietal lobe

The parietal lobe is involved in a number of complex tasks involving attention, integration of information such as recognition, visuospatial abilities and appreciation of environmental cues and the appropriate connection of sensory input to action. Hence, whilst patients with parietal lobe impairment are not visually blind to a visual stimulus, they cannot interpret the stimulus, particularly its spatial attributes or use visual information to guide movements of the body. The parietal lobe syndrome consists of constructional apraxia, visuospatial agnosia, topographical disorientation (getting lost, inability to learn new routes), visual inattention and cortical sensory loss, when objects can be felt but not fully interpreted or discriminated.

Lesions in the dominant lobe result in motor aphasia if the lesion is anterior, or sensory aphasia if the lesion is posterior. Other consequences include agraphia with alexia, motor apraxia and bilateral tactile agnosia. Visual agnosia occurs if the parieto-occipital region is affected.

A specific syndrome, Gerstmann's syndrome, is associated with lesions of the dominant parietal lobe. This consists of dyscalculia, agraphia, finger agnosia and right-left disorientation. Lesions in the nondominant hemisphere result in anosognosia, hemisomatognosia, dressing apraxia and prosopagnosia.

Occipital lobe

The occipital lobe is involved in processing visual information. Although all of the following can occur with dysfunction of either hemisphere, the more common associations are described. Lesions in the dominant lobe result in alexia without agraphia, colour agnosia and visual object agnosia. Lesions in the non-dominant lobe result in visuospatial agnosia, prosopagnosia, metamorphosia (image distortion) and complex visual hallucinations.

The occipital lobe syndrome consists of contralateral homonymous hemianopia, scotomata and simultagnosia.

Specific signs and syndromes seen with cortical lobe dysfunction

Apraxia

Apraxia is the inability to carry out purposeful voluntary movements. This cannot be accounted for by paresis, incoordination, sensory loss or involuntary movements. The same movements can, however, be performed in another context such as part of a reflex. The different types of apraxia and associated site of dysfunction are listed in Table 2.1.

Agnosia

Agnosia is the inability to recognize an object through sensation, however it is presented, e.g. touch, sight, smell. The impairment cannot be attributed to sensory defects, mental deterioration, disorders of consciousness or attention or to non-familiarity with the object. Some different types of agnosia are listed in Table 2.2. Examples of various agnosias and apraxias are described in Table 2.3.

CEREBELLUM

The cerebellum develops from the metencephalon and lies posteriorly to the pons and medulla. It is concerned with coordination of movement, maintenance of muscle tone and equilibrium. Increasingly, the role of the cerebellum in cognition is being recognized. There are two hemispheres flanking the midline vermis.

Phylogenetically, there are three parts to the cerebellum. The archicerebellum is the inferior portion of vermis and receives efferents from and sends efferents to the vestibular nuclei. Lesions here result in a broad-based gait. The paleocerebellum is the anterior lobe and receives afferents from the anterior and posterior spinocerebellar tracts and sends efferents to vestibular and reticular nuclei. The role of the paleocerebellum is concerned with muscle tone and lesions here affect extensor tone. The neocerebellum consists of the posterior lobe and the tonsil. Afferents come from the pontine nuclei, which is a relay for cortical information. Thus this part of the cerebellum is concerned with skilled voluntary movements.

Cellular constituents of the cerebellar cortex

The cerebellar cortex is three-layered (Table 2.4). The ascending fibres to the cerebellum all terminate in specific parts of the cortex and send collaterals to one or more of the cerebellar nuclei. They are all excitatory. Mossy fibres are

Table 2.1 Types of apraxia and their associated dysfunctional area	
Type	Site of dysfunction
Ideomotor apraxia	Parieto-temporal
Ideational apraxia	Temporo-parietal
Dressing apraxia	Parieto-occipital
Constructional apraxia	Parieto-occipital

Table 2.2 Types of agnosia and their associated dysfunctional area	
Type	Site of dysfunction
Visuospatial agnosia, e.g. prosopagnosia, simultagnosia	Parietal (especially right) Right-sided lesions result in left-sided neglect
Visual identification problems, e.g. hemisomatognosia, anosognosia, autotopagnosia	Temporal lesions (especially right)

Table 2.3   Glossary of apraxias and agnosias

Constructional apraxia/visuospatial agnosia*	Inability to construct or copy figures
Dressing apraxia	Difficulty putting clothes on
Agraphia	Inability to write
Alexia	Inability to read
Dyscalculia	Inability to calculate
Topographical disorientation	Getting lost, inability to learn new routes
Autotopagnosia	Inability to name, recognize or point to parts of own or someone else's body
Hemisomatognosia	Part of body felt to be absent
Prosopagnosia	Inability to recognize faces
Anosognosia	Failure to recognize a disabled limb
Finger agnosia	Inability to name/number fingers
Simultagnosia	Inability to recognize complex pictures
*There is considerable overlap in the signs of these two syndromes.	

Table 2.4   Layers of the cerebellar cortex

Superficial	Cell type	Function
Molecular layer	Basket cell Stellate cell	Inhibitory on Purkinje cell
Purkinje layer	Purkinje cell	Predominant cell type, receives all afferent information and provides only efferent pathway; contains GABA
Granular layer	Granule cell Golgi cell	Axon ascends to molecular layer and bifurcates to run parallel to surface; synapses on dendrites of Purkinje cell
Deep		

excitatory fibres that are the terminal projections of spinocerebellar, pontocerebellar and vestibulocerebellar tracts. The fibres terminate in glomeruli, which are synaptic arrangements involving a granule cell, its dendrites and Golgi cells. Climbing fibres provide excitatory input from the olivocerebellum and reticulocerebellum. These fibres terminate on the GABA-containing Purkinje cells, in a 1:1 arrangement, wrapped around their dendrites. Descending fibres from the cerebellum all originate from Purkinje cells and end in cerebellar nuclei where they exert an inhibitory influence. The cerebellar nuclei are the dentate, emboliform, globose and fastigial nuclei.

Connections of the cerebellum

The cerebellar peduncles contain the afferent and efferent tracts of the cerebellum. The inferior cerebellar peduncle contains four afferent tracts (posterior spinocerebellar,

vestibulocerebellar, olivocerebellar and reticulocerebellar) and one efferent tract (the cerebellovestibular tract). The middle cerebellar peduncle is the largest and contains only afferent fibres from the pontine nucleus. This pontocerebellar tract provides an important connection between the cerebral cortex and cerebellum and modulates skilled activities of hands and fingers. The superior cerebellar peduncle contains one afferent, anterior cerebellar tract and one efferent tract from the cerebellar nuclei to the red nucleus, thalamus and medulla.

Cerebellar function

The cerebellum receives information from eyes, ears, proprioceptors, brainstem, cerebral cortex and reticular formation, which is integrated and relayed to other centres involved in controlling movement in the brain. The result of this integration is smooth, coordinated motor function.

Patients with cerebellar dysfunction may show truncal ataxia and dysequilibrium. Muscle tone will be reduced, muscles will tire easily and decreased reflexes will be present. Incoordination of movements will be manifest by poor ability to perform rapid alternating movements (dysdiadochokinesis), past-pointing in finger–nose testing (dysmetria) and intention tremor. Speech may be slurred, jerky, explosive and intermittent. Nystagmus will prevent visual fixation on an object, and gait will be that of a wide-based ataxia.

Until relatively recently, the cerebellum has only been thought of in terms of its key role in motor control. Functional neuroimaging studies have shown that the cerebellum is also involved in working memory, implicit and explicit learning and memory and language. However there are no clinical tests that specifically probe this aspect of its function.

DIENCEPHALON

The diencephalon is comprised of the thalamus, hypothalamus, epithalamus and subthalamus (Box 2.4).

Thalamus

The thalamus is a collection of many nuclear groups and hence consists largely of grey matter. It is a relay station for both sensory and motor information. The connections and functions of the nuclei, with particular reference to psychiatry, are described in Table 2.5.

Hypothalamus

Like the thalamus, the hypothalamus consists of groups of nuclei, involved in endocrine control, neurosecretion, regulation of autonomic function, regulation of body temperature, the biological clock, food and water intake and

Box 2.4 Constituents of the diencephalon
Thalamus
Hypothalamus
Epithalamus
Subthalamus

Table 2.5 Thalamic nuclei, connections and functions

Nucleus	Afferents	Efferents	Function
Anterior	Mammillothalamic	Cingulate gyrus	Part of limbic system, connects hypothalamus, hippocampus, and corticolimbic regions to thalamus
Dorsomedial	Hypothalamus Prefrontal cortex	Prefrontal cortex	Stimulation produces anxiety and dread; cut in lobotomy
Dorsolateral	Cingulate gyrus Parietal cortex (association areas)	Cingulate gyrus Parietal cortex	
Lateral posterior	Occipital cortex	Parietal cortex	Synthesis of higher-order sensory perception
Ventral anterior Ventral lateral	Basal ganglia Cerebellar nuclei via via inferior peduncle	Premotor cortex Motor cortex	Cortical motor mechanisms are continuously updated
Ventral post. medial Ventral post. lateral	Trigeminothalamic medial lemniscus, i.e. ascending sensory inputs	Primary sensory cortex	Processing centres for general sensory input
Med. geniculate body Lat. geniculate body	Lateral lemniscus Optic tract	Primary auditory area Primary visual area	
Pulvinar	Occipital cortex Temporal cortex Parietal cortex	Visual cortex	Visual processing
Intralaminar	Midbrain Basal ganglia Motor, prefrontal cortex	Basal ganglia	Part of reticular system

sexual function. It is also part of the limbic system and is involved in mediating emotion, rage, fear, pleasure and reward.

In addition to being named (Table 2.6), the nuclei of the hypothalamus are also described by their anatomical location within the hypothalamus. Thus the ventromedial nucleus which controls satiety and feeding has a lateral feeding centre and a medial satiety centre. Ablation of the satiety or feeding centres leads to hyperphagia and aphagia respectively. The control of water intake is similarly located. A major role of the hypothalamus in controlling endocrine function is to release hypothalamic releasing factors which stimulate or inhibit the release of hormones from the anterior pituitary. The hypothalamic releasing factors and their corresponding anterior pituitary hormones are described in Table 2.7.

Connections of the hypothalamus

Many of the connecting pathways of the thalamus are part of a two-way system projecting between the midbrain and limbic lobe (Fig. 2.2).

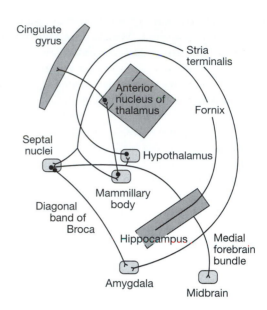

Figure 2.2 Stylized diagram of connections within the limbic system. The stria terminalis and medial forebrain bundle contain fibres travelling in both directions.

Table 2.6 Hypothalamic nuclei and their function		
Nuclear region	*Subnucleus*	*Function*
Preoptic		Produces gonadotrophic hormones
Supraoptic	Supraoptic, paraventricular	Secrete antidiuretic hormone (vasopressin), oxytocin
	Anterior hypothalamic	Parasympathetic – decreases heart rate, secretion in gastrointestinal tract
	Suprachiasmatic	Secretes antidiuretic hormone
Tuberal	Ventromedial	Control of hunger, satiety – terminates feeding on stimulation
	Dorsomedial	Emotional behaviour, rage when ablated
Arcuate		Contributes neurosecretory fibres to vascular portal system of anterior pituitary
Mammillary	Mammillary bodies	Integrates information from limbic system via fornix
		Memory – affected in Korsakoff's psychosis
Posterior		Sympathetic responses

Table 2.7 Hypothalamic releasing factors and the associated anterior pituitary hormone	
Hypothalamic releasing factor	*Anterior pituitary hormone*
Corticotrophin (CRF)	Adrenocorticotrophin (ACTH)
Gonadotrophin releasing factor	Follicular stimulating hormone (FSH)
	Luteinizing hormone (LH)
Growth factor releasing hormone	Somatotrophin, growth hormone (GH)
Growth factor inhibiting factor, somatostatin	
Melatonin stimulating hormone release inhibiting factor (MSHRIF)	Melatonin stimulating hormone (MSH)
Prolactin releasing factor	Prolactin
Prolactin inhibiting factor (dopamine)	
Thyrotrophin	Thyroid stimulating hormone (TSH)

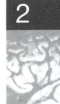

Afferent pathways

There are a number of pathways that connect the hypothalamus with other components of the limbic system, the medial forebrain bundle, fornix and stria terminalis. The medial forebrain bundle consists of projections from the olfactory part of forebrain and septal nuclei and passes through the hypothalamus, to the tegmentum in the midbrain. Fibres from the medial forebrain bundle project into the lateral hypothalamus.

The fornix arises from the hippocampus and projects to the mammillary bodies, and is more fully described in relation to the hippocampus. The stria terminalis arises in the amygdala, a nuclear complex with a key role in the formation and processing of emotional content. In addition to terminating in the nucleus of stria terminalis, projections terminate in the preoptic, tuberal and anterior nuclei of the hypothalamus.

Other afferent fibres arise in the forebrain, upper brainstem, thalamus and visual pathways.

Efferent pathways

Many of the pathways described above also carry efferent projections from the hypothalamus. The medial forebrain bundle carries fibres from the lateral hypothalamus to the septal nuclei and tegmentum of the midbrain. The stria terminalis carries fibres from the ventromedial hypothalamic nucleus to the amygdala.

Other efferent pathways include the projections from the supraoptic and paraventricular nuclei, which secrete antidiuretic hormone and oxytocin, to the posterior lobe of pituitary gland or neurohypophysis. The tubero-infundibular tract arises in the arcuate nucleus and terminates near the hypophyseal portal system. Releasing hormones diffuse into blood vessels of the portal system to enter the pituitary and stimulate the release of hormones from the anterior lobe.

Other pathways include those that arise in the mammillary bodies and the mammillotegmental and mammillothalamic tracts, and project to the tegmentum and anterior nucleus of the thalamus respectively.

Epithalamus

The epithalamus contains the medial and lateral habenular nuclei, the pineal gland and the stria medullaris. Light regulates the synthesis of melatonin, allowing the pineal gland to modulate the circadian rhythm.

Subthalamus

The subthalamus contains several nuclei and is concerned with motor control.

THE LIMBIC SYSTEM

The limbic system is concerned with memory and behavioural and emotional expression. The limbic system or Papez circuit was initially described as comprising the hippocampus, mammillary bodies of the hypothalamus, anterior nucleus of the thalamus and cingulate gyrus and their connecting pathways. Since then other regions have been included in the limbic system, but different authorities list different components (Box 2.5). Generally, however, the limbic system includes the hippocampal formation, the parahippocampal, cingulate and subcallosal gyri, the anterior nucleus of the thalamus, the hypothalamus, amygdala, septal area and areas associated with mediating olfaction. The hippocampal formation comprises the hippocampus, dentate gyrus and the parahippocampal gyrus, which includes the entorhinal cortex. The alveus, fimbria, fornix and mammillothalamic tracts provide the intralimbic and external communication pathways of the limbic system (Fig. 2.2).

Box 2.5 Constituents and pathways of the limbic system	
Hippocampus	Cingulate gyrus
Mammillary bodies	Parahippocampal gyrus
Hypothalamus	Amygdala
Anterior nucleus of the thalamus	Nucleus accumbens
Septal nuclei	
Fornix	Mammillothalamic tract

Hippocampus

The hippocampus is a curled structure within the medial aspect of the temporal lobe, lying in the floor of the inferior horn of the lateral ventricle. It interlocks with the dentate gyrus like two capital C's facing each other. The dentate gyrus lies between the hippocampus and parahippocampal gyrus. It is continuous with the uncus at its anterior margin and with the indusium griseum posteriorly. The indusium griseum is a strip of grey matter over the corpus callosum. The parahippocampal gyrus, which includes the entorhinal cortex or secondary olfactory cortex, is also continuous with the uncus anteriorly.

Connections of the hippocampus
Afferent pathways

The hippocampus receives afferent fibres from the cingulate gyrus, the dentate gyrus, the contralateral hippocampus, parahippocampal gyrus, the septal area, indusium griseum and the diencephalon.

Efferent pathway: the fornix

Efferent fibres from the hippocampus converge in the alveus, which then join together in the fimbria. The fimbria further converge to form the fornix, which is the major efferent tract from the hippocampus. Some fibres from the fornix terminate in the anterior nucleus of thalamus. At the anterior commissure, the fornix bifurcates into pre- and post-commissural fibres that terminate in the septal nuclei and mammillary bodies respectively. Other regions innervated include the anterior hypothalamus, habenular nuclei and tegmentum.

There are a number of other reciprocal pathways linking the hippocampus to other limbic regions. The amygdala and hippocampus are connected via the stria terminalis and also via the septal nuclei. Another pathway is from the hippocampus via the fornix to the septal nuclei from which the diagonal band of Broca relays information to the amygdala.

Amygdala

The amygdaloid complex contains many nuclei involved in both sensory and motor functions. It is an important component of the limbic system. The amygdala plays a key role in emotional processing and associative learning, making emotional memories easier to recall than non-emotional events. Damage to the amygdala can result in impaired emotional processing of stimuli such as increased threshold, e.g. degree of fear, threat, disgust, and anger, impaired emotional learning, and deficits in emotional perception and expression. Stimulation of the amygdala produces aggressive behaviour in animals, while ablation causes placidity.

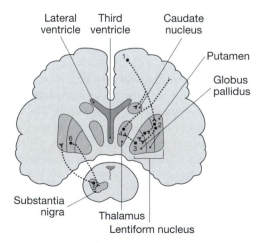

Figure 2.3 Basal ganglia and its connections: coronal stylized section. Pathway 1→4 is the mechanism by which voluntary movement is modulated. Pathway 5→6 is the nigrostriatal/striatonigral pathway.

Nucleus accumbens

The nucleus accumbens is contained within the ventral striatum in man but is not visible as an anatomically separate division within this part of the striatum. The nucleus accumbens is part of the mesolimbic system and receives dopaminergic projections from the ventral tegmental area (VTA) in the brainstem. Release of dopamine in the nucleus accumbens is critical in mediating positive reinforcement or pleasure for both natural rewards such as food or sex and also substances of abuse such as alcohol and cocaine. Dopamine-dependent processes are involved in recognizing stimuli and in 'labelling' them with appetitive value, predicting and detecting rewards and signal alerting and novel events. More recently, it has been recognized that release of dopamine here also occurs in response to aversive stimuli.

BASAL GANGLIA

Components of the basal ganglia

The basal ganglia consist of the corpus striatum, globus pallidus, claustrum and specific nuclei of the amygdaloid complex (Fig. 2.3 and Box 2.6). The corpus striatum comprises the caudate nucleus and putamen. The combination of the putamen laterally and globus pallidus medially is referred to as the lentiform nucleus. The claustrum is the strip of grey matter lateral to the lentiform nucleus.

Connections of the basal ganglia

The caudate and putamen receive afferent fibres from all parts of the cerebral cortex and topographically project onto the globus pallidus. Efferent fibres from the globus pallidus project to the ventral nuclei of the thalamus and brainstem. The ventral nuclei of the thalamus also project to the premotor cerebral cortex, completing a circuit whereby motor activity arising in the motor cortex can be monitored and modulated by the basal ganglia. The other major reciprocal connection is between the striatum and the

Box 2.6   Components of the basal ganglia

Corpus striatum
  caudate nucleus
  putamen

Lentiform nucleus
  globus pallidus
  putamen

Claustrum
Amygdala

substantia nigra, the nigrostriatal and striatonigral pathways (see Fig. 2.3).

Functions of the basal ganglia

The basal ganglia are responsible for programming, integration and termination of motor activity. Motor activity controlled by the basal ganglia forms a significant part of the extrapyramidal motor system (see below). However, the traditional view that the basal ganglia are simply involved in the control of movement has been challenged in recent years. Activity in some parts of the basal ganglia is higher during cognitive or sensory functions and circuits exist between the basal ganglia and cognitive areas of the cerebral cortex. The basal ganglia appears to be involved in fundamental aspects of attentional control (often covert), in the guidance of the early stages of learning (especially reinforcement-based learning, but also in encoding strategies in explicit paradigms), and in the associative binding of reward to cue salience and response sequences via dopaminergic mechanisms.

Basal ganglia dysfunction

Dysfunction involving the basal ganglia results in a number of motor disorders. The resulting typical signs and symptoms are described in Table 2.8. The nigrostriatal projection to the globus pallidus and striatum from the substantia nigra contains dopamine. Degeneration of this pathway, due to loss of neurons in the substantia nigra and consequent loss of dopamine, underlies Parkinson's disease. The symptoms of Parkinson's disease or so-called parkinsonism can be reproduced by blockade of dopamine D_2 receptors in the basal ganglia. This is commonly seen secondary to the use of typical antipsychotic medication.

Other disorders associated with dysfunction of the basal ganglia include Huntington's chorea, caused by degeneration of the caudate, and Wilson's disease, caused by copper deposition in the basal ganglia and liver. In Huntington's chorea, loss of caudate function causes choreiform movements and neuropsychiatric symptoms such as depression, psychosis and dementia. Huntington's chorea is an autosomal dominant disease, with the gene on

chromosome 4. In addition to dysfunction of the basal ganglia, the classic sign of Wilson's disease is the Kayser–Fleischer ring – a brown coppery ring around the cornea. Wilson's disease is due to an inborn error of copper metabolism.

BRAINSTEM

The brainstem ascends from the spinal cord through the medulla, pons, and midbrain and into the diencephalon (Box 2.7).

SPINAL CORD

The spinal cord consists of a number of ascending and descending tracts that convey sensory and motor information between the periphery and the brain (Fig. 2.4).

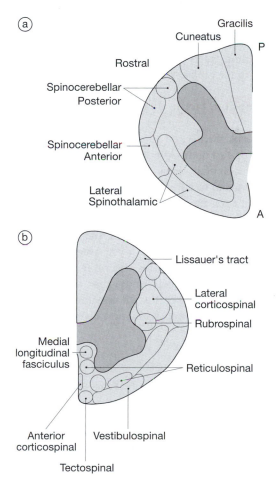

Figure 2.4 Spinal cord tracts. (a) Ascending tracts. (b) Descending tracts. A = anterior; P = posterior.

Table 2.8 Basal ganglia dysfunction	
Disturbance of muscle tone	Rigidity – cog-wheeling
Loss of automatic associated movement	Swinging arms when walking, facial expression
Unwanted movements, uncontrollable, purposeless, usually distal	Choreiform – 'fidgety' movements Hemiballismus Athetoid – slow, writhing movements of arms and legs Resting tremor

Box 2.7   Contents of the brainstem

Medulla	Pons	Midbrain
Decussation of pyramids – corticospinal tracts	Corticobulbar, rubrospinal tracts	Mesencephalic nucleus of V
Rubrospinal, vestibulospinal, tectospinal tracts	Medial longitudinal fasciculus	Nucleus of IV
Medial longitudinal fasciculus – ascending and descending fibres (involves eye movements – III, IV, VI)	Spinal trigeminal nucleus and tract	Oculomotor nucleus (III) (Edinger–Westphal)
	Mesencephalic nuclei of V	Medial longitudinal fasciculus
	Nucleus of VI	Reticular formation
Inferior olivary nucleus – projects to cerebellum	Nucleus of VII	Raphe nuclei (serotonin)
Nucleus gracilis and cuneate	Trapezoid body	Periaqueductal grey matter
Decussation of medial lemniscus – fibres from gracilis and cuneus to thalamus	Superior olivary nucleus – auditory	Superior cerebellar peduncle
	Lateral and superior vestibular nuclei	Medial and lateral lemniscus
	Reticular formation	Crus cerebri
Nuclei of cranial nerves XII and spinal root of XI	Locus coeruleus (noradrenaline)	Substantia nigra
Spinal root of cranial nerve V	Floor of fourth ventricle	Inferior colliculi – auditory
Medial, lateral, superior and inferior vestibular nuclei	Middle and superior cerebellar peduncles	Superior colliculi – visual
Anterior and dorsal cochlear nuclei		Red nucleus – afferents from cerebellum and cerebral cortex and efferents to spinal cord, cranial nuclei
Dorsal motor nucleus of cranial nerve X		Cerebral aqueduct
Solitary nucleus		
Nucleus ambiguus – motor – for IX, X, XI		
Reticular formation		
Fourth ventricle		
Inferior cerebellar peduncle		

Ascending tracts

The ascending tracts carry sensory information from the periphery to the central nervous system.

Proprioception, tactile discrimination and vibration sense

The fasciculus gracilis and cuneatus constitute large tracts in the posterior part of the spinal cord. Fibres in these tracts are organized such that those from sacral to cervical spinal nerves lie medial to lateral respectively. They carry sensory information regarding proprioception, tactile discrimination and vibration sense. The tracts are ipsilateral until they reach the medulla, where they synapse in their respective nuclei. Fibres project from here, cross over, ascend as the medial lemniscus and terminate in the ventral posterior nucleus of thalamus. Fibres project from the thalamus to the somatosensory, parietal cortex, via the internal capsule. The body is mapped somatotopically and inverted with the face most inferior.

Pain and temperature

The lateral spinothalamic tract carries information about pain and temperature. The anterior spinothalamic tract carries sensory information regarding light, poorly localized touch. This information is carried in slow-conducting fibres (Aδ and C fibres) in contrast to the rapidly conducting fibres carrying information about pain and temperature. After joining the spinal cord, the fibres cross after ascending 1-2 segments and synapse in Lissauer's tract. From there the fibres ascend as the lateral or anterior spinothalamic tract,

and terminate in the ventral posterior nucleus of the thalamus. Fibres are also given off to the reticular formation and periaqueductal grey matter. The sensory cerebral cortex receives the final projections as described above.

Since the dorsal columns and spinothalamic tracts contain ipsilateral and contralateral fibres respectively, transection of one-half of the spinal cord leads to a characteristic pattern of sensory loss. This is known as Brown–Sequard syndrome or sensory dissociation. Below such a lesion, there is loss of two-point discrimination and proprioception ipsilaterally and loss of pain and temperature sensation contralaterally.

Muscle and tendon function

The spinocerebellar tract relays information from muscle spindle or tendon–organ receptors. It is an ipsilateral tract.

Descending tracts

The descending tracts relay information from cortical and subcortical regions and the brainstem to the periphery to initiate and modulate movement.

Corticospinal or pyramidal tracts

The corticospinal tracts mediate voluntary movements and arise from the cerebral cortex as described previously. The lateral corticospinal tract is present throughout the entire length of the spinal cord. The anterior corticospinal tract is different in two respects from the lateral corticospinal tract in that it is ipsilateral and terminates at the level of the thoracic vertebrae.

The extrapyramidal tracts

There are several tracts that constitute the extrapyramidal motor system. The vestibulospinal tract arises from the vestibular nuclei and terminates on the anterior horn cells. Information in this tract facilitates activity in all anti-gravity (extensor) muscles. The rubrospinal tract arises from the red nucleus in the midbrain and terminates on interneurons. This tract terminates in the thoracic part of the spinal cord and controls flexor tone. The tectospinal tract arises from the superior colliculus and terminates on interneurons. This tract relays information to the cervical level about postural reflexes to do with visual and auditory stimuli. The reticulospinal tract arises from brainstem nuclei and also terminates on interneurons.

Mixed ascending and descending tract

The medial longitudinal fasciculus contains both ascending and descending fibres. It relays information regarding visual tracking of a moving object through coordinated movements of eyes, head, neck and trunk. The descending fibres arise from the superior colliculus, motor nucleus of the third cranial nerve (visual, visual tracking), and pontine and vestibular nuclei (balance). The fibres terminate on anterior horn cells. Ascending fibres arise from vestibular nuclei and terminate in the third, fourth and sixth cranial nerve nuclei.

OVERVIEW OF SENSORY AND MOTOR SYSTEMS

Sensory system

Conscious appreciation of sensation occurs in the post-central gyrus, of the parietal lobe, of visual stimuli in the occipital lobe and of auditory stimuli in the temporal lobe. The sensory nerve for all of these modalities arises in the dorsal root ganglion, the processes of which terminate at the peripheral receptor in the tissue and centrally at nuclei specific to the information being carried. A projection then relays the information topographically to the thalamus, from which the final projection to the parietal cortex arises.

Receptors

There are a number of different peripheral receptors. Flower-spray and anulospiral endings in muscle spindle organs and Golgi tendon organs register stretching or movement. Thus they play an important role in proprioception, perception of limb position and control of posture and muscle tone.

Touch, temperature and pain are detected by unencapsulated receptors such as free or Merkel's discs. The encapsulated receptors, the Pacinian and Meissner corpuscles, detect pressure and vibration and two-point discrimination, respectively. Sensory information is carried in myelinated Ad and Ab fibres and in unmyelinated C fibres. Touch is mediated by Ad and Ab, pain by Ad, and temperature by C fibres. Each spinal nerve carries information from a specific dermatome, or area of cutaneous and subcutaneous tissue. The pathways running within the spinal cord to the brainstem and associated with each sensory modality are described above.

Motor system

Voluntary movement is initiated in the primary motor cortex of the frontal lobe. The body is mapped somatotopically and inverted, with the face most inferior on the lateral surface and lower limbs represented on the medial surface of the frontal lobe. The pyramidal cells of this region give rise to fibres that run through the internal capsule, decussate in the midbrain and travel down the spinal cord as the corticospinal tract. The tracts terminate on the anterior horn cells and also on interneurons within the spinal cord.

In addition, collaterals are given off to the basal ganglia – predominantly the putamen – and to the cerebellum. This allows modulation and coordination of voluntary movement. These systems constitute part of the extrapyramidal system (see description of extrapyramidal tracts above).

The corticospinal tract provides an excitatory input to the anterior horn cells, whereas the extrapyramidal system tends to be inhibitory. All projections onto the anterior horn cell are referred to as upper motor neuron, and from the anterior horn cell to the muscle as lower motor neuron. The effects of lesions of lower and upper motor neurons are described in Table 2.9.

AUTONOMIC NERVOUS SYSTEM

The autonomic nervous system (Fig. 2.5) is that part of the peripheral nervous system that innervates and regulates smooth and cardiac muscles and glands. The autonomic system and the central nervous system, including the hypothalamus and limbic system, interact in order to integrate activity appropriately. However, many autonomic responses are at an unconscious level and are governed through reflexes.

Table 2.9 Effects of lower and upper motor neuron lesions	
Lower motor neuron	*Upper motor neuron*
Hypotonia	Hypertonia
Flaccid paralysis	Spastic paralysis
Hyporeflexia	Hyperreflexia
Wasting of muscles with fasciculation, fibrillation	Babinski sign

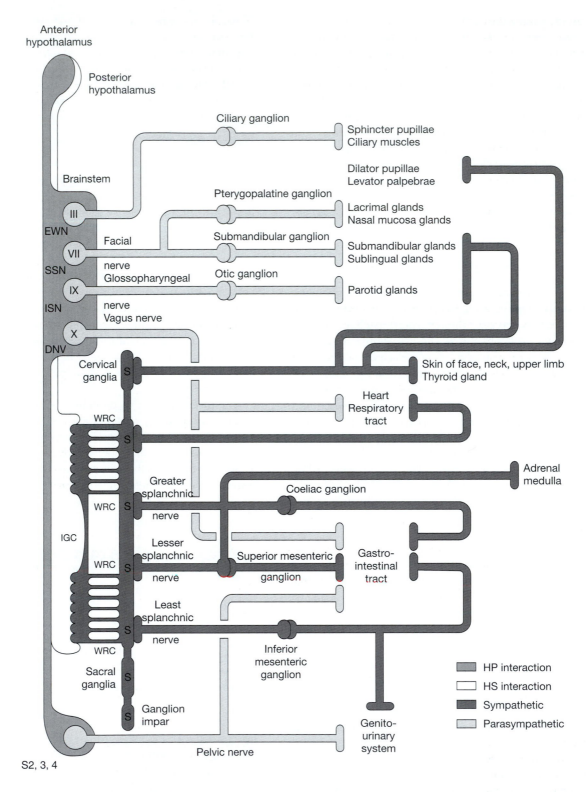

Figure 2.5 Schematic diagram of the autonomic nervous system showing sympathetic and parasympathetic supplies to major glands and organs. Sympathetic nerves leave the sympathetic chain at all levels but only the major nerves are shown. EWN: Edinger–Westphal nucleus, SSN: superior salivary nucleus, ISN: inferior salivary nucleus, DNV: dorsal nucleus of vagus, III, VII, IX and X: cranial nerves, IGC: interomediolateral grey column of segments T1–L2, S: sympathetic chain, WRC: white rami communicantes, HP: hypothalamo–parasympathetic, HS: hypothalamo–sympathetic, S2, 3, 4: sacral segments, 2, 3 and 4. (From original drawing by Pádraig Wright.)

The autonomic nervous system comprises sympathetic and parasympathetic systems. These nervous systems tend to have the opposite effect on target organs such that parasympathetic stimulation leads to increased gut motility, for example, while sympathetic stimulation causes reduced motility.

The peripheral target organ is reached through a two-neuron relay in the autonomic system. The preganglionic neuron is located in the spinal cord or brainstem and terminates in a peripheral ganglion. Arising from this ganglion, the postganglionic neuron innervates the target organ. In the sympathetic nervous system, the postganglionic fibres are much longer than the preganglionic fibres. The reverse is true in the parasympathetic system. Thus the ganglia in the sympathetic system lie close to the central nervous system while the ganglia of the parasympathetic lie close to the target organ. Another difference between these two systems is the neurotransmitter released by the postganglionic fibres. Parasympathetic postganglionic fibres release acetylcholine while sympathetic fibres release noradrenaline with the exception of those that terminate in sweat glands which release acetylcholine. In both parasympathetic and sympathetic systems, the preganglionic neurons release acetylcholine.

The site of origin of the sympathetic and parasympathetic nervous systems also differ anatomically. The sympathetic nervous system arises from the interomediolateral grey column of thoracolumbar segments T1–T12 and L1–L2 of the spinal cord. The preganglionic cell bodies of the parasympathetic system are located in the brainstem, and in the intermediate grey matter of sacral segments S2–S4 of the spinal cord. Brainstem parasympathetic nuclei include the Edinger–Westphal nucleus (IIIrd cranial nerve), the superior and inferior salivatory nuclei (VIIth and IXth cranial nerves) and the dorsal motor nucleus of the vagus (Xth cranial nerve) (see Cranial Nerves and Fig. 2.5).

Sympathetic nervous system

Anatomy
The sympathetic myelinated preganglionic fibres leave the spinal column within the motor nerves, but soon separate to form the white rami communicantes, which terminate in the sympathetic chain of ganglia. On entering this chain, the nerve fibres may synapse at the level of entry, or ascend (particularly in the cervical region) or descend (particularly in the lumbar region) to synapse with cell bodies of postganglionic neurons. Alternatively, the nerve fibres pass through the chain, form the thoracic or lumbar splanchnic nerve and synapse in the prevertebral ganglia of the abdomen and pelvis (see below).

The ganglia in the sympathetic chain are paired and extend either side of the vertebral column from the cervical region to the coccyx. This chain is also referred to as the paravertebral ganglion. There are generally three cervical ganglia, namely superior, middle and inferior, which lie on the posterior wall of the carotid sheath. If the inferior cervical ganglion is fused with the first thoracic ganglion, it is called the stellate ganglion. There are usually eleven thoracic, four lumbar and four sacral ganglia. At the level of the coccyx there is a single ganglion called the ganglion impar.

Postganglionic fibres leave the chain forming the grey rami communicantes and enter the spinal nerve. These fibres are non-myelinated. Grey rami communicantes are found at all levels of the sympathetic chain. The postganglionic fibres are distributed to the blood vessels, sweat glands and erector pili muscles throughout the dermatome supplied by the spinal nerve associated with each ramus communicante. Thus there are 31 pairs of grey rami communicantes, accompanying each spinal nerve. However, there are only 14 white rami communicantes, limited to the thoracic and upper lumbar segments. Therefore ganglia situated in the cervical, lower lumbar, sacral or coccygeal levels receive their preganglionic fibres after they have travelled within the sympathetic chain.

Divisions and functions
Generally, sympathetic stimulation prepares the body for 'fight or flight', hence pupils are dilated, cardiac and respiratory performance increases and peripheral vasoconstriction, sweating and piloerection occurs. By contrast, gut activity is lessened, sphincters are contracted and blood is diverted from the splanchnic bed.

Cervical ganglia
The superior cervical ganglion gives rise to the carotid plexus whose fibres run with the carotid arteries and provide sympathetic innervation to the head. This includes supplying the dilator muscles of the iris, lacrimal glands, salivary glands, levator palpebrae, erector pili muscles and small blood vessels. In addition, postganglionic fibres from this ganglion join the cardiac plexus as the cardiac nerve, or join the IXth, Xth and XIth cranial nerves and also form the grey rami communicantes of spinal nerves C1–C4.

The medial cervical ganglion gives rise to fibres that innervate the thyroid gland, oesophagus and trachea, and contribute to the cardiac plexus and the grey rami communicantes of spinal nerves C5–C7. The inferior or stellate ganglion also contributes to the cardiac plexus in addition to the grey rami communicantes of spinal nerves C7 and T1.

The cardiac plexus supplies organs within the thorax. In addition, postganglionic fibres from the upper five thoracic levels contribute to a pulmonary plexus. Sympathetic stimulation results in easier breathing by relaxing the bronchial smooth muscle and inhibiting bronchial secretions and in increased cardiac output by increasing the rate and contractility with vasodilation of the coronary arteries.

Mesenteric ganglia

The greater splanchnic nerve is formed from the preganglionic fibres of T5–T9, which traverse the paravertebral ganglion and terminate in the coeliac and superior mesenteric ganglia. The lesser and least splanchnic nerves are similarly formed from levels T10 and T11 and from T12 respectively, which terminate in the superior and inferior mesenteric ganglia respectively. These three ganglia are known collectively as the prevertebral ganglia and are located at the root of the arteries of the same name. The postganglionic fibres supply the gut, and generally inhibit motility and secretion and result in contraction of sphincters such as the pyloric and ileocaecal.

Preganglionic fibres of the lesser and least splanchnic nerves terminate directly on cells in the adrenal medulla that secrete adrenaline and noradrenaline. The medullary cells are derived from embryonic nerve tissue and are akin to a modified sympathetic ganglion. Various stimuli, including pain, rage and fear, evoke the fight or flight response by stimulating release of adrenaline.

The inferior mesenteric ganglion also receives fibres from L1 and L2 preganglionic neurons, known as the lumbar splanchnic nerve. The large intestine and kidney are the target organs from this ganglion in addition to a contribution to the pelvic plexus. This pelvic plexus also contains parasympathetic nerves.

The lumbar splanchnic nerves arise from the upper lumbar levels and terminate in the inferior mesenteric and hypogastric ganglia. From these prevertebral ganglia, the postganglionic fibres supply organs in the pelvis, lower abdomen and lower limb.

Parasympathetic nervous system

Anatomy

As described above, the cell bodies of the preganglionic fibres of the parasympathetic system are located in the brainstem and sacral part of the spinal cord. The anatomy and function of the nerves from the brainstem are also described more fully with their associated cranial nerve (III, VII, IX, X).

Divisions and functions

Preganglionic fibres arise in the Edinger–Westphal nucleus, run with the oculomotor (III) nerve and terminate in the ciliary ganglion. Stimulation results in constriction of the pupils via contraction of the ciliary muscle and sphincter.

The pterygopalatine and submandibular ganglia are associated with the facial (VII) nerve and innervate the lacrimal glands, mucous glands of the nose, sinuses, mouth and pharynx and the submandibular and sublingual glands respectively. Stimulation of the submandibular and otic ganglia results in the production of a watery secretion by all salivary glands.

The vagus (X) nerve supplies a great number of organs over an extensive area, including the heart, lungs, gut and other abdominal organs. The ganglia from which the postganglionic fibres arise are sited usually in the walls of the target organ. Vagal stimulation results in reduced heart and respiratory rate, constriction of bronchi and increased bronchial secretion, and increased gut motility and secretions therein.

The sacral component of the parasympathetic nervous system arises in the neurons of the lateral horn of sacral segments S2–S4 of the spinal cord. The preganglionic fibres are termed the pelvic splanchnic nerves. The target organs include the colon, rectum, urinary bladder and reproductive organs. Stimulation results in emptying of the bladder, increased gut motility and erection of the penis or clitoris. In addition, vaginal secretions are increased in women.

CRANIAL NERVES

There are 12 pairs of cranial nerves. Their exit foramina from the skull are described in Table 2.10. Each cranial nerve is described as to whether it has sensory or motor, or somatic or autonomic components.

Table 2.10 The cranial nerves and the skull foramina through which they exit

Olfactory nerves	I	Cribriform plates of ethmoid bone
Optic nerve	II	Optic canal with ophthalmic artery
Oculomotor nerve	III	Superior orbital fissure
Trochlear nerve	IV	Superior orbital fissure
Ophthalmic (1st) of trigeminal nerve	V	Superior orbital fissure
Maxillary (2nd) of trigeminal nerve	V	Foramen rotundum
Mandibular (3rd) of trigeminal nerve	V	Foramen ovale
Abducens nerve	VI	Superior orbital fissure
Facial nerve	VII	Internal auditory meatus
Vestibulocochlear nerve	VIII	Internal auditory meatus
Glossopharyngeal nerve	IX	Jugular foramen
Vagus nerve	X	Jugular foramen
Both roots of accessory nerve	XI	Jugular foramen
Spinal roots of accessory nerve	XI	Foramen magnum
Hypoglossal nerve	XII	Hypoglossal canal

Olfactory nerve

The Ist cranial nerve is the olfactory nerve, a sensory nerve arising peripherally in the mucous membrane of the nasal cavity. The nerve passes through the cribriform plate of the ethmoid bone and synapses in the olfactory bulb. The second-order neurons form the olfactory tract and project to the septal area, and from there to the hippocampus and hypothalamus. The primary (amygdaloid complex and piriform cortex) and secondary (entorhinal cortex) olfactory areas are the final projection areas.

Optic nerve

The retina

This sensory cranial nerve arises from the retinal ganglion cells. The outermost layer of the retina comprises pigmented epithelium under which lie the rods and cones. These are sensitive to light. The rods are more sensitive to light than the cones and hence are responsible for night vision. The cones contain one of three different pigments that are maximally sensitive to light in the blue, green or orange range. They are concentrated in the fovea centralis. Both rods and cones synapse with bipolar cells, cones in a 1:1 relationship, while rods may synapse with many bipolar cells. The bipolar cells then synapse with ganglion cells, whose axons form the optic nerve.

The optic nerve and radiation

The medial fibres of the optic nerve, which represent the temporal visual fields, cross in the optic chiasma to join the contralateral optic tract (Fig. 2.6). The lateral fibres of the optic nerve, representing the nasal visual field, pass through the optic chiasma to the ipsilateral optic tract. The fibres of the optic tract synapse in the lateral geniculate body of the thalamus. From here, the optic radiation runs within the posterior part of the internal capsule. The optic radiation terminates in the visual cortex, which is part of the occipital lobe, with fibres also going to association areas of the parietal cortex. Myer's loop is part of the optic radiation that loops anteriorly from the lateral geniculate ganglion into the temporal lobe before travelling posteriorly to terminate in the occipital cortex. Fibres in Myer's loop carry information from the top half of the visual field. In the occipital cortex, the visual fields are inverted such that the inferior cortex receives information from the upper visual field.

Effects of lesions of the visual pathway

Lesions within the visual pathway produce characteristic visual defects that pinpoint the site of the lesion (Fig. 2.6). A lesion anterior to the optic chiasma results in loss of the visual field to that eye. Any lesion of or posterior to the optic chiasma will result in visual defects in both eyes. A pituitary tumour compressing the optic chiasma and hence the temporal visual field fibres as they cross will result in bitemporal heteronymous hemianopia. Homonymous hemianopia results from loss of the optic tract or radiation on one side. Damage to Myer's loop results in homonymous superior quadrantanopia and may be the first indication of a lesion within the temporal lobe. Papilloedema is characterized by blurring of the optic disc on fundoscopy and can be caused by a number of different conditions (see Table 2.11).

Oculomotor nerve

The oculomotor nerve is a motor nerve containing both somatic and parasympathetic components.

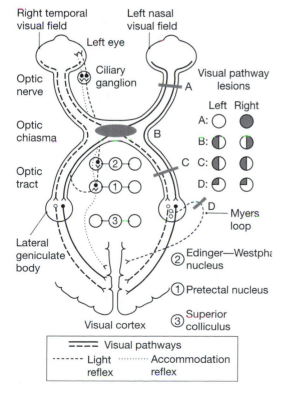

Figure 2.6 The visual pathway and its reflexes.

Table 2.11 Common causes of papilloedema	
Intracranial mass lesion	Optic neuritis (MS)
Encephalitis	CO_2 retention
Subarachnoid haemorrhage	Chronic anoxia
Accelerated hypertension	Optic neuropathy
Disc infiltration	
Retinal vein obstruction	

Motor somatic

The oculomotor nuclei are within the midbrain, next to the periaqueductal grey matter and superior colliculus, and give rise to a nerve that ascends and passes through the superior orbital fissure. The eye muscles innervated by the oculomotor nerve are the inferior rectus, medial rectus, superior rectus, inferior oblique and levator palpebrae. The role of these muscles and their innervation is described in Table 2.12.

The motor nuclei of the IIIrd, IVth and VIth nerves are linked through the medial longitudinal fasciculus, which coordinates movement of the eyes. Fixation to a target or searching the visual fields involves involuntary and voluntary movement of the eyes respectively. The former involves a reflex arc including the occipital association areas. Visual search or saccadic eye movements involves a projection from the occipito–parietal cortex to the frontal eye fields in the frontal lobe.

Motor parasympathetic

The parasympathetic motor nucleus of the third nerve is the Edinger–Westphal nucleus, which sends preganglionic fibres to the ciliary ganglion. The short ciliary nerves comprise the postganglionic fibres and project to the ciliary and sphincter pupillae muscles of the iris. Stimulation results in pupillary constriction and focusing for near vision or accommodation.

Pupillary reflexes

Light reflex
The pupillary light reflex functions to allow the size of the pupil to respond to light conditions by contracting and dilating and also allows both pupils to react together or consensually. The afferent limb consists of the optic nerve, projecting through the optic chiasma and optic tract bilaterally to the pretectal nucleus and the parasympathetic Edinger–Westphal nucleus. The efferent limb consists of parasympathetic preganglionic fibres from the Edinger–Westphal nucleus which accompany the oculomotor nerve and synapse in the ciliary ganglion. From there, postganglionic fibres innervate the ciliary and constrictor muscles of the iris. The light reflex does not involve the visual cortex (Fig. 2.6).

Accommodation reflex
The accommodation reflex functions to allow the eye to focus on near objects. Projections from the primary visual cortex via the superior colliculus and/or pretectal nucleus terminate in the Edinger–Westphal nucleus. From here, parasympathetic nerves follow the same pathway as for the light reflex and project to the ciliary muscle. On contraction of this muscle, lens convexity increases, facilitating near vision (Fig. 2.6).

Effects of lesions

Lesions of the oculomotor nerve result in ptosis and deviation of the eye downwards and outwards. If parasympathetic innervation is also lost, the pupil will be dilated. Argyll-Robertson pupils occur in neurosyphilis and are small, unequal, irregular pupils that do not react to light. The convergence reflex, however, is normal. In Horner's syndrome, the pupil is constricted due to the loss of sympathetic innervation. Ptosis, anhydrosis and eno-phthalmos also occur.

Trochlear nerve

The trochlear or IVth cranial nerve is a motor nerve that supplies the superior oblique muscle of the eye (Table 2.12).

Abducens nerve

The abducens nerve (VI) is also solely a motor nerve and supplies the lateral rectus muscle of the eye (Table 2.12). This nerve emerges at the cerebellopontine angle and has the longest intracranial course, both of which make this nerve particularly vulnerable to damage. Loss of nerve function results in 'cross-eye'. This nerve is the most commonly affected in ophthalmoplegia associated with Wernicke–Korsakoff's syndrome.

Trigeminal nerve

The trigeminal nerve is the largest cranial nerve and contains both motor and sensory, and somatic and autonomic components. It emerges at the cerebellopontine angle, along with cranial nerves VI, VII, VIII and IX.

Motor-somatic
The motor nucleus lies close to the sensory nucleus, and fibres run within the mandibular branch. Thus, unlike the other two branches of the trigeminal nerve, the mandibular branch contains both sensory and motor nerve fibres. It supplies the muscles of mastication, which are temporalis,

Table 2.12 Movements of the eye and the muscles responsible		
Muscle	Nerve	Movement
Medial rectus	III	Horizontally inwards
Inferior rectus	III	In abduction: depresses eye
Superior rectus	III	In abduction: elevates eye
Inferior oblique	III	In adduction: elevates eye
Superior oblique	IV	In adduction: depresses eye
Lateral rectus	VI	Horizontally outwards
Levator palpebrae	III	Lifts eyelids

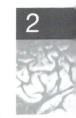

masseter and pterygoids, and in addition supplies tensor tympani of middle ear, tensor veli palatini of pharynx and digastric muscles of mouth. A lesion involving this nerve results in loss of the jaw jerk.

Sensory somatic

The cell bodies of primary sensory somatic neurons are located in the trigeminal ganglion and give rise to three peripheral divisions or branches:

- The ophthalmic division enters the orbit through the superior orbital fissure with the ophthalmic artery and IIIrd, IVth and VIth cranial nerves. This branch innervates skin on top of the head and scalp and is involved in the corneal reflex, via the nasociliary branch.
- The maxillary branch innervates skin on the cheek area.
- The mandibular branch innervates skin on the lower part of the face, buccal cavity, external ear, lower teeth and lip.

Centrally, fibres from these sensory nerves convey impulses to three sensory nuclei:

- The spinal trigeminal nucleus mediates facial touch, temperature and pain via the spinal trigeminal tract.
- The main sensory nucleus mediates touch, position sense and two-point discrimination.
- The mesencephalic nucleus of the Vth nerve mediates proprioception of muscles of mastication.

From the spinal trigeminal nucleus and main sensory nucleus fibres relay information to the sensory cortex of parietal lobe via the ventral posterior nucleus of the thalamus.

Autonomic

While it has no parasympathetic nucleus, as seen with the IIIrd nerve, various branches of the trigeminal nerve include autonomic – both parasympathetic and sympathetic – components.

Facial nerve

The VIIth nerve contains motor somatic and parasympathetic, and sensory somatic and autonomic components. Like the Vth nerve, it emerges at the cerebellopontine angle.

Motor somatic

The motor somatic component supplies the facial muscles. Its course runs through the ear, giving off a branch to the stapedius muscle, and it emerges from the facial canal into the parotid gland. There it divides into the temporal, zygomatic, buccal, mandibular and cervical branches, which supply all the muscles of facial expression. Other muscles innervated include the posterior belly of digastric and the stylohyoid.

There are a number of sites on its course where the facial nerve is particularly vulnerable to damage. These include the internal auditory meatus (by a tumour of the VIIIth nerve), in the facial canal (by infection of the middle ear) or within the parotid gland (by tumour or surgery). Peripheral lesions result in paralysis or weakness ipsilaterally, i.e. Bell's palsy. Central lesions, which are upper motor neuron lesions, result only in the contralateral muscles in the lower part of the face being affected. Since forehead muscles are supplied by crossed and uncrossed fibres, there is seldom any objective paralysis of these muscles.

Motor parasympathetic

The secretomotor parasympathetic nerves arise from the superior salivary nucleus and supply the nasal, palatine, sublingual, submandibular and parotid glands. The parasympathetic nerves run in the greater and lesser petrosal nerves. The lacrimal nucleus supplies the lacrimal gland.

Sensory somatic

The cell bodies of the sensory somatic nerves arise in the geniculate ganglion and terminate in the spinal trigeminal nucleus. Touch, pain and temperature from a small area of skin on the external ear are mediated through these nerves. The spinal trigeminal nucleus subserves these modalities for a number of cranial nerves (V, VII, IX and X).

Sensory autonomic

The cell bodies of the autonomic nerve lie in the nucleus solitarius and convey taste from the anterior two-thirds of the tongue in the greater petrosal nerve. The nucleus solitarius also sends fibres to the IXth and Xth cranial nerves.

Vestibulocochlear nerve

The VIIIth nerve is solely sensory and subserves both hearing and balance. This nerve also emerges at the cerebellopontine angle and is vulnerable to damage.

Cochlea – hearing

Fibres from the cochlea terminate in the superior and inferior cochlear nuclei, situated at the inferior cerebellar peduncle. Fibres then ascend ipsilaterally to the superior olivary nucleus or cross in the trapezoid body to the contralateral superior olivary nucleus in the pons. From here fibres constitute the lateral lemniscus and terminate in the inferior colliculus, where some fibres also cross. The final part of the pathway is via the auditory radiation, which is part of the internal capsule, to the superior temporal or Heschl's gyrus (auditory cortex). Since the fibres cross, lesions within the auditory cortex cause minimal deafness. However, a lesion of the peripheral nerve will cause unilateral deafness.

Vestibular – balance

The vestibular nerve mediates balance and its projections terminate within the cerebellum and nuclei of the oculomotor nerves.

Glossopharyngeal nerve

The IXth nerve is both motor sensory and parasympathetic, and sensory somatic and autonomic. The nerve emerges at the cerebellopontine angle.

Motor somatic

This component supplies stylopharyngeus and superior constrictor muscles of pharynx and hence lesions result in ipsilateral paralysis and difficulty in swallowing. The cell bodies are in the nucleus ambiguus, which also gives rise to motor fibres for the Xth and XIth cranial nerves.

Motor parasympathetic

Cell bodies for the motor parasympathetic division lie in the inferior salivatory nucleus and terminate in the parotid gland. Stimulation results in watery secretions, rich in amylase.

Sensory somatic

The somatic sensory nerve innervates the skin of the external auditory meatus and the back of the ear. Fibres terminate in the spinal trigeminal nucleus.

Sensory autonomic

The autonomic sensory nerve mediates:

- pain and poorly localized sensation from palate, pharynx, tonsils
- carotid sinus – pressure receptors at bifurcation of carotid artery
- carotid body – chemoreceptor for hydrogen ion, CO_2 and O_2, and
- taste on the posterior third of the tongue.

All fibres join together in the inferior (petrosal) ganglion and the central processes terminate in the nucleus solitarius. This nucleus also receives fibres from the VIIth and Xth cranial nerves and projects to the ventral posterior nucleus of the thalamus.

Vagus nerve

The Xth nerve is both motor somatic and parasympathetic, and sensory somatic and parasympathetic.

Motor somatic

The motor somatic nerve fibres arise in the nucleus ambiguus and innervate muscles of pharynx and palate. A branch, the recurrent laryngeal nerve, innervates the laryngeal muscles. Unilateral lesion of this nerve results in a partially obstructed airway and dysphonia while a bilateral lesion results in closed vocal cords and a narrowed airway. This nerve is particularly vulnerable to damage in thyroid surgery.

Motor parasympathetic

Postganglionic fibres arise from ganglia in cardiac, pulmonary, gastric and intestinal walls. Stimulation results in contraction of smooth muscle, slowed heart rate and secretomotor activity in all glands including liver, pancreas and gall bladder.

Sensory somatic

This is a small branch that innervates the skin of the external ear and whose fibres terminate in the spinal trigeminal nucleus.

Sensory parasympathetic

These fibres arise from the full length of the gastrointestinal tract from the oesophagus to the proximal descending colon, including the liver, pancreas and gall bladder. They assemble in cardiac, oesophageal, pulmonary and pharyngeal plexi. Afferents from the larynx form the superior laryngeal nerves and terminate in the nucleus solitarius.

Accessory nerve

The XIth nerve contains only motor nerves and is divided into cranial and spinal parts. The fibres of the cranial root arise from the nucleus ambiguus and innervate intrinsic muscles of the soft palate. The spinal root arises from motor neurons in the anterior horn of C1 through C5 or C6 and innervate the sternocleidomastoid and trapezius muscles. Lesion of the nerve supply to these muscles results in paralysis such that the head cannot turn to the affected side and the ipsilateral shoulder is dropped.

Hypoglossal nerve

The XIIth nerve is motor only and innervates intrinsic and extrinsic muscles of the tongue. Peripheral lesions result in ipsilateral deviation of the tongue on protrusion, while central lesions above the level of the nucleus result in contralateral deviation on protrusion.

BLOOD SUPPLY OF THE BRAIN AND SPINAL CORD

Arterial

The external and internal carotid and vertebral arteries supply the head and neck. The external carotid artery supplies the facial and anterior neck region. The internal carotid artery passes through the carotid foramen and the large cavernous sinus and into the medial cranial fossa. At this point a branch, the ophthalmic artery, supplies the eyeball. The internal carotid enters the circle of Willis (Fig. 2.7) and divides into the anterior cerebral and middle cerebral arteries. Blood is also supplied to the circle of Willis from the posterior cerebral arteries, which are linked via the posterior communicating artery. The rest of the circle is made up by anterior communicating arteries, between left and right anterior cerebral arteries, and posterior communicating arteries, between middle and posterior arteries. The circle is rarely functionally a circle due to atrophic posterior communicating arteries.

The posterior cerebral arteries arise from the basilar artery, which in turn is formed at the level of the pons by the left and right vertebral arteries. Branches of the basilar artery as it ascends include the anterior, inferior and superior cerebellar arteries, and the pontine arteries. The vertebral arteries arise from the subclavian arteries and ascend through the transverse foramina, giving branches to the spinal cord. The vertebral arteries pass through the foramen magnum and lie on the ventral aspect of the medulla and give off the anterior and posterior spinal arteries, and medullary and posterior inferior cerebellar arteries.

Blood supply to the cerebral hemispheres is shown in Figure 2.8 and to the deep forebrain in Table 2.13. The anterior cerebral artery supplies the medial and superior lateral aspects of the cerebral cortex to the parietal/occipital border. Loss of this artery results in loss of sensation and spastic paresis of the foot, but other subtle changes indicative of frontal lobe dysfunction will also be present (see above). The greater part of the lateral aspect of the cerebral cortex is supplied by the middle cerebral artery. Thus this artery supplies the primary sensory and motor

cortices, except for the lower leg. It also supplies Wernicke and Broca's areas in the dominant hemisphere. The posterior cerebral artery supplies the inferomedial temporal lobe and the occipital lobe.

Venous

Venous drainage from the brain occurs via the cavernous sinus, which is located in the medial cranial fossa. This sinus is traversed by the internal carotid artery, the IIIrd, IVth and VIth cranial nerves and the ophthalmic division of the Vth nerve.

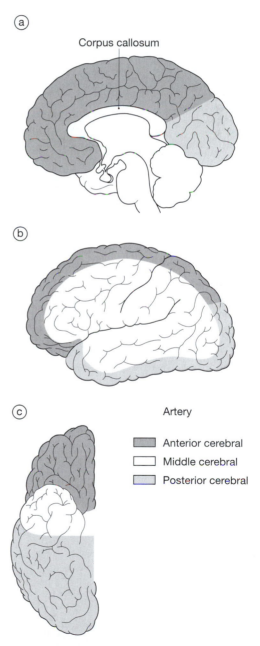

(a)

Corpus callosum

(b)

(c)

Artery

Anterior cerebral
Middle cerebral
Posterior cerebral

Figure 2.8 Blood supply of the cerebral hemispheres. (a) Medial view. (b) Lateral view. (c) Inferior view.

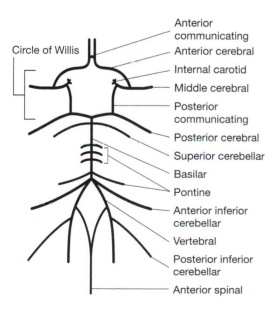

Circle of Willis

Anterior communicating
Anterior cerebral
Internal carotid
Middle cerebral
Posterior communicating
Posterior cerebral
Superior cerebellar
Basilar
Pontine
Anterior inferior cerebellar
Vertebral
Posterior inferior cerebellar
Anterior spinal

Figure 2.7 Arteries of the brain and spinal cord.

Table 2.13 Blood supply to the deep forebrain

Artery	Area supplied
Anterior cerebral artery	Anterior limb of internal capsule Head of caudate
Anterior communicating and anterior medial arteries	Hypothalamus Head of caudate Anterior limb of internal capsule
Medial cerebral artery to lenticulostriate arteries (prone to thrombosis resulting in contralateral hemiplegia)	Basal ganglia Internal capsule
Posterior cerebral artery (occlusion results in contralateral anaesthesia and hemiplegia)	Posterior thalamus, including geniculate bodies Posterior limb of internal capsule
Posterior inferior cerebellar artery	Cerebellum – vermis
Anterior inferior cerebellar artery (prone to occlusion at cerebellopontine angle)	Cerebellum – inferior surface
Superior cerebellar artery	Most of cerebellar hemispheres, superior and middle cerebellar peduncles Cerebellar nuclei
Anterior inferior cerebellar artery Pontine arteries Superior cerebellar	Pons

THE VENTRICULAR SYSTEM AND CEREBROSPINAL FLUID

Cerebrospinal fluid (CSF) is formed at a rate of approximately 300 ml/day within the choroid plexus, in the lateral, IIIrd and IVth ventricles. Each lateral ventricle is divided into anterior, posterior and inferior (temporal) horns, which project into the frontal, occipital and temporal lobes respectively (Fig. 2.9). Anteriorly the septum pellucidum divides the lateral ventricles. CSF circulates from the lateral to the IIIrd ventricle via the interventricular foramina of Munro, then into the IVth ventricle via the cerebral aqueduct to Sylvius and finally via the foramina of Magendie (midline) and Luschka (two, lateral) into the subarachnoid space where it is reabsorbed passively from the subarachnoid space by arachnoid villi within the dural venous sinuses.

Obstruction of CSF flow in the IIIrd or IVth ventricles or their communicating pathways leads to non-communicating hydrocephalus. Raised intracranial pressure is associated with non-communicating hydrocephalus and the symptoms and signs reflect this: nausea and vomiting, headache made worse on lying down, reduced pulse, raised blood pressure and papilloedema.

Obstruction to CSF flow in the subarachnoid space leads to communicating or normal pressure hydrocephalus. The symptoms associated with this condition are ataxia, urinary incontinence and nystagmus with impaired cognition.

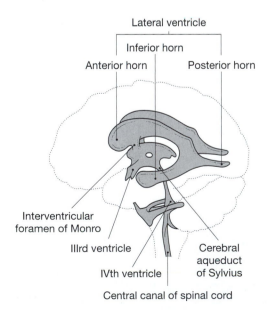

Lateral ventricle
Inferior horn
Anterior horn   Posterior horn
Interventricular foramen of Monro
IIIrd ventricle
IVth ventricle
Cerebral aqueduct of Sylvius
Central canal of spinal cord

Figure 2.9 The ventricular system.

FURTHER READING

Diamond MC, Scheibel AB & Elson LM (1985) *The Human Brain Coloring Book*. HarperPerennial.
Gilam S & Newman SW (1987) Manter & Gatz's *Essentials of Clinical Neuroanatomy and Neurophysiology*. Philadelphia: FA Davis.
Lishman WA (1998) *Organic Psychiatry*. Oxford: Blackwell Science.
Talley N & O'Connor S (1989) *Clinical Examination*. Oxford: Blackwell Scientific Publications.
Williams PL (1995) *Gray's Anatomy*, 38th edn. Edinburgh: Churchill Livingstone.

Psychiatric genetics

Aiden Corvin and Michael Gill

INTRODUCTION

Genetics is the scientific study of the inheritance of physical and behavioural traits. Genes, the units of inheritance, provide an assembly code for the complex molecules that make up life and enable reproduction of living organisms. Genes are located at varying intervals on chromosomes, which are highly compacted linear molecules of deoxyribonucleic acid (DNA) housed in cell nuclei. Within species they pass from generation to generation providing familial resemblance and individual variation, which through evolution, is responsible for the diversity of life. This chapter describes the basic principles of genetics and their relevance to psychiatric practice.

GENETICS

The history of genetics

Knowledge of heredity has been exploited in the breeding of animals and plants since prehistoric times. The first recorded reference and response to genetic disease (haemophilia) was recorded 1500 years ago. Although the term 'genetics' was coined in 1906 by the British biologist William Bateson, the science of genetics began 40 years earlier. In 1866 an Austrian monk, Gregor Mendel described the pattern of inheritance of seven simple, bimodal traits including seed shape (round or wrinkled) and colour (yellow or green) in pea plants. Mendel suggested that each parent plant had a pair of units of inheritance for each trait but contributed only one unit from each pair to its offspring. He developed two laws to account for his observations and noted that all possible combinations of the seven traits could occur:

- Mendel's first law (the law of segregation) states that one of an individual's two genes (alleles) at any locus is randomly distributed to each gamete.
- Mendel's second law (of independent assortment) states that the segregation of the alleles for any one trait to a gamete occurs independently of the segregation of the alleles for any other trait to that gamete.

The significance of Mendel's work was only realized at the turn of the 20th century, and the laws he derived became the foundation of modern genetics. Mendel's research informed the work of Thomas Hunt Morgan, an American geneticist who studied fruit flies. He demonstrated that genes were arranged linearly on chromosomes within cell nuclei, so that, contrary to Mendel's second law, genes on the same chromosomes could be inherited together depending on the physical distance between them and the frequency of recombination (see below) in the region. Genes inherited in this way are said to be linked, and the phenomena of genetic linkage (departure from Mendel's second law) has enabled genetic maps to be constructed and used to locate genes responsible for diseases. Morgan also demonstrated that linkage is rarely complete and that some traits are sex-linked.

In 1944 Oswald Avery, a Canadian bacteriologist, confirmed that genes were composed of DNA by transferring DNA from one strain of bacteria to another and showed that the second strain acquired traits from the first, and could pass these traits to future generations. Also in the 1940s the American geneticists George Beadle and Edward Tatum discovered that specific genes produced specific polypeptide enzymes. In 1953 geneticists James Watson and Francis Crick, American and British respectively, discovered that the DNA molecule was composed of two long strands in the form of a double helix (Watson & Crick 1953). Their deduction of the structure of DNA was made from X-ray photographs taken by a British scientist, Rosalind Franklin, and a New Zealander, Maurice Wilkins. Crick & Watson determined that DNA resembled a long, spiral ladder with a sugar-phosphate backbone and rungs composed of pairs of complementary nucleotide bases. This proposition immediately suggested that genetic information could be transmitted across generations if the two strands of DNA unwound and separated at the nucleotide bases and the new complementary nucleotide bases linked to each separated strand. Such a mechanism would result in the production of two identical double helices.

By this time it was known that genes produced proteins and scientists speculated that a genetic code, encrypted in the order of nucleotide bases, must determine the sequence of amino acids in proteins. Only four different nucleotides had been identified in DNA, but at least 20 different amino acids were known to occur in proteins. In 1962 Crick found that the coding sequence was a series of three nucleotide bases and that each amino acid was specified by at least one of these sequences (a codon). Recent developments have made significant contributions to the new science of molecular genetics. The British biochemist Fredrick Sanger developed methods for analysing the molecular structure of proteins and for rapidly determining the nucleotide sequence of nucleic acids. The American biochemist Kary Mullis developed the polymerase chain reaction (PCR), which allowed rapid enzymatic synthesis in vitro of specific DNA sequences.

Chromosomes, cell division and genes

The nucleus of a human cell has 23 homologous pairs of chromosomes (46 in all), one member of each pair being inherited from each parent. Each chromosome consists of a single molecule of DNA, and the total DNA complement in a cell is referred to as its genome. The human genome is over 2 m long and contains approximately 3.9×10^9 base pairs. Only 2–3% of the genome contains the complement of approximately 30 000 genes: the remainder of the genome is not entirely 'junk' but has many functions including regulation of DNA structure, repair and expression.

A gene is a length of DNA that codes for a sequence of amino acids. Each gene is located at a specific site on a chromosome called a locus. Because chromosomes exist in homologous pairs there are a pair of genes at any given locus. The DNA base sequence throughout the genome, including within genes, varies considerably between individuals and between the two copies possessed by an individual. These different forms are called alleles and are often denoted by letters such as A or a, B or b. As stated in Mendel's first law, only one allele for each gene may be inherited from each parent. Individuals who inherit the same allele for a gene from both parents are said to be homozygous (e.g. AA or BB) while those who inherit different alleles for a gene from their parents are termed heterozygous (e.g. Aa or aA). This means that an individual has two genes for every trait. At a locus the alleles of the two genes constitute the individual's genotype. The expression of the trait coded for by the genotype is called the phenotype. If AA and Aa individuals have the same phenotype, the allele A is said to be dominant over allele a (or allele a is recessive to allele A). If the Aa phenotype is intermediate between AA and aa phenotypes, the alleles A and a are termed codominant.

The nucleus of the human cell generally contains 46 chromosomes (23 pairs). This is termed the diploid state and applies to somatic cells, but sex cells (gametes) have only 23 chromosomes and are termed haploid. These differences in chromosome number, on which sexual reproduction depends, arise because somatic cells replicate by mitosis and gametes by meiosis. In mitosis chromosomes are duplicated in the prophase stage of the cycle. The duplicated chromosomes join at a constricted chromosomal region called the centromere to form sister chromatids. In *metaphase*, a spindle forms from a centriole at each cell pole to the centromere. During *anaphase* the spindles retract, pulling a chromosome to each pole and distributing the chromosomes equally between two daughter cells identical to the parent cell (*telophase*).

In contrast, gametes are produced by meiosis in which daughter cells receive only half the number of chromosomes (see Fig 3.1). During the prophase stage of meiosis, each chromosome of each homologous pair duplicates itself, and the resulting sister chromatids are joined at the centromere. Each homologous pair of chromosomes produces a tetrad consisting of four chromatids. Non-sister chromatids pair together, and recombine (cross over) exchanging genetic information. On average one recombination occurs per chromosomal arm in meiosis. This means that genes originally on different members of a pair of parental (non-recombinant) chromosomes may become located on a single daughter (recombinant) chromosome. The cell now divides into four daughter cells, each haploid and each containing a single chromatid from the tetrad. At fertilization when gametes fuse the normal diploid state of 46 chromosomes is restored. These two processes, recombination and random assortment of chromosomes at fertilization, contribute to individual differences and diversity within species.

Human chromosomes can be easily visualized by microscope in cells undergoing mitosis obtained from a stained buccal smear. For chromosomal studies the chromosomes are paired and sorted in roughly decreasing length from 1–22 and called autosomes. The remaining two chromosomes are the sex chromosomes X and Y. Females have two X chromosomes (genotype XX) and males have an X chromosome and a shorter Y chromosome (XY). Early in female development one of these X chromosomes is inactivated and is known as the Barr body (or sex chromatin); whether the active X chromosome is of maternal or paternal origin is a random event. Healthy females are therefore mosaics of cells with active X chromosomes of either maternal or paternal origin (mosaicism is described more fully below).

Each chromosome is divided by the centromere into two arms, usually of different lengths. The shorter arm is designated the p (for petit) arm and the longer is designated q (because q comes after p in the alphabet). Some chromosomes (8–11 for example) are of similar length, and with a homogenous stain it may not be possible to

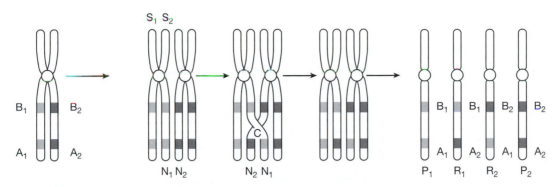

Figure 3.1 Meiosis and crossing over. (1) Pairing of homologous chromosomes. A_1 and A_2 are different alleles of the same gene A. Similarly, B_1 and B_2 are different alleles of the same gene B. (2) Duplication of homologous chromosomes to form 4 chromatids (referred to as the tetrad). S_1 and S_2 are sister chromatids while N_1 and N_2 are non-sister chromatids. (3) Crossing over of non-sister chromatids N_1 and N_2 at the chiasma, C. (4) For clarity, only one crossing over is illustrated. However, for any pair of non-sister chromatids, crossing over occurs at numerous chiamata; genes that were originally on the same chromosome are dispersed to separate chromosomes (and vice versa) at each crossing over. (5) Separation of the tetrad to chromatids. R_1 and R_2 are recombinant chromatids while P_1 and P_2 are parental chromatids. The four daughter cells resulting from this meiosis will each contain a chromatid. (From original drawings by Pádraig Wright.)

distinguish them. Additional staining procedures produce pale or dark bands of varying thickness specific to each chromosome, allowing individual chromosomes or chromosomal regions to be consistently identified. A standard nomenclature is used when studying chromosomal regions. For example, a locus in the second subdivision of the first band on the p arm of chromosome 8 would be termed 8p1.2.

MOLECULAR GENETICS

Molecular genetics is the branch of genetics that investigates the chemical and physical nature of genes and the mechanisms by which genes control development, growth and physiology.

Basic molecular genetics

Each chromosome contains a molecule of DNA composed of a backbone of sugar (deoxyribose) and phosphate, the purine bases adenine (A) and guanine (G), and the pyrimidine bases cytosine (C) and thymine (T). These repeating units of 5-carbon sugar, phosphate and organic bases are called nucleotides. The DNA molecule resembles a spiral ladder, where each side is composed of alternating deoxyribose and phosphate molecules with pairs of bases as rungs. Because bases can only pair by forming hydrogen bonds between T and A, or G and C, the sequence of one DNA strand is dependent on the sequence of the other, so the strands are complementary, one being orientated in a 3′ to 5′ direction and the other in a 5′ to 3′ direction. The DNA molecule unwinds during cell division and each strand acts as a template for the production of a new strand with a complementary sequence of nucleotides. As this new

sequence forms, DNA polymerase enzymes bind deoxyribonuclueotides and fit them in place with the phosphate group of each incoming nucleotide being joined enzymatically to the 3′-deoxyribose group of the previous nucleotide. Because of the number of base pairs in a chromosome, replication is initiated at many different sites along each template and the segments of newly formed DNA are joined together with phosphodiester bonds by ligase enzymes. A special replication enzyme called telomerase is used to complete the chromosomal ends. In mammalian chromosome replication, approximately 3000 nucleotides are added per minute, with an estimated accuracy of greater than 99.98%. Errors in this process are called mutations; these can occur naturally but are also induced by external agents (called mutagens) such as radiation, ultraviolet light, and various chemicals.

The information for protein production contained in DNA is decoded (transcribed) by a similar molecule (RNA) and transported from the nucleus to ribosomes in the cytoplasm for translation into amino acids and protein construction (see Fig 3.2).

Transcription

Transcription begins when a section of the DNA molecule unzips and one of the DNA strands acts as a template for the synthesis of an RNA transcript. The DNA gene sequence is preceded by a 5′flanking (upstream) signal region that initiates transcription and succeeded by a 3′flanking (downstream) region containing a termination sequence. The DNA sequence is 'read' in a 5′ to 3′ direction, so that one or other DNA strand may be transcribed. In certain instances both strands can produce RNA transcripts, which being of different sequence will form different genes. RNA differs from DNA by being single stranded, having ribose instead of deoxyribose as its sugar and uracil (U) instead of the

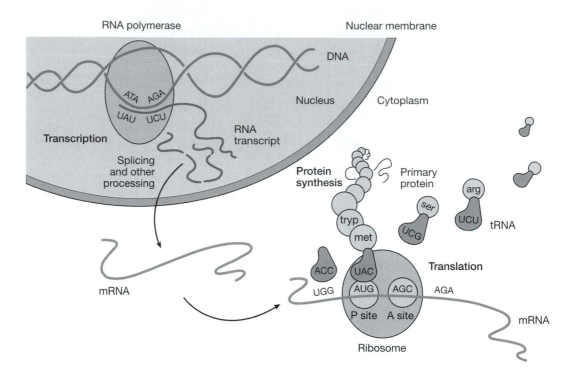

Figure 3.2 Transcription, translation and protein synthesis. Transcription occurs in the nucleus. The DNA molecule unwinds and, in the presence of RNA polymerase, a complementary strand of ribonucleic acid (RNA), termed an RNA transcript, is synthesized. RNA transcripts undergo splicing (removal of introns and other non-functional sequences of RNA) and other processing, and are then termed messenger RNA (mRNA) because they convey the message (the amino acid sequence) from the nucleus to the ribosomes in the cytoplasm.

Translation occurs in the cytoplasm at ribosomes, protein/ribosomal RNA strtctures capable of decoding mRNA. Amino acids in the cytoplasm are brought to the ribosome by transfer RNA (tRNA). Each molecule of tRNA includes a three base sequence or anticodon which is complementary to the codons of mRNA and a corresponding amino acid. The codon AUG on the mRNA strand, for example, complements the tRNA anticodon UAC with its associated amino acid, methionine.

Protein synthesis occurs in the cytoplasm as follows. The mRNA sequence is translated when tRNA anitcodons line up along mRNA codons (forming cistrons) and construct the amino acid sequence specified by the mRNA. Peptide bonds hold the amino acids together until the protein specified by the original DNA sequence in the gene has been produced. Following this, mRNA is degraded. (From original drawings by Pádraig Wright.)

pyrimidine base thymine. As the transcript forms the DNA helix reconstitutes. Within a DNA gene sequence there may be redundant, noncoding regions (introns) as well as coding regions (exons). After transcription the introns are enzymatically removed and the exons spliced together in the correct order to form functional messenger RNA (mRNA). Exons can be spliced together in many different ways so that different gene products can be generated in different tissues from the same structural gene. The Human Genome Project has demonstrated that it is the complexity of gene regulation and alternative splicing rather than a large increase in the number of genes that largely explains the evolution of more complex organisms.

Translation

This involves transfer of genetic information from mRNA into a sequence of linked amino acids to form proteins. As described above, specific three-base sequences (codons) individually code for each amino acid and this code is the same in all living organisms. The functional mRNA transcript initially attaches to a ribosome, which is composed of a large and small subunit each made from ribosomal RNA and proteins. Amino acids are brought to the ribosomes by transfer RNA (tRNA) molecules that also have specific three-base sequences (called anticodons) complementary to the codons of mRNA. For example, the codon AGA on the mRNA strand attracts the tRNA anticodon UCU with its associated amino acid, arginine. Thus mRNA is translated when tRNA anticodons line up along mRNA codons (together referred to as the cistron) and construct the amino acid sequence specified by the mRNA. As each codon is read peptide bonds are formed between consecutive amino acids in a growing protein chain and the tRNA molecule that is no longer 'charged' to an amino acid is ejected from the ribosome. The ribosome continues to move along 'reading' the mRNA until the protein specified by the original DNA sequence has been produced. The mRNA transcript can be translated simultaneously by many ribosomes, offering further potential sources of control over gene expression. It is degraded enzymatically over a variable period of time.

Regulation

Cells require ongoing transcription of certain genes to maintain cell function, but also the ability to activate or repress transcription of genes during development or in response to the environment. Proteins called transcriptional factors can bind to DNA to activate or repress transcription, but extracellular factors such as hormonal activity can also influence transcription. The regulation of gene transcription is complex and an individual gene can be activated by different signals in different cell types at different developmental stages.

Inheritance of disease

A mutation during mitotic division in cells that do not give rise to gametes is called a somatic mutation and is not heritable. Mutations in cell precursors of gametes are called germinal mutations and may be transmitted to the next generation. A mutation can involve a single base-pair (a point mutation), or a sequence of base pairs (a chromosomal mutation).

- **Point mutations:** a mutation can be understood as an event leading to a change in the sequence or structure of DNA, for example, a base-pair substitution producing a codon that specified a different amino acid (missense mutation) or which changes the sequence to a stop codon, causing production of an incomplete protein (a nonsense mutation). The term mutation is generally taken to mean a sequence or structural difference that causes or contributes to a disease or abnormal phenotype. If the DNA variant created by a mutation event becomes, through many generations, common in the population (found at a frequency of >1%) it is known as a polymorphism.
- **Chromosomal mutations:** these involve a change in the number of chromosomes or rearrangement of sequences during DNA replication. Chromosomal mutations are often lethal but embryos in which chromosomes are rearranged by deletions (e.g. 22q11 deletion syndrome), translocations (where a DNA sequence is displaced to a non-homologous chromosome), duplications or inversions may be viable. The condition where the number of chromosomes is different to the normal diploid complement of 46 is called aneuploidy. This is caused by nondisjunction, a failure of the normal segregation of chromosomes at meiosis that in most cases is lethal. Where development is possible the phenotypic effects of aneuploidies are so severe that many were clinically recognized before cytogenetic diagnosis was possible. Down's syndrome (caused by an extra chromosome 21 or, more rarely, a translocation at chromosome 21), Edwards' syndrome (trisomy 18) and Patau syndrome (trisomy 13) are examples of autosomal aneuploidies. Aneuploidies that involve extra sex chromosomes often have less biological impact although distinct phenotypes are recognized such as Turner's syndrome (XO, females with one X chromosome) and Kleinfelter's syndrome (XXY). Chromosomal abnormalities do not always occur in all cells of an individual. Mitotic chromosomal error occur rarely in early development. In this case, tissues or organs of an individual may have two or more cell populations with different chromosomal or genetic constitution. This is known as mosaicism, the effect of which usually results in less abnormal phenotypic expression or, if it occurs late in development, may be negligible.

DNA variation and genetic markers

In any two randomly selected human genomes 99.9% of DNA sequence is identical, the remainder accounts for population diversity and individuality including susceptibility to disease. Molecular genetics seeks to correlate differences between this DNA polymorphism/variation (genetic markers) and phenotypic differences (such as having a disease or trait). Many different types of polymorphisms can be used as genetic 'markers', including small deletions or insertions, variability in small (1–5bp) repeat sequences (microsatellite markers), or single nucleotide polymorphism (SNPs), the commonest form of polymorphism. To date many thousands of microsatellite markers and more than four million SNPs have been identified and are publicly available to researchers (www.ncbi.nlm.nih.gov/SNP) seeking to map disease or trait genes.

Mendelian inheritance

The patterns of inheritance described by Mendel are due to the relative effects of complementary genes on both members of a pair of autosomes or the sex chromosomes. Where a mutation interferes with the function of one gene it is likely that the complementary gene will be unaffected and in this case gene expression may occur but at a reduced level that may or may not influence cell function or phenotype. Mendelian inheritance applies to the bimodal traits described by him in pea plants, but also to human diseases caused by single mutations, where the mutation is both necessary and sufficient to cause the disease and is said to have a major gene effect:

- **Autosomal dominant disorders:** the most common Mendelian disorders (7 per 1000 live births), apparent in individuals having one (heterozygous) or two (homozygous) mutant genes. Such conditions will, on average, affect half of all individuals in a sibship. If a proband has a dominant disorder one of their parents will also be affected, unless the disorder represents a new mutation. The extent to which a heterozygote shows features of the disorder is described as the penetrance of the condition, e.g. the Huntington's mutation has a penetration of almost 100%.

- **Autosomal recessive disorders:** these are less common (<3 per 1000 live births), partly because the disorder is expressed only in homozygotes. As with dominant disorders, the extent of expression depends on the penetrance of the mutations. If both parents are haeterozygous for the mutant gene then, on average, one in four children will be affected. These conditions are rare as it is less likely that both parents will have a copy of the mutant gene unless they are related (e.g. in a geographically or ethnically isolated population) or the mutant is common in the general population (e.g. haemochromatosis or cystic fibrosis in the European population). For this reason recessive disorders may appear to 'skip' generations.

- **X (or sex)-linked disorders:** these arise from mutations of the sex chromosomes and follow different inheritance patterns because males can only pass on their Y-chromosomes to sons. Most X-linked conditions are recessive. A heterozygotic mother may pass on the mutant gene to her son and he will be affected, while a heterozygote sister will be a carrier. Affected males transmit the carrier state to half of their daughters but do not transmit the disease to their sons. Examples include Duchenne muscular dystrophy and haemophilia A and B. In pedigrees with a dominant X-linked disorder, each generation usually has an affected individual as all daughters of affected males are affected and both sons and daughters of an affected heterozygous female may be affected. Dominant X-linked disorders, such as nephrogenic diabetes insipidis, are extremely rare.

- **Mitochondrial disorders:** rare single gene disorders caused by mutations in a mitochondrial gene. They follow a distinct inheritance pattern because mitochondrial DNA in fertilized embryos is exclusively acquired from the ovum, as sperm do not contain mitochondria. Similarly, Y chromosomes are exclusively inherited through sperm in males. For mitochondrial disorders, the children of an affected woman, but none of the children of an affected man, are affected depending on disease penetrance.

Inheritance of complex genetic disorders

Most common biological traits or behaviours are in the statistical sense, distributed normally in the general population and are likely to be determined by the interaction between multiple genes of minor effect and the environment, rather than by the effects of single genes of major effect. Within the normal distribution of biological traits, offspring of parents who are at the extremes of a continuously distributed trait (e.g. very tall individuals) tend to be closer to the population mean, a phenomenon called regression to the mean. Genes or locations on the genome that contribute to biological traits or behaviours that display these characteristics are called quantitative trait loci (QTLs). Biometrical analysis and quantitative genetics study the contribution that QTLs and environmental effects make to phenotypes that approximate to a continuous normal distribution within the population.

Some common disorders may be due to genes of major effect, but the bulk of cases are due to genes of minor effect, which are neither necessary nor sufficient to cause the disorder but increase risk. Each minor or risk gene may have an effect independent of all other genes (an additive component); effects that are dependent on the other allele at that locus (a dominant interaction) or effects that are influenced by genotype at other loci (epistatic interactions). The proportion of the total variance of a trait in a population explained by additive genetic effects is called its narrow heritability (h^2). (The genetics of complex disorders is covered in greater detail by Plomin et al. 1994.)

Molecular genetics: techniques and terminology

Recombinant DNA technology

Also called molecular cloning, this is an umbrella term for the process of introducing a gene from an organism into a host cell, where it can be replicated and studied. This technology developed from the discovery in the 1970s of restriction enzymes produced by various bacteria that recognize particular short nucleotide sequences (4–8 base pairs) and cut the DNA molecule specifically at such a location. This enables the bacteria to 'restrict' which foreign DNA could incorporate into the bacterial genome. Using these enzymes in vitro, lengths of DNA could be cut to manageable sizes, and could be ordered into fragments of varying lengths as part of a restriction 'map'. These fragment lengths, called restriction fragment length polymorphisms (RFLPs), could be used to detect DNA polymorphism/variation if, as a consequence of the polymorphism, a restriction site is created or removed.

Vectors and cloning

When two different DNA samples are treated with a specific endonuclease enzyme to produce a staggered cut and then mixed together in the presence of another enzyme (DNA ligase) the two ends anneal forming a new DNA sequence, which can be inserted into a cloning vector, often a plasmid. This vector, when inserted into a host bacterial cell, replicates with the bacteria when cultured, allowing millions of copies of the original DNA sequence to be obtained (cloned). Cloning vectors include extrachromosomal bacterial elements (plasmids), bacterial viruses (bacteriophages), combinations of sequences from both these sources (cosmids), and phage, bacterial or yeast artificial chromosomes (PACs, BACs or YACs).

Polymerase chain reaction – enzymatic DNA amplification
DNA can be caused to unwind when heated to over 90°C; cooling causes the double helix to reform. In polymerase chain reactions (PCR) small pieces of DNA, called oligonucleotide primers, are chemically synthesized to be complementary to the DNA on either side of the sequence to be amplified. Mixing these primers with DNA containing the sequence to be amplified, a supply of individual nucleotides, and a heat-stable DNA polymerase enzyme at a suitable temperature, these primers bind to their complimentary sequences on each strand. Next, the individual DNA bases extend along the strand reforming the double helix. Returning to over 90°C the strands separate and the process begins again with twice the number of molecules at the target. This procedure is automated by machines that cycle the reaction mixture through at the different temperatures to produce a very large number (many millions) of copies of the target DNA sequence.

Visualization
Fragments of DNA produced by cloning and/or other methods may be electrophoretically separated in agarose or acrylamide gels according to size, and visualized using dyes or radiolabelling. Further analysis is possible if DNA fragments are transferred and attached to a membrane (Southern blotting). Specific single-stranded DNA molecules can be detected by immobilizing the DNA molecule on a membrane and testing it with a DNA molecule complementary to that sought. This technique (using cDNA to hybridize RNA transcripts) has been extended so that expression levels of thousands of genes can be simultaneously investigated using microarrays of probe sequences immobilized on glass or silicon (Bunney et al. 2003).

Genotyping
Newer methods of detecting DNA variation (genotyping), using hybridization with allele-specific probes or single nucleotide primer extension, have superceded the traditional enzyme cleavage RFLP method. These modern methods detect DNA sequence differences using a range of chemistry and detection devices. Such innovations mean that thousands or millions of individual genotypes can now be rapidly produced using automated procedures.

Human Genome Project
The completed draft of the sequence of the human genome sequence has recently been released. It has already produced insights into the collective history of humans, our shared identity and our individuality. It will also open up exciting possibilities for the understanding, identification, treatment and prevention of disease. Sequencing the genome involved its fragmentation using site-specific restriction endonucleases. Each segment (of approximately 150 bp in length) was inserted and replicated using a BAC vector, and the resulting clones were restricted to produce small fragments called 'fingerprints'. A physical map of overlapping fingerprints was assembled and sequenced using computer technology to assemble the raw sequence. At 3.2 gigabases (Gb), the human genome is 25 times larger than any previously sequenced genome. What is now available is a map of the genome encompassing most of the 'euchromatin' (2.95 Gb of the genome, where most genes are found). The task underway is to annotate the sequence with all its elements including genes, regulatory elements, repeats and duplications. Additional tasks include the comparison between the human sequence and that of other organisms.

As mentioned above, one of the most surprising findings is that the estimated number of genes is much smaller, at 30–40 000, than previously predicted. Proteins encoded by these genes can be grouped into families on the basis of their similarity to one another, and it turns out that humans share most of the same protein families with worms, flies and plants. However, humans generally have many more genes in a particular family than other organisms. For example, humans have 765 genes with immunoglobulin subunits, while the fly has 140 and the worm 64. The increased complexity in humans seems to be due to a number of factors, including additional genes within families, more complex regulatory mechanisms and alternative splicing of RNA. Around 60% of human genes have two or more alternatively spliced transcripts, compared, for example, with only 22% in the worm. Humans have twice as many proteins that switch genes on and off as the fly and nearly five times as many as the worm.

Genomics and bioinformatics
Genetics is the study of single genes and their effects. Genomics is the study of the functions and interactions of all the genes in the genome. Genomics as a science has been driven by the increased availability of entire genomes for comparison between species and the application of human genome information to common conditions. Bioinformatics is a new science that has evolved to cope with the growing banks of molecular sequence data. This involves computational methods for retrieval and analysis of data, including algorithms for sequence similarity searches, and prediction of the structure and function of genes.

Confirming a genetic contribution to disease: family, twin and adoption research

Family studies
If a disease is genetic it should be familial, i.e. it should be more common in first-degree relatives of an affected proband (who share on average 50% of their DNA) than in

second-degree relatives (who share 25% of their DNA) and more common in this group than in the general population. This information can be collected either by taking a detailed family history from affected individuals or their relatives (the family history method), or more rigorously by using a family study approach, where all affected individuals are directly interviewed. Many psychiatric disorders including schizophrenia, bipolar affective disorder and autism cluster in families.

Family studies by themselves are insufficient to define an illness as genetic because families share common environments – more so than unrelated individuals. Shared effects reflect the environmental influences, which make family members similar for a trait. Nonshared influences are the effects that cause members of a family to be different and in psychiatry reflect how different individuals cope with the same stressors.

Two natural forms of biological and social experiment, namely, twin births and adoption, allow some separation of genetic and environmental effects.

Twin studies

Monozygotic (MZ) twins arise from a single fertilized ovum and thus have identical genes; dizygotic (DZ) twins develop from different ova and like any full siblings share an average of 50% of their genes. Twin research assumes that twins share environmental effects equally. If both twins have a disease, they are said to be concordant for that condition, but if only one twin is affected they are described as discordant. Higher concordance of disease in MZ than DZ twins is strong evidence of a genetic contribution to disease.

Early twin studies measured pair-wise concordance, where the total number of concordant twins is divided by the total number of twins studied. However, if twins have been ascertained independently, they may be counted twice and MZ concordant twins will be over-represented. Another method, proband-wise concordance, is now more common as it avoids this problem by dividing the number of affected co-twins of an affected proband by the total number of co-twins in the study. Ascertainment bias at recruitment is also a potential flaw, but researchers in the US, UK, Denmark and Sweden have overcome this problem by exploiting national or local twin registers to systematically screen all twin births. Twin studies assume that twins within a family share the same environment. This may not be completely true:

- environmental factors including prenatal nutrition or birth trauma may differ between twins
- MZ twins may share a different microenvironment to DZ twins
- being a twin, in itself, may contribute to illness.

Despite these caveats, twin studies remain a powerful tool in the elucidation of the genetic component of behavioural and psychiatric phenotypes. Twin studies have also proved valuable by exposing different aspects of gene expression in identical individuals. A study by Gottesman & Bertelsen (1989) of twin pairs discordant for schizophrenia showed that, for MZ twins, offspring had the same increased rate of schizophrenia, whether their parent was the affected co-twin or not. This finding suggested that the genetic risk, although unexpressed in one of the MZ twins, is nonetheless passed on to offspring. Apart from environmental differences, a number of genetic factors have been proposed to account for discordance including DNA methylation, somatic mutations, and imprinting (discussed below).

Adoption studies

These studies examine the effect of being adopted into, or out of, a family with a specific disorder using a variety of designs. In the Danish adoption study of schizophrenia (Kety 1988), adopted children who become ill are ascertained and rates of illness are compared in their adoptive and biological families (the adoptee family method). Adoption can also be studied prospectively, by using the parent as proband. In this adoptee study method, the rates of illness in adopted offspring of affected individuals are compared with rates in adopted offspring of individuals without the disorder. A third method is the cross-fostering design where rates of illness are compared between adoptees of affected biological parents raised by healthy adoptive parents and adoptees of unaffected biological parents raised in a family where an adoptive parent has become affected. As with twin studies, there are caveats:

- a child having affected biological parents may influence potential adoptive parents
- adopted children may experience particular intrauterine effects
- age at adoption is often overlooked
- adoption is a rare event.

Mode of inheritance

Family, twin and adoption studies may each have their limitations, but if independent evidence from all three methods points to a significant genetic component to a disease or trait then it is not unreasonable to assume that one exists. Other methods are required to identify the mode of inheritance involved.

Mode of inheritance can be investigated by examining the recurrence risk of disorder in different classes of relatives and in the general population. A rapid decrease in risk from MZ co-twins to first-degree relatives to the general population is inconsistent with single gene models of inheritance. An alternative method of investigating inheritance patterns is segregation analysis, where the segregation of phenotypes within pedigrees is observed and statistically compared to expected patterns for known models of inheritance. Analyses of many common psychiatric disorder phenotypes including schizophrenia, depression, and bipolar affective disorder indicate that the observed patterns of inheritance in most families are not compatible with Mendelian inheritance. Ruling out a simple Mendelian model is a much simpler proposition than distinguishing between more complex genetic models. It is becoming apparent that some psychiatric disorders, such as Alzheimer's disease, Attention Deficit Hyperactivity Disorder (ADHD) and possibly schizophrenia are oligogenic, where a small number (5–20) genes account for most of the genetic risk. For other conditions, the genetic risk may be attributable to many genes, each of very small effect. This is the polygenic model, which better fits continuous traits, although with the addition of a threshold, may also account for categorical diagnoses. To complicate matters further, different genes may account for illness in different families. This is known as genetic heterogeneity. The reality is that for a given disorder some or all of the models may apply.

Quantitative and mathematical aspects of genetics

Hardy–Weinberg law

The English mathematician Godfrey Harvey and the German obstetrician Wilhelm Weinberg independently formulated this law in 1908. This states that the frequencies of alleles will, in the presence of random mating and in the absence of disturbances including mutation, natural selection, migration, inbreeding or random genetic drift, remain constant from generation to generation. Thus let two alleles A and a exist in a population. If their frequencies of occurrence (expressed in decimals) are p and q respectively than $p + q = 1$, and if mating between individuals is random, after one generation the frequencies of the three genotypes will be p^2, $2pq$ and q^2. This generation will produce gametes (A and a) with frequencies p and q, similar to the previous generation. A sample of individuals is said to be in Hardy–Weinberg equilibrium if the frequencies of the observed genotypes AA, Aa and aa are not statistically different from the expected frequencies derived from allele frequencies using the above formula.

Recombination fraction

We have already described the process of recombination during meiosis. Genetic markers on separate chromosomes will segregate independently of each other and statistically therefore parental versions of the markers are as likely to transmit together into gametes as not. Even on the same chromosome, many markers will segregate independently. The recombination fraction is defined as the number of recombinant gametes divided by the total number of gametes and for independently segregating markers takes the value 0.5. This means that if the recombination fraction (θ) between two loci is less than 0.5 they are not independently segregating and instead are linked, meaning in physical terms that they lie close together on the same chromosome.

Genetic distance

Where two loci are linked the probability of recombination occurring between them (θ) is proportional to the physical distance between them. This fraction is expressed in Morgans (M), where 1 M corresponds to the length of DNA on which 1 recombination is expected on average (roughly equivalent to 100 million base pairs), but is usually written as centiMorgans (cM), where 1 cM is the genetic distance corresponding to a recombination fraction of 0.01. This is roughly equivalent to 1 million base pairs of DNA, but the relationship between genetic and physical distance is imprecise as recombination rates vary across the genome.

Linkage analysis

Linkage studies investigate possible cosegregation of genetic markers and disease in one or more families. This process of genetic tracking or mapping follows the descent of DNA markers down generations in pedigrees and their segregation with illness. Large multiply affected pedigrees or many small families or even multiple pairs of affected siblings may be studied, and each approach has advantages and disadvantages (further details are provided in Lander & Kruglyak 1995). Now that sufficient genetic markers are available, most linkage studies take a genome-wide approach using regularly spaced genetic markers or polymorphisms to locate the disease gene on the map of the genome. Linkage studies have two aims:

- To establish whether two loci (genetic locations, eg. genes or polymorphic markers) segregate independently during meiosis.
- If there is a departure from independent segregation, to estimate the amount of recombination between the marker and the putative disease gene.

The value of θ is less than 0.5 when two loci are co-inherited more often then expected by chance and generally means they are physical located close together on the same chromosome. If two loci are physically close, crossing-over is unlikely to occur between them during the small number of meioses that might be observed in a family. Linkage analysis estimates θ and tests whether $\theta = 0.5$. The conventional statistical method of doing this is to calculate a LOD (log of the odds) score. This is the common logarithm of the probability that the recombination fraction has some given value, divided by the probability that the value is 0.5. Where the mode of inheritance is known and the phenotype can be clearly defined a LOD score of 3.0 (odds in favour of linkage 1000:1) is accepted of proof of linkage and a score of −2.0 (odds against of 100:1) as proof of exclusion of linkage. However, the LOD score takes Bayesian theory into account whereby the prior odds that two loci are linked is ~1:50. The observed odds ratio of a LOD score of 3 is 1000:1 leading to a posterior probability of about 20:1, roughly equivalent to a p-value of 0.05.

Genetic association methods and linkage disequilibrium (LD)

In their simplest form, association studies look for differences in allele frequencies between populations of patients and healthy controls. If the patient population has a specific allele more frequently then the control population that allele is said to be associated with the disorder. It is important to match populations carefully for studies of this type, because different allele frequencies among ethnic groups, called population stratification, can cause false positive results. To avoid this difficulty many studies use ethnically homogenous populations or a family based approach including the non-transmitted parental allele as the control group (haplotype relative risk or transmission disequilibrium test methods). Association studies may be hypothesis-driven and select potential candidate genes or polymorphisms based on genes associated with known biological systems. An example of a candidate gene is the ApoE gene in late-onset Alzheimer's disease, which is described in the next section.

Evidence of association may also be found where a marker is closely linked to an involved gene. This can occur because of linkage disequilibrium (LD), which is a form of linkage where the 'pedigree' selected is the entire population and the number of generations is unknown. If two genetic variants are in close proximity they are said to be in LD when recombination between them is rare, even over many generations. The extent of LD is variable throughout the genome for many reasons including the local rate of recombination and age of the original mutation. Association/LD studies are a powerful way of identifying even small genes effects, but to date, they have been confined to candidate genes. This is because the likely extent of LD at a local level may be small meaning a huge number of markers would be required to produce a genome map. Neither the density of markers required or the variation in LD between populations is fully understood. For this reason, a public collaboration, the International HapMap Project, was formed in 2002 to characterize LD across the human genome.

CLINICAL AND MOLECULAR GENETICS OF PSYCHIATRIC DISORDERS

The importance of diagnosis

Operationalized diagnostic systems such as DSM-IV and ICD-10 have considerably improved the reliability of diagnosis. Using these systems a more consistent pattern of results has emerged from genetic epidemiology confirming a heritable component to many psychiatric and behavioural phenotypes. Although reliable the biological validity of psychiatric diagnoses is yet to be established.

Neuropsychiatric genes of major effect

Neuropsychiatric disorders caused by a single mutation are uncommon but include fragile X syndrome, Huntington's disease, and early onset familial Alzheimer's disease. In total, over 100 rare single gene disorders, which clinically present with mental retardation or neuropsychiatric symptoms are recognized. For these disorders the mutant gene is both necessary and sufficient to cause the disorder and is described as a gene of major effect. Information about each specific human genetic disorder is available from a catalogue called Online Mendelian Inheritance in Man (OMIM) available at: http://www.ncbi.nlm.nih.gov/Omim/. Details about clinical aspects of specific genetic learning disability phenotypes such as Fragile X syndrome and Down's syndrome are discussed elsewhere in this volume.

Single gene/chromosomal abnormalities in psychiatry

As is the case with much of medicine, single gene/chromosomal abnormalities account for a small percentage of total psychiatric morbidity. Illustrative examples are velo-cardio-facial syndrome (VCFS), Prader–Willi syndrome and the heritable dementias. This group of dementias includes Familial Alzheimers disease (FAD), Huntington's disease (HD), Creutzfeldt–Jakob disease (CJD) and Cerebral Autosomal Dominant Arteriopathy with Subcortical Infarcts and Leuko-encephalopathy (CADASIL).

Velo-cardio-facial syndrome (VCFS)

VCFS (also known as diGeorge syndrome and 22q11 deletion syndrome) affects 1/4000 live births and is caused by a common chromosomal microdeletion in the q11 band of chromosome 22. The syndrome has a complex phenotypic expression affecting multiple organs. Typical features are facial dysmorphology (long face, narrow palpebral fissures, flattened malar eminences, prominent nose and small mouth); palate abnormalities (cleft palate or hypernasal speech); borderline learning disability; congenital heart disease; and psychiatric disorders. In particular, psychotic disorders are much more common in VCFS populations (affecting ~30% of patients), and VCFS may be over represented in schizophrenia samples (Murphy 2002).

Prader–Willi/Angelman syndrome

These learning disability syndromes are discussed here because they exhibit the phenomenon of imprinting. Imprinting, also known as a parent-of-origin effect, is where different phenotypes are associated with paternal and maternal inheritance of a disorder. The changes involved are known as epigenetic phenomena as they are inherited but involve phenotypic but not genotypic change. The mechanism is uncertain but it is assumed that activation or inactivation of genes from one parent occurs in the germline DNA. Prader–Willi syndrome follows an autosomal dominant pattern of inheritance and is caused by deletion of several paternally inherited genes at 15q11–13. This results in mild or moderate learning disability with short stature, overeating and hypogonadism. In contrast, inactivation of the maternally inherited genes at the same locus results in Angelman syndrome. This disorder is less common, and presents with severe learning disability, lack of speech, epilepsy and ataxia.

Huntington's disease (HD)/trinucleotide repeat expansion diseases (TREDs)

HD is a progressive, fatal, neuro-degenerative disorder with an incidence of 1 in 100 000. The condition commonly presents between ages 35 and 50 with impaired muscle coordination, choreiform movements, psychiatric symptoms and progressive subcortical dementia. Almost all cases are familial with an autosomal dominant mode of inheritance. In 1993 the HD mutation was identified as an expansion of a CAG trinucleotide repeat coding for glutamine in exon 1 of the HD gene. Non-HD individuals have less than 35 CAG repeats, those with 36–39 repeats may have phenotypic expression of HD and those with higher numbers of repeats are more severely affected. Expansions of more than 55 repeats frequently cause a juvenile form of the disease. Unlike other mutations trinucleotide repeats are unstable and vulnerable to dynamic mutation, meaning that longer repeat sequences are more likely to undergo further expansion. This effect, called anticipation, explains why the disease tends to become more severe and have an earlier onset in successive generations of HD families

Studies using a transgenic mouse model that expresses exon 1 of the human HD gene have found that mice with lengthy CAG repeats develop progressive neurological symptoms and other HD features. These mice develop cerebral interneuronal aggregates of huntingtin similar to those reported in human HD brains at post mortem. The method of accumulation, cellular function and pathological effects of these protein aggregates are as yet unclear. However, it has recently been demonstrated that pharmacological interventions to inhibit polyglutamine aggregate formation in a mouse model for HD have neuroprotective effects (Sanchez et al. 2003).

Since the early 1990s more than 20 trinucleotide expansion diseases have been identified. Many of these are developmental or degenerative neuropsychiatric disorders and, in common with HD, exhibit the phenomenon of anticipation. TREDs can be due to expansions within exonic or intronic regions. All identified exonic expansions are caused by CAG and include spinocerebellar ataxia (SCA) types 1–3, 6, 7 and spinobulbar muscular atrophy (SBMA). Those with intronic expansions include CGG repeats in fragile X site A (FRAXA) and fragile X site E (FRAXE); CTG repeats in myotonic dystrophy; and GAA repeats in Friedreich's ataxia.

Familial Alzheimer's disease (FAD)

Most cases of Alzheimer's disease develop after the age of 65 (late onset) and are sporadic. Familial Alzheimer's disease represents a small subset of all AD cases, and typically several generations of a family will be affected with early onset disease (<55 years). The first gene linked to the disease was the gene coding for amyloid precursor protein (APP) on chromosome 21. Although at least five common mutations have been identified they only occur in a small number of families. By contrast, mutations of the presenilin-1 gene on chromosome 14q24.3 account for 40–50% of all early onset familial cases with mutations at the related presenilin-2 gene on chromosome 1 accounting for a further small percentage of early onset cases. Both genes produce membrane proteins highly expressed in CNS neurons and other cell types, but only recently has presenilin-1 been linked to our biological understanding of the disorder. It appears to be the secretase enzyme (or a cofactor of the enzyme) involved in APP processing (Xia et al. 2000). At present, a DNA diagnosis is possible in ~80% of people with FAD, but in the absence of preventive treatment the take-up for testing is likely to be low, as has been the case for HD. The contribution of genes to general AD risk will be considered below.

CJD and prion diseases

Familial CJD represents ~15% of cases of reported human spongioform encephalopathies. The presentation of familial CJD is similar to the spontaneous form, but inherited prion diseases are associated with at least 20 distinct coding mutations in the prion protein gene (PRNP), which are absent in sporadic or acquired forms of the disease. Inherited prion diseases can be diagnosed by PRNP analysis, and the use of these definitive genetic diagnostic markers has enabled recognition of a wider phenotypic spectrum of human prion disease, including fatal familial insomnia (FII) and a range of atypical dementias. A common prion protein (PrP) polymorphism at residue 129 (where methionine or valine can be encoded) is a key determinant of genetic susceptibility to acquired and sporadic prion disease in homozygous individuals. For example, new variant CJD (vCJD) appears only to have been transmitted to people who have the PRNP codon 129-methionine homozygous genotype (which represents 38% of Caucasians). Heterozygosity for this polymorphism appears protective even in some of the inherited prion diseases. The clinical presentation and pathology of prion disorders are discussed in Chapter 26.

Psychiatric disorders with a genetic contribution

The most important chromosomal loci and susceptibility genes for the major psychiatric disorders are presented in Table 3.1.

Alzheimer's disease

Many patients with late onset Alzheimer's disease also have affected relatives with AD although mutations of presenilin-1 or 2 are not responsible. Within families with late-onset AD linkage was observed between AD and chromosome 19q13.2, a region known to include the apolipoprotein E gene (APOE). Apolipoprotein E is synthesized primarily in astrocytes and transports cholesterol and triglycerides from cellular debris to neurons where they are used for synaptic membrane formation. The APOE gene is polymorphic for three common alleles, each of which encodes a distinctive isoform: APOEε2, APOEε3, and APOEε4. Candidate gene studies have found significant evidence that the APOEε4 allele is associated not only with normal age-related cognitive change but also with late-onset AD. The association between APOE4 and AD is additive – ε4/ε4 genotype has a greater risk than ε4/ε3. The APOE2 allele has been shown to be protective. The ε4 allele has a minor gene effect, meaning that it is neither necessary nor sufficient to cause AD, but does increase the relative risk of developing the disease. Neither is the ε4 allele predictive of AD, as many individuals who are heterozygous or homozygous for the ε4 allele will never develop the disease. In fact, 50% of those homozygous for ε4 who survive to 80 show no evidence of AD.

Genome-wide linkage scans of late-onset Alzheimer's disease have recently indicated susceptibility loci on chromosomes 10 and 12. Plasma Aβ42 (amyloid β42 peptide) levels are elevated in brain and serum in early-onset familial AD, but also in late-onset cases and their unaffected first-degree relatives. A recent investigation (by Ertekin-Taner et al. 2000) found linkage between extreme levels of Aβ42 (a QTL) and a marker within the chromosome 10 susceptibility locus. The locus specific relative risk to siblings associated with the chromosome 10 finding is significant (equivalent to the risk with APOE) and this may be due to modification of Aβ42 metabolism.

Schizophrenia

The biggest risk factor for schizophrenia is the sharing of genes with someone who is affected, as evidenced by family, twin and adoption studies. Segregation analysis supports a polygenic, complex genetic aetiology in most affected families. In general, identifying genes for complex disorders has proved to be a difficult task. The standard linkage approach to identify susceptibility loci of moderate effect may lack statistical power even for samples with thousands of families. Association studies of schizophrenia had a low

Table 3.1   Chromosomal loci and susceptibility genes for major psychiatric disorders

Major psychiatric disorder	Chromosomal locus	Susceptibility gene
Alzheimer's disease	19q13 10, 12	Apolipoprotein E (APOE) –
Recurrent depressive disorder	–	–
Schizophrenia	6p 8p 13q 1q,2q,3p,5q,11q,14p,20q,22q	Dysbindin-1 (DTNBP-1) Neuregulin-1 (NRG-1) G72/G30
Bipolar affective disorder	4p,12q,15q,17q,18p,18q,21q	G72/G30, BDNF
Anxiety/Panic disorder	9q31, 13q	–
Obsessive-compulsive disorder	–	–
Attention deficit hyperactivity disorder	–	DRD4, DRD5, DAT1
Alcohol dependence	1,4,7,11,16	ADH2
Autism	2q, 7q, 15q, X	NLGN3, NLGN4
Anorexia nervosa	1,4	–
Bulaemia nervosa	10p	–
Specific language impairment	7q	FOXP2
Specific reading disorder	2, 6p, 15q	

prior-probability because the neuropathology of schizophrenia is unknown (meaning that thousands of genes were potentially plausible candidates). All molecular studies are dependent on accurate phenotype definition, but the diagnosis of schizophrenia is clinical. Despite these problems a number of schizophrenia susceptibility genes and loci have now been identified using a combination of linkage, association, cytogenetic and gene expression studies.

Cytogenetic studies have reported numerous associations between schizophrenia and chromosomal mutations such as translocations, inversions, deletions and trisomies. Because schizophrenia is relatively common, many may have been co-incidental. However, chromosome 22q deletions are more common in individuals with schizophrenia and expression of the chromosome 22q deletion phenotype (VCFS) increases risk of psychosis. Strong evidence for linkage has also been reported for a balanced (1;11)(q42.1;q14.3) translocation which segregates with schizophrenia and related psychiatric disorders in a large Scottish pedigree (St Clair et al. 1990).

More than 20 genome-wide linkage scans of schizophrenia have been performed. Individually these have provided suggested evidence of linkage to many different loci. A meta-analysis of these studies (n ~2000 affected individuals) provided statistical evidence that a number of these loci (including chromosome 6p, 8p and 22q) are true positive findings (Lewis et al. 2003). Gene expression studies have also contributed to advances in the molecular genetics of schizophrenia. This approach looks for differences in expression of genes in postmortem brain tissue between affected individuals and controls. Advances in microarray technology mean that the expression profiles of thousands of genes can be investigated simultaneously. Reproducible differences in expression have been demonstrated for a number of genes, some of which map to known susceptibility loci.

From these complementary research strategies putative schizophrenia susceptibility genes have been identified. These include neuregulin-1 (NRG-1); dysbindin-1 (DTNBP-1); regulator of G-protein signalling-4 (RGS4); catechol-o-methyltransferase (COMT); proline hydroxylase (PRODH); G72; D-aminoacid oxidase (DAOO); disrupted in schizophrenia-1 (DISC-1); dopamine DRD3 and serotonin 5HT2a receptor genes. As predicted, individually these genes are of small to moderate effect (having an odds ratio (OR) = 1.2–2.0). Some of these genes (e.g. PRODH and DISC-1) may be risk factors in particular families or patient subgroups. Others (e.g. DTNBP-1 and NRG-1) may influence the development, plasticity and signalling of neural networks. Much work is still to be done in identifying pathogenic variants at these genes, exploring their functional relationships, and in identifying interactions with environmental risk or different aspects of phenotype (such as treatment response, course of illness and neuropsychological deficit).

Affective disorders
Recurrent depressive disorder
Evidence from family, twin and adoption studies in European and US community and clinical samples support a genetic component to major depressive disorder. There also appears to be genetic overlap between depression and anxiety disorders. The odds ratio for depression in first-degree relatives of depressive probands when compared to relatives of unaffected probands is 2.8 and heritability has been estimated to be ~40%. Several studies have suggested that more severe depressive disorder may have a substantially higher heritability (McGuffin et al. 1996). A complex aetiology involving both genetic liability and a major environmental component is most likely. Indicators of familial liability include recurrence of depression, early age at onset and more severe functional impairment. Research points to the environmental effects being unique to the individual rather than due to common effects within families (such as poverty or parenting style). It has been suggested that individuals at low genetic risk develop depressive episodes in response to stressful life events, in contrast to individuals at higher genetic risk who are more likely to develop spontaneous depressive episodes (Kendler et al. 2001). A number of large collaborative linkage studies of recurrent depressive disorder and early onset depressive disorder are now underway.

Bipolar Affective disorder (BP)
The mean population risk for BP is approximately 0.5% and at least 30 published family studies report an increased risk of BP in the relatives of affected probands. The relative risk to first-degree relatives of bipolar probands (measured in odds ratios) is OR = 7 (CI 5–10), equivalent to a population risk of 10–18%. A meta-analysis of six twin studies indicates an average MZ concordance for BP of 50% with an average DZ concordance of 7%. There is also an increased risk of unipolar depression within the families of bipolar probands, which may represent shared genetic susceptibility (see Table 3.2). The lifetime risk is increased for probands with early age of onset, and in families with more affected members, but risk does not seem to be influenced by either the sex or type of affected relative. The only adoption study of sufficient size to provide statistically meaningful results showed a significantly greater risk of affective disorder (bipolar, unipolar and schizo-affective disorder) in the

Table 3.2 Risk of BP disorder

	Risk of BP (%)	Additional UP risk (%)
MZ co-twin	50	15–25
First degree relative	5–10	10–20
Population controls	0.5–1.5	5–10

biological parents of bipolar adoptees compared with adoptive parents.

BP linkage studies in the 1980s focused on rare, large pedigrees where the disorder appeared to follow an autosomal dominant pattern. Early promising linkage results were later retracted as key unaffected members of pedigrees became ill and examination of new members reduced linkage evidence. It is now apparent that for a majority of BP cases, the genetic aetiology is more complex and may involve epistatic interaction of multiple genes. Large-scale genome-wide studies have reported a number of possible susceptibility loci, including 4p, 12q23–24, 15q11–13, 17q, 18p, 18q, and 21q22. Interestingly, a number of these susceptibility loci overlap with potential susceptibility loci for schizophrenia.

Most genetic association studies of BP have targeted genes involved in monoamine neurotransmission or metabolism. Both the serotonin transporter gene (5-HTT) and a common functional variant (*val108/158met*) of the COMT gene are associated with BP. In each case the contribution to genetic susceptibility is small (OR < 1.2). Recent evidence provisionally suggests that variation at the 5-HTT may have a more significant effect in the subgroup of BP females with bipolar puerperal psychosis (OR = 4). In the UK population the 'risk' allele is present in 75% of individuals, meaning that other allele variants could be seen as protective (Coyle et al. 2000).

The COMT enzyme metabolises dopamine and has an important role in regulation of dopamine neurotransmission in the prefrontal cortex (PFC). The mutation associated with BP causes a valine to methionine substitution that results in a fourfold reduction in COMT activity and hence increased dopamine neurotransmission. Interestingly, association with COMT has been reported for a number of psychiatric disorders including schizophrenia and OCD. The role of the COMT genotype in memory function is discussed below. Evidence from two recent studies suggests that another gene, which appears to be involved in memory function, the brain derived growth factor (BDNF) is associated with BP. The putative schizophrenia susceptibility genes G72/G30 map to a chromosome locus also linked to BP (chromosome 13q32–33). Following from speculation that SZ and BP may share common genes and common biology, association has recently been reported between these genes and BP.

Anxiety and panic disorder

There is significant co-morbidity between individual anxiety disorders and between anxiety disorders and depression. In most cases the clinical phenotypes do not run true in families. The most robust genetic epidemiological data is in relation to panic disorder (PD). Numerous worldwide studies indicate that PD is more prevalent in first-degree relatives of affected probands (~8%) than in relatives of controls (1–3%). Twin studies provide evidence for a heritability estimate in the 40–48% range. The processes that underlie anxiety disorders are also substantially heritable. For example, twin research indicates a significant genetic component to the habituation, acquisition and extinction of fear stimuli.

Most molecular studies of anxiety have focused on the PD phenotype, although individual studies have defined this phenotype differently. An Icelandic study of anxiety disorders identified significant evidence of linkage (LOD = 4.18) to chromosome 9q31 in a subgroup of 25 families where at least one proband was affected with PD (Thorgeirsson et al. 2003). Because most affected individuals did not have panic disorder, the authors comment that this finding may represent susceptibility to anxiety in general, rather than specifically to PD. Two linkage studies of PD have also suggested a region of possible interest on chromosome 13 (Knowles et al 1998; Crowe et al 2001). A broader 'panic syndrome' phenotype that includes medical co-morbidity (e.g. bladder/kidney conditions) has also been investigated. In a study of 587 individuals from 60 families with panic syndrome, significant evidence of linkage (MLS = 3.57) to a chromosome 13q locus was reported.

Few human molecular studies of anxiety/fear have been conducted. Because anxiety/fear is readily reproduced across species and appears to share common neurophysiology, many animal studies have been performed. Artificial selection has been used to create mouse strains with heritable differences in anxiety behaviour. QTL mapping of these mice has identified susceptibility loci for mouse 'anxiety'. This information may prove valuable in identifying candidate loci for molecular studies of human anxiety.

Attention deficit hyperactivity disorder (ADHD)

ADHD is a common condition of childhood affecting 3–6% of school age children worldwide with males being affected three times more commonly than females. Its clinical features include excessive motor activity, impaired attention and impulsivity. ADHD causes marked educational, social and family difficulties for sufferers and their relatives. The condition is of early onset (usually before age seven) and tends to persist throughout childhood. A substantial genetic element has been implicated by family, twin and adoption studies. The heritability (h^2) of ADHD has been estimated to be between 0.50 to 0.98

Abnormalities of dopamine neurotransmission have been implicated in ADHD. The mainstay of treatment for ADHD is methylphenidate and other psychostimulant medications (dextroamphetamine, pemoline) that are known to inhibit the dopamine transporter. These drugs ameliorate hyperactivity, inattention and impulsivity in ADHD cases. Animal models also support a dopaminergic hypothesis in ADHD. Mice without a functioning dopamine transporter (DAT1 knockout mice) have high extracellular striatal dopamine levels, a doubling of the rate of dopamine synthesis, and a nearly complete loss of functioning of dopamine autoreceptors. They display markedly increased locomotor and stereotypic activity compared to normal (wild-type) mice. Structural brain imaging studies in affected children have shown abnormalities in the frontal lobe and subcortical structures (globus pallidus, caudate, corpus callosum), regions known to be rich in dopamine neurotransmission and important in the control of attention and response to organisation. Thus, unlike many other psychiatric disorders, reasonable candidate genes exist.

Many genetic association studies have been conducted and for the dopamine system, the receptors DRD4 and DRD5 and the dopamine transporter (DAT1) have shown strong evidence for association in many but not all samples examined. A meta-analysis of DRD4 studies (Faraone et al. 2001) showed strong support for association with an odds ratio (OR) of 1.4 for family based designs ($p = 0.02$) and a stronger OR of 1.9 for case control studies ($p = 0.08 \times 10^{-6}$). A more recent joint analysis of a DRD5 polymorphism (Lowe et al. 2003) showed association with the *DRD5* locus ($p = 0.00005$, OR = 1.24, 95% CI 1.12–1.38). Interestingly, this association appears to be confined to the predominantly inattentive and combined clinical subtypes. Other dopamine-related candidate genes showing positive results are dopamine β-hydroxylase (DBH) and the synaptic vesicle docking fusion protein, SNAP-25. Candidate genes within the serotonergic and adrenergic system are being examined but with no clear pattern emerging as yet. Work directed toward a biological hypothesis is underway and is attempting to integrate the genetic findings together with emerging neuropsychological and neuroimaging data. In turn, a better understanding of the underlying biology will facilitate the validation and refinement of the ADHD phenotype.

Obsessive-compulsive disorder (OCD)

More than 20 family studies of OCD have been performed, but individual studies have differed in ascertainment, methodology and diagnostic criteria. A recent meta-analysis of these data (including studies that used operationalized diagnostic criteria, direct interviews and case-control designs) indicated familial aggregation of OCD. Rates of OCD were significantly greater in 1209 first-degree relatives of affected probands (8.2%) than in 746 control relatives (2%) (Hettema et al. 2001). A small twin study based on clinical OCD cases ascertained from the Maudsley twin register indicated higher concordance in 15 MZ twin pairs (33%) than in 15 DZ twin pairs (7%). Other small OCD twin studies have been reported but may have over-emphasized MZ concordant pairs because of ascertainment bias. Obsessional traits and symptoms in the general population are also heritable. Two large studies of normal twins indicate heritability in the 25–50% range (Clifford et al. 1984; Jonnal et al. 2000). It is yet to be determined whether such traits/symptoms in the general population share genetic risk with clinical OCD.

Two OCD linkage studies have reported suggestive findings. The first study ascertained probands through a tic-disorder phenotype (Gilles de la Tourette syndrome – see below) and found suggestive evidence for linkage to a chromosome 4q locus for a 'hoarding' phenotype. The second study investigated paediatric probands and identified suggestive evidence for linkage to a locus on chromosome 9p. However, both studies were small (<100 probands) and will require independent confirmation. A larger OCD study (which will collect 500 pedigrees) is now underway. Associations with the COMT and BDNF genes have been reported, but require further investigation (see above).

Gilles de la Tourette syndrome (TS)

TS is a familial neuropsychiatric disorder of childhood onset characterized by both motor and vocal tics. Individuals with TS and their relatives often have symptoms of OCD that may be an alternative expression of the TS gene (s) in TS families. Some studies of TS have included other tic disorders and OCD as part of the phenotype, although tic disorders may be genetically heterogeneous. Three genome-wide linkage scans of TS have been completed. These have provided suggestive evidence for linkage to several loci, with two studies reporting linkage to chromosome 11q23. Most candidate gene studies of TS have reported negative findings.

Autism/autistic spectrum disorders

Autism is a complex neurodevelopmental disorder characterized by significant disturbances in social, communicative, and behavioural functioning. Initially described by Leo Kanner (1943), the core features of autism have remained consistent since this early formulation. Onset is typically before age three and symptoms are chronic. Autism is one of a group of disorders called Pervasive Developmental Disorders (PDDs), which include Asperger syndrome, Rett syndrome, childhood disintegrative disorder, and Pervasive Developmental Disorder Not Otherwise Specified (PDDNOS). A recent review of multiple epidemiological surveys estimates the prevalence of autism at ~1 per 1000 children, with the prevalence for all PDDs at ~7 per 1000 (Fombonne 2003).

Autism is considered by many to be the most strongly genetically influenced multifactorial childhood psychiatric disorder. The rate among siblings (called the sibling recurrence risk ratio (λ_s)) is at least 50 times higher than in the general population. Four twin studies have reported increased MZ:DZ twin concordance, averaging 73:7 across studies. Adopted away children have been identified, but formal adoption studies have not been possible because the condition is so rare. From family and twin data heritability has been estimated at ~90%. The mode of inheritance is unknown but likely to be complex and involve multiple genes of small effect with epistatic interactions. Autism appears genetically related to the more common pervasive developmental disorders/autistic spectrum of disorders (ASDs), so both narrow and broad definitions of the disorder have been suggested for use in genetic studies. Both autism and ASDs are more common in males. Data from a large twin study also indicates that some autistic traits may be continuously distributed in the general population.

Genome-wide linkage studies of autism have provided suggestive, but not significant linkage evidence, to loci on chromosomes 2q, 7q, 15q and X. Cytogenetic abnormalities have also been reported in autistic individuals at each of these loci. Analysis of subsets of autistic individuals with (i) delayed speech increased linkage evidence at chromosomes 2 and 7, and (ii) insistence on sameness increased evidence at 15q. Candidate genes at these loci are now being investigated. Functional mutations of the neuroligin gene family (on chromosome X) have been identified in autistic individuals. These genes, NLGN3 and NLGN4 encode postsynaptic cell adhesion molecules that may have a role in the formation of functional synapses (Jamain et al. 2003). How this relates to the neurobiology of autism is not yet understood.

Alcohol abuse/dependence

Family, twin and adoption studies indicate that 40–60% of the individual variation in alcohol preference and vulnerability to alcohol dependence syndrome (ADS) is genetic in origin. The largest proportion of this genetic vulnerability is substance-specific although nicotine addiction may be co-inherited. All studies point to a large and complex environmental contribution as the prevalence differs widely between cultures; in the same culture over time (e.g. due to the effect of prohibition in the US); and between the sexes within the same culture. Indeed the lifetime rates in partners of affected women are similar to rates in male relatives, suggesting that learned behaviour and assortative mating may have an important role.

Polymorphisms of two major enzymes of alcohol metabolism are well established as genetic factors for differential susceptibility to ADS. Both alleles are found in half the population of South Eastern Asian countries but are rare in Caucasian and African populations. The alcohol dehydrogenase allele (ADH2 His47) increases metabolism of alcohol to acetaldehyde and the aldehyde dehydrogenase allele (ALDH2 Lys487) decreases the rate of acetaldehyde removal. Both lead to an accumulation of acetaldehyde after alcohol intake and a flushing reaction similar to that produced by disulfiram. Even for Japanese people with one ALDH2 Lys487 allele (30–40% of the population) the risk of alcoholism is reduced 5- to 10-fold. Studies of alcoholism in Americans of Asian ancestry imply that the protective effect of both polymorphisms varies across different environmental backgrounds.

Rodent models of alcohol sensitivity are being used to increase our molecular understanding of ADS. For example, differences in $GABA_A$ receptor function appear to be a critical determinant of ethanol sensitivity. QTL mapping in rodents has identified candidate genes and loci for alcohol-related behaviour for further investigation in humans. In such models withdrawal severity is attributable primarily to loci at chromosome 1, 4 and 11; the chromosome 11 locus contains a $GABA_A$ gene cluster that may contribute to this differential alcohol response. Animal models are also indicating potential candidate genes. Dopaminergic neurons in the ventral tegmental region mediate reinforcement of continued alcohol consumption, suggesting a potential role for DRD2 receptor polymorphisms. Two independent genome scans in humans have provided suggestive evidence that chromosomes 1, 4, 7, 11, and 16 may carry genes contributing to alcohol dependence. Some investigators are applying intermediate clinical phenotypes to identify specific subgroups for genetic analysis. For instance, a low level of response to the socially desirable effects of alcohol at age 20 years has been shown to be a strong predictor of later ADS in families with a history of alcohol dependence. In this case it is thought that low level of alcohol response encourages heavier drinking, exposure to which increases risk of alcohol dependence. The Collaborative Study on the Genetics of Alcoholism (COGA) also recently reported that the chromosome 1 locus may predispose some individuals within a family to alcoholism and others to depression (Nurnberger et al. 2001).

Eating disorders

Eating disorders are significantly more common in relatives of affected probands. In the absence of adoption data, twin studies support a significant genetic component. Concordance rates are higher in MZ (55%) than DZ (5%) twin pairs with anorexia nervosa (AN), but similar in MZ (35%) and DZ (30%) twin pairs with bulimia nervosa (BN). Although this might suggest a greater genetic contribution to AN than other forms of eating disorder, diagnostic boundaries are not absolute, and patients migrate between the AN, BN and atypical eating disorder categories over time (Fairburn & Harrison 2003). Population-based twin studies indicate a substantial genetic contribution to specific eating behaviour (including self-induced vomiting and binge eating) as well as self reported eating disorder in the general population. Eating disorders are associated with significant co-morbidity and depression, substance abuse and obsessional/perfectionistic traits are also more common in families of eating disorder probands. It is yet to be established to what extent this represents common genetic or environmental liability.

Several linkage studies of eating disorders have now been reported. An affected sibling pair study of 192 AN families suggested linkage to chromosome 4 (Grice et al. 2002). This study also found evidence that a chromosome 1p susceptibility locus contributes to the restricting subtype of AN (RAN), which is characterized by severe limiting of food intake without binging or purging behaviour. Using a similar strategy an investigation of BN in 308 families provided suggestive evidence of linkage to a chromosome 10p (maximum Lod score (MLS) = 2.92) (Bulik et al. 2003). When this analysis was restricted to the subset of families with at least two family members with self-induced vomiting (n = 133) the MLS observed at this locus increased (MLS = 3.39). Independent replication of these promising findings is required.

Speech, language and reading disorders

Specific language impairment (SLI) and dyslexia/specific reading disability (SRD) are frequent childhood disorders, which appear to be related. They are defined by a significant difficulty in acquiring language (SLI) or learning to read/write (SRD), after appropriate educational exposure and in the absence of sensory, developmental or intellectual disability. The familial nature of these deficits has long been recognized (see Williams 2002 for review). The risk of SLI in first-degree relatives of affected probands is ~28% compared to 4% in the relatives of controls. Family studies of SRD indicate a recurrence rate in siblings of ~40% although the general population prevalence of SRD is 5–10%. Twin studies indicate a substantial genetic component. A meta-analysis of SLI twin studies found that concordance was higher among the 188 MZ twin pairs (73%) than among the 94 DZ pairs (35%), and estimated a heritability of 0.76. Two large twin studies of SRD, with different methodologies, have been performed. The Colorado study (deFries & Fulker 1987) included twin pairs where one member was reading disabled. In contrast the London study (Stevenson et al. 1987) investigated reading ability in 285 twin pairs from the general population. Both provided strong evidence for the role of genes in SRD. In particular, deficits in awareness, decoding, storage and retrieval of small segments of speech (termed phonemes) were substantially heritable (h^2 ~80%).

Molecular genetic studies of SLI have already identified the first gene contributing to language impairment (Lai et al. 2001), FOXP2. This gene is expressed in the brain and is involved in regulation of embryo development. The observed mutation in the FOXP2 gene appears to interfere with the development of neural systems regulating speech and language. Although this finding may be important in understanding the biology of language processing, the mutation itself is rare and the resultant language disorder phenotype is not typical of SLI. Progress is also being made in the molecular genetics of SRD with studies producing strong statistical evidence of linkage to chromosome 6p, 15q and 2.

Genetics and behaviour, treatment response and research ethics

Intelligence, memory and cognition

Intelligence is one of the most controversial areas in behavioural genetics. Meta-analyses based on 10 000 twin pairs estimate that ~50% of the variance in general cognitive ability (g) scores can be attributed to genetic factors. Measuring cognitive ability by IQ produces a normal distribution and suggests multiple minor QTLs, each of small effect in combination with environmental effects. A large UK study, the IQ QTL project, would appear to confirm this. This study performed a genome wide scan to investigate individuals with very high IQ and a sample of average IQ individuals. None of the 1800 markers investigated were linked to general cognitive ability. This suggests that contribution of individual genetic effects to general cognitive ability is small, although the study may have failed to identify larger effects because of insufficient marker density. An association analysis performed as part of the IQ QTL project did find evidence for association with insulin-like growth factor-2 (IGF2R). This is a plausible candidate gene, as it appears to be active in brain regions involved in memory.

Several other potential candidate genes for memory function have been investigated. The BDNF gene (see above) has a significant neurodevelopmental role but also a role in hippocampal long-term potentiation (LTP), a process of synaptic change involved in learning and behavioural adaptation. A mutation causing an amino acid substitution (val/met) reduces BDNF secretion. In a study of healthy human subjects the met allele was associated with deficits in episodic memory and in particular with impaired information acquisition. An extension of this study found functional imaging evidence of diminished hippocampal response in individuals with the met allele during memory tasks.

The enzyme COMT is important in dopamine breakdown and may be particularly relevant to regulation of dopamine function in prefrontal cortex (PFC) and subcortical structures. A valine/methionine (val/met) substitution of COMT has been identified. The met allele results in a fourfold reduction in COMT activity, increasing dopamine neurotransmission. It has recently been demonstrated that the COMT genotype is associated with variation in executive cognition and PFC physiology during working memory in healthy human subjects (Goldberg et al. 2003). These findings suggest that individual gene variants can have significant impact on memory and cognitive function. The impact of BDNF and COMT gene variation on cognitive function may explain reported associations between these genes and a variety of psychiatric disorders (including OCD and BP). These and other variants may have an effect on cognitive function, which could influence the expression or severity of individual psychiatric disorders.

Personality and behaviour

Personality traits are relatively enduring individual differences in behaviour that are stable across time and across situations. Such traits are not strongly predictive, as individual behaviour will also depend on particular environmental situations. For this reason, 'personality' phenotypes may be difficult to measure, particularly as most measures use self-report data. However, measures have been developed which show test-retest reliability and have been validated by collateral information or laboratory testing. One such measure is the five-factor model of personality traits (extraversion v introversion, agreeableness v antagonism, conscientiousness v lack of direction, neuroticism v emotional stability, openness v closedness). Heritability in the 20–40% range has been demonstrated for each of these five factors. A genome scan of personality indicated, not surprisingly, that the genes contributing to personality are likely to be of small effect. Several studies have reported association between the dopamine D4 receptor gene (*DRD4*) and novelty seeking. Variation at this receptor alters receptor structure, and the receptor's efficiency in vitro. In this case, shorter alleles code for a receptor variant that is more efficient at binding dopamine than the larger alleles. It has been suggested that there is a reward mechanism whereby novelty seeking promotes dopamine release, and that individuals with larger alleles have to engage in more novelty-seeking behaviour to increase dopamine release. Although such a mechanism may contribute to novelty-seeking behaviour, this genetic effect only accounts for about 4% of the variance in this trait. Candidate genes studies suggesting association between functional variants of the serotonin transporter gene and a number of disparate traits (neuroticism, shyness and aggression), if confirmed are likely to be of similar small effect. It has also been suggested that genotype may influence response to environmental risk. In a large epidemiological study of male children, those with a genotype conferring high levels of monoamine oxidase A expression were less likely to develop antisocial problems. In this study, individuals having a combination of maltreatment and the low-activity *MAOA* genotype represented 12% of the birth cohort but accounted for 44% of those convicted of violence (Caspi et al. 2002). Further studies are required to confirm the attributable risk fraction and predictive sensitivity suggested by this finding.

Pharmacogenetics

Genetic variation may explain differences in drug treatment response or the development of side effects. Many drugs target proteins such as enzymes and neuroreceptors and changes in the structure or function of these target proteins will affect the interaction between drug and protein. Pharmacogenetic studies investigate genetic variation in genes that encode proteins that interact with drugs, with the aim of establishing predictive relationships between polymorphisms and treatment response or side effects. A more recent advance is pharmacogenomics where whole genome information is used to identify susceptibility loci that influence inter-individual differences in treatment, and to use this information to identify novel drug targets.

Many typical antipsychotic drugs are significantly metabolized by the polymorphic cytochrome P450 2D6 enzyme, which shows large variation in activity between individuals. Because of this genetic variation certain individuals have poor or extremely rapid metabolism for substrates of this enzyme, which can lead to an increased risk of side effects or lack of treatment response. Data indicates that variation at the 5-HT_{2A} receptor gene is probably associated with clozapine response in patients with schizophrenia. Several studies also indicate that variation at the DRD3 gene is associated with risk for tardive dyskinesia. However, in neither instance is the polymorphism involved predictive of treatment response or movement disorder so as yet the goal of individually tailored treatment has yet to be realized.

Ethics and public understanding

In this chapter, we have made it clear that both the genes we inherit and the environment in which we live influence human behaviour and the risk of developing psychiatric disorder. Advances in genetics are likely to have an important impact on scientific understanding of psychiatric disorders and human behaviour. This will undoubtedly affect public perception and raise ethical questions (Nuffield Council on Bioethics 2002).

Employers already use psychometric testing to assess personality and intelligence of potential employees. In the future will employers and potential insurers wish to know about an individual's genetic susceptibility to traits such as aggression or novelty seeking? Might individuals with risk factors for certain behaviours be selected, and discriminated against as genetically abnormal, or in need of corrective treatment? Selection on the basis of genetic tests might also include prenatal testing, the streaming of children in schools on IQ or aptitude, the screening by employers, and the use of genetic information for insurance purposes. Is this type of selection acceptable? Is an individual with a genotype known to be associated with impulsiveness, for example, less responsible for their behaviour? Could this have legal implications? Could the study of normal behavioural traits contribute adversely to their medicalization? If so, the boundaries between normal variation and disorder may shift towards the centre and social tolerance for previously normal traits may be undermined and the role of the environment undervalued. Are there dangers in the widening of diagnostic boundaries?

It is likely that the predictive value of individual genetic tests will be so low as to be of no value for screening purposes, for determining optimal treatment, or for attributing diminished responsibility. However, the potential value of a combination of many genetic tests and environmental information has yet to be determined and will require careful consideration. Currently, public opinion supports the use of legislation to prevent the misuse of genetic information but this may vary between nations and with the proposed use of the information. Legal opinion suggests that tests for traits within the normal range fall outside of the current legal definitions of insanity and diminished responsibility and cannot, therefore, be used as a defence. However, many issues remain to be resolved and new ethical issues will undoubtedly arise in the future. These ethical questions and dilemmas will require debate. It is important that the scientific community takes part in that debate, and provides accurate and unbiased information to help construct reasonable guidelines.

REFERENCES

Baron M. (2001) Genetics of schizophrenia and the new millennium: progress and pitfalls. *American Journal of Human Genetics* 68: 299–312

Bulik CM, Devlin B, Bacanu SA et al. (2003) Significant linkage on chromosome 10p in families with bulimia nervosa. *American Journal of Human Genetics* 72(1): 200–7.

Bunney WE, Bunney BG, Vawter MP et al. (2003) Microarray technology: a review of new strategies to discover candidate vulnerability genes in psychiatric disorders. *American Journal of Psychiatry* 160(4): 657–66.

Caspi A, McClay J, Moffitt TE et al. (2002) Role of genotype in the cycle of violence in maltreated children. *Science* 297: 851–4

Clifford CA, Murray RM & Fulker DW (1984) Genetic and environmental influences on obsessional traits and symptoms. *Psychological Medicine* 14: 791–800.

Coyle N, Jones I, Robertson E et al. (2000) Variation at the serotonin transporter gene influences susceptibility to bipolar affective puerperal psychosis. *Lancet* 356(9240): 1490–1.

Crowe RR, Goedken R, Samuelson S, Wilson R, Nelson J & Noyes R Jr. (2001) Genomewide survey of panic disorder. *American Journal of Medical Genetics* 105(1):105–9.

deFries JC, Fulker DW & LaBuda MC (1987) Evidence for a genetic aetiology in reading disability of twins. *Nature* 329(6139): 537–9.

Ertekin-Taner N, Graff-Radford N, Younkin LH et al. (2000) Linkage of plasma Abeta42 to quantitative locus on chromosome 10 in late-onset Alzheimer's disease pedigrees. *Science* 290(5500): 2303–4.

Fairburn CG & Harrison PJ (2003) Eating disorders. *Lancet* 1361(9355): 407–16.

Faraone SV, Doyle AV, Mick E et al. (2001) Meta-analysis of the association between the 7-repeat allele of the dopamine D(4) receptor gene and attention deficit hyperactivity disorder. *American Journal of Psychiatry* 158(7): 1052–7.

Fombonne E (2003) The prevalence of autism. *Journal of the American Medical Association* 289(1): 87–9.

Goldberg TE, Egan MF, Gscheidle T et al. (2003) Executive subprocesses in working memory: relationship to catechol-o-methyltransferase Val158Met genotype and schizophrenia. *Archives of General Psychiatry* 60: 889–96.

Gottesman II & Bertelsen A (1989) Confirming unexpressed genotypes for schizophrenia. Results in the offspring of Fisher's Danish identical and fraternal twins. *Archives of General Psychiatry* 46: 867–72.

Grice DE, Halmi KA, Fichter MM et al. (2002) Evidence for a susceptibility gene for anorexia nervosa on chromosome 1. *American Journal of Human Genetics* 70(3): 787–92.

Hettema JM, Neale MC & Kendler KS (2001) A review and meta-analysis of the genetic epidemiology of anxiety disorders. *American Journal of Psychiatry* 158: 1568–78.

Jamain S, Quach H, Betancur C et al. (2003) Mutations of the X-linked genes encoding neuroligins NLGN3 and NLGN4 are associated with autism. *Nature Genetics* 34(1): 27–9.

Jonnal AH, Gardner CO, Prescott CA & Kendler KS (2000) Obsessive and compulsive symptoms in a general population sample of female twins. *American Journal of Medical Genetics* 96: 791–6.

Kendler KS, Thornton LM & Gardner CO (2001) Genetic risk, number of previous depressive episodes, and stressful life events in predicting onset of major depression. *American Journal of Psychiatry* 158(4): 582–6.

Kety SS (1988) Schizophrenic illness in the families of schizophrenic adoptees: findings from the Danish national sample. *Schizophrenia Bulletin* 14(2): 217–22.

Knowles JA, Fyer AJ, Vieland VJ, Weissman MM, Hodge SE et al. (1998) Results of a genome-wide genetic screen for panic disorder. *American Journal of Medical Genetics* 81(2): 139–47.

Lai CS, Fisher SE, Hurst JA et al. (2001) A forkhead-domain gene is mutated in a severe speech and language disorder. *Nature* 413: 519–23.

Lander E & Kruglyak L (1995) Genetic dissection of complex traits: guidelines for interpreting and reporting linkage results. *Nature Genetics* 11: 241–7.

Lewis CM, Levinson DF, Wise LH et al. (2003) Genome scan meta-analysis of schizophrenia and bipolar disorder, part II: schizophrenia. *American Journal of Human Genetics* 73(1): 34–48.

Lowe N, Kirley A, Hawi Z, Sham P, Wickham H et al. (2004) Joint analysis of the DRD5 marker concludes association with attention-deficit/hyperactivity disorder confined to the predominantly inattentive and combined subtypes. *American Journal of Medical Genetics* 74(2): 348–56.

McGuffin P, Katz R, Watkins S, Rutherford JA (1996) Hospital-based twin register of the heritability of DSM-IV unipolar depression. *Archives of General Psychiatry* 53(2): 129–36.

Murphy KC (2002) Schizophrenia and velo-cardio-facial syndrome. *Lancet* 359(9304): 426–30.

Nuffield Council on Bioethics (2002) *Genetics and Human Behaviour, the Ethical Context*. Online. Available at: www.nuffieldbioethics.org/publications/pp_0000000015.asp [accessed 1 May 2004].

Nurnberger JI Jr, Foroud T, Flury L, Su J, Meyer ET et al. (2001) Evidence for a locus on chromosome 1 that influences vulnerability to alcoholism and affective disorder. *American Journal of Psychiatry* 158(5): 718–24.

Plomin R, Owen MJ & McGuffin P (1994) The genetic basis of complex human behaviours. *Science* 264: 1733–9.

Sanchez I, Mahlke C & Yuan J (2003) Pivotal role of oligomerization in the expanded polyglutamine neurodegenerative disorders. *Nature* 421: 373–9.

St Clair D, Blackwood D, Muir W et al. (1990) Association within a family of a balanced autosomal translocation with major mental illness. *Lancet* 336(8706): 13–6.

Stevenson J, Graham P, Fredman G & McLoughlin V (1987) A twin study of genetic influences on reading and spelling ability and disability. *Journal of Child Psychology and Psychiatry* 28(2): 229–47.

Thorgeirsson TE, Oskarsson H, Desnica N et al. (2003) Anxiety with panic disorder linked to chromosome 9q in Iceland. *American Journal of Human Genetics* 72: 1221–30.

Watson JD & Crick FHC (1953) Molecular structure of nucleic acids. *Nature* 171: 737–8.

Williams J (2002) Reading and language disorders. In: McGuffin P, Owen MJ & Gottesman II (eds) *Psychiatric Genetics and Genomics*, pp. 129–146. Oxford: Oxford University Press.

Xia W, Ray WJ, Ostaszewski BL et al. (2000) Presenilin complexes with the C-terminal fragments of amyloid precursor protein at the sites of amyloid beta-protein generation. *Proceedings of the National Academy of Sciences of the United States of America* 97(16): 9299–304.

Human personality development

Nick Goddard

INTRODUCTION

Development is a complex process, involving physical, cognitive, personality and social changes and adaptations throughout life. Attention is often focused on the early years of life, but development continues throughout life and a lifespan developmental approach will encompass not only the major changes in infants, but also the adjustments made in adolescence, in adult life and in old age, that occur as well as the major events that impact on life, e.g. bereavement, chronic illness.

Human development is clearly a diverse topic, which has given rise to many models and theories. The main areas are covered in this chapter.

NATURE VERSUS NURTURE

Conceptualizing development has led to several polarized approaches and the nature/nurture or genetics/environment debate has a long history.

The nurture argument was perhaps first articulated by John Locke in the 17th century. He contended that at birth children were blank slates (*tabula rasa*) and that what they became was dependent on learning and experience. Therefore, their environment determines their development.

In contrast, Jean Jacques Rousseau supported the nature argument, believing that development was an invariant sequence of Nature's plan and that all a child required was guidance.

This argument has been repeated in various forms, more recently as the environment versus genetics debate. Whilst there has been no clear resolution to the debate, at best it is reductionist. More recent research has focused on the interaction of genes and environment, giving rise to behavioural genetics. Of interest here is how the genetic developmental plan is dependent on environmental factors (both protective and adverse) for its expression. Genes can also influence the environment through reactive, evocative and proactive interactions.

COGNITIVE DEVELOPMENT

Jean Piaget, a Swiss born psychologist, brought a new approach to cognitive development. He moved away from environmental or biological components of development to how a child's naturally developing abilities interact with the environment.

Piaget proposed a 'stage' model in which a child passes through development in an *invariant sequence*, through a process of *assimilation* (taking in new information) and *accommodation* (modifying existing information or *schema*). Such information requires *organization* and the whole process involves active participation (Piaget & Inhelder 1969).

Piaget, through his observations and discussions with children, including his own, proposed the following four-stage process of development:

- **Period I (0–2 years): sensorimotor intelligence.** During this time the baby recognizes self as an agent and begins to act in an intentional way. Through the organization of its actions, e.g. sucking and grasping, the baby becomes prepared to deal with the outside world. *Object permanence* also develops in this period. This is the realization that objects still exist even if not in the baby's sight, e.g. if a toy is covered with a cloth, a 2-month-old will not look for the toy, whereas by 10–12 months an infant will look under the cloth for the toy.
- **Period II (2–7 years): preoperational thought.** A child begins to think in symbolic terms, e.g. playing with a box pretending that it is a car, though thought is not yet organized in a logical manner. There are no learnt rules or *operations*. Typically, thinking is egocentric and the classification of objects depends on one feature, e.g. colour.
- **Period III (7–11 years): concrete operations.** Thought becomes increasingly more logical in this period. The child achieves *conservation* – the ability to perform mental operations with various qualities, e.g. in conservation of liquid a child presented with two

containers, one tall and thin, one short and wide, both containing the same amount of liquid, will be able to recognize this. A younger child would pick the thin container as having more liquid, as the level appears higher. Conservation also occurs with number, substance, weight and volume. Classification occurs according to several features.

- **Period IV (11 years to adulthood): formal operations.** The ability to think about the future, abstract propositions and about hypothetical situations develops.

Piaget's work has received much criticism and more refined studies have found that he underestimated babies' abilities. Additionally, many adults only function at the formal operations level for a proportion of the time! However, Piaget does capture the essential characteristics of cognitive development.

MORAL DEVELOPMENT

Piaget developed a basic two-stage theory of moral judgements. Children under 10–11 years based their moral judgements on the consequences of actions and viewed rules as fixed and absolute. At around the age of 10–11 years, moral thinking changes and judgements are made on intentions, with rules being more flexible.

Lawrence Kohlberg (1927–1987) developed this theory further. Kohlberg interviewed children of various ages, giving them a series of dilemmas. In one example, a man whose wife is dying requires a medicine he cannot afford. He asks the pharmacist to sell the medicine at a cheaper price and when the pharmacist refuses the man steals the drug. By analyzing the answers, in terms of the reasoning behind the answer, Kohlberg suggested six stages of moral development (Kohlberg 1976):

- Level I (to 10 years): preconventional morality
  Stage 1 – obedience and punishment orientation: rules are obeyed to avoid punishment.
  Stage 2 – individualism and exchange: conformity in order to obtain rewards or return favours.
- Level II (10–13/14 years): conventional morality
  Stage 3 – good interpersonal relations: conform to avoid disapproval of others, often at the level of family/friends.
  Stage 4 – maintaining the social order: laws are obeyed and authority respected in order to uphold the social order.
- Level III (13/14 years – adult) post-conventional morality
  Stage 5 – social contract and individual rights: uphold principles agreed as essential for society, but recognize the view points of others and the need to have means of changing laws.

Stage 6 – universal principles: justice is valued above rules, i.e. a recognition of universal principles respecting the basic dignity of all individuals (e.g. the thinking of Gandhi).

Approximate age ranges are attached to the different levels of morality, though these are tentative. Only a small proportion of the adult population function at stage 5 and less than 10% at stage 6, which even then may be transitory.

The theory has also been criticized for being culturally and sexually biased, presenting a 'masculine' style of reasoning. Despite the criticisms, Kohlberg presented a framework beyond Piaget's for studying and understanding moral development.

LEARNING THEORY

Learning theory emphasizes development as a function of the external environment through a process of conditioning. The two major approaches are classical conditioning and operant conditioning. These theories are considered in more detail in Chapter 5.

SOCIAL LEARNING THEORY

Whilst learning theorists propose that the same principles apply to learning in social situations as to experiments in physical settings, social learning theorists argue that development occurs from *imitation* of behaviour. Of the many social learning theorists, Albert Bandura's work generates a large amount of research.

Bandura suggests that there are four components to observational learning (Bandura 1977):

1. **Attentional processes:** subjects need to pay attention to actions around them and attention is attracted by models because of their distinctiveness, success, power and prestige.
2. **Retention processes:** models' actions can be remembered in symbolic form through *stimulus contiguity*, e.g. the use of verbal codes to remember a route – second right, straight on, etc.
3. **Motor reproduction processes:** observation of a pattern also requires the motor skills to perform it, e.g. an infant imitating a carer playing with a puzzle may lack the motor development to reproduce the action.
4. **Reinforcement and motivational processes:** Bandura distinguishes between acquisition of new responses and their performance. Performance is governed by reinforcement, either direct or vicarious, and motivation.

Social learning theory becomes more complex as abstract modelling is considered, but offers valuable insights into one component of development and how certain influences (e.g. television) could effect behaviour (e.g. aggressive behaviour.)

Social learning has been criticized because of its emphasis on the environment and overlooking the importance of cognitive structures. Also, whilst the area is well researched, studies have often been carried out in artificial laboratory conditions and it is not clear how these apply to everyday life.

Social learning however, demonstrates the importance of models in development.

PSYCHODYNAMIC THEORY

The emphasis of many developmental theories is on motor or cognitive development. Psychodynamic theory looks at the world of feelings and impulses.

Sigmund Freud pioneered this area, though his work was later extended and adapted by a variety of therapists, e.g. Jung, Adler, Klein. Further details of the concepts behind this approach are contained in Chapter 35.

Erik Erikson adapted a lifespan approach to this area, enlarging the picture of child development and extending the developmental process into adulthood in his 'Eight Stages of Man' (Erikson 1963; see Table 4.1).

Erikson's model is a stage model, which proposes that an individual will pass through all the stages propelled by biological maturation and social expectations. Each stage can be negotiated to different degrees of success and the outcome of each stage may effect the outcome of subsequent stages.

The main criticism against Erikson's model is its lack of specificity: it is vague.

ATTACHMENT THEORY

John Bowlby (1907–1990) noted from his work with children in institutions that they frequently developed emotional problems and an inability to form intimate, lasting relationships with others. He drew upon ethological theories to develop *attachment theory* (Bowlby 1969).

Attachment behaviours are gestures and signals to promote and maintain proximity to care-givers, e.g. crying, babbling, grasping. Babies therefore form attachments to their carers, whilst carers *bond* to babies.

Bowlby proposed four phases of attachment:

- **Phase 1 (0–3 months): indiscriminate responsiveness.** Babies, in the first few months of life, react in similar ways to different people.
- **Phase 2 (3–6 months): focusing on familiar people.** Responses become directed to selective people, particularly the principal carer.
- **Phase 3 (6 months–3 years): intense attachment and proximity seeking.** Infants become intensely attached, usually to the principal carer, showing distress if left (separation anxiety) and a wariness of strangers (fear of strangers). As mobility increases babies begin to attempt to follow the carer.
- **Phase 4 (three years to adulthood): partnership behaviour.** The child becomes more aware of the carer's actions, allowing them to leave and working more in partnership.

Table 4.1 Erikson's Eight Stages of Man		
Age (years)	*Erikson's stage*	
0–1	Trust versus mistrust	Through dependence on carers, the infant experiences trust and mistrust, developing *hope*
1–3	Autonomy versus shame and doubt	Adjustment to social regulations without the loss of too much independence leads to *will*
3–6	Initiative versus guilt	Children's wishes and plans can lead to failure and by developing a balance of goals, restrictions and tolerance of failure, the child develops *purpose*
6–11	Industry versus inferiority	Children remain vulnerable to feelings of inadequacy. Resolution leads to *competence*
Adolescence	Identity versus confusion	Adolescence is a time for establishing a new sense of identity, which, when formed, establishes *fidelity*
Young adult	Intimacy versus isolation	Whilst people are different, an ability to tolerate others and periods of isolation leads to *love*
Adult	Generativity versus self-absorption/stagnation	The ability to look after others without becoming too self-focused, generates *care*
Old age	Ego-integrity versus despair	Old age is a time for reviewing life's successes and failures, leading to *wisdom*

The main emphasis of Bowlby's work is on early infancy and while there is little on phase 4 or attachments in later life, more recent work is attempting to examine these periods.

Bowlby had a major impact on child-rearing practices. He described that separation leads to a process of *protest*, followed by *despair* and then *detachment*. The adverse effect of such separations was one factor influencing the attitudes of hospitals to parents staying with their children during paediatric admissions.

Attachment work has been furthered by Mary Ainsworth. She was interested in how babies used mothers as a secure base from which to explore. Their reactions were investigated using the *Strange Situation Procedure*. Baby and carer enter an unfamiliar room, containing a one-way viewing screen. A stranger enters and the carer leaves the baby for a predesignated period of time, then returns. The baby's reactions are observed at each stage. From this work, Ainsworth described three patterns of attachment (Ainsworth et al. 1978), later adding a fourth:

- **Securely attached:** these infants use mother as a base from which to explore. When mother leaves their play decreases and they look upset. On mother's return they greet her, remain close and then begin to re-explore. About 60–70% of infants demonstrate this pattern of attachment.
- **Insecure–avoidant:** infants in this category look independent and do not check with mother while exploring. When mother leaves they do not appear upset. As mother returns they seek proximity to her though avoid her if picked up. This pattern is present in about 20% of infants.
- **Insecure–ambivalent:** infants are clingy and preoccupied with mother, exploring little. They appear upset when left, but are ambivalent on mother's return, reaching out to mother but pushing her away at the same time. Around 10% of infants show this pattern.
- **Disorganized:** this category, added at a later date, describes a subgroup whose behaviour lacked any coherent pattern. Some 10–15% of infants fall into this category.

There is increasing interest in the implications of attachment for adult life. The *Adult Attachment Interview* developed by Mary Main seeks to examine adults' perceptions of their early relationships. Four categories of adult attachment have been described which in turn have been linked with childhood attachments (Table 4.2).

This is an on-going area of research in development. Research suggests that the pattern of attachment expressed by mothers may determine the attachment of infants. Attachment styles are also being examined in relation to specific mental illnesses, though as yet there are few robust connections.

LANGUAGE DEVELOPMENT

Language development is a complex phenomenon, acting as a means of developing reasoning, thought and communication. The development of language is a mixture of learning and innate processes.

Learning processes

Imitation plays some role in learning language, but cannot be the only means of developing language. Conditioning may also help the process, but adults do not pay attention to every detail of speech uttered by infants.

Children also appear to learn a set of operating principles, which allows them to generalize certain constructions, e.g. the addition of '-ed' to a verb to form the past tense – 'walk, walked'. Children learn gradually not to over-generalize, e.g. 'go, goed', and to recognize irregular verbs.

Innate processes

All children, regardless of culture, seem to go through the same sequence of language development, implying an innate knowledge. Language development also has critical

Table 4.2 Patterns of adult attachment and their relationship to childhood attachment		
Adult attachment	*Childhood attachment*	
Autonomous	Secure attachment	Typically, such adults are self-reliant, coherent in describing their early experiences, objective and not defensive. They give a history of good supportive relations or have come to terms with their absence
Dismissing	Insecure–avoidant	Adults with this pattern of attachment appear to have few emotional memories of childhood. Caregivers are often idealized and the effect of traumatic experiences are minimized
Pre-occupied	Insecure–ambivalent	These adults appear to be still caught up in childhood events, often expressing anger towards the parents
Unresolved	Disorganized	The narrative of adults in this group is characterized by lapses or gaps, particularly around traumatic events

periods when it is easier to learn languages, such as the early years of life.

One of the foremost theorists in this area is Noam Chomsky, whose work has spawned a new science of neuro-linguistics. He suggests that language development is built in (Chomsky 1972). The theory then becomes very dense, but a summary is shown in Table 4.3.

Chomsky has been criticized on the grounds of reading adult meanings into children's speech. He also believes that language should be studied separately to other aspects of development!

FAMILY DEVELOPMENT

Development is not confined to individuals but also applies to the social units in which individuals live.

Defining the exact nature of what constitutes a family is difficult. One definition is to consider the family to be everyone living in a household, but also to extend this to others important to members of that household, e.g. extended family members, estranged parents.

In Western society the nuclear family of husband, wife and children has tended to be regarded as normal. This view has been challenged. The following types of family have been defined:

1. Nuclear.
2. Childless couple.
3. One-parent families – widows/widowers, divorced/separated, non-married.
4. Adopted – husband, wife, plus adopted children.
5. Communal – groups of families.
6. Reconstituted – with eight combinations:
   - (i) divorced man – single woman
   - (ii) divorced man – widowed woman
   - (iii) divorced man – divorced woman
   - (iv) single man – widowed woman
   - (v) single man – divorced woman
   - (vi) widowed man – single woman
   - (vii) widowed man – widowed woman
   - (viii) widowed man – divorced woman.

Family lifecycle

Development may vary because of the different forms of families. Classically, family development is described in the form of the family lifecycle. McGoldrick & Carter (1982) described six stages:

1. Unattached young adult – between families.
2. Joining of families through cohabitation or marriage.
3. Family with young children – adults become parents.
4. Family with adolescents– child becomes more independent.
5. Launching children – children leave and may begin their own family lifecycle, leading to the 'empty nest'.
6. Family in later life – parents become grandparents and acquire new interests.

The above is a simplistic model as many other events can occur, such as death, divorce, illness and other life events. Families may get into trouble at these points of stress or transition. Barnhill & Longo (1978) defined nine 'transition points':

1. Commitment – two people decide to form a relationship.
2. Developing parent role – man/woman becomes father/mother.
3. Accepting new personality – adapting to child's development.
4. Introducing child to institutions outside of family – such as school.
5. Accepting adolescence – parents come to terms with adolescent changes.
6. Allowing experimentation with independence – late adolescence.
7. Preparations to launch – as young adult moves into outside world.

Table 4.3 Language development		
Age	*Theory of Chomsky*	
0–12 months	Early language	Babies respond to speech. At 1 month they gurgle and coo and by 6 months babble
1 year	One-word utterances	Single, simple words
1 year–18 months	Two-word utterances	Connecting words, e.g. 'good boy'
2–3 years	Grammar development	Begin to make noun phrases, e.g. 'I making tea', and over-generalize rules, e.g. 'I runned'
3–6 years	Transformations	Increasingly complex grammar. Form questions using transformations, i.e. changing a sentence around, e.g. 'I can put it where?' → 'Where can I put it?'
5–10 years	Near-adult grammar	Develop more subtle aspects of grammar, e.g. the passive voice

8 Letting go –facing each other – father/mother face each other again as partners without child-rearing responsibility.

9 Accepting retirement/old-age.

Family functioning

Families adopt their own styles of getting along together. In working with families a normative model is used based on the characteristics of well-functioning families. Difficulties can arise because of:

- **Discord:** family discord refers to arguments, hostility and criticism in the family setting. Discord often relates to poor and inconsistent discipline in the home. An association has been established between child psychiatric disorders and exposure to family discord.
- **Over-protection:** parents seeking to prevent exposing the child to the stressors of daily life can become over-protective. Overprotection is part of a group of four patterns of family interaction (enmeshment, over-protection, rigidity and lack of conflict resolution) described by Minuchin as characterizing family functioning in families with children presenting with psychosomatic disorders.
- **Enmeshment:** families can be considered as systems, where boundaries operate to demarcate one system from surrounding systems or parts of the system from each other, e.g. parents from children. Enmeshment occurs if boundaries are not clear enough, leading to the functions of child and parent becoming blurred and overlapping. Such a situation can reduce autonomy and lead to difficulties in separation.

PARENTING

Parents use a variety of styles in rearing their children. Some may be relaxed and warm, others aloof and cold. *Child-centred* parenting refers to being involved with the child and aware of their needs, whilst *parent-centred* parents are more preoccupied with their own needs and interests.

Several models of parenting have been described. Maccoby & Martin (1983) divide parenting into two areas: the amount of control exerted and responsiveness. This produces four styles of parenting:

- **Authoritative:** these parents are responsive, warm, accepting and child-centred. They have expectations about behaviour and exert control and authority when required, whilst also being responsive to the child's needs. Children of such parents tend to be independent, make good peer and parental relationships. Also, they tend to be well motivated.
- **Authoritarian:** parents in this class also exert control but in a parent-centered manner, attempting to control the behaviour of the child without responding to the child's needs. Children from this category can be responsible and contented, but boys may be more aggressive and girls less motivated.
- **Indulgent:** here, parents are child-centred but make few demands on children, exerting little authority. Children are often positive but can be immature and the lack of authority contributes to increased aggressive behaviour.
- **Neglecting:** this is not used in the abuse sense, but to describe parents who are parent-centred, unresponsive and exert little control. Children may be more likely to be impulsive, with poor concentration and prone to temper outbursts.

While these four parenting styles are convenient, parents do not always fall into one category and may use different styles at different times.

ADOLESCENCE AND DEVELOPMENT

The physiological changes marking the onset of puberty also herald a period of social development. Resolution of this period involves:

- attainment of separation
- establishment of a sexual identity
- commitment to work
- development of a moral system
- development of the capacity to form lasting relationships
- establishment of a relationship with parents based on relative equity.

During this time adolescents often work hard at understanding themselves and shaping further their sense of self.

Identity

One of the fundamental tasks of adolescence is to establish this sense of self or identity. Marcia (1966, 1980) suggests four identity statuses:

- **Identity achievement:** this follows a period of active questioning and self-definition.
- **Foreclosure:** an identity may develop, though often without an active period of questioning. Adolescents may just adopt family values without question.
- **Moratorium:** during this period, adolescents may be actively seeking answers and an identity. During this time adolescents can be open and sensitive or anxious and self-righteous.
- **Identity diffusion:** the adolescent has no sense of self and is not taking steps to test out ideas.

These are not necessarily distinct stages, though there is some progression to identity achievement with age. It is also possible to be in one status with respect to one set of beliefs, e.g. religious values, and not to have formed any opinion in other areas, e.g. occupational interests.

Adolescent turmoil

The classic picture of adolescent–parent relationships is of highly charged atmospheres and stormy arguments, with adolescents in a state of emotional flux or 'turmoil'. Research suggests that major difficulties are not common and may be more characteristic of the small proportion referred to psychiatric services. Family conflict may be more common, but usually revolves around everyday matters – housework, homework, curfew times. Resolution occurs by negotiating a new working relationship with parents and the adolescent being granted more autonomy in return for increased responsibility.

'Turmoil' may be slightly more common. Around one fifth of adolescents report feeling miserable and depressed, though this may be mild and transient. However, adolescence is the time when rates for depression and deliberate self-harm do begin to mirror adult patterns.

SEXUAL DEVELOPMENT

Sexual development is also complex, representing an interplay of biological, psychological and social influences. The three main components are:

- **Gender (anatomical) identity:** an awareness of the two different categories, male or female, like father or like mother. By the age of 2, 80% of children can correctly answer the question 'are you a boy or girl?'. By age three, 80% can pick an appropriately sexed doll.
- **Sex-typed behaviour:** refers to activities considered by society to be appropriate. Sex differences in play are evident by the age of 3–4 years, though even one-year-olds may show toy preferences (girls prefer soft toys and dolls; boys mechanical toys).
- **Sexual orientation:** the direction of emotional/romantic and erotic interests. Typically evident in early adolescence, though probably present at a much earlier age.

Much research is based on 'atypical' development with competing claims for genetic and environmental influences.

ADULTHOOD AND DEVELOPMENT

Physical changes continue through adulthood, e.g. hair loss, slowing of reflexes, etc., and social development also continues. Less work has been done on formalizing patterns of development in adulthood. Levinson et al. (1978) suggest the following stages:

- Early adult life:
  22–28: entering adult world – a period of stability, developing careers and families
  28–33: 'age 30 transition' – decisions about where life will go
  33–40: settling down – stable and become more autonomous
- Middle adulthood:
  40–45: mid-life transition – 'mid-life crisis', re-evaluation of life, which can result in changes of jobs, re-marriage, etc.
  45–50: entering mid-adulthood – either develop a more compassionate, wise view of life or stagnate
  50–55: transition – similar to 'mid-life crisis' at age 40, if no crisis at earlier stage
  55–60: culmination – preparing for late adulthood
- Late adulthood
  60+: retirement and late life.

These stages are not comprehensive and there may be sex differences, but they give a flavour of the changes in adult life.

LATE ADULTHOOD AND DEVELOPMENT

Late adulthood is a time of great physical change and also of cognitive decline. A reappraisal of life is required with retirement from work. Older people on the whole feel just as satisfied with life, though this is dependent on physical health. Many adjust well, though others have difficulties. Those who are more positive are more likely to be financially comfortable, healthy, to have planned their retirement, and not to consider work as central to their lives.

Death

Late adulthood inevitably leads to the end of life. Older people's attitudes to death depend more on the degree of control they feel they can exert on the environment rather than number of years lived.

A 'dying trajectory' has been described, tracing the process of anticipation of death. Kubler–Ross (1969) describes the following stages:

- **Denial and isolation:** the prospect of death is initially denied. The individual may appear calm and carry on with life in the usual manner.
- **Anger and resentment:** angry feelings can surface, directed against others or one's self.
- **Bargaining:** this may represent partial acceptance, though often immediate problems are denied. Miracle 'cures' can be looked for.
- **Depression:** sadness at understanding that death will occur.
- **Acceptance:** coming to terms with the inevitable.

These phases do not always occur in the same sequence, and some may not be experienced at all. Individuals may move backwards and forwards through the stages depending on their state of health, their personality and the support they receive.

Development is not necessarily a straight pathway. Events can occur along the way that add or change the process, e.g. pregnancy, illness and bereavement. Human development is therefore a lifelong process.

FURTHER READING

Atkinson RL, Atkinson RC, Smith E, Bem D & Nolen–Hoeksema S (1999) *Hilgard's Introduction to Psychology*, 13th edn. New York: Thomson Learning.

Barnes P (ed.) (1995) *Personal, Social and Emotional Development of Children*. Oxford: Open University, Blackwell Publishers.

Oates J (ed.) (1995) *Foundation of Child Development*. Oxford: Open University, Blackwell Publishers.

REFERENCES

Ainsworth MDS, Blehar M, Waters E & Wall S (1978) *Patterns of Attachment: a Psychological Study of the Strange Situation*. Hillsdale, NJ: Lawrence Erlbaum.

Bandura A (1977) *Social Learning Theory*. New Jersey: Prentice Hall.

Barnhill LH & Longo D (1978) Fixation and regression in the family life cycle. *Family Process* 17: 469–78.

Bowlby J (1969/1982) *Attachment & Loss: Attachment*. New York: Basic Books.

Chomsky N (1972) *Language and Mind*. New York: Harcourt Brace Jovanovich.

Erikson E (1963) *Childhood and Society*, 2nd edn. New York: Norton.

Kohlberg L (1976) Moral stages and moralisation: the cognitive–developmental approach. In: Lickong T (ed.) *Moral Development and Behaviour*. New York: Holt, Rinehart & Winston.

Kubler–Ross E (1969) *On Death and Dying*. New York: Macmillan.

Levinson DJ, Darrow C, Klein E, Levinson M & Mckee B (1978) *The Seasons of a Man's Life*. New York: Knopf.

Maccoby EE & Martin JA (1983) Socialisation in the context of the family: parent–child interaction. In Mussen P.H. (ed.) *Handbook of Child Psychology*, vol 4. New York: Wiley.

Marcia JE (1966) Development and validation of egoidentity status. *Journal of Social Psychology* 3: 551–8.

Marcia JE (1980) Identity in adolescence. In: Adelson J (ed.) *Handbook of Adolescent Psychology*. New York: Wiley.

McGoldrick M & Carter EA (1982) The family life cycle. In: Walsh F (ed.) *Normal Family Processes*. New York: Guildford.

Piaget J & Inhelder B (1969) *The Psychology of the Child*. New York: Basic Books.

Schlesinger LB (1980) Distinctions between psychopathic, sociopathic and anti-social personality disorders. *Psychol Rep* 47(1): 15–21.

5

Psychology

Sarah L Helps and Nick Goddard

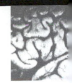

INTRODUCTION

Psychology is the scientific study of behaviour and cognitive processes. The scientific method was first applied to the study of the mind and mental processes at the start of the 20th century. Early methods of inquiry involved introspection; these were soon replaced by behaviourist theories which focused on only what can be measured or observed. Later, the Gestalt psychologists (mainly interested in perception) became prominent. From the the 1950s onwards, cognitive theorists dominated; initially the brain was seen as analogous to a computer: a sequential, serial processor. Today cognitive theorists still dominate the research field in understanding mental processes.

A number of branches of applied psychology exist today: occupational, educational, clinical and counselling being the most prominent. Psychiatrists are most likely to encounter clinical psychologists in their work, based in mental health settings, or educational psychologists who work primarily within the education system. While clinical practice has moved far from the basic theories outlined here, it is these that represent the building blocks of knowledge in psychological treatment approaches such as cognitive therapy, behaviour therapy and broader clinical practice.

LEARNING THEORY

Learning is a hypothetical construct representing a relatively permanent change in observable behaviour, which results from prior experience. It is not the result of maturational factors or reversible influences such as hunger or fatigue. There are three main forms of learning:

- **Associative learning:** refers to the behavioural approach and covers classical and operant conditioning.
- **Cognitive learning:** relates to the cognitive processes of perception and language.
- **Social learning**: relates to learning from observations and modelling.

Forms of associative learning

Classical conditioning

Classical conditioning is the pairing of two stimuli, usually a reflex behaviour (e.g. blinking when air hits the eye) with a neutral response. The work of Pavlov, an influential physiologist and behaviourist, in the early 1900s, was extremely valuable in demonstrating this phenomenon. Interested initially in the process of digestion in dogs, he noticed that the dogs would often start salivating (the *unconditioned response*) not only before food was given to them (the *unconditioned stimulus*), but also when they heard the bell that signalled mealtimes (a *conditioned stimulus*). The dogs were pairing a stimulus usually unconnected with a salivatory response (the bell) with another stimulus, which was associated with that response (i.e. food). The three stages of classical conditioning are shown in Figure 5.1.

Pavlov (1927) demonstrated different types of classical conditioning based on relationships between the conditioned and unconditioned stimuli:

- **Delayed/forward conditioning**: the conditioned stimulus (CS) is presented before the unconditioned stimulus (UCS) and remains 'on' whilst UCS is presented until the unconditioned response (UCR) appears. Strongest learning occurs when the delay is no more than 0.5 seconds. The longer the interval the poorer the learning.
- **Simultaneous conditioning**: CS and UCS are presented together and conditioning occurs when the CS has produced the CR alone.
- **Trace conditioning**: CS is presented and removed before UCS is presented; only a 'trace memory' of the CS remains to be conditioned. The shorter the interval, the stronger the conditioning. Usually this tends to be a weaker pairing than in delayed or simultaneous conditioning.
- **Backward conditioning**: CS is presented after the UCS. Used widely in advertising, i.e. set the sunny scene, then introduce the drink to be drunk in the sunny scene.

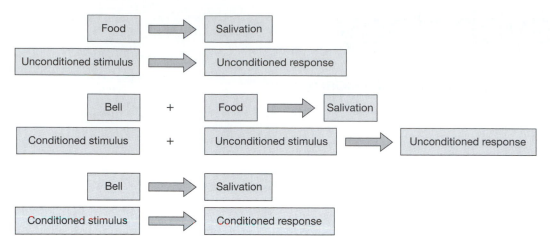

Figure 5.1 The three stages of classical conditioning.

- **Stimulus generalization**: where a similar CS can generate the same CR, e.g. different bells give rise to the CR. The further the stimulus differs from the original CS, the weaker the response. The case of Little Albert, (described by Watson, often referred to as the founder of behaviourism, who attempted to apply Pavlov's work with dogs to humans), an 11-month-old infant who developed a generalized fear of white fluffy things after touching a white rabbit that had been paired with a loud scary noise, is one of the most famous examples of this (Watson & Rayner 1920).
- **Higher order conditioning**: CS can be paired with another stimulus (CS^2) to produce a further CR, e.g. once the CR (salivation) had been paired with the bell, the bell could be paired with a light, which then when presented alone elicits the CR. The original CS (the bell) serves as a UCS for the new association, in the same way as did the food originally. Higher order conditioning tends to be fairly weak, as the CS^2 is never actually paired with the UCR. Third and fourth order conditioning are possible, but become weaker with each pairing.
- **Extinction**: when the CS (bell) is continually presented without the UCS (food) the CR (salivation) stops. Through presentation of the CR without CS the response becomes 'unlearnt'. If after a time the pairing is repeated, the association appears again and the CR will again bring on the CS. Spontaneous recovery of the response may occur after a period of time but in a weaker form.

Operant/instrumental conditioning

Operant Conditioning was clearly demonstrated by Skinner, working a little before Pavlov, through his work with rats in mazes. He was the first behaviourist to make a distinction between respondent behaviour (that which is triggered auto-matically) and operant behaviour (that which occurs voluntarily). Skinner believed that most animal or human behaviour is not elicited by a specific stimulus, but is a voluntary, active process. He argued that people 'operate' on their environment and that behaviour is 'instrumental' in leading to certain 'consequences,' which lead to the behaviour being repeated. Contingent upon the consequences of the action, responses that bring pleasure or satisfaction are likely to be repeated, those that bring discomfort or pain, are not (Skinner 1938).

Thorndike's Law of Effect

Skinner's work was much influenced by Thorndike, who had carried out experiments with cats in puzzle boxes (Thorndike 1898). These boxes had a latch, which opened a door enabling the cat to get out. The cat's task was to open the latch to escape the box and get to the waiting fish outside. Thorndike found that the more times the cats attempted to get out of the box, the quicker they became at opening the latch. Thorndike explained their quicker responses in terms of trial and error learning, so proposing a link between the stimulus (the puzzle box and latch) and the response (getting out). He called this the *Law of Effect* showing that what happens as a result of a behaviour will affect that behaviour in the future. In classical conditioning, it is what happens before the behaviour that is said to determine the behaviour.

A variety of terms for clarifying behaviours has been developed:

- **Reinforcement:** there are two types of reinforcers:
  (a) primary reinforcers are those stimuli that meet biological needs, e.g. hunger, thirst, etc.
  (b) secondary reinforcers are those which one has to learn the value of. These do not rely on basic needs

but tend to be those that we have chosen to value, e.g. self-esteem, money, etc.

- **Consequences of conditioning:** the consequences of operant conditioning may be positive reinforcement, negative reinforcement or punishment:
  - (a) positive reinforcement – refers to the presentation of something pleasant to make the behaviour stronger, in order that the behaviour will be repeated
  - (b) negative reinforcement – relates to acting or behaving in order that an aversive stimulus is removed. Both positive and negative reinforcement serve to strengthen behaviour
  - (c) punishment – refers to pain or annoyance administered to decrease or weaken behaviour, i.e. electric shocks given to those who respond in an unwanted way to a certain stimulus. Punishment tends not to be as effective in learning situations as positive or negative reinforcers which increase the probability of the desired behaviour.
- **Reinforcement schedules**: how often and how regularly the reinforcement is presented will effect behaviour:
  - (a) continuous reinforcement – reinforcing every occurrence of the response. Very easily extinguished
  - (b) partial reinforcement – reinforcement is given to only some responses
  - (c) fixed interval – reinforcement is given regularly, for example every 30 seconds. The response rate will increase, as the next reinforcement becomes available. Extinction achieved fairly easily
  - (d) variable interval – reinforcement is given regularly but the interval varies from trial to trial, it is unpredictable. Extinction takes a long time to occur
  - (e) fixed ratio – reinforcement given for a fixed number of responses. Extinction occurs fairly easily
  - (f) variable ratio – reinforcement given regularly but the number of responses required changes from trial to trial. Extinction is extremely hard to achieve.

Applications of conditioning today are found in basic behavioural management schedules, for example in fears and phobias, in biofeedback and in programmed learning.

Observational learning

This refers to learning by watching rather than by doing and stems from social learning theory. Bandura, a major proponent of these theories, posited that while both classical and operant conditioning are important, they cannot account for novel behaviour, (behaviour which has not been displayed before) and therefore that novel behaviour must develop from observational learning (Bandura 1977). Bandura also argued that a variety of cognitive factors mediate the learning process:

- attention
- perception
- memory

- reproduction of the seen motor activities
- motivation.

This kind of learning is especially relevant to the development of children with their expanding repertoire of behaviours. Observational learning is discussed in greater depth in Chapter 4.

Insight learning

From this theoretical viewpoint, learning is seen as a purely cognitive process. The Gestalt theorists, of whom Kohler was a major author (Kohler 1947) argued that all psychological theory should be treated holistically, looking at the whole rather than only certain relationships. These theorists, best known for their work on perception, saw learning as a process involving the perceptual restructuring of elements that constitute a problem situation, with the addition of a piece of information that was previously missing. Whereas in stimulus–response theories learning is said to occur by trial and error, in insight learning cognitive processes are put into play and the situation thought about. Then a solution will suddenly become evident when the missing piece of information becomes 'seen' and therefore available for use in solving the problem. It is the cognitive relationship between the means and the end that is learned, not a specific set of conditioned associations, thus ensuring easier application to similar problems in the future. Kohler did not believe that past experience had an impact on learning processes, and this is one major weakness of the theory.

Linking stimulus–response and cognitive theories: learning sets

Harlow argued that stimulus–response (s–r) learning and insight learning are based along a continuum, where stimulus–response learning dominates early on and cognitive or insight learning appears later (Harlow 1949). He argued for a learning set, or a way of *learning to learn*; this is a process that occurs somewhere between S–R and insight learning. A set comprises a general rule or skill applicable to a whole class of problems and demonstrates the transfer of learning, in that earlier learning influences later learning. The more sets a person has, the better equipped they are to learn new information.

MOTIVATION

Motivated behaviour is goal-directed, purposeful behaviour. The study of motivation is highly dependent upon one's theoretical approach, whether:

- psychoanalytic (examining unconscious motives and desires)
- behaviourist (based on learning and reinforcement schedules)

- humanist(related to self-actualization, as described above)
- cognitive (looking for appraisal and attribution)
- neurobiological (looking at nervous system, endocrine system and other bodily systems).

There are two broad categories of motivational drives – survival or physiological motives and competence or cognitive motives. Social motives are an occasionally used third category.

- **Homeostatic or primary drives**, described by Cannon (1929) are those that are guided by a physiological need, i.e. hunger or thirst. The drive leads to behaviour aimed at reducing a tissue deficiency need, i.e. finding food or something to drink, leading to the restoration of the internal balance of homeostasis. The primary reinforcers for primary drives are food, water and sex.
- **Drive reduction theory** (Hull 1943) relates to his theory of learning and the notion of reinforcement described earlier. Here a physiological need is noted, along with a drive to reduce that need; behaviour is then directed to reduce the drive and this drive reduction reinforces the drive reducing behaviour.
- **Competence or secondary drives** are those things that people seek out that do not fulfil a physiological need. These are continuous motives, unlike primary motives that come and go. Play is an example of a competence motive. It is now clear that behaviour is much more complex than simple reactions to physiological or even secondary drives. These motives tend to involve the search for stimulation, through curiosity and exploration, without any extrinsic reward.

PERCEPTION

An understanding of the sensory processes is important in building a full picture of cognitive learning. Perception is an effortless but active process involving the selection, inference, organization and interpretation of information received by the senses at any one time in conjunction with prior knowledge and memory. It is an immediate discriminatory response of an organism to energy-activating sense organs. By means of perception it is possible to build up a mental representation of the world, a process that occurs from birth. The process of perception encompasses a variety of processing systems, including the physiological systems of each sensory modality and central brain processes.

Visual perception

It has been estimated that about 90% of the information received about the world comes through the eyes. Vision is therefore the most widely researched sensory system.

Given the vast amount of information available to the sensory systems at any one time, it is possible to use only a small percentage of it. The brain has limited capacity to process the information and is able to attend or select some things and not others. At times, the information received is incomplete and the whole picture may not be seen. It is therefore necessary to supplement the incoming information with previous experience and knowledge of the world, in order to infer the whole picture. The notion of *constancy* describes this.

Constancy is the ability to perceive objects as they are, rather than as they may be seen. Constancy can be found in:

- shape – a cup may appear, due to perspective, as an ellipse but is still known to be round; a tree will be perceived as vertical even when one's head is tilted to the side
- size – whether an object is 1 or 10 metres away, we are able to judge its approximate breadth and height
- colour – whatever the availability of light, the colour or hue of an object can be perceived
- brightness – regardless of the brightness of the light in which it is seen, coal is seen as black
- location – even if a person spins round, kinaesthetic feedback ensures that the person knows they, rather than the world, is spinning.

Pattern recognition is a key feature of visual perception. It involves assigning meaning to visual input by identifying objects in the visual field. Three main theories exist:

- **Template matching theories** suggest that pattern recognition involves a comparison between the information held in the sensory register and miniature copies or templates of previously seen information, held in long-term stores. If this theory were true there would have to be an infinite number of templates in the long-term storage facility and the search for a match would take a very long time; it also does not explain how the search would happen.
- **Prototype theories** suggest that each stimulus belongs to a category, and shares key attributes with the other stimuli in that category, so a smaller number of pieces of information are stored than with template theories. In order to recognize a pattern, the basic elements or features are compared with the stored prototypes. Whilst this theory is better substantiated than template theories, it does not explain how the matching process works.
- **Feature detection theories** are the best-developed theories. They suggest that each stimulus pattern represents a specific organization of certain basic attributes or features. Perception involves extracting these attributes from the presented stimuli, which are then compared with previously stored information. Whilst these theories are better able to explain the

complexities of pattern recognition, and much support has been generated from behavioural and neurological studies, they still have inherent weaknesses.

Set and schema

Allport (1955) described a *set* as a perceptual bias, predisposition or readiness to perceive particular features of a stimulus; a way of selecting some parts of information and ignoring others. A *schema* is a persistent well-organized classificatory system of perceiving, thinking and believing. The set first works as a selector based on the expectations formed by the schema and then as an interpreter, using information from the schema to classify, understand and infer from the information. Set is influenced by both organismic or perceiver variables and situational variables.

Perceptual organization: figure–ground differentiation

Visual information is almost always organized into a way that makes sense of the information presented. Figure–ground differentiation is a clear example of how this organization works, and can make mistakes. Distinct parts of a visual field are said to stand out from other parts; this has been called the figure–ground relationship. A classic example of this is the Rubin vase, where some part of a stimulus always stands out at any one time. The vase also demonstrates how the part that stands out can change (Fig 5.2).

Figure–ground organization appears to be an automatic process, and Gestalt psychologists have argued that it reflects an important part of the innate organizational ability of the visual system. Other organizational principles relate to proximity (elements perceived to be close together are seen as linked), closure (the perceptual system tends to try and 'close' objects to make them whole), similarity (the perceptual system will draw out and focus on commonalties) and part/whole relationships (i.e. the whole is greater that the sum of its parts). It is these principles that at times lead to mistakes by the perceptual system.

When the visual perceptual system makes mistakes

Although the perceptual system is highly accurate, due to the principles described above, it can misinterpret the information is receives. Attempts to make sense of data, given prior knowledge and experience, may lead to perceptual errors:

- **Illusions** are examples of mistaken perception and show how the perceptual system can sometimes go beyond the information received by the senses and perceive something, which is not in the stimulus. Gregory (1983) argues that as the perceptual system is actively involved in interpreting the information it receives, it creates a hypothesis that is at times incompatible with all the presenting information. Illusions can be distortions (as with the Rubin vase), ambiguous figures, paradoxical figures and fictions.
- **Hallucinations** are apparent sensory experiences generated by the brain in the absence of stimulation from the environment. They are most frequently auditory but may affect any sensory modality. These are discussed in greater depth in relation to the abnormal perceptual experiences associated with mental illnesses such as schizophrenia, in Chapter 18.
- **Agnosias** represent higher order perceptual disorders, where the individual experiences difficulties in recognizing and classifying objects. These disorders are often described in terms of the individual being unable to put meaning to their perceptions, demonstrating the (at times faulty) interaction between the visual perceptual systems, higher brain regions and the learning and memory systems.

Developmental perspectives on visual perception

The study of visual perception provides a good example of constitutional/environmental or nature–nurture interactions.

Fantz examined the eye movements of babies when placed in a cot and presented with a choice of visual objects (Fantz 1961). He demonstrated clear perception of form within a few days of birth, showing that infants spent more time looking at complex as opposed to simple figures, favouring checkerboards to a blank square, a bull's eye to stripes. He also showed that as infants grew, they preferred looking at narrower and narrower stripes, showing a developing capacity for differentiation of stimuli and an increased ability to scan.

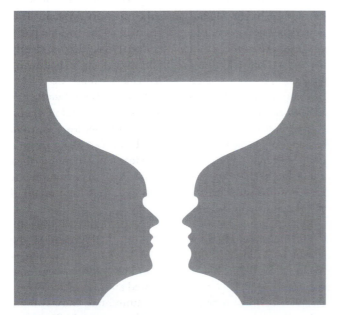

Figure 5.2 The Rubin vase.

Face preferences

Using similar methods, Fantz showed that babies as young as four days old prefer pictures of human faces to drawings of the same shape with the features muddled up or with no features. Findings are however more consistent for babies of over four weeks of age. Infants over two months of age appear to prefer three rather than two-dimensional representations of a face.

Visual acuity

New-borns have about 1/10 the visual acuity of adults but the preference for clear images is present in infants of one to three months of age. This has been demonstrated in a study of infants, in which the babies' sucking response was linked to a dial controlling the focus of the lens of a projector. When the image projected was blurred, infants would change their sucking rates in order to make the image clearer. By six to 12 months a baby's acuity will be within adult ranges, but within a very broad range of individual differences, and may not reach 20:20 until 10 or 11 years of age.

Depth perception

If babies can perceive depth when they are born, then it can be assumed that this is an innate ability. Gibson and Walk (1960) built a miniature Grand Canyon: a platform with a patterned surface under glass on one end (the shallow end) and plain glass on the other (the deep end). Under the plain glass there was a 'drop' giving the appearance of a large drop or cliff. Babies of between six and 14 months would not crawl onto the 'deep end' side of the glass where there was a 'drop'. Further indications of the ability to perceive depth in infants aged two months were shown by placing a baby at the 'deep end' and monitoring their heart rates. The heart rate would decrease compared with being on the shallow side, representing greater interest and more attention to what was underneath them. As these infants did not show distress on the 'deep end', it has been concluded that the *distress* from depth perception is a learnt rather than an innate behaviour.

This evidence suggests that certain features of perception are innate. Other parts are definitely learnt, for example, if young animals are deprived of stimulation by patterned light, or by having the extra-occular muscle cut, they show deficiencies in form perception and binocular vision.

The simple nature–nurture dichotomy is clearly a gross oversimplification of the process of perception. A more modern (interactionist) perspective is that while humans are born with certain capacities to perceive the world, environmental or learnt experiences are vital in determining whether and how these innate capacities develop (Bornstein 1988).

Auditory perception

Much more is known about visual perception than about auditory perception, although the organizational principles of visual perception described apply to auditory stimuli as well. Whereas the perception of a visual stimulus instantly provides a great deal of information, with auditory information it has to be received and analyzed sequentially. Attention is an important concept to consider in relation to auditory perception. It can be defined as the concentration of mental effort on sensory or mental events (Solso 1995).

There are two main methods of studying attention: shadowing or dichotic listening experiments and dual task techniques (Eysenck 1984).

Shadowing, or dichotic listening experiments

If each ear receives a different auditory stimulus through headphones, it is easily possible to concentrate on one stimulus and understand nothing of the other. This suggests that it is possible to *selectively attend* to only one source at a time, i.e. that there is a selective filter attenuating what is processed by auditory perception system. However, if a stimulus in the background or information unattended to suddenly becomes salient, e.g. you hear your name being said, it is possible to tune into that stimulus, suggesting low-level processing of background information also (the '*cocktail party effect*').

Dual task techniques

Dual task techniques ask people to respond to both or all messages, so dividing attention between the incoming information sources.

The filter model of attention

At some point in the auditory processing system there is a bottleneck; some information is processed further and the rest is either dropped or is processed in only a cursory way.

Broadbent's (1958) theory suggests that information enters the senses, is sent to a *sensory buffer* system, and from this is selectively filtered into the memory system. This model does not account for effects such as the cocktail party effect, where some of the attentional resource is clearly directed at the background stimuli, suggesting a shadowing ability.

Many models have been put forward since Broadbent's early work, such as Treisman's attenuator model (1954) and the pertinence model of Deutsch & Deutsch (1963). Current thinking suggests that although attention is likely to be a finite resource, some tasks require more attention than others, hence allowing more than one thing to be done at one time. Arousal and alertness will further affect the amount of attentional resources available.

Factors such as task similarity, practice and task difficulty will affect how attention is divided. This suggests the existence of some kind of central processor, which is dynamic and flexible in its allocation of attentional resources.

Other theories view attention as modular, comprising a number of different processing mechanisms (Allport 1980).

Synthesis theories explain how these modules might fit together. The best known of these is Baddely's theory, also referred to as a theory of working memory, described below.

MEMORY

Memory is the hypothetical construct of three specific but inseparable and interrelated processes – registration, storage and retrieval – that process information received by the senses:

- **Registration** represents the input of any stimulus into the memory system. Registration is necessary but not sufficient for storage to take place. Memories may last here for just a fraction of a second. Here, information needs to be encoded. Information is extracted from stimuli under the condition in which it is experienced. This is closely related to selective attention, described earlier.
- **Storage** is the process by which information is organized and stored. It is necessary but not sufficient for retrieval.
- **Retrieval** is the process of accessing the information logged into the system. One can only recover information that has been stored, but the fact that it has been stored does not mean that it can be retrieved when required.

Memory storage

There has been ongoing debate as to the number of memory stores. It is now clear that two stores exist, one processing information in the here and now and one processing information which is stored in the longer term. The work of Atkinson & Shiffrin (1968, 1971) was most influential in the description of the two-part memory store. Baddely's more recent work has led to greater understanding of the short term or working memory system (Baddely 1990).

Inputs to the memory system: sensory memory

Sensory memory (or sensory buffer store), represents the entrance to the memory system. It contains relatively unprocessed memory traces, which last only slightly longer than the stimulus itself. Sensory memory is modality specific: information is stored in the modality by which it entered. Less than one hundredth of the information which touches the human senses reaches the short-term memory (STM) store (Lloyd et al. 1984).

Visual (iconic) stimuli

These represent the brief visual memory system, where images may rest for up to half a second. Even if visual information is presented for a very short period of time, not long enough for any deep encoding to occur, it is possible to recall certain aspects of that information, suggesting that the trace of the information left in the iconic memory can be utilized.

Auditory (echoic) stimuli

Echoic memory is similar to iconic memory, in that the stimulus persists for longer than it is presented for, and probably for longer (2–3 seconds) than in iconic memory but with a lower capacity due to sequential processing. The notion of playback is interesting here: if someone asks a question and you ask them to repeat it, while they are repeating the question, you can 'play back' what you first heard and give them an answer before they have finished repeating themselves.

Short-term memory storage

Short-term or primary memory (STM) is a temporary storage facility where the memory trace lasts up to 30 seconds. It has long been known that the capacity of STM is limited to seven 'chunks' of information, plus or minus two (Ebbinghaus 1885). A chunk may be a single letter, a word or a phrase. Chunking is the process of reducing a large amount of information into a smaller amount, so that it becomes a familiar unit that is based on previous learning and experience. Information can be held in STM for longer than 30 seconds by using techniques of auditory rehearsal or repetition, which 'refresh' the memory trace. Coding in the STM tends to be acoustic, whether information was primarily visual or verbal.

Forgetting and short-term memory

There has been much debate as to whether information held in STM disappears due to trace decay (i.e. the memory trace disintegrates and is lost from the memory system) or interference/displacement of old information by new information entering the system. As might be expected, short-term forgetting seems to be a combination of the two, the trace weakens over time and becomes harder to be retrieved or be discriminated from other competing traces.

Working memory

Alan Baddely and colleagues proposed that STM should be replaced with working memory (Baddely & Hitch 1974), a system which could hold and manipulate information and that was vital in performing a range of cognitive tasks comprising three parts:

- **Central executive:** has a limited capacity and is used when dealing with cognitively demanding tasks. It closely resembles attention.
- **Articulatory or phonological loop:** temporally and serially, encodes phonemic information. It is used to supplement the storage capacity of the central executive in verbal tasks.
- **Visuospatial scratch pad:** less well understood, but appears to manipulate visuospatial images, managing

visual information, again feeding into the central executive. It seems to be useful in tasks involving visuospatial manipulation.

The early model has been expanded, now comprising a central executive controlling the articulatory loop, visuospatial scratch pad and primary acoustic store (Salame & Baddely 1982).

Long-term memory storage

Long-term memory (LTM) is thought to have an unlimited capacity, in which memories can last from a few minutes to many years. The LTM store is highly organized around a central store. Information tends to be stored semantically (i.e. verbal meaning is encoded) or in visually (i.e. in pictures). There also appears to be an episodic memory store, demonstrated by patients who have suffered brain damage, who may forget personal information (episodic memory) but do not forget their native language (semantic memory).

Mnemonics: one example of long-term memory organization

Mnemonics are rules of learning that aid recall by providing a fast way of learning new information with the help of existing memory structures. A common example would be trying to visualize a new piece of information displayed in every room of a familiar house. As one visualizes the rooms of the house, the new information is recalled as well.

Retrieval from the long-term memory

Retrieval of information relies of information being stored in a logical, rational order. There are several forms of remembering:

- **Recognition:** involves being able to recognize but not spontaneously recall an answer to a question, e.g. when presented with a multiple choice of answers to a problem, it is easy to pick out the correct one, whereas it would not have been possible to spontaneously generate the correct response.
- **Recall:** involves actively searching the memory stores and reproducing something that was learnt. Retrieval clues are sparse here.
- **Relearning:** involves learning something which been learnt and then forgotten. It takes less time the second time around, as the existing memory, although inaccessible, is likely to have left some trace.
- **Reconstructive memory:** the type of remembering involved in the passing on of information from one person to another, often involving distortion of the information received. It is this kind of memory that is implicated in eye witness testimony, described in Chapter 30.
- **Confabulation:** a memory error often made at times of high arousal, where if a full memory cannot be found, pieces are added to make the story seem more

appropriate. Confabulation is frequently found in patients with Korsakoff's syndrome.

- **Redintegration:** recollection of past experiences based on certain cues, e.g. a perfume, an unusual sound. A small amount of the memory is triggered and then a systematic search of memory stores gives rise to the whole memory.

Context and memory storage

Context and state-dependent memory are concerned with:

- the state of the person (e.g. under the influence of alcohol)
- the place in which the memory was initially encoded for the retrieval of information.

Retrieval of information is generally better given similar rather than different contextual cues.

Motivational and emotional factors

These are also likely to effect recall and forgetting. Freud argued that painful or emotionally salient memories can be repressed and placed out of conscious access as a protective mechanism. Clinically, this may be seen in amnesia in patients following severe emotional trauma. Motivated forgetting is however hard to assess empirically. Some research suggests that high levels of arousal may lead to enhanced recall under certain circumstances, due to the positive effect of arousal on memory trace consolidation.

Mood and retrieval

A person in a gloomy mood is more likely to recall gloomy information, a person in a happy mood is more likely to remember cheerful information. Patients with clinical depression have been found to recall more negatively focused information than nondepressed controls. However, stress and anxiety states may distort the attentional processes rather than the memory processes and hence may lead to distorted encoding of a stimulus due to heightened attention to salient aspects of a traumatic scene.

Forgetting in long-term memory

It is impossible to say that information can be forgotten from LTM, rather that it is not accessible or available at the present time.

- **Passive decay theory:** as time goes by, memory traces may decay unless maintained. It has been suggested that this may in part be due to metabolic processes or neural decay, although there is little evidence for this (Solso 1995).
- **Systematic distortion of the memory trace:** the longer the memory is stored, the more subject to distortions it becomes. Evidence now suggests that distortions may occur at all points of the memory system.

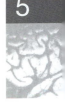

- **Interference theories:** The greater the similarity between two things, the more likely they are to interfere with the memory trace. Thus, as more is learnt over time, forgetting is more likely to occur due to increasing competition between similar memories. What is learnt will be influenced by pro-active (prior learning) and retroactive (future learning) interference.

A full understanding of the memory system has not as yet been reached and further exciting work is continuing especially with regard to understanding the development of memory in children.

INTELLIGENCE

Intelligence represents one of the most widely studied and controversial areas in psychology today. Many theories have been developed to try and explain it. Many methods for measuring intelligence have been developed, the most influential being the psychometric approaches, which rely on factor analysis. Definitions of intelligence refer to it either as a biological construct, (related to adaptation to the environment), a psychological construct, (related to the measurement of individual differences), or an operational construct, (intelligence defined as what intelligence test measure). In general it is seen as a multidimensional cognitive ability, comprising an individual's capacity to understand, reason and problem solve.

Factor analytic approaches

These approaches are based on the analysis of large amounts of data from individuals using factor analysis.

1. **Spearman's two-factor theory.** Spearman carried out a factor analysis of the results of children's performance on a number of tests, and found many positive correlations between the tests. From this he concluded that all tests measured both a common factor of general intelligence (g) and a specific factor (s). He believed that individual differences were due to differences in g. His theory of g, although nowadays held to be inaccurate, was extremely influential.

2. **Cyril Burt**, a student of Spearman, expanded the two-factor model and developed the Hierarchical model, where g is what all tests measure. He and a colleague Vernon, proposed that between g and s were major and minor group factors. The major group factors (divided into verbal–educational ability and spatial–mechanical ability) were what all tests measure; the minor group what particular tests measure. They then saw specific factors as what particular tests measured on specific occasions (Vernon 1960).

3. **Guilford** (1967) rejected the notion of g and classified cognitive tasks along three dimensions:

- content (what is the problem?)
- operations (how does the subject need to approach the task?)
- products (what kind of answer is needed?).

From the different kinds of operations needed in each of these dimensions he calculated at least 120 mental abilities. Results on tests designed using this model often correlated well, suggesting far fewer distinct mental abilities (Brody & Brody 1976).

It is now widely accepted that intelligence is a combination of general mental and specific mental ability. Theorists relying on factor analytic studies to define intelligence have proposed very different theories. This is in part because they used differing subject pools, of different ages with different factor analytic techniques and different tests. A further danger with factor analytic methods is that the factor described (e.g. verbal ability) becomes a reality (the process of reification) rather than simply a statistic.

Other models of intelligence

Fluid and crystallized intelligence

Cattell & Horn (Cattell 1963; Horn & Cattell, 1967) using factor analysis again, proposed that g should be divided into two parts:

- **Fluid intelligence** relates to untaught abilities, relatively free of cultural bias, e.g. abstract problem-solving abilities. It was argued that this ability peaked during adolescence, then plateaued and decreased after young adulthood, although recent research has not demonstrated this decline.
- **Crystallized intelligence** relates to cumulative learning experiences and is based on acquired knowledge and skills from school and life experiences. It is said to increase throughout the life span and there is some evidence to support this claim.

Measurement of intelligence

The intelligence quotient

Intelligence quotient (IQ) refers to mental age (MA) expressed as a ratio of chronological age (CA) multiplied by 100. For IQ to remain stable, MA must increase with CA over time. This is true until around 18 years, when intellectual abilities are usually fully developed. As stated above, it was erroneously thought that intellectual ability started to decline after young adulthood. It now appears that although fluid intelligence may start to decrease, crystallized intelligence continues to develop throughout the lifespan. Intelligence is said to be normally distributed with a slight 'bump' at the lower end of the normal distribution curve, representing those with severe learning difficulties.

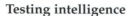

Testing intelligence

It is now said that intelligence tests assess a range of cognitive abilities, rather than the more abstract concept of intelligence. Intelligence tests are said to measure the level of performance upon specific tests. While it is then suggested that, due to the fact that the test are standardized, reliable and valid, they measure IQ, the debate continues as to whether this is so and indeed whether tests of intelligence are indeed useful (Kaufman 1994).

The Stanford–Binet test

Generally said to be the first intelligence test, Binet & Simon (1905) developed a measure to identify those school children who would not benefit from mainstream education due to low levels of cognitive ability. The test was modified by an American, Terman, who was working at Stanford University. It then became known as the Stanford–Binet test. It has been revised many times but is not now widely used.

The Wechsler scales

The most widely used tests of intelligence are the Wechsler scales, initially developed for adults in the 1940s and revised many times for different ages and cultural groups. The most commonly used versions in the UK are (Wechsler 1991, 1999a, 1999b, 2003):

- Wechsler Adult Intelligence Scale – R (WAIS-R), for people of 16 years and over
- Wechsler Intelligence Scales for Children – III-UK (WISC-III-UK), for 7- to 16-year-olds
- Wechsler Pre-School and Primary Scales of Intelligence (WPPSI-III-UK) for 3- to 7.3-year-olds.

The raw scores obtained from all Wechsler subtests are converted into scale scores. Scale scores range from 1 to 19, the average range being 8–12.

The Wechsler tests all contain a variety of subtests, which are divided into two domains of verbal and performance abilities (verbal IQ and performance IQ). The combined standardized scores of the subtests on these two domains give an overall intelligence quotient (IQ). WISC-III-UK scores are also commonly organized into factor indexes, of verbal comprehension, perceptual organization, processing speed and freedom from distractibility (Kaufman 1994). For the IQ and index scores the mean is 100, with 15 points representing 1 standard deviation. So 68% of the population will score between 85 and 115, 14% between 70 and 84, or 116 and 130, and 2 % less than 70 or more than 130.

The Wechsler Abbreviated Scale of Intelligence (Wechsler 1999b) has also been introduced to screen a wide age-range using 2–4 subtests. This measure is primarily used in research rather than in clinical practice.

Differences between subtest scores provide important diagnostic information: for example, children with attention deficit hyperactivity disorder may perform better on verbal than performance subtests and children with autism may do better on specific performance subtests compared with verbal subtests. While much clinical information can be obtained from an analysis of the cognitive profile, it is rare that an IQ test on its own will yield sufficient information to make recommendations about the care of a person who has demonstrated either global or specific difficulties. Further testing using a variety of attainment and neuropsychological measures is usually indicated.

Other tests such as the British Ability Scales (BAS II) are also widely used by educational and clinical psychologists. This measure comprises 24 subscales that measure 24 distinct aspects of cognitive abilities in 2.1- to 17-year olds and gives standardized scores in order that the results can be compared between measures.

Raven's progressive matrices

In order to overcome cultural biases prevalent in intelligence tests, i.e. biased in favour of white, middle-class children and adults, tests like the Raven's progressive matrices were developed (Raven et al. 1983). This test comprises a series of non-verbal pattern-matching exercises. The object of the test is evident without much understanding of language. However, the test is still considered to be culture-dependent as the skill of pattern matching is more commonly used in some cultures than in others.

Cultural and racial factors

Jensen, an American psychologist argued that there were intellectual differences between different races (Jensen 1980). His research has been shown to be biased and it is now clear that there are not actual differences in the intellectual abilities of different racial or cultural groups but that environmental factors, test bias and genetic differences all play a part in any individual's performance.

Factors affecting test performance

A test result is meaningless unless it is evaluated together with all other relevant information about the person (social and medical history, school or work reports, information from family and significant others) including the following variables:

- **Arousal and anxiety:** can impinge on a person's ability to perform as well as they otherwise might on these tests. People with depression tend to perform more poorly due to motor and thought slowing.
- **Ability to plan and organize one's approach to test materials:** these factors can affect the speed with which a person can complete a task and give clues as to how they may approach tasks in everyday life.
- **Lack of motivation:** may reduce the overall score.
- **Changes in neurological functioning:** may be responsible for decreases in functioning, as might changes in psychiatric status.

- **Physical difficulties:** such as motor difficulties, visual field deficits, may impair performance, especially on timed tests.
- **Linguistic and cultural background:** if English is not fluent, the person may not be able to demonstrate their true ability. As stated above, different stimuli may be applicable to different cultural groups.
- Familiarity with the test material: if a test is repeated frequently, practice effects will occur and the person will be seen to improve. The Wechsler tests should not be repeated within less than six months in order to avoid this.

Indications for testing

The testing of cognitive ability has a variety of uses in clinical practice and should be carried out only when the result is likely to influence clinical practice, for example:

- in the assessment and diagnosis of specific and global learning difficulties
- in examining the effect of a brain injury or systemic illness upon a person's functioning
- to aid in rehabilitation planning following a brain injury.

EMOTION

Emotions

There have been many attempts to classify emotions; recently Plutchick (1980) proposed the existence of eight primary emotions, composed of four pairs of opposites. These are arranged in a wheel and are surrounded by eight complex emotions (Fig. 5.3). Plutchik argues that the primary emotions are biologically and subjectively distinct.

However the spectrum of emotions interrelate, it is argued that there are three components to every emotional response:

1. **Subjective experience:** the experience of joy, sadness, anger, etc.
2. **Physiological changes:** changes in the autonomic nervous system and endocrine system, over which the individual has little control such as sweating.
3. **Behavioural associations:** specific patterns associated with specific emotions such as smiling when happy.

Theories of emotion

Initial theories of emotion focused purely on physiological reactions, later theories include the importance of cognitive aspects into the understanding of emotional experience.

1. **The James–Lange theory** (originally described by James in 1890) viewed the emotional response to a situation as the result of physiological reactions, i.e. we feel frightened because we are running away from something, not because something makes us scared. It is the notion of feedback from bodily changes that is key to this theory. The theory suggests that each emotion results from a different physiological state. Critics of the theory argue that as emotion is felt instantly (without time for physiological responses to begin), physiological arousal might not even be necessary for the experience of emotion. Furthermore, they point out that similar physiological reactions can occur when no emotion is felt, e.g. exercise may bring about the same physiological changes as those experienced in fear.
2. The **Cannon–Baird theory** (Cannon 1929) suggested that the autonomic nervous system responds in the same way to all emotional stimuli, so emotional experience must be more than basic physiological arousal. The thalamus was seen as central in emotional regulation, in sending impulses to the sympathetic nervous system and to the cerebral cortex. Whilst this theory also has weaknesses, it is clear that physiological factors play a large, interdependent role in emotional experience.
3. In the **two-factor theory of emotion**, Schachter (1964) argued that an emotional reaction involves initial peripheral physiological changes, such as heart rate and blood pressure and the interpretation or appraisal of those changes. Emotional specificity is therefore based on what the arousal is attributed to, i.e., the cognitive appraisal of the arousal.

More recently, there has been much work on the role of cognition in the experience of emotion, especially by Lazarus & Folkman (1984).

Emotion and performance

An important relationship between the level of emotional arousal and performance is demonstrated by the

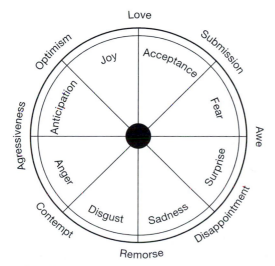

Figure 5.3 Plutchik's wheel.

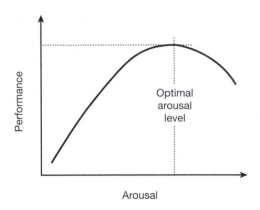

Figure 5.4 Yerkes–Dodson curve.

Yerkes–Dodson curve (Yerkes & Dodson 1908; Fig. 5.4). The theory suggests that there is an inverted U-shaped relationship between arousal (or motivation) and performance level. As the level of emotional arousal increases, so does performance efficiency, to an optimal level. As emotional arousal increases above this point, performance starts to deteriorate. The optimal level is not a fixed point and depends upon factors such as task complexity. In order to do well in an exam a degree of arousal, or anxiety, is needed. Too much arousal and performance will suffer.

The experience of stress demonstrates what happens when negative emotions become too much to manage. While there is no single accepted definition of stress, there are three main views as to what it is:

1 **Stimulus models** (Cox 1978). Developed from engineering models, such as Hooke's Law of Elasticity (involving the deformation by loads of metals that have passed a critical level), stress is seen as a stimulus in the environment that acts upon and is disturbing to the adaptive ability of the organism. In humans, a certain amount of stress is needed to maintain alertness, to explore, and to adapt to the environment, but when the 'load' becomes too much, harm is caused. This is an extremely simplistic theory and takes no account of the person interacting with their environment.

2 **Response models** (Seyle 1956). Here, stress is viewed as the non-specific response of the body to the demands placed upon it. Seyle argued that no matter what the stressor, the body has a set pattern of physiological reactions, based upon principles of homeostasis and described as the general adaptation syndrome (GAS):

   - Alarm reaction – activation of the sympathetic nervous system, which stimulates the adrenal medulla to secrete increased levels of adrenaline and noradrenaline, which stay in the system for longer than the stressor is present.

   - Resistance – sympathetic activity is decreased and autonomic activity increases.
   - Exhaustion – if the autonomic activity goes on for too long, the body becomes exhausted, the adrenals no longer function properly, blood glucose levels drop and could result in hypoglycaemia and possibly death.

   Whilst the GAS takes into account the physiological reactions to stress, it does not account for the psychological reactions to stress.

3 **Transactional models** (Lazarus & Folkman 1984) blend the first two models and view stress as an individual perceptual phenomenon rooted in psychological processes. The individual is seen as an active participant in the process of emotional appraisal. Stress is said to arise when there is an imbalance between the perceived demands of a situation and the person's perceived abilities to deal with those demands.

Causes of stress

Stress may, as the models suggest, arise from the environment, or from one's own biological or psychological responses to it.

- **Life events:** Holmes & Rahe (1967) created the Social Readjustment Rating Scale (SRRS), a list of 43 life events of varying severity collected from analysis of data from 5000 patient records. Death of a spouse was arbitrarily rated as the most serious life event, minor violations of the law rated as the least serious. The measure aimed to quantify the impact of a life event, but did not account for individual differences and personal appraisal of the event.
- **Daily hassles and uplifts:** whereas the SRRS is concerned with major life changing events, an alternative measure was developed based on daily hassles, such as concerns about weight and the rising price of food. It was found that concern about such hassles was positively related to undesirable psychological symptoms. Uplifts (e.g. relating well to spouse/lover) were found to be negatively related to such symptoms.
- **Trauma:** one well-documented clinical reaction to stressors outside the range of usual human experience, is post-traumatic stress disorder. This is a syndrome of persistent symptoms of increased arousal, re-experiencing elements of the trauma and avoidance of stimuli associated with the trauma. Post-traumatic stress disorder is described in detail in Chapter 15.

Coping

Cultural or ethnic background, gender and personality have been found to mediate the experience of stress. Coping (the process by which an individual attempts to manage or deal with the stress they experience) also mediates the experience. The aim of the GAS is to cope with the physiological aspects of stress. Other psychological strategies against stress are:

- **Defence mechanisms:** unconscious processes, which occur in the individual as a way of coping with anxiety, and work by altering the individual's perception of reality (see Chapter 36).
- **Coping mechanisms:** conscious ways of attempting to resolve stress. These tend to be problem-focused, e.g. trying to do something about the problem by getting information, or emotion-focused, e.g. thinking about how the problem makes one feel, rather than looking for solutions (Lazarus & Folkman 1984). Each coping mechanism is appropriate in different situations, often dependent upon the amount of control the individual has over the situation.

Cohen & Lazarus (1979) describe five general categories of coping strategies:

1. Direct action – directly trying to change the situation.
2. Information seeking – trying to understand the situation better to predict what might happen next.
3. Inhibition of action – doing nothing. This may work especially well if the individual has no control whatsoever over the situation.
4. Intrapsychic or palliative coping – changing a person's view of the situation, through drugs, alcohol, relaxation or meditation.
5. Turning to others – for help and/or emotional support.

Personality and stress

Certain personality (or behaviour pattern) types are at relatively greater risk for diseases associated with stress, such as high blood pressure and coronary heart disease. The Type A personality is characterized by enhanced aggressiveness and competitive drive, a preoccupation with deadlines and chronic impatience and at greater risk while the Type B personality is seen as calmer, more laid-back and relaxed, and appears to be less at risk of these kinds of disorders (Friedman & Rosenman 1974). It seems to be the way in which people with Type A personalities respond to the experience of stress, rather than the notion that they experience different stressors, which increases their vulnerability.

Locus of control

Locus of control (Rotter 1966) refers to an individual's beliefs about the extent of control that they have over things that happen to them. The more anxious or depressed a person is, the more external their locus of control tends to be and a

greater external locus of control is associated with a greater vulnerability to physical illness. Over the course of a psychotherapeutic intervention, the locus of control tends to become more internalized.

Stress management interventions incorporate parts of the theories described above. Biofeedback aims to change the physiological state directly, as does progressive muscular relaxation. Cognitive restructuring changes the way individuals think, which then leads to alterations in emotions and behaviour (the basis for cognitive behavioural therapy).

PERSONALITY

Personality is a hypothetical construct of the dynamic organization within the individual of those systems that determine their characteristic behaviour or thought. It has been said that there are as many definitions of personality as there are personality theorists. There are two main groups, the *nomothetic* (looking for specified dimensions and traits common to all) and the *idiographic* (interested in individual's unique characteristics).

Nomothetic theories

These theories construe personality as a set of stable fixed traits (a stable covariant set of behavioural acts, which organize a person's behaviour, e.g. sociability, impassivity) or dimensions that are present in everyone to varying degrees and which can be compared between people, by using psychometric questionnaires. The main proponents of these theories are Eysenck and Cattell.

Eysenck

Eysenck (Eysenck 1947, 1965, 1980) argued that two uncorrelated dimensions could represent personality: extroversion and neuroticism. These are both normally distributed. In his later work, he developed a third trait, psychoticism, that is not normally distributed. Eysenck's theory is founded on a biological basis, stating that extroversion exists as a balance between excitation and inhibition processes in the ascending reticular activating system, and that neuroticism is connected to the reactivity of the autonomic nervous system. The biological basis for psychoticism has as yet not been so clearly identified but is hypothesized to be related to hormone levels, especially androgen. Eysenck developed the *Eysenck Personality Inventory*, a self-report questionnaire to assess the three personality dimensions he espoused (Eysenck & Eysenck 1975). In order to account for people 'faking good' by responding in a certain manner, an index assessing response bias was included.

Cattell

Cattell (1965) used factor analytic studies to produce 16 source factors, which he considered to be the fundamental dimensions of personality. Cattell referred to surface traits as the common-sense ways of describing people's behaviour and described these as representing interactions between the source traits. Further factor analysis of the 16 source traits yielded second-order factors, the two most important being exvia-invia and anxiety, which correspond to Eysenck's dimensions of extraversion and neuroticism. On the basis of his theory, Cattell developed the 16PF Questionnaire to tap the 16 source traits.

It is now commonly held that there are five main personality dimensions or traits; however, further research is still needed to allow proper evaluation of these:

- Factor 1 extroversion
- Factor II agreeableness
- Factor III conscientiousness
- Factor IV neuroticism
- Factor V openness to experience.

Idiographic theories

Here the focus is upon individuals over time rather than on between-group comparisons. Idiographic theorists see personality as changeable and without fixed traits. The main proponents of the theories are Allport, Rogers, Kelly and Maslow. Rogers and Maslow are also described as humanistic psychologists.

Allport

Allport (Allport & Odbert 1936) believed in the study of individuals rather than of large-scale experimental statistical studies. He saw each person as unique, and described two kinds of traits:

- **Common traits:** the basic blocks of adjustment, applicable to all members of a cultural or linguistic background, such as levels of acceptable aggression.
- **Individual traits:** unique sets of personal dispositions based on life events and unique ways of organizing the world. These are not dimensions that could be applied to all people. These individual traits take three forms:
  - (a) cardinal traits – all pervading, directing most of an individual's behaviour
  - (b) central traits – blocks that make up the core personality
  - (c) secondary traits – refer to tastes, preferences, political views, etc.

It has been argued that Allport's idiographic methods are basically nomothetic theories applied to individuals.

Kelly and personal construct theory

Kelly (1955) described the person in terms of their own experiences and view of the world (the phenomenological approach). He proposed that an individual has their own concepts or ideas which are used to understand the world, and make predictions about future events. He defined the way in which one sees the world through constructs, (each person's construct system being hierarchically organized; based on broad (superordinate) and narrow (subordinate) constructs).

The *Repertory Grid Technique*, devised to test construct systems, involves choosing elements (e.g. the most important figures in the person's life) and describing in what way these elements are alike or different from a third element. These differences or similarities (the constructs) are then applied to all other elements. This process is reproduced until the person has produced all the constructs they can. The information is presented in a grid, which can be analyzed statistically to enable a person to gain a clearer sense of the way they see the world. Kelly (1955) and Bannister & Fransella (1980) produced a thorough review of Personal Construct Theory, which is helpful in understanding the complexities of the theory (Bannister and Fransella 1980, 1981).

Rogers and client-centred therapy

Rogers (1951) (who, along with Maslow, was one of the most influential humanistic psychologists), saw people as rational, whole beings who know about their feelings and reactions. He argued that self-knowledge is the basis of personality and that it develops from interactions with the world. It aims for consistency but can change as a result of its interactions. The basic need for positive regard is one of Rogers' key arguments. Difficulties arise if there is a discrepancy between an individual's self-concept and their experiences.

The *Q-Sort Technique*, developed from this theory, involves a person sorting cards with statements on them, into piles. They may be asked to sort the cards into piles indicating how they think of themselves presently, or indeed how they would like to be. The task can then be repeated over the course of therapy in order to monitor the person's changing views of themselves.

Maslow and the hierarchy of needs

Maslow's approach was also phenomenological in that he was concerned with individuals' experiences of their world. He postulated a hierarchy of needs (Fig 5.5), factors that need to be fulfilled in order that one can become 'self-actualized', the highest form of personal growth. In order to reach the higher levels, the lower levels (involving basic survival needs) must be satisfied (Maslow 1943). Maslow's hierarchy of needs is in essence more about needs and motivation so is not a 'pure' theory of personality, such as that of Eysenck or Cattell.

Freud and psychoanalytic approaches

Freud construed personality as having three main components:

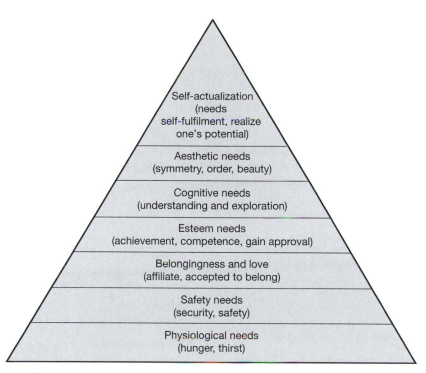

Figure 5.5 Maslow's hierarchy of needs.

1. **Id**: responds directly to impulses and biologically based needs, e.g. food, warmth, shelter
2. **Ego**: that part of the id that has been modified by the direct influence of the external world through the medium of conscious perception
3. **Superego**: this develops once a person has absorbed moral values which determine the acceptability of behaviour, representing the moral or judicial part of the personality.

These concepts are covered in depth in Chapter 36.

It is now generally accepted that attempting to explain all behaviour in terms of personality is unwise: behaviour in any one situation is a reflection of both person and situation variables and even these situational variables have to do with the psychological meaning of the situation to the person.

CONSCIOUSNESS

Whilst psychodynamic theorists may see consciousness as described in Chapter 36, i.e. the conscious, the preconscious and the unconscious, psychologists tend to see it more as a continuum from being fully conscious to being totally unconscious. Different amounts of thoughts, feelings, memories can be accessed, often referred to as the subjective awareness of actions and of the world around us (Rubin & McNeil 1983). Consciousness also has links with attention, and is often described as what we pay attention to.

Arousal

Arousal relates to the level of alertness of the individual and refers to a continuum of possible behavioural and physiological states. Levels of arousal are influenced by circadian rhythms, (the 24-hour patterns of biological change). Sleep represents the common, daily change in levels of arousal, and is described further in Chapter 34.

Hypnosis and suggestibility

Hypnosis has been described as an altered state of consciousness, where the hypnotized subject can be influenced to behave and to experience things differently than he or she would have in the ordinary waking state (Rubin & McNeil 1983). Others would argue that it is not an altered *state* of arousal. It was first demonstrated by Mesmer, who showed that when hypnotized, a patient could be instructed to change their behaviour when the hypnotic session was finished. The Stanford hypnotic suggestibility scales can measure suggestibility, relating to how readily hypnotizable the subject is (Weizenhoffer & Hilfard 1959). Suggestibility is highest in children, reaching a peak at around age 10 and declining with age.

Uses of hypnosis

Hypnosis is commonly used to help people overcome habits such as smoking, and in the treatment of pain. The subject is hypnotized and then receives instructions that the quality or intensity of the pain they are experiencing is altered, turned down or transferred in location. A typical experiment to demonstrate the efficacy of hypnosis is the *cold pressor* response, where a patient is asked to immerse their arm in a bucket of cold water. Patients who have been hypnotized will report less pain or discomfort than those who have not (Hilgard 1978). Hilgard also refers to the *hidden observer* phenomenon: when the hypnotized person is asked about the pain or discomfort, they report low levels, but when the 'hidden observer' (i.e. another part of the person's consciousness) is asked, levels almost the same as a non-hypnotized subject are reported. This is referred to as Hilgard's neo-dissociation theory.

The debate as to whether hypnosis is a real state of altered consciousness continues and studies abound trying to prove or disprove its existence and its mechanisms (Wagstaff 1995).

Meditation and trances

Meditation refers to a technique of clearing the mind through focused thought. It represents a way of trying to alter consciousness to achieve inner calm. There are two main forms of meditation:

- Concentrate meditation as practised by some Hindus, which seeks an alteration of consciousness through detachment from the external environment and from internal thought processes, by concentrating on a mandala (a visual image on which all attention is focused) or a mantra (a single word, repeated silently to oneself).
- Mindfulness meditation, as practised by Zen Bhuddists, where all mental attention is directed at the thoughts that pass through the mind, the object of the exercise being to observe these things in a detached manner rather than challenge them or direct the mind in any way.

Through meditation, thought to be mainly a right-hemisphere activity, people have been able to control their bodily processes, slow down heart rate and reduce the amount of oxygen capacity used, akin to the aims of biofeedback.

SOCIAL PSYCHOLOGY

Social psychology is the study of how people perceive, think and feel about the social world and how we interact and influence one another. Behaviour is then determined according to the power of the situation and a person's interpretation of the situation.

Attitudes

Attitudes are a set of beliefs (favourable and unfavourable evaluations) that predispose an individual to particular behaviours. There are three components:

1. **Cognitive:** beliefs based on information, e.g. exercise is good for your health.
2. **Affective:** (often very hard to change), e.g. 'I love long-distance running'.
3. **Behavioural:** e.g. 'I run every day'.

In general people hold similar attitudes on a range of subjects.

Measurement of attitudes

There are several ways of measuring attitudes, e.g. projective tests such as Rorshach inkblots, physiological tests, e.g. Galvanic skin response, and questionnaires. The following are the main three forms of questionnaire:

1. **Likert scales:** agree/disagree on a five-point scale. Such scales are relatively sensitive and simple to design, though similar scores can be obtained with different answers.
2. **Thurstone scales:** a range of statements is presented and you pick those you agree with. These scales are less sensitive than Likert scales and can have value-laden biases.
3. **Semantic-differential:** a visual analogue scale with polarized adjectives separated by a line. Subjects mark their attitude between the two. These are easy to complete and reliable but may be subject to positional response bias.

Social effects may also impact on measurements of behaviour:

- **Response set:** tendency to always agree/disagree to a set of questions.
- **Bias to middle:** avoidance of extreme responses.
- **Halo effect:** the observer allows preconceptions to influence responses.
- **Hawthorn effect:** positive social interactions between experimenter and subject affects response.

Attitudes and behaviour

A major reason for studying attitudes is expectation that they will predict a person's behaviour. Attitudes predict behaviour best if they are:

1. strong and consistent
2. based on experience
3. related to the behaviour being predicted.

Behaviour may also determine attitudes as expressed in cognitive dissonance theory.

Cognitive dissonance theory (Festinger 1957)

Individuals strive for consistency in their attitudes with discomfort or dissonance arising if two cognitions are held that are inconsistent.

This was demonstrated in an experiment where subjects were recruited for a very dull task and paid $20 or $1. They were then asked to tell others how interesting and fun the task was. Those paid $1 did change attitudes and said the task was fun, whilst the $20 group were less enthusiastic. Cognitive dissonance theory implies that $20 was sufficient reason to take part, while receiving $1 and doing a boring task was harder to justify leading to the subjects decreasing dissonance by changing attitudes.

Dissonance is increased if there is:

- low pressure to comply
- increased choice of options
- awareness of responsibility for consequences
- expected unpleasant consequences of behaviour to others.

Dissonance is decreased by:

- changing behaviour
- dismissing information/cognitions
- adding new cognitions.

The theory has little predictive power as to what course of action will be chosen.

Attitude change

Advertising attempts to change/influence attitudes using new information (cognitive), appealing to emotions and offering rewards (behaviour). Similar processes are used in persuasive communication. There are three main areas to consider:

1. **Communicator factors.** More persuasive if:
   - expert or leader of opinions
   - motivation clear (no vested interest)
   - attractive/likeable
   - uses non-verbal cues – attention paid to body language, etc.
2. **Recipient factors.** These are influenced by:
   - self-esteem – increased co-operation if simple message in low self-esteem
   - intelligence – though relationship not simple.
3. **Message.**
   - an interactive personalized discussion – with a two-sided discussion to a neutral audience and a more one-sided discussion to an already favourable audience
   - fear – excess fear may be counter-productive but also depends on anxiety levels. Low anxiety requires a higher fear content, with medium fear in highly anxious states.

Self-psychology

Self-concept refers to a set of attitudes that an individual holds about themselves, e.g. 'I am popular', 'I am thin'.

Self-esteem is a sense of contentment and self-acceptance arising from a process of appraisal of one's own worth, significance, attractiveness, etc., and one's ability to satisfy aspirations. Increased self-esteem is associated with social activity, fulfilling relationships, etc. Decreased self-esteem is associated with mental illness, a vulnerability to depression and some physical illnesses.

Self-image is a descriptive view of self, derived from experiences of success and the content of social interactions.

Self-perception theory (Bem 1972) proposes that we make judgements about ourselves using the same inferential processes and errors that we use for making judgements of others (see below). Specifically, individuals form their attitudes by inferring them from the observation of their behaviours and situations. If internal cues are weak, then we rely on external cues. *Fundamental attribution errors* (see below) also mean that self-perception is affected by the tendency to give too much weight to personal characteristics rather than situations, e.g. in a conversation someone who selects topics for discussion will feel and be seen as more knowledgeable than others who follow the conversation flow.

Self-concept is influenced differently by various characteristics, e.g. gender, age:

- Gender:
  (a) males – predominance of activity, dominance
  (b) females – affection, sensitivity.
- Age:
  (a) childhood – physical characteristics, kindness
  (b) adolescents – interests
  (c) adults – occupation, family role.

Interpersonal psychology

Of all attitudes, one of the most interesting is the attitudes of others and factors that influence interpersonal attraction. Attraction is mediated by:

- **Physical attractiveness:** while individuals do not rate this as important, research suggests it does play a major part. People are rated more favourably if with an attractive partner and photos of attractive people are rated as being more popular.
- **Proximity:** research suggests that one of the best predictors is how close people live to each other. Being in close proximity to someone is likely to promote friendship.
- **Familiarity:** proximity also promotes familiarity and familiarity also increases liking for something or someone.

- **Similarity:** couples tend to have similar interests or outlooks, similar psychological characteristics, e.g. intelligence and physical attributes – *assortative mating*.

Social exchange theory

This theory suggests that people like their partner more according to the rewards received compared to those given. Relationships can be divided into 'exchange' relationships (rewards exchanged predominantly) and 'communal' relationships (rewards given out of concern for other). 'Exchange' relationships are characterized by insecurity and dissatisfaction.

Stereotypes

A limited amount of information about an individual will result in them being fitted into a specific group and other behavioural characteristics will be ascribed to that individual even with no evidence to support them, e.g. age. In general the first information received has the greatest effect on the overall impression: the *primacy effect* or *first impressions count!*

Stereotypes persist, even if data does not confirm them and cause us to interact with people we have stereotyped in ways that cause self-fulfilling stereotypes.

Attribution theory

Attribution theory (Heider 1958) suggests that we develop attitudes based on what we observe. If we infer something based on a belief that it is due to that individual's characteristics, then this is an internal or *dispositional* attribution. If we conclude that an external cause is responsible, e.g. money, then this is a *situational* attribution.

The *fundamental attributional error* suggests a bias towards dispositional attributions, e.g. in a debate. If people are randomly allocated to each side of the debate, people will still estimate the debater's own personal attitudes to be close to the position argued, despite clear evidence that the situation was responsible.

Social interaction and influence

Interacting with others helps determine our actions and beliefs, while the influence of others attempts to change these for positive or negative reasons. Such influence can be direct or indirect and unintentional. Social norms (implicit rules) also influence behaviour, e.g. standing face forward in a lift.

Presence of others

Being part of a group can determine actions through several processes:

- **Audience effect:** activity levels can be increased by the presence of a crowd, e.g. an athletics race. If the task is more complex or novel then an audience can impede behaviour.
- **De-individuation:** being an anonymous member of a group can reduce self-awareness and decrease social restraints. In such a situation people may act in a less inhibited fashion.
- **Bystander intervention:** this describes the tendency not to intervene in a situation, due to the presence of others, e.g. a man lying in the street is more likely to be offered help if there is only one passer-by, than if he is in a crowded street. This is partly due to *pluralistic ignorance*, where members of a group convince each other that there is no problem, and *diffusion of responsibility*, where people feel that is not their responsibility and that someone else will do something.

Conformity

Normative social influences can lead to an individual acquiescing with a group view even if the individual holds a different personal view. Asch (1952) demonstrated this by placing a subject in a group of stooges and asking them to judge the length of a line. When all the stooges gave patently wrong answers, the subject was also more likely to agree with this view even though the correct answer was obvious.

Conformity pressures increase with group size up to a maximum of three, unanimity of the group decision, and perceived high status of other group members. Also, vulnerability to conform is decreased by intelligence, self-esteem and self-reliance. Traditionally, females were felt to be more vulnerable to conform than males, though more recent evidence suggests no difference.

Obedience

The potential to comply with authority is powerful. Milgram (1963) demonstrated that in certain situations individuals would obey orders, even if these broke the limits of their normal beliefs. Subjects were instructed to administer electric shocks to stooges who were supposedly failing in a learning experiment. The experimenter encouraged the subject to increase the voltage to almost lethal levels. The stooge acted out the pain of the mock shocks, but two-thirds of subjects continued despite the apparent inflicted suffering.

Obedience is affected by the proximity to the victim (increased obedience with distance) and the authority of the instructor.

Group decision-making

Many everyday decisions are not made by individuals but by groups. This process contains its own dynamics.

Group polarization

Group decisions were traditionally viewed as being cautious. However, various experiments have demonstrated that group decisions are often more extreme than individual views. If an individual is prone to risk-taking then the group decision will be riskier, conversely conservative individuals will result in a more conservative group decision. This tendency is termed group polarization.

Groupthink

Groupthink is the desire to achieve consensus and avoid dissent in group decisions (Janis 1982). It occurs when a group of decision makers meet in isolation from outside influences, without systematic procedures for looking at the advantages and disadvantages of a course of action. It is promoted by having a directive leader, who favours a course of action, and high stress levels.

The symptoms of groupthink are:

- an illusion of invulnerability and morality
- pressure on dissenters to agree
- self-censorship of dissent
- collective rationalization
- 'mindguards' – individuals who are self-appointed to prevent the group from considering information that would challenge the effectiveness of the group.

Groupthink leads to decisions that:

- are based on incomplete information;
- have failed to fully examine all the risks and appraise alternative plans.

Such decisions can lead to disastrous implementation of plans. Groupthink can be guarded against by:

- being aware of it
- having open debates
- appointing a 'devil's advocate' or using external experts to challenge the group's decisions.

In mixed-sex groups, males will talk more, interrupt more and raise topics for discussion more than female members.

FURTHER READING

Atkinson RL, Atkinson RC, Smith E, Bem D & Nolen-Hoeksema S (1999) *Hilgard's Introduction to Psychology*, 13th edn. New York: Thomson Learning.

Gross R (2001), *Psychology, The Science of Mind and Behaviour*, 4th edn. London: Hodder Arnold.

Gross R (2003), *Key studies in psychology*, 4th edn. London: Hodder Arnold.

Radford J & Gover E (eds) (1992) *A Textbook of Psychology*, 2nd edn. London: Routledge.

REFERENCES

Allport GW (1955) *Becoming – Basic Considerations for a Psychology of Personality*. New Haven, CT: Yale University Press.

Allport GW (1980) Attention and performance: In: Claxton G (ed.) *Cognitive Psychlogy: New Directions*. London: Routledge, Kegan Paul.

Allport GW & Odbert HS (1936) Trait names: a psycho-lexical study. *Psychological Monographs: General and Applied*, **47** (whole no. 211).

Asch SE (1952) *Social Psychology*. Englewood Cliffs, NJ: Prentice-Hall.

Atkinson RC & Shiffrin RM (1968) Human memory: a proposed system and its control processes. In: Spence KW & Spence JT (eds) *The Psychology of Learning and Motivation*, vol. 2. London: Academic Press.

Atkinson RC & Shiffrin RM (1971) The control of short term memory. *Scientific American* **224**: 82–90.

Baddely AD (1990) *Human Memory*. Oxford: Oxford University Press.

Baddely AD & Hitch G (1974) Working memory. In: Bower GH (ed.) *Recent Advances in Learning and Motivation*, vol. 8. New York: Academic Press.

Bandura A (1977) Self efficacy: toward a unifying theory of behaviour change. *Psychological Review* **84**: 191–215.

Bannister D & Fransella F (1980) *Inquiring Man: The Psychology of Personal Constructs*, 2nd edn. Harmondsworth: Penguin.

Bem DJ (1972) Self-perception theory. In: Berkowitz L (ed.) *Advances in Social Psychology*, vol. 6. New York: Academic Press.

Binet A & Simon T (1905) New methods for the diagnosis of the intellectual level of subnormals. *Annals of Psychology* **11**: 191.

Bornstein MH (1988) Perceptual development across the life cycle. In: Borstein MH & Lamb ME (eds.) *Perceptual, Cognitive and Linguistic Development*. Hove, East Sussex: Lawrence Erlbaum Associates.

Brody EB & Brody N (1976) *Intelligence: Nature, Determinants and Consequences*. New York: Academic Press.

Broadbent DE (1958) *Perception and Comunication*. London: Pergamon.

Cannon WB (1929) *Bodily Changes in Pain Hunger, Fear and Rage*. New York: Appleton-Century-Crofts.

Cattell RB (1965) *The Scientific Analysis of Personality*. Harmondsworth, Middlesex, Penguin

Cohen F & Lazarus R (1979) Coping with the stresses of illness. In: Stone CG, Cohen F & Ader NE (eds.) *Health Psychology: A Handbook*. San Fransisco, CA: Jossey-Bass.

Cox T (1978) *Stress*. London: MacMillan Education.

Deutsch JA & Deutsch D (1963) Attention: some theoretical considerations. *Psychological Review* **70**: 80–90.

Ebbinghaus H (1885) *On Memory*. Leipzig: Dunker.

Eysenck HJ (1965) *Fact and Fiction in Psychology*. Harmondsworth: Penguin.

Eysenck HJ (1980) The biosocial model of man and the unification of psychology. In: Chapman AJ & Jones DM (eds.) *Models of Man*. Leicester: British Psychological Society.

Eysenck HJ & Eysenck SBG (1975) *Manual of the Eysenck Personality Questionnaire*. London: Hodder & Stoughton.

Eysenck MW (1984) *A Handbook of Cognitive Psychology*. London: Lawrence Erlbaum Associates.

Fantz R.L (1961) The origin of form perception. *Scientific American* **204**(5): 66–72.

Festinger L (1957) *A Theory of Cognitive Dissonance*. Standford, CA: Stanford University Press.

Friedman M & Rosenman RH (1974) *Type A Behaviour and your Heart*. New York: Knopf.

Geen RG (1995) Social motivation. In: Parkinson B & Colman AM (eds) *Emotion and Motivation*. London: Longman.

Gibson EJ & Walk PD (1960) The visual cliff. *Scientific American* **202**: 64–71.

Gregory RL (1983) Visual illusions. In: Miller J (ed.) *States of Mind*. London: BBC Publications.

Guilford JP (1967) *The Nature of Human Intelligence*. London: McGraw-Hill.

Harlow HF (1949) Formation of learning sets. *Psychological Review* **56**: 51–65.

Heider F (1958) *The Psychology of Interpersonal Relationships*. New York: Wiley.

Hilgard ER (1978) Hypnosis and consciousness. *Human Nature* January: 42–9.

Holmes TH & Rahe RH (1967) The social readjustment rating scale. *Journal of Psychosomatic Research* **11**: 213–18.

Horn JL & Cattell RB (1967) Age differences in fluid and crystallised intelligence. *Acta Psychologica* **26**: 107–29.

Hull CL (1943) *Principles of Behaviour*. New York: Appleton-Century-Crofts.

James W (1890) *Principles of Psychology*. New York: Holt.

Janis IL (1982) *Groupthink: Psycholgical Studies of Policy Decisions and Fiascoes*, 2nd edn. Boston: Houghton Mifflin.

Jensen AR (1980) *Bias in Mental Testing*. New York: Free Press.

Kahneman D (1973) *Attention and Effort*. Englewood Cliffs, NJ: Prentice Hall.

Kaufmnan AS (1994) *Intelligent Testing with the WISC-III*. New York: Wiley.

Kelly GA (1955) *A Theory of Personality – The Psychology of Personal Constructs*. New York: Norton.

Kohler W (1947) *Gestalt Psychology*. New York: Harcourt Brace.

Lazarus RS & Folkman S (1984) *Stress, Appraisal and Coping*. New York: Springer-Verlag.

Lloyd P, Mayes A, Manstead ASR, Mendell PR & Wagner HL (1984) *Introduction to Psychology – An Integrated Approach*. London: Fontana.

Maslow AH (1943) A Theory of human motivation. *Psychological Review* **50**: 370.

Milgram S (1963) Behavioural study of obedience. *Journal of Abnormal and Social Psychology* **67**: 371–8.

Pavlov IP (1927) *Conditioned Reflexes*. London: Oxford University Press.

Raven JC, Court JH & Raven J (1983) *Manual for Raven's Progressive Matrices and Vocabulary Scales (Section 3) – Standard Progressive Matrices*. London: Lewis.

Rogers CR (1951) *Client Centred Therapy – Its Current Practices, Implications and Theory*. Boston: Houghton Mifflin.

Rotter JB (1966) Generalised expectancies for internal versus external control of reinforcement. *Psychological Monographs* **30**(19): 1–26.

Rubin Z & McNeil EB (1983) *The Psychology of Being Human*, 3rd edn. London: Harper & Row.

Salame P & Baddely AD (1982) Disruption of short term memory by unattended speech: implications for the structure of of working memory. *Journal of Verbal Learning and Verbal Behaviour* **21**: 150–64.

Schachter S (1964) The interaction of cognitive and physiological determinants of emotional state. In Berkowitz L (ed.) *Advances in Experimental Social Psychology*, Vol 1. New York: Academic Press.

Seyle H (1956) *The Stress of Life*. New York: McGraw-Hill.

Skinner BF (1938) *The Behaviour of Organisms*. New York: Appleton-Century-Crofts.

Solso RL (1995) *Cognitive Psychology*, 4th edn. Boston: Allyn & Bacon.

Thorndike EL (1898) Animal intelligence: an experimental study of the associative processes in animals. *Psychological Review, Monograph Supplement* **2** (whole no. 8).

Triesman A (1969) Strategies and models of selective attention. *Psychological Reviews* **76**: 282–99.

Vernon PE (1960) *The Structure of Human Abilities,* rev. edn. London: Methuen.

Wagstaff GF (1995) Hypnosis. In: Colman AM (ed.) *Controversies in Psychology*. London: Longman.

Watson JB & Rayner R (1920) Conditioned emotional reactions. *Journal of Experimental Psychology*, **3**: 1–14.

Wechsler D (1991) *Wechsler Intelligence Scale for Children*, 3rd UK edn. London: The Psychological Corporation.

Wechsler D (1999a) *Wechsler Adult Intelligence Scale*. London: The Psychological Corporation.

Wechlser D (1999a) *Wechsler Abbreviated Scale of Intelligence*. London: The Psychological Corporation.

Wechsler D (2003) *Wechsler Pre-School and Primary Scales of Intelligence*, 3rd UK edn. London: The Psychological Corporation.

Weitzenhoffer AM & Hilgard ER (1959) *Stanford Hypnotic Susceptibility Scale, Forms A and B*. Palo Alto, CA: Consulting Psychologists' Press.

Yerkes R.M & Dodson JD (1908) The relation of strength of stimulus to rapidity of habit formation. *Journal of Comparative and Neurological Psychology* **18**: 459–82.

6

Descriptive psychopathology

Sadgun Bhandari

INTRODUCTION

Descriptive psychopathology is the method of precisely describing and categorizing abnormal experiences as recounted by psychiatric patients and observed in their behaviour. It eschews explanations and is atheoretical. The uses of descriptive psychopathology are (adapted from Sims 1991):

1 **Diagnostic:** facilitates communication of the clinical features to other professionals.
2 **Scientific:** allows precise observations and deductions to be made.
3 **Therapeutic:** facilitates the establishment of an empathic relationship.
4 **Forensic:** medico-legal evaluation of the patient is largely based upon psychopathology.

The term phenomenology is often inaccurately used interchangeably with descriptive psychopathology. According to Jaspers (1959), phenomenology is the description of the actual experiences of the patient without reference to the sources of these experiences, to the emergence of one psychic phenomenon rather than another, nor to theories of underlying cause. Psychic phenomena should be elicited empathically in an attempt to render the patient's experience understandable.

When eliciting and describing psychiatric signs and symptoms one should heed a note of caution from Schneider (1959) who commented that clinical diagnosis often precedes enquiry and that symptoms tend to be subsequently evaluated in the light of the diagnosis. Ideally unbiased observation and description of symptoms should precede diagnosis.

The principal symptoms encountered in clinical psychiatry occur in the realm of perception, thinking, affect, motor activity, consciousness, sense of self and memory. Disorders of consciousness and memory will be discussed in Chapter 26.

DISORDERS OF PERCEPTION

Disorders of perception are classically divided into sensory distortions, in which real objects are perceived as altered in some way, and false perceptions, in which non-existent objects are perceived (Box 6.1).

Sensory distortions

In sensory distortion a real perceptual object is perceived as distorted. The intensity of a perception can become heightened or diminished and qualitative changes can occur. This commonly affects the visual modality when toxicity from certain drugs alters colour vision (e.g. santonin causing violet or yellow vision). Quantitative changes include micropsia, macropsia or dysmegalopsia, in which objects are seen as smaller or larger than they really are, or as altered in shape, respectively. Such phenomena may be due to end-organ disease or to acute organic disorders and epilepsy.

False perceptions

Illusions are thought to occur when stimuli from a perceived object are combined with mental images to produce a false perception. Illusions are associated with inattention when external sensory stimuli are meagre or when attention is impaired due to delirium. Illusions are also associated with prevailing affect, thus shadows may appear like human figures to a frightened individual. Illusions almost always disappear when sensory stimuli increase or when attention improves.

Box 6.1 Disorders of perception	
Sensory distortions	*False perceptions*
(i) Altered intensity of perception	(i) Illusions and pareidolia
(ii) Qualitative alteration of perception	(ii) Hallucinations
(iii) Quantitative alteration of perception	

Pareidolia is a type of illusion that occurs when imagination is used to create images from ill-defined sensory stimuli such as clouds or flames. It is a normal phenomenon (especially in children) that does not disappear when attention is focused, and the images are recognized as unreal by the individual.

Hallucinations are the most clinically significant false perceptions. Hallucinations are not distortions of real perceptions but arise de novo and occur alongside real perceptions (Jaspers 1959). Hallucinations are not experienced in inner subjective space, but occur in the individual's external environment. They have the substantiality of a normal perception and are not under voluntary control.

As summarized by Slade (1976), a hallucination is:

1. a percept-like experience in the absence of an external stimulus
2. a percept-like experience that has the full force and impact of a real perception
3. a percept-like experience that is unwilled, occurs spontaneously, and cannot be readily controlled by the percipient.

Hallucinations may occur due to disorders of peripheral sense organs, sensory deprivation and while falling asleep or awakening (these are referred to as hypnagogic hallucinations or hypnopompic hallucinations respectively). Pathologically significant hallucinations occur most commonly in patients with organic psychoses, schizophrenia or affective disorders. Hallucinations should be differentiated from illusions, pseudohallucinations, hypnagogic and hypnopompic images, and from vivid imagery. Hallucinations may be classified as shown in Box 6.2.

Auditory hallucinations

Auditory hallucinations may range from elementary noises to fully formed voices. Voices may be single or multiple and may talk to or about the person. When eliciting auditory hallucinations the interviewer should ensure that the patient is not stating that he hears actual voices. Furthermore auditory hallucinations need to be clearly distinguished from the patient's own thoughts.

Box 6.2 Classification of hallucinations	
Modality specific	*Special types*
Auditory	Functional
Visual	Reflex
Bodily senses	Extracampine
Gustatory	Autoscopic
Olfactory	

Diagnostic significance

Auditory hallucinations are one of the most important symptoms for the diagnosis of psychosis, especially schizophrenia. Schneider (1959) included three particular types of auditory hallucinations as symptoms of the first rank for the diagnosis of schizophrenia. These particular hallucinations are part of the diagnostic criteria for schizophrenia in both the ICD 10 and DSM IV. The three types are *thought echo* (which is also known as *gedankenlautwerden* and *echo des pensées*), *running commentary hallucinations*, and *third person hallucinations* of two or more voices arguing about or discussing the patient (see Chapter 18). Other types of auditory hallucinations can also occur in schizophrenia, including voices commanding the patient and voices talking directly to him. Paraphrenia may also present with prominent auditory hallucinations (see Chapter 31).

Auditory hallucinations occur in affective disorder in which case the content often reflects the underlying mood; these hallucinations are referred to as mood congruent hallucinations.

Alcoholic hallucinosis is characterized predominantly by auditory hallucinations with a derogatory or persecutory content. Delirium due to any cause is also associated with auditory hallucinations, as is cerebral dysfunction, even when consciousness is not impaired.

Visual hallucinations

Visual hallucinations can range from elementary flashes of light through fully formed visions of animals, objects and persons, to complex scenes. It is sometimes difficult to distinguish between internal images, illusions and clear visual hallucinations.

Diagnostic significance

Visual hallucinations characteristically occur in delirium of any cause, but dementia due to Alzheimer's disease, Pick's disease and Lewy bodies disease is also associated with visual hallucinations. Intoxication with hallucinogenic drugs like lysergic acid diethylamide (LSD) and mescaline is a relatively common cause of visual hallucinations. Visual hallucinations are very uncommon in patients with schizophrenia and affective disorders (Sims 1995) and if present, suggest an organic disorder.

Charles–Bonnet syndrome

The Charles–Bonnet syndrome is a condition in which individuals, mostly female, experience extremely vivid visual hallucinations. These occur persistently and repetitively without any delusions or hallucinations in any other modality, and without disturbance of consciousness. Insight is preserved. The condition is most often associated with low visual acuity and advanced age (Teunisse et al. 1995). It is believed that they represent release phenomena due to de-afferentation of the visual association areas of the cerebral cortex (Manford & Andermann 1998).

A similar phenomenon has been described in impaired hearing and presents as musical hallucinations (Ali 2002).

Bodily senses

These hallucinations include those affecting the skin, muscle and joint sense and inner organs (Sims 1995), and can include sensations of heat or cold, electric shocks, sexual experiences and visceral sensations. The term tactile hallucinations is used commonly to describe hallucinations affecting the skin (another term commonly used, haptic hallucinations refers to hallucinations of being touched). Tactile hallucinations are unique in that they are invariably delusionally elaborated, the commonest delusions are those of being controlled. This is somatic passivity, which is a Schneiderian first rank symptom. Possibly deriving from this, the term somatic hallucination is also used to describe hallucinations of bodily senses.

Diagnostic significance

Hallucinations of bodily senses along with delusional elaboration occur in schizophrenia. In certain acute organic psychoses and cocaine intoxication tactile hallucinations occur in the form of formication, which is the sensation of animals crawling all over the body. This differs from Ekbom's syndrome, the delusion of infestation (see Chapter 22).

Gustatory hallucinations

Gustatory hallucinations refer to false perceptions of taste and are often difficult to diagnose. They may sometimes present with changes in taste, which may be persistent.

Diagnostic significance

Gustatory hallucinations may occur in schizophrenia where they may be delusionally elaborated, for example a change in taste may be elaborated as a delusion of being poisoned. They may also present as a feature of temporal lobe epilepsy (see Chapter 26).

Olfactory hallucinations

Olfactory hallucinations are not common and may range from the experience of something smelling to the patients complaining that they themselves smell unpleasantly. This needs to be distinguished from the rare olfactory reference syndrome where a person is preoccupied with emitting foul odour (Stein et al. 1998).

Diagnostic significance

Olfactory hallucinations are a feature of temporal lobe epilepsy. They have also been described in schizophrenia and depression, and in the latter they may reflect the underlying mood.

Functional hallucinations

In functional hallucination the hallucination is provoked by a stimulus and occurs in the same sensory modality as the stimulus. Both the stimulus and the hallucination are perceived simultaneously but they are also perceived as being distinct. Thus a patient may hear a voice only when a tap is turned on and then hears both the sound of the voice and the sound of running water.

Reflex hallucinations

In reflex hallucinations a stimulus in one sensory modality provokes a hallucination in another modality. This is thought to be a morbid form of synaesthesia. Synaesthesia is a normal phenomenon, in which a stimulus in one modality produces an image in another modality, for example the feeling of discomfort caused by seeing and hearing somebody scratch a blackboard with their finger nails (Sims 1995).

Extracampine hallucinations

These are hallucinations that are outside the normal limits of the sensory fields. Thus an individual at one location may see or hear another individual miles away.

These variations of hallucinations – functional, reflex and extracampine – are not of themselves indicative of any specific diagnosis.

Autoscopy (the Doppelganger phenomenon)

This is the experience of seeing an image of oneself and knowing that it is oneself (Sims 1991). Usually the image is in front of the patient and may be a fleeting image or an image that persists throughout the day.

Diagnostic significance

Autoscopy can occur during epileptic seizures, with migraine or drug intoxication and in some organic psychoses.

Pseudohallucinations

Pseudohallucinations differ from hallucinations by lacking the reality of a true perception and by being experienced in inner subjective space. In this respect they are like images. They share some characteristics of a true hallucination in that they are vivid and are not under voluntary control.

The term pseudohallucination has also been applied when patients do not consider their hallucinations to be real, i.e. they have insight.

Diagnostic significance

Pseudohallucinations are not indicative of mental illness and are known to occur in healthy individuals during times of crises such as bereavement.

DISORDERS OF THINKING

The disorders of thinking will be discussed under the following headings:

- delusions
- overvalued ideas
- disorders of control of thinking
- disorders of the flow of thought
- formal thought disorder.

Delusions

A delusion is a false, unshakeable idea or belief that is out of keeping with the patient's social and cultural background. The main features of delusions according to Jaspers (1959), besides their being false, are (1) they are held with an extraordinary conviction and subjective certainty; (2) there is imperviousness to other experiences and to compelling counterargument; and (3) their content is impossible. As Sims (1995) suggests, the absurdity or erroneousness of their content is manifest to other people.

According to Kraupl-Taylor (1983) delusions are:

1. absolute, because they are held beyond a shadow of doubt
2. idiosyncratic, because they are unshared
3. ego-involved, because they are of sensitive personal significance
4. incorrigible, because they resist all powers of persuasion
5. often preoccupying, because they monopolize the patient's mind.

Delusions are traditionally divided into two groups usually referred to as primary and secondary (see Box 6.3).

Primary delusions are not understandable and are psychologically irreducible, while secondary delusions are understandable in the context of preceding affects or other experiences. The emphasis in primary delusions is on the form of the symptom, i.e. how they originate rather than the content. Jaspers termed primary delusions as delusions proper and secondary delusions as delusion-like ideas. He suggested four types of primary delusions: delusional atmosphere; delusional perception; delusional ideas; and delusional awareness.

Box 6.3 Subdivision of delusions	
Primary (autocthonous)	*Secondary*
Delusional mood	Secondary to hallucinations, affect or other experiences
Delusional perception	
Sudden delusional idea	

Similarly, Schneider (1959) divided delusions into delusional perception and delusional notion. He described delusional perception as a two-stage process, in which abnormal self-referential significance is attached to a genuine perception without any comprehensible rational or emotional justification (i.e. it is not understandable). Perception itself is not altered but the meaning attached to what is perceived is altered.

Delusional perception may arise out of delusional mood (also known as delusional atmosphere). Delusional mood is akin to a predelusional state or a 'precursor phenomena' during which the person has a vague feeling that something odd is going on. Delusions arising out of delusional mood are considered primary delusions because they are vague, their content does not refer to the delusional mood and they are not understandable. The notion of a primary delusion arising from a preceding primary delusion (delusional mood) is confusing but as Sims (1995) points out, the core of a primary delusion is that it is not understandable (and not any temporal relationship). Sudden delusional ideas are also classified as primary delusions (Fish 1967).

Secondary delusions are easier to understand as they arise from an abnormal affect such as depression and from phenomena such as hallucinations. Thus secondary delusions are always interpretations, and are psychologically reducible, for example grandiose delusions in mania or persecutory delusions secondary to hallucinations.

According to cognitive therapy theory, delusions are not impervious to change as they share certain cognitive characteristics. These include an egocentric bias, by which patients become locked into an egocentric perspective and construe even irrelevant events as self-relevant; an externalizing bias, in which internal sensations or symptoms are attributed to external agents; and an intentionalizing bias, which leads the patient to attribute malevolent and hostile intentions to other people's behaviour (Rector & Beck 2002). For further information refer to Chapter 37.

Delusional memories

This term has been used to denote two types of experiences: (1) a delusion is suddenly remembered, or as defined in the Present State Examination (Wing et al. 1974), 'experiences of past events which clearly did not occur but which the subject equally clearly remembers'; and (2) where delusional interpretation is applied to a normal memory. In the latter the experience is akin to a delusional perception in which the memory is the normal perception to which abnormal significance is attached.

Systematization

When a delusion is elaborated, it is said to be systematized when there is one basic delusion upon which the remainder of the system is logically built. Systematized delusions are more likely in persistent delusional disorders than in schizophrenia.

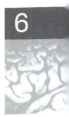

Bizarre delusions

This is a commonly used term in clinical descriptions. The DSM IV makes a distinction between bizarre and non-bizarre delusions based on plausibility of the content. Bizarre delusions are those that are clearly implausible and not understandable and do not derive from ordinary life experience, for example the belief of being controlled by aliens through radio waves as compared to delusions of infidelity. The distinction is diagnostically important as bizarre delusions occur in schizophrenia and the presence of non-bizarre delusions in the absence of other symptoms is suggestive of delusional disorder.

Classification of delusions by content

Delusions are often classified by their content, as follows:

- delusions of reference
- delusions of persecution
- delusions of guilt
- delusions of grandeur
- religious delusions
- hypochondriacal delusions
- delusions of love (erotomania, De Clarambault's syndrome)
- delusions of infidelity (delusional jealousy, Othello syndrome)
- nihilistic delusions (Cotard syndrome)
- delusion of doubles (Capgras syndrome)
- shared delusions (*folie a deux*).

Stompe et al. (2003) have shown that, despite the incorporation of new technologies in the content of delusions and cultural influences on them, historically and across cultures the basic themes have remained remarkably stable.

Delusions of reference

Objects and events are considered to have obvious significance to the patient who may think he is being talked about, being discussed on the radio or television, etc. When eliciting this symptom it must be determined that the patient is not misinterpreting auditory hallucinations.

Diagnostic significance
Delusions of reference occur commonly in schizophrenia and can also occur in affective disorder. Ideas of reference, in which the criteria for a delusion are not met, i.e. they may be short-lived or not firmly held, can also occur in sensitive self-conscious people and those with paranoid personality disorder.

Delusions of persecution

This is one of the commonest types of delusion. The person believes that he is being harmed by others or is being poisoned, infected or influenced by external agencies. The term 'paranoid' is often used as a substitute for persecutory in everyday clinical use but is best avoided.

Diagnostic significance
Persecutory delusions occur in schizophrenia, affective disorders, and both acute and chronic organic disorders.

Delusions of guilt

These delusions are characterized by beliefs of personal wickedness and sinfulness.

Diagnostic significance
Delusions of guilt are common features of depression.

Delusions of grandeur

The themes of grandiose delusions include those of exalted birth, ability and status or wealth.

Diagnostic significance
Delusions of grandeur occur in mania, schizophrenia, delusional disorder and organic disorder. These delusions were classically described in general paresis of the insane (i.e. neurosyphillis).

Religious delusions

Delusions with a religious content are common and reflect the patient's predominant concerns and interests. It may be important to clarify unfamiliar religious beliefs (by reference to the patient's peers) before concluding that the belief is a delusion.

Diagnostic significance
Religious delusions occur in schizophrenia, mania and depression.

Hypochondriacal delusions

These are also referred to as delusions of ill-health. They range from the belief that something vague and generalized is wrong, to beliefs in the presence of specific diseases. Delusions of infestation are also included under the category of hypochondriacal delusions (see Chapter 22).

Diagnostic significance
Hypochondriacal delusions can present as single systematized delusions in delusional disorders or as symptoms of depression and schizophrenia.

Delusions of love, delusions of infidelity, nihilistic delusions, the delusion of doubles, delusions of infestation and shared delusions are discussed in Chapter 22.

Overvalued ideas

Overvalued ideas are isolated, preoccupying beliefs, accompanied by a strong affective responsef. The ideas tend to dominate the sufferer's life, often indefinitely. They are generally associated with an abnormal personality and grow out of adverse experience in a way that is comprehensible. They may be distinguished from obsessions because the patient does not view them as senseless, i.e. they are ego-syntonic, and from delusions proper because they arise comprehensibly from a given personality and situation, and also do not lead to repeated action considered to be justified. Judgement regarding the presence of an overvalued idea depends somewhat on the absence of other psychopathology (McKenna 1984; Veale 2002).

Diagnostic significance
Disorders which are characterized by overvalued ideas include the querulous paranoid state, morbid jealousy, hypo-chondriasis, dysmorphophobia, parasitophobia, anorexia nervosa, pseudocyesis and apotemnophilia (McKenna, 1984, Veale 2002). Apotemnophilia is a rare disorder in which a person feels that one or more limbs do not seem to belong to them. Overvalued ideas may also be features of an emerging psychosis or an organic disorder.

Dysmorhophobia
The term *body dysmorphic disorder* is used in the DSM IV and this describes the development of an excessive concern with the imagined unsightly appearance of a single, often facial, feature. (Hay 1970). The DSM IV also describes a delusional subtype. The commonest features affected are nose, hair and complexion. The disfigurement is believed to be noticeable to other people but the actual appearance lies within the normal range. Patients more often consult plastic surgeons than psychiatrists. Usually dysmorphophobia is the only complaint, though personality disorders may coexist, or the complaint may be an early symptom of schizophrenia or, less often, depression (McKenna 1984).

Disorders of control of thinking

Normally a person is in control or possession of his thinking but some symptoms are characterized by a dysfunction of this control. The two main phenomena discussed here are obsessions and thought alienation (passivity of thought).

Obsessions
These are recurrent ideas, thoughts, impulses or images that are experienced as being intrusive and senseless but are recognized as the person's own thoughts. The experience is distressing and attempts to resist its content or form are not successful.

Compulsions include actions or cognitions such as praying or counting and are also referred to as rituals.

Thought alienation
This is characterized by the experience of one's thoughts being alien, not emanating from one's own mind, and not being under voluntary control. Three forms of this passivity phenomenon in relation to thinking were described by Schneider (1959) and included as symptoms of first rank for the diagnosis of schizophrenia. These are *thought broadcasting* (*diffusion of thought*), *thought insertion* and *thought withdrawal* (*interruption of thought*). Thought withdrawal may be responsible for thought blocking. In both thought blocking and thought withdrawal the patient describes his/her thoughts as being controlled or influenced by an external agency, therefore these experiences are delusions of control, and are also ego-alien.

Other passivity experiences described by Schneider (1959) are those in which feelings, impulses and will are believed to be the product of others or to be under the direct control of others and are referred to as 'made' phenomena. The term 'made action' has been used interchangeably with 'made impulse'. These experiences represent disturbances of the sense of identity and are delusions of control. Schneider (1959) considered these to be symptoms of first rank for schizophrenia. Somatic passivity is also a first-rank symptom. It consists of somatic hallucinations associated with the belief that outside influences are responsible. Thus again, a hallucination is accompanied by a delusion of control and is considered to be a passivity experience. Clinically, it is essential to ensure that the patient is not using a figure of speech for example 'as though' their arms feel electrified. First-rank symptoms are important diagnostic criteria for schizophrenia in both ICD 10 and DSM IV and are summarized as follows:

- thought echo (*gedenkenlautwerden* and *echo de la pensée*)
- running commentary hallucinations
- voices discussing the patient in the third person (voices arguing)
- delusional perception
- thought broadcast
- thought insertion
- thought withdrawal
- made feeling (emotion)
- made impulse
- made volition (action)
- somatic passivity.

First-rank symptoms were described by Schneider (1959) who suggested that, in the absence of any organic symptoms, the presence of a first-rank symptom suggests a diagnosis of schizophrenia. Further studies have suggested that they are not exclusive to schizophrenia, but there is evidence that when narrower definitions are used they are exclusive to schizophrenia. They lack predictive value with regard to the prognosis and are not inherited. One of their major advantages is their reliability. This has been demonstrated by studies such as the International Pilot Study of Schizophrenia (IPSS), which used the Present State Examination, which relies on the first-rank symptoms.

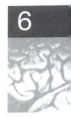

Disorders of the flow of thought

These include flight of ideas, retardation, thought blocking, perseveration and circumstantiality.

Flight of ideas

Flight of ideas occurs when thoughts follow each other rapidly, the connections between successive thoughts are understandable and clang associations, alliterations and other similar phenomena occur. Flight of ideas often occurs in the context of pressure of speech.

Diagnostic significance
Flight of ideas is typical of mania. It can also occasionally occur in schizophrenia and in some organic disorders, especially those resulting from lesions of the hypothalamus (Fish 1967).

Retardation

In retardation, thinking is slowed down and the number of ideas entering consciousness is decreased. This is experienced as difficulty making decisions, loss of concentration and lack of clarity of thinking.

Diagnostic significance
Retardation of thinking is typical of depression.

Thought blocking

This refers to the complete interruption of speech before a thought or an idea has been completely expressed. Occasional loss of the train of thought may be due to poor concentration or distractibility. Thought blocking should only be accepted as present when the patient voluntarily describes it or when on questioning it is clear that a pause in speech is due to the experience of thoughts breaking off or ceasing.

Diagnostic significance
Thought blocking occurs in schizophrenia. It may occur in the context of thought withdrawal.

Perseveration

Perseveration refers to the adherence of an individual to the same concepts and words beyond the point at which they are relevant.

Diagnostic significance
It is characteristically an organic symptom and occurs when consciousness is impaired as in acute organic disorders as well as chronic organic disorders such as dementia.

Circumstantiality

In circumstantiality, speech is very indirect and delayed in reaching its goal due to the inclusion of tedious details.

Diagnostic significance
It is a feature of obsessional personality disorder and probably of temporal lobe epilepsy. Milder forms may be encountered in the absence of any psychiatric or organic disorder.

Formal thought disorder

The term formal thought disorder refers to abnormalities of thought expressed in language, most commonly in speech but also in writing. The term 'thought disorder' may be used to convey the same meaning, but can cause confusion because it is also used to describe all aspects of disordered thinking in psychoses. Historically, formal thought disorder has been described in various ways:

- akataphasia (Kraeplin 1919)
- loosening of associations, condensation, displacement, misuse of symbols (Bleuler 1911)
- asyndesis, metonyms, overinclusion (Cameron 1939)
- derailment, substitution, omission, fusion, drivelling (Shneider 1930)
- other terms: knight's-move thinking, paraphasia, neologisms, tangentiality, circumstantiality.

It is clear that different terms have been used to describe the same abnormalities. These have often been defined rather vaguely making them difficult to elicit. The concept of thought disorder is problematic. Thought disorder is inferred on the basis of disordered speech, that is, an assumption is made that speech directly mirrors thought, but language is self-contained and has a structure independent of thought. Some language for example greetings and introductions does not convey thought (Chaika 1982). Andreasen (1979) has suggested that formal thought disorder is not a homogenous entity but is a multi-level disturbance involving abnormalities of thinking, language and social cognition. She has therefore proposed the use of the term 'communication disorders'.

Some of the commonly used terms and their definitions (adapted from Andreasen 1994) are as follows (some terms are included in parentheses to highlight the overlap in definition):

- **Derailment (loose associations, flight of ideas):** a pattern of spontaneous speech in which ideas slip from one track to another that is either clearly but obliquely related or completely unrelated.
- **Incoherence (word salad, jargon aphasia, paragrammatism):** a pattern of speech that is essentially incomprehensible at times due to several different mechanisms. The difference between derailment and incoherence is based on the abnormality in derailment occurring within the level of sentences and clauses
- **Neologism:** a completely new word or phrase whose derivation cannot be understood.

- **Poverty of speech:** a restriction in the amount of spontaneous speech so that replies to questions tend to be brief, concrete and unelaborated.
- **Poverty of content of speech:** occurs when speech is adequate in amount but tends to convey little information. Language tends to be vague, overabstract, repetitive and stereotyped.
- **Tangentiality:** involves replying to a question in an oblique, tangential or irrelevant manner.

Explanations for thought disorder

Explanations for thought disorder derive from: association psychology (Bleuler 1911); overinclusive thinking (Cameron 1939), which may be studied using object sorting tests; concrete thinking (Goldstein 1944), which may be studied with proverb tests; and personal construct theory (Bannister 1963).

Diagnostic significance

Historically, formal thought disorder has been always associated with the diagnosis of schizophrenia and this is reflected in the ICD 10 and the DSM IV. However thought disorder is not exclusive to schizophrenia (Andreasen 1979) and frequently occurs in mania. It is not a common feature of depression. Thought disorder tends to persist in schizophrenia and patients tend to exhibit negative thought disorders such as poverty of speech in addition to positive thought disorders such as derailment (Andreasen 1994).

DISORDERS OF MOTOR ACTIVITY

Abnormal motor behaviour is a feature of many psychiatric illnesses, either as a disorder of movement intrinsic to the illness or, more commonly, as side effects of commonly prescribed drugs. In addition several neurological motor disorders (Huntington's chorea, Parkinson's disease) also present with psychiatric symptoms (see Chapter 26).

Psychiatric motor disorders include increased or decreased motor activity and catatonic symptoms.

Increased motor activity

This manifests as hyperactivity and agitation. In hyperactivity the increased motor activity is goal directed and is associated with pressured speech and distractibility usually in the context of mania.

In agitation the increased activity is non-goal directed and the subject is distressed. Agitation occurs in depression, schizophrenia, organic disorders and anxiety states. In cases where antipsychotic medication has been commenced agitation should be distinguished from akathisia.

The term *excitement* is also used to describe markedly increased motor activity. Excitement occurs in a variety of disorders but catatonic excitement occurs predominantly in schizophrenia and consists of senseless and purposeless overactivity (Fish 1967).

Decreased motor activity

This manifests as retardation or stupor and is usually a symptom of depression with melancholic symptoms (endogenous depression), and organic disorders. The term *psychomotor retardation* implies a slowing down of both psychic and motor activity. Clinically, motor activity is also slowed down due to parkinsonian side effects of antipsychotics.

Stupor is a state of extreme motor retardation characterized by akinesis and mutism in a setting of preserved consciousness. Tumours of the third ventricle also cause stupor or akinetic mutism. It can occur in schizophrenia, affective disorders (usually depression but occasionally mania) and hysteria. Stupor, also referred to as 'catatonic stupor', always merits careful investigation.

Catatonic symptoms

These may be separated into spontaneous and induced movement disorders.

Spontaneous movement disorders

- **Posturing:** the maintenance of strange and uncomfortable postures for long periods of time
- **Schnauz-krampf:** a characteristic facial expression in which the nose and lips are drawn together
- **Stereotypies:** unusual repetitive, non-goal directed movements
- **Mannerisms:** unusual, repetitive, goal directed movements
- **Obstruction:** the person stops while carrying out a normal activity
- **Mutism:** the absence of speech in preserved consciousness.

Induced movement disorders

- **Waxy flexibility (flexibilitas cerea):** the patient may be placed in strange uncomfortable positions and will maintain them for a minute or more.
- **Automatic obedience:** the patient carries out every command in a literal concrete fashion.
- *Mitmachen* **(cooperation):** passive bodily movements initiated by the examiner, for example a light touch on the inner arm will result in patient raising arm.
- *Mitgehen* **(extreme cooperation):** an extreme form of mitmachen.
- **Echolalia/echopraxia:** the patient repeats the actions or speech of the examiner.

- **Negativism:** the patient actively resists all attempts to make contact during the examination.
- *Gegenhalten* (opposition): the patient opposes all passive movements with the same degree of force as that applied by examiner.

Other catatonic symptoms include psychological pillow (the patient maintains their head a few inches off the bed or couch by sustained contraction of the sternomastoid muscles); mannerisms and stereotypies of speech; and catatonic excitement and stupor (see above).

Diagnostic significance

Catatonia has always been associated with the diagnosis of schizophrenia. However, catatonic presentations may occur with focal neurological lesions, intoxications, metabolic disturbances and in affective disorders, particularly bipolar disorder (Fien and McGrath 1990). When eliciting catatonic features such as waxy flexibility, automatic obedience, echophenomena and cooperation, the patient must be told clearly to resist the examiner's commands and attempts to move their limbs.

DISORDERS OF EMOTION

Describing mood and feelings and eliciting their associated symptoms is one of the most important skills of clinical examination because mood disorders are extremely common.

The terms used to describe this aspect of psychopathology are often employed interchangeably and overlap with everyday words (example, 'feeling' which has multiple meanings). Definitions of these terms vary, and sometimes they are differentiated on the basis of duration and intensity:

- *feeling* describes a positive or negative subjective reaction to an experience
- *affect* is used to describe the overall emotional state, inferred objectively
- *mood* is a prolonged emotional state.

In practice the terms are often used interchangeably.

Abnormal moods

- depression
- elation
- emotional lability
- euphoria
- ecstasy
- apathy
- affective blunting/flattening
- anxiety
- irritability.

Depression

Depression of mood is common and subjective experience may include feeling sad, despondent, dejected, despairing, hopeless, apathetic or indifferent. Anxiety is a common concomitant symptom. Depressed mood may be accompanied by slowing of thoughts and actions (psychomotor retardation), occasionally by stupor, and by agitation and restlessness. Concentration and decision making are impaired. Feelings of guilt hopelessness, helplessness and unworthiness occur, and suicidal thoughts are common. Depression is also associated with anhedonia, the loss of ability to experience pleasure (Snaith 1993).

Elation

Elation of mood, the subjective experience of feeling happy and cheerful, is often accompanied by overactivity, rapid thoughts, distractibility, pressure of speech and flight of ideas. It is a classic feature of mania. Elation may turn to irritability if attempts are made to curtail the patient's overactivity. Elation may occur in schizophrenia and organic disorders and is distinguished from mania on the basis of the lack of communicability of the mood and the absence of associated features such as flight of ideas or grandiosity.

Emotional lability

This is characterized by rapid changes of mood from one extreme to the other. Lability of affect occurs in personality disorders, the manic phase of bipolar affective disorder and in mixed affective states.

Affective incontinence is characterized by a complete loss of control over emotions, the patient crying or laughing for long periods of time with no provocation. It occurs in multi-infarct dementia, pseudobulbar palsy and multiple sclerosis.

Euphoria

This is a state of excessive, unreasonable cheerfulness. It can be a normal phenomenon but more often occurs in mania and organic conditions such as multiple sclerosis and general paresis of the insane. In frontal lobe syndrome a silly euphoria with lack of foresight and general indifference may occur. This is called moria or *Witzelsucht*.

Ecstasy

This is a state of extreme wellbeing associated with a feeling of bliss and grace. It can occur in healthy individuals and during religious experiences, but more often occurs in schizophrenia and organic states, especially temporal lobe epilepsy.

Apathy

This is the absence of feeling and is often associated with anergia (the person lacks physical energy and is inactive, sitting around for long periods of time) and lack of volition (the person shows no internal drive). Apathy and the related symptoms are characteristic of schizophrenia and with other symptoms such as poverty of speech and social withdrawal, are often referred to as the negative symptoms of schizophrenia (see Chapter 18).

Affective blunting

Blunting of affect refers to a lack of emotional sensitivity, which overlaps with inappropriate affect, which refers to affect that is strikingly inconsistent with the patient's thoughts or environmental circumstances. The term 'incongruent' is sometimes used to refer to affect that is not in keeping with the patient's stated mood.

Flattening of affect refers to a less marked limitation of the usual range of emotions.

Anxiety

This describes the subjective experience of fear and is usually accompanied by subjective bodily discomfort such as a sense of constriction in the chest leading to difficulty in breathing, and overactivity of the autonomic nervous system with tachycardia, piloerection, pallor and sweating. Anxiety may be a state or trait, and may be generalized or situational.

Panic attacks are characterized by hyperventilation with subsequent hypocapnia and its symptoms and an overwhelming fear of death or becoming insane, and depersonalization. Attacks usually last several minutes. Depersonalization may be classified as a disorder of the awareness of self. The most prominent feature is a feeling of change involving the inner and/or outer worlds associated with a vague but uncomfortable sense of unfamiliarity. The experience may be described as 'unreal' or 'detached' but patients characteristically find it difficult to provide a comprehensible account. The experience has an 'as if' quality. When the environment is felt to be unreal the term derealization is used. Four features of depersonalization have been described by Acker (1954):

1. Feelings of unreality; unreality is used as a generic term.
2. Unpleasant quality.
3. Nondelusional nature.
4. Loss of affective response.

Diagnostic significance

Depersonalization may occur in healthy individuals but is most commonly described in association with agoraphobia, panic disorder and other phobic states. It has also been described in depression and as a separate syndrome. Depersonalization may also occur in temporal lobe epilepsy and drug intoxication. Clinically it must be distinguished from passivity experiences in schizophrenia.

Irritability

Irritability is a common feature of psychopathological disorder that is not confined to diagnostic categories (Snaith 1991). It is characterized by reduced control over temper, which usually results in irascible verbal or behavioural outbursts, but irritable mood may be present without observable symptoms. Irritability may be experienced as brief episodes in particular circumstances, or may be prolonged or generalized. The experience of irritability is always unpleasant for the individual and overt manifestation lacks the cathartic effect of justified outbursts of anger (Snaith and Taylor 1985).

Diagnostic significance

Irritability is associated with premenstrual syndrome, depression (particularly in young depressed patients) and in postnatal depression.

INSIGHT

Insight is included in the current chapter as assessment of insight is a very important aspect of clinical examination. It is a commonly used term and its meaning differs according to the professionals using it or the situations it is used in. In psychotherapy for instance the emphasis is on subjective understanding and determining and differentiating emotional and intellectual insight. In clinical psychiatry, especially in psychotic disorders, it is useful to concentrate on the practical aspects of insight and as suggested by David (1990), assess insight on the following three dimensions: (1) awareness of illness; (2) the capacity to relate psychotic experiences as abnormal; and (3) treatment compliance. These features are important as they relate to the patient engaging in treatment and the future course of treatment.

REFERENCES

Ackner B (1954) Depersonalization I. Aetiology and phenomenology. *Journal of Mental Science* **100**: 838–53.

Ali JA (2002) Musical hallucinations and deafness: a case report and review of the literature. *Neuropsychiatry Neuropsychology and Behavioural Neurology* **15**: 66–70.

Andreasen NC (1979) Thought language and communication disorders: 2. diagnostic significance. *Archives of General Psychiatry* **36**: 1325–30.

Andreasen NC (1994) Thought disorder. In: Winokur G. & Clayton PJ (eds) *The Medical Basis of Psychiatry*, 2nd edn. Philadelphia: WB Saunders.

Bannister D (1963) The genesis of schizophrenic thought disorder. A serial invalidation hypothesis. *British Journal of Psychiatry* **109**: 680–6.

Bleuler E (1911) *Dementia Praecox*. Leipzig: Franz Deuticke.

Cameron N (1939) Schizophrenic thinking in a problem solving situation. *Journal of Mental Science* **85**: 1012–1035.

Chaika, E. (1982). Thought disorder or speech disorder in schizophrenia? *Schizophrenia Bulletin* **11**: 8–14.

David AS (1990) Insight and psychosis. *British Journal of Psychiatry* **156**: 798–808.

Fien S & McGrath MG (1990) Problems in diagnosing bipolar disorder in catatonic patients. *Journal of Clinical Psychiatry* **51**: 203–10.

Fish F (1967) *Clinical Psychopathology*. Bristol: John Wright.

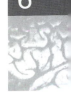

Goldstein K (1944) Methodological approach to the study of schizophrenic thought disorder. In: Kasanin JS (ed.) *Language and Thought in Schizophrenia*. Berkeley: University of California Press.

Hay GG (1970) Dysmorhophobia. *British Journal of Psychiatry* **116**: 399–406.

Jaspers K (1959) *General Psychopathology*, 7th edn (trans. J Hoenig & MW Hamilton 1963). Manchester: Manchester University Press.

Kraupl–Taylor F (1983) Descriptive and developmental phenomenology. In: Speherd M & Zangwill OL (eds) *Handbook of Psychiatry*, Vol. 1. Cambridge: Cambridge University Press.

Kraeplin E (1919) *Dementia Praecox and Paraphrenia* (trans. Barclay, M.). Edinburgh: Churchill Livingstone.

Manford M & Andermann, F. (1998) Complex visual hallucinations. Clinical and neurobiological insights. *Brain* **121**: 1819–40.

Mckenna PJ (1984) Disorders with overvalued ideas. *The British Journal of Psychiatry* **145**: 579–85.

Rector NA & Beck AT (2002) Cognitive therapy for schizophrenia from conceptualization to intervention. *Canadian Journal of Psychiatry* **47**: 39–48.

Schneider C (1930) *Psychologie der Schizophrenen*. Leipzig: Thième.

Schneider K (1959) *Clinical Psychopathology* (trans. BW Hamilton). New York: Grune & Stratton.

Sims A (1991) Delusional syndromes in ICD-10. *British Journal of Psychiatry* **159**(suppl. 14): 46–51.

Sims A (1995) *Symptoms in the Mind*, 2nd edn. London: WB Saunders.

Slade PD (1976) Hallucinations. *Psychological Medicine* **6**: 7–13.

Snaith P (1991) *Clinical Neurosis*, 2nd edn. Oxford: Oxford University Press.

Snaith RP (1993) Anhedonia: a neglected symptom of psychopathology. *Psychological Medicine* **23**: 957–66.

Snaith RP & Taylor CM (1985) Irritability: definition, assessment and associated factors. *British Journal of Psychiatry* **147**: 127–36.

Stein DJ, Le Roux L, Bouwer C & Van Heerden B (1998) Is olfactory reference syndrome an obsessive-compulsive spectrum disorder?: two cases and a discussion. *Journal of Neuropsychiatry and Clinical Neurosciences* **10**: 96–9.

Stompe T, Ortwein-Swoboda G, Ritter K & Schanda H (2003) Old wine in new bottles? Stability and plasticity of schizophrenic delusions. *Psychopathology* **36**: 6–12.

Teunisse RJ, Cruysberg JRM, Verbeek A & Zitman G (1995) The Charles-Bonnet syndrome: a large prospective study in The Netherlands. *The British Journal of Psychiatry* **166**: 254–8.

Veale D (2002) Overvalued ideas: a conceptual analysis. *Behaviour Research and Therapy* **40**: 383–400.

Wing JK, Cooper JE & Sartorius N (1974) *The Description and Classification of Psychiatric Symptoms: An Instruction Manual for the PSE and Calego System*. London: Cambridge University Press.

Social psychiatry and sociology

Claire Henderson and Michael Phelan

INTRODUCTION

Social psychiatry is the study of: (1) social factors associated with the onset, course and outcome of psychiatric disorders; (2) social influences on the nature and availability of treatment; and (3) the social implications of mental illness for patients, their carers and their families. All of these areas are discussed in this chapter, along with the sociological theories and concepts that underpin social psychiatry.

SOCIAL FACTORS ASSOCIATED WITH THE ONSET, COURSE AND OUTCOME OF PSYCHIATRIC DISORDERS

Epidemiology is the main tool used for examining the influence of social and demographic factors on psychiatric disorder. Data from large populations can provide evidence for possible aetiological theories and guide rational service planning. This section summarizes the research findings on rates of psychiatric morbidity within the general population and highlights the populations most at risk. Some of the aetiological theories explaining these findings are considered and specific psychosocial factors such as life events and expressed emotion are discussed. Epidemiological methodology is described in Chapter 9.

Social and demographic factors associated with mental disorder

Social class

Definition and measurement

Social class has traditionally been defined in the UK on the basis of occupation using the Registrar General's classification introduced in 1911 (Box 7.1).

The shortcomings of this system are increasingly recognized. For instance, non-working mothers are classified according to their husband's occupation, and there are difficulties in rating those who work part-time, are retired or

are unemployed. Also, the status and pay of individuals engaged in various occupations changes over time, and some job titles, for example 'engineer', may be applied to a wide range of occupations, with very different levels of qualifications and pay. In the USA, a broader concept of socio-economic status (SES) is usually used. This combines measures of education and income, and sometimes of occupation and area of residence.

Sociologists are increasingly moving away from hierarchical models of social class to models involving a core and peripheries. The core is composed of full-time employees; moving away from the centre are part-time, temporary and self-employed workers, and beyond them are the short- and long-term unemployed. Outside this is the 'underclass', including homeless people and refugees.

Despite the problems inherent in defining and measuring social class, there are clear and consistent social class gradients in morbidity and mortality for all ages and for nearly all diseases. Thus, individuals classified as social class V are twice as likely to die before retirement and have twice the neonatal mortality compared to those in social class I.

Social class and mental illness

In Britain, the National Psychiatric Morbidity Study (NPMS) (e.g. Meltzer et al. 1995) demonstrated that rates of non-psychotic disorders are highest among people in social classes IV and V, and that functional psychotic disorders and drug and alcohol dependence are commonest in social class

Box 7.1	Registrar general's classification of social class
I	Professional, landowners and higher managerial
II	Intermediate
III	Skilled workers
IV	Semi-skilled workers
V	Unskilled workers
O	Students, retired

95

V. When the individual components of social class were examined, having no educational qualifications increased the risk of a depressive episode, while being economically inactive or unemployed increased the risk of most disorders (see below on unemployment). Similar findings have been reported from the USA. The Epidemiological Catchment Area (ECA) study demonstrated that the association between SES and mental disorder is strongest for schizophrenia, intermediate for alcohol abuse and dependence, and weakest for depression (Holzer et al. 1986). Studies on the true prevalence and treated incidence of schizophrenia, suggest that low class confers a relative risk of 2–3. Other studies, which have included less developed countries, have not replicated these findings consistently (World Health Organization 1979).

Two hypotheses have been proposed to explain the differing rates of schizophrenia in industrialized countries. The social causation theory suggests that exposure to social stressors induces the onset or relapse of schizophrenia. The selection/drift model, in contrast, proposes that schizophrenia itself causes a reduction in social status compared to the parental generation, and a progressive deterioration in the patient's socio-economic status. These processes are not mutually exclusive, and the relative importance of each may vary over time and place. Social selection is most visible before any process of social drift has started. However, the onset of social drift relative both to the parental status and to expectations based on early academic performance may begin very early, often before admission to hospital (Goldberg & Morrison 1963). After many years during which the drift theory held sway, it is now being challenged by the suggestion that social deprivation and city life (e.g. Lewis et al. 1992) are mainly responsible for the social class gradient (see Chapter 18 also).

Age

Psychiatric disorders common to children and adolescents show the same patterns for risk by social class and geographical location as those in adults (Rutter 1989). The group at highest overall risk of mental illness includes children and adolescents in care.

In elderly people, depression is not more common, but is more severe and more likely to require hospital admission. Admission is related not only to severity but to the higher rates of living alone (50% over the age of 75 years), coexistence of physical disorder and risk of suicide. Among the elderly, those at greatest risk of depression are those in residential homes and medical wards, where the rate of depression, at 20–30%, is two or three times higher than that of the background population.

Sex

In the UK, the NPMS showed a one-week prevalence for neurotic disorders of 19.5% in women, compared to 12.3% in men. Men had considerably higher rates of alcohol and drug dependence. In this survey, there were no sex differences in the overall rates of psychoses. However, service use appears to be higher in men with schizophrenia; the onset of illness is earlier; and the course, outcome and treatment response are less favourable when compared to women.

Marital status

For both sexes, the prevalence of non-psychotic disorders is lowest for married individuals and highest for those who are divorced or separated (Meltzer et al. 1995). A similar pattern exists for schizophrenia, although heavy service users are more likely to be unmarried.

Ethnic group

In countries with large immigrant populations, some ethnic groups have similar rates of mental illness as exist in the general population (e.g. people from South Asia in Britain), whereas other groups have higher rates. In Britain, for example, particular attention has been paid to African Caribbeans, who are 3–5 times as likely to be admitted to hospital with schizophrenia, compared to the native population (London 1986). A study in Nottingham found that rates of hospitalization for schizophrenia may be even higher among second-generation African Caribbeans (Harrison 1988), and these individuals are also more often compulsorily treated (Davies et al. 1996) and are less satisfied with mental health services than other patients (Parkman et al. 1997).

Employment status

Unemployment can impair physical and mental health and increase the risk of suicide and deliberate self-harm. Unsatisfactory and insecure employment may have a similar impact. The extent to which this is due to the resulting impoverishment versus the non-financial benefits of working may vary with individual circumstances.

At an ecological level, the unemployment rate was the most effective predictor of psychiatric admissions in Bristol (Kammerling & O'Connor 1993), while at the individual level, the NPMS showed that unemployment, rather than economic inactivity (including due to disability), was the variable most consistently associated with mental illness. Only living alone or in rented accommodation approached a similar level of impact (Meltzer et al. 1995).

Geographic variation

Area level factors

In recent years there has been a resurgence of research into the effects of residential environments on the risk of mental disorder and suicide for all or certain groups of residents, regardless of their individual characteristics. Broadly, the hypothesis is that contextual features of residential environments, usually referred to as area level factors, may be related to health outcomes even after individual factors are taken into account. This adjustment for individual level factors represents a refinement of the ecological study where only area level factors are studied (see Chapter 9), as well as an improvement on surveys of individuals, which ignore their context. The influence of context may be exerted for example through chronic stressors related to neighborhood characteristics or aspects of neighborhoods that affect social support and access to goods and services; at a wider level public policies may exert an effect. The geographic areas investigated have ranged from large regions of countries with populations of several million to neighborhoods of a few thousand people.

One example of an area level effect is that of group density. This has been studied most extensively for ethnic density; it is suggested that, for people from a specific ethnic group, rates of mental disorder decrease if the proportion of people from the same ethnic group increases in the local population (Halpern 1993). A similar protective effect has also been described for density of occupation and religious affiliation. The effect is thought to be mediated through increased levels of social support and reduced levels of stress, and has been shown for rates of psychiatric hospitalization (e.g. Faris & Dunham 1939), treated rates of psychoses (Boydell et al. 2001), suicide (Neeleman & Wessley 1999) and nonfatal self-harm (Neeleman et al. 2001). With respect to common mental disorder (anxiety and depression), the ethnic density hypothesis has been supported in a sample from England and Wales (Halpern & Nazroo 1999). For ethnic minorities, the protective relationship of ethnic density on mental health found by these authors remained after adjustment for language fluency, and was strengthened by adjusting for economic hardship.

Intra-urban patterns

For 60 years ecological studies have shown higher rates of admission for schizophrenia in inner city populations, when compared to populations from suburban areas (e.g. Faris & Dunham 1939). These patterns are stable over time and to some degree independent of the ethnicity, housing status or age composition of the local population.

Urban–rural differences

Dohrenwend (1975) reported that overall prevalence rates of psychosis showed little rural–urban difference, but that the prevalence of schizophrenia appeared higher and manic-depressive psychosis lower, in cities. More recent work has demonstrated that being born in a city is associated with a higher risk of developing schizophrenia, indicating that social drift cannot explain this variation entirely (Lewis et al. 1992). For non-psychotic disorders, the NPMS discovered higher rates of generalized anxiety disorder, depressive episodes and phobias in urban compared to semirural and rural populations.

Residential mobility

Higher rates of schizophrenia in areas of high residential mobility were suggested by the work of Faris & Dunham in

Chicago (1939) and reinforced by further research in Los Angeles (Dear & Wolch 1987).

Accommodation

Individuals who live alone, and those who live in overcrowded and/or council housing are more likely to have a mental disorder. The NPMS (Meltzer et al. 1995) demonstrated that living in rented accommodation in contrast to occupier-owned accommodation increased risk for functional psychosis and for most non-psychotic disorders (Box 7.2).

Box 7.2 Summary of sociodemographic factors that influence psychiatric morbidity rates	
Strong research evidence for	*Reasonable evidence for*
Unemployment	Inner city residence
Social class	High residential mobility
Sex	
Ethnic group	
Living situation	
Marital status	

Homelessness

Homeless individuals are a heterogeneous group, found in a variety of accommodation settings:

- 'roofless' (e.g. sleeping in parks)
- hostels for the homeless
- emergency accommodation
- precariously housed (e.g. squatting, staying with friends)
- institutional (e.g. prisons, hospitals).

People who are street homeless (roofless) are the visible minority of the overall homeless population. It is difficult to count the homeless, and routine indicators of psychopathology such as social withdrawal, suspiciousness and poor personal hygiene may erroneously suggest the presence of mental illness in a population in whom these features may be the norm. Estimating the rate of mental disorder among homeless people is therefore difficult. But while estimates vary, they are universally high when this population is compared to the general population. High rates of suicide and childhood adversity are also reported in young homeless people (Craig & Hodson 1998).

Closure of large mental hospitals does not appear to have increased the number of homeless mentally ill people directly because few patients discharged after long-stay hospitalization ('the old long stay') become homeless. However, 'new long stay' (NLS) patients (defined as those in acute hospital beds for over 6 months) accumulate in hospitals because of the difficulty in finding them suitable accommodation. About 10% of patients admitted to psychiatric wards are of no fixed abode (Box 7.3).

Box 7.3 Groups at high risk for mental illness
Children in local authority care
Homeless individuals
Elderly people no longer living independently
Refugees and asylum seekers

Understanding the associations between social factors and psychiatric morbidity

Several authors interpret the above results in terms of constructs presumed to mediate the relationships. Thus it is proposed that poverty, social isolation and social disorganization, all of which have been suggested to explain physical health inequalities, are responsible for mental health inequalities. These constructs themselves present challenges in measurement due to a lack of data and difficulty of definition.

Poverty

The observation that reductions in absolute poverty in developed countries have not reduced social class gradients in health has stimulated two variations on the basic concept that poverty causes these gradients. Wilkinson (1989) suggests that the extent of inequality between social classes is now the most significant factor contributing to health inequalities in developed countries. Income inequality is a variable only measurable at the group level. However, when individual income is also controlled for, the results of studies focusing on income inequality and deprivation or neighborhood socio-economic status (SES) have been conflicting.

The second suggestion is that social mobility has decreased, at least for the American poor, such that poverty is now 'chronic rather than episodic, more intractable and more concentrated' (Rogler 1996). This may increase the incidence of psychiatric disorders by increasing the likelihood of 'cumulative adversity', i.e. the lifetime exposure to traumatic events (including life events as described below) and stressors that are more enduring than for other groups.

Social isolation

Social isolation as a cause for inequalities in mental health was suggested by Hare (1956), who found an ecological correlation between schizophrenia admission rates and districts with a high proportion of the population living alone. The alternative, Hare suggested, was that affected individuals clustered in poorer, isolated households. Whatever the causal relationship, it appears that psychiatric patients who are isolated or who lack social support – the unmarried, the unemployed, those living alone and those without religious affiliations – are disproportionately heavy users of the mental health services.

Social disorganization

Studies in Chicago led to the view that urban areas with high psychiatric morbidity suffered social disorganization, another factor only measurable at the area level. This is characterized by excessive residential mobility, ethnic conflict, communication breakdown and a lack of consensus (Dunham 1965). These ideas are representative of the Chicago school of sociology, which drew parallels between individual pathology and social disorganization, and which greatly influenced contemporary social psychiatric literature. Thus, recent studies of the relationship between community disorder (defined as a lack of social control reflected by residents' reports of noise, litter, vandalism, graffiti, drug use and trouble with neighbors; Ross 2000) and depressive symptoms have found a small but consistent relationship after adjustment for individual level characteristics.

Psychosocial risk factors

Life events

'Life events' (LEs), can be defined as occurrences that happen to most people at some time during their lives, but which are nevertheless extraordinary occurrences for the individual (Dohrenwend 1975). LEs include bereavement, birth of a first child, physical illness, redundancy and marriage. Such stressful events taken singly may be opportunities for the development of adaptive coping behaviours; the assumption in LEs research is that certain types of event in certain circumstances, or an excess of events, are likely to cause psychiatric disorder in certain people.

Early attempts to study the aetiological role of LEs used a simple checklist of potential events. Based on surveys of the general population, events were ranked according to their perceived impact. Scores were then added for events over a given time reported by an individual to estimate the amount of stress experienced. Subsequently, it was pointed out that combining scores for these events could confound any causal relationship, as some events such as divorce or losing a job could occur as a result of pre-existing psychiatric illness. This led to the distinction between independent and possibly independent LEs (Brown & Birley 1968). If a man loses his job because his firm closes, this is most likely independent; however, if he is sacked shortly prior to being diagnosed as having schizophrenia, independence cannot be assumed. A similar concept is that of 'fateful loss' (Shrout et al. 1989), defined as 'any adverse event that is outside of the control of the person and causes significant negative disruption in the person's life'. Detailed information is required to determine the fatefulness and disruptiveness of the event.

The likelihood that a specific LE would have different implications for different people led to the term 'contextual threat', referring to the total threat considering the psychosocial features of the individual (Brown & Harris 1978). This concept and the research that has used it has been criticized for combining variable and unsystematized information rather than measuring several social and psychological constructs independently. However, the Brown and Harris Life Events and Difficulties Scale remains the most reliable and established measure for recording LEs themselves.

A further problem of much LEs research is that it is retrospective and is thus potentially subject to bias. Events intervening between the index LE and collection of data may influence the respondent's perception of the index event, while 'effort after meaning' may cause difficulties in establishing temporal relationships between LEs and onset of disorder. These same factors may cause relative under-reporting in the control group.

Requirements to establish a causal role for life events in psychiatric disorder

- clear correlation between LE and onset of disorder
- LE must lead to disorder, not vice versa
- satisfactory theoretical construct
- confounding variables must be excluded
- relationship should hold across different populations at different times.

As the majority of individuals do not become depressed following a LE, Brown & Harris (1978) developed the idea of 'vulnerability factors' in an attempt to explain why some individuals were more vulnerable to the effects of LEs than others. They identified four factors in women living in an inner city area, which increased risk for depression:

- loss of mother before age 11 years
- not working outside the home
- lack of a confiding relationship
- three or more children under age 15 at home.

A problem with these factors is that all but loss of mother before age 11 years would also be included in the rating of contextual threat, used to decide on the severity of the LEs. The resulting association between LEs and vulnerability could therefore overestimate the causal role of LEs. This may explain why attempts to replicate these findings have shown only loss of mother before age 11 years to be a relatively consistent vulnerability factor (Brown & Prudo 1981). However, the remaining factors are of importance in that their presence is inversely related to treatment seeking.

The study of the contribution of LEs to schizophrenia suggests that they are more important with respect to relapse than onset (Tennant 1985). When compared with depression, the LEs related to relapse of schizophrenia are less severe and occur within a shorter interval prior to the psychotic illness.

Trauma/extreme situation

LEs research was stimulated by observations of the effects of combat on soldiers during the Second World War. A range of psychiatric disorders, including psychoses, were diagnosed in soldiers suffering from 'battle fatigue'. A similar process followed the Vietnam War, and led to the description of post-traumatic stress disorder (PTSD) in veterans, and to its subsequent recognition in survivors of civil disasters. More recently PTSD has been diagnosed following events that increasingly overlap those events studied in LEs research. The marked comorbidity between PTSD and depression, anxiety and substance abuse is perhaps a reflection of an artificial separation in terms of both classification and research between an aetiologically defined disorder such as PTSD and non-aetiologically defined disorders such as depression.

SOCIAL FACTORS AND TREATMENT

Provision and resource allocation

In Britain, proxy measures of social deprivation are used to try and distribute mental health resources equably. The Jarman Under Privileged Area (UPA) score and the Mental Illness Needs Index (MINI) are two of the measures commonly used (Box 7.4).

There is a strong association between measures of deprivation and psychiatric admission rates (Thornicroft

Box 7.4 Proxy measures for resource allocation	
Census data used in Jarman UPA score	*Census data used in Mental Illness Needs Index (MINI)*
Rate of unemployment	Social isolation
Overcrowding	Poverty
Proportion of single-parent families	Unemployment
Number of children under age 5	Permanent sickness
Proportion of elderly living alone	Temporary housing
Residential mobility	
Poor housing	
Crime rates	

1991); the highest positive associations are found with notification of drug addiction and standardized mortality rates, and the highest negative associations with levels of car ownership. Such associations probably reflect an increased likelihood of being admitted to hospital with a given disorder, as well as an absolute increase in the rates of disorders. As the relationship between deprivation and rates of psychiatric disorder is complex, service planners need precise data about their local population, as well as epidemiological data collected nationally.

Access and pathways into care

Goldberg & Huxley (1980) have described the 'filters' to be passed through before an individual reaches psychiatric care. First, a person must decide whether he/she has a disorder or not, and then decide whether to consult their general practitioner (GP). At the next stage the GP may or may not recognize that the patient has a psychiatric disorder, and may or may not decide to refer the person to specialist services. Social and demographic characteristics of the patient and the GP influence the recognition and referral rates; features of the local service, such as waiting times for outpatient appointments, will also influence referral rates.

The Epidemiological Catchment Area (ECA) study (Shapiro et al. 1984) showed that the following factors predict greater likelihood of receiving psychiatric treatment:

- higher social class
- young adult age
- male gender
- city residence
- divorced or separated status
- geographically accessible services.

The NPMS found that 18% of adults with a psychotic disorder and living in private households had received no relevant services in the previous year, while a further 18% had received care only from their GP.

Black patients in the UK suffer access barriers in that they are less likely than whites and Asians to have mental health problems recognized by their GP (Commander et al. 1997). For Asians, the difficulties in accessing mental health care occur both at the level of under-recognition compared to whites and at the level of relative under-referral from primary to secondary care. Mixed-sex wards also create a barrier to inpatient service use for women, especially those from certain ethnic and religious groups. Refugees, asylum seekers, children in care, elderly people no longer living independently and homeless people are all among the groups at high risk of mental illness. Many of these individuals are already in contact with a range of statutory services but nonetheless, their psychiatric illness is often undertreated. Improved inter-agency working should facilitate the identification and treatment of those in need. The nature of the disorder will also influence access to

specialist care, with the most severe psychiatric disorders being the most likely to be treated (Table 7.1).

Nature of care

There are particular problems with service provision in relation to individuals from ethnic minority groups. Black patients in Britain are not only over-represented among hospitalized patients, but are also more likely to be detained under the Mental Health Act (Davies et al. 1996), to be admitted to psychiatric intensive care facilities and to have been imprisoned. In one study, the proportion of African-Caribbeans with poor outcome at one year was 2.5 times that of white individuals with schizophrenia (Bhugra et al. 1997). Behind these findings lies the problem that black patients find statutory service provision unacceptable and thus are less likely to seek help. The development of voluntary sector services supported by the statutory sector may be an appropriate alternative, particularly since the numbers of black patients in a given area will usually not warrant the provision of an entire sectorized mental health team.

An important subgroup of patients requiring care in certain areas of most countries is refugees and asylum seekers. People who have been forced to migrate, especially those who have been subjected to organized violence or torture, have a particularly high prevalence of mental disorder, but local mental health services are often ill-equipped to identify and manage psychiatric problems in this context. Linguistic and cultural differences can further impede access to care and, additionally, individuals who are detained while their refugee status is investigated are often suspicious of government agencies and may therefore be unwilling to seek or accept help (see Chapter 8).

SOCIAL IMPACT OF MENTAL ILLNESS

Stigma

Stigma is the attribution of prejudicial characteristics to a whole class of people. Those with chronic mental illness are viewed with distaste and fear (e.g. Link et al. 1987), which has a profound impact upon them. Stigma operates both through discrimination by others and through 'self-stigmatization', resulting in loss of self-esteem and confidence to participate in activities that might facilitate

Table 7.1 Proportion of patients receiving treatment

Diagnosis	Median % of true cases ever in treatment
All psychiatric diagnoses	27
All psychoses	60
Schizophrenia	83

recovery. Mechanic et al. (1994) demonstrated that patients who do not attribute their problems to mental illness (and thus reject the label 'mentally ill') have a higher measured quality of life, lower sense of stigma and higher self-esteem, than those who perceive themselves as mentally ill. Furthermore, the consequences of stigmatization, such as loss of social support and unemployment, are themselves powerful risk factors for mental illness (see above). Stigma also impacts on families who have to cope with 'stigma by association' (for a more detailed discussion see Chapter 11).

Impact of mental illness on social roles

The direct impact of mental illness and its associated stigma will often reduce the number of social roles (e.g. mother, housewife, employee, friend) undertaken by an individual. However, Greenberg et al. (1994) have highlighted the positive roles played by many patients with a mental illness within their families, particularly in the provision of companionship and help around the house.

The 'sick role' was first described by Parsons (1951). When ill, an individual is relieved of occupational and domestic obligations and becomes entitled to care and sympathy. At the same time such an individual is expected to demonstrate a desire to recover, for example by accepting the doctor's diagnosis and complying with treatment. The 'sick role' concept is less applicable in the context of rehabilitation for chronic illness during which the patient is encouraged to resume his or her normal duties to as great an extent as possible. It is also less applicable to illness that is regarded as self-induced (such as addictions), and illness that is stigmatized and thus does not attract care and sympathy. Furthermore, disagreements between patients and psychiatrists about the cause and meaning of their symptoms or behaviour are frequent, and may lead to patients being described as without insight or non-compliant with treatment. The resolution of such difficulties by reattribution therapy has become an important part of treatment for individuals with psychogenic physical symptoms, while compliance therapy seeks to change the attitudes and illness behaviour of patients by education about the nature of their illness and its treatment.

For many patients mental health professionals and fellow patients may be the only people who do not automatically reject them. This can lead to an understandable unwillingness on the part of patients to reduce contact with services when deemed appropriate by professionals. This may on occasion lead to a worsening of symptoms or to problematic behaviours. This may frustrate professionals, and may result in rejection or pejorative labeling. However, this sequence of events has also been described in a more constructive manner in terms of attachment theory by Adshead (1998), who has considered mental health professionals as attachment figures.

The rejection or acceptance of a psychiatric diagnosis and treatment may be described as facets of 'illness behaviour', a term introduced by Mechanic (1968) to describe people's responses to illness (or at least to what many regard as illness). This commences with the perception of a problem on the part of the sufferer (or those close to him or her), followed by decisions as to whether this problem represents illness or not, and if so, future decisions about advice and treatment (usually from family or friends initially). Different patterns of consulting with doctors, e.g. a higher frequency among women when compared to men, has been suggested to result from differences in illness behaviour rather than in actual morbidity. In addition to sociodemographic factors, prior experience of health services is also likely to play a role in deciding whether or not to seek help from the same source again.

The specific social roles of the mentally ill within the context of the mental health care system have been described by sociologists and anthropologists such as Goffman (1961). Recently, the roles of many patients have broadened through membership of user groups. Such groups are beginning to play a part in the selection of mental health professionals, the training of students and junior psychiatrists and in influencing priorities and methods in mental health research. They also campaign for improvements in mental health services.

Social networks

Social networks are formed by the connections between people who frequently communicate with each other. Such communication involves the exchange of emotional, physical, economic and informational support and involves family members, colleagues, friends and neighbours. Beyond the emotional and practical support that social networks provide, they also give a sense of belonging to individuals, in turn promoting self-esteem, self-worth and self-confidence (Greenblatt et al. 1982).

The quality and quantity of social networks experienced by people with severe long-term mental illness differ from those experienced by members of the general population. Healthy individuals can usually list around 22 to 25 people who are important to them, with five or six in each of the categories of family, other relatives, friends and neighbours, and social and work associates. By contrast, people with chronic psychiatric disorders can only list around half this number, of whom about two-thirds are relatives. Thus such individuals have few links to other social groups. This finding has led to the emphasis on enlarging and strengthening a patient's social network as part of a treatment plan. This can be undertaken within institutions and with outpatient populations, and may utilize social skills training and other group activities. The increasing use of hostels in the community facilitates social contacts, and family work such as psycho-education may be useful in strengthening pre-existing connections. The social networks of carers also become diminished over time, often as a result of giving up work or other activities in order to look after an ill relative, but also because of 'stigma by association'. Communication between carers through relatives' support groups and other organizations may allow new contacts to be made and these may provide particularly salient emotional and informational support.

Carers

Unlike the families of patients with other chronic illnesses, the families of those suffering chronic mental illnesses have in the past been seen as having a causal role (Tsiegel et al. 1991). This was particularly the case with respect to mothers of patients with schizophrenia. In 1948 Fromm-Reichmann published a theory that hostile and rejecting feelings expressed by mothers were responsible for schizophrenia in the child. Bateson et al. (1956) described the 'schizophrenogenic mother' who, by behaving in a rejecting manner while verbalizing affection, placed the infant in a 'double-blind'. Lidz et al. (1965) broadened the aetiology to marital partners, using the terms 'marital skew' and 'marital schism' to describe pathogenetic relationships thought to cause schizophrenia (see Chapter 18).

These ideas have fallen from favour, as they were based on uncontrolled and subjective studies. However, there is sound evidence that some forms of family interaction may precipitate relapse in people with schizophrenia (see below). It is also true that there is greater than average psychopathology in the relations of people with schizophrenia, probably due both to the strain of caring and to genetic loading (Schulz et al. 1990).

The concept of 'burden' (Tsiegel et al. 1991), is used to encompass the broad effects on a family of caring for a sick relative. These include effects on income and employment, social and leisure activities, domestic routine, caring for children at home, health of household members and relationships with neighbours. Many standardized instruments exist to measure burden, but these have been criticized for not being based on an explicit theory of care-giving, for using predominantly white, middle-class respondents and for being beset by the difficulty of measuring burden objectively (Szmukler et al. 1996). The study of care-giving, more established in the relatives of patients with dementia and the concept of 'stress-appraisal-coping' that has been widely used in this field, is now being applied to carers of people with major mental illness. The most common problems experienced by carers are:

- difficult behaviours exhibited by patient
- negative symptoms exhibited by patient
- inaccessible services
- bereavement
- patient dependency
- impact on other family members
- stigma.

Expressed emotion

The observation that patients with schizophrenia discharged from hospital to live with parents or spouse appeared to relapse more often than those discharged to live with other relatives or non-relatives, prompted an examination of various factors correlated with relapse. This led to the concept of *expressed emotion* (EE) (Brown et al. 1972), a composite variable with high and low values, that may be determined by the semi-structured Camberwell Family Interview. This rates the number of critical comments, hostility and emotional over-involvement on the part of patient's relatives. These factors each predict the liability for relapse, and give the interview its validity. A number of studies have demonstrated the overall impact of EE, the importance of the amount of time that patients spend in contact with 'high EE' relatives, and the partial role of medication in mitigating these effects.

On the basis of studies on EE and relapse, a number of intervention packages have been designed to reduce the level of EE and, where relevant, the amount of face-to-face contact with relatives. Treatment involves family psycho-education addressing the symptoms, course and treatment of schizophrenia, and the development of alternative coping strategies for dealing with problem behaviours (which may be based on the strategies adapted by low EE families). Interventions have involved meetings with individual families and/or the formation of relatives' groups. Further work is necessary to identify which patients will most benefit from which treatments and to isolate the 'active' ingredients of family interventions (Penn & Mueser 1996). Evaluations of these interventions need to show first whether the intervention has reduced EE and face-to-face contact and, second, whether the relapse rate has decreased. A meta-analysis of family interventions (Mari & Streiner 1994) showed that changes in EE status between experimental and control groups combining 9-month and 1-year follow-ups were marginally significant, in favour of the experimental group. In addition, the experimental group showed a significant increase in compliance with pharmacotherapy and a reduction in hospitalization during the period studied. The authors calculate that between two and five patients must be treated to avert one episode of relapse during a 9-month treatment period.

CONCLUSIONS

This chapter has attempted to outline the marked interplay between social factors and mental illness, and to emphasize the importance of considering social factors in the management of patients. As our understanding of the biology of our patients grows, we must never forget their sociology – patients will always be influenced by others, and will always themselves influence others.

REFERENCES

Adshead G (1998) Psychiatric staff as attachment figures: understanding management problems in psychiatric services in the light of attachment theory. *British Journal of Psychiatry* **172**: 64–9.

Bateson G, Jackson DD, Haley J & Weakland JH(1956) Toward a theory of schizophrenia. *Behavioural Science* **1**: 251–64.

Bhugra D, Leff J & Mallett G (1997) Incidence and outcome of schizophrenia in whites, African Caribbeans and Asians in London. *Psychological Medicine* **27**: 791–8.

Boydell J, van Os J, McKenzie K, Allardyce J, Goel R, McCreadie RG & Murray RM (2001) Incidence of schizophrenia in ethnic minorities in London: ecological study into interactions with environment. *British Medical Journal* **323**: 1336–8.

Brown GW & Birley JLT (1968) Crises and life changes and the onset of schizophrenia. *Journal of Health and Social Behaviour* **9**: 203–14.

Brown GW, Birley JLT & Wing JK (1972) Influence of family life on the course of schizophrenic disorder, a replication. *British Journal of Psychiatry* **121**: 241–58.

Brown GW & Harris T (1978) *Social Origins of Depression*. New York:Free Press.

Brown GW & Prudo R (1981) Psychiatric disorder in a rural and an urban population: I. Aetiology of depression. *Psychological Medicine* **11**: 581–99.

Commander MJ, Sashi Dharan SP, Odell SM & Surtees PG (1997) Access to mental health care in an inner city health district. II: Association with demographic factors. *British Journal of Psychiatry* **170**: 317–20.

Craig TK & Hodson S (1998) Homeless youth in London: 1. Childhood antecedents and psychiatric disorder. *Psychological Medicine*, **28**, 1378–88.

Davies S, Thornicroft G, Leese M, Higginbotham A & Phelan M (1996) Ethnic differences in risk of compulsory admission among representative cases of psychosis in London. *British Medical Journal* **312**: 533–7.

Dear M & Wolch J (1987) *Landscapes of Despair*. Oxford: Polity.

Dohrenwend B (1975) Socio-cultural and social-psychological factors in the genesis of mental disorders. *Journal of Health and Social Behaviour* **16**: 365–92.

Dunham W (1965) *Community and Schizophrenia*. Detroit: Wayne State University Press.

Faris R & Dunham H (1939) *Mental Disorders in Urban Areas*. Chicago: University of Chicago press.

Fromm-Reichmann F. (1948) Notes on the development of treatment of schizophrenics by psycho-analytic therapy. *Psychiatry*, **11**, 263–73.

Goffman E (1961) *Asylums*. New York: Doubleday Anchor.

Goldberg D & Huxley P (1980) *Mental Illness in the Community*. London: Tavistock.

Goldberg E & Morrison S (1963) Schizophrenia and social class. *British Journal of Psychiatry* **109**: 785–802.

Greenberg KS, Greenley JR & Benedict P (1994) Contributions of persons with serious mental illness to their families. *Hospital and Community Psychiatry* **45**: 475–80.

Greenblatt M, Becera RM & Serafetinides EA (1982) Social networks and mental health: an overview. *American Journal of Psychiatry* **139**: 977–84.

Halpern D (1993) Minorities and mental health. *Social Science & Medicine* **36**:597–697.

Halpern D & Nazroo J (1999) The ethnic density effect: results from a national community survey of England and Wales. *Internation Journal of Social Psychiatry* **46**: 34–46.

Hare E (1956) Mental illness and social conditions in Bristol. *Journal of Mental Science* **102**: 349–57.

Harrison G (1988) A prospective study of severe mental disorder in Afro-Caribbean patients. *Psychological Medicine* **18**: 643–57.

Holzer CE, Brent MS, Swanson JW et al. (1986) The increased risk for specific psychiatric disorders among persons of low socioeconomic status. *American Journal of Social Psychiatry* **5**: 259–71.

Kammerling RM & O'Connor S (1993) Unemployment rate as predictor of rate of psychiatric admission. *British Medical Journal* **307**: 1536–9.

Lewis G, David A, Andreasson S & Allebeck P (1992) Schizophrenia and city life. *Lancet* **340**: 137–40.

Lidz T, Fleck S & Corneilson AR (1965) *Schizophrenia and the Family*. New York: International Universities Press.

Link BG, Cullen FT, Frank J & Wozniak JF (1987) The social rejection of former mental patients: understanding why labels matter. *American Journal of Sociology* **92**: 1461–1500.

London M (1986) Mental illness among immigrant minorities in the United Kingdom. *British Journal of Psychiatry* **149**: 265–73.

Mari JJ & Streiner DL (1994) An overview of family interventions and relapse on schizophrenia: meta-analysis of research findings. *Psychological Medicine* **24**: 565–78.

Mechanic D (1968) *Medical Sociology: A Selective View*. New York:Free Press.

Mechanic D, McAlpine D, Rosenfields & Davis D (1994) Effects of illness attribution and depression on the quality of life among persons with serious mental illness. *Social Science and Medicine* **39**: 155–64.

Meltzer H, Gill B, Petticrew M & Hinds K (1995) *The Prevalence of Psychiatric Morbidity Among Adults living in Private Households*. London: HMSO.

Neeleman J & Wessely S (1999) Ethnic minority suicide: a small group are study in South London. *Psychological Medicine* **29**: 429–36.

Neeleman J, Wilson-Jones C & Wessely S (2001) Ethnic density and deliberate self harm; a small area study in south east London. *Journal of Epidemiology and Community Health* **55**: 85–90.

Parkman S, Davies S, Leese M, Phelan M & Thornicroft G (1997) Ethnic differences in satisfaction with mental health services among representative people with psychosis in South London. *British Journal of Psychiatry* **171**: 260–4.

Parsons T (1951) *The Social System*. Glencoe, IL: Free Press.

Penn DL & Mueser KT(1996) Research update on the psychosocial treatment of schizophrenia. *American Journal of Psychiatry* **153**: 607–17.

Rogler L (1996) Increasing socioeconomic inequalities and the mental health of the poor. *Journal of Nervous and Mental Diseases* **184**: 719–22.

Ross C (2000) Neighborhood disadvantage and adult depression. *Journal of Health and Social Behavior* **41**: 177–87.

Rutter M (1989) Isle of Wight revisited: twenty-five years of child psychiatric epidemiology. *Journal of the American Academy of Child and Adolescent Psychiatry* **28**: 633–53.

Schulz R, Visintainer P & Williamson GM (1990) Psychiatric and physical morbidity effects of caregiving. *Journal of Gerontology* **5**: 181–91.

Shapiro S, Skinner E, Kessler L & Von Korff M (1984) Utilization of health and mental health services. Three epidemiologic catchment area sites. *Archives of General Psychiatry* **41**: 971–8.

Shrout PE, Link BG, Dohrenwend B et al. (1989) Characterising life events as risk factors for depression: the role of fateful loss events. *Journal of Abnormal Psychology* **98**: 460–7.

Szmukler GI, Burgess P, Herrman H et al. (1996) Caring for relatives with serious mental illness: the development of the Experience of Caregiving Inventory. *Social Psychiatry and Psychiatric Epidemiology* **31**: 137–48.

Tennant C (1985) Stress and schizophrenia: a review. *Integrative Psychiatry* **3**: 248–61.

Thornicroft G (1991) Social deprivation and rates of treated mental disorder. *British Journal of Psychiatry* **158**: 475–84.

Tsiegel DE, Salls E & Schulz R (1991) Caregiving in chronic mental illness. In: *Family Caregiving in Chronic Illness*. Newbury Park, CA: Sage, 164–98.

Wilkinson RG(1989) Class mortality differentials, income distribution and trends in poverty, 1921–1981. *Journal of Social Policy* **18**: 307–35.

World Health Organization (1979) *Schizophrenia: an International Follow-up Study*. Chichester: Wiley.

Wyatt R, Alexander R, Egan M & Kirch D (1988) Schizophrenia, just the facts. What do we know, how well do we know it? *Schizophrenia Research* **1**: 3–18.

8

Cultural psychiatry

Kamaldeep Bhui

INTRODUCTION

The culturally capable psychiatrist requires a number of skills (Box 8.1). These skills can only be developed in clinical practice, with support in training and education. However, *core knowledge* and an evidence base are needed to exercise these skills. This chapter provides this core knowledge: it outlines how culture, in relation to race and ethnicity, influences the presentation and treatment of mental disorders. The chapter does not address all cultural groups or all treatments in their specific details. This chapter aims to equip the practitioner with general principles for a better understanding of the clinical management of mental disorders across cultures. Some specific examples are given, for example, data on ethnic inequalities in incidence and prevalence of disorders and service use are outlined. As the

Box 8.1   Skills of the culturally capable psychiatrist
To be able to use interpreters effectively and consider the translations in a cultural and psychopathological context.
To be able to recognize an absence of personal cultural knowledge, or contextual knowledge, necessary to deliver a precise diagnosis.
To be able to ask about cultural identity and explanatory models.
To be able to complete a cultural formulation, taking full account of the transference and counter-transference issues related to race, ethnicity and culture, as well as mental distress.
To be able to work with families, couples, or groups when gathering information or delivering psychiatric interventions and reviewing progress.
To be able to work effectively with voluntary and independent services which offer specialist care to black and minority ethnic groups.
To take account of well-established evidence showing cultural variations of psychopathology, pharmacokinetics and pharmaco-dynamics.
To be active in research and audit of areas of practice identified locally to be poorly understood and undermine effective treatments.

chapter does not offer a comprehensive literature review, key papers are recommended for specific contemporary debates.

The work on culture and mental health has passed through several phases, from being entirely political, and aimed at exposing and addressing racism, to exploring anthropologically what constitutes culture and how this influences mental health. Within a cultural framework, the practitioner is not seen as neutral or scientifically objective, but an active player in the cultural exchanges, bringing to bear his or her own cultural assumptions and stereotypes. The practitioner's age, gender, cultural origins, biography and personality characteristics all play a part in his or her aptitude for work with culturally dissimilar groups. A reflexive and active listening approach to the consultation is essential for the culturally capable psychiatrist to identify the unspoken gaps in their own knowledge. Cultural psychiatry does not demand or expect every mental health professional to know about every cultural group they may encounter. Cultural psychiatry encourages professionals to develop ways of thinking about the presentation and clinically effective management of mental illness for patients from any cultural group. This inevitably means having a process in the consultation in which cultural knowledge is gathered, and a process in which cultural issues are explicitly explored.

DEFINITIONS

There is often confusion about the meaning of the word 'culture'. For example, it can be used in the institutional sense of an organizational culture more akin to a social system; culture is often also equated with civilization or cultured behaviour or higher tastes of people of high social status. In this chapter I use the term culture to refer to cultural aspects of thinking, feeling and behaviour to do with nation, heritage, place of birth and ethnicity. Cultures construct distinct ethnic groups and give meaning to attributes such as skin colour rather than the other way around. How does a cultural group differ from an ethnic group? Even here different perspectives are taken by distinct disciplines (see Box 8.2).

Box 8.2   Definitions

Ethnic group

A community whose heritage offers important characteristics in common between members, and which makes them distinct from other communities. The boundary between us and them is recognized by peoples on both sides of the boundary (Peach 1996).

A social group characterized by distinctive social and cultural tradition, maintained within the group from generation to generation, a common history and origin, and a sense of identification with the group. Members of the group have distinctive features in their way of life, shared experiences, and often a common genetic heritage (Last 1995).

Culture

Culture is that complex whole which includes knowledge, belief, art, morale, law, customs and other capabilities and habits acquired by man as a member of society (Tylor 1871).

A set of guidelines which individuals inherit as members of a particular society, and which tells them how to view the world, how to experience it emotionally, and how to behave in it in relation to other people, supernatural forces or gods, and to the natural environment (Helman 1990).

A broader analysis of culture allows practitioners and researchers to truly explore the cultures of all people, and not only black and minority ethnic groups. Thus, the mental health care needs of the Irish or Welsh, if different, would receive no specific attention if we restricted cultural psychiatry to a psychiatry of racial or ethnic groups. Black and minority ethnic groups' cultural worlds can only be considered separate and distinct and in need of a unique form of psychiatry if cultures were truly independent and geographically isolated. However, with ever-increasing travel and globalization, there are few cultures that are or will remain separate and isolated. Therefore cultural psychiatry is becoming ever more important in the face of cultural mixing and given that ethnic groups are highly prevalent in the world's largest cities, sometimes being the majority.

Cultural psychiatry challenges the assumptions of established good clinical practice, and raises some philosophical, theoretical and technical dilemmas for practitioners. Cultural psychiatry has not emerged in a vacuum. Much can be learnt from the discipline of cultural studies, which asserts that our understanding is always unstable and influenced by context; one main aim of cultural studies is to explore power relationships and their expression in modern society. The academic discipline of cultural psychiatry draws on sociology, anthropology, epidemiology, statistics, philosophy, psychoanalysis and health services research to unravel the relationship between culture and mental health. Cultural studies generally, and cultural psychiatry specifically, examines power relationships, and how they are manifest in therapeutic

encounters. It does not restrict itself to one discipline or one approach but deploys any method or model to better understand the relationship between culture and mental health care. Any study of cultures has to be focused on understanding the limitations of our knowledge and skills while questioning our assumptions (often more common in social sciences); this approach contrasts with making positive scientific statement (more often found in medicine and epidemiology). This tension between discovering scientific data and recognizing and accepting uncertainty and the limitations of our knowledge has been one of the main sources of controversy and debate among psychiatrists studying culture and mental disorders.

CULTURE, SOCIETY AND MENTAL HEALTH

Culture determines which social behaviours and institutions are sanctioned and which are prohibited. Culture determines our everyday behaviours and attitudes towards each other, and towards the supernatural world. Through living in a culture we are informed about how to live, and more specifically, how to react to experiences of dysfunction or disability or distress. Culture influences and is the substance of beliefs, attitudes, behaviours, social and family systems within which we live. Illness behaviour – the way individuals experience, appraise and respond to an episode of illness – is both shaped by culture and constitutes culture. Thus help-seeking patterns, as well as the ascriptions of normality are all defined by cultural norms. These norms are, on the whole, implicit rules for living, experiencing and seeing the world. Each culture has 'rites of reversal' (Helman 1990), when these rules are temporarily flouted. For example, carnival, Christmas celebrations, attending football matches in large crowds, being possessed by spirits during a Zar possession in Ethiopia, or speaking in tongues during religious ceremonies. Each of these is normal, even though the rituals and behaviours may seem abnormal to an outsider. However, they are normal only if the behaviours adhere to cultural rules and codes. If speaking in tongues continued for too long, or happened too frequently, or not in a church at all, the peer group that is familiar with these rituals would recognize this as abnormal.

People from different cultural groups will have different norms of behaviour, dress, and attitudes towards family, sexuality, relationships, education, religion, state and society. Cultures are characterized by distinct family and kinship patterns, marriage ceremonies and other ritualized social activities. Tseng (2003) summarizes the evidence showing how child development also varies across cultures, and indeed, specific personality types have been ascribed to particular nations. National language films and books, for example, capture these national stereotypes (Bhugra 2003) and can be used to teach cultural psychiatry, although it is recognized that these stereotypes are representations of real but subtle differences in national and cultural characteristics.

Culture can be said to consist of personality dispositions, collective and individual beliefs, knowledge, attitudes and values, and the impact of these on interpersonal relationships, social organizations, ancestors, spirits and supernatural forces. People of any culture implicitly know how to behave when distressed or when suffering ill-health, and this knowledge determines how they appraise their experiences of distress and, ultimately, from whom they seek help. The carer they seek out then further informs them how to relieve their suffering or misfortune. Kleinman (1980) considers that the majority of mental distress (60–70%) is remedied within the folk and popular sectors of health care, rather than by formal health care services. In the popular and folk arena, healing can take place within families, informal groups such as prayer groups, social clubs, and practically any shared interest group. Within such gatherings individuals seek out opinion and advice, and explain the measures they have taken to remedy their distress. They may not even consider or experience their difficulties as being 'mental' in nature, or that they reflect a 'health' problem. Psychological forms of distress are often contrasted with somatized expressions of distress, but the mind–body dichotomy exists in Euro-American societies, and the industrialized and developed world. Consequently, it is often forgotten that this is not necessarily how people experience distress first hand. Somatic complaints may reflect true physical illness or co-morbid mental distress that takes a physical symptom form. The physical complaint may be an idiom of distress, or a metaphorical means of communicating distress, or distress may actually be truly experienced subjectively as having physical origins. Kirmayer (2001) argues that, contrary to the claim that non-Westerners are prone to somatize their distress, somatization is ubiquitous. Somatic symptoms serve as cultural idioms of distress in many ethno-cultural groups and, if misinterpreted by the clinician, may lead to unnecessary diagnostic procedures or inappropriate treatment. Clinicians must learn to decode the meaning of somatic and dissociative symptoms, which are not simply indices of disease or disorder but part of a language of distress with interpersonal and wider social meanings. Although early studies suggested that somatic symptoms were common in South and East Asians, more recent data show that this does not mean that such groups are not aware of the emotional or psychological component to their distress. Such distinct ways of experiencing and responding to distress can be better understood using theories about 'explanatory models'.

Explanatory models

An explanatory model sets out the patient's own way of naming their problem, describes the patient's explanation of

causation, cure and prognosis, as well as who is equipped to help. Explanatory models (EMs) are not fixed cognitive representations or maps of how to behave (Bhui & Bhugra 2002). They are unstable and fluctuate, and are context dependant. They are assessed using a process of mini-ethnography, whereby the practitioner discovers cultural narratives and discourses around health, illness and their mental distress. However, any one individual's set of inter-related EMs constitute their total approach and ways of relating to distress and healers. EMs are operationalized as a set of beliefs about the identity of the problem, and the causes of their distress, as well as what they should do to remedy their difficulties. Thus some EMs include 'misfortune, breaking a taboo, black magic, karma' and 'an act of God' as forms of identity. More familiar models to the West include 'cold' and 'damp weather', 'stress', 'working too hard', and 'depression'. Causal explanations are patterned by culture; for example: stormy love affairs and the break-up of relationships, loss of status by a job loss, complaints of discrimination, food poisoning and a weak constitution. The veracity of the causal explanation is, in cultural terms, not essential, if the explanation serves a purpose of giving an individual some meaning and also influences their behaviour. A complication to this way of understanding culture is that in the West, and in more medicalized societies, medical models of health and dysfunction are more likely to penetrate the social imagination and lay explanations for problems. Therefore 'ME, stress, blood pressure, headache, back pain, a virus' might all be more readily used as explanations for dysfunction in the West, whereas in South Asia, explanations may include ghosts, spirits, Gods, or the natural elements. Lay understanding about how the body works, and how dysfunction arises include 'blockages, wearing out of parts, or tensions or nerves'. In a health-conscious and medically informed society, such explanations may be more accurate, than in societies that are isolated, or which do not have access to the Internet, television or modern medicine. Alternatively, some societies steeped in religious and strong cultural traditions sustain alternative explanatory frameworks for misfortune, unexpected events and health problems.

Box 8.3 gives an account of an in-depth research interview in which a woman's explanatory model for her depression was explored. This woman was not psychotic and, although depressed, remained relatively functional in the nursing home where she lived after having to leave her family home as her children were not prepared to live in an extended family and continue to support her in the way she expected.

Acculturation and cultural identity

Acculturation is defined as 'the phenomena that results when groups of individuals having different cultures come

Box 8.3   Case history

Mrs H A is a Muslim woman (Agha Khan group of Muslims) who speaks Hindi, Gujerati and Urdu. She is 70–75 years of age, and has hemiplegia due to stroke. She needed an interpreter.

When asked about worry and depression, she said she was depressed due to her family. 'When the family becomes your enemy you inevitably become depressed'. She related family problems as the primary cause of worry and depression. When pressed, she added money shortages to the difficulties with her family.

I asked, 'Why do people become depressed or develop worry?' She then said that her daughter-in-law had practised magic and used 'Taveez' against her. God, she said, had intervened and she was therefore OK. When asked more about this, she said that her daughter-in-law had used magic water, that one daughter-in-law had asked the second to place it in her food, in her curry. Since then she had not been well. However, they also had suffered and had had major financial worries. Anyone who ate the curry would be affected and she was worried as her name 'was written on the water' and thus if anyone else was affected by it , this would be her fault in some way also.

She did not see doctors as having any role to play as it was a 'family problem' and as such it had to be resolved within the family. She said that the doctor could not change things to do with the family and indeed 'family problems' were not shared. 'Doctors give medication only'. She proceeded to explain how the doctor could help identify causes of physical problems and give medication, but she did not see that the doctor had a role to play in financial or family problems whether they caused her terrible worry or not.

into continuous first-hand contact with subsequent changes in the original cultural patterns of either or both groups' (Redfield et al. 1936). Acculturation is the term given to the changes in everyday practices, attitudes and beliefs that take place when two relatively isolated cultures come into contact. This is influenced not only by the individual biographies of the people meeting each other, but also by the social, cultural and contextual differences between the host and original society (Fig. 8.1).

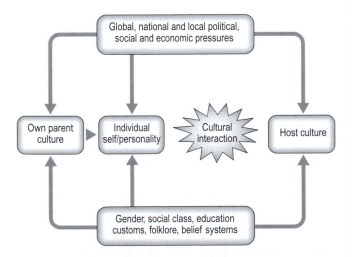

Figure 8.1 Acculturation as a function of group identity, national and social policy as well as individual demographics. (*after Bhugra & Bhui 2001*)

Cultural adaptations are seen in changes in language dominance, dress preference, food and leisure pursuits, topics of conversation, attitudes to religious worship, marriage partner selection, child rearing and the balance between work, home and family life. Use of health services and attitudes to illness and mental health may also change. This can lead to tensions between the individual and their immediate family, social group and society.

The identity of an individual is in part determined by their culture of origin, but also by their identification with different social groups, such as older people, women, black people, speakers of another language, etc. However, the preoccupation with identifying ethnic identity, although assessing subjective identity, can be misleading, as people may be forced to give their identification with one of a number of cultural groups to which they relate. Identification with either host or original culture were originally seen as mutually exclusive processes. However, more sophisticated models of identity suggest people can be identified with host and original culture on independent domains (Berry 1980). That is they can be biculturally proficient, or traditional by only identifying with culture of origin; they may be considered 'assimilated' if they give up their original culture and adopt the host culture; those considered marginalized give up their culture of origin and don't adopt the new culture.

The identities that an individual adopts carry with them explanatory models, expectations of health care, linguistic metaphors for describing distress, stigma about mental illness, and experiences of mental health care. Berry (1980) argues that biculturally proficient identities are the most healthy, with the marginalized group being least healthy. However, a great deal of empirical work on cultural identity and acculturation experiences show this to be a methodologically complex field, with too many value-laden assumptions about what constitutes culture, and how to remedy ill health, which is seen to be either generated by immigrant or foreign culture or exacerbated by it. Research studies have reached differing conclusion about the consequences of acculturation. Separate studies have described it increasing, decreasing and having no impact on rates of mental health problems. In part, such studies are limited by trying to draw generalizations across too many subcultural populations as if they were a single group.

THE CULTURAL FORMULATION

The American Psychiatric Association recommends that all psychiatrists assess cultural identity and explanatory models of their patients (Griffith 2002). This should take place alongside an assessment of the impact on the therapeutic relationship of culture of the professional and/or patient. Cultural factors related to the sociocultural environment (discrimination, unemployment, asylum laws) should also be considered as factors that impact on mental health. Finally, there should be an overall statement outlining any culturally relevant aspects of diagnosis and treatment. Professionals should take particular care to ensure that the rationale for the treatment is understood, and does not break any cultural taboos or undermine any cherished cultural beliefs, as this may lead to potential non-compliance. Most importantly, any further investigations to improve an understanding of the cultural aspects of presentation should be stated explicitly. For example, talking to family or friends of a patient enables the professional to consider their views about psychopathology and ensures that cultural phenomena are not considered as pathology due to a lack of familiarity with the cultural norms of patients. Although the Royal College of Psychiatrists in the UK has not formulated any specific recommendation, there are now capability indicators for trainees reflecting the multicultural nature of the population (Moodley 2002).

Psychopathology and culture

It is known that first-rank symptoms are not specific to schizophrenia and are not uncommon in mania. They are also present to varying degrees in different cultural groups and do not always carry the same diagnostic significance across cultures (see Bhugra & Bhui 2001). Breaching individual ego boundaries in some non-Western cultures is not as pathologically regarded as it is in Western societies. In societies with a more socio-centric or diffuse sense of self, where connectedness, dependency and shared communications are not considered immature, incursions from ancestors or family members into the personal space (social or body or mind) of a person are common. For example, in India spirit possession and exorcisms are not automatically considered abnormal or needing a psychiatrist for treatment. Helman (1990) suggests that all societies allow temporary abnormally behaviours if they obey culturally coded rules. If the rules are broken, then they may be seen as pathology. For example, spirit possession or talking in tongues can be normal experiences, but if they persist or are associated with experiences that people from the reference group consider atypical, then they may be indicators of abnormality. Tseng (2003) has summarized the many ways in which culture affects mental health (Box 8.4).

All of these make the mental state assessment more difficult to interpret in terms of normal or abnormal phenomena. Although psychotic phenomena are often considered to be due to the same universal neuro-chemical changes in brain which influence perceptions, the same phenomena cannot be assumed to have the same trigger factors, aetiology or meaning for the patient. Furthermore, susceptibility to hallucinations is determined by the relative significance of hallucinations as ordinary events in societies. Van Os et al.(2000) found that 17.5% of a population sample experienced hallucinations and only 4.5% of these subjects had a diagnosed mental disorder. This presence of non-clinically-significant psychotic symptoms may explain cultural variations if psychotic symptoms can exist in response to social and psychological events compounded by general distress and preparedness to express distress through psychosis. Although visual hallucinations are considered to be rare in schizophrenia, they are not that rare in presentations of schizophrenia in Asian and some African countries. A recent study by Suhail & Cochrane (2002) explored the content of psychotic symptoms among Pakistanis in Pakistan, Pakistanis in Britain and White British patients. They found greater differences in phenomenology between Pakistani Pakistanis and British Pakistanis than between British White and British Pakistani patients. This suggests that immediate environment also influences the expression of distress and the content of psychosis. Can culture influence the form of psychosis? This study also reported that visual hallucinations are more common in Pakistani Pakistanis where religious doctrine encourages 'visions'. They also report more grandiose symptoms among Pakistani Pakistanis, where there is marked poverty and a greater gap between rich and poor.

These studies challenge a universalistic application of knowledge to all cultural groups, and argue that cultural relativism is necessary and real. There is an active debate about the cultural universality of diagnostic categories. Psychiatric epidemiological studies generate diagnoses

---

Box 8.4 Psychopathology and culture (after Tseng 2003)

Patho-plastic: shaping the content of symptoms or the overall picture. For example, 'sinking heart' as metaphor for depression and social isolation and interpersonal distress among Punjabi Asians. Also the content of delusions, hallucinations, etc., can vary.

Patho-selective: personality and psychological make up can also recruit specific styles of expressing distress. Deliberate self-harm and anorexia were seen as typical of a Western expression of distress. Personality dispositions influence how people select specific behaviours as expressions of distress.

Patho-genic: distress can be generated by cultures, for example, by demands for role fulfilment, or prohibitions on certain behaviours.

Patho-facilitative: this suggests that culture does not generate or determine specific psychopathology, but facilitates or makes more likely specific expressions of distress. Thus the frequency of certain disorders varies across societies depending upon availability of means, and social sanctions for specific expressions of distress.

Patho-elaborative: the exaggeration of certain behaviours in specific societies. Latah in the Far East, for example, is an exaggerated startle reaction and is manifest as posturing and taking up stances, after unexpected prodding or startle.

Patho-reactive: culture influences how people react to illness. The meaning of the symptoms may be interpreted, or there may be stigma or fear about specific manifestations of distress.

Patho-discriminative: this indicates which behaviours a culture identifies as normal or abnormal.

using structured interview schedules, so diagnoses are certainly reliably made. Are they as valid? It appears that psychiatric disorders occur around the world, but their recognition as illness varies, and the expectation that doctors can intervene also varies. The more biological the aetiology of specific mental disorders, the more likely it is that these disorders take the same form in different societies. Therefore common mental disorders such as depression and anxiety are more subject to cultural variation, and any psychopathological phenomena that psychiatrists label as abnormal (delusions, hallucinations, aggression and paranoia) occur to varying extents in different societies, and may not always be thought of as a mental illness. Such symptoms must be understood in the context of the patient's dominant cultural frame of reference and belief system (Bhugra & Bhui 2001).

Psychopharmacology and culture

Lin (1995) has outlined how different ethnic and cultural groups physiologically handle and respond to psychotropic medication in distinct ways. These findings are explained by distinct pharmacodynamic and pharmacokinetic profiles, and variation in pharmaco-genetic vulnerabilities across cultures (see Bhugra & Bhui 2001 for summary). Essentially, the studies indicate that lower doses of benzodiazepines and antidepressants are necessary for similar therapeutic effects among South Asian and East Asian patients. Black people appear to need lower doses of lithium and antipsychotics, and may suffer more adverse effects. Regrettably, general statements about any one ethnic group cannot be made with confidence as the genetic variation in metabolic pathways is inherited in a complex manner and is vulnerable to the interplay of multiple factors. However, it can be said that some specific populations, on average, are more likely to suffer from inherited variations in metabolic enzyme activity. Furthermore, it is known that other cultural factors influence medication metabolism, for example alcohol consumption, smoking, dietary factors, and herbal remedies that may be taken from the folk and popular sectors (see Bhugra & Bhui 2001: p. 65 for a summary). The clinical relevance of such studies is that psychotropics should be initiated with more caution, and complaints of adverse effects at unexpectedly low doses should not be ignored or considered a psychological response or resistance, or lack of insight.

Psychotherapy and culture

Common themes to all healing are those first identified by Frank (1989): a healing place, a ritual, a myth, rationale or conceptual system, and finally an emotionally charged confiding relationship with a *helpful* person (see Chapter 36). Tseng (2003: 291) suggests that when adapting psychotherapy to other cultural groups, the therapist needs to revisit philosophical and theoretical limitations, before adapting technical aspects of a therapy. Often therapists try and improve their use of interpreters, or take a greater number of sessions to educate the patient about therapy, or offer more flexibility by giving social interventions to engage the patient before therapeutic work is possible. All of these are helpful strategies in modification of 'delivery'. Family therapies are thought to be more acceptable to some families, and group processes may also be more attractive and less stigmatizing for people from socio-centric societies, or where the manifestations of their distress include interpersonal fears and avoidance. This requires therapists to be courageous and to modify, experiment and innovate with sensitivity, while always taking care not to make assumptions about the patients' expectations or use of language, especially where English is a second language. Ethnic matching, although often advocated, has not been proved to improve outcomes, and in some instances people from specific ethnic groups may distance themselves defensively from their emotional world by seeking a therapy in a second language. Alternatively, some are fearful of breaches of confidentiality if they see the therapist as coming from their social and cultural group in a small community with intimate social networks.

The greater challenges facing therapists are the philosophical and theoretical issues that limit the simplistic transportation of one model of therapy from one culture to another. Do all societies accept talking about a problem as a solution? Do all cultures assume therapists help with depression and physical symptoms? Mrs HA (Box 8.3) did not want formal help with her depression, but sought to sort out her family problems. Clearly, therapists need to be cautious not to be heroic in prematurely rescuing ethnic minorities from distress by offering ill-adapted therapeutic paradigms. Therapist may find themselves 'lost' and 'perplexed' about how to intervene if their specific skill or treatment modality is not well understood or received. Therapists must also attempt to understand the basis of culturally determined coping strategies, for example, prayer, social gatherings, and maybe even magico-religious solutions for misfortune. If these are supported by therapists, not only will they add to resilience, but they may also become the basis of mutual understanding and the beginning of a therapeutic alliance. Clearly, this will take more time than is standard for a short-term therapy, but early education about the therapeutic modality on offer is essential. An exploration of the patient's natural ways of coping, alongside their cultural identity and explanatory models for distress, can begin a therapeutic process by ensuring understanding and trust. Conducting a therapy through interpreters is not impossible, but makes the authentic communication of material more challenging, and use of non-verbal gestures and shared efforts to overcome a difficulty should not be underestimated, especially where the therapeutic paradigm involves the family or a partner.

HEALTH SERVICE RESEARCH AND MINORITY ETHNIC PEOPLE: RESEARCH DATA

Over two decades of British psychiatric research demonstrates ethnic inequalities of service utilization, experiences and benefit from services (Department of Health 2003). Similar studies of health services in the USA also find disparities in access to services, interventions, and outcomes (Snowden 2003; van Ryn & Fu 2003; US Dept of Health & Human Services 2001). The differences vary in each ethnic group. Explanations for the inequalities might be found in the cultures of the ethnic groups and their impact on help-seeking behaviour and the expression of distress; or in the cultures of organizations and professional practice which may reduce access to desired interventions and impose undesired interventions. Furthermore, social inequalities are closely linked to migration and ethnic status, and to mental health risk factors, making the disentangling of such contributions a complex process that remains open to criticism (Nazroo 2003).

The main findings in the British context indicate higher rates of non-affective psychosis among black Caribbean people, with the highest rates in the second generation, so dismissing genetic or predispositional risks as explanations (Harrison 1988; Sharpley 2002). Few studies have examined first incidence data among other groups, although some studies indicate that South Asians in the UK are less likely to use inpatient care; they may also be developing a similar risk of incident schizophrenia (Gupta 1991; King et al. 1994). A consistent finding is a higher rate of psychiatric admissions, both compulsory and voluntary, and over-representation in psychiatric forensic services (Bhui 1995; Coid 2000, 2002a, b). This contrasts with similar rates of psychosis across population samples of ethnic minorities (Nazroo 1997), although this study used a screening instrument to generate a psychosis diagnosis and this may account for the discrepancy. However, the suggestion, if the method is considered valid, is that the discrepancy between hospital contact data and population data may reflect a process of over-engaging black people with psychoses in mental health services. This may be mediated through less social support (Cole 1995), more adverse life events, which prevent restitution from psychosis in the community (Myin-Germeys 2003), or perceptions of greater risk if black people are not engaged or detained within mental health services (van Ryn 2003). This tendency not to reach an alliance may be fed by mistrust of mental health services (Sainsbury Centre for Mental Health 2002) or diagnostic uncertainty due to ethnic variations in affective and non-affective symptoms (Hickling 1999; Hutchinson 1999; Kirov & Murray 1999). Actual differences in levels of violence, crime or threat preceding admission could also explain less voluntary treatment (Bhugra 2000; Wessely 1998), yet recent data on mental health act admissions showed that Caribbeans were no more likely to have violent presentation or substance misuse problems when admitted to prison or to secure psychiatric facilities (Bhui 1998; Lelliot et al. 2001).

Black people are more dissatisfied with consecutive contacts with inpatient admission environments (Parkman et al. 1997), and so may fear voluntary engagement with agencies of which they are suspicious and in which they have little confidence (Mclean 2003; Sainsbury Centre for Mental Health 2002). This may explain more absconding from inpatient care (Falkowski et al. 1990) and less likelihood of engaging in community programmes of mental health care. Furthermore, recent evidence suggests that there are ethnic variations in perceptions of what constitutes mental illness. For example, Pote & Orrell (2002) report that African-Caribbean people were less likely to view thought disorder as pathological, and Bangladeshis were less likely to conclude that hallucinations and suspiciousness were mental health problems. Consequently, where there are different explanatory models for distress, distrust can emerge and compromise collaborative treatment plans (Bhui & Bhugra 2002), perhaps leading to more restricted bio-medical explanations and interventions if sociological and culturally specific explanations are not forthcoming (Cooper-Patrick 1999).

A systematic review of the evidence on ethnic variations in access to specialist psychiatric care concluded that African-Caribbean groups are more likely to be compulsorily detained, admitted to hospital, referred to specialist care by GPs, and least likely to be recognized to have a mental disorder in primary care (Bhui et al. 2003). South Asians are less likely to use inpatient care, more likely to visit their general practitioners, are considered to present somatic manifestations of mental distress more commonly than other groups, and are less likely to be recognized to have a mental disorder than white groups; even when recognized to have a mental disorder they are the least likely to be referred to specialist care by GPs (Bhui et al. 2003). There is little data on other groups such as white subgroups, Africans, South and East Asians. There are no British surveys looking at service structures and clinical practice, and how this may generate or perpetuate inequalities. Such data are limited to small local studies or case reports that are rarely judged to offer generalizable understandings. Van Ryn (2003), using data from the USA, describes a useful schema for cognitive distortions of actual facts presented in vignettes or real clinical scenarios, and how these distortions affect perceived clinical needs and risks when ethnic groups are compared. Specifically, two patterns emerge: overstating risks and clinical needs or underestimating them (van Ryn 2003). These errors of judgement are influenced by provider beliefs about help-seeking and providers' interpretation of symptoms, which influences diagnosis and decision making and recommendations. The authors reported that, in making recommendations, moral judgements appear to influence assessment of clinical needs, sometimes in an explicit manner to justify resource allocation.

Doescher and Corbie-Smith, in two independent studies, demonstrated distrust of physicians by African-Americans, although physician characteristics other than race also influenced satisfaction (Corbie-Smith 2002; Doescher 2000). A study of primary care presenters found that South Asian GPs were poorer at recognizing mental disorders among South Asian patients, than were GPs of other cultural backgrounds (Odell 1997). Similarly, Bhui (2001) demonstrated that, from a pool of South Asian GPs, Punjabi and non-Punjabi GPs were equally able to recognize common mental disorder irrespective of the patient's culture (Punjabi or non-Punjabi), but Punjabi GPs were less effective in recognizing common mental disorders among English women (Bhui et al. 2001). Such disparities are often equated with discriminatory behaviour on the part of the physicians and heath care providers, without attention to cultural influences on interpersonal communication processes.

Coid (2000) has consistently demonstrated an over-representation of black people in forensic units. Why this arises remains the subject of controversial debate, but escape behaviours in response to legal detention, faulty appraisal of dangerousness or risk, or socio-economic disadvantage contributing to risk factors for personality disorders all seem plausible. However, studies exploring personality disorders and culture find that black and minority ethnic groups are less likely to suffer from these. This may reflect caution in making personality disorder diagnoses across cultures, especially as personality norms do vary by nation and culture (see Tseng 2003) or that common personality typologies vary between ethnic groups, so making any diagnostic decision-making more uncertain.

MENTAL HEALTH POLICY

Two policy frameworks were recently launched in Britain: *Inside/Outside* and *Delivering Race Equality: a Framework for Action* (Department of Health 2003a, b). These documents emerged from extensive discussion with community groups and working parties exploring how to eradicate ethnic inequalities in service users' experiences of services, and in clinical outcomes. It was clear that these documents were not aimed at eradicating the causes of ethnic inequalities, which include socio-economic disadvantage, poverty, unemployment, migration and possibly discrimination in society. They were not aimed at influencing any physiological mechanisms proposed to explain higher rates of psychosis among Caribbean black people (Sharpley 2001). The aims of the policy reform were to eradicate inequalities in service users' experience of services and outcomes, to ensure the emergence of a culturally capable workforce, and

to develop communities by proposing a new professional called a community development worker. *Delivering Race Equality* proposed a strategic framework driven by the Race Relations Amendment Act, and proposed more specific action around in-patient care, pathways to care, and suicidal behaviour. These documents, at the time of writing, are out to consultation, but pose challenges for the future of mental health care.

CONCLUSIONS

This chapter has set out some basic evidence for cultural variation in the presentation and expression of mental disorders, and described the key aspects of assessment and management for clinicians. The chapter has also proposed methods by which clinicians can improve their assessment, and develop ways of undertaking ethnographic analyses of patients presenting from cultural groups that are unfamiliar to the practitioner. A brief review of the evidence on inequalities in access to mental health care, and an outline of two recent policy documents that set out a plan of action to eradicate inequalities have also been included.

To complement the chapter, the Further Reading section offers key reading on contemporary debates/questions as well as key textbooks for further information.

FURTHER READING

Key readings on contemporary debates in cultural psychiatry

Why do black Caribbean people more often suffer with schizophrenia?
Sharpley M, Hutchinson G, McKenzie K & Murray RM (2001) Understanding the excess of psychosis among the African-Caribbean population in England. Review of current hypotheses. *British Journal of Psychiatry Supplement* 40: s60–8.

Should we have specialist mental health services for specific ethnic minority groups?
Bhui K & Shashidharan SP (2003) Should there be separate psychiatric services for ethnic minority groups? *British Journal of Psychiatry* 182:10–12.

Does racism cause mental disorder?
Chakraborty A & McKenzie K (2002) Does racial discrimination cause mental illness? *British Journal of Psychiatry* 180: 475–7.

What do we know about ethnic variations in access to mental health care?
Bhui K, Stansfeld S, Hull S, Priebe S, Mole F & Feder G (2003) Ethnic variations in pathways to and use of specialist mental health services in the UK. Systematic review. *British Journal of Psychiatry* 182: 105–16.

Are mental health practitioners racist?
Minnis H, McMillan A, Gillies M & Smith S (2001) Stereotyping: survey of psychiatrists in the United Kingdom. *British Medical Journal* 323(7318): 905–6.

Key textbooks

Bhui, K (ed.) *Racism & Mental Health*. London: Jessica Kingsley Publishers.

Bhugra D & Bhui K (2001) *Cross Cultural Psychiatry: A Practical Guide*. London: Arnold.

Tseng WS (2003) *Clinician's Guide to Cultural Psychiatry*. San Diego, CA: Academic Press.

Helman C (2000) *Culture, Health & Illness*. London: Butterworth-Heinemann Medical.

REFERENCES

Berry W (1980) *Acculturation as Varieties of Adaptation in Acculturation: Theory, Models and Some New Findings* (ed. by A Padilla). Bolder, CO: Westview.

Bhugra D & Bhui K (2001) *Cross Cultural Psychiatry: A Practical Guide*. London: Arnold.

Bhugra D (2003) Using film and literature for cultural competence training. *Psychiatric Bulletin* 27: 427–8.

Bhui K, Stansfeld S, Hull S, Priebe S, Mole F & Feder G (2003) Ethnic variations in pathways to and use of specialist mental health services in the UK. Systematic review. *British Journal of Psychiatry* 182: 105–16.

Bhui K, Christie Y & Bhugra D (1995) The essential elements of culturally sensitive psychiatric services. *International Journal of Social Psychiatry* 41: 242–56.

Bhui K, Brown P, Hardie T, Watson JP & Parrott J (1998) African-Caribbean men remanded to Brixton Prison. Psychiatric and forensic characteristics and outcome of final court appearance. *British Journal of Psychiatry* 172: 337–44.

Bhui K & Bhugra D (2002) Explanatory models for mental distress: implications for clinical practice and research. *British Journal of Psychiatry* 181: 6–7.

Bhui K, Bhugra D, Goldberg D, Dunn G & Desai M (2001) Cultural influences on the prevalence of common mental disorder, general practitioners' assessments and help-seeking among Punjabi and English people visiting their general practitioner. *Psychological Medicine* 31(5): 815–25.

Coid J, Kahtan N, Gault S & Jarman B (2000) Ethnic differences in admissions to secure forensic psychiatry services. *British Journal of Psychiatry* 177: 241–7.

Coid J, Petruckevitch A, Bebbington P, Brugha T, Bhugra D, Jenkins R et al. (2002a) Ethnic differences in prisoners. 1: criminality and psychiatric morbidity. *British Journal of Psychiatry* 181: 473–80.

Coid J, Petruckevitch A, Bebbington P, Brugha T, Bhugra D, Jenkins R et al. (2000b) Ethnic differences in prisoners. 2: risk factors and psychiatric service use. *British Journal of Psychiatry* 181: 481–7.

Cole E, Leavey G, King M, Johnson-Sabine E & Hoar A. (1995) Pathways to care for patients with a first episode of psychosis. A comparison of ethnic groups. *British Journal of Psychiatry* 167: 770–6.

Corbie-Smith G, Thomas SB & St George DM (2002) Distrust, race, and research. *Archives of Internal Medicine* 162: 2458–63.

Department of Health (2003a) *Inside/Outside*. London: Department of Health.

Department of Health (2003b) *Delivering Race Equality: A Framework for Action*. London: Department of Health.

Doescher M, Saver BG, Franks P & Fiscella K (2000) Racial and ethnic disparities in perceptions of physician style and trust. *Archives of Family Medicine* 9(10):1163.

Falkowski J, Watts V, Falkowski W & Dean T (1990) Patients leaving hospital without the knowledge or permission of staff – absconding. *British Journal of Psychiatry* 156: 488–90.

Frank JD (1993) *Persuasion and Healing: A Comparative Study of Psychotherapy*. Baltimore, MD: Johns Hopkins University Press.

Gupta S (1991) Psychosis in migrants from the Indian subcontinent and English-born controls. A preliminary study on the use of psychiatric services. *British Journal of Psychiatry* 159: 222–5.

Harrison G, Owens D, Holton A, Neilson D & Boot D (1988) A prospective study of severe mental disorder in Afro-Caribbean patients. *Psycholical Medicine* 18: 643–57.

Helman C (2000) *Culture, Health and Illness*. Oxford. Oxford University Press.

Hickling FW, McKenzie K, Mullen R & Murray R. (1999) A Jamaican psychiatrist evaluates diagnoses at a London psychiatric hospital. *British Journal of Psychiatry* 175: 283–5.

Hutchinson G, Takei N, Sham P, Harvey I & Murray RM.(1999) Factor analysis of symptoms in schizophrenia: differences between white and Caribbean patients in Camberwell. *Psychological Medicine* 29(3): 607–12.

King M, Coker E, Leavey G, Hoare A & Johnson-Sabine E (1994) Incidence of psychotic illness in London: comparison of ethnic groups. *British Medical Journal* 309: 1115–19.

Kirmayer L (2001) Cultural variations in the clinical presentation of anxiety and depression: implications for diagnosis and treatment. *Journal of Clinical Psychiatry* 62: 22–8.

Kirov G & Murray RM (1999) Ethnic differences in the presentation of bipolar affective disorder. *European Psychiatry* 14: 199–204.

Kleinman A (1980) *Patients and their Healers in the Context of Culture*. Berkeley, CA: University of California Press.

Last JM (1995) *A Dictionary of Epidemiology*, 3rd edn. Oxford: Oxford University Press.

Lelliott P, Audini B & Duffett R. (2001) Survey of patients from an inner-London health authority in medium secure psychiatric care. *British Journal of Psychiatry* 178: 62–6.

Lin KM, Anderson D & Poland RE. (1995) Ethnicity and psychopharmacology. Bridging the gap. *Psychiatric Clinics of North America* 18: 635–47.

Littlewood R & Lipsedge M (1998) *Alients & Alienists: Ethnic Minorities and Psychiatry*. London: Unwin Hyman.

Mclean C, Campbell C & Cornish F (2003) African-Caribbean interactions with mental health services in the UK: experiences and expectations of exclusion as (re)productive of health inequalities. *Social Science & Medicine* 56: 657–69.

Moodley P (2002) Building a culturally capable workforce – an educational approach to delivering equitable mental health services. *Psychiatric Bulletin* 26: 63–5.

Myin-Germeys I, van Os J, Schwartz JE, Stone AA & Delespaul PA (2001) Emotional reactivity to daily life stress in psychosis. *Archives of General Psychiatry* 58(12): 1137–44.

Nazroo JY (2003) The structuring of ethnic inequalities in health: economic position, racial discrimination, and racism. *American Journal of Public Health* 93: 277–84.

Nazroo J (1997) *Ethnicity & Mental Health*. London: Policy Studies Institute.

Odell SM, Surtees PG, Wainwright NW, Commander MJ & Sashidharan SP (1997) Determinants of general practitioner recognition of psychological problems in a multi-ethnic inner-city health district. *British Journal of Psychiatry* 171: 537–41.

Parkman S, Davies S, Leese M, Phelan M & Thornicroft G (1997) Ethnic differences in satisfaction with mental health services among representative people with psychosis in south London: PRiSM study 4. *British Journal of Psychiatry* 171: 260–4.

Peach C (1996) Introduction. In: Peach C (ed.) *Ethnicity in the 1991 Census*. Vol 2: *The ethnic minority populations of Great Britain*. London: HMSO, Office of National Statistics.

Pote HL & Orrell MW (2002) Perceptions of schizophrenia in multi-cultural Britain. *Ethnicity & Health* 7(1): 7–20.

Redfield R, Linton R & Herskovits MJ (1936) Memorandum on the study of acculturation. *American Anthroplogist* 38: 149–52.

Sainsbury Centre for Mental Health (2003) *Circles of Fear*. London: Sainsbury Centre for Mental Health.

Sharpley MS, Hutchinson G, Murray RM & McKenzie K (2001) Understanding the excess of psychosis among the African-Caribbean population in England: Review of current hypotheses. *British Journal of Psychiatry* 178: S60–8.

Snowden LR (2003) Bias in mental health assessment and intervention: theory and evidence. *American Journal of Public Health* 93: 239–43.

Suhail K & Cochrane R (2002) Effect of culture and environment on the phenomenology of delusions and hallucinations. *International Journal of Social Psychiatry* 48(2): 126–38.

Tseng WS (2003) *Clinician's Guide to Cultural Psychiatry*. San Diego, CA: Academic Press.

Tylor EB (1871) *Primitive Culture. Research into the Development of*

Mythology, Philosophy, Religion, Art and Customs. London: John Murray.

US Department of Health and Human Services (2001) *Mental Health, Culture, Race & Ethnicity: A Supplement to Mental Health: A report of the Surgeon General*. Washington, DC: US Dept. Health and Human Services.

van Ryn M & Fu SS (2003) Paved with good intentions: do public health and human service providers contribute to racial/ethnic disparities in health? *American Journal of Public Health* **93**: 248–55.

van Os J, Hanssen M, Bijl RV & Ravelli A (2000) Strauss (1969) revisited: a psychosis continuum in the general population? *Schizophrenia Research* **45**(1–2): 11–20.

Wessely S. (1998) The Camberwell Study of Crime and Schizophrenia. *Social Psychiatry and Psychiatric Epidemiology* 33(Suppl 1): S24–8.

9

Epidemiology

Martin Prince

INTRODUCTION AND OVERVIEW

What is epidemiology?

Last's Dictionary of Epidemiology defines epidemiology as:

> The study of the distribution and determinants of health-related states or events in specified populations, and the application of this study to the control of health problems (Last 2001).

What is the purpose of epidemiology?

Epidemiology is concerned with the health states of populations, communities and groups. The health states of individuals is the concern of clinical medicine. Epidemiology may simply describe the distribution of health states (extent, type, severity) within a population. This is *descriptive epidemiology*. Alternatively it may try to explain the distribution of health states. This is *analytical epidemiology*. The basic strategy is to compare the distribution of disease between groups or between populations, looking for *associations* between hypothesized *risk factors* (genes, behaviours, lifestyles, environmental exposures) and *health states*. These associations may or may not indicate that the hypothesized risk factor has caused the disease (Fig. 9.1).

What do epidemiologists do?

Epidemiological studies are generally not controlled experiments. Observations are made on individuals living freely in the 'real world'; these non-experimental studies are referred to as 'observational'. There is much background noise, so it is difficult to make clear-cut inferences from the resulting data. Observed associations between risk factors and diseases may represent the effects of chance (random error), or bias or confounding (nonrandom error) (Box 9.1). Occasionally the apparent risk factor may be a consequence rather than a cause of the disease. This is called 'reverse causality'.

Two key functions for epidemiologists are therefore to design and analyse their studies in such a way as to maximize the *precision* and *validity* of their findings.

Maximizing precision reduces random error. The two main sources of random error are sampling error and measurement error. Precision may be increased by ensuring an adequate sample size and by maximizing the accuracy of the measures.

Maximizing validity implies the avoidance of non-random error. Non-random error arises from bias and confounding. These concepts will be dealt with in more detail later in this

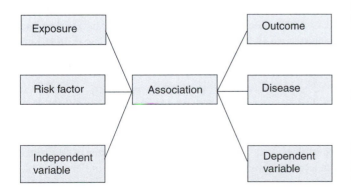

Figure 9.1   Some terminology used in analytical epidemiology

Box 9.1   Possible explanations for an observed association
Chance
Bias
Confounding
Reverse causality
Valid association (may or may not be causal)

chapter. The error is nonrandom, because its effects are unequal (differential) between the two or more groups which are being compared.

If precision and validity of epidemiological studies are adequate, and the effects of chance, bias, confounding and reverse causality can be confidently excluded, then and only then can tentative causal inferences be made from observed associations. Identification of causal factors may lead to strategies for prevention.

For ethical reasons, it is generally not possible to study under experimental conditions in human populations the effects of factors thought likely to increase the risk of disease. However causal inferences made from observational (non-experimental) studies can be assessed further by testing the disease-preventing effects of reducing or eliminating exposure to potential risk factors under experimental conditions. Thus epidemiologists have tested the effects of:

- laying babies on their backs on sudden infant death syndrome (cot death)
- reducing dietary fat on coronary heart disease
- iodine supplementation on cretinism.

The optimal experimental design is the randomized controlled trial, in which the allocation to either the active intervention or the control or placebo arms is randomly determined.

Epidemiology has been described as the basic science of public health medicine; in reality these are complimentary disciplines. Without epidemiology there can be no evidence-based direction to public health policy. Without public health medicine, epidemiological findings cannot be prioritized and converted into practical policies.

MEASUREMENT IN PSYCHIATRIC EPIDEMIOLOGY

The science of the measurement of mental phenomena, psychometrics, is central to quantitative research in psychiatry. Without appropriate, accurate, stable and unbiased measures, research is doomed to fail. Most measurement strategies are based on eliciting symptoms, either by asking the subject to complete a self-report questionnaire, or by using an interviewer to question the respondent. Some are long, detailed, comprehensive clinical diagnostic assessments. Others are much briefer, designed either to screen for probable cases, or as scalable measures in their own right of a trait or dimension such as depression, neuroticism or cognitive function.

Researchers in other medical disciplines sometimes criticize psychiatric measures for being vague or woolly, because they are not based on biological markers of pathology. For this very reason, psychiatry was among the first medical disciplines to develop internationally recognized operationalized diagnostic criteria. At the same time the research interview has become progressively refined, such that the processes of eliciting, recording and distilling symptoms into diagnoses or scalable traits are now also highly standardized. These criticisms are therefore mainly misplaced.

Our confidence in our measures is based on our understanding of their psychometric properties, principally their *validity* and *reliability*. Validity refers to the extent to which a measure really does measure what it sets out to measure. Reliability refers to the consistency of a measure when applied repeatedly under similar circumstances. Put simply, a measure is reliable if you use it twice to measure the same thing and arrive at the same answer. A measure is valid if you measure the same thing twice using two different measures, one known to be valid, and come to the same answer. The reliability and validity of all measures needs to be cited in research grant proposals and research publications. If they have not been adequately established, particularly if the measure is new, then the investigators need to do this themselves in a pilot investigation.

Types of measure

Binary or dichotomous variables are measures of exposure or outcome that have only two levels, exposed or unexposed, and case or non-case. Examples would include gender, recent bereavement (yes/no), current DSM major depression (yes/no). Some variables are reduced to binary form to simplify an analysis. For example, data on lifetime smoking habit could be reduced to a binary variable, ever smoked (yes/no).

Categorical variables may have two or more levels that describe categories to which no meaningful numerical value can be ascribed. Examples would include ethnicity, eye colour and marital status (married, never married, widowed, separated, divorced). These measures describe types rather than quantities.

Ordered categorical variables still describe discrete categories, but with some meaningful trend in the quantity of what is being described from level to level of the variable. Examples would include current smoking status (classified as non-smoker, 1–10 cigarettes daily, 10–20 cigarettes daily, > 20 cigarettes daily) and number of life events (classified as none, one, two or more)

Continuous variables are, strictly speaking, measures of attributes that can be indexed at any point along a scale. Thus weight can be measured as 70 kg or 70.1 kg or even more precisely as 70.09 kg. Age and temperature are other examples of true continuous variables. Number of children is not a continuous variable, as only integer values are possible. Such measures, and many scales used in psychiatric research have this property, are discrete quantitative variables sometimes referred to as ordinal scales.

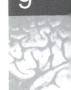

Domains of measurement

Measures in common use in psychiatric epidemiology can be thought of as covering six main domains:

1. **Demographic status:** age, gender, marital status, household circumstances, occupation.
2. **Socio-economic status:** social class, income, wealth, debt.
3. **Social circumstances:** social network, social support.
4. **Activities, lifestyles, behaviours:** a very broad area, its contents are dictated by the focus of the research – examples would include tobacco and alcohol consumption, substance use, diet, and exercise. Some measures such as recent exposure to positive and negative life events may be particularly relevant to psychiatric research.
5. **Opinions and attitudes:** an area of measurement initially restricted to market research organizations, but increasingly being adopted by social science and biomedical researchers.
6. **Health status:** measures can be further grouped into:
   (a) specific measures of 'caseness', i.e dichotomous diagnoses such as schizophrenia, or dimensions, i.e continuously distributed traits such as mood, anxiety, neuroticism and cognitive function
   (b) global measures, e.g.subjective or objective global health assessment, disablement (impairment, activity and participation) and health-related quality of life
   (c) measures reflecting the need for, or use of health services.

Caseness and dimensions

Measures of 'caseness'

At first sight, the concept of psychiatric caseness can seem arbitrary, confusing and possibly even unhelpful. For example, a recent review of 40 community-based studies of the prevalence of late-life depression concluded that there was wide variation in reported prevalence, but that the most important source of variation seemed to be the diagnostic criteria that were used to identify the cases. Thus the 15 studies that measured DSM major depression had a weighted average prevalence of 2% (range 0–3%). Twenty-five studies using other criteria gave a weighted average prevalence of 13% (range 9–18%). Is the correct prevalence of late-life depression 2% or 13%? Surely both these contrasting estimates cannot be right. In our confusion, we are led to ask the question 'What is a case of depression?'. The answer will depend always on the purpose for which the measurement is being made. The question should therefore not be 'What is a case?' so much as 'A case for what?'.

Diagnostic criteria can be classified as broad or narrow, and as more or less operationalized. Broader criteria include diffuse and less severe forms of the disorder, narrow criteria exclude all but the most clear-cut and severe cases. Operationalized criteria make explicit a series of unambiguous rules according to which people either qualify or do not qualify as cases. DSM-IV major depression criteria (American Psychiatric Association 1994) are both narrow and strictly operationalized. In the other studies included in the review late-life depression was both more broadly and more loosely defined. Operationalized criteria were not used; for these studies the threshold was defined in terms of the concept of 'clinical significance', a level of depression that a competent clinician would consider merited some kind of active therapeutic intervention.

The narrow criteria for major depression define a small proportion of persons with an unarguably severe form of depressive disorder, implying strong construct validity. Since the criteria are strictly operationalized they can also be applied reliably. This might then be a good case definition for the first studies investigating the efficacy of a new treatment for depressive disorder. Major depression might also be a good 'pure' case definition for a genetic linkage study, aiming to identify gene loci predisposing to depression in a multiply affected family pedigree. However, these criteria will not suit all purposes. One cannot presume for instance that the findings from the drug efficacy studies will generalize to the broader group of depressed patients whom clinicians typically diagnose and treat, but who do not meet criteria for major depression. Also, major depression criteria arguably miss much of the impact of depressive disorder within a community population. Depressed persons are known to be heavy users of health and social services. However, the very small number of cases of major depression account for a tiny proportion of this excess, which is mainly made up of cases of 'common mental disorder'.

Measures of dimensions

The idea of a psychiatric disorder as a dimension can be difficult for psychiatrists to grasp. They are used to making a series of dichotomous judgements in their clinical practice. Is this patient depressed? Does he need treatment? Should he be admitted? Does he have insight? Is he a danger to himself? As Pickering commented (when arguing that hypertension was better understood as a dimensional rather than a dichotomous disorder) 'doctors can count to one but not beyond'. It is important to recognize that a dimensional concept need not contradict a categorical view of a disorder. As with the relativity of the concept of 'a case', it may be useful under some circumstances to think categorically and in others dimensionally. There is for instance a positive correlation between the number of symptoms of depression experienced by a person and:

- the impairment of their quality of life
- the frequency with which they use GP services
- the number of days they take off work in a month.

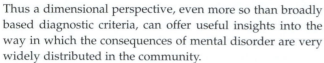

Thus a dimensional perspective, even more so than broadly based diagnostic criteria, can offer useful insights into the way in which the consequences of mental disorder are very widely distributed in the community.

From a technical point of view, continuous measures of dimensional traits such as depression, anxiety, neuroticism and cognitive function offer some advantages over their dichotomous equivalents, major depression, generalized anxiety disorder, personality disorder and dementia. These diagnoses tend to be rather rare; collapsing a continuous trait into a dichotomous diagnosis may mean that the investigators are in effect throwing away informative data; the net effect may be loss of statistical power to demonstrate an important association with a risk factor, or a real benefit of a treatment.

Validity

Construct validity

This refers to the extent to which the construct that the measure seeks to address is real and coherent, and then also to the relevance of the measure to that construct. Construct validity cannot be demonstrated empirically, but evidence can be sought to support it. For example, the scope and content of the construct can be identified in open-ended interviews and focus group discussions with experts or key informants. These same informants can review the proposed measure and comment on the appropriateness of the items (face validity).

Concurrent validity

This is tested by the extent to which the new measure relates, as hypothesized, to other measures taken at the same time (hence concurrent). There are four main variants: criterion, convergent, divergent and known group validity.

Criterion validity is tested by comparing measures obtained with the new instrument to those obtained with an existing *criterion* measure. The criterion is the current 'gold standard' measure and is usually more complex, lengthier or more expensive to administer, otherwise there would be little point in developing the new measure! In psychiatry there are generally no biologically based criterion measures as, for example, bronchoscopy and biopsy for carcinoma of the bronchus. The first measures developed for psychiatric research were compared with the criterion or 'gold standard' of a competent psychiatrist's clinical diagnosis. More recently, detailed standardized clinical interviews such as SCAN have taken the place of the psychiatrist's opinion.

Convergent and divergent validity should be tested in relation to each other. A measure will be more closely related to an alternative measure of the same construct than it will be to measures of different constructs. Thus the general health questionnaire (GHQ – a measure of psychiatric morbidity) should correlate more strongly with the Beck Depression Scale than with a physical functioning scale, or with a measure of income.

Known group validity can be assessed where no established gold standard external criterion exists. Thus a new questionnaire measuring the amount of time parents spend in positive joint activities with their children could be applied to two groups of parents, identified by their health visitors or teachers as having contrasting levels of involvement with their children.

Predictive validity

This assesses the extent to which a new measure can predict future variables. Thus depression may predict time off work, or use of health services; cognitive impairment may predict dementia.

Measuring validity

Concurrent validity of a continuous measure against another continuous measure as criterion is measured with a Pearson's (parametric) or Spearman's (non-parametric) correlation coefficient. Concurrent validity against a dichotomous criterion is usually expressed in terms of the validity coefficients, *sensitivity*, *specificity*, and *positive* and *negative predictive value*. When the same subjects have been assessed using the new measure and the 'gold standard' criterion measure, the results can be summarized in a 2×2 table (Table 9.1).

The *sensitivity* of the new measure is the proportion of true cases correctly identified:

$$\text{Sensitivity} = a / a + c.$$

The *specificity* of the new measure is the proportion of non-cases correctly identified:

$$\text{Specificity} = d / b + d.$$

The *positive predictive value (PPV)* of the new measure is the proportion of respondents it identifies as cases that actually are cases according to the 'gold standard':

$$\text{PPV} = a / a + b.$$

The *negative predictive value (NPV)* of the new measure is the proportion of respondents it identifies as non-cases that actually are non-cases according to the 'gold standard':

$$\text{NPV} = d / c + d.$$

Table 9.1   Validity assessment: a 2×2 table

New measure	Gold standard	
	Case	Non-case
Case	a	b
Non-case	c	d

Likelihood ratios

The overall predictiveness of a given test result can be conveniently summarized as the *likelihood ratio*. The likelihood ratio is easily calculated:

LR = Probability of a given test result in diseased persons / Probability of that test result in non-diseased persons.

Using Bayes' theorem we can calculate the post-test probability of disease given knowledge of the pre-test probability (in this case disease prevalence) and the likelihood ratio (LR) associated with different test results.

For example, the apolipoprotein E ε4 genotype is strongly associated with risk for Alzheimer's disease (AD). A typical finding for the association is given in Table 9.2. Use of these prevalence rates, and the presence of any apoE ε4 allele as the test criterion, suggests a test with 78% specificity and 63% sensitivity for a diagnosis of AD.

The LRs derived from the ApoE ε4 frequencies given in Table 9.2 are:

$$\text{Homozygous (two } \varepsilon4 \text{ alleles)} = 0.13 / 0.03 = 4.3$$

$$\text{Heterozygous (one } \varepsilon4 \text{ allele)} = 0.50 / 0.19 = 2.5$$

$$\text{No } \varepsilon4 \text{ alleles} = 0.37 / 0.78 = 0.48$$

The likelihood ratio for a positive test result (e.g. one or two ε4 alleles) is sometimes known as a likelihood ratio positive and that for a negative test result (e.g. no ε4 alleles) as a likelihood ratio negative.

The LR for a given test result is related to the pre-test and post-test probability of disease, for:

$$\text{Pre-test odds of disease} \times \text{LR} = \text{Post-test odds of disease}$$

If the pre-test probability of Alzheimer's disease is 0.10 (a generous estimate for the eventual lifetime prevalence for those who have already survived into their sixties) then the pre-test odds are $0.1 / (1 - 0.10) = 0.11$. If a subject is then found to be homozygous for apoE ε4 their post-test odds, given this additional information, become $0.11 \times 4.3 = 0.47$. This translates into a post-test probability of disease (Positive Predictive Value for the test) of: $0.47 / (1 + 0.47) = 0.32$. The post-test probabilities for heterozygosity and for no apoE ε4 allele are 0.22 and 0.05 respectively. The positive predictive values (0.32 and 0.22)

therefore encompass too much uncertainty to be of use to screened subjects and their clinicians. One reason for this shortcoming is the low prevalence of AD. For a test with given predictive power the post-test probability of disease is crucially dependent on the pre-test probability. Rarely can a single test be used as an early indicator of a disease with as low a population prevalence as AD. This demonstrates in another way the impact of disease prevalence upon PPV mentioned above. It can be shown that a test with a given LR will provide a maximum 'gain' of post-test diagnostic probability when the pretest probability is in the region of 0.4–0.6. One solution then might be to apply the test to a target population with a known high lifetime prevalence of the disease; in the case of apoE ε4 and AD for instance the test might work satisfactorily in those with a strong family history of AD. Alternatively, Bayes' theorem can be used to combine a number of moderately predictive tests into a more effective package. Given the assumption of conditional independence (that is, that the results of the second test do not depend on the results of the first) then:

$$\text{Pre-test odds} \times \text{LR (test 1)} \times \text{LR (test 2)} =$$
$$\text{Post-test odds (tests 1 and 2)}.$$

Reliability

Test–retest reliability (intra-measurement reliability)

Intra-measurement reliability tests the stability of a measure over time. The measure is administered to a respondent, and then after an interval of time is administered again to the same person, under the same conditions (e.g. by the same interviewer). The selection of the time interval is a matter of judgement. Too short and the respondent may simply recall and repeat their response from the first testing. Too long, and the trait that the measure was measuring may have changed, e.g. the respondent may have recovered from their depression.

Inter-observer reliability

Inter-observer reliability tests the stability of the measure when administered or rated by different investigators. Administering the measure to the same respondent under the same conditions by first one and then the other interviewer tests interinterviewer reliability. Having the same interview rated by two or more investigators tests inter-rater reliability.

Measuring reliability

Intra-measurement and inter-observer reliability are assessed using measures of agreement. For a continuous scale measure the appropriate statistic would be the intra-class correlation. For a categorical measure the appropriate statistic is Cohen's kappa; this takes into account the agreement expected by chance, and is independent of the prevalence of the condition in the test population.

Table 9.2 The association of the apolipoprotein E ε4 genotype with Alzheimer's disease		
	Controls	*AD cases*
Homozygous (two ε4 alleles)	3%	13%
Heterozygous (one ε4 allele)	19%	50%
No e4 alleles	78%	37%

The internal consistency of a measure indicates the extent to which its component parts, in the case of a scale the individual items, address a common underlying construct. This is conventionally considered a component of reliability. For a scale it is usually measured using Cronbach's coefficient alpha, which varies between 0 and 1. Coefficient alpha of 0.6 to 0.8 is moderate but satisfactory, above 0.8 indicates a highly internally consistent scale. Another measure of internal consistency is the split-half reliability, a measure of agreement between subscales derived from two randomly selected halves of the scale.

EPIDEMIOLOGICAL STUDY DESIGNS

As with the plots of Hollywood movies, there have only ever been a limited number of epidemiological designs in general use. However, the details of the study designs, and the conduct and analysis of these studies has become increasingly refined and sophisticated. Studies may be experimental or nonexperimental (observational). Observational studies may use observations made on individuals, or aggregated data from groups or populations. They may be descriptive or analytic in purpose and design. Figure 9.2 summarizes the main types of study design.

On the following pages, the essentials of these basic types of study design are illustrated with reference to their application to the epidemiology of schizophrenia.

Studies of disease frequency (population prevalence and incidence)

Prevalence is defined as the proportion of persons in a defined population that have the disease under study at a defined time period. This may be point prevalence (prevalence at the instant of the survey), one month prevalence (prevalence at any time over the month before the study) and so on. The one year prevalence for schizophrenia has been reported generally to lie between 0.3 and 0.8 per cent (Jenkins et al.1997a).

Incidence risk is defined as the probability of occurrence of disease in a disease free population (population at risk) during a specified time period. The annual incidence risk for schizophrenia lies between 7 and 14 per 100 000 (Sartorius et al. 1986).

Note that the 1-year prevalence of schizophrenia is approximately 50 times greater than the annual incidence risk. Prevalence (P) is approximately equal to the product of incidence (I) and disease duration (T): $P = I \times T$. Disease is terminated either by death or recovery. For conditions with high short-term mortality rates (lung cancer) or short-term recovery rates (common cold) prevalence and incidence rates are similar. Schizophrenia is evidently a chronic condition.

Descriptive studies of disease frequency can be used to generate hypotheses about disease aetiology, particularly where the prevalence and incidence of a disease varies by geographical region (geographic variation) or over time (secular variation).

Geographic variation

Some early individual studies of schizophrenia prevalence have reported unusually low rates (e.g.among the Hutterite Anabaptist sect in the USA) or unusually high rates (e.g.in north-western Yugoslavia, and among the Tamils of southern India). Such unusual findings may be used to generate hypotheses about aetiology. However, the US–UK Diagnostic Project (Cooper et al. 1972) indicated that the higher rates of schizophrenia observed in New York compared with London could be accounted for by diagnostic bias – a much broader concept of schizophrenia was being used by US psychiatrists. The WHO International Pilot Study of Schizophrenia (WHO 1973), and the later WHO Collaborative Study on Determinants of Outcome of Severe Mental Disorders (Sartorius et al. 1986) demonstrated that when both clinical interview techniques and case criteria were standardized, there was little variability in prevalence and incidence rates between different centres, in North and South America, Europe, Africa, Asia and the Far East. However, 2-year outcome did still seem to be better in developing than developed countries (Sartorius et al. 1977; Sartorius et al. 1986). The WHO findings illustrate some important points to bear in mind when making comparisons between studies in different regions:

Non-experimental					Experimental
Descriptive	Analytic				
1. Population prevelance/ incidence (a) geographic variation (b) temporal ('secular') variation	2. Ecological correlation	3. Cross-sectional survey	4. Case-control study	5. Cohort study	6. Randomized controlled trial

Figure 9.2 Types of study design

1. Diagnostic procedures for psychiatric disorders that have been standardized in one setting may not be applied indiscriminately to another. They may turn out to be culturally biased, giving a misleadingly high or low estimate of the prevalence of the disease.
2. Other methodological differences between studies, for example in sampling procedures and in inclusion and exclusion criteria, may have important effects on prevalence estimates.
3. Low prevalence may be accounted for either by selective out-migration of susceptible persons, or by in-migration of those unlikely to develop the disorder, and vice versa for high prevalence.
4. As prevalence is the product of incidence and duration, low prevalence rates may indicate a high recovery rate or a low survival rate for those with the disorder, rather than a true difference in incidence. Longitudinal studies measuring disease incidence and duration are needed if valid comparisons are to be made between settings.

Temporal (secular) variation

Der et al. (1990) reported that UK first contact rates for schizophrenia and related disorders had been falling over the previous two decades. Their paper was entitled 'Is schizophrenia disappearing?'. The decline in first contacts with psychiatric services may have reflected an underlying decline in the incidence of schizophrenia over the same period. As with geographic variation, secular changes in the incidence of disease can give important clues about aetiology. However, first admissions may have fallen in this case because of changes in the organization of psychiatric services, or, for example, an increasing tendency for new cases to be managed more extensively in primary care. Responses to this paper (Graham 1990; Prince & Phelan 1990) discuss some of the reasons why administrative data on first admission may have been an unreliable and unstable (hence biased) indicator of the underlying incidence rate for schizophrenia in the general population.

Ecological correlations

It has long been recognized that there is a correlation at the ecological level between the prevalence of schizophrenia in populations and the socio-economic status of the populations (Faris & Dunham 1939; Hare 1956), with higher rates among residents of more deprived areas. There are three main problems with ecological correlations. In the first instance both exposure and outcome are aggregate measures at the level of populations. We do not know if the people with schizophrenia are necessarily those with low socio-economic status. Thus, an ecological correlation need not imply a correlation at the level of individuals within the population. This problem is referred to as the 'ecological fallacy'. Secondly, even if the ecological correlation does

reflect an association at the level of individuals, a third factor, correlated with socio-economic status (for instance diet in childhood) may be the real causal factor. This factor would be a confounder (see later in the chapter), but since data on this exposure has not been collected, we have no way of controlling for its effects. Thirdly, we do not know if the low socio-economic status of the neighbourhood has caused the schizophrenia (the social causation theory), or whether people about to develop schizophrenia lose social status and move into areas of relative socio-economic deprivation (the social drift theory)(Gerard & Houston 1953). The social drift theory would be an example of reverse causality in action – the disease causing the 'exposure' rather than vice versa. For all these reasons it is difficult to make causal inferences from ecological correlations. They may however be used to develop hypotheses for further investigation.

The cross-sectional survey

In a cross-sectional survey, all members of a population are surveyed simultaneously for evidence of the disease under study (the outcome) and for exposure to potential risk factors.

Uses of a cross-sectional survey

Cross-sectional surveys can be used to measure the prevalence of a disorder within a population. This may be useful for:

- planning services – identifying need, both met and unmet
- drawing public and political attention to the extent of a problem within a community
- making comparisons with other populations or regions (in a series of comparable surveys conducted in different populations)
- charting trends over time (in a series of comparable surveys of the same population).

They can also be used to compare the characteristics of those in the population with and without the disorder, thus:

- identifying cross-sectional associations with potential risk factors for the disorder
- identifying suitable (representative) cases and controls for population-based case-control studies.

Findings from population-based cross-sectional surveys can be generalized to the base population for that survey, and to some extent, to other populations with similar characteristics. The main drawback of cross-sectional surveys for analytical as opposed to descriptive epidemiology, is that they can only give clues about aetiology. Because exposure (potential risk factor) and outcome (disease or health condition) are measured simultaneously one can never be sure, in the presence of an association, which led to which. The technical term is 'direction of causality'.

Base populations and sampling frames

Cross-sectional surveys survey a defined base population. This could be, for instance:

- all in-patients in a hospital
- all hospital in-patients in a given country
- all residents of a city borough aged 65 and over
- all residents of a country (aged 18-60).

First it is necessary to identify a sampling frame of all eligible persons. Criteria for eligibility need to be thought through carefully, but usually include a place of residence criterion and a period criterion; thus all residents of a defined area, resident on a particular day or month. Participants may (rarely) need to be excluded from the survey because of health or other circumstances that render their participation difficult or impossible. These exclusion criteria should ideally be specified in advance. Every effort should be made to be as inclusive as possible, in order to maximize the potential for generalization of the survey findings. Sampling frames for population-based surveys require an accurate register of all eligible participants in the base population. In most countries, such registers are drawn up and updated regularly for general population censuses, for taxation and other administrative purposes, and for establishing voting entitlement in local and national elections. However, there are problems associated with using such registers. Some may not contain all of the information (e.g. age, sex and address) that is needed to identify and contact a sample with a specified age range. Many governments will either not allow researchers to have access to these registers, or will set limits on the information that can be gleaned from them, or will limit the way in which the data is used. Also many administrative registers are surprisingly inaccurate, particularly in the case of highly mobile urban populations. Thus people move address without informing the relevant agency, or move or die in the interval between regular updates of the register. Because of these deficiencies, some population-based surveys draw up their own register by carrying out a door-knock census of the area to be surveyed. While this is practical for a small catchment area survey, a survey of a larger base population such as the population of a whole country would need a different strategy. Often investigators draw a random sample of households, which are then visited by researchers who interview either all eligible residents, or individuals selected at random from among the eligible residents in the household.

Rare conditions

The cross-sectional survey is an inefficient design for a rare disorder such as schizophrenia. With a population prevalence of less than 1%, noncases will outnumber cases

by more than 100 to 1. However, all participants need to be screened for the presence of the disorder. If all the true cases are to be identified, many false positives will also have to be processed. Cases will be over-represented in in-patient facilities, in hostels and among the homeless. These populations may be difficult to access by standard community survey techniques. Unless special attempts are made to sample these subpopulations there is a clear risk that an unrepresentative sample of cases would have been identified, leading to bias. For all these reasons cross-sectional surveys of schizophrenia are relatively uncommon (Jenkins et al. 1997b). The case-control study is a much more efficient design (see below).

Case-control studies

Case-control studies are relatively quick and cheap, and are particularly appropriate for the initial investigation of the aetiology of rare conditions. Schizophrenia is a rare disorder, and case-control studies have been widely used. Case-control studies aim to recruit, from a notional base population, a random sample of all persons with the disease under study (cases) and a random sample of persons without the disease (controls). The odds of being exposed for cases is compared with the odds of being exposed for controls. The resulting measure of effect, an odds ratio (OR), will approximate to the relative risk (RR) if the disease is rare. The OR begins to depart significantly from the RR when the prevalence of the disease in the population reaches 10% (Table 9.3).

Bias (see also p. 126) can be a particular problem in case-control studies unless particular care is taken with the study design. Selection of cases and controls is crucial. The chances of being selected as a case or as a control must not depend on exposure, as this would lead to *selection bias*. Since cases have already developed the disease, inquiry into exposure to risk factors is generally retrospective. The methods used to ascertain exposure must be applied symmetrically to both cases and controls in order to reduce *information bias* (observer bias or recall bias).

The case-control design has been used to investigate the relationship between obstetric complications and the onset of schizophrenia in later life. Lewis et al. (1987) compared

Table 9.3 Case-control studies		
	Cases	*Controls*
Exposure[+]	a	b
Exposure[−]	c	d
Odds of being exposed if a case = a / c		
Odds of being exposed if a control = b / d		
Odds ratio = (a / c) / (b / d) = (a d) / (b c)		

the birth circumstances of their case series of patients with schizophrenia with those of a large control group of patients with other psychiatric diagnoses, from the same case register. This was probably a reasonable choice of control group. However, exposure was ascertained retrospectively from relatives who may well have been influenced in their recall of obstetric complications by the subsequent knowledge that their relative had gone on to develop schizophrenia. Dalman et al. (2001) largely avoided the problem of recall bias by ascertaining exposure from maternity records made at the time of birth.

Cohort studies

Cohort studies compare the incidence of new cases of the disease under study in groups of persons free of the disease at outset but who are (1) exposed and (2) not exposed to a hypothesized risk factor. The ratio of incidence risk between the two groups gives a risk ratio (RR), which is the measure of effect for a cohort study (Table 9.4).

Cohort studies have two principal advantages over case-control studies. Firstly, the longitudinal perspective allows direction of causality to be established. Since exposed and unexposed are both free of the disease at the outset of the study, an increased risk of *disease onset* among the exposed, implies that the exposure has led to the disease rather than

Table 9.4 The cohort study

	Cases	Non-cases	Total
Exposure$^+$	a	b	a + b
Exposure$^-$	c	d	c + d
Incidence risk in exposed = a / (a + b)			
Incidence risk in non-exposed = c / (c + d)			
Risk ratio = (a / (a+ b)) / (c / (c + d))			

vice versa. Secondly, information bias is limited, for at the time when the exposure is ascertained neither the respondent nor the investigator should be influenced by the disease outcome, which has not yet occurred. However, cohort studies can be lengthy and costly, as the sample size needs to be large enough, and the period of follow-up long enough to accumulate sufficient numbers of incident cases of the disease to make a statistically meaningful comparison between the two groups. For these reasons they are not the first choice of study design for rare conditions. However, many of these obstacles can be removed where a cohort with appropriate baseline exposure measures already exists, and the outcome may be cheaply and conveniently ascertained. These studies are called historical cohort studies. There are two good examples of such opportunistic designs within the schizophrenia literature. David et al. (1995) used data routinely gathered on handedness, hearing and epilepsy among male conscripts to the Swedish army, and related it to their future risk of developing schizophrenia, by linking the army conscription data to the Swedish National Register of Psychiatric Care. Jones et al. (1994) used data on child development gathered during the UK National Survey of Health and Development, based on a representative sample of all babies born in one week in 1946, and again related it to the participants' future risk of developing schizophrenia. The continuing regular surveillance of the birth cohort helped to identify those who had developed the disorder. In the UK there is no national register of schizophrenia cases but the 1946 cohort could also be cross linked with the Mental Health Enquiry, a central register of all admissions to psychiatric hospitals, with ICD diagnoses on discharge.

The defining characteristics of case-control and cohort studies are described and compared in Table 9.5.

Randomized controlled trials

Randomized controlled trials are experimental studies. Given the tightly controlled experimental conditions, it may

Table 9.5 Case-control and cohort studies: characteristics, advantages and disadvantages

	Case-control	Cohort
Subjects selected according to	Caseness	Exposure
Perspective	Retrospective (subjects recall exposure)	Prospective (usually) (observers attend outcome)
Sources of bias	Selection Information (recall and observer)	Information (observer only). Non response
Resources	Quick Relatively cheap	Lengthy Relatively expensive
Useful for	Rare outcomes Single exposures Multiple exposures	Rare exposures Single exposures Multiple outcomes
Measure of effect	Odds ratio	Relative risk

be possible, for once, to make direct causal inferences from effects observed to be associated with a particular treatment condition. The ability to make these inferences relies on two essential conditions for a well-conducted trial; blinding and randomized allocation.

Blinding

A trial is double-blind if neither the participant nor the investigator know the treatment condition to which the subject has been randomized, single blind if the investigator knows but the participant does not. Blinding is an essential condition for a rigorous trial. Information bias may otherwise be a problem. A participant who believes themselves to be receiving an effective treatment may report a falsely positive outcome, and an investigator may also bias their assessment of outcome if they know the treatment condition. The adequacy of blinding can be assessed by asking participant or investigator, as appropriate to guess the participant's random allocation. Blinding the participant can be difficult, or impossible where psychological rather than pharmacological therapies are being trialled. Blinding the investigator should still be feasible.

Randomized allocation

Assuming that randomization is carried out properly and that the trial is large, then all potential confounding factors, anticipated and unanticipated, should be evenly distributed between the different treatment conditions. Any difference in outcome between the groups should then be attributable to the treatment alone. Confounding should not be a problem unless randomization procedures have failed. This may occur through chance alone, particularly if the trial is small, or through non-random interference with the allocation procedure. The advantages of randomization can also be lost if the data analysis is restricted to those participants who complete the trial. An *intention to treat analysis* analyses all on the basis of their initial randomized allocation, regardless of whether they initiated, complied with or completed the intervention as planned.

One consistent finding in the schizophrenia literature has been that high levels of expressed emotion (EE) among relatives and co-residents of persons with schizophrenia tends to increase the relapse rate in the short to medium term. The validity of this finding has been enhanced by the demonstration in well-conducted randomized controlled trials that family interventions designed to reduce EE lower the relapse rate (Leff et al. 1982). Several such trials have been published and the results have been brought together in a meta-analysis demonstrating a convincing and consistent effect (Mari & Streiner 1994). This was one of the first such reviews in clinical psychiatry published by the Cochrane Collaboration. The Cochrane Collaboration aims to encourage and disseminate evidence-based practice by sponsoring meticulous and comprehensive reviews and judicious meta-analyses of accumulated data.

INFERENCE

Inference is the 'process of passing from observations to generalizations'. As such, this is a key activity in epidemiological investigation. We have seen already that the observation of an association need not signify that the risk factor *causes* the outcome with which it is associated. The role of chance, bias, confounding and reverse causality first need to assessed. Only if these competing explanations can be confidently excluded may a causal attribution be considered.

Chance

Statistical inference involves generalizing from sample data to the wider population from which the sample was drawn. Inferences are made by calculating the probability that, given the size of the sample, chance alone might have accounted for a given observation.

Sampling error and sampling distributions

Chance operates through sampling error. If we wanted to know the average height of boys aged 16 in the United Kingdom, we would not go to the trouble of measuring the height of every male of that age. We would instead draw a representative sample from a population register. Random selection of participants should ensure representativeness. However, if the sample was relatively small, say 100 boys, then it is quite likely that, by chance, we would happen to sample those who were on average slightly taller or slightly shorter than 16-year-olds in general. If we repeat the study over and over again, drawing each time a sample of 100 boys, and measuring the mean height on each occasion we would end up with a *sampling distribution* as in Figure 9.3. The observed means from repeated sampling are normally distributed. This tends to be true even if the trait itself is not normally distributed in the population (the proof is referred to as the central limit theorem). The mean (and median and mode) of the sampling distribution are equal to the population mean; sample estimates for the mean that

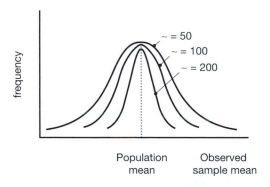

Figure 9.3 Sampling distribution for different sample sizes

deviate considerably from the true population mean are observed much less commonly, and are represented in the tails of the distribution. Note that if the size of the samples is increased, then the variance of the means obtained through repeated sampling decreases. This is because larger samples tend to give more precise estimates.

Standard errors and confidence intervals

The standard deviation for the sampling distribution is known as the standard error of the mean, and has the property that 95% of sample means obtained by repeated sampling lie ±2 (actually 1.96) standard errors above or below the population mean. This information can therefore be used to construct limits of uncertainty around an observed sample mean, giving the range of likely values for the population mean. These limits of uncertainty are referred to as 95% confidence intervals. The standard error of the mean is the standard deviation of the population (usually estimated as the standard deviation of the sample) divided by the square root of the sample size. Thus the observed mean height of the sample of 100 boys might be 160 cm with a standard deviation of 40 cm. The standard error of the mean would then be $40 / \sqrt{100} = 4$ cm. The 95% confidence intervals would then be 160 cm $\pm 4 \times 1.96$, or 152–168 cm. This would signify that given the sample size and the variance of heights in the sample, there would be a 95% probability that the true mean height of the whole population of 16-year-olds would lie between 152 cm and 168 cm, with only a 5% probability that it lay outside. In descriptive studies, statistical inference therefore allows us to estimate the precision of sample estimates of measures such as mean anxiety score or prevalence of depression.

In analytical epidemiology, however, we test hypotheses; for example, that those exposed to obstetric complications are more likely to go on to develop schizophrenia than those not so exposed. Statistical inference still works in much the same way as with descriptive studies. Now we are using a *sample* of a certain size to estimate the real relative risk for the association between obstetric complications and schizophrenia *in the general population*. Sampling error may lead us to observe a relative risk (RR) that is lower or higher than the real population effect. We can calculate the standard error of the RR, and use it to construct 95% confidence

intervals around our observed value. Again there will be a 95% probability that the true RR lies within these confidence intervals, and a 5% probability that it lies outside. Thus in the study of OCs and schizophrenia, an observed RR of 2.0 with 95% confidence intervals of 1.4 to 2.6 would suggest that a true RR less than 1.4 or more than 2.6 would be extremely unlikely (less than 2.5% probability in each case).

Statistical tests and p-values

Statistical tests test whether a hypothesis about the distribution of one or more variables should be accepted or rejected. In the case of a hypothesized association between a risk factor and a disease, we can estimate the probability (p) of the observed or an even greater degree of association being observed if the null hypothesis were true, i.e accounted for by chance alone, there being no association. Conventionally, the threshold for statistical significance is taken to be 0.05. This means that, for a population in which two factors were *not* associated, if the same study, with the same sample size were to be repeated a hundred times, then on average an association of at least the size observed might be recorded five times. It is important to remember that there is nothing magical about the p = 0.05 threshold. It represents nothing more than a generally agreed acceptable level of risk of making what is known as a Type I error, i.e. falsely rejecting a null hypothesis when it is true. The probability of rejecting the null hypothesis when it is indeed false (i.e detecting a true association) is the study's statistical power. The converse scenario, accepting a null hypothesis when it should have been rejected (i.e. failing to detect a true association) is referred to as a Type II error, and the probability of committing this error is clearly (1 – power) (Table 9.6).

The relationship between p-values and confidence intervals

If we return to the example of the study assessing the association between obstetric complications and schizophrenia we can see that confidence intervals convey all of the information given by p-values, and more besides. The 95% confidence intervals for the RR of 1.4 to 2.6 tell us immediately that the null hypothesis RR of 1.0 is implausible given the observed value of 2.0, and thus that the null

Table 9.6 Type I and Type II errors		
Null hypothesis	True	False
Accepted	No association Null hypothesis correctly accepted	True association, but null hypothesis mistakenly accepted Type II error Probability = 1 – power
Rejected	No association, but chance observation mistakenly leads to rejection of null hypothesis Type I error Probability = significance	True association, correctly identified Probability = power

hypothesis can be rejected with reasonable confidence. The probability of a true RR of 1.0 is certainly less than 5% and thus the association is 'statistically significant' at $p < 0.05$. However, the confidence intervals also give us a range of plausible values, both upper and lower, for the true RR.

Bias

Bias is a special type of error. Most error is random, arising either from sampling error or simple lack of precision in measurement. Such error is equally likely to result in higher or lower estimates. Bias, however is non-random or systematic error. In the case of simple descriptive measurements bias may arise because, for example a doctor taking blood pressure rounds up every measurement to the next 5 mmHg mark. The estimate of the mean blood pressure level for the population will clearly be biased upwards. In the case of estimating associations, bias occurs where error operates differentially with respect to both exposure and outcome. Thus in a case-control study addressing the hypothesis that depressed people had low blood pressure, the doctor taking the blood pressure measurements might round up the blood pressure levels of controls but round *down* the blood pressure levels of depressed cases. This bias would overestimate the strength of any true association, or perhaps produce a wholly spurious association between depression and low blood pressure.

Bias is an entirely undesirable feature that cannot be adjusted for once data has been gathered (contrast with confounding below). The epidemiologist's only hope is to limit the scope for bias in the way in which the study has been designed.

There are several different types of bias. The most common are

- selection bias
- non-response bias
- information bias including:
  (a) recall bias
  (b) observer bias.

Selection bias

Selection bias is a potential problem wherever individuals are selected for inclusion in a study because of the presence or absence of certain characteristics. This is particularly an issue in case-control studies, where controls are selected to be as similar as possible to the cases who are included in the study, except that they do not have the disease. The golden rule in designing case-control studies is that a control should be eligible to be included as a case should they develop the disease, and a case should be eligible to be a control if they did not have the disease. A case-control study seeking to identify risk factors for Alzheimer's disease, found that arthritis was more common among controls than among cases. This finding might have been taken to suggest that

arthritis was in some way protective against AD. However, this case-control study recruited its cases from among new cases of AD recently referred to specialist dementia clinics. Its age and sex-matched controls were selected at random from among patients *attending* primary care surgeries. The flaw in this selection procedure, as the authors of the study acknowledged, was that the controls needed some reason to visit their doctor. One of the most common reasons in this age group was arthritic aches and pains. Had the dementia cases not developed Alzheimer's disease they might not have been eligible to be controls, because they may not have needed to visit their doctor. The cases, simply because of the different selection procedures for cases and controls, were less likely than the controls to have had to have a history of arthritis. This is selection bias.

Selection bias can be minimized by following the 'golden rule' cited above. Selection of cases and controls is a critical component of case-control studies. It needs to be attended to very carefully, and inclusion and exclusion criteria described in detail in published papers.

Non-response bias

Non-response bias can occur when subjects who refuse to take part in a study, or who drop out before the study can be completed, are systematically different from those who participate. In simple descriptive epidemiology for example, the prevalence of depression in a community may be underestimated if those with depression are less likely to participate in the cross-sectional survey than those without depression. An association between lack of social support and depression may be overestimated if either those with good social support are less likely to take part if they are depressed, or if those with poor social support are less likely to take part if they are not depressed. Again, note that when an association between an exposure and a disease is being estimated, bias will only occur if the error operates differentially with respect *to both*.

Non-response bias can be minimized by minimizing non-response. Non-response becomes a critical issue when response rates fall below 70%, but significant non-response bias can still occur even at these levels of participation. The likelihood of non-response bias having occurred can be assessed (although not quantified) by comparing the characteristics of responders and non-responders. Usually some basic socio-demographic information such as age and gender is available from the register or database from which the subjects have been recruited. Similarity of responders and non-responders in terms at least of these basic characteristics is reassuring but does not exclude the possibility that bias has occurred.

Information bias

Recall bias occurs when participants in a study are systematically more or less likely to recall and relate information on exposure depending on their outcome status, or to recall information regarding their outcome dependent on their exposure. This form of bias can be a particular problem in case-control studies. Thus cases with multiple episodes of major depression as an adult may be more likely to recall and report childhood abuse than controls with no history of mental health problems. Often the experience of having the disease that is being studied encourages an 'effort after meaning' whereby the person who is a case has already gone over his/her life history in an attempt to understand why he/she had become ill. This clearly predisposes to recall bias.

Observer bias is another form of information bias caused by an investigator incorrectly ascertaining or recording data from a participant in a study. Again, for bias to be a problem, the error must be systematic with respect to both exposure and outcome. The example given above of the investigator selectively rounding up and rounding down blood pressure measurements is an example of observer bias. Alternatively, an investigator who believes that child sexual abuse does cause major depression in adulthood might put extra effort into obtaining disclosure of abuse from subjects whom they knew to be in the depression case group.

Information bias can be reduced in case-control studies by keeping participants and observers blind to the hypotheses under investigation. This can be difficult, and some would argue may challenge the ethical principal of informed consent. However, biased research results are wrong, misleading and a waste of subject's time. Blinding can be encouraged by making the title of the study non-specific, and by including irrelevant questions in the risk factor questionnaire to distract subjects from the central hypothesis under investigation. Information bias will be less of a problem in cohort studies because neither exposed nor unexposed participants or the investigators know who will go on to develop the disease that is being studied, when their exposure status is ascertained at the beginning of the study.

Confounding

The term confounding derives from the latin *confundere*, meaning to mix up. Confounding describes a situation in which a measure of the effect of an exposure is distorted because of the association of that exposure with other factors that influence the disease or outcome under study. A confounding variable can cause or prevent the outcome of interest, is not an intermediate variable and is independently associated with the exposure under investigation.

The concept of confounding is best illustrated with an example. Clearly, there is an association between grey hair and the risk of dying. Some imaginary but plausible data is given in Table 9.7. While there is an association between grey hair and risk for dying, this association is a spurious one, accounted for entirely by the confounding effect of a third variable, age. Thus older people are more likely to have grey

hair, and independently (i.e for reasons entirely unconnected with the grey hair) are at greater risk of dying (Fig. 9.4).

When we carry out a *stratified analysis*, we find that the strong association between grey hair and dying is no longer apparent in each of the different age strata. This example illustrates some of the ways in which we may control for confounding in both the design and the analysis of our studies.

In the design, if we had *matched* our grey-haired and non grey-haired subjects for the suspected confounding variable (age), then we would have been able to make a fair comparison of the death rates of the two groups. Matching could have been carried out on a one-to-one basis, i.e. for every grey-haired person recruited, we recruit a non-grey-haired person of a similar age, or by restriction matching, i.e we only recruit those aged 40–60. Randomization is the ultimate technique for control of confounding. Where an intervention can be randomly assigned then *all* other factors should be evenly distributed between the intervention group and the control group. Any difference between the two groups can be reasonably confidently attributed to the intervention. The virtue of the randomized design is that all potential confounders measured and unmeasured,

Table 9.7 An imaginary example of confounding

	Annual mortality rate		
	Grey hair	No grey hair	RR
All ages	20/1000	5/1000	4.0
20–40 years	1/1000	1/1000	1.0
40–60	10/1000	10/1000	1.0
60+ years	40/1000	40/1000	1.0

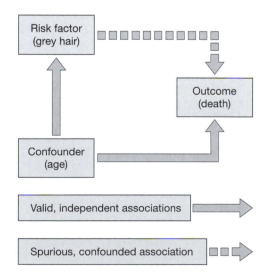

Figure 9.4 An example of confounding.

suspected and unsuspected are automatically controlled for in the design. Of course, ethically, we can only randomize interventions that we believe may benefit, but where no strong evidence exists one way or the other.

In the analysis of the data, where matching has not been carried out, a stratified analysis of the kind seen in Table 9.7 clearly demonstrates the presence or absence of confounding. There are also more complicated forms of statistical analysis, collectively referred to as multivariate analysis, which can adjust simultaneously for the effects of several potential confounding variables. These are multiple regression and analysis of variance (ANOVA) for continuous outcomes, and logistic regression for dichotomous outcomes. Note that confounding differs in this respect from bias. A biased study is irretrievably flawed. With confounding, as long as the confounding variable has been measured, we can adjust for its effects (Box 9.2).

Causation

The refutationist approach to the study of causation, advanced by Karl Popper, holds that 'the criterion of the scientific status of the theory is its falsifiability or refutability or testability'. Thus, in its purest form a theory regarding causation should lead to an observational prediction (a hypothesis). An experiment is then designed with the express purpose of showing that the prediction *will not be fulfilled*. If that happens, the theory from which the prediction was deduced must be wrong. On the other hand, if the prediction is borne out by the experiment, then the theory from which the prediction was deduced is not, thereby, confirmed but merely corroborated. That is, it has survived one attempt to falsify it, but may not avoid others in the future. In short, hypotheses can be definitively refuted, but never proved.

When the effects of chance, bias, confounding and reverse causality have been excluded, we have demonstrated a valid statistical association. This is not the same as demonstrating that a risk factor has caused a disease. Austin Bradford Hill, one of the originators of the modern epidemiological method laid down some further criteria to be considered before making a causal attribution:

- strong associations
- consistency with findings from other studies
- plausibility given our understanding of possible underlying biological mechanisms
- dose–response relationships.

In fact none of these criteria, with the exception of temporality, is a necessary condition for a causal association. Each of them individually, and in particular several of them combined, can bolster the case for considering an association to be causal. The process is not unlike a judge and jury weighing the evidence against a defendant and convicting 'beyond reasonable doubt'. Furthermore, each scientific study provides a mere brick in the wall of a carefully constructed characterization of a causal process. Pursuing the doctrine of refutationism, the most carefully constructed edifice can come tumbling down in the face of superior evidence for the absence of an association. As Bradford Hill remarked, 'All scientific work is incomplete – whether it be observational or experimental. All scientific work is liable to be upset or modified by advancing knowledge. This does not confer upon us a freedom to ignore the knowledge we already have, or to postpone the action that it appears to demand at a given time.'

FURTHER READING

Prince M, Stewart R, Ford T & Hotopf M (2003) *Practical Psychiatric Epidemiology*. Oxford: Oxford University Press.
Hennekens CH, Buring JE & Mayrent SL (eds) (1987) Epidemiology in Medicine. Boston/Toronto: Little Brown.
Kirkwood BR (1998) *Essentials of Medical Statistics*, 2nd edn. Edinburgh: Churchill Livingstone.
Lewis G & Pelosi AJ (1990) The case-control study in psychiatry. *British Journal of Psychiatry* 157: 197–207.
Mari JJ & Streiner D (1997) Family intervention for schizophrenia. Schizophrenia module of the Cochrane Database of Systematic Reviews. Available in the Cochrane Library disk and CD-ROM. The Cochrane Collaboration; Issue 4. Oxford: Update Software. (Originally published as Mari J & Streiner D (1994) An overview of family interventions and relapse on schizophrenia: meta-analysis of research findings. *Psychological Medicine* 23: 565–78.)

REFERENCES

American Psychiatric Association (1994) *Diagnostic and Statistical Manual of Mental Disorders*, 4th edn. Washington, DC: APA.
Cooper JE, Kendall RE, Gurland BJ, Sharpe L, Copeland JRM & Simon R. (1972) *Psychiatric Diagnosis in New York and London*. Maudsley Monograph No 20. London: Oxford University Press.
David A, Malmberg A, Lewis G, Brandt L & Allebeck P (1995) Are there neurological and sensory risk factors for schizophrenia? *Schizophrenia Research* 14: 247–51.
Dalman et al. (2001) Signs of asphyxia at birth and risk of schizophrenia. *British Journal of Psychiatry* 179: 403–8.
Der G, Gupta S & Murray RM. (1990) Is schizophrenia disappearing? *Lancet* 335: 513–16.
Faris R & Dunham W (1939) *Mental Disorders in Urban Areas* (reprinted 1960). New York: Hafner.
Gerard DL & Houston LG (1953) Family setting and the social ecology of schizophrenia. *Psychiatric Quarterly* 27: 90–101.

Box 9.2   Controlling for confounding
In the design of a study:

Matching
   One-to-one
   Restriction matching

Randomization
In the analysis of a study:
Stratified analysis
Multivariate analytical techniques

Graham P (1990) Trends in schizophrenia [letter]. *Lancet* **335**: 852.

Hare EH (1956) Mental illness and social conditions in Bristol. *Journal of Mental Science* **102**: 349–57.

Jenkins R, Lewis G, Bebbington, P, Brugha T, Farrell M, Gill B & Meltzer H (1997a) The National Psychiatric Morbidity Surveys of Great Britain – initial findings from the Household Survey. *Psychological Medicine* **27**: 775–89.

Jenkins R, Bebbington P, Brugha T, Farrell M, Gill B, Lewis G, Meltzer H & Petticrew M. (1997b) National Psychiatric Morbidity Surveys of Great Britain – strategy and methods. *Psychological Medicine* **27**: 765–74.

Jones P, Rodgers B, Murray R & Marmot M (1994) Child development risk factors for adult schizophrenia in the British 1946 birth cohort. *Lancet* **344**: 1398–402.

Last JM (2001) *A Dictionary of Epidemiology*. New York: Oxford University Press.

Leff J, Kuipers L, Berkowitz R, Eberlein-Vries R & Sturgeon D. (1982) A controlled trial of social intervention in the families of schizophrenic patients. *British Journal of Psychiatry* **141**: 121–34.

Lewis G, David A, Andreasson S & Allebeck P (1992) Schizophrenia and city life. *Lancet* **340**: 137–40.

Lewis SW & Murray RM. (1987) Obstetric complications, neurodevelopmental deviance and risk of schizophrenia. *Journal of Psychiatric Research* **21**: 413–22.

Mari J & Streiner D (1994) An overview of family interventions and relapse on schizophrenia: meta-analysis of research findings. *Psychological Medicine* **23**: 565–78.

Prince MJ & Phelan MC (1990) Trends in schizophrenia [letter]. *Lancet* **335**: 851–2.

Sartorius N, Jablensky A & Shapiro R (1977) Two-year follow-up of patients included in the WHO International Pilot Study of Schizophrenia. *Psychological Medicine* **7**: 529–41.

Sartorius N, Jablensky A, Korten A, Ernberg G, Anker M, Cooper JE & Day R. (1986) Early manifestations and first-contact incidence of schizophrenia in different cultures. *Psychological Medicine* **16**: 909–28.

World Health Organization (1973) *Report of the International Pilot Study of Schizophrenia*. Geneva: WHO.

Critical appraisal: reading academic papers and reviewing scientific evidence

Matthew Hotopf

INTRODUCTION

The medical literature is vast, complex and contradictory. There has been an exponential rise in the number of journals and the volume of research published over the past 30 years. Doctors are expected to keep abreast of this literature, but may find themselves unable to balance the competing demands of clinical and managerial work. Textbooks such as this attempt to help by distilling this knowledge into manageable information, yet there are many reasons why much of the knowledge accumulated and presented as 'fact' may be incorrect (even here!). Examinations that use multiple choice questions require candidates to answer complex questions with simple yes/no responses, when many of these answers require careful qualification.

Evidence-based medicine

Evidence-based medicine (EBM) has grown out of these concerns. A recent handbook on EBM (Sackett et al. 1997) described the process as follows:

> The practice of EBM is a process of life-long, self-directed learning in which caring for our own patients creates the need for clinically important information about diagnosis, prognosis, therapy and other clinical and health care issues.

The description then outlines five stages by which EBM is practised: (1) identifying the information needs of the practitioner; (2) identifying the literature that can fulfil those needs; (3) checking how good that literature is; (4) applying the literature to clinical practice and (5) checking on progress.

The emphasis of this chapter will mainly be on the third stage – namely, critical appraisal of published literature. The chapter starts with a general guide on how to read and interpret the results of scientific papers. This will be followed by worked examples of the four main epidemiological study designs. These examples describe fictitious studies whose methodological flaws are explored in a questions and answers format. The aim is to introduce the reader to typical methodological concerns that arise with each study design, and to indicate how well-designed studies may be able to address these concerns. The final section of the chapter covers the methodologies of systematic reviews and meta-analysis. There are numerous websites that discuss aspects of evidence-based medicine, and some of these are listed in Box 10.1.

Box 10.1 Useful websites related to evidence-based medicine	
Cochrane Collaboration:	http://www.cochrane.org/
UK Department of Health National Research Register:	http://www.update-software.com/National/
Oxford Centre for Evidence-Based Medicine:	http://www.cebm.net/
Bandolier:	http://www.jr2.ox.ac.uk/bandolier/
Centre for Health Evidence:	http://www.cche.net/che/home.asp
Health Information Research Unit:	http://hiru.mcmaster.ca/
NHS Centre for Reviews and Dissemination:	http://www.york.ac.uk/inst/crd/
Evidence-Based Medicine Resource Center:	http://www.ebmny.org/

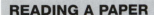

READING A PAPER

In contrast to reading a novel, reading academic papers is an active process. When reading a novel the reader is a relatively passive recipient of a stream of narrative. Unless the reader cheats (for example, checking who the murderer is in a 'whodunit') he/she usually starts at the beginning and reads to the end. When reading academic papers this approach is usually too time consuming. It is better to approach the paper as an active process: the reader becomes a researcher in his/her own right setting out with a number of questions to be answered. This chapter is structured around the sorts of questions which are helpful to ask before, during and after reading an academic paper. A number of texts are available that cover these issues in more depth (Crombi.e. 1996; Greenhalgh 1997; Prince et al. 2003).

1. What are your aims in reading the paper?

The intensity with which a paper is read depends on why you are reading it in the first place. It may be for no more than passing curiosity, or because you are setting up a research project on a related topic. You may want to find out the best treatment for a patient you are seeing, or to assess whether a previous experience reported by a patient (for example sexual abuse or delayed milestones) has any bearing on his/her current condition. Each of these are legitimate reasons for setting out to read the literature, but in each case the information required from it differs.

Even if you are simply skimming the literature, it is important not to be too easily impressed by a paper's 'take home message'. The temptation in reading it is to seek the final definitive answer such as 'non-directive counselling doesn't work', 'passive smoking causes lung cancer' or 'depression increases mortality'. Approaching a paper in this simple way leads to a number of problems. The 'message' requires substantial qualification before it can be accepted, let alone generalized to clinical practice.

In order to address this problem a number of journals have attempted to break complex information presented into more readily digested chunks. One approach to this is the structured abstract, where the summary of the aims, methods, results and conclusions of the paper allows the reader to extract the salient points quickly. In journals such as the *British Medical Journal* the study design and participants form separate headings, making the information available in the abstract still more explicit. *The British Journal of Psychiatry* breaks down the 'take home message' by asking the authors to have three conclusions to the paper balanced by three of its limitations. In order to get used to extracting information from papers in a meaningful way it is worth reading a number of journals regularly – these may include the major psychiatric journals (*Psychological Medicine, British Journal of Psychiatry, Archives of General Psychiatry, American Journal of Psychiatry*) and some general medical journals (*Lancet* and *British Medical Journal*).

2. What were the authors' aims?

Good papers always state explicitly why the authors set out to do what they have done. The aims should usually be obvious from three sources: the title, the abstract, and at some point in the introduction (usually in the last paragraph). Broadly speaking, the aims of the paper will depend upon whether it is a *descriptive* or *analytical* study.

Descriptive studies

The aim of much research is to describe. In epidemiology this is often a measure of the frequency of a disorder, e.g. 'We aimed to determine the prevalence of schizophrenia in a rural Nigerian population'. In qualitative research it may be to describe the attitudes of a small group, e.g. 'We aimed to describe attitudes of carers of patients with psychiatric disorder regarding the use of the Mental Health Act'. In both cases the authors try to tell us something about how things are in the world, which may be useful in order to answer questions like 'What provision would be required to provide care for people with schizophrenia in rural Nigeria' or 'What changes would users of mental health services like to see in Mental Health Legislation?'. Note that these sorts of questions are unlikely to be answered with statistical testing: they are not trying to prove or disprove anything, only to describe.

Analytical studies

In analytic studies the aim is to test a hypothesis. By convention the researcher starts with a null hypothesis, e.g. 'Active treatment is no more effective than placebo'. The study then sets out to test this hypothesis. If at the end of the study 20% more patients on active treatment have recovered compared to those on placebo, one may be tempted to reject the hypothesis, and state that active treatment is more effective. Analytic studies often assess causal relationships between risk factors and illness, or treatments and recovery. In doing so they usually use statistical testing to assess the degree to which the observed association could be explained by chance.

3. What study design was used?

The next question is to determine what broad approach was used in the research. The previous chapter has described the main epidemiological study designs. It is striking how well the quality of a paper correlates with how clearly and explicitly the study design is described. The design should be described in full in the methods section, but is often also given in the title and abstract.

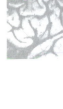

A useful test of the adequacy of a paper's methods section is whether another researcher would have a chance of replicating the study on the information provided. Would they be sure how the participants were recruited, what questions they were asked, or treatments they received? In much clinical research the study design is not explicitly stated. This is especially true of biological research which, for example applies a new technology (imaging, neuro-endocrine challenge tests and so on) to a series of patients and compares the results with a control group. This sort of research rests on the same assumptions as case-control studies, and is susceptible to the same flaws. For example, a study that uses functional magnetic resonance imaging on 20 patients with schizophrenia and compares the results with 20 healthy controls can still suffer from selection bias (see below), especially if the researcher has twisted the arms of his highly educated colleagues to act as controls!

4. What are the main results?

The next step is to examine the main results of the paper. These are usually to be found in the abstract, in the results section (including tables) and at the start of the discussion section. Results can be presented in many different ways depending on the study design, outcomes and statistical techniques used.

Good research should always give the reader a feel for the data. You should expect to see a table where the data are described in a simple way, without complicated statistics. For example, in a cohort study it is reasonable to see how those exposed to the risk factor compare to those not exposed to it. Are they similar in terms of their main socio-demographic characteristics? Always be suspicious if the only results you see are the results of sophisticated statistical models. Data presentation should be transparent.

Another consideration in digesting the results is the exact form they take. Consider a hypothetical case-control study of obstetric complications in schizophrenia. The paper found that 20% of cases (with schizophrenia) and only 10% of controls (without schizophrenia) had a history of obstetric complications. Leaving aside alternative explanations for this association (which are discussed below), then each of the following statements could describe these results:

1. 'Individuals with schizophrenia were more likely to report obstetric complications than were controls.'
2. 'Individuals with schizophrenia had a statistically significant (< 0.05) higher level of reported obstetric complications than controls.'
3. 'Some 20% of our participants with schizophrenia had obstetric complications as opposed to 10% of controls.'
4. 'Schizophrenia was associated with more reported obstetric complications (odds ratio 2.0; 95% confidence interval 1.1–3.5).'
5. 'Schizophrenia was associated with more reported obstetric complications (odds ratio 2.0; 95% confidence interval 1.1–3.5). Given a population rate of obstetric complications of 10% the population attributable fraction was 9.1%.'

Each statement is describing the same result, but with increasing sophistication. There are five components to these results:

1. The simple result (schizophrenia is associated with obstetric complications).
2. The level of statistical significance (described as a p-value).
3. The effect size (i.e. the fact that 20% of those with schizophrenia versus 10% of those without it had obstetric complications. The odds ratio is also an expression of effect size).
4. The *precision* of the estimate of effect size (described as the confidence intervals around the odds ratio).
5. The population impact of the exposure. This is the population attributable fraction, which is described in the previous chapter, and is the proportion of cases of schizophrenia that would be avoided if obstetric complications were directly causal and could be eradicated.

Note that the effect size is much more interesting than the level of statistical significance. In older studies it is very common to see results presented almost solely as p-values, but it is very difficult to understand what this means. With a sufficiently large sample size it is possible for even very small effect sizes (for example odds ratios of 1.1) to become highly statistically significant. However, it is the effect size, rather than the level of significance, that usually determines how much faith the reader will have in the results. As a rule of thumb for observational studies (cross-sectional, case-control and cohort), an odds ratio or relative risk of less than 2 is very easily produced as a result of bias or confounding. Unless the study is remarkably large and well conducted this sort of effect size should be interpreted with caution. Randomized controlled trials are by no means immune to bias and confounding, but are less susceptible, and therefore smaller effect sizes can be reliably identified.

5. What alternative explanations are there for any reported results?

Good papers explicitly point their readers to potential flaws in the research. This is usually done in the discussion section. In some journals authors are now required to provide a list of shortcomings for their paper. Usually the main shortcomings may be addressed by thinking of the list of alternative explanations of reported associations. These were covered in the previous chapter and are briefly revised here:

1 chance

2 bias

3 confounding

4 reverse causality.

Chance

Type I and Type II error

Most studies aim to describe reality by taking a *sample* of the total population. However the sample will not exactly describe the true underlying population distribution: there is always a degree of *sampling error*. This is akin to the fact that tossing a coin 10 times will yield different combinations of heads and tails. Statistically the *most likely* result would be five heads and five tails, but any combination of heads and tails is possible. More extreme results (e.g. all tails or all heads) become less probable with increasing tosses of the coin. In other words, increasing the sample size increases the precision with which the underlying 'true' situation can be estimated. In the example of schizophrenia and obstetric complications described above, we *assume* that the study is representing reality. Nevertheless, if 10 identical studies were performed they would all come up with slightly different results. The size of the difference would depend upon the size of the sample in each study.

Studies that report a positive finding (i.e. they find an association between obstetric complications and schizophrenia) may either be describing the true underlying situation, or by chance have committed a Type I error. Type I error occurs where an association is detected by chance. This is assessed by statistical testing. By convention the Type I error rate is usually set at $p < 0.05$, in other words the probability of the association being false is 1 in 20. It is easier for a study to detect a true association if that association is a very powerful one. In other words, it is considerably easier to detect the ten-fold increase in lung cancer among smokers than it is to detect the 1.1-fold increase in schizophrenia among those born in winter months.

Studies that report a negative finding (i.e. they find no association between obstetric complications and schizophrenia) may either be describing the true underlying situation, or by chance have committed a Type II error. Type II error occurs when a genuine association is missed by chance. Type II error is dealt with in the design of the study by performing a power calculation. This usually sets the Type II error rate at 10–20%. In other words, most studies that perform a power calculation accept that there is a 10–20% chance that they will fail to detect a true difference. Statistical power is the converse of the Type II error rate: usually set at 80–90%. Statistical power is increased with larger sample sizes. Type I and Type II errors are shown in tabular form in Table 10.1.

Points to consider if a study reports one or more positive associations:

1. It could still be chance There is no p-value that can 'prove' an association, but by convention we often take 'statistical significance' to mean $p < 0.05$. This means that one time in 20 we expect to detect the difference by chance, and there is no way of knowing whether the study we are reading is that one time. This is why cautious researchers will often make comments such as 'our findings require replication'. It may be that the finding simply was a fluke, even with 'statistically significant' results.

2. *Multiple statistical testing* The more hypotheses tested, the greater the likelihood of finding a significant association. If researchers performed a case-control study of risk factors for dementia, and collected data on 40 possible risk factors, they might expect two such risk factors to be associated at $p < 0.05$ *just by chance*. This leaves researchers and their readers with genuine dilemmas. On the one hand it seems wasteful not to report all possible associations. On the other, it would be misleading to pretend that some of the results reported couldn't have occurred by chance.

The best way to overcome this dilemma is for the researcher to set out with one or two main hypotheses to be tested. These would form the centre of the research proposal, and the sample sizes would be determined on these hypotheses. All additional findings can be labelled 'secondary analyses', and be seen as a useful by-product of the main research. This consideration is especially important in randomized trials of new treatments as the results of the research may have direct impact on patients. Of course it is up to the reader to decide whether the '*a priori*' hypotheses described by the researchers really were proposed before the results were analysed. There is a move to publish protocols to research projects in advance, and this improves the transparency of the reporting of the completed study.

3. *Publication bias* Publication bias is another problem that may lead to chance positive findings being more evident than a true underlying negative relationship. Publication bias occurs when the likelihood of research being published

Table 10.1 The relationship between the results of a study and 'true life'		'True life'	
		Association exists	No association exists
Study	Association demonstrated	✓	Type I error
	No association demonstrated	Type II error	✓

✓ indicates the study results represent 'true life'.
Most studies set the Type I error rate (α) at 0.05 or less, and the Type two error rate (β) at 0.1 – 0.2. The *power* of a study is $1 - \beta$ (i.e. 80–90%).

is influenced by the results of that research. Journals may prefer to publish results that back up an association, rather than those that report a negative finding. This is discussed further in the section on systematic reviews.

4. *Subgroup analyses*   In subgroup analyses the researcher breaks down the statistical analysis according to certain characteristics of the subjects. For example, imagine you had performed a randomized trial of clomipramine and placebo in the treatment of obsessive compulsive disorder. To your disappointment you find no overall difference. What many researchers go on to do is find a difference in special groups and end up making statements like 'While our findings indicated clomipramine was no better than placebo for the majority of patients with OCD, it does appear to have a useful effect in females over the age of 55 with a family history of the disorder'. This statement implies that they have made a number of different comparisons and ended up squeezing the data to detect a significant result in this small group. Subgroup analyses are very common (Pocock et al. 1987), and very deceptive.

Points to consider if the study reports a 'negative finding'
Imagine an antidepressant drug trial assessing two antidepressants in the treatment of depression. The investigators chose a reference compound (imipramine) and compared it with a new drug (hypexine). They recruit 50 patients with depression and compare the treatment effects of the two drugs on the change in Hamilton Depression Rating scores. In presenting their results they state 'We detected no difference between the two compounds in terms of changes in the Hamilton scores. This results indicates that hypexine is as potent and effective as imipramine'. This sort of study is extremely common (Hotopf et al. 1997), and frequently comes to this sort of conclusion.

In this example the investigators pit two drugs against one another, both which may be effective in depression. If a true difference existed between the two treatments it is likely to be a small one. Note that placebo-controlled trials of antidepressants indicate that one-third of people treated with a placebo will be better at six weeks. Two-thirds of people treated with imipramine get better. Now imagine that people treated with the new drug experience an efficacy rate somewhere between that of imipramine and placebo – say a 50% recovery rate. Table 10.2 shows the numbers of people who would have to be randomized to detect these differences setting power at 80% and confidence at 95%.

Table 10.2 indicates that it is not really surprising that the study failed to show a difference between the two treatments. If the investigators had performed a power calculation before embarking on their study it would have shown that they needed at least 320 subjects to show 50% of people recovering on hypexine. These sorts of small trials are common in psychiatry and the rest of medicine. The main thing to be aware of is the interpretation of the results: an

underpowered study that demonstrates no difference between two treatments *does not* indicate that the treatments have similar efficacy!

Bias

Bias is a result of study design, and takes two main forms: selection bias and information bias. Selection bias is a particular problem of case-control studies and is most likely to occur in situations where cases are derived from highly specialized clinical settings. An example of the role of selection bias is given in the worked example of case-control studies.

Information bias occurs in two main ways: recall bias and observer bias. In recall bias the disease status of subjects affects their likelihood of reporting the exposure. For example, a patient with cancer may be more likely to recall being a smoker. In schizophrenia research the disease status may reduce the likelihood that the sufferer will recall an exposure. Recall bias is best avoided either by using cohort studies or by gaining information from alternative sources (such as hospital records).

Observer bias occurs where the disease status or treatment of the subject leads the researcher to ask questions or assess the subject differently. This is the main reason why double blinding of clinical trials is so important, especially when subjective symptoms (e.g. depression) are used as an endpoint.

Confounding

Confounding was described in Chapter 9. The difference between confounding and bias is that confounding is a property of 'real life' situations, whereas bias is an error the researcher introduces into the design of the study. Confounding occurs where an *additional* factor causes the outcome of interest and is associated with the exposure under study. For example, if a study found that alcohol consumption was associated with lung cancer, the obvious

Table 10.2 Effect size and power: note how ever increasing numbers are required as the effect size gets smaller	
Recovery rate on hypexine (%) (compared with 66% improvement on imipramine)	Number required to be randomized
33	82
40	128
50	320
55	654
60	2096

confounder would be smoking, because heavy drinkers are more likely to be heavy smokers.

In reading a paper it is worth considering first: 'Could any confounder have accounted for the association reported?' and second: 'Have the researchers controlled for any of the confounders that I have thought of?'.

In the example of alcohol and lung cancer, you will already have identified smoking as an important potential confounder. The researchers could have dealt with this in a number of ways:

1. **Restriction:** they could have only included people who had *never smoked* into the study. In other words they deal with the confounder by excluding anyone who could be affected by it.
2. **Matching:** in a case-control study they may have matched those with lung cancer and those without according to how much they reported smoking, and then assessing alcohol consumption between groups.
3. **Stratifying:** they may have collected the data and then broken down the sample into *strata* according to how much they reported smoking. The association between alcohol and lung cancer is then examined in never smokers, past smokers, light smokers and heavy smokers.
4. **Statistical modelling:** a number of statistical approaches exist whereby confounders are added into a regression equation to determine whether accounting for them reduces the association between the exposure and the disease.

If you can think of a potential confounder and the researchers have not dealt with it using one of these methods, it may be the reason for the association.

Reverse causality

Reverse causality occurs when the exposure is caused by the disorder rather than the disorder being caused by the exposure. In the life event literature one possibility would be that patients with depression are more likely to suffer life events. Their depression may lead to an under-performance at work that may cause them to lose their job. Much of the research on life events has sought to address these concerns.

Sometimes reverse causality may be quite subtle. For example, obstetric complications are associated with schizophrenia. The usual assumption is that this is because obstetric complications lead to subtle brain damage which predisposes to schizophrenia. An alternative view, however, is that individuals who later develop schizophrenia already have developmental brain abnormalities *in utero* that make them more prone to difficult deliveries, since childbirth requires the active participation of the foetus as well as the mother.

Having satisfied yourself that the reported association was not due to chance, bias, confounding or reverse causality, you are then in a position to take the association at face value. The next section will use a number of worked examples to look at specific study designs in greater detail.

WORKED EXAMPLES OF FOUR STUDY DESIGNS

Cross-sectional study

A cross-sectional study aims to estimate the prevalence of dementia in a community sample of adults aged 65 years or over. The investigators used a database of addresses available from a telephone company in order to identify their sampling frame. They then sent a letter to a random sample of 1000 adults over 65 inviting them to participate. Those who agreed were seen by a researcher. Those who did not reply were sent a second letter, and later visited by the research team. In the final report the response rate was reported to be 56%. The estimated prevalence of dementia was 5%.

Questions and answers
These are:

1. **How might the sampling procedure have biased the estimate of prevalence?**
   Cross sectional studies aim to measure prevalence. They therefore need to be representative of the population under study. The sampling frame chosen in this example may not have been representative because:
   (i)   Not everyone has a telephone. This sampling procedure would not have identified people who did not own a telephone. If people with dementia are less likely to have a telephone, this method would have underestimated dementia prevalence.
   (ii) Related to the first point is the fact that a high proportion of people with dementia will be in long term residential care. If the homes they live in did not have individual telephones for each resident, it is likely that they would have again underestimated the prevalence of dementia.
   (iii) If the telephone company was a relatively new one, people with dementia may have been less likely to have changed company.

These sorts of concerns are especially important in psychiatric disorder where, for many reasons, those affected may be less likely to live at a private residential address. Similar points could be made about surveys of prevalence of schizophrenia that do not consider the homeless population.

2. **Is the response rate likely to have affected the estimated prevalence of dementia?**
   The reported response rate was low – just over one-half of those eligible were contacted. It is not hard to see how in this sort of survey could get the estimate of

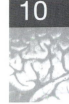

prevalence wildly wrong, if those having the disorder under study were more or less likely to participate. In this example, dementia is likely to affect the ability of sufferers to agree to participate. Those with dementia may be unable to understand the letter, or unlikely to have the wherewithal to answer it. Again this sort of problem is common for many psychiatric disorders: one could imagine how people with severe depression may feel less motivated to participate in community surveys of prevalence of depression. Similarly such research might feed into the paranoid delusions of people with psychotic illness.

3   **What techniques can be used to assess the impact of nonresponders on surveys?**
Any cross-sectional study should give details of the characteristics of nonresponders. For example, in the example given above of prevalence of dementia, it would be worth knowing whether the nonresponders were older than the responders. Age is an important risk factor for dementia, thus if those contacted were, on average five years younger than those not contacted, we would be even more concerned about the effects of non response bias.

Another useful technique is to guess how far the prevalence estimate could be out by. In the example given above the estimate could vary enormously. If *all* the nonresponders had dementia, the prevalence would rise to 46.8%. Of course it is very unlikely that all nonresponders had dementia. However, it is not inconceivable that the rate of dementia was increased three-fold in the nonresponders, in which case the total population prevalence would rise to 9.4%. This example illustrates how essential full response rates are for cross-sectional studies.

Case-control study

A group of virologists were interested to know whether a viral infection (coxsackie B virus) was a risk factor for chronic fatigue syndrome (CFS). They ran a clinical service that had attracted patients with debilitating fatigue for some years, and had previously published an influential paper suggesting this hypothesis. They decided to perform a case-control study comparing patients with post-viral fatigue syndrome and healthy controls. They devised a clinical diagnosis of post-viral fatigue syndrome that included the following criteria:

- debilitating fatigue lasting at least six months
- history of viral infection preceding the onset of fatigue.

They decide to measure exposure by estimating viral antibodies (IgG). The healthy control group was identified by asking cases to identify a friend or neighbour who was not fatigued. The research group found that 50% of those with post-viral fatigue had IgG to the infection, whereas only 15% of those without fatigue had antibodies.

Questions and answers
These are:

1   **How might the case definition used affect the prevalence of viral antibodies in the cases?**
The case definition of those affected is not independent of exposure. In other words, in order to be a case you have to have reported the exposure under study (i.e. viral infection). This is called *ascertainment bias*: the way in which the study population is ascertained has biased the results of the study. Note the circularity in this: in order to be a case, you have to have recalled exposure to a viral infection. It is therefore not surprising that the cases have higher rates of antibodies.

2   **Could the selection of patients into the clinic have affected the results?**
The clinic was run by enthusiasts who were wedded to a certain hypothesis. This means that local GPs may have been especially keen to refer patients who reported fatigue, and whom they also knew had a history of the infection. In other words there was *selection bias*. It is probably unusual to refer patients to see virologists if there is no history of viral infection!

3   **Could the selection of healthy controls have affected the results?**
The patients may have selected controls whom they knew had not been exposed to a recent viral infection. It is improbable that the patients would have chosen someone just recovering from influenza, hence the controls are not random members of the population. Thus there could have been a selection bias operating to reduce the chances of exposure among controls.

4   **Selection bias is a common problem in case-control studies. What techniques may be used to reduce selection bias?**
Selection bias is most likely to occur in the rarefied atmosphere of tertiary referral centres which may represent very unusual populations and where a suitable control group may be difficult to identify. Case control studies are best when they are 'nested' in cross-sectional or cohort studies or where the means of sampling cases is based on some population-based register. In selecting controls, ask 'If the control had got the disorder, would he/she have got into the study as a case?' In the example demonstrated above, a control who had chronic fatigue but who had not had a history of viral infection may not have been included.

Cohort study

A study examined the effect of depression as a risk factor for myocardial infarction. Patients with a history of depression

137

were recruited from a psychiatric service and compared with nondepressed individuals identified from general practice lists. The two cohorts were then followed for 10 years, at the end of which those who have died are identified from death certificates. The remaining sample were sent a questionnaire in the post asking whether they had suffered a heart attack or stroke in the past 10 years.

Seventy-five per cent of the survivors with depression responded, whereas 60% of the nondepressed survivors responded. The study found that the rate of nonfatal myocardial infarction was twice as high in the depressed group compared to the nondepressed.

Questions and answers

1   **Could the result have arisen from reverse causality?**
    This is possible, even though a cohort design was used. Cohort studies normally exclude people with the outcome of interest (i.e. heart disease) at the outset. However, there is no evidence that this happened from the above description. Some cohort studies in this area have taken *retrospective* samples of people with depression. This means they may not have been thoroughly assessed at the start of the study. Because heart disease (for example angina) is associated with depression, the depressed group may have started off with higher rates of heart disease than the non-depressed, and the result could simply reflect this relationship.

2   **Why might the response rate have differed for the depressed versus the non-depressed?**
    As in the discussion of cross-sectional studies, people with psychiatric disorders may be more or less likely to participate in research. In this case the people with depression were more likely to be followed up. This may reflect less mobility among the depressed group (in other words they remained at the same address and were therefore easier to contact at follow up) or greater interest in participating in research due to their experience of illness.

3   **Could the differential response rate have caused a problem?**
    It certainly is a potential problem. The overall follow up rate is not especially good. If the non-depressed non responder had a systematically higher rate of myocardial infarction than the depressed non responders this would suggest the reported association is exaggerated.

4   **Are there any additional explanations for the association?**
    Apart from chance, the other possibilities are recall bias, observer bias, and confounding. Recall bias could occur if subjects with depression may be more likely to experience chest pain of non-cardiac origin, and to interpret this as a heart attack. Confounding could

occur if those with depression had more risk factors for heart attack (smoking, high serum cholesterol or demographic risk factors such as coming from more deprived backgrounds). Observer bias could occur if either group were more assiduously investigated for heart disease.

Randomized controlled trials

You read a report of a multicentre randomized controlled trial of 'problem solving' versus antidepressants in the treatment of depression. Participants were recruited from primary care and were randomly assigned to receive either problem solving (five weekly sessions) or amitriptyline. The outcome is assessed by the general practitioner using the Hamilton Rating Scale for Depression at six weeks.

Questions and answers

1   **What problems could occur with the randomization and what descriptions would you like to see covered?**
    The main point about this study is that the treatments cannot be given blind. Both the doctor and patient are obviously aware that the patient has been prescribed an antidepressant or been enrolled into problem solving. This is in contrast with the usual double blind drug trials where patients are randomly assigned to receive one of two or more identical tablets. This has an impact on both the randomization, and how it is carried out, and the assessment of outcome.
    The problem in randomizing in this trial is that the doctor may have strong views about who would and who would not benefit from problem solving or antidepressants. If the doctor was also delivering the problem solving intervention they might only want the most cooperative patients to be allocated into this group. The randomization must *conceal allocation* adequately, such that it is impossible for the doctor to *predict* which patient would go into which group. For example, in some *quasi randomized* designs patients would get one treatment if randomized on an odd day of the month, or another treatment if randomized on the even days. It is thus easy to put the randomization off one day, and give the patient the treatment the investigator thinks will be best for them.
    In the above example there is another opportunity to cheat. If the doctor was randomizing patients him- or herself, and the patient was randomized to what he/she saw as the 'wrong' group, the doctor might 'forget' that the patient had been randomized, and try again, hoping that this time they would go into the 'right' group! Such fraudulent practice has happened, and therefore clinical trialists spend much time and energy making sure cheating cannot occur. Good randomized trials will report exactly how the randomization was performed.

It is worth noting that the adequacy of randomization is related to whether 'positive' findings are reported. Trials that use inadequate methods of randomization are far more likely to report 'positive' findings than those that do not, indicating that cheating the randomization may impact upon the research findings (Schulz et al. 1995). Improper randomization is akin to selection bias: there is a systematic bias whereby one group is likely to have a worse outcome than the other group.

2 **What problems might arise with the assessment of the outcome?**
The danger of using the assessment described is that it could introduces observer bias. The Hamilton Rating Scale for Depression is unstructured: it gives the clinician guidelines on how to assess the severity of depression based on their clinical interview. When the researcher is not blinded to the treatment group the patients have been allocated there is considerable room for observer bias.

3 **What techniques could reduce such observer bias?**
There are two main techniques. One would be to blind the rater to the treatment group. The other would be to use an assessment that is structured or even to use a written questionnaire. This would reduce the latitude the researcher had to ask leading questions.

REVIEWS

Clinicians with an unusual patient, or researchers about to explore a new field, often rely on reviews of the literature to describe what is known. Such reviews (which are common in medical journals and book chapters) are usually written by an expert with a special interest who distils a series of papers on the field into a summary of available evidence.

There has been a growing disquiet with this sort of *narrative review*. The main problem is that the process of data gathering (where data are now defined as published articles) may be haphazard. Narrative reviews often miss important articles, overemphasize others and are likely to show a bias towards research published by colleagues from similar backgrounds and nationalities. In other words, narrative reviews tend to include research reviewers know and agree with, but ignore work that comes from disciplines they are unfamiliar with or which contradict their point of view (Joyce et al. 1998).

The alternative approach is the *systematic review*, which may be loosely defined as a review where a systematic effort has been made to identify all relevant literature, to apply inclusion and exclusion criteria to that literature and to extract results in a systematic way (Lewis et al. 1997). As such, systematic reviews have a 'methods' section that should include the search strategy. This approach at least increases the likelihood that the reviewer will see a representative sample of all relevant literature. Systematic reviews may be done on all kinds of topics and all kinds of study designs including studies on screening and prognosis (Altman 2001; Deeks 2001); however, they have been most strongly associated with randomized controlled trials of treatments.

One component of systematic reviews is the methodology of meta-analysis. Whilst systematic reviews aim to identify, summarize and critically appraise all available literature, meta-analysis is a statistical synthesis of the main findings of the reviews. Meta-analysis is therefore a subsection of systematic reviews, and the two terms are not synonymous. The Cochrane Collaboration has in recent years provided an infrastructure for researchers to perform systematic reviews. Box 10.2 describes some of the work of the Collaboration.

Box 10.2   The Cochrane Collaboration

The Cochrane Collaboration is a non-profit making international organization that aims to assist researchers perform systematic reviews and disseminate their results. It is named after the British epidemiologist Archie Cochrane, who noted the failure of medicine to systematically gather data regarding the efficacy of medical treatments. The Collaboration has centres in Europe, Australasia, and North and South America. The centres support local researchers. The collaboration also has review groups that focus on specific illnesses. In psychiatry these include the Schizophrenia Group and the Depression Anxiety and Neurosis Group. Each group has several editors and one coordinating editor who assist researchers setting out with new projects, and ensure a high quality work.

The Cochrane Collaboration has several databases that are publicly available via libraries and the internet:

- The Cochrane Database of Systematic Reviews (CSDR) – a database of all completed reviews and protocol reviews.
- Cochrane Controlled Trial Register (CCTR) – a database of identified trials.
- The Database of Abstracts of Reviews of Effectiveness (DARE) – this is produced by the UK NHS Centre for Reviews and Dissemination and describes:
- The Cochrane Review Methodology Database – this is a database of research papers into the methodology of systematic reviews.

The Cochrane Collaboration produces computer software to assist meta-analysis, and runs an annual conference, the International Cochrane Colloquium.

The website for the Collaboration is http://www.cochrane.org/.

The main components of systematic reviews are:

1 The aims of the review (including hypotheses to be tested).
2 The search strategy.
3 Describing the inclusion and exclusion criteria for studies.
4 Critically appraising the quality of studies.
5 Summary of the results of included studies including meta-analysis.

Aims

Just as with primary research, systematic reviews should aim to answer specific questions, such as 'Is hormone replacement therapy associated with breast cancer?' or 'Are atypical antipsychotics more effective than typical antipsychotics for first episode psychosis?'

The search strategy used

There are numerous databases of the medical literature. Familiar ones are MEDLINE and EMBASE, which are generic medical databases. These two databases have different coverage, and only around one-third of the references on each are included in both. They are available on the internet and through academic libraries, and searching them is a basic skill. For psychiatrists and psychologists PsycINFO is a specialized database, one of whose advantages is that it contains many older studies. The Cochrane Collaboration has developed a database of randomized controlled trials, CENTRAL (The Cochrane Central Register of Controlled Trials).

Good systematic reviews go beyond electronic searches in a number of ways. Reference lists from the identified literature should be examined for citations of further relevant studies. Existing review articles (both systematic and narrative) that address overlapping subject matter can be used. Experts in the field should be contacted to see whether they have information on unpublished research. Pharmaceutical companies should be contacted for information on trials using their compounds. The 'grey literature' (unpublished theses, conference abstracts and the like) should also be identified where possible.

Description of inclusion and exclusion criteria

The systematic review should state explicitly which studies are included and which excluded. For reviews of treatment, the commonest exclusion criteria will be non randomized studies, or studies where the concealment of allocation is inadequate (see above). However, there may be additional reasons why studies are excluded: for example, they did not provide sufficient information on certain outcomes in which the reviewer is interested.

Critical appraisal of included studies

One of the most useful products of systematic reviews is a description of common problems in research methodology in a particular field. Systematic reviews should inform researchers in the future regarding weaknesses of previous studies, and especially why previous studies have not been able to answer burning clinical questions (Hotopf et al. 1997).

Presentation of results and meta-analysis

The results section will usually contain some information on the number of studies identified from the literature search, the number excluded and included, and the characteristics of the studies included (where they were done, and who was included).

Meta-analysis involves pooling together the results of a number of (usually) randomized controlled trials simultaneously. The main advantage of the approach is to improve statistical power. Because the majority of randomized trials in psychiatry are too small to give useful information, pooling the results of many studies should improve the precision of the effect size. The exact statistical methodology of meta-analysis is outside the scope of this chapter, but a few points are worth bearing in mind.

Not all studies are the same

Meta-analyses have been criticised for lumping together 'apples and oranges'. For example, different trials of the same intervention may take place in very different settings (outpatient, in-patient, primary care) with patients of differing severities or chronicity of the disorder. For pharmacological treatments the drug prescribed in different trials may have been identical, but the dosage is likely to be different. For non-pharmacological treatments such as psychotherapy or trials of the way in which community care is delivered, the treatment may differ radically between trials.

This *heterogeneity* between trials should be explored in meta-analyses (Thompson 1994). It is possible to use a statistical test of heterogeneity to assess whether all the trials included in a meta-analysis are 'pulling the same way'. If this test indicates that significant heterogeneity between trials exists, the investigators should be expected to investigate further. This would involve testing whether the effect size differs according to the type of study included.

Publication bias

Another serious problem with meta-analysis is publication bias. It is a fact of life that researchers and journal editors like to have 'positive' results. There is considerable evidence that papers that show one treatment has a clear advantage over another are more likely to be published than those that do not. Publication bias is the result: papers that are negative end up in the desk drawer of the researcher. This is equivalent to selection bias in observational epidemiology: it is as though all subjects who reported smoking but had not developed lung cancer were excluded from the study.

Meta-analysis assumes that no publication bias has occurred. It is not difficult to see how substantial publication bias could radically alter the conclusions of a meta-analysis. This has been one of the most serious criticisms of meta-analysis and has led to considerable efforts being made to avoid publication bias.

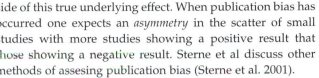

Registration of trials and medical trials amnesty
Randomized controlled trials now have to be registered, and this should mean that studies that would otherwise have remained unpublished are included in systematic reviews.

The search strategy
Good reviews attempt not to rely solely on published literature and go to considerable efforts to include unpublished work or work that has only been published in the 'grey literature' – for example, conference abstracts and university theses. To identify such literature the researchers may contact a number of key researchers in the field. The pharmaceutical industry sometimes does not publish research that has been used as submission data for licensing authorities. Reviews should therefore contact the makers of the drugs being studied and request such data.

Using a funnel plot
The funnel plot is a method to assess the potential role of publication bias (Egger et al. 1995). It relies on the fact that small studies are more likely to be susceptible to publication bias than large ones. If a researcher completes a large randomized trial they are likely to want to see it published even if the result is negative because of the effort involved. For small trials, however, the situation may be different. If publication bias does exist, it is most likely to be due to small negative trials not being published.

The funnel plot is a graphical representation of the size of trials plotted against the effect size they report (see Fig. 10.1) As the size of the trial increases trials are likely to converge around the true underlying effect size. For the large trials one would expect to see an even scattering of trials either

side of this true underlying effect. When publication bias has occurred one expects an *asymmetry* in the scatter of small studies with more studies showing a positive result that those showing a negative result. Sterne et al discuss other methods of assesing publication bias (Sterne et al. 2001).

SUMMARY

This chapter has aimed to describe some of the common flaws in research designs in psychiatry that readers of academic papers need to be aware of. I have attempted to cover some of the common flaws in a number of epidemiological study designs, and although I have not covered some of the more specialized areas of psychiatric research (for example neuroimaging, neuropsychological or endocrine studies), many of these principles still apply. In critical appraisal it is important to strike a balance between gullibility and cynicism. Most research has some flaws. Good critical appraisal involves recognizing those flaws, and pitting them against the main findings of the research.

REFERENCES

Altman DG (2001) Systematic reviews in health care: systematic reviews of evaluations of prognostic variables. *British Medical Journal* **323**(7306): 224–8.
Crombie IK (1996) *The Pocket Guide to Critical Appraisal*. London: BMJ Publishing Group.
Deeks JJ (2001) Systematic reviews in health care: systematic reviews of evaluations of diagnostic and screening tests. *British Medical Journal* **323**(7305): 157–62.
Egger M & Davey Smith G (1995) Misleading meta-analysis. *British Medical Journal* **310**: 752–4.
Greenhalgh T (1997) *How to Read a Paper. The Basics of Evidence Based Medicine*. London: BMJ Publishing Group.
Hotopf M, Lewis G & Normand C (1997) Putting trials on trial: the costs and consequences of small trials in depression: a systematic review of methodology. *Journal of Epidemiology and Community Health* **51**: 354–8.
Joyce J, Rabe-Hesketh S & Wessely S (1998) Reviewing the reviews: the example of chronic fatigue syndrome. *Journal of the American Medical Association* **280**(3): 264–6.
Lewis G, Churchill R & Hotopf M (1997) Systematic reviews and meta-analysis. *Psychological Medicine* **27**: 3–7.
Pocock SJ, Hughes MD & Lee RJ (1987) Statistical problems in the reporting of clinical trials. A survey of three medical journals. *The New England Journal of Medicine* **317**: 426–32.
Prince M, Stewart R, Ford T & Hotopf M (2003) *Practical Psychiatric Epidemiology*. Oxford: Oxford University Press.
Sackett DL, Richardson WS, Rosenberg W & Haynes RB (1997) *Evidence-based Medicine. How to Practice and Teach EBM*. New York: Churchill Livingstone.
Schulz KF, Chalmers I, Hayes RJ & Altman DG (1995) Empirical evidence of bias *Journal of the American Medical Association* **273**: 408–12.
Sterne JAC, Egger M & Smith GD (2001) Systematic reviews in health care: investigating and dealing with publication and other biases in meta-analysis. *British Medical Journal* 323(7304): 101–5.
Thompson SG (1994) Why sources of heterogeneity in meta-analysis should be investigated. *British Medical Journal* **309**: 1351–5.

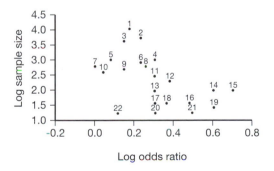

Figure 10.1 Example of a funnel plot. Each point represents an individual randomized trial. The *y*-axis is the log of the sample size of the trials. The *x*-axis is the log of the odds ratio of a good outcome. Trial 1 is the largest and estimates the odds ratio to be 1.5. Trials 2–10 are large and are evenly scattered around this value. Trials 11–22 are much smaller and tend to be more scattered around larger effect sizes. Note that there is an area in the lower left quadrant of the graph with only one trial (22). This represents possible publication bias, indicating that smaller 'negative' trials are less likely to be published.

Challenges to psychiatry: antipsychiatry, the user movement and stigma

Joanna Moncrieff, Peter Byrne and Michael Crawford

THE ANTIPSYCHIATRY MOVEMENT

Introduction

The aim of this first section is to to provide an introduction to some of the ideas of the antipsychiatry movement. Antipsychiatry is usually taken to refer to ideas expressed by some philosophers, sociologists and psychiatrists that first became widely recognized during the 1960s. Although there had been criticism of psychiatry before this, the ideas of antipsychiatry were new in the sense that they presented a fundamental critique of psychiatry from a philosophical and political perspective (Crossley 1998). They became popular and influential and converged with many of the wider changes in social attitudes and behaviour that occurred during the 1960s. Although there are differences between the ideas of individual antipsychiatrists, certain themes emerged as central to a common theory of what psychiatry was really concerned with.

The myth of mental illness

> Mental illness is a myth, whose function it is to disguise and render more palatable the bitter pill of moral conflict in human relations.
> (Szasz 1970: 24)

In his many publications, the psychiatrist Thomas Szasz has argued that the concept of mental illness is a myth, or a 'metaphor.' By this he means that mental illnesses are not the same as physical diseases, and only resemble them by virtue of the fact that 'we call people physically ill when their body functioning violates certain physiological and anatomical norms: similarly we call people mentally ill when their personal conduct violates certain ethical, political and social norms.' (Szasz 1970: 23). The brain can be diseased, for example in neurological disorders, such as epilepsy, brain tumours and degenerative brain diseases, but the mind cannot. Diagnosis of physical disorders is quite different from the way in which mental disorders are characterized. In physical diseases there are characteristic pathological findings or objective signs. In contrast, mental illnesses are ascribed on the basis of behaviours that deviate from social norms. Diagnosis of mental disorder is therefore an inherently subjective process, involving normative judgements that will vary depending upon the particular social and cultural context.

Szasz' challenge includes biological models that assume that mental illnesses are actually types of neurological or brain disorder, differing from most other neurological conditions only in the fact that their unique neuropathology has not yet been firmly identified. He argues that regardless of findings of some minor pathological deviations, major mental illnesses such as schizophrenia are still diagnosed on the basis of behavioural criteria, and hence are still defined by deviation from social and ethical norms. If specific and consistent neuropathology is uncovered, then the condition would cease to be a 'mental illness' and would become a neurological condition instead.

Szasz prefers to describe the behaviours that are labelled as mental illnesses as 'problems in living.' They arise from conflict between the individual concerned and the demands of society or the social network around him or her. Psychiatry is thus a 'moral and social enterprise' dealing with 'problems of human conduct' (Szasz 1970: 47). The conflicts may concern low-level antisocial behaviour, which may fail to reach the threshold of criminal activity. But often the conflict is about dependency. In a later work Szasz describes how psychiatry has arisen to provide a solution to the problem of adult dependency: 'the business of psychiatry is distributing poor relief (concealed as medical care) to adult dependents' (Szasz 1994: 149).

R.D. Laing, a Scottish psychiatrist, described the problems labelled as mental illness in slightly different, although not contradictory terms. Laing's main concern was to render the symptoms and behaviours associated with mental illness as meaningful experiences, not merely as the products of pathological processes. His first book, *The Divided Self* (Laing 1960), is a detailed examination of how the 'symptoms' of long-term institutionalized patients could be understood with reference to their lives and histories. His later work is a celebration of the experience of psychosis and its possibilities for expanding consciousness and transcending the alienation of everyday life. These ideas have been much criticized for minimizing the suffering of people with psychotic illnesses, but should be seen as the product of their time. The late 1960s was a time when experimenting with drug-induced altered forms of consciousness was much valued by the large counter-cultural movement. Some modern accounts of the experience of mental illness also attempt to reclaim the notion that there is positive value in psychotic and other extreme mental states.

Psychiatry and social control

> Psychiatry is a moral practice overlaid by the myths of positivism . . .
> (Foucault 1965: 276)

Michel Foucault was a French philosopher who was associated with the ideas of postmodernism. His first published book was about the evolution of society's response to madness from the Middle Ages through to the 19th century. Foucault's thesis is that up to the medieval period, madness was public and recognized as something to be feared and respected. In contrast, from the enlightenment onwards, madness came to be seen simply as an absence of reason or rationality that needed correcting. First attempts to achieve this involved confinement and discipline, but later a medical approach was adopted which disguised the fact that the management of the mad remained an essentially moral and political enterprise. These developments came about because of social changes wrought by the bourgeois and industrial revolutions that problematized idleness and demanded a strong work ethic and strict discipline. Hence psychiatry is seen as an institution that helps the modern state to create and maintain a disciplined work force by controlling behaviour that threatens that discipline. Foucault describes early psychiatric institutions as 'instruments of moral conformity and social denunciation' (Foucault 1965: 259).

Foucault's work on madness and psychiatry was part of his wider endeavour to uncover the development of methods of control and authority in modern societies. Over the last two centuries, there has grown a belief that social problems and conflicts could be effectively dealt with by experts exercising technical solutions. Handing over these problems to experts or professionals has allowed modern governments to shed some of their thorniest problems and to present themselves as more liberal than they might otherwise appear. For example, in England, it was the government who took the leading role in medicalizing the issue of psychiatric confinement over the 20th century (Moncrieff 2003).

Szasz also takes up this theme extensively. He has argued that 'The mandate for contemporary psychiatry . . . is

precisely to obscure, indeed to deny, the ethical dilemmas of life and to transform these into medicalized and technicalized problems susceptible to "professional" solutions' (Szasz 1970: 11). Szasz is a long-time passionate advocate of the complete abolition of involuntary psychiatric hospitalization and treatment. He argues that psychiatric coercion is equivalent to imprisonment without trial. If someone is not breaking the law they should remain free. He challenges the paternalism that is the basis for much psychiatric intervention. Paternalism is the assumption that others, usually professionals, are in a better position to judge someone's best interests than they are themselves. Szasz argues that paternalism subverts democracy and the rule of law, which rest on the assumption that human beings are autonomous agents that can make their own decisions. It is also easily abused, as people are apt to define other's interests in ways that are actually expressions of their own interests.

Protests and alternatives

The antipsychiatry movement was not just intellectual. In the 1970s protest groups sprung up in parts of Europe and North America, foreshadowing the more recent rise of the psychiatric users movement (see below). In the USA and the Netherlands large demonstrations were held against ECT and biological psychiatry.

Projects offering alternative forms of management of the mentally disordered were also established. In 1965 R.D. Laing and associates David Cooper and Aaron Esterson set up the Philadelphia Association, a charitable trust that ran a number of therapeutic communities, the first being Kingsley Hall in London. The principle of these communities was that people with psychosis should be encouraged to live through their psychotic episode with the hope that this would lead to an enlightened recovery. There was also an emphasis on breaking down distinctions between staff and patients.

Franco Basaglia, an Italian psychiatrist, established an organization called *Psichiatria Democratica*. This group successfully campaigned for the passing of a law that shut down all psychiatric hospitals in Italy. The benefits or otherwise of this action have been hotly disputed since.

Loren Mosher, an American psychiatrist, set up the Soteria project in the 1970s, which was designed to treat people with severe psychotic illnesses in a small therapeutic environment with no or minimal psychotropic drugs. He conducted a randomized controlled trial of the project comparing it to routine care in a hospital ward. The original project survives to this day, and other similar projects have been developed in the United States and Europe.

Influence of antipsychiatry

The 'antipsychiatrists' have been criticized from many different perspectives and their popularity and influence has declined since their heyday of the 1960s and 1970s. Philosophers and psychiatrists have defended the notion of mental illness, sometimes by pointing to the difficulties of defining physical illness. Others have accused the antipsychiatrists of giving fuel to right-wing political imperatives to cut spending on mental health care. However, the ideas of antipsychiatry were influential in several respects.

The development of diagnostic criteria, with which we are now so familiar, started in the 1970s partly in response to the challenge posed by antipsychiatry. The Rosenhan (1973) experiment, in which normal volunteers were diagnosed as having schizophrenia, created a furore and seemed to confirm the idea that psychiatric diagnosis had no objective validity. International research at this time also highlighted large discrepancies in rates of diagnosis of schizophrenia between different countries. Since the publication of DSM III in 1980, diagnosis has become an increasingly detailed, quantitative and apparently objective exercise, although there are still those who doubt its reliability and validity (Kutchins & Kirk 1997).

Psychiatric legislation is another area where the ideas of antipsychiatry can be seen to have had some influence. In England and Wales the 1959 Mental Health Act had given doctors more powers than any previous piece of legislation. This Act was drafted and passed in an atmosphere of great optimism about the potential of psychiatry to solve all the problems posed by mental illness. However, antipsychiatric ideas suggested this optimism was misplaced and gave fuel to the civil rights movement's arguments that there should, at the very least, be more restrictions on the powers of doctors to admit and forcibly treat mental patients. The 1983 Mental Health Act reflected these concerns. By narrowing definitions of certain categories of mental disorder, shortening periods of maximum detention and placing restrictions on circumstances in which compulsory treatment can and cannot be given, it limited medical power and increased patients' rights.

The ideas of antipsychiatry were influential far beyond psychiatry and were taken up by the media, the arts and the political and social sciences (Crossley 1998). Within psychiatry, they were rarely addressed directly, but their influence and popularity elsewhere must have presented a challenge to the psychiatric establishment. The shift towards a more biologically based psychiatry that has occurred over the last three decades may represent a tactical response to this challenge. Groups and ideas that challenge orthodox views of psychiatry still exist, both within and outside of organized psychiatry and have inherited to greater or lesser degrees the ideas of antipsychiatry. The Critical Psychiatry Network is a group of psychiatrists in the United Kingdom, who have united around issues such as questioning some of the assumptions of biological psychiatry, and opposition to the introduction of increased coercion in psychiatric legislation and the influence of the pharmaceutical industry.

In the United States the Institute for the Study of Psychiatry and Psychology started by the psychiatrist Peter Breggin unites radical professionals and service users. Current ideas such as critical psychiatry, post-psychiatry and the limits of psychiatry have all inherited much from their antipsychiatry predecessors.

THE USER MOVEMENT

This second section aims to provide an introduction to the history of the psychiatric user movement and its influence.

Over the last 50 years people on the receiving end of psychiatric services have played a central role in the debate about the nature of, and appropriate response to, mental distress. While the word 'patient' continues to be the preferred term for many during contact with mental health services, it has generally been rejected by those seeking to challenge the passive role that traditional doctor–patient relationships have assigned to patients. The term 'service user' provides a less value-laden term for describing this role. Others favour terms such as 'service survivor' to indicate the damaging effect they feel psychiatric services have had on their health. More recently user groups such as 'Mad Pride' in the UK have started to reclaim the language of others as a sign of refound self belief in the face of widespread discrimination.

While the term used to describe people who have experienced mental distress may at first seem unimportant, it has been argued that by choosing a term that best describes one's experiences, a person can take an important step towards regaining some of the confidence that mental distress and its treatment may have eroded (Campbell 1998).

Origins of the user movement

Notable examples of user involvement in the development of mental health services have occurred ever since the development of institutional responses to mental illness. Protests by inmates of mental institutions occurred in Britain during the 17th and 18th centuries, and in 1845 the Alleged Lunatics Friends Society was set up in support of those treated in asylums (Barnes & Bowl 2001). The development of a large-scale user movement did not occur until the 1970s and 1980s. This movement, which came to the fore in North America and Western Europe, grew in parallel with other social movements of the age that championed the rights of women, ethnic minorities, lesbians and gay men, and other groups. In Britain groups such as the Federation of Mental Patients Union campaigned against compulsory treatment and the overuse of psychotropic drugs.

During this period service users worked with others in mental health charities such as MIND in the UK and the National Mental Health Association in the US to campaign for improved services for people with mental health problems. These organizations provided logistical support which enabled service users to campaign successfully around issues such as the over-prescription of benzodiazepines and changes to employment legislation.

Parallel campaigns by users of other medical services, notably the 'natural child-birth movement', contributed to changes in other medical services and drew attention to what was seen as an increasing tendency to medicalize the human state. Partly as a result of these activities, national governments began to put in place official bodies that could represent the views of users in the development of services. These included Community Health Councils (CHC) in Britain and more radical attempts to give members of the public control over the budgets of Health Systems Agencies in the USA and Canada. The impact of these institutional attempts to give service users a say in the development of health care are difficult to assess. While it is clear that some decisions were made in response to the views of service users, many Health Systems Agencies found it impossible to enact changes unless these were supported by local health care professionals. CHCs frequently reported that health care planners either failed to consult local people about service changes or ignored their views.

Consumerism and public health care

In the latter part of the 20th century a variety of attempts were made in Europe and elsewhere to develop a more market-orientated approach to the management of publicly funded health care. The rationale for this approach was complex but involved Government attempts to curb the influence of professional groups and exert greater control over the increasing costs of health care. Government-sponsored enquiries into the organization of health care by those with backgrounds in the commercial sector led to calls for greater involvement of 'consumers' in the development and delivery of health care (e.g. Social Services Committee 1984).

More recent changes to the management of health care have seen further increases in the range of activities to which service users are asked to contribute. This is particularly the case in relation to mental health services. For instance in England, national guidelines for the development of mental health services call for user involvement in a range of activities including monitoring the effectiveness of service, staff training and attempts to develop more culturally sensitive services (Department of Health 1999). Service users have contributed to other tasks within health care including staff selection procedures (through sitting on appointments committees), clinical governance and audit. It has been argued that successful audit requires the involvement of users in order to ensure that standards are set that are meaningful to those who receive care (Kelson 1996). Service users have also been directly involved in service provision through employment as support workers and advocates.

Evaluation of such interventions suggests that service users employed in these roles help to improve clinical outcomes and may be better able than non-service users to engage patients with services (Simpson & House 2002). Such findings stand in contrast to reports of health care professionals who have experienced mental health problems and have reported that employers and colleagues can be unsympathetic and unsupportive of their attempts to continue their work.

Evaluating the impact of user involvement is a complex task. Multiple factors may lead to the adoption of a change in practice and eliciting the contribution that service users play in change may not be possible. While there are many examples of changes being made to services that have been attributed to the role played by service users, surveys of users who have collaborated with service providers reveal that many suggestions go unheeded (Crawford et al. 2003).

New directions

Just as professional groups such as psychiatrists include people with diverse opinions, service users are not a homogenous group and include those with differing views about the causes and appropriate management of mental distress. Campaigning groups of service providers, service users and carers in the United States, such as the National Alliance for the Mentally Ill, advocate a medical model of mental distress. This is seen as challenging stigma by promoting the view that people with mental illness are the same as those who suffer from any other medical condition. This argument is being used to encourage greater spending on psychiatric services and the development of improved drug treatments, a position supported by the pharmaceutical industry in the US who are keen to provide financial support for users who express these views. Other service users have highlighted the negative effects of medication, including withdrawal effects of selective serotonin reuptake inhibitors. The initial apathy and subsequent acceptance of these problems by psychiatrists echoes the response of service providers to concerns about benzodiazepines in the 1970s.

Despite these differences, most service users are keen to continue to press for a holistic understanding of mental disorder that requires that personal meanings of mental distress are considered when planning care. The importance of personal meaning is emphasized in peer support groups for those hearing voices. 'Hearing voices groups' seek to provide a space where service users can meet, find out about others' experiences, and use these as the basis for mutual understanding (Romme & Escher 2000). Psychiatrists treating people with psychosis expect most people to continue to experience symptoms and disability. In contrast, hearing voices groups emphasize the role that individual services users can play in actively attempting to recover from their illness. While the outcome of such interventions is unclear, the aims of these groups resonate with the wider aim of empowerment that lies at the heart of the user movement.

Service users are currently involved in a broad range of activities at a local and national level. These include independent activities aimed at self expression and peer support, and collaborative work with service providers aimed at improving the quality of service provision. In medicine in general, but especially in psychiatry, these developments are further evidence that the definition of illness and decisions about its management are no longer the preserve of doctors and other service providers.

MENTAL ILLNESS AND STIGMA

Introduction

This section aims to (1) explain the theoretical basis for, and effects of, stigma from different perspectives; (2) examine the way in which the media reinforce negative stereotypes; and (3) identify levels of intervention that will reduce stigma-discrimination

Link & Phelan (2001) have set out the current sociological context for understanding stigma. Stigma exists when the following four components converge:

- distinguishing and labelling differences between people
- the association of some human differences with negative attributes
- the separation of 'us' from 'them'
- status loss and discrimination against the out-group.

Table 11.1 sets out each of these components, using two general stigma examples, and with specific reference to the stigma of mental illness. Almost all researchers have divided the world into good and bad. The stigmatized out-group are passive victims of prejudice. Stigmatizers are *bad people*, holders of prejudicial belief systems and/or people who use their powerful positions to mark and maintain stigma. But Link & Phelan argue beyond this: 'by itself the standard model that asks "what-makes-person-A-discriminate-against-person-B" is inadequate for explaining the full consequences of stigma processes.' Discrimination need not be overt or conscious, and frequently it is the loss of status (by the stigmatized or labelled person) that is the source of other (social, economic, political, etc.) discriminations. For these to occur, the (previously neglected) fifth dimension of *power* must exist in the relationship between potential stigmatizer and stigmatized (Link & Phelan 2001).

Definition of stigma

The dictionary definition is helpful here: 'a mark of disgrace or discredit that sets a person apart from others'. In the context of the discussion above, we can better define stigma as a *prejudice*, based on *stereotypes*, that results in *discrimination*. Stigma is about 'them and us' or social exclusion. The full clinical impact of mental illness stigma is presented as Table 11.2. This lists the consequences of stigma from four different perspectives, from the first onset of 'psychiatric' symptoms onwards.

How does stigma-discrimination operate?

Link & Phelan (2001) conclude by asking four questions of potential stigmatizers:

1. Do they have the power to ensure that the human difference they recognize is broadly identified in the culture?
2. Do they have the power to make sure the dominant culture accepts the stereotypes they connect to labelled differences?

Table 11.1	The five components of the stigma process	
Components from Link & Phelan (2001)	Examples of other stigma	The stigma of mental illness
(1) Labelling differences	A: Physical deformity B: Different ethnic origin	Excess sedation or Parkinsonian symptoms (medication) Person seen leaving a psychiatric hospital or clinic
(2) Association with negative attributes	A: Less attractive B: Racist stereotypes	Beliefs that people with mental illness are weak, self-indulgent Perceptions that people with schizophrenia are violent
(3) Separation of 'us' from 'them'	A: Physical barriers B: Racial segregation	Locking people up, or 'asylum in the community' Loss of social networks after diagnosis/admission
(4) Status loss and discrimination	A & B: Barriers to employment, tenancy and education	See Table 11.2 for full list of stigma-discrimination: only 17% of people with severe mental illness are in (full or part-time) employment
(5) Power differential between stigmatizer (member of dominant in-group) and stigmatized (out-group member)	Dominant culture is A (of different ethnic origin) and B (able-bodied, etc.)	Potential stigmatizers: health professionals (including psychiatrists), social services, educationalists, police and judiciary, landlords

Table 11.2 The clinical impact of the stigma of severe mental illness

	Presentation	Course	Outcome
Person	Denial of symptoms Other explanations sought Self-medication (alcohol/drugs) Declines referral to psychiatric clinic	Rejection of diagnosis Self-stigmatization Incomplete disclosure of symptoms Non-adherence to treatments Increase in involuntary admissions	Lack of insight Poor therapeutic relationships Intermittent medication use Loss to follow up Isolation: loss of relationships, unemployment, homelessness, suicide
Family/carers	Denial of symptoms Other explanations: 'lazy' Divisions within families Blaming, scapegoating	Denial of diagnosis: 'doctor shopping' Minimization of symptoms Ambivalence to medications Loss of earnings	Poor relations with professionals 'All-or-nothing' consultations Chronic illness of family member Economic consequences
Neighbours	Unaware that person is becoming ill	Isolation of individual who is ill Exclusion of family of ill person See only the illness, not the person: 'them and us' reinforced Increase in calls to police if notice problems	Blame person and family Abuse/bullying of ill person Aversive prejudice/nimbyism ('not in my back yard') Poor opinions of mental health services: 'only act in extreme emergencies, need to be prodded into action'
Health and social services	Increase in untreated mental illness in the community Late presentation of illness Increase in duration of untreated psychosis Decreasing possibilities for early intervention	'Difficult to engage' patients Social factors more difficult to control if job/supports lost Frustrations at non-compliance Increased ratio of involuntary to voluntary inpatients (more people on Sections, possible increase in ward violence)	Cycle of low morale and recruitment, loss of trained staff, lack of resources, perception of being undervalued, and reacting only to emergencies and serious incidents: 'take it or leave it' psychiatry Combination of work pressures, more losses to follow up and isolation make (rare) violence more likely

3 Do they have the power to separate us from them, and to make the designation stick?

4 Do they control access to education, employment, health care, and housing?

If the answers here are yes, we can expect stigma to result. If no, 'what we generally mean by stigma would not exist' (Link & Phelan 2001). Put simply, for any act of stigma-discrimination against any group (people with mental or physical disabilities, or of minority ethnic status), a powerful dominant culture needs to identify (label) and act (discriminate). Discrimination can occur at a structural level (think of institutional racism), a group level (residents objecting to a group home in their locality) or an individual level (bullying, and verbal and physical abuse).

Stigma and the media

Another approach to understanding stigma is through the media. For some, the media are *the* cause of mental illness stigma, yet this is impossible to prove: various media produce snapshots of stigma, and these are an interesting way to reveal aspects of stigma (Byrne 2000). Characters with mental illness are common in television fiction, and far more frequently violent (than in reality) to capture the ratings. Their currency is the stereotype, at its most extreme in media representations of the psychokiller. The movie psychokiller, with (usually) *his* roots in Victorian horror and

melodrama, is both mad and bad, and frequently returns to familiar surroundings to effect a terrible revenge for real or imagined wrongs (Byrne 1998). Porter (1991) describes how, in 1793, Philippe Pinel 'struck off the chains from his charges' at Salpêtrière and Bicêtre asylums in Paris, preceding even the enlightened *York Retreat* of Samuel Tuke. Yet it was Pinel who defined madness in stark black and white terms:

> Of all the afflictions to which human nature is subject, the loss of reason is at once the most calamitous and interesting. Deprived of this faculty, by which a man is principally distinguished from the beasts that perish, the human form is frequently the most remarkable attribute that he retains of his proud distinction. His character, as an individual of the species is always perverted, sometimes annihilated. His thoughts and actions are diverted from their usual and natural course. The chain which connected his ideas in just series and mutual subserviency is dissevered. His feelings for himself and others are new and uncommon. His attachments are converted into aversions, his love into hatred.
> Pinel (1806) (cited in Porter 1991, ch. 1, p. 12.)

Though undoubtedly progressive for its time, Pinel demonstrates the common habit to divide the world into good/evil, sane/insane, human/inhuman, moral/immoral, love/hate, etc. It is this division, crystallized by Robert Louis

Stevenson when he wrote *The Strange Case of Dr Jekyll and Mr Hyde* in 1885, that drives the psychokiller stereotype (Byrne 1998). There are parallels between stereotypes of mental illness and ethnic stereotypes. By definition, stereotypes are one-dimensional caricatures that manage limited information efficiently. It is also important to note that recognition of a stereotype (ethnic, racist, ageist, sexist, etc.) is often a neutral finding, in that recognition does not imply agreement with the stereotype. Banner headlines and movie psychokillers do not in themselves prove that there is a stigma of mental illness: they prove that the writer/producer is at least aware that society recognizes the motifs and, on occasions, endorses them as having some basis in reality. Three other stereotypes of mental illness are the pathetic mad, the comedic and the weak. Glasson (1996) makes the point that current media excesses should be seen in the context of wider public concerns about community care. Along with other commentators, she identifies many failures of community care, and cites poor liaison between health and social services, closure of hospitals before development of community facilities, and inadequate community support as important additional considerations (Glasson 1996). In other words, don't shoot the messenger.

Sociological theories

Erving Goffman (1963) first articulated the theoretical concept of stigma from a sociological perspective. It is important to note that stigma is a theoretical concept: Goffman did not discover stigma, rather he invented it. For Goffman (1963), a stigmatized person:

- is disqualified from full social acceptance (p. 9)
- is a blemished person, ritually polluted, to be avoided especially in public places (p. 11)
- has a discrepancy (stigma) between his actual social identity and his virtual social identity . . . that virtual social identity is formed by certain expectations and normative expectations (by others about the stranger) (p. 12)
- has a character blemish . . . (and) we construct an ideology to explain difference using language (p. 15).

From the perspective of the in-group, we do not wish to define ourselves as prejudiced: we idealize our responses ('Some of my best friends have mental illness') and seek to minimize acts of discrimination and omissions ('I'd like to hire someone with schizophrenia, but the job would be too stressful for him'). For people with mental illness stigma, shame and secrecy maintain equilibrium until (for some) it can no longer be denied. Equally, the coping mechanisms listed by Goffman (denial, displacement, projection and search for sympathetic others) all make stigma harder to find and to quantify. Such reactions to mental illness by people who become ill, are exactly the same as those found in

general public samples (who do not), namely denial, isolation and insulation of mental illness. Although Goffman had considerable expertise about the plight of people with mental illness (an earlier book, Asylums, described the experience of being mentally ill with great precision), his work on stigma was intended to cover all possible stigmata within a unified theory.

After Goffman

A second influential sociologist, Thomas Scheff, wrote specifically about people with mental illness: for Scheff, the process of deviance and its labelling overrode other concerns (Scheff 1966). Scheff rejected the psychiatric 'slogan' that mental disorders were an illness like any other, arguing that none of the four components of the medical model (cause, lesion, symptoms and outcome) applied to psychiatry (Scheff 1975). Labelling Theory assumed societal conceptions of mental illness would cause deviant behaviour to be so labelled; others' reactions to the behaviour were based on these conceptions; and the person then adopted the 'role of mental illness'. Scheff (1966) believed that 'labelled deviants may be rewarded for playing the stereotyped role . . . and are punished when they attempt to return to conventional roles'. He concluded: 'when the individual internalizes this role, incorporating it as a central identity, chronic mental illness is the consequence' (Scheff 1966). Scheff's Labelling Theory has often been cited as implying that there is no mental illness, but he later argued that he did not wish the theory to replace psychiatry, and regretted stating that societal reaction was the *most important single cause* (of mental illness), but perhaps accounted for 5 to 10% of cases (Scheff 1975).

Modified Labelling Theory (MLT) proposed an alteration to the intermediate stage in Scheff's labelling theory: it was not the response of others, but rather the response of the labelled individual that predicted consequences for future vulnerability to relapse of illness and damaged self-esteem (Link et al. 1989). MLT allowed for multiple relapses in severe mental illness where the person was unaware of the label (insightless about the diagnosis) and it accepted circumstances where psychopathology alone led to negative outcomes.

Social psychology

Social psychology recognizes that all behaviour takes place within a social context, and that even when alone, our actions and inaction are influenced by others. Gross (2000) defines prejudice as an extreme attitude with cognitive, affective and behavioural components, though the third part may not be manifested. Because stigma is a social construct, we must firstly distinguish between interpersonal and intergroup processes: there are similarities, but the two processes need to be studied within separate frameworks. Crocker et al. (2000) have produced a comprehensive review of social stigma, of which mental illness is one example. While there are aspects of the stigmatization of people with mental health problems unique to these labels and processes, they provide a useful conceptualization of the power of situations to shape experiences and esteem. One aspect, stereotype threat, occurs where a stigmatized person is aware both of the negative stereotypes (about their status/condition) and that their behaviour will be judged on these grounds. They also conclude that for stigmatizers, 'stigma is about sustaining the belief that I am and we are good (or at least better than they are), maintaining our belief that we are just, fair and deserving' (Crocker et al. 2000).

The psychiatric literature

It is worth noting that stigma became a major subject in psychiatric journals only in the last decade, as a direct result of anti-stigma campaigns. Current diagnostic manuals for mental disorders do not include provision for the effects of any kind of stigma or discrimination in the course of someone's illness. Textbooks of general or social psychiatry have only recently included references to, let alone sections on, stigma-discrimination. In these respects, the medical model has failed to address stigma.

It has been argued that the institution of psychiatry has contributed to *increasing* the stigma attached to mental illness (Byrne 2000; Porter 1991; Sayce 2000). There is also evidence that psychiatrists are not good at highlighting or understanding the effects of stigma. For example, during the asylum era, patient characteristics that we now recognize as the effects of *institutionalization* were then described as part of the syndrome of schizophrenia (Byrne 2000). One would expect that, recently, the profession would have heightened awareness of stigma in severe mental illness, namely schizophrenia. Yet a recent extensive review based on meta-analysis (152 references) in a major journal (*Acta Psychiatrica Scandinavica*) failed to consider *any* role for stigma-discrimination in the differential diagnosis of low mood in people with schizophrenia (Hausmann & Fleischhacker 2002). They concluded that depressed mood unrelated to medication, substance misuse, organic pathology, negative symptoms or active psychosis, could be explained by either primary process schizophrenia (prodrome/postpsychotic depression), schizoaffective disorder or *demoralization*. 'Chronic demoralization should be considered when patients present with a chronic and persistent state of hopelessness and existentialist distress in the absence of somatic features of depression' (Hausmann & Fleischhacker 2002). The concept of demoralization, in contrast to stigma or discrimination, implies that the problem is located within the individual and fails to highlight the role of wider social processes.

What about *discrimination*?

Service users' surveys measure discrimination by asking people directly about their experiences (Mental Health Foundation 2000; Read & Baker 1995) but have had low response rates (17% and 13% respectively), and are therefore open to the charge of overreporting acts of discrimination by a self-selected group. That said, their findings are not easy to ignore. Read & Baker (1995) reported that 47% had been abused or harassed in public, 26% had moved home because of harassment, with physical assault in 14%. Other sources of discrimination were the workplace (47%), seeking employment (37%), from friends (26%) and access to housing (10%) (Mental Health Foundation 2000). Of course a major focus on any work should be to measure the consequences of stigma (Table 11.2), and one cannot study stigma without studying discrimination, but addressing discrimination alone will not answer the why and how questions, or uncover hidden (indirect) discriminations. Put another way, discrimination is the behavioural consequence of prejudice and stigma, but limiting studies to discrimination alone is problematic in underestimating the totality of stigma-discrimination.

Stigma includes indirect discrimination

Examination of all aspects of stigma-discrimination is especially important in Western societies where anti-discrimination legislation has unintended consequences in driving discrimination underground. Taking just two examples of this, the workplace and health services, we can identify several aspects of stigma: indirect discrimination, value judgements, prejudice, and social exclusion. Goldberg & Steury (2001) identify employers' misconceptions about effective treatments for depression, untreated depression as a workplace disability, and its economic consequences including lower wages, different insurance supports, and a discriminatory workers' compensation system. Levenson & Oldbrich (1993) have measured medical staff opinions as to the suitability of people with schizophrenia for organ transplantation, given the rationing and high costs of these procedures. They report that 'active schizophrenia' (sic) is an *absolute* contraindication to transplant in 92% of cardiac, 67% of liver and 73% of renal units; when the condition is described as 'controlled schizophrenia', staff believe this to be either an absolute or relative contraindication: 85%, 80% and 68% respectively. Phipps (1997) has described 11 years of cardiac transplantation ($n=706$) in Canada: 28 people were denied transplants on 'psychiatric grounds'. These included drug and alcohol misuse (7), non-compliance (3), multiple suicide attempts (2), unrealistic expectations (2), and borderline personality disorder (2) (Phipps 1997). In doctors' daily practice, there are more subtle ways (short of denying life) in which psychiatric patients are discriminated against.

Solutions at individual level/clinic-based

One of the unique benefits of detailed psychosocial assessment is the ability to understand the meanings of symptoms and events for *that patient* at this time. We can therefore note the interaction of reduced social networks and stigma experiences on service users. It is no more 'dangerous' to enquire about stigma/victimization events than it is to enquire about suicidal ideation. Without assigning blame onto the service user, are there ways in which the outward signs of mental illness can be better disguised? Each day, reflect on the mental health service you provide, and ask yourself: 'Is this how I, or a member of my family, would like to be treated?' Mind your language: describing someone as 'a schizophrenic' gives little information to his or her situation or humanity. Better again, is the growing practice of increasing service user participation at every stage of service delivery, teaching and research. More than any other intervention, direct contact with service users in a context of equality (not across the clinic table) will reduce the 'them and us' of Table 11.1. There is also a growing evidence base for a cognitive-behavioural approach to stigma, with an emphasis on the problems that can be solved. Equally, everyone who has been or could be stigmatized could do a 'cost–benefit analysis' of the benefits and risks of disclosing the secret of mental illness to others including family, employers and landlords.

Solutions at group-based and structural levels

These are much harder. This section of the chapter began with two different stigma examples, physical disability and race. At every level of society, discrimination against these two *broad* groups is negatively sanctioned. There are laws (disability and race relations acts) to prevent overt discrimination, verbal abuse and exclusion. Many governments practise positive discrimination: in Italy, firms of a certain size are legally bound to employ people with disabilities (physical or mental) as 15% of the workforce. Companies who fail to do this pay fines into a social fund. It is also true that people with disabilities and from ethnic minorities are well-represented by government and non-governmental agencies, and that as (historical) out-groups, they have united in a common cause. The fact that mental illness, unlike physical disability and race, can be concealed poses particular problems: secrecy may work as a strategy for the stigmatized individual, but makes collegiality more difficult. In the UK, our culture has changed to such a degree that words such as 'cripple, spastic, nigger, wog, etc.' have been driven underground. By contrast, the media continue to use terms such as 'loony, bonkers, maniac, psycho, etc.' that dehumanize people and make a complex problem inaccessible to the public. In their desire to sell newspapers and fill airtime, the (rare) homicides where mental illness is a factor are sensationalized. The challenge is to engage with the media and explain the context even of those instances that could be characterized as psychiatry's failures. Recent successes with target groups such as police, doctors, teachers and schoolchildren have made anti-stigma research one of the most exciting areas of mental health.

REFERENCES

Barnes M & Bowl R (2001) *Taking Over the Asylum: Empowerment and Mental Health*. Palgrave, Basingstoke.

Byrne P (1998) The fall and rise of the movie psychokiller. *Psychiatric Bulletin* **21**: 173–5.

Byrne P (2000) The stigma of mental illness and ways of diminishing it. *Advances in Psychiatric Treatment* **6**: 65–72

Campbell P (1998) The service user/survivor movement. In: Newnes C, Holmes G & Dunn C (eds) *This is Madness*. Ross-on-Wye: PCCS Books.

Crawford MJ, Aldridge T, Bhui K et al. (2003) User involvement in the planning and delivery of mental health services: A cross-sectional survey of service users and providers. *Acta Psychiatrica Scandinavica* **107**: 410–14.

Crocker J, Major B & Steele C (2000) Social stigma and the self. In: Heatherton TF, Kleck RE, Hebl MR & Hull JG (eds) *The Social Psychology of Stigma*, pp. 504–553. London: Guildford Press.

Crossley N (1998) R.D. Laing and the British anti-psychiatry movement: a socio-historical analysis. *Social Science & Medicine* **47**: 877–89.

Foucault M (1965) *Madness and Civilisation*. London: Tavistock.

Department of Health (1999) *A National Service Framework for Mental Health*. London: Department of Health.

Glasson J (1996) The public image of the mentally ill and community care. *British Journal of Nursing* **5**: 615–17.

Goffman E (1963) *Stigma: Notes on the Management of Spoiled Identity*. Engelwood Cliffs, NJ: Prentice-Hall.

Goldberg RJ & Steury S (2001) Depression in the workplace: costs and barriers to treatment. *Psychiatric Services* **52**: 1639–43.

Gross R (2000) Prejudice and discrimination. In: [anonymous] *Psychology*. London: Hodder and Stroughton.

Hausmann A & Fleischhacker WW (2002) Differential diagnosis of depressed mood in patients with schizophrenia: a diagnostic alogorithm based on a review. *Acta Psychiatrica Scandinavia* **106**: 83–96.

Kelson M (1996) *Consumer Involvement in the Audit Activities of the Royal Colleges & Other Professional Bodies*. London: College of Health.

Kutchins H & Kirk SA (1997) *Making us Crazy*. New York: The Free Press.

Laing RD (1960) *The Divided Self*. Tavistock: London.

Levenson JL & Oldbrisch ME (1993) Psychosocial evaluation of organ transplant candidates. *Psychosomatics* **34**: 314–23.

Link BG, Cullen FT, Struening EL, Shrout PE & Dohrenwend BP (1989) A modified labeling theory approach to mental disorders: an empirical assessment. *American Sociological Review* **54**: 400–23.

Link BG & Phelan JC (2001) Conceptualizing Stigma. *Annual Review of Sociology* **27**: 363–85.

Mental Health Foundation (2000) *Pull Yourself Together: a survey of the stigma and discrimination faced by people who experience mental distress*. London: Mental Health Foundation.

Moncrieff J (2003) The politics of a new Mental Health Act. *British Journal of Psychiatry* **183**: 8–9.

Phipps L (1997) Psychiatric evaluation and outcomes in candidates for heart tansplantation. *Clinical Investment Medicine* **20**: 388–95.

Pinel P (1806) *A Treatise on Insanity*. London: Cadell and Davies.

Porter R (1991) *Faber Book of Madness*. London: Faber and Faber.

Read J & Baker S (1996) *Not Just Sticks and Stones: a survey of the stigma, taboos and discrimination experienced by people with mental health problems*. London: MIND Publications.

Romme M & Escher S (2000) *Making Sense of Voices: a guide for mental health professionals working with voice-hearers*. London: MIND Publications.

Rosenhan DL (1973) On being sane in insane places. *Science* **179**: 250–8.

Sayce L (2000) From *Psychiatric Patient to Citizen*. London: Macmillan.

Scheff T (1966) *Being Mentally Ill: A Sociological Theory*. Chicago: Aldine.

Scheff T (1975) Labelling theory: reply to Chauncery and Gove. *American Sociological Review* **40**: 252–7.

Simpson E & House A (2002) Involving users in the delivery and evaluation of mental health services: systematic review. *British Medical Journal* **325**: 1265.

Social Services Committee (1984) *Griffiths NHS Management Inquiry Report*. London: HMSO.

Szasz T (1970) *Ideology and Insanity*. New York: Anchor books.

Szasz T (1994) *Cruel Compassion*. New York: John Wiley.

Clinical psychiatry

Psychiatry of learning disability

Jean O'Hara

INTRODUCTION

What is learning disability? The UK Government's policy document *Valuing People* (Department of Health 2001a) defines it as 'a significantly reduced ability to understand new or complex information, to learn new skills (impaired intelligence), with a reduced ability to cope independently (impaired social functioning), which started before adulthood, with a lasting effect on development'.

Whilst the psychiatry of learning disability is a specialist field, *Valuing People* makes it explicit that the NHS should be able to accommodate the needs of people with learning disabilities in mainstream services, with specialist support as appropriate. This 'integration' and 'social inclusion' has meant that the needs of people with learning disabilities must feature in the undergraduate and postgraduate training of all health care professionals (Box 12.1).

This chapter provides a core text to the understanding of learning disabilities and the generic and specialist mental health needs of this population.

DEFINITIONS AND TERMINOLOGY

In the UK, the Department of Health has adopted the term 'learning disability', although people themselves prefer 'learning difficulty'. (The reader should also be aware that 'learning difficulty' is used in education to cover a wider group of specific learning problems, such as dyslexia.) In the USA the official term is 'mental retardation'; in developing countries it is 'mental handicap' whilst in international literature the term 'intellectual disability' has emerged. Older terms like 'defective', 'idiot' and 'moron' have become common terms of abuse.

International classification systems such as ICD-10 and DSM-IV refer to 'mental retardation'. Mental impairment and severe mental impairment, as defined in the Mental Health Act (1983) are not synonymous with learning disability.

> **Box 12.1   The MRCPsych curriculum**
>
> The MRCPsych curriculum (Royal College of Psychiatrists 2001a) expects the following core subjects to be examined in the Part II examinations with regard to learning disability psychiatry:
>
> 1. Aetiology and development of learning disability – including neurobiology of brain development and effects of genetic, environmental and social factors
> 2. Psychiatric disorders in learning disability – including aetiology, epidemiology, classification and concepts of impairment, disability and handicap
> 3. Assessment of people with learning disability – demonstrating a multi-axial perspective and a working knowledge of ethical issues
> 4. Principles of treatment options – including pharmacotherapy, psychological and behavioural treatments, and the treatment of uncomplicated psychiatric disorders and epilepsy
> 5. Service provision – models of service, history of provision, and how policy and philosophy have shaped services

The World Health Organization (1980) makes a distinction between impairment, disability and handicap (see Box 12.2).

HISTORICAL OVERVIEW

> ... even if the nature went wrong, yet nothing has been wrong with the soul and the spirit.
> (Paracelsus, 16th century Swiss physician)

Societies and historical periods have dealt with disability and handicap in different ways. In European history, the

---

> **Box 12.2   WHO definitions of impairment, disability and handicap**
>
> **Impairment:** a loss or abnormality of structure or function, including psychological functioning
>
> **Disability:** a restriction or lack of ability to perform an activity within the range considered normal for a human being
>
> **Handicap:** a disadvantage resulting from an impairment or disability that limits or prevents the fulfilment of a normal role

Spartans allowed weak infants to perish, while the Romans killed malformed children, and used 'defectives' for amusement. In the Middle Ages, witchcraft and belief in changelings often resulted in cruel treatment of 'idiots'. It was during the reign of Edward I (1272–1307) that a distinction was made between the 'born fool' (learning disability) and the 'lunatic' (mental illness). Eighteenth-century education theories led to attempts to educate the deaf and the 'wild boy of Averyon'. In 1846, Seguin declared that 'while waiting for medicine to cure idiots, I have undertaken to see that they participate in the benefit of education'.

By the mid-nineteenth century, there was a greater scientific interest in the nature and the inheritance of abilities, clinical and behavioural symptoms and syndromes. The development of the IQ test was hailed as a great scientific advance, and led to the 'discovery' of many 'mentally deficient people' who would not fit into the education system of the time.

In an attempt to provide more humane and protective care for those afflicted, and to prevent a 'national degeneracy', Victorian England created the first workhouses and asylums. An Idiots Act was passed in 1886 to care for 'idiots and imbeciles'. The 1910 General Election included a vigorous campaign 'discouraging parenthood in feeble-minded and other degenerate types' and for the building of separate institutions. The Mental Deficiency Act (1913) introduced compulsory certification for people admitted to institutions as 'mentally defective' (Ryan 1980).

Ideas of degeneration persisted, with the Nazi extermination of thousands of 'mentally handicapped' people, and the 'voluntary' sterilization of 'mentally defective' women in the UK, while such sterilizations became compulsory in many US states.

UK GOVERNMENT POLICIES AND PHILOSOPHY OF CARE

In 1948 in post-war Britain, asylums were incorporated in the newly formed National Health Service. It resulted in the 'medicalization' of learning disability: residents became patients, 'treated from cradle to grave' by nurses and doctors, often in institutions far away from the local community. Over the years it led to appalling physical and material conditions, as well as chronic understaffing. Scandals reached the public awareness in 1967/8 through two newspaper articles. The government responded with the publication of its policy document, *Better Services for the Mentally Handicapped*, in 1971. Its core premise was that people with learning disability should not 'necessarily' be segregated from others. 'Normalization' of the physical environment and a normal living routine were essential components to care. Treating the person as an individual, and valuing his/her role within society (social role valorization) underpinned this social philosophy. However, the blanket adoption of normalization and ordinary life principles led, in some cases, to a denial of difference. Health needs were ignored or neglected in an 'antimedical' stance, while community teams (community team for people with learning disabilities otherwise known as CTLD, or community learning disability team otherwise known as CLDT) adopted a social model of care where specialist skills were often denied and medical or psychiatric involvement marginalized.

Thirty years later, the Government published *Valuing People* (Department of Health 2001a), with its emphasis on valuing the person with a learning disability: upholding their human rights; their right to live as ordinary citizens, to live in the community and access ordinary services and to have a family life. It recognized the barriers to accessing the same health care as others and acknowledged that people with learning disabilities may have complex health needs requiring specialist knowledge and intervention. It also acknowledged their increased vulnerability to mental illness.

AETIOLOGY AND PREVENTION

While much has been published on the causes of learning disability and interventions to prevent the birth of such an afflicted child, it is important to consider how society's 'pursuit for perfection' may impact on the life of an individual with learning disability and his/her family.

Globally, learning disability is associated with poverty, malnutrition and environmental factors (Box 12.3). In the UK, 90% of the learning disabled population are only mildly disabled, and up to 60% will not have an identifiable cause for their disability. They are, however, more likely to have parents belonging to lower socio-economic groups and to have experienced a socially disadvantaged environment.

Box 12.3   Some examples of environmentally-mediated intellectual decline (EMID) (Williams 2002)

Protein energy malnutrition (PEM) affects the intellectual ability of a third of all poor-nation children

Lead pollution is a well-known cause of EMID. It may impair intellectual intelligence in 17% of children in the US, and up to 90% in some African cities

1.6 billion people are at risk, globally, of iodine-deficiency disorders. In China, it reduces IQ levels by 10–15 points in 8 million people, and affects 22% of the population of Bhutan

The incidence of intellectual disability in polluted Soviet cities has increased twice as fast as in rural areas

Malnutrition has been an accepted cause of intellectual decline since the 1970s

---

It is customary for textbooks to list examples of the many prenatal, perinatal and postnatal causes of learning disability, including:

- infective and inflammatory agents – e.g. the ToRCH infections (toxoplasmosis, rubella, cytomegalovirus and herpes)
- toxic/metabolic factors – e.g. lead, maternal smoking in pregnancy, maternal alcohol consumption in pregnancy, drugs – prescribed and illicit
- traumatic events pre- and perinatally – e.g. assisted deliveries, hypoxic events, prematurity, very low birth weight
- chromosomal and genetic causes (see Box 12.4)
- endocrine disorders
- maternal factors – e.g. anaemia, hypertension, bleeding during pregnancy
- postnatal factors
  - e.g. encephalitis, meningitis, severe dehydration and electrolyte imbalance, head injuries, non-accidental injuries (violent shaking), hypoxia.

Box 12.4 Some chromosomal and genetic causes of learning disability

Chromosomal disorders	
Autosomal	Down's syndrome (trisomy 21)
Deletion/microdeletion	Prader–Willi syndrome (long arm – chromosome 15)
	Cri du Chat syndrome (short arm – chromosome 5)
Sex-linked	Klinfelter's syndrome (47XXY)
	Turner's Syndrome (45XO)

Genomic imprinting	
	Prader–Willi syndrome (chromosome 15 – paternal origin)
	Angelmann syndrome (chromosome 15 – maternal origin)

Single-gene disorders	
Dominant	Neurofibromatosis
	Tuberous sclerosis
Recessive	Inborn errors of metabolism (e.g. phenylketonuria)
X-linked	Lesch–Nyhan (hyperuricaemia)
	Fragile X syndrome (Xq27) – CGG repeats

Psychological or reversible causes include maternal and sensory deprivation, neglect and sexual abuse, leading to a failure to thrive in an infant or developmental delay in a child. Such experiences can lead to a 'secondary handicap'– a psychological defence that protects the self from unbearable memories. It may be the primary cause of the disability, or may exacerbate the experience of 'handicap' (Sinason 1992).

EPIDEMIOLOGICAL ASPECTS AND THE IQ TEST

The total learning-disabled population in England is about 1.2 million; 210,000 have severe or profound disabilities.

Intelligence is believed to follow a normal distribution, with the average at 100, although this is increasing. There is a smaller peak towards the lower end of the bell-shaped curve, to take account of those with severe learning disability caused by clear organic factors. Two standard deviations above and below the mean would encompass 95% of the population, i.e. 95% of the population would score between 70 and 130 on an IQ test. A score below 70 is defined as 'intellectual impairment', and below 50 is defined as severe. Clearly these are arbitrary cut-offs, but they give a prevalence rate of mild (2-3%) and severe (0.2-0.3%) intellectual impairment in the population.

However, impaired intellectual functioning is only one factor in the definition of learning disability. It is important to assess social/adaptive skills, particularly in those with mild intellectual impairment, and to be clear about the person's educational opportunities and personal history. In practice, this consideration is not of diagnostic importance in those presenting with severe disabilities.

IQ scores must therefore be interpreted with care, particularly as there are many different profiles of ability that give the same total IQ score. Nonverbal tests are used where English is not the primary language, but cultural sensitivity cannot be assumed. Performance is also affected by medication/drugs, mental state, concentration, motivation and the ability to complete tasks within a time frame.

COMMUNICATION

The GMC's publication *Tomorrow's Doctors* (2002) highlights the importance of being able to communicate effectively with individuals, regardless of their disability (Box 12.5). People with learning disabilities may have cognitive difficulties such as slow reaction times, difficulty sustaining attention, and long- and short-term memory problems. Their language development may either be:

- delayed – smaller vocabulary, limited grammar resulting in difficulty understanding and using the full range of tenses, and difficulties understanding and expressing abstract concepts, such as time, 'before' and 'after', or
- disordered – in addition to a delayed pattern, there may be difficulties of perception, sequencing, word finding, understanding precise meaning of words, correct use of pronouns, echolalia and the social use of language (Ambalu 1997)

What is verbalized may be a reflection of the person's own experiences, whether it be previous contacts with doctors,

---

Box 12.5   Good clinical communication

Prepare for the interview

Identify yourself

Make contact with the person – find out how best to communicate, approach from the 'better' side, use an interpreter/signer if necessary

Explain purpose of the meeting/consultation

Allow the person to express him/herself if at all possible

Use short, simple sentences; speak more slowly; use open ended and either/or questions, use probes as necessary, and repeat questions with small changes

Consider the use of prepared materials (e.g. *Books Beyond Words* series)

Have pen and paper ready – pictures may help describe experiences and aid understanding

Concepts of time can be very difficult— link symptoms to an 'index event' (e.g. birthday, holiday, party)

Remember that the person's understanding of the full range of tenses may be limited

Check the person's understanding

Watch and observe – for non-verbal clues and signs of anxiety or distress

Sum up at the end and explain what will happen next

---

social exclusion or limited life opportunities. There are also different aspects to look out for when communicating with someone who has autism, cerebral palsy or sensory impairments. The expression of psychological and emotional distress is of particular importance to the psychiatrist as well as the ability to localize and communicate pain. Assessment of capacity to consent or withhold consent to treatments and the whole issue of medication concordance is part of everyday clinical practice.

HEALTH NEEDS

People with learning disabilities are more prone to chronic health problems, yet receive suboptimal health care. Apart from the specific health needs that might be associated with various syndromes, people with learning disabilities have a higher prevalence of additional health needs compared to the general population. These include:

- visual impairments (12–57%)
- hearing impairments (5–60%)
- dental disease (11–29%)
- epilepsy (16–34%, rising to 67% in those with severe disability)
- neurological and orthopaedic problems
- mobility problems (particularly associated with cerebral palsy)

- psychiatric disorders (10–39%)
- severe 'challenging behaviours' (6–7%)
- communication difficulties (50–?%).

Not only is it important to identify and 'treat' these conditions in their own right, but they may also have an impact on the person's behaviour and mental state, and the ability of psychiatrists to make a proper psychiatric assessment.

Sensory impairments

Visual and hearing impairments have educational, health and social implications. They may be overlooked, particularly in people with limited communication skills. Diagnostic overshadowing may lead to behavioural symptoms being dismissed as part of the person's learning disability.

Behavioural and developmental problems are more common in visually impaired children compared to children with normal sight. The recognition of 'I' as a separate entity can be delayed in blind children, by up to 5 years. Children with visual impairment often engage in stereotyped behaviours such as eye-pressing, eye-poking and prolonged light gazing, perhaps because of sensory under-stimulation. The combination of a delayed concept of 'self', stereotypies, and a preference to be left alone may lead to a 'schizoid' presentation in adulthood or difficulties distinguishing between this and autistic symptoms (Carvill 2001).

Epilepsy

Epilepsy is commonly associated with learning disability. In many cases the same damage or maldevelopment of the brain that has lead to the learning disability causes epilepsy. Formation and closure of the neural tube is normally complete by 3–4 weeks' gestation. Abnormalities in this developmental process lead to anencephaly or cephalocoeles. Expansion of the forebrain into the cerebral hemispheres and thalami occurs between 5–10 weeks gestation, while cortical development with neuronal and glial proliferation, migration and organization occurs until the age of 18 years. Disruptions to this process may give rise to a range of generalized or focal causes of epileptic seizures. Thus the prevalence of epilepsy increases with severity of disability, with multiple and/or unclassified seizure types in those with profound disabilities.

Epileptic syndromes with early onset are associated with a poorer outcome. West syndrome (infantile spasm) and Lennox–Gastaut syndrome are of particular importance as they may lead to severe learning disabilities. Prolonged or inadequately managed epilepsy may also lead to brain hypoxia and cognitive decline.

The diagnosis of epilepsy is essentially a clinical one and can be difficult to make. People with learning disabilities may not be able to describe the experiences associated with the aura before a generalized seizure, or during a complex partial seizure. A developmental history is important, as well as establishing whether or not there is a relationship between seizures and any behavioural disorder – i.e. in the prodromal, pre-ictal, peri-ictal or post-ictal phase. (Epilepsy is discussed further in Chapter 26.)

The diagnosis of epilepsy is often perceived as an additional blow to families already trying to come to terms with having a disabled child. Management often involves a multi-disciplinary approach, with input from carers, day centre and respite care staff, as well as clinicians within learning disability teams and doctors specializing in epilepsy and/or psychiatry of learning disability.

VULNERABILITY ISSUES

Research suggests that people with learning disabilities are at increased risk of personal violence, neglect, exploitation and abuse. Possible reasons for this include their own difficulties in understanding or communicating, the way they receive services (institutionalized settings, their need for support and assistance) and the fact that they may be actively targeted (Brown 1997).

No Secrets (Department of Health 2000) requires all local authorities to have an interagency 'vulnerable adults policy' in place, as often it is the threshold of seriousness which practitioners find difficult to interpret.

Categories of abuse that are covered by the vulnerable adults procedures include:

- **Physical abuse:** bruising, finger marks, bite marks, over-medication or misuse of procedures such as enemas.
- **Sexual abuse:** direct or non-direct sexual behaviours where the individual does not, or cannot consent, or where he/she has been unduly pressured. The law distinguishes between adults with mild and severe learning disabilities.
- **Psychological/emotional abuse:** as in elder abuse, it often involves verbal assault, insults, humiliation and threats of abandonment. It may be akin to 'failure to thrive' in child protection.
- **Financial or material abuse:** often not reported within the framework of adult protection; financial motivation may be at the root of a preferred care arrangement or an unwillingness to 'allow' the learning disabled adult to leave home.
- **Neglect:** where the individual's basic physical, social and health care needs are not being met.

CHALLENGING NEED/BEHAVIOURS

Challenging behaviour is a social construct and not a clinical diagnosis. Behaviours commonly identified include aggression, self-injury and property damage. The term 'challenging behaviour' is often used to describe:

> 'behaviours of such intensity, frequency or duration that the physical safety of the person or others is likely to be placed in serious jeopardy, or behaviour that is likely to seriously limit or delay access to or use of ordinary community facilities'
> (Emerson et al. 1987)

Studies suggest between 12–17% of those identified as having learning disabilities will display challenging behaviour, 40–60% of them to a severe degree (Health Evidence Bulletin, Wales 2000).

Most behaviours are functional, i.e. they achieve an important, immediate outcome for the individual, at least some of the time. They are the result of many contributory environmental factors and/or individual variables, of which some will be unknown or beyond control. A functional analysis may be important: this includes a description of the target behaviour, identification of antecedents, consequences and maintaining factors for the behaviour, and collection of observational data to test out hypotheses which link the behaviour to specific triggers or consequences.

Assessment of challenging behaviours needs to be wide-ranging and comprehensive. It should include assessment of:

- cognitive abilities
- communicative abilities
- perceptual and motor abilities
- social skills
- domestic, self-care and community skills
- family history
- social history and living arrangements
- health and medical status
- mental health
- behavioural phenotypes and syndromal cause for learning disability.

Positive behavioural approaches aim to change the behaviour by environmental manipulation and teaching alternative, more adaptive responses that serve the same function as the target behaviour.

BEHAVIOURAL PHENOTYPES

Behavioural and cognitive aspects may be so striking as to be almost characteristic of some syndromes associated with learning disabilities. This has become of increasing interest in clinical research and practice (Table 12.1).

AUTISM

Autism/autistic spectrum disorder is a developmental disorder covered in Chapter 13. It is mentioned here because

Table 12.1 Examples of behavioural phenotypes (adapted from Deb 1997)

	Clinical features	Learning disability	Behavioural phenotype
Prader–Willi syndrome (PWS)	1 in 5–10 000 live births Neonatal hypotonia Age 1–4: gradual development of hyperphagia leading to gross obesity Short stature Obesity Cryptoorchidism	40% have IQ between 70–90 60% have mild to moderate learning disabilities	Abnormal speech Sleep disturbance with excessive daytime sleepiness Behavioural problems around hyperphagia SIB, spot picking, temper tantrums Motor slowness, stereotypies, ritualistic behaviours Specific pattern of cognitive deficit – visual-spatial skills remain particularly strong while short-term memory reduces
Phenylketonuria (PKU)	Fair hair, fair skin and blue eyes due to lack of skin pigment precursor, tyrosine Low birth weight Microcephaly Non-specific neurological signs Epilepsy (26%)	Corrective diet in childhood appears to prevent developmental delay and maladaptive behaviours	Hyperactivity, irritability, episodes of screaming, noisiness and uncontrolled temper tantrums SIB – biting, head banging Clumsiness, poor motor control
Rett syndrome (RS)	1 in 5–10 000 live births Fatal for male foetuses Affects girls exclusively No gene has yet been identified	Severe to profound learning disability Normal development up until 18 months – 2 years Loss of skills Age 4-5: development of epilepsy in 59-72%	Mood changes Episodes of anxiety characterized by hyperventilation, screaming, self-injury SIB – hand biting, head banging, hair pulling Stereotyped motor movements 'Autistic' features
Fragile X syndrome (FRAX)	1 in 1200 males 1 in 2000–5000 females Most common inherited cause of learning disabilities: 50% of all X-linked causes 2–5% of learning disabled population	Range from normal intellectual functioning to profound disability No correlation between level of disability and proportion of fragile-X positive cells Decline of mean IQ with age	Language delay – with perseveration and 'litany-like' speech Hyperactivity, restlessness and lack of concentration Mood swings Psychotic features – paranoia, hallucinations, ritualistic behaviours and other autistic features SIB Active gaze avoidance Delay in initiative and symbolic play
Tuberous sclerosis complex (TSC)	1 in 10 000 births 70% due to new mutations TSC1 9q34 (coding for hamartin) TSC2 16p13 (coding for tuberin)	Normal intellectual functioning to profound disability with multiple seizure types	(Possible phenotype): Autistic features – aloofness, non-communicative and obsessional behaviours Overactivity, aggression and destructive outbursts Schizophrenic-like psychosis that may or may not be related to epilepsy

(SIB = self-injurious behavior)

70% of people with autism function within the learning disabled range. Those adults who do not are in danger of falling between services designed to meet the needs of adults with severe mental illness and those that meet the needs of adults with learning disability.

The lack of a developmental history and an understanding of the core symptoms and behaviours associated with autism can lead to a misdiagnosis of schizophrenia and non-recognition of depressive illness and suicide risk.

It is important that the diagnosis of autism is made as early as possible in childhood, so that the special educational and communication supports required are identified and put in place.

MENTAL HEALTH NEEDS

Prevalence rates for psychiatric illness range from 10–50%, depending on sample selection, definition of caseness (e.g. some studies exclude behavioural and pervasive developmental disorders), diagnostic criteria and the diagnostic method used. This increased vulnerability is thought to be the result of a complex interaction between organic (e.g. brain damage), psychological (e.g. poor coping mechanisms, low self-esteem) and social factors (e.g. social isolation, adverse life events). Learning disability itself is considered to be a risk factor.

Behavioural disturbance is often a presenting symptom, and may or may not be due to an underlying psychiatric illness. Whether one presents to specialist health services or not often depends on the ability of others to recognize symptoms. Behaviours that are aggressive, antisocial or self-injurious are therefore more likely to reach services.

People with learning disability show the same range of mental health needs as the rest of the population, and are entitled to the same range of services with local specialist provision as needed (Box 12.6).

The psychiatric assessment

Specific factors may influence the diagnostic process (Box 12.7). A reliable, longitudinal history is important but often difficult to achieve in practice.

The psychiatric history should include:

- obstetric history – e.g. hypoxia, birth injury, low Apgar scores
- family history – of learning disability, epilepsy and psychiatric illness
- developmental history – motor and developmental milestones, language, play
- aetiology of learning disability – if known
- how parents/family were told and what supports were offered
- premorbid level of functioning – do not assume that the current level of functioning is due to the learning disability
- communicative style and communicative environment
- life events – loss, bereavement, staff changes, abuse, moving home

- history of change – e.g. of mental or social functioning
- social history – institutionalization, support networks, activities, hobbies
- treatment history – interventions and outcome, allergies and side effects
- physical health – including epilepsy, sensory impairments
- precipitants or maintaining factors
- behavioural equivalents – e.g. level of activity/interest, biological symptoms.

Attention must be paid to enabling the person with the learning disability to tell their story in their own way. Apart from using good communicative techniques, the clinician should pay attention to environmental factors (such as background noise) and the power imbalance that exists in the discourse between patient and doctor. The degree of suggestibility and acquiescence will be minimized by an experienced clinician. Observation of nonverbal behaviours can provide important insights into the person's mental state. If necessary, be prepared to conduct a series of short interviews over a period of time, and in different settings.

The interpretation of any symptom or sign must take into account the person's developmental level and experiences. For example, echolalia is a normal developmental phase and not necessarily indicative of schizophrenia. Carers often report that the person is seen talking to him/herself either alone or in the company of others. It is much more likely that

---

Box 12.6 What *Valuing People* (Department of Health 2001a) says about mental health services

The National Service Framework for Mental Health applies to all adults of working age

People with learning disabilities should be able to access and benefit from mainstream mental health service, with specialist support if needed

There should be access to local acute assessment and treatment resources for those who are unable to access mainstream services even with specialist support

Out-of-borough placements should rarely be used

CPA 'care coordinators' should have expertise in both learning disabilities and mental health

Local protocols need to be established for those with borderline learning disabilities and those with autism/Asperger's syndrome, as they often fail to meet eligibility criteria for either service

---

Box 12.7 Some factors that may affect the diagnostic process

Sovner (1986)

Intellectual distortion – the person may be unable to label their experiences or moods, or to communicate them

Psychosocial masking – simple and naïve symptoms go unrecognized as psychopathology

Cognitive disintegration – non-specific stress response leading to misdiagnosis of psychosis

Baseline exaggeration – severity of pre-existing cognitive deficits and maladaptive behaviours may cloud the diagnostic process

Reiss (1994)

Diagnostic overshadowing – the presence of learning disability overshadows the diagnostic significance of a symptom or behaviour

Others

Establishing a reliable, longitudinal history

Limited verbal abilities

Reliance on others to recognize symptoms as significant

Physical illnesses/disorders and pain presenting with behaviour disturbance

Side effects of medication presenting as psychiatric, behavioural or epileptic disturbance

The importance of life events and changes in routine, day care, residence and care staff/keyworker

The importance of changes in staff approach and management within care homes

such behaviours are due to limitations in social skills, and the person is remembering or fantasising about a conversation (Einfeld 2001). Similarly, grandiose ideas are more likely to be an attempt to compensate for poor self-esteem.

Clarifying the nature of behaviours requires time with the patient. Behavioural baseline recordings can be extremely useful. Records of the target behaviours identified for treatment (such as disturbed sleep, aggressive outbursts) can be used as a way of monitoring treatment efficacy.

The need for multi-disciplinary assessments, particularly in those with complex needs, is not only helpful but necessary.

Multi-axial classification/diagnosis

Diagnostic criteria for psychiatric disorders for use with adults with learning disabilities (DC-LD) was published to complement ICD-10 manuals for people with mild learning disabilities, as well as being a stand-alone classificatory system for those with moderate to profound learning disabilities. It provides operationalized diagnostic criteria, which reflects current practice and opinion amongst psychiatrists practising in the field (Royal College of Psychiatrists 2001b). It recognizes that:

- the range of psychopathology experienced by a person with learning disability may be different from someone of average ability
- current diagnostic criteria are weighted towards verbal items
- subdivisions in DSM-IV and ICD-10 are likely to introduce inaccuracy and lessen validity in a population where eliciting psychopathology and communication may be difficult.

A single diagnostic label often does not do justice to the complexity of the presenting problems. As well as a psychiatric diagnosis (see BOX 12.8) it is often useful to think of other important areas, which not only influence presentation but management options.

A hierarchical approach to diagnosis is adopted within learning disability psychiatry, in accordance with ICD-10 (mental retardation):

Axis I: Severity of learning disabilities
Axis II: Cause of learning disabilities; other associated medical conditions
Axis III: Psychiatric disorders –
    DC-LD Level A: Developmental disorders
    DC-LD Level B: Psychiatric illness
    DC-LD Level C: Personality disorders
    DC-LD Level D: Problem behaviours
    DC-LD Level E: Other disorders
Axis IV: Global assessment of psychosocial disability
Axis V: Associated abnormal psychosocial situations

Treatment issues

The range of investigations and treatments available to the general population should also be made available to people with learning disabilities. It is important to acknowledge that access to healthcare is often dependent on others, and referrals may be made to services without the person's knowledge or agreement. Particular issues to consider include:

- person-centred approach
- consent and incapacitated adults
- physical treatments
- psychological treatments.

The decision to prescribe medication should follow a comprehensive assessment of the person's emotional and behavioural disturbance. The psychiatrist should try to resist 'knee-jerk' responses despite the pressure of crises presentations (Einfeld 2001). It is unusual for medication alone to be sufficient; drug treatment should be part of an

---

Box 12.8 Specific psychiatric conditions in adults with learning disabilities

Schizophrenia

Prevalence 3–4 times higher than the general population

Cannot be reliably diagnosed in someone with an IQ below 45

Negative symptoms may pose particular diagnostic difficulties

Nature or content of hallucinatory experiences may be difficult to elicit

Passivity phenomena must be interpreted with care, as people with learning disability often have and experience little control over their lives

Some people with learning disability have problems separating fact from fantasy

Affective disorders

Prevalence ranges from 0.9–6%

Diagnosis often missed, particularly unipolar depression

Symptoms are not markedly different from the general population

Anhedonia, changes in activity levels, appetite or other biological symptoms can easily be elicited with a good history

Increases in pre-existing maladaptive behaviours, hypochondrical or somatic symptoms, irritability or agitation may be suggestive of the diagnosis

Presentation often dependent on degree of disability, with more atypical symptoms in the more severely disabled

Dementia

As life expectancy increases, so does prevalence of psychiatric disorders associated with old age

Neuro-pathological changes of Alzheimer's found at post-mortem in most adults with Down's Syndrome over 35 years. Clinically, it is found in 8% of adults between 35–49, and in 60% of those over 60.

The diagnosis is often difficult in the absence of premorbid levels of functioning

It is important to exclude and treat other causes of apparent deterioration in skills – such as depression, hypothyroidism, sensory impairments—in practice, however, these frequently occur at the same time as signs or symptoms of dementia

Potentially treatable pseudo-dementias and other types of dementia need to be excluded

integrated multidisciplinary care plan. Proper consideration needs to be given to informed consent (see below).

Antipsychotics

- Atypical antipsychotics are now the first drug of choice in the treatment of schizophrenia.
- There is no good evidence that antipsychotic medication helps in managing challenging behaviour (systematic review of RCTs).
- Lower-level evidence suggests antipsychotic medication can reduce challenging behaviours but with significant side effects. Approximately 25% can be treated effectively, 50% fairly effectively and the remaining 25% with intermittent success or not at all.
- Akathisia is an important side effect to consider particularly as the person may be unable to describe the sense of restlessness and irritability. The resultant increase in agitation may lead the psychiatrist to increase the dose of antipsychotic medication inappropriately.
- The fatality rate of neuroleptic malignant syndrome is twice that of the general population.

Antidepressants

- SSRIs have largely supplanted tricyclic antidepressants in the treatment of depression in people with learning disability.
- SSRIs are widely used to treat repetitive behaviours, including ritualistic/stereotypic behaviours associated with autism and self-injurious behaviours (SIB).
- In practice, the availability of a liquid preparation often makes it easier to accept and administer, and may be the deciding factor in the choice of one SSRI over another.

Anxiolytics

- No specific studies available on the treatment of anxiety in people with learning disabilities.
- Use of medication is similar to the general population, with the assumption that it acts in the same way and with the same results.
- Benzodiazepines are commonly used in the treatment of epilepsy, but is not used for behavioural or emotional disturbance as it frequently causes disinhibition and irritability in people with organic brain impairment.

Mood stabilizers

- Lithium, carbamazepine and valproate are used as mood stabilizers in the treatment of bipolar affective disorder.
- The difficulties of monitoring side effects of lithium, as well as serum lithium levels, in this population make carbamazepine and valproate the drugs of choice.
- Lithium and carbamazepine have also been used in the treatment of impulsive, aggressive behaviours.

Other drugs

- People with learning disabilities are frequently taking antiepileptic drugs. These may have psychiatric side effects.
- Stimulants are used in the treatment of attention deficit hyperactivity disorder (ADHD).
- Antilibidinal drugs are sometimes used as a last resort in the treatment of inappropriate sexual behaviours in men with learning disabilities who have sexually offended.
- As in the general population, hypnotics may help with sleep problems in the short term, but it is more important to assess the reasons why sleep is disturbed, to establish good sleep hygiene and to treat any underlying physical, emotional, psychiatric or environmental cause.

PARENTS WITH LEARNING DISABILITY

The reproductive rights of women with learning disabilities have been at risk for much of the 20th century. They are now enshrined in human rights legislation, and reflected in *Valuing People*. Parents with learning disabilities have special needs whilst acknowledging that the needs of their children are paramount. Until the last decade, the literature tended to concentrate on risk factors, the inadequacies of parenting skills, parenting assessments and the provision of parenting skills programmes to those at the mild or borderline range of intellectual functioning.

Children of learning-disabled parents are particularly vulnerable to removal from their natural parents. Care proceedings are often inaccessible to parents with learning disabilities. Research suggests that an IQ score below 65 means that children are invariably placed into care, whilst above this score the outcome depends on the network of support available. All too often services are patchy and constrained by resources.

GROWING OLDER WITH LEARNING DISABILITY

People with learning disabilities are an ageing population. This increased lifespan is in part due to advances in medical treatments, better nutrition and healthier lifestyles. It is reasonable to speculate that many older people with learning disabilities will experience significant psychiatric health needs, but there is little research data available (Cooper 1997). However, studies have shown that the prevalence of dementia is much higher than in the age-matched general population. This has been a relatively neglected area as much clinical and research attention has been given to the dementia of Down's syndrome.

The barriers to accessing appropriate health care for people with learning disabilities are compounded when one is older in part due to forced 'retirement' from day centres and loss of contact with care managers as they 'transfer' into mainstream elderly services.

LEARNING DISABILITY AND THE LAW

People with learning disabilities and the Criminal Justice System

Intellectual impairment (i.e. low IQ, but not necessarily learning disabilities) is a risk factor for offending in both adults and juveniles. There is little evidence to suggest that the presence of learning disability predisposes to criminal behaviour. There are particular difficulties looking at the numbers convicted; it is generally considered that the prevalence rates for offenders with learning disabilities may be higher than the general population, especially amongst those convicted of arson or sexual offences. There is also a predominance of males amongst offenders with learning disability.

People receiving specialist learning disability services are unlikely to offend, partly because the offending behaviour is relabelled as 'challenging behaviour' and therefore decriminalized. However, in the UK, people with learning disabilities are over-represented amongst those arrested and taken to police stations, especially those with mild disability. The Police and Criminal Evidence Act 1984 (PACE) seeks to protect vulnerable people during the interview process, and requires the presence of an appropriate adult.

People with learning disabilities are also victims of crime. The fact that they have learning disabilities may prejudice their chances of being judged to be a reliable witness. Prosecutions are therefore not very common. Consideration has been given to making the process more sensitive to the special needs of this group.

The Mental Health Act (1983): England and Wales

Admission to hospital for assessment and treatment under the Mental Health Act applies if the person with learning disabilities fulfils the criteria for compulsory admission. As with psychopathic disorder, those who are admitted under the category of mental impairment or severe mental impairment do so on the proviso that medical treatment is likely to alleviate or prevent deterioration of their condition. Patients admitted under this category have learning disabilities (i.e. arrested or incomplete development of mind), which is associated with 'abnormally aggressive or seriously irresponsible conduct'. Therefore, this definition will only apply to a minority of people with learning disability needing hospital treatment because of a severe behavioural problem.

Guardianship allows an individual to receive community care where it cannot be provided without the use of compulsory powers. It requires the person to reside in a specified place, attend for education, training and day care and gives access to any medical practitioner, social worker or other person specified by the guardian. It cannot be used for compulsory medication.

The Bournewood Gap refers to the situation where a person who lacks the capacity to consent can be admitted to hospital provided he/she does not actively object or dissent. This action is taken in his/her 'best interests' and does not require formal admission. However, neither does it provide the reviews, appeals and safeguards afforded to others under the Mental Health Act. This situation may change in the future when the European Courts announce their ruling.

The Mental Capacity Bill has been in draft form for the past few years. It is hoped that it will become law, thus providing a clear framework for the provision of health care to individuals who are unable to consent to admission, care or treatment.

The Care Programme Approach (CPA) and supervised discharge

The use of CPA in learning disability services is variable across the country, yet all those with mental health needs must be assessed for CPA. The situation is partly due to the current fragmentation and organisation of learning disability services, some within a partnership trust, others within a primary care or mental health trust.

It is obvious that CPA would benefit people with learning disabilities who have mental health needs and additional health needs and vulnerability factors (Roy 2000). Features of an integrated CPA and care management include a single operational policy; joint training for health and social care staff; common risk assessment and management processes; shared information systems across health and social care; and agreement on the allocation of budgets. The National Service Framework for Mental Health also sets a standard that those entitled to CPA should be able to access services 24 hours a day, 365 days a year (Roy 2000). *Valuing people* states that CPA coordinators must be trained in both learning disabilities and mental health.

Consent to treatment

Assessments, investigations and treatments are sometimes not offered to people with learning disability because of anxiety and difficulties over issues of consent. The anticipated legislation of the Mental Capacity Bill will go some way towards ensuring that people who lack capacity will not be neglected or receive sub-standard healthcare.

The definition of incapacity includes:

- inability to make a decision
- inability to understand or retain relevant information
- inability to use the material information
- inability to communicate a decision.

Currently, no one is able to give consent on behalf of another adult. Parents, relatives or members of the multidisciplinary team cannot give consent for the adult with learning disabilities because:

- the ethics of consent is to encourage autonomy
- consent must be voluntary, competent and informed
- capacity is presumed – if there is doubt, a functional approach to the assessment of capacity must be made by the health professional proposing the treatment or care
- there is no automatic relationship between most mental disorders and capacity
- capacity may be temporarily affected by other factors such as confusion, panic, shock, pain, fear, drugs/medicines
- capacity is not concerned with the reasonableness of the individual's decision.

As useful guide with accompanying consent forms and patient leaflets, including one designed for people with learning disabilities, has been published by the Department of Health (2001b) and can be found on their website (http://www.doh.gov.uk/consent).

THE NEEDS OF CARERS

The majority of people with learning disabilities in the UK live with their families, usually with their parents. In recognition of this, *Families Matter: Counting Families In* was published to accompany *Valuing people* (Department of Health 2001c). It acknowledged the lifelong commitment of families in caring for their learning-disabled relative and the difficult transitions to be negotiated in the caring relationship. It stressed the importance of understanding this relationship, of partnership working between families and professionals, the disadvantages and discrimination carers often face, the emotional and practical supports required and the extra burden of care often experienced by family carers from minority ethnic groups. The needs of elderly carers is a distinct group requiring extra consideration and support because of their particular needs (Hubert & Hollins 2000).

ADVOCACY AND SELF-ADVOCACY

Nothing About Us Without Us (Department of Health 2001d) was also published with *Valuing People*. It puts the person with learning disabilities at the centre of the network of services. It is important therefore, to involve people with learning disabilities at every stage of the planning and delivery of services.

SERVICE PROVISION

... the wider NHS has failed to consider the needs of people with learning disabilities. This is the most important issue the NHS needs to address.
(Department of Health 2001b)

Mainstream services – primary care, community, accident and emergency, hospital outpatient and admission wards – must all be able to meet the health needs of people with learning disabilities, with specialist support if necessary. Such services also need to be sensitive to the cultural and ethnic diversity of their local community (O'Hara 2003). Where health care cannot be met in these settings, local specialist resources need to be available. It will no longer be acceptable to send people out of borough, to admission facilities away from their homes and families and friends. This requires mainstream services, including mental health, to invest in making sure their services are comprehensive and accessible (Box 12.6). Local protocols are required to ensure that people do not fall between services, and that health care is not delayed while different agencies and organizations argue over funding.

All strategic plans and developments now rest with a local multi-agency Learning Disability Partnership Board, chaired by the local authority, charged with the task of implementing the considerable challenges contained in *Valuing people*. The Board is made up of the usual statutory stakeholders as well as having membership from housing, leisure, ethnic minority groups, people with learning disabilities and their carers.

FURTHER READING

Fraser W & Kerr M (eds) (2003) *Seminars in the Psychiatry of Learning Disabilities*, 2nd edn. London: Gaskell Publications, Royal College of Psychiatrists.
O'Hara J & Sperlinger A (eds) (1997) *Adults with Learning Disabilities: A Practical Approach for Health Professionals*. Chichester: John Wiley.
Ryan J with Thomas F (1980) *The Politics of Mental Handicap*. London: Penguin.

REFERENCES

Ambalu S (1997) Communication. In: O'Hara J and Sperlinger (eds) *Adults with Learning Disabilities: A Practical Approach for Health Professionals*. Chichester: John Wiley.
Brown H (1997) Vulnerability issues. In: O'Hara J and Sperlinger (eds) *Adults with Learning Disabilities: A Practical Approach for Health Professionals*. Chichester: John Wiley.
Carvill S (2001) Sensory impairments, intellectual disability and psychiatry. *Journal of Intellectual Disability Research* **45**(6): 467–83.
Cooper, S-A (1997) Learning disabilities and old age. *Advances in Psychiatric Treatment* **3**: 312–20.

Deb S (1997) Behavioural phenotypes. Chapter 4. In: Read SG (ed.) *Psychiatry in Learning Disability*. London: WB Saunders.

Department of Health (2000) *No Secrets: The Protection of Vulnerable Adults. Guidance on the Development and Implementation of Multi-agency Policies and Procedures*. London: HMSO.

Department of Health (2001a) *Valuing People: A Strategy for Learning Disabilities for the 21st Century*. London: HMSO.

Department of Health (2001b) *Reference Guide to Consent for Examination and Treatment*. London: HMSO. Available at: http://www.doh.gov.uk/consent

Department of Health (2001c) *Families Matter: Counting Families In*. London: HMSO.

Department of Health (2001d) *Nothing About Us Without Us*. London: HMSO.

Einfeld SL (2001) Systematic management approach to pharmacotherapy for people with learning disabilities. *Advances in Psychiatric Treatment* **7**: 43–9.

Emerson E, Barrett S, Bell C, Cummings R, McCook C, Toogood A & Mansell J (1987) *Developing Services for People with Severe Learning Difficulties and Challenging Behaviours*. Canterbury: Institute of Social and Applied Psychology.

General Medical Council (2003) *Tomorrow's Doctors: Recommendations on Undergraduate Medical Education*. London: GMC. Also available at http://www.gmc-uk.org/med_ed

Health Evidence Bulletins, Wales (2000) Available at: http://www.hebw.uwcm.ac.uk/learningdisability

Hubert J & Hollins S (2000) Working with elderly carers of people with learning disabilities and planning for the future. *Advances in Psychiatric Treatment* **6**: 41–8.

O'Hara J (2003) Learning disability and ethnicity: achieving cultural competence. *Advances in Psychiatric Treatment* **9**: 166–74.

Reiss S (1994) Psychopathology in mental retardation. In Bouras N (ed.) *Mental Health and Mental Retardation: Recent Advances and Practices*. Cambridge: Cambridge University Press.

Roy A (2000) The Care Programme Approach in learning disability psychiatry. *Advances in Psychiatric Treatment* **6**: 380–7.

Royal College of Psychiatrists (2001a) *Council Report 95: Basic Specialist Training and the MRCPsych*. London: RCP.

Royal College of Psychiatrists (2001b) *Diagnostic Criteria for Psychiatric Disorders for use with Adults with Learning Disabilities/Mental Retardation. DC-LD*. Occasional Paper OP 48. London: Gaskell Publications.

Ryan J (1980) *The Politics of Mental Handicap*. London: Penguin.

Sinason V (1992) *Mental Handicap and the Human Condition: New Approaches from the Tavistock*. London: Free Association Press.

Sovner R (1986) Limiting factors in the use of DSM-III criteria with mentally ill/mentally retarded persons. *Psychopharmacology Bulletin* **24**(4): 1055–9.

Williams C (2003) *The Environmental Causes of Intellectual Disabilities*. Available at: http://www.intellectualdisability.info

World Health Organisation (1980) *International Classification of Impairment, Disabilities and Handicaps*. Geneva: WHO.

APPENDIX

Useful websites

http://www.intellectualdisability.info

A regularly updated web-based learning resource for medical and health care students and practitioners. Developed in collaboration with the Downs' Syndrome Association and the Department of Mental Health–Learning Disabilities at St. George's Hospital Medical School, University of London, UK.

http://www.hebw.uwcm.ac.uk

Health Evidence Bulletins – Wales: acts as signposts to the best evidence across a broad range of evidence types and subject areas, including learning disabilities and mental health.

Child and adolescent psychiatry

Nick Goddard

INTRODUCTION

An understanding and knowledge of child and adolescent psychiatry is important not just for prospective child psychiatrists, but for all psychiatrists. Adults with mental health problems were once children and it is therefore necessary to know the relevance of problems in childhood. Additionally, many adults will also be parents and parental illness can adversely effect children.

EPIDEMIOLOGY

Several studies have looked at the epidemiology of child and adolescent mental health. As the child and adolescent population contains subjects at different stages of development, studies have focused on age groups of children. Broadly, the young population can be divided into: pre-school children, middle childhood and adolescence.

Pre-school children

One of the most informative studies in this age group is the pre-school to school study by Richman et al. (1982). One in four three-year-olds from a north-east London borough were selected randomly. The study involved an initial screening interview with assessments at 3, 4 and 8 years for those found to be 'positive' (i.e. above the cut-off point for a mental health problem) and a sample of screen 'negative' children.

- **Findings at 3-years-old:** 7% had moderate–severe problems with a further 15% having mild problems. There was a slight excess of boys. Factors associated with psychiatric problems were learning delay, marital discord, low warmth and high criticism in the family, living in a large tower block, large family size and maternal depression.
- **Findings at 8-years-old:** of the 3-year-olds with problems, 75% of the boys still had problems and about

50% of the girls. Hyperactivity and low intelligence predicted persistence in boys, though not in girls.

With age, the nature of the problems changed. At 3-years-old fears, sleep problems, soiling and overactivity were more common. These decreased with age and worries became more common in older children.

The study has implications for early intervention as early childhood problems can persist, therefore intervention at an early stage seems indicated. It can be difficult, however, to detect problems at this age and predict which ones will persist.

Middle childhood

One of the main sources of information on problems in this age group comes from an elegant study carried out on the Isle of Wight by Rutter et al. (1976). All 10- to 11-year-olds living on the Isle of Wight and attending a state school were included. Screening interviews were carried out with teachers and parents. Further assessments were then done on all children who scored above the cut-off point or who were known to have attended child and adolescent mental health services (CAMHS).

Findings of the Isle of Wight study were as follows:

1. The prevalence of psychiatric problems was 6.8%.
2. Emotional disorders accounted for 2.5% of the prevalence with a similar rate amongst boys and girls (boy:girl = 0.7:1). There were more only children and children from small families in the group.
3. Mixed emotional and conduct disorders were more similar in characteristics to pure conduct disorder.
4. Conduct disorder (CD) was present in 4% with an excess of boys (boy:girl = 4:1). Children from large families (more than 4 children) were over-represented.
5. Specific reading difficulties (SRD) overlapped with CD, though mixed SRD/CD was more similar to pure SRD in its presentation.
6. Physical disorders were a risk factor for psychiatric problems. In children with a physical disorder not

affecting the brain, the proportion with psychiatric problems was 12%; in children with epilepsy the figure was 29% and 44% in those with cerebral palsy.

7. Only 10% of children with psychiatric problems were attending child psychiatric services, with a further 10% receiving help from other services.

A similar study was later carried out in an inner London borough, in a deprived area of London. Compared to the IoW study, rates of psychiatric problems were double in the inner London borough study. This is believed to be due to increased rates of marital discord, parental illness, social disadvantage and a high pupil/teacher turnover in schools (Rutter et al. 1975).

Adolescence

Epidemiological studies in adolescence are hard to compare because of differences in defining the age range e.g. 11–19, 13-18. Therefore studies often examine adolescents of a particular age.

The Isle of Wight study was extended to follow-up children at the age of 14–15 years and still living in or around the area. The findings were:

1. Prevalence of problems was around 9% (2% more than at age 10), with a further 10% of adolescents self-reporting feelings of misery.

2. Depressive disorders rose to 2% (an increase from 0.2% at age 10). School refusal also increased.

3. Of adolescents who had a problem, about 50% had a problem at the age of 10. New problems were not associated with educational difficulties, were slightly more common in males and had fewer adverse family factors.

Similar studies have been carried in Dunedin (New Zealand), Christchurch (New Zealand) and Ontario (Canada). Some studies have found rates of psychiatric problems from 10–40%, though these high rates may be a product of diagnosis based on symptoms without a measure of the impact of the problem.

CLASSIFICATION

Both ICD-10 and DSM-IV have a multiaxial framework for child and adolescent psychiatric diagnoses. ICD-10 has six axes and DSM-IV five axes. Axis 1 in DSM-IV allows multiple diagnoses and encompasses both specific developmental disorders and psychiatric diagnoses (Box 13.1).

Where conditions occur in both childhood and adult life, then the main ICD-10 diagnostic category is used, e.g. depression, obsessive compulsive disorder (OCD). ICD-10 contains a section relating to conditions specific in their onset to childhood e.g. hyperkinetic disorder, enuresis.

HYPERACTIVITY

Hyperactivity, like depression, is a term with a variety of uses and meanings. To parents, it may mean that their child is always in trouble or has excess energy. Child psychiatrists view it as implying a difficulty with restlessness, poor concentration and impulsive behaviour. These conceptual difficulties have also been mirrored in ICD-9 and DSM-III, leading to Americans diagnosing *attention deficit disorder with hyperactivity* (ADDH) more frequently than the narrower *hyperkinetic disorder* previously used in Britain. ICD-10 (hyperkinetic disorder) and DSM-IV (attention deficit hyperactivity disorder ADHD) are now closer in their diagnostic guidelines. ADHD has perhaps become the most commonly used term.

ICD-10 lists:

- hyperkinetic disorder with a disturbance in attention and activity
- hyperkinetic disorder with conduct disorder.

Epidemiology

Hyperkinetic disorder has a prevalence of 1–2%, occurring more frequently in boys (male:female = 3:1) (Taylor et al. 1991).

Features

1. **Chronicity:** 6 months of symptoms are required for diagnosis. Onset has to be in childhood (before age 7), though usually there are symptoms before 5 years and frequently before 2 years. Although a long history of symptoms may be present, the problem may not be recognized until the start of schooling when the difficulties in attention and disruptive behaviour become more apparent.

Box 13.1 ICD-10 axis		
1. Psychiatric diagnosis	e.g.	conduct disorder
2. Specific developmental disorder	e.g.	autism
3. Intellectual level	e.g.	moderate learning disability
4. Medical diagnosis	e.g.	diabetes
5. Psychosocial adversity	e.g.	sexual abuse
6. Level of functioning	e.g.	moderate social disability

2 **Behaviour:** characterized by restlessness (unable to sit still, fidgeting); poor attention (frequent changes of activity); and impulsive behaviour.

3 **Pervasive across settings:** behaviour is evident in all settings, i.e. both at home and school.

Associated features

1 Defiant, aggressive and antisocial behaviour.
2 Poor social relations, this includes rudeness to adults.
3 Below average IQ and specific learning problems.
4 Developmental delay, e.g. speech delay and sometimes clumsiness.

Aetiology

1 **Biological:** twin studies suggest a genetic component, though this may be mediated through other risk factors. Dietary factors may be important in a small proportion.

2 **Psychosocial:** deprivation, institutionalized upbringing. Attachment problems.

Treatment

1 **Support:** general advice, education and support to parents and school.

2 **Behaviour modification:** careful behavioural assessment of problem behaviours at home and school. Requires positive reinforcement and appropriate negative feedback for unacceptable behaviour.

3 **Medication:**
(a) stimulants – methlyphenidate, dexamphetamine. Stimulant medication has a growing evidence base for its efficacy, though the use of medication remains a source of controvesy. Pressure groups opposed to medication use, argue that many of the troubles faced by young people with ADHD are due to the medication and use of stimulants leads to increased substance misuse (see Timimi & Taylor 2004, for an example of the debate). A key study in this area was the MTA trial, which looked at the outcome of young people treated pharmacologically compared with behavioural interventions (MTA cooperative group 1999 a, b). The findings suggest that combined treatment (medication and behaviour) may be most effective (68%), followed by medication alone (56%); behavioural treatment only (34%); and standard community treatment (25%) (Swanson et al. 2001; Connors et al. 2001). Side-effects of stimulant medication include loss of appetite, insomnia, stomach aches and dysphoria. Side-effects are often transitory. Stimulants can exacerbate tics and are therefore not usually the first-line treatment if present. Controversially,

stimulants may slightly decrease growth. Height and weight should be recorded at least 6 monthly.
(b) other agents:
- imipramine
- clonidine – used as an adjunct or second line treatment
- neuroleptics – usually third-line treatment.
(c) new developments (see Chapter 38):
- long-acting preparations – stimulants have short half-lives and need to be given two to three times a day. Longer-acting once-a-day preparations have been developed and one of these (Concerta®) is licensed in the UK
- transdermal preparations – a once-a-day patch for methylphenidate is in development
- non-stimulant preparations – atomoxetine (a specific noradrenaline [norepinephrine] reuptake inhibitor) is a promising non-stimulant treatment. Work is also being undertaken with nicotine patches.

4 **Diet:** often very popular with parents though can be very time-consuming. Some children may respond to a selective diet.

Prognosis

Hyperactive behaviour decreases in adolescence, though there may be a residual degree of restlessness and impulsivity. Many children will suffer from poor educational attainment, particularly if untreated. The main risk is antisocial behaviour in late adolescence/adulthood and higher rates of substance misuse have been reported.

CONDUCT DISORDER

Conduct disorder (CD) is essentially a persistent difficulty in behaviour (i.e. behaving outside of the usual social rules). Whilst epidemiological studies suggest this is the most common child and adolescent psychiatric problem, there is some controversy as to whether CD should be thought of as a psychiatric problem or as a social or educational problem.

ICD-10 divides CD into:

- socialized conduct disorder (i.e. involving peers)
- unsocialized conduct disorder (i.e. on own)
- oppositional defiant disorder (ODD)

DSM-IV requires CD to have been present for 12 months and makes no sub-division of socialized/unsocialized. ODD is a separate category.

Epidemiology

The Isle of Wight study found a prevalence of 4%, with an increased rate in inner city areas. The disorder is more common amongst boys (male:female = 3:1), and is associated with psychosocial deprivation.

Features

1. Fighting or bullying.
2. Cruelty to animals or other people.
3. Destructiveness or fire-setting.
4. Truancy and running away from home.
5. Stealing.
6. Persistent disobedience, defiant behaviour and temper tantrums.

Associated features

1. Hyperactivity.
2. Emotional symptoms – unhappiness and misery.
3. Educational failure– one-third have specific reading difficulties.
4. Poor interpersonal relationships.

Aetiology

1. **Genetic:** there is some support from monozygotic (MZ) twin studies of a genetic contribution, though concordance rates are also high in dizygotic twins. Adoption studies imply that environmental factors may have a strong effect.
2. **Environmental:** there are associations with parenting and school environment. An overly punitive type of parenting, with poor supervision and inconsistent setting of boundaries, can contribute to behaviour problems, along with rewarding dysfunctional behaviour. Parental psychiatric problems and criminality have also been implicated.

Treatment

1. **Assessment:** a thorough assessment is required, including parenting style, family dynamics and school performance (obtain school report).
2. **Parent training:** several models of parent training have been developed and evaluated as being effective. The aim is to promote prosocial behaviour and develop more effective techniques to deal with antisocial behaviour.
3. **Family therapy:** can be effective in addressing dysfunctional dynamics, except in the most chaotic, disorganized families.
4. **Individual therapy:** focused individual therapies, using problem-solving or behaviour modification can be effective.

Prognosis

Forty per cent of children with CD become delinquents in adolescence. Poor outcome is predicted by early onset of CD, severity and pervasiveness, along with adverse family factors, family psychiatric history, criminality and family discord. (Robins 1978).

PERVASIVE DEVELOPMENTAL DISORDER

Pervasive developmental disorder (PDD) refers to autism and autistic spectrum disorders. Autism was previously called *infantile psychosis*, a misleading term as there is no connection with psychosis or schizophrenia. (see Volkmar et al. 2004 for recent review).

ICD-10 divides PDD into:

- childhood autism
- atypical autism
- Asperger's syndrome – similar to autism with no cognitive or language delay, but often clumsy. More common in boys (male:female = 8:1)
- Rett's syndrome – present in girls, with arrest of development between 7–24 months, hand-wringing stereotypies and severe learning difficulty.

Autism is generally thought of as the core problem, with others as less severe variants not fulfilling the full criteria for autism. A very small proportion may have islets of ability, like mental calculation or drawing ability (as shown in the film *Rain Man*). This is not a typical picture of what is a very disabling condition.

Epidemiology

The prevalence is 2–12/10 000, with 10–20/10 000 for broader definitions. Autism is more common amongst males (male:female = 3:1). Despite early studies, there is no evidence of a socio-economic status link (previous supposed links being due to bias).

Features

1. **Onset before 36 months:** problems are often present from a very young age, though not always noticed.
2. **Social impairment:** children are aloof, with little interest in others and difficulties in forming relationships. If social interest does develop then it is characterized by poor empathy with the feelings of others and a deficit in social responsiveness. Autistic children usually have few peers. The deficits are not always present in all areas and children can have one or more behaviours for a period of time or even seem quite social in certain settings.

3. **Communication:** early babble is decreased and 50% have a language delay or never develop language. When language does develop it lacks, or has an unusual, social quality, characteristically talking at people. Some children can talk at length, though this is often repetitious or like a monologue. Specific abnormalities include: echolalia (repeating words/phrases); pronominal reversal (referring to themselves as you or he/she); there are also abnormalities in rhythm, intonation and pitch.

4. **Restricted and repetitive repertoire:** a strict routine is often followed, reacting strongly to any change. Play is characterized by a lack of fantasy or creativity. Children can demonstrate stereotypies, hand-flapping or other repetitive movements of the hands. Preoccupations with restricted subjects occur (e.g. birth dates, shoe sizes).

Associated features

1. **Learning disability:** most children with PDD have a lower than average IQ with verbal IQ less than non-verbal IQ, because of the associated language problems. Fifty per cent have an IQ <50, 70% <70 and approximately 100% (95%) <100.

2. **Seizures:** 10–30% develop seizures, usually in adolescence.

3. **Hyperactivity:** hyperactive behaviour is common, with temper tantrums and aggressive behaviour. Food fads are also common and deliberate self-injurious behaviour (biting self) also occurs.

Differential diagnosis

1. **Hearing impairment:** the unresponsiveness and language difficulties can be confused with deafness. Hearing tests should be carried out.

2. **Asperger's syndrome:** sometimes regarded as 'mild autism'. Asperger's differs in that there is little language delay, an absence of the early aloofness and no stereotypies. There may be narrow or pedantic interests and often marked clumsiness.

3. **Rett's:** occurs in girls only. Typically, development regresses at 12 months with decreased head growth and characteristic hand-washing movements. The illness is progressive and affected individuals die by the age of 30 years.

4. **Disintegrative psychosis (Heller's syndrome):** onset is usually between 3–8 years with regression, autistic features and mental retardation.

5. **Learning difficulty ± autistic features:** can be very similar, though lacks all the essential features.

6. **Severe deprivation:** studies on deprived orphanage children, later adopted, suggest some continue to demonstrate autistic features.

7. **Fragile X:** can present with similar features of gaze avoidance and social anxiety.

8. **Developmental language disorder:** even with profound language problems, communication exists with gestures and reasonable social interaction, though there are overlapping cases.

Aetiology

1. **Genetic:** twin studies suggest a concordance of up to 90%. There is a recurrence rate of 3% in families with one affected child. Whilst several genes are of interest, current research suggests that a broader phenotype of social, communication and/or behavioural difficulties is transmitted in a familial manner.

2. **Neurobiology:** most structures of the brain have been implicated, though there is as yet no clear pathology, interest has focused on the medial temporal lobe structures and the cerebellum. Affected individuals do have larger brains and head circumference (Bailey 1993).

3. **Psychology:** several competing theories exist:
   (a) 'Theory of mind' – this describes the ability to think of other people's points of view and understand and predict their actions. Various stories are related or acted out, characteristically autistic individuals are unable to predict the actions of others (Baron-Cohen 1989).
   (a) Inborn error in the ability to communicate and relate to others – this suggests that autistic children are less able to respond to social or affect-related information (e.g. tones of voice) than non-social input (e.g. train whistles).
   (c) Deficit in executive function – an inability to plan and organize.

4. **Immunization:** recent controversy has centred on the role of immunization (in particular the MMR vaccine) as a causative agent for autism. The area remains highly controversial.

Treatment

1. **Parental support:** parents require support and education. Voluntary support groups can be helpful as can planned respite care.

2. **Education:** autistic children do well in a well-structured environment that has experience with autistic children.

3. **Behaviour modification:** a functional analysis of problem behaviour can then lead to modification using behavioural techniques, e.g. reducing temper tantrums.

4. **Medication:** anticonvulsants are required for seizure control. Stimulants may decrease the hyperactivity but can increase stereotypies. Low-dose atypical

neuroleptics may decrease problem behaviours but can be harmful if used long-term. There was a flurry of interest in the gut hormone secretin, but a series of RCTs has failed to demonstrate a significant benefit over placebo.

Prognosis

About half of sufferers acquire speech, though if there is no language development by the age of 5 years, then it is unlikely to develop. Ten per cent of autistic adults are working and living independently. A poor prognosis is associated with lack of language development and an IQ <60.

SCHOOL REFUSAL

School refusal is very common, accounting for around 5% of referrals to child psychiatry. In itself, school refusal is not a diagnosis (i.e. not in ICD-10), but a reflection of underlying problems (Hersov & Berg 1980).

Epidemiology

School refusal has three age peaks:

1. **5–7 years:** school-starting age (may be associated with separation anxiety)
2. **11 years:** transfer to secondary school
3. **14–16 years old**.

The Isle of Wight study found no cases at age 10, but by age 15 there were 15 cases (0.7% prevalence). The sex incidence is equal.

Features

Children refuse to go to school or return home after leaving. Not going to school can be upsetting for them (ego-dystonic) and there may be overt anxiety or somatic complaints. Such complaints are usually absent in holidays and at weekends (though they may return on Sunday evenings). Parents are aware of the non-attendance. The onset can be abrupt or gradual with a range of precipitants – bullying, reading difficulties, etc.

Associated features

1. **Intelligence:** usually of average intelligence and ability.
2. **Family organization:** families can be ineffective in ensuring a return to school. This may be related to over-involvement with the children (e.g. over-enmeshed mother), lack of consensus on behaviour

management (e.g. ineffectual father) or the child may be considered 'special' (e.g. because of difficulties at birth).
3. **Family size:** there is no family size effect, though the youngest child may be at increased risk.
4. **Underlying psychiatric problems:**
   (a) separation anxiety – in younger children, often unable to go anywhere without one or both parents
   (b) phobia – may be specific phobia (e.g. of buses, or fear of being bullied)
   (c) depression
   (d) substance misuse – characterized by a change of behaviour, apathy
   (e) schizophrenia – a rare cause in adolescence.

Differential diagnosis

1. **Truancy:** differs from school refusal in that it is ego-syntonic (i.e. the child is not upset about not attending school) and wilful; the parents are often unaware; and it is associated with other antisocial behaviour (and therefore linked with associated features of CD – male sex, social disadvantage, marital discord, etc).
2. **Physical illness:** a genuine physical illness may exist.

Treatment

1. **Behavioural:** if acute onset, then should aim for a rapid reintroduction to school. If chronic, then a graded programme of exposure to school life may be needed. Close liaison with education services is essential, and tuition units may help.
2. **Family therapy:** may change the family dynamics and empower the parents to aid the return to school. If a two-parent family, both parents working together are required.
3. **Medication:** generally of little value, unless there is an underlying psychiatric condition.

Prognosis

Two-thirds of school refusers return to school, with return being more likely if the child is younger, if less severe and there is early intervention. One-third may have persisting neurotic problems, and a very small proportion may develop agoraphobia in adulthood, though the link with school refusal is less than conclusive.

ELIMINATION DISORDERS

Difficulties in toileting are not uncommon and may be due to underlying developmental problems.

Encopresis

Strictly speaking, encopresis is the passage of normally formed stools in abnormal places, while soiling is the passage of semi-solid faeces. Practically speaking, they are synonymous.

Epidemiology

Bowel control is usually achieved by the age of 4 years. At age 7–8, the prevalence is 1.5% (2.3% boys, 0.7% girls) and at age 10, 1.0% (1.3% boys, 0.3% girls). By the age of 16, soiling is extremely rare. At all ages, soiling is more common in boys.

Aetiology

Various classifications of soiling have been devised (primary/secondary, retentive/non-retentive), though rarely does soiling occur in such a clear pattern. Failure to go to the toilet may result in constipation with overflow of semi-soiled faeces. More important is to determine what may be causing the problem:

1 **Physical cause:** where bowel control has never been achieved an underlying physical cause should be considered, e.g. Hirschsprung's disease.
2 **Phobia:** a fear of sitting on the toilet or of monsters in the toilet is not uncommon among young children; careful questioning may be required to elicit the problem.
3 **Family difficulties:** chronic discord and chaotic family organization may lead to soiling in strange places. Also lack of appropriate toilet training can contribute.
4 **Stress:** stressful life-events, e.g. bereavement, parental separation, can precipitate regression to soiling behaviour.

Treatment

1 **Assessment:** joint assessment involving paediatrician may be required.
2 **Medication:** laxatives can be used to soften the stool and promote bowel opening.
3 **Behaviour management:** the use of star-charts and behavioural regimes promotes a normal toilet routine. Appropriate steps and goals should be decided upon.
4 **Family therapy:** involving the whole family may help decrease anxiety and ensure consistency of approach.

Prognosis

Soiling usually resolves by adolescence. It can take up to six months to retrain the bowel wall.

Enuresis

Enuresis is the involuntary passage of urine in the absence of physical abnormalities after the age of five years. In *primary* *enuresis* children have never acquired bladder control. In *secondary enuresis*, bladder control was achieved for at least 6 months and then lost. The prognosis is worse for secondary enuresis, though otherwise the two have similar characteristics.

Nocturnal enuresis (bed-wetting) is more common and associated with boys; 10–30% also have diurnal enuresis. *Diurnal enuresis* (day-time wetting) is associated with girls; 60–80% also have nocturnal enuresis.

Epidemiology

Nocturnal
At age 5 the prevalence is 10% (male : female = 1:1), at age 10, 2.5% (male : female = 1.6:1), and at age 15, 1% (male : female = 1.8:1)

Diurnal
Two per cent of all 5-year-olds, with a female excess.

Associated features

1 **Urinary tract infections (UTI) in girls:** 1% of all 5-year-olds have asymptomatic UTI, but in children with enuresis 5% have UTIs.
2 **Family history:** 70% have a positive family history.
3 **Stress:** life events at the age of 3 to 4 years double the likelihood of enuresis.
4 **Late toilet training:** training after the age of 20 months is associated with enuresis.
5 Enuresis is not associated with deep sleep, and is not an epileptiform equivalent.

Treatment

1 **Bedtime routine:** general advice on a night-time routine (going to the toilet before sleep, restricting fluids) may help.
2 **Behavioural:** a star chart reward system is effective in 20–30% of cases. Most effective is the 'bell & pad' or enuresis alarm. Success rates of 50–100% within 2 months are reported, although 35% then relapse, which can be offset by 'over-learning' – repeating the procedure with a pre-bedtime fluid load.
3 **Medication:** desmopressin (DDAVP) – usually as a nasal spray – is effective, but relapse rates are high when discontinued. Tricyclic antidepressants also achieve dryness, but tolerance can develop and relapse rates are high. There is also the potential for toxicity.

Prognosis

Most children fully recover. Approximately 3% of enuretics are still wetting at age 20. Poor prognosis is associated with boys, low social status and nightly wetting.

TICS AND TOURETTE'S SYNDROME

Tics are rapid, involuntary, repetitive, stereotyped, motor movements or phonic productions. ICD-10 classifies tics as:

- transient tic disorder
- chronic motor or vocal tic disorder
- combined vocal and multiple motor tic disorder (de la Tourette's syndrome).

Simple tics

Simple tics such as blinks, grunts or sniffs are usually transitory, occurring in 10% of children, with an excess of boys. They resolve spontaneously.

Tourette's syndrome

Tourette's syndrome (TS) combines both motor and phonic tics. Motor tics usually start first, with a mean age of 7 years (range 2–15 years) and vocal tics from 8–15 years. A small proportion may exhibit coprolalia (swearing), echolalia, echopraxia and copropraxia.

Associated features

1. Obsessive-compulsive disorder: found in 30–60% of cases.
2. Hyperactivity: present in 25–50%.

Aetiology

TS runs in families along with obsessive compulsive disorder, possibly due to a dominant gene with incomplete penetrance.

Treatment

1. **Support:** families may require support and education to understand the condition.
2. **Behavioural:** relaxation may help, particularly with the stress associated with chronic tics.
3. **Medication:**
   - low-dose haloperidol or pimozide decreases tic frequency
   - more recent interest has fixed on atypical neuroleptics
   - clonidine
   - chlomipramine or SSRI.

Prognosis

Tics usually decrease in frequency in adolescence/adulthood, although they can persist (Bruun 1988).

ELECTIVE MUTISM

Electively mute children demonstrate a marked, emotionally determined selectivity in speaking. Speech occurs in some situations and not in others, e.g. at school. The disorder occurs in early childhood with an equal sex frequency.

Epidemiology

Around 1% in children of school-starting age, and 2–5/10 000 at age 7–8 years.

Associated features

1. **Language difficulties:** the diagnosis presupposes a near-normal level of comprehension and expression. A history of some speech delay is not uncommon, but the diagnosis requires fluent speech in some situations.
2. **Socio-emotional problems:** often present, particularly social anxiety. Tics, depression, enuresis, encopresis and oppositional behaviour may also be present.

Aetiology

The cause of the mutism is not clear. Inherent personality factors such as shyness may interact with psychosocial factors. However, there is often a family history of social anxiety. The role of trauma, e.g. sexual abuse, may also contribute.

Treatment

1. **Speech therapy** assessment and intervention may help, particularly where articulation problems are present.
2. **Behavioural work**, usually in the school setting, aims to decrease social anxiety.
3. **Medication:** SSRIs may help, though further studies are required.

Prognosis

Mutism usually resolves, but the prognosis is worse if no improvement occurs in 6–12 months.

SUICIDE AND DELIBERATE SELF-HARM

Suicide

Suicide is rare under the age of 12 and increases thereafter with age. Although suicide rates in adolescents are well beneath rates in adults, it is the second most common cause of death in adolescents. It occurs more commonly in males (male:female = 4:1) and there may be differences between ethnic groups.

Epidemiology

- 5–14 years 0.8/100 000
- 15–19 years13/100 000

Official figures may under-report the true rate of suicide deaths.

Associated features

1. **Method:** males tend to use more violent means – hanging, vehicle exhaust fumes, shooting (particularly in the USA). Females are more likely to overdose (particularly paracetamol).
2. **Psychiatric disorder:** high rates of depression, anxiety and eating disorders.
3. **Family history:** increased rates of deliberate self-harm, depression and alcohol or substance misuse.
4. **Substance misuse:** alcohol and drug misuse found in one study to be a predictive factor for eventual suicide following deliberate self-harm.
5. **Precipitant:** often a recent crisis, e.g. school or police trouble, or arguments with parents or boy/girl friends.
6. **Imitation:** some inconsistent evidence that recent exposure to suicide, either directly or in media may lead to similar acts. In residential settings, e.g. boarding schools, one suicide may lead to several other attempts by fellow pupils (so-called 'contagion').

Prevention

1. **Discussion:** up to 50% may discuss suicidal thoughts with someone, or be in contact with health professionals in the 24 hours before death. All such contacts should be viewed as potential pre-suicide consultations.
2. **Education:** several 'suicide curricula' have been tried in schools, aiming to increase awareness, indirectly find cases and provide information. Results have been mixed.
3. **Crisis services:** telephone help lines, e.g. the Samaritans, provide point of contact at time of crisis.
4. **Limiting access to methods:** e.g. decreasing availability of paracetamol, fitting catalytic converters to vehicles.
5. **Postvention:** this refers to an intervention after a suicide with the family and peers. By acting as a 'de-briefing', postvention helps increase understanding and prevent imitation.

Deliberate self-harm

There is no current consensus on best terminology. Deliberate self-harm (DSH) refers to *parasuicide* and *attempted suicide,* and includes self-poisoning (overdose) and self-injury (cutting). DSH is much more common than suicide (up to 100 times more frequent), with self-poisoning being the most common method.

Epidemiology

Rates vary between studies. The incidence increases with puberty (before then it is more common in boys). Community studies suggest 8% of adolescents have made a DSH attempt, though only 2% receive medical attention. Up to 20% of adolescents may have had serious suicidal ideation. After puberty it is more common in females (female:male = 7:1).

Associated features

1. **Method:** overdose most common. Tablets used by children and adolescent may vary enormously from psychotropics to antibiotics. Most common is paracetamol. DSH is often impulsive and therefore any medication easily available may be used.
2. **Precipitant:** often interpersonal conflicts – boy/girlfriend rows, family arguments and school problems. One-third cannot identify any precipitant.
3. **Past history:** around 20% have made previous attempts.
4. **Psychiatric problems:** some studies suggest that over 50% have depression. Usually this is transient and the majority are not severely depressed.
5. **Abuse:** previous abuse may be more common.
6. **Intent:** can be difficult to assess in young people. Attempt is often impulsive, but can be a way of coping with a difficult situation. Should not be seen as a 'cry for help' from professionals. Intent should be assessed in terms of the amount of planning, precautions taken about being found, knowledge about the lethality of the method and leaving a suicide note.

Treatment

1. **Assessment:** of reasons, precipitants, intent, current suicidality, etc. The assessment of adolescents after DSH differs from adult assessments in that parents/carers should also be seen. Engaging the young person in the assessment process may also take some time.
2. **Outpatient treatment:** family therapy is often offered, though it is often hard to engage families. Individually, cognitive therapy or solution-based brief therapies may help. Longer term psychotherapy may occasionally be required. Compliance with follow-up is notoriously low (Brent 1997).

Outcome

Follow-up studies are very difficult. Up to 10% may repeat, usually within one year and 1% may eventually commit suicide. Some studies suggest that this group are more prone to depression in adult life (e.g. Pfeffer et al. 1994).

SCHIZOPHRENIA

Schizophrenia in childhood and adolescence is uncommon, and when it does occur the symptomatology is similar to that in adults. Incidence increases in puberty, though cases in younger children are recorded. Diagnosis may be difficult initially, not least because the onset is often insidious. (See Chapter 18 for further details on management.)

Differential diagnosis of schizophrenia in children/adolescents

1. **Alcohol and substance misuse:** may present with a similar picture of change of behaviour.
2. **Depression.**
3. **Schizoaffective disorder, other psychoses:** can be difficult to differentiate.
4. **Autism:** not very similar, with onset before three years, social impairment, language delay and ritualized behaviour. Neuroleptics are rarely useful in the treatment of autism.

DEPRESSION

Feeling miserable is not uncommon among children and even more so with adolescents. Depression, when present, is diagnosed using the same criteria as for adults. There have been protracted arguments over whether children can be depressed. Generally, from around the age of 8–9 years, children exhibit depressive symptomatology and the rate increases with adolescence. Somatic complaints may be more common, along with irritability. Appetite and sleep problems are less common, with less evidence of hopelessness.

Epidemiology

The rare is 1–2% for pre-pubertal children and 2–5% for adolescents. In prepubertal children the sex ratio is equal, but a similar pattern to adults occurs after puberty, with a female excess.

Treatment

1. **Family therapy.**
2. **Individual therapy:** cognitive behaviour therapy (CBT) and interpersonal therapy (IPT) have shown some benefits.
3. **Medication:** the evidence for the role of antidepressants is equivocal. Tricyclic antidepressants

in one study were found to be as effective as placebo. Additionally, there is their potential toxic side-effects. SSRIs may have a role, though further studies are required; only fluoxetine is currently indicated for use in young people under the age of 18 years.

Prognosis

True depressive episodes can last up to 9 months and may recur. There is a subsequent increased risk for depression in adulthood (Harrington et al. 1990).

BIPOLAR AFFECTIVE DISORDER

More recently there has been a series of publications, mainly from the USA on early-onset bipolar disorder. The literature in this area is confusing, mainly arising from the application of diagnostic criteria designed for adults to children and adolescents. The blurring of diagnostic boundaries has led to the suggestion that bipolar disorder in children may present as disruptive behaviour, irritability and temper tantrums (Biederman 1998).

Adult studies suggest that between 20% to 54% of people with bipolar disorder report symptoms in childhood. The lifetime prevalence of bipolar disorder for adolescents is about 1%.

Treatment can involve lithium, sodium valproate or carbamazepine, with some evidence for atypical neuroleptics. Mood stabilizers are being used in the USA on younger children who in the UK may receive alternative diagnoses and non-medication treatments.

Compared to adults, adolescents with bipolar disorder have a longer early course and can be more resistant to treatment. In a 5-year follow-up, 4% of young people remained ill, 44% had a relapse and 21% had a further two or more episodes (Strober et al. 1995).

CHILD ABUSE

Child abuse is not a new phenomenon, though only more recently has it been seen as a child-health or welfare problem. Previously abuse was restricted to physical abuse ('the battered baby syndrome'), but now includes physical, sexual and emotional abuse plus neglect.

The epidemiology of abuse is difficult due to definitional issues and sources of information. Around 4% of children under the age of 12 are brought to the attention of social services each year because of suspected abuse. In 1988 3.5/1000 children under 18 years were on Child Protection Registers in England, with 1 in 4 registered for physical abuse and 1 in 8 for emotional abuse.

Rates of child sex abuse vary even more according to the definition used, with studies finding incidence rates of 6 to

62% in females and 3 to 31% in males. Most studies find higher rates of abuse in girls (female : male = 2.5–5 : 1). Studies into ethnic differences are few; the available evidence suggests no differences in rates of sexual abuse between white and black women.

Physical abuse

Physical abuse usually presents with some form of injury, which is inferred to be nonaccidental (NAI) in nature. Injuries consist of fractures, head injuries, burns, bruising, deliberate poisoning and sometimes deliberate suffocation.

Signs of NAI are not exact, but may include:

- a vague account of the accident
- the account is not compatible with the observed injury
- a delay in seeking help
- parental affect does not reflect the level of anxiety expected
- the child's affect may be sad, withdrawn and frightened and the child may say something to arouse suspicion.

Characteristics of abused children and their families include:

- unwanted pregnancy
- low birthweight/separation from mother in neonatal period
- mental or physical handicap
- restless baby, sleepless or crying non-stop
- physically unattractive.

Parental risk factors include:

- young, single parent
- abused themselves as children
- inconsistent or punishment-orientated discipline
- adverse social circumstances – low income, social isolation, social stressors
- large family.

Munchausen syndrome by proxy

First described by Meadow (1977), this syndrome describes a parent, usually mother, who fabricates illness in her child/children and presents to medical attention. Presentations are usually persistent, though symptoms end when separated from the parent. Other children in the family are often, or have often been, presented with similar problems. Forms of presentation include seizures, smotherings, poisoning, apparent bleeding, temperatures and rashes.

Sexual abuse

The definition of child sexual abuse ranges from acts of exhibitionism to fondling to forced penetration. Cases that come to clinical attention are more likely to be severe. Children of all ages are abused, though studies suggest a peak onset between the ages of 8 to 12.

Most sexual abuse is committed by men, with 5–15% perpetrated by females. Often the perpetrator is known to the child. In intrafamilial abuse, fathers are the most common perpetrator. Stepfathers are over-represented in the figures and a girl living with a stepfather is reported as being six times more likely to be abused compared to one living with her biological father. Many of the studies into stepfathers are old and the findings may not apply to today's families.

Abuse outside the family often occurs with individuals known to the child. Stranger abuse also occurs (though is under-represented in studies) and is more likely to be directed at boys (Finkelhor 1979).

Neglect

Neglect includes a lack of providing for a child's physical needs and also not fulfilling his or her developmental and cognitive needs. Children may be inadequately fed, dressed and bathed or may be deprived of satisfactory contact with the parent or other children/adults.

Neglect may be evident on direct observation, though usually is noticed by other family members or a teacher, or is inferred from the child's behaviour. Other forms of abuse often accompany neglect.

Emotional abuse

Physical abuse can result in visible injury, whereas emotional abuse is much harder to quantify. Emotional abuse is diagnosed if there is observable impairment in a child's mental or emotional functioning, evidenced by emotional or behavioural disorders and there is evidence that this is a result of rejection, deprivation of affection, exposure to domestic violence, inappropriate criticism or threats to the child.

Emotional abuse is not usually the only reason for seeking child protection. In extreme cases it has been proposed that emotional abuse can effect growth and weight gain – non-organic failure to thrive (NOFT).

Management of abuse

Broadly speaking, the management of abuse occurs in three stages:

- **Stage 1:** detection and disclosure
- **Stage 2:** child protection and legal proceedings
- **Stage 3:** support and therapeutic intervention.

Detection and disclosure
This is usually the responsibility of social services and involves interviewing the child, family and possibly

perpetrator. Interviewing the child has to occur with some skill, though there is good evidence that even young children's recall of past events is well developed. In cases of sexual abuse, anatomical dolls may be used, though this can be controversial.

Child protection and legal proceedings

A decision to undertake legal proceedings may then be made. Children may be removed from their families either pending further investigations or with a view to long-term fostering or adoption. Psychiatric reports may be requested about the child, the parent's ability to parent or about the parents.

Support and therapeutic intervention

Work may be required to rehabilitate children with their families, or in cases where rehabilitation is not possible to work to a new family placement. Therapeutic input may also be required to deal with the consequences of the abuse. Various models of abuse work have been tried including individual, family and group therapy. In sexual abuse, working with the whole family including the perpetrator has had some success.

Outcome

In the short-term, abuse can result in a change in a child's behaviour and emotional state. Children may be prone to mood swings, temper tantrums, wariness of strangers, etc. They can feel isolated, anxious and depressed. With sexual abuse, sexualized behaviour may develop. The specific consequences of physical abuse depend on the nature of the injury.

In the longer-term, abuse can have profound consequences on self-esteem, the ability to form satisfactory adult relationships and may also impact on parenting abilities. Sexual abuse in childhood, in particular, has been linked with the development of eating disorders, self-injury and depression in adults (see Chapter 24).

CHILD AND ADOLESCENT MENTAL HEALTH SERVICES

The Department of health recommends that child and adolescent mental health services (CAHMS) are delivered according to the following 'tiered' model:

- **Tier 1:** services delivered at the primary care level by GPs, health visitors, school nurses, teachers, etc.
- **Tier 2:** unidisciplinary mental health services, i.e. a professional working alone without backup of a team, e.g. psychologists, nurses.
- **Tier 3:** multidisciplinary team, usually located in the community or attached to a hospital; can consist of a child psychiatrist, child psychotherapist, social worker, psychologist, etc.

- **Tier 4:** specialist services, includes adolescent in-patient units and highly specialized regional services.

CAMHS are therefore not just the province of the child psychiatrist, but delivered in a wide variety of settings, including voluntary agencies. Ideally, referrals should pass between the tiers as required and the main agencies – health, education and social services – should work together in the best interest of the child or adolescent.

The Royal College of Psychiatrists recommends that there should be 1.3 whole time equivalent (wte) consultants in child and adolescent psychiatry per 100 000 total population. In a population of 250 000, the British Psychological Society recommends 3.5 wte psychology posts. One psychotherapist is recommended per 100 000 and recommendations exist for other members of the multidisciplinary team.

FURTHER READING

Goodman R & Scott S (1997) *Child Psychiatry*. Blackwell, London.

MTA cooperative group (1999a) A 14 month randomized clinical trial of treatment strategies for attention-deficit/hyperactivity disorder. The MTA cooperative group multi-modal treatment study of children with ADHD. *Archives of General Psychiatry* **56**: 1073–86.

MTA cooperative group (1999b) Moderators and mediators of treatment response for children with attention-deficit/hyperactivity disorder; the multi-modal treatment study of chidren with attention-deficit/hyperactivity disorder. *Archives of General Psychiatry* **56**: 1088–96.

Rutter M & Taylor E (eds) (2002) *Child and Adolescent Psychiatry*, 4th edn. Oxford: Blackwell.

REFERENCES

Bailey AJ (1993) The biology of autism. *Psychological Autism* **23**: 7-11.

Baron-Cohen S (1989) The autistic child's theory of mind: a case of specific developmental delay. *Journal of Child Psychology and Psychiatry* **15**: 315-21.

Biederman J (1998) Resolved: mania is mistaken for ADHD in prepubertal children: affirmative. *Journal of the American Academy for Child and Adolescent Psychiatry* **37**: 1091-3.

Brent DA (1997) Practitioner review: the aftercare of adolescents with deliberate self-harm. *Journal of Child Psychology and Psychiatry* **38**: 277–86.

Bruun R (1988) The natural history of Tourette's syndrome. In: Cohen D, Bruun R & Leckman J (eds) *Tourette's Syndrome and Tic Disorders*. New York: Wiley.

Connors CK, Epstein JK, March JS et al. (2001) Multi-modal treatment of ADHD in the MTA: an alternative outcome analysis. *Journal of the American Academy of Child and Adolescent Psychiatry* **40**: 159–67.

Finkelhor D (1979). 'What's wrong with sex between adults and children? Ethics and the problem of sexual abuse'. *American Journal of Orthopsychiatry* **49**: 692–7.

Harrington R, Fudge H, Rutter M, Pickles A & Hill J (1990) Adult outcome of childhood and adolescent depression. I. Psychiatric status. *Archives of General Psychiatry* **47**: 465–73.

Hersov L & Berg I (eds) (1980) *Out of School*. Chichester: Wiley.

Meadow R (1977) Munchausen syndrome by proxy. The hinterland of child abuse. *Lancet* **ii**: 343–5.

MTA cooperative group (1999a) A 14-month randomized clinical trial of treatment strategies for attention-deficit/hyperactivity disorder. The MTA cooperative group multi-modal treatment study of children with ADHD. *Archives of General Psychiatry* **56**: 1073–86.

MTA cooperative group (1999b) Moderators and mediators of treatment response for children with attention-deficit/hyperactivity disorder; the multi-modal treatment study of chidren with attention-deficit/hyperactivity disorder. *Archives of General Psychiatry* **56**: 1088–96.

Pfeffer CR, Hurt SW, Kakuma T, Peskin JR, Siefker CA & Nagabhairava S (1994) Suicidal children grow up: suicidal episodes and effects of treatment during follow-up. *Journal of the American Academy of Child and Adolescent Psychiatry* **33**: 225–30.

Richman N, Stevenson JE & Graham P (1982) *Pre-school to School: A Behavioural Study*. London: Academic Press.

Robins LN (1978) Sturdy childhood predictors of adult antisocial behaviour: replications from longitudinal studies. *Psychological Medicine* **8**: 611–22.

Rutter M, Cox A, Tupling C, Berger M & Yule W (1975) Attainment and adjustment in two geographical areas – I. The prevalence of psychiatric disorder. *British Journal of Psychiatry* **126**: 493–509.

Rutter M, Tizard J, Yule W, Graham P & Whitmore K (1976) Isle of Wight studies 1964–1974. *Psychological Medicine* **6**: 313–32.

Strober M, Schmidt-Lackner S, Freeman R, Bower S, Lampert C & DeAntonio M (1995) Recovery and relapse in adolescent with bipolar affective illness: a naturlistic study. *American Journal of Psychiatry* **147**: 457–71.

Swanson J, Kraemer HC, Hinshaw SP et al. (2001) Clinical relvance of the primary findings of the MTA; success rates based on the severity of ADHD and ODD at the end of treatment. *Journal of the American Academy of Child and Adolescent Psychiatry* **40**: 168–79.

Taylor E, Sandberg S, Thorley G & Giles S (1991) *The Epidemiology of Childhood Hyperactivity*. Maudsley Monographs no. 33. Oxford: Oxford University Press.

Timimi S & Taylor E (2004) ADHD is best understood as a cultural construct. *British Journal of Psychiatry* **184**: 8–9.

Volkmar FR, Lord C, Bailey A, Schulz RT & Klin A (2004) Autism and pervasive developmental disorders. *Journal of Child Psychology and Psychiatry* **45**(1): 135–71.

Personality disorder

Martin Feakins

So God created man in His own image; in the image of God created He him.

Genesis 1 : 27

INTRODUCTION

Not all bizarre behaviour is due to functional psychiatric illness. Most psychiatrists are familiar with patients who present at A & E with repeated self-harm, with lifelong unhappiness or with behaviour which brings them to the attention of hospitals or the police but which does not meet the diagnostic criteria for psychiatric illness.

Management of these patients is different from that of patients with functional psychiatric illness. Where admission is appropriate for a depressed, suicidal patient who has self-harmed, it may be harmful for a patient with borderline personality disorder who has taken 10 paracetamol tablets.

Knowledge of the personality disorders is essential to the practice of clinical psychiatry because:

- Personality disorder may be the primary diagnosis. In this case, the diagnosis is in clinical practice most likely to be borderline or dissocial personality disorder.
- There may be a personality disorder complicating a diagnosis of functional illness. Examples are drug dependence combined with dissocial or borderline personality disorder, depression with dependent personality disorder, anxiety neurosis with avoidant personality disorder.
- Underlying personality *traits* might be detected, which complicate another diagnosis.

HISTORY

Classification of personalities is an old concept. Hippocrates, for example, described four: choleric, phlegmatic, sanguine, and melancholic.

In this century, numerous approaches to personality and its disorders have been offered (see Box 14.1).

Box 14.1   Concepts of personality in the 20th century
Kretschmer Endomorph (fat and relaxed) Ectomorph (aloof and thin) Mesomorph (sturdy)
Sheldon Viscerotonic Cerebrotonic Somatotonic (correlate broadly with Kretschmer's concepts)
Jung Introvert Extrovert
Eysenck Axes of extroversion–introversion Neuroticism–psychoticism Stability Intelligence
Rotter Internal/external 'locus of control'
Freud Id, ego, superego Conscious and unconscious mind Fixations at oral, anal or phallic stages Repression of traumatic experiences
Maslow Hierarchy of needs, self-actualization Man needs to progress through a hierarchy of needs, from food and shelter to fulfilment of his full potential (self-actualization)
Friedman and Rosenman Type A (coronary-prone, high-achieving) Type B (relaxed)
Schneider Hyperthymic, depressive, anankast, formatic, attention-seeking, labile, explosive, affectionless, weak-willed, asthenic

DEFINITION

Personality disorder

The ICD-10 (WHO 1992) offers a lengthy definition of personality disorders, from which the following are the critical points. Personality disorders are:

- enduring and deeply ingrained ways of behaving, thinking, feeling and relating
- which deviate significantly from the norm
- are sufficient to cause significant personal and social distress and disruption
- are usually present since adolescence or childhood and persist throughout most of adult life.

The ICD-10 emphasizes the importance of excluding functional psychiatric illness and organic illness. It also emphasizes the long-term nature of the symptomatology, dating at least from adolescence, if not from childhood. Although everyone has a unique personality, the point at which personality becomes a disorder is clarified as the point at which 'significant personal and social distress and disruption' occurs. The ICD-10 and DSM-IV also provide a classification of personality disorders (Table 14.1).

Personality traits

A personality trait is said to be present when a patient exhibits some symptoms of a personality disorder, but these symptoms are not sufficient to make a diagnosis of a personality disorder. Everyone has personality traits. Life brings us into contact with colleagues or friends who are, for example, obsessionally tidy, or who are theatrical, flamboyant and attention-seeking. These are anankastic and histrionic personality traits, respectively.

Personality disorder may be diagnosed when *three or more* of the ICD-10 diagnostic criteria for a particular personality disorder are present. These criteria will be discussed in the section dealing with individual disorders. Alternatively,

Table 14.1 ICD-10 and DSM-IV classification of personality disorders

ICD-10	DSM-IV	
Paranoid Schizoid	Paranoid Schizoid Schizotypal	'Cluster A'
Dissocial Emotionally unstable Histrionic Other	Antisocial Borderline Histrionic Narcissistic	'Cluster B'
Anxious (avoidant)	Avoidant	
Dependent	Dependent	
Anankastic	Obsessive-compulsive	

more than three criteria may be present, but 'significant personal and social distress and disruption' do not exist. In this situation also, personality trait, and not disorder, should be diagnosed. Hence, it is the breadth and enduring nature of personality disorder, and its ability to cause personal and social distress, that are requisite for the diagnosis.

PREVALENCE OF PERSONALITY DISORDERS

This depends upon the diagnostic criteria used. Several studies have looked at prevalence, yielding figures ranging from 5–25%. Casey (1986), found that 7% of a community sample had personality difficulties, 7% personality disorders, and 4% severe personality disorders.

The Epidemiological Catchment Area (ECA) Study in the USA (Regier et al. 1984) found a 6% prevalence of personality disorder. Unsurprisingly, surveys of prison populations find high prevalences of dissocial personality disorder.

The prevalence of personality disorder in psychiatric hospitals has been estimated at between 36% and 67%.

AETIOLOGY

There is a consensus that personality disorder in general arises from dysfunctional family dynamics and upbringing. A pattern of dysfunctional behaviour usually begins in childhood and emerges into personality disorder in adulthood.

Dissocial personality disorder has been widely investigated and the findings are summarized in the following section. For the aetiology of the other personality disorders, however, there is a wealth of theories but a dearth of evidence. Individual authorities formulate theories on aetiology in terms of their own approaches – Kleinian, Freudian, and so on. A knowledge of these concepts (Chapter 36) provides a helpful theoretical framework that facilitates an understanding of the pathological mechanisms underlying, and used by, patients with personality disorder.

GENERAL PRINCIPLES OF MANAGEMENT

The following are general guidelines. The management of individual personality disorders will be addressed later.

First, a thorough history and mental state examination are essential with particular emphasis on:

- personalities of parents
- family dynamics
- family history of psychiatric illness, alcoholism or imprisonment

- perinatal trauma
- a detailed account of childhood and adolescence
- history of physical or sexual abuse
- relationships with friends and relatives
- truanting and delinquent behaviour
- previous episodes of self-harm
- previous admissions, and whether helpful
- contact with professionals and whether helpful
- drug and alcohol use and abuse
- medication and what helped
- physical examination for signs of self-harm and drug abuse
- mental state examination
- functional and/or organic illness must be excluded.

Collateral history is *essential* for a valid diagnosis of personality disorder. Gather as much information as possible from friends, relatives, other professionals and hospital records, and any others involved. When considering treatment, remember that progress will be slow and that the goal should be to reduce distress and improve functioning, rather than to hope for a radical change in personality.

Mental health legislation is rarely appropriate for treatment of personality disorder, with the exception of dissocial personality disorder if deemed treatable, and some cases of borderline personality disorder. This will be discussed further in this chapter.

A number of questionnaires are available for the evaluation of personality. Some of these are briefly described in Box 14.2.

Treatment of personality disorders

Just as there is a wealth of theories on aetiology, virtually every psychological approach has been used to treat personality disorder, including psychoanalysis, milieu therapy, cognitive behavioural therapy, supportive psychotherapy and more recently dialectical behavioural therapy. Results are difficult to analyze due to lack of control groups, confusion about the natural history of the various disorders, and use of inconsistent outcome parameters: when does one say that the patient is 'better'?

Drug treatment lends itself to more rigorous investigation, but the lack of randomized double-blind, placebo controlled trials is still striking. Such evidence as there is, however, suggests that low-dose neuroleptics are effective in reducing a broad range of symptoms in a number of patients with personality disorders, including agitation, aggression, impulsivity, and depression. Mood stabilizers appear to have a similar effect, but have mostly been investigated only in dissocial and borderline personality disorders.

The lack of good quality research into treatment of the other personality disorders is profound, though there is an abundance of open trials and theories.

In all cases, consider carefully whether it is wise to intervene at all: 'First do no harm'. Many patients with personality disorder never come into contact with psychiatric services. As discussed by Castillo (2003), of those who do, many describe highly negative experiences and would choose in retrospect never to have met psychiatrists.

Management is discussed further under individual personality disorders.

COMORBIDITY

Any personality disorder or trait can coexist with any functional psychiatric illness. Box 14.3 lists the most common codiagnoses. As a rule, personality disorder coexisting with functional illness is a bad prognostic factor. It is also frequent for traits of more than one personality disorder to coexist. It is much more common for a combination of different personality traits to be present in one individual than a single personality disorder. This makes research difficult, and contributes to therapeutic uncertainty.

Box 14.2   Standard questionnaires used in assessing personality disorder

Minnesota Multiphasic Personality Inventory (MMPI) (Hathaway & McKinley 1951)
- The most widely used
- Long and thorough self-rating scale
- Takes at least 1 hour to complete
- 550 statements about personality to which subject answers: true/false/cannot say

Personality Assessment Schedule PAS (Tyrer et al. 1979)
- Observer-rated
- 24 personality variables (e.g. aloofness, callousness, rigidity) are rated over three interviews

Cattell's 16 Personality Factor Questionnaire (Cattell & Butcher 1968)
- 'Factor' is synonymous with trait. Uses factor analysis to provide a graph representing the subject's personality. Factors include 'happy go lucky', 'very serious', 'tense' versus 'relaxed'.

Eysenck Personality Questionnaire (EPQ)
- Supersedes the Maudsley Personality Questionnaire (MPQ) and the Eysenck Personality Inventory (EPI)
- Based on the four dimensions described by Eysenck (Box 14.1)

Box 14.3   Comorbid diagnoses

Drug/alcohol abuse/dependence	borderline dissocial dependent
Mood disorders	borderline dissocial
Psychotic disorders	borderline

INDIVIDUAL PERSONALITY DISORDERS

Diagnostic criteria vary between different authorities. There is more variation for those personality disorders which have been recognized for longer. The diagnostic criteria given in this chapter are drawn mostly from the ICD-10.

Borderline personality disorder

Diagnostic criteria for borderline personality disorder are:

- unstable emotions and mood
- impulsivity, including impulsive self-harm and violence
- unstable self-image
- unstable sexual preferences
- chronic feelings of emptiness
- unstable, intense relationships
- fear of abandonment
- in times of stress, pseudopsychotic or dissociative symptoms may emerge.

This diagnosis is also known as 'emotionally unstable personality disorder, borderline type' in the ICD-10. It is more common in females.

The recurrent theme to the diagnostic criteria is instability. 'Unstable mood' means that the patient is subject to episodes of depression or elation that may mimic functional illness, but are of shorter duration or lesser intensity. 'Unstable sexual preferences' refers to homosexuality and sexual behaviour such as sado-masochism, fetishism, and trans-sexuality. With regard to relationships, these tend to be multiple, intense and abusive. Exploring relationships in the history is therefore particularly helpful in making the diagnosis.

Although impulsive self-harm is a frequent cause of admission to hospital, this is usually inappropriate. Most patients are honest in stating that they are likely to self-harm again, and this results in admission, with the best of intentions, to provide protection from further episodes. Pseudo-psychotic symptoms also result in admission when the disorder may be mistaken for a functional psychotic illness.

Difficulties in discharging these patients arise from their fear of abandonment. Having been briefly accepted into the hospital environment, which provides them with safe asylum, they experience discharge as abandonment, which is intolerable. This leads to distress, with greater instability as a result, and further self-harm. Often the experience of relieving distress by self-harm is described. Paradoxically, the end result of admission is in this case an escalation of the patient's instability, with the result that the patient is made worse, not better, by admission.

Aetiology

De La Fuente et al. (1998) found abnormal diffuse slow wave activity in the electroencephalographic readings of 40% of a sample of 20 patients with borderline personality disorder (Chapter 26).

Many patients with borderline personality disorder have suffered physical and sexual abuse and chaotic parenting as children. They exhibit delinquent behaviour during adolescence, such as drug abuse, truancy and promiscuity. It is reasonable to assume that these experiences are in some way formative, but there is a lack of evidence supporting this. Associations have been found between reported child sexual abuse and subsequent deliberate self-harm by Romans et al. (1995), but proving that childhood experiences cause subsequent personality disorder is impossible (and this applies to all personality disorders) as obtaining proof would require randomizing infants to abusive and non-abusive parenting.

Management

- Full history, mental state examination, physical examination, maximum collateral history.
- Stable therapeutic relationship with one authority figure.
- Manage crises conservatively.
- Advise the patient to avoid drugs and alcohol.
- Consider use of:
  - (a) selective serotonin reuptake inhibitors (SSRIs) for depression, anxiety and phobias
  - (b) low-dose anti-psychotics for impulsivity, agitation, anxiety and pseudo-psychotic symptoms.

Collateral history is especially important. The patient's medical notes will confirm the diagnosis, and state what treatment is helpful. The patient may be unwilling to discuss a traumatic childhood, but this may be indicated by the notes. Previous episodes of deliberate self-harm will be documented. Patients with borderline personality disorder are often only seen at times of crisis, following an episode of self-harm. Frequently, the presentation is accompanied by a sense of great urgency and anxiety, with immediate action demanded by hospital staff, patient and relatives. In this situation, the patient's distress is so great that he/she is using primitive defence mechanisms, such as splitting and projective identification (see Chapter 36) to undermine the professionalism of staff. The psychiatrist must use his/her skills to defuse this tension, while gathering the history and collateral history. The key to this is to create a sense of 'containment' by being calm and professional, to convey to the patient that although he/she cannot contain his/her distress, the psychiatrist can.

As well as establishing the diagnosis, the psychiatrist needs to explore any other diagnoses, particularly psychosis or depression. Drug or alcohol abuse needs to be explored, as either contributes to instability.

If the psychiatrist is not normally responsible for the patient's care, efforts should be made to discuss the patient's case history with the psychiatrist who is. Because of the anxiety and disturbance these patients engender, it is not infrequent for two consultants to have opposite views about management.

It has already been stated that admission to hospital is not helpful in the long term. In some circumstances, however, it is inevitable. Patients are sometimes so desperate for containment that they overwhelm the psychiatrist, who then feels that the only safe option is to admit. Admission may be warranted if the circumstances of the current presentation are exceptional, for example if an unusually severe life event has happened. In this scenario, exceptional self-harm or instability is likely, and containment might only be provided by an admission, despite the drawbacks.

Admission may also be appropriate where the patient has a superimposed illness, such as an affective or psychotic disorder, which has relapsed. It is important not to allow the personality disorder to 'blind' one to the presence of a superimposed illness that needs treatment.

With regard to drug therapy, depressive episodes should be treated with an anti-depressant, preferably one which is safe in overdose such as an SSRI (Rinne et al. 2002). SSRIs will also help reduce the anxiety and phobias experienced by some patients. They are not suitable for recurrent brief depression (i.e. episodes lasting less than two weeks) (Montgomery et al. 1994).

Other patients may benefit from low doses of an antipsychotic, such as olanzapine, risperidone, chlorpromazine, promazine or fluphenazine. This can be effective across a broad spectrum of symptoms, including anger, anxiety, dissociation, depression, and paranoia.

A number of literature reviews, including one by Tyrer and Seiveright (1988), found that mood stabilizers reduce aggression, impulsiveness and affective instability, but many of the studies reviewed had small numbers or were open trials.

There is some evidence that depressive symptoms respond to monoamine oxidase inhibitors (MAOIs) but these will be unsuitable for most patients because of their dangers.

Hori (1998) reviewed only double-blind, placebo-controlled trials. The outcome of these trials was consistent with earlier evidence for the efficacy of low-dose neuroleptics, mood stabilizers and monoamine oxidase inhibitors (MAOIs). It was remarked that amitriptyline and alprazolam were detrimental. Some evidence has emerged that a newer agent, divalproex sodium, may also have a beneficial effect (Hollander et al. 2001).

A recent development has been the introduction of a type of cognitive-behavioural therapy, called dialectical behaviour therapy (DBT). Linehan et al. (1993) found significant reductions in parasuicide, global functioning, anger and in-patient days among borderline patients over a 12-month period. They have replicated their results in further studies, but questions remain over the longevity of the improvement.

The most stable patients may be suitable for psychoanalysis or psychoanalytical psychotherapy. The majority, however, fare better if their follow up is centred on a single individual who is sufficiently qualified and experienced to deal with them, such as a psychiatrist or psychotherapist. Any other professional seeing them should make it clear to the patient that significant changes in treatment can only be made by this person. This reduces the problem of splitting.

Therapeutic communities such as the Henderson and Cassel Hospitals in the UK are helpful for some patients, but they require a high level of insight and willingness to change. The psychotherapy department for the patient's locality can provide further details of the referrals procedure. Usually, there is a long waiting list (6–12 months) and rigorous assessment before the patient is accepted. Funding the placement can also be an obstacle. Nevertheless, Dolan et al. (1997), for example, found that the Henderson Hospital was effective in reducing symptoms, as measured by the Borderline Symptoms Index.

Bateman & Fonagy (1999) also found that an 18-month period of 'partial hospitalization' improved many outcome variables of the disorder when compared to standard treatment, in a study group of 19 patients, as compared to an equal control group. Partial hospitalization meant attendance for five days a week at a programme of group and individual psychotherapy based on attachment theory. They also demonstrated (2001) that patients maintained their improvement over the subsequent 18 months, and (2003) that the treatment was cost effective.

Dissocial personality disorder

Diagnostic criteria are:

- callous unconcern for the feeling of others
- disregard for rules and obligations
- inability to experience guilt
- inability to learn from punishment and experience
- inability to maintain relationships but no difficulty in establishing them
- low tolerance for frustration, resulting in violence
- tendency to blame others.

This is synonymous with psychopathic, antisocial and sociopathic personality disorder. It is more common in males.

These patients usually come to attention as a result of law-breaking activities. The presentation is often complicated by drug or alcohol abuse, or by depression, which tends to occur later in life. Typically, the history will include a long forensic history of thefts and assaults, multiple relationships, and a tendency not to learn from experience.

Dissocial personality trait or disorder is a common additional diagnosis to drug or alcohol dependence and their psychiatric sequelae.

Aetiology
EEG findings of patients with dissocial personality indicate the following:

- Around 50% have generalized, widespread slow waves.
- Almost 50% display 'positive spike' phenomena, i.e. bursts of activity over the temporal lobe. It has been postulated that this is associated with outbursts of aggression. The same phenomenon occurs in 10% of healthy individuals.
- Hill (1952) found abnormal slow-wave activity over the temporal lobes of 14% of severely aggressive patients with anti-social personality disorder. Children also show more slow waves than normal adults. Links have been postulated in terms of 'cortical immaturity'.

Evoked potentials studies have found evidence for autonomic under-arousal. It has been suggested that dissocial behaviour is designed to compensate for this, by providing more stimulation.

About 40% of conduct-disordered children become antisocial adults (Robins 1966). Family studies have shown that:

- Dissocial behaviour runs in families. It is associated with chaotic family dynamics, alcohol abuse in the family, and social problems in the family. Twin studies have shown higher monozygotic than dizygotic concordance for dissocial behaviour, but the difference is not huge.
- Adoption studies have shown that adopted children of antisocial, natural parents have a higher incidence of anti-social behaviour than the general population.

Management

- Full history, mental state examination, physical examination, and collateral history
- Assess dangerousness
- Explore any additional diagnoses
- Establish what treatment is appropriate, if any.

The history should lay particular emphasis on:

- family history of violence
- violent childhood
- conduct disorder or delinquency as a child
- forensic history, including outstanding charges which may have precipitated
- the presentation
- relationships
- incapacity to feel remorse.

It is essential to assess dangerousness (see also Chapters 30 and 35). The most useful index for dangerousness is a past history of dangerousness. A patient who always hits out when frustrated can be expected to hit out again when frustrated again. If assaults always occur in the context of alcohol or drug intoxication, further use of these substances can be expected to precipitate further assaults. Dangerousness is the most important index of severity of the disorder. The following have also been put forward as ominous prognostic signs for future violence:

- use of disinhibiting substances
- lack of remorse
- early onset
- family history
- fear engendered in the examining psychiatrist.

Whether a patient is suitable for treatment depends on several variables, including:

- how severe the disorder is
- whether the patient is willing to accept treatment
- if not, whether he/she is 'treatable'.

Treatability refers to the likelihood of a patient responding to treatment. There are no clear guidelines for assessing this. Different psychiatrists will form differing opinions as to the treatability of the same patient. If the patient has had treatment previously, evaluate whether or not it has helped. If it has, it is reasonable to assume that further similar treatment will also help. If not, and if a reasonable range of options was explored, the patient may not be treatable.

In the UK, treatability is important because patients with dissocial disorders may only be treated under current mental health legislation if they are deemed 'treatable'. If the patient has no previous psychiatric history, insight and willingness to change are important determinants for treatability. However, if these are present, the patient is unlikely to require detention under mental health legislation.

The following treatment options are available:

- **Psychotherapeutic:** treatment strategies in dissocial personality disorder include:
  (a) individual and group psychodynamic psychotherapy
  (b) therapeutic community
  (c) behaviour modification
  (d) cognitive behavioural therapy

  The effectiveness of these treatments is reviewed by Bluglass & Bowden (1990). They conclude that there is evidence that all of these treatment methods improve antisocial behaviour to some extent, in some patients, but none can be claimed to work for all patients. The main index of improvement was incidence of re-offending in patients who had already been convicted of violent disorders. There was little evidence of underlying change in personality as a result of these interventions.
- **Drug treatment:** antipsychotic drugs reduce arousal levels and often reduce the frequency of aggressive outbursts. Mood stabilizers may calm the more aggressive patients. Antidepressants are likely to be helpful only when there is an element of depression, and carry a risk of precipitating a manic state, with worse violence if the patient has a tendency to bipolar disorder. Benzodiazepines can cause disinhibition and rebound irritability on withdrawal, so are best avoided.

Mental health legislation and dissocial personality disorder

In the UK, the Mental Health Act 1983 (MHA) defines psychopathic disorder as 'a persistent disorder of mind (whether or not including significant impairment of intelligence) which results in abnormally aggressive or seriously irresponsible conduct on the part of the person concerned'.

The MHA states that patients with this disorder can only be detained if they are treatable, as already discussed. Considerable differences exist between different psychiatrists as to what treatability means, and Bluglass & Bowden (1990) have remarked that it appears to depend, to some extent, on how many beds are available to the psychiatrist.

In the UK, if the patient is not seen in the context of legal proceedings, Section 2 or 3 of the MHA will be appropriate. If he/she has been charged with an offence, and is appearing in court, a hospital order, such as a Section 36 for assessment and treatment, may be appropriate to clarify treatability.

If the patient is not treatable, as determined by a psychiatrist, hospital disposal is not an option. In this case, he/she must be dealt with by the penal system.

Changes are pending in the management of patients with dissocial personality disorder in the UK, and a useful review is offered by Eastman (1999). He reviews the 1997 Labour government's intention to allow 'preventive detention of even the unconvicted' in 'new specialist institutions which would be hybrids of prison and hospital and would house only people with severe personality disorder'. He comments that the Fallon inquiry into the Personality Disorder Unit at Ashworth High Security Hospital found it to be a 'deeply flawed creation'. Eastman remarks that the government's intention 'contrasts with the solution proposed by Fallon of specialized personality disorder units in both prisons and high security hospitals, with transfer to hospital according to prisoner/patient consent and treatability'.

Eastman also highlights that the prediction that only 2700 individuals will require such a service, 'looks suspect, given both surveys of morbidity in prisons and the continuing public appetite for protection from people with mental disorder'.

To detain people in this new way, 'there will be an indeterminate reviewable order imposed by a Court', which will apply not only to the treatable and those who have committed an offence, but also to the untreatable and the unconvicted. This move would appear to be a response to perceived public pressure to exclude from society those who might pose a threat, and poses ethical, moral, clinical, political and practical questions.

Dependent personality disorder

Diagnostic criteria for this disorder include:

- encouraging others to take decisions about one's life
- excessive compliance with other people's wishes
- not making demands on others
- fears of inability to cope alone
- fears of abandonment
- need for reassurance
- feelings of incompetence, helplessness and lack of stamina.

This is also known as passive personality disorder.

Dependent patients often come to psychiatrists' attention through their unwillingness to live independently. Dependence is a recognized symptom of institutionalization, and is often seen in patients with schizophrenia or depression who have had several long admissions and whose ability to live independently has been eroded by their illness.

Dependent personality disorder, however, must by definition begin at childhood or adolescence. Such patients present to psychiatrists with complaints of inability to cope. Further history reveals feelings of sadness (rather than depression), and low self-esteem. The diagnosis will be aided by excluding a depressive disorder, and by collateral history. Characteristically, the psychiatrist is presented with the inability to cope in a way that suggests he/she must find the solution without any help from the patient.

Depressive personality *traits* can accompany any psychiatric disorder, but will be seen more often where the history is long, with multiple hospitalizations, and in drug and alcohol abuse.

Aetiology

This disorder has not provoked much research. Learned behaviour in childhood is important, whether by modelling on others, or as a result of over-protective behaviour by a parent.

Management

- full assessment
- diagnosis and treatment of coexisting illness
- simple methods, e.g. refusing to take decisions on patient's behalf
- consider rehabilitation unit, group home, etc., if coexisting schizophrenia
- psychotherapy
- community mental health team.

It is not necessarily within psychiatrists' responsibility to offer any intervention to patients with dependent personality disorder. However, if it has become so extreme that the patient cannot continue without help, or if it complicates management of a coexisting illness, intervention is needed.

The focus of such intervention is to enable the patient to learn, or re-learn, the ability to take his/her own decisions. Thus, the psychiatrist should:

- articulate for the patient that he/she has difficulty in taking decisions, which is perpetuating his/her problems
- advise that the patient must take the decision with which he/she is faced for him/herself,
- assure him/her that he/she will be supported in what is chosen.

Patients who find it unbearable to be more independent – for example, when told they are to be discharged from hospital – may express their distress in depression, self-harm or violence. Sympathy and support will help, but if their distress does not abate, other options must be explored. These include sheltered or group homes, rehabilitation and psychotherapy. Rehabilitation aims to train patients to live more independently. Rehabilitation programmes can take months or years, and are designed mostly for patients with chronic schizophrenia. Psychologists may provide suggestions regarding behavioural management, or explore with the patient reasons for their dependence. Finally, support from the community mental health team may also be helpful where there is an additional diagnosis of functional illness, especially schizophrenia.

Paranoid personality disorder

Diagnostic criteria include:

- sensitiveness
- bearing grudges
- suspiciousness, including doubt about partner's sexual fidelity
- misinterpretation of events as persecutory
- strong sense of personal rights
- self-importance
- fondness for conspiratorial explanations of world events.

These patients may be referred with a tentative diagnosis of schizophrenia. Full assessment without collateral history will be particularly difficult as the patient, by definition, is suspicious and will be guarded about giving a full history.

There will be a lack of first-rank symptoms. The patient will feel generally hard-done-by and aggrieved, but will hold none of his/her beliefs with delusional intensity.

Apart from excluding functional psychiatric illnesses, the differential diagnosis of a prodromal phrase of schizophrenia must be explored. This may present quite similarly in a snapshot view, but a long-term view will show that the personality disorder is of much longer duration, and does not change over time.

It should also be borne in mind that relatives of personality disordered patients frequently have disordered personalities themselves, and may therefore give dysfunctional interpretations of the patient's behaviour.

Aetiology

A genetic component has been established by the finding that first degree relatives of schizophrenics have a higher incidence of paranoid personality disorder than the general population.

Cassady et al. (1998) also found a higher than normal prevalence of dyskinetic movement in a sample of 34 neuroleptic-naïve patients with paranoid, schizotypal or schizoid personalities ('schizophrenia spectrum personality').

Freud regarded paranoia as abnormal primary narcissism, stating that sufferers were incapable of forming empathic relationships. He also described paranoia as a symptom of repressed homosexuality, and he believed that such patients were unsuitable for analysis.

Management

- full history, mental state examination and collateral history
- anti-psychotics
- consider psychotherapy.

Paranoid personality disorder, like dependent-personality disorder, does not require treatment unless it is causing significant problems. If it is, a low dose of an antipsychotic will reduce arousal levels. If well tolerated and symptoms persist, a higher dose can be tried, but the success seen with psychotic illnesses should not be expected and most patients will be suspicious of any medication offered. Referral for psychotherapy may be considered if the patient displays good insight and willingness to change.

The literature on both psychotherapy and antipsychotics in paranoid personality disorder is too sparse to form an opinion as to their effectiveness.

Schizoid personality disorder

Diagnostic criteria include:

- detachment, aloofness, coldness, solitude
- little interest in sexual relationships
- fondness for fantasy and introspection
- indifference to others
- lack of close friends
- insensitivity to social norms.

This personality disorder was thought by Kretschmer to predispose to schizophrenia, but there is no evidence for this. It can be distinguished from paranoid personality disorder by the lack of paranoia, but it is not infrequent for the patient with paranoid personality disorder to lead a solitary life.

History-taking is easier than from patients with paranoid personality disorder, which is fortunate as it is unlikely that there will be anyone who knows the patient well enough to give a collateral history. The lack of sexual relationships is a striking finding.

A coexisting illness will make assessment of personality difficult, and the personality should be assessed when this illness is in remission.

The disorder must also be distinguished from the prodromal phrase of schizophrenia, and, as with paranoid personality disorder, the distinction will be helped by evidence of long duration without change.

Aetiology

(See paranoid personality disorder.) Theories abound but there have been few other significant findings.

Management

Diagnosis depends on full history, mental state examination and collateral history where possible. Coexisting illnesses should be treated appropriately but little research has been carried out into what is helpful for patients who seek help.

There is some evidence that psychotherapy is more helpful than in paranoid and schizotypal disorders.

Histrionic personality disorder

Diagnostic criteria are:

- theatrical, dramatic behaviour
- shallowness
- seeking attention and excitement
- seductiveness and vanity
- suggestibility
- manipulative and demanding behaviour.

This diagnosis is also known as hysterical personality disorder. Hysteria is one of the oldest terms in psychiatry and, as such, has acquired a number of different meanings, few or none having positive connotations.

Aetiology

The term 'hysteria' was already in use in Freud's time, when it was thought to stem from the uterus. Freud believed that the syndrome stemmed from repressed traumatic experiences. This theory is still held by some psychotherapists.

Management

- full history, mental state examination and collateral history
- consider psychotherapy
- trial of low-dose antipsychotic.

It is essential to explore the history fully. The main differential diagnosis is mania, where similar sexual behaviour, expansiveness and irresponsible behaviour are seen. Mania will have a shorter and more fluctuating course.

If treatment is sought, or if the patient is no longer capable of continuing his/her life without help, intervention should be considered. If the patient is psychologically minded, a referral to psychotherapy may be worthwhile. Alternatively, the arousal level of those who are over-active will be reduced by a low dose of antipsychotic medication.

Anankastic personality disorder

The diagnostic criteria for this disorder are:

- preoccupation with order, routine, lists, details and rules
- perfectionism and conscientiousness
- rigidity and stubbornness
- demands that others do things the same way
- intrusive thoughts or impulses as described for obsessive-compulsive disorder.

This disorder has also been called obsessive-compulsive personality disorder. It tends to cause fewer problems than the disorders already described and may be of benefit to students, cleaners, architects and those in similar professions where total application to the task, and successful completion, is required.

Aetiology

Freud viewed obsessive compulsive symptoms as part of the syndrome of 'anal fixation'. His case study was of the 'Rat Man' (see Chapter 36) who displayed obsessive-compulsive symptoms and was fascinated by a Chinese torture involving the rectum. This patient's symptoms were greatly alleviated by psychoanalysis but he unfortunately died soon afterwards during the First World War.

Management

- full history, mental state examination and collateral history
- low doses of an antipsychotic in some cases
- psychotherapy in some cases.

Obsessive-compulsive disorder must be excluded. In contrast to the early years of this century, this disorder is now rarely seen as requiring treatment. If treatment is sought, or if the patient is no longer capable of continuing his/her life without help, psychotherapy should be considered. An antipsychotic in low doses may reduce arousal and distress. Once again, these measures are unproven by research.

Anxious (advoidant) personality disorder

Diagnostic criteria are:

- persistent symptoms of anxiety
- feeling socially inept, unappealing and inferior
- preoccupation with social rejection
- tendency to avoid relationships unless acceptance is certain
- restrictions to lifestyle as a result of the above.

This personality disorderly is broadly similar to shyness of an extreme nature. Differential diagnoses are social phobia, generalized anxiety disorder and depression.

Aetiology

Psychologists link shyness with over-protective parents, especially mothers. Freud believed that symptoms of anxiety resulted from repressed conflicts and traumatic events, and linked these to sexual frustration. Other analysts express broadly similar views. Behavioural therapy, on the other hand, emphasizes the importance of learned behaviour, especially from parents.

Management

- full history and mental state examination and collateral history
- simple measures, e.g. self-help books and explanation
- psychotherapy referral
- antipsychotics or SSRIs
- avoid drugs and alcohol.

In a few cases, full history-taking will uncover childhood traumas or other issues that may be suitable for an analytical approach. In the majority, simple measures such as self-help books, explanation and instructions to carry out a basic programme of gradually increasing social contact will help. Psychologists use the same techniques, but more intensively. High motivation for change is a prerequisite for these treatment methods.

Functional illness, such as an anxiety disorder or depression, should be excluded, as should physical disorders such as hyperthyroidism and phaeochromo-cytoma.

Because of the long-standing nature of the disorder, benzodiazepines must be avoided. Where anxiety symptoms are prominent, an SSRI or antipsychotic may help some patients. There is little evidence that they will help the majority, however.

The patient who uses alcohol or drugs should be warned of their dangers. Alcohol and benzodiazepines cause rebound anxiety on withdrawal, and are therefore not helpful in the long term.

Other personality disorders

A number of other personality disorders have been described, but with the exception of the first, these are not ICD-10 diagnoses. Their use is therefore best avoided as they are subsumed within the eight disorders described above.

Emotionally unstable personality disorder, impulsive type

This appears to be a 'cross-over' category between dissocial personality disorder and borderline personality disorder, having some characteristics of both.

Narcissistic personality disorder

This is recognized by DSM-IV. Individuals with this disorder display grandiosity, lack of empathy, and hypersensitivity to evaluation by others. It is said to be similar to borderline personality disorder, but without the same instability.

Inadequate personality

This is thought to describe a patient's general inability to behave and think in a mature adult way. It is a highly pejorative term and should be avoided.

Immature personality

This is self-descriptive. It is less pejorative than inadequate personality, but still should be avoided.

Sensitive personality

This is also self-explanatory. In 1918 Ernst Kretschmer published the monograph *Der sensitive Beziehungswahn*. He was convinced that an interaction of specific personality traits and environmental conditions played a vital role in the formation of delusional symptoms.

He stated that subjectively shameful and humiliating experiences of everyday life could in some individuals give rise to an enduring feeling of being subject to increased attention by people around them.

The projection onto the external world of the individual's feelings of contempt and being under threat was termed 'inversion' and would effectively result in the transformation of an understandable reaction into a delusional experience (see Chapter 18).

Dysthymia and cyclothymia

See Chapter 19.

Schizotypal disorder

This is analogous to prodromal or prepsychotic schizophrenia, and is classified by the ICD-10 in schizophrenia, schizophreniform and delusional disorders, rather than as a personality disorder. In DSM-IV it is included with the personality disorders (see Chapter 18).

FURTHER READING

[Anonymous] (2002) *Personality Disorder: No Longer a Diagnosis of Exclusion*. National Institute for Mental Health in England. Includes a useful treatment review by Bateman and Tyrer.

Castillo H (2003) *Personality Disorder: Temperament or Trauma?* London: Jessica Kingsley.

Roth A & Fonagy P (1996) *What Works for Whom? A Critical Review of Psychotherapy Research*. New York: Guilford Press.

REFERENCES

American Psychiatric Association (2001) Practise guidelines for the treatment of patients with borderline personality disorder. *American Journal of Psychiatry* **158**(10 suppl): 1–52.

Bateman A & Fonagy P (1999) Effectiveness of partial hospitalization in the treatment of borderline personality disorder: a randomized controlled trial. *American Journal of Psychiatry* **156**(10): 1563–9.

Bateman A & Fonagy P (2001) Treatment of borderline personality disorder, with psychoanalytically oriented partial hospitalization: an 18-month follow-up. *American Journal of Psychiatry* **158**(1): 36–42.

Bateman A & Fonagy P (2003) Health service utilization costs for borderline personality disorder patients treated with psychoanalytically orientated partial hospitalization versus general psychiatric care. *American Journal of Psychiatry* **160**(1): 169–71.

Bluglass R and Bowden P (1990) *Principles and Practice of Forensic Psychiatry.* Edinburgh: Churchill Livingstone.

Casey PR & Tyrer PJ (1986) Personality, functioning and symptomatology. *Journal of Psychiatric Research* **20**: 363.

Casey PR & Tyrer P (1990) Personality disorder and psychiatric illness in general practice. *British Journal of Psychiatry* **156**: 261–5.

Cassady SL, Adam H, Moran M, Kunkel R & Thaker GK (1998) Spontaneous dyskinesia in subjects with schizophrenia spectrum personality. *American Journal of Psychiatry* **155**(1): 70–5.

Castillo H (2003) *Personality Disorder: Temperament or Trauma?* London: Jessica Kingsley.

De La Fuente JM, Tugendhaft P & Mavroudakis N (1998) Electroencephalographic abnormalities in borderline personality disorder. *Psychiatry Research* **77**(2): 131–8.

Dolan B, Warren F & Norton K (1997) Change in borderline symptoms one year after therapeutic community treatment for severe personality disorder. *British Journal of Psychiatry* **171**: 274–9.

Eastman N (1999) Public health psychiatry or crime prevention? *British Medical Journal* **318**: 549–51.

Hollander E, Allen A, Lopez RP, Bienstock CA , Grossman R, Siever Merkatz L & Stein DJ (2001) A preliminary double-blind, placebo-controlled trial of divalproex sodium in borderline personality disorder. *Journal of Clinical Psychiatry* **62**(3): 199–203.

Hori A (1998) Pharmacotherapy for personality disorders [review]. *Psychiatry and Clinical Neurosciences* **52**(1): 13–19.

Linehan MM, Heard HL & Armstrong HE (1993): Naturalistic follow-up of a behavioural treatment for chronically parasuicidal borderline patients. *Archives of General Psychiatry* **50** 971–4.

Markovitz P & Schulz S (1993) Drug treatment of personality disorders. *British Journal of Psychiatry* **162**: 122–3.

Montgomery DB, Roberts A, Green M et al. (1994) Lack of efficacy of fluoxetine in recurrent brief depression and suicidal attempts. *European Archives of Psychiatry and Clinical Neuroscience* **244**(4): 211–15.

Moran P (1999) *Antisocial Personality Sisorder – An Epidemiological Perspective.* London: Gaskell.

Regier DA. Myers JK, Kramer M et al. (1984) The NIMH epidemiologic catchment area program. *Archives of General Psychiatry* **41**: 934–41.

Rinne T, van den Brink W, Wouters L & van Dyck R (2002) SSRI treatment of borderline personality disorder. *American Journal of Psychiatry* **159**(12): 2048–54.

Robins LN (1966)Ä*Deviant Children Grown Up.* Williams & Wilkins. Baltimore

Romans SE, Martin JL, Anderson JC, Herbison GP & Mullen PE (1995) Sexual abuse in childhood and deliberate self-harm. *American Journal of Psychiatry* **152**(9): 1336–42.

Soloff PH (1987) Neuroleptic treatment in the borderline patient: advantages and techniques. *Journal of Clinical Psychiatry* **48**(suppl): 26–31.

Stein G (1992) Drug treatment of the personality disorders [review]. *British Journal of Psychiatry* **161**: 167–84.

The Quality Assurance Project [no authors listed] (1990) Treatment outlines for paranoid, schizotypal and schizoid personality disorders. *Australia New Zealand Journal of Psychiatry* **24**(3): 339–50.

Tyrer P & Seivewright N (1988) Pharmacological treatment of personality disorders [review] *Clinical Neuropharmacology* **11**(6) 493–9.

World Health Organization (1992) The ICD-10 classification of mental and behavioural disorders. In: [anonymous] *International Classification of Diseases*, 10th revision. Geneva: Division of Mental Health, WHO.

Anxiety disorders

James V Lucey and Aiden Corvin

INTRODUCTION

Anxiety disorders are common, disabling and treatable. Although they account for the bulk of patients with psychological conditions presenting to primary care practitioners, they remain under-recognized and frequently undertreated. Most anxious patients have combinations of symptoms in which clinical phenomena overlap, frequently with secondary depressive symptoms or substance abuse. Consequently, there is no single effective treatment method and none that is exclusively related to a specific disorder. Thus dual diagnoses and dual treatment modalities – psychological and pharmacological – are common.

HISTORY

Anxiety disorders are grouped together because of their historical association with the concept of neurosis and because a proportion of their aetiology is thought to involve stress. In *The Anatomy of Melancholia* (1621) Robert Burton described fear of death, fear of loss of a loved one, fear associated with depersonalization, hypochondriasis, anticipatory anxiety, agoraphobia and specific fears, such as fear of heights, public speaking or claustrophobia. The term neurosis was first used in a medical context by William Cullen in 1769, and was later adopted by psychiatry to distinguish anxiety disorders from melancholia and from the psychoses.

Westphal (1872) was the first to use the term *agoraphobia* in a technical sense, stating that patients' dizziness was caused by their anxiety. By contrast, the erroneous James–Lange theory proposed that bodily changes caused feelings and emotions. Clinical observation soon contradicted this view. Beard (1890) proposed the concept of *neurasthenia* in which patients suffered a *deficiency of nervous energy*, expressing itself in symptoms across the central nervous system, digestive system and reproductive tract. Although not predominant among these symptoms, morbid fear and phobia were recognized as the most refractory to treatment.

In 1903 Pierre Janet proposed the term *psychasthenia* for what we now refer to as anxiety disorders. This was characterized by three groups of neurotic experience: obsessive thoughts; irresistible movements (compulsions, tics, outbursts of temper); and visceral anxiety (generalized anxiety, panic, phobias and pain syndromes). Janet noted that suppression of one symptom type often led to the emergence of another; for example, blocking obsessions might heighten anxiety and induce compulsive behaviour, while resisting compulsion might lead to palpitations and fear of suffocation. Anxiety's fluctuating manifestations continue to strain attempts to place these disorders in rigid diagnostic categories (Glas 1996).

CLASSIFICATION OF ANXIETY DISORDERS

In 1895 Sigmund Freud proposed the separation of anxiety neurosis from neurasthenia. In his view, the origins of *anxiety neuroses* including phobic anxiety, obsessive-compulsive neurosis and hysteria, were different from the origins of the *actual neuroses* of neurasthenia. Freud implicated sexual repression in the aetiology of unconscious 'conflict', maladaptive defence mechanisms and anxiety symptoms. This separation of anxiety neurosis from neurasthenia represented the first major step towards the modern concept of anxiety disorder. Anxiety neuroses are conditions characterized by symptoms that are ego-dystonic (distressing and out of keeping with the patient's character). During neurotic illness the ability to test reality remain intact, and social norms are not grossly violated. Neuroses tend to be enduring or recurrent, and demonstrable organic factors are absent. Despite patients' psychological pain, reality testing remains intact, a fact that distinguishes neurosis from psychosis. The neurotic label is now largely redundant because modern operational diagnostic systems refer to anxiety neuroses or *anxiety disorders* characterized by a variety of disabling manifestations of anxiety (Glas 1996).

DSM-IV and ICD-10

A series of descriptive subdivisions within anxiety neurosis lead to the modern non-theoretical, operational approach used in DSM-IV (American Psychiatric Association 1994) and in ICD-10 (World Health Organization 1992). Dual diagnoses are possible. In ICD-10 the presumption of shared stress-related aetiology is stated; in contrast, DSM-IV makes no presumption as to aetiology. In DSM-IV the term 'anxiety neurosis' is abandoned altogether and replaced by *anxiety disorders*.

In ICD-10, anxiety disorders are categorized under *neurotic stress-related and somatoform disorders* under seven separate headings:

- phobic anxiety disorders
- anxiety disorders (including panic disorder and generalized anxiety)
- obsessive-compulsive disorders
- reactions to severe stress and adjustment disorders
- dissociative (conversion) disorders
- somatoform disorders
- other neurotic disorders.

In DSM-IV 12 distinct anxiety disorders are listed as follows:

- panic disorder without agoraphobia
- panic disorder with agoraphobia
- agoraphobia without a history of panic disorder
- specific phobia
- social phobia
- obsessive-compulsive disorder
- post-traumatic stress disorder
- acute stress disorder
- generalized anxiety disorder
- anxiety disorder due to general medical condition
- substance-induced anxiety disorder
- anxiety disorder not otherwise specified.

PHENOMENOLOGY

Phobias are disproportionate irrational fears of situations or circumstances. Fear is recognized by the subject as unwarranted and yet leads to avoidance of the precipitating circumstance.

Panic is a crescendo of overwhelming anxiety with somatic symptoms of autonomic hyperactivity such as palpitations, sweating, pallor, breathlessness, dizziness and vertigo. In addition there may be feelings of depersonalization, derealization, or fear of collapse or of becoming insane or even fear of death. Panic is not necessarily induced by an environmental stimulus.

Obsessions are recurrent unwanted distressing (egodystonic) ideas, thoughts or images that are resisted (at least initially) but are recognized as products of the subject's own mind.

Compulsions are repetitive, stereotyped and often trivial motor behaviours. Patients experience an overwhelming need to complete these behaviours, which forces itself into consciousness even though the subject does not wish to complete the act. These compulsive rituals are obsessions in action. Failure to complete them generates anxiety, while completion of the ritual attenuates anxiety, at least temporarily (see Box 15.1).

EPIDEMIOLOGY

Epidemiological data on anxiety disorders acquired prior to the era of operational diagnoses are of little value. Earlier studies were confounded by inconsistent methodologies and differing diagnostic criteria, and especially by different attitudes to the inclusion of mood disorder in the data. The Epidemiological Catchment Area (ECA) study (Myers et al. 1984) used DSM-III criteria and lay assessors, trained in the Diagnostic Interview Schedule, to produce a massive database of more than 15 000 home and institutional assessments. They found a six-month prevalence rate of 18% for at least one anxiety disorder, the most common being

Box 15.1	The symptoms of anxiety
Psychological	restlessness irritability poor concentration fear of death, heart attack or nervous breakdown
Respiratory	dyspnoea tachypnoea
Gastrointestinal	nausea vomiting dry mouth weight loss
Cardiovascular	chest pain palpitations flushing pallor
Neurological	dizziness headache vertigo paraesthesia tremor tinnitus blurred vision
General	tiredness insomnia loss of libido sweating increased frequency of urination muscle aches

phobic disorders. Comorbid alcohol abuse or dependence, dysthymia and major depression were also frequent. Overall morbidity rates were equal for the sexes, but females had an increased prevalence of phobias and depression and males had an increased prevalence of alcoholism. The peak incidence was between 24 and 44 years. Racial differences were not significant but anxiety disorders other than phobias were more common in urban than in rural settings. See Table 15.1 for approximate lifetime prevalences of individual anxiety disorders.

In European primary care settings, anxiety disorders have been reported as the main reason for contact by 4.6% of patients, thus accounting for nearly 80% of all psychiatric patients treated by general practitioners.

Outcome studies suggest that the prognosis for patients with a dual diagnosis of anxiety and depression is worse than for those with anxiety alone. There are few outcome studies comparing the different anxiety disorders with each other, but in general these disorders have an enduring or relapsing course with an increased risk for secondary alcohol or substance abuse, and for depression and potential suicide. Moreover, when compared to those with depression alone, patients with comorbid anxiety and depression have a poorer prognosis.

AETIOLOGY OF ANXIETY DISORDERS

Just how the mammalian brain mediates anxiety, or fear, is unknown. Learning-based theories build on the literature of classic and operant conditioning. Anthropological, sociological and analytical theories are also well developed. Analytical theorists suggest that the classic defense

mechanisms that may underlie anxiety disorders include avoidance, magical undoing and reaction formation. Family studies have demonstrated an increased risk for panic disorder/agoraphobia, OCD and phobic disorders in families of affected probands. These studies suggest a significant role for genetic and environmental influences in the aetiology of anxiety disorders. Molecular genetic studies are now being performed for specific anxiety disorders and are discussed elsewhere in this volume.

Both genetic and environmental risk factors are also likely to contribute to the acquisition, habituation and extinction of fears. Genetic epidemiological research also indicates extensive overlap between anxiety disorders, depression and substance/alcohol abuse. At this point it is uncertain to what extent this represents common aetiology/biology or more complex effects. Much of the variance in liability to anxiety disorders is due to environmental factors. Exposure to stressful life events throughout development (from early parental loss to marital disharmony) increases the likelihood of an anxiety disorder. The effects of early attachments may also be important, particularly consistency and support for a child in developing a sense of control over events.

Biological theories concentrate on specific abnormalities within noradrenaline (NA) (Charney & Henninger 1986a, b), gamma-aminobutyric acid (GABA) (Roy-Byrne et al. 1989), corticotrophin-releasing factor (CRF) (Yehuda 2001), glutamate, tachykinins and serotonin (5HT) neurotransmitter systems (Charney & Henninger 1986a, b).

Increasingly, the neuropsychology and functional anatomy of anxiety and fear is emerging, and it is becoming apparent that certain deep brain structures are involved in both normal and abnormal fear responses. The amygdala has long been implicated in the mediation of emotional behaviour and is now thought to play a central role in the mediation of anxiety and conditioned fear (Davis et al. 1997). This central role is suggested by the extensive afferent connections to the amygdala from thalamic and cortical exteroceptive systems, as well as by subcortical visceral afferent pathways. Neuronal interactions between the amygdala and other structures enable the individual to initiate adaptive behaviours in response to threat based upon the nature of the threat and prior experience (Charney & Deutch 1996). Input to the amygdala from the medial prefrontal cortex is thought to play a vital role in governing emotional response, for example by reducing the fear response when a threatening stimulus has passed. The hippocampus supplies the amygdala with information about the context in which threatening stimulus are presented and can be matched with experience from explicit memory. Hippocampal dysfunction has been shown to result in poor recognition of the context of stimuli and may result in the overgeneralization of fear responding, typical of anxiety disorders. Projections from the amygdala to autonomic, neuroendocrine and motor systems generate behavioural responses.

Table 15.1 Anxiety disorders and their lifetime prevelance	
Anxiety disorder	Lifetime prevalence (%)
Panic disorder	1–2 (female more than male)
Phobic disorders	2–7
agoraphobia	3–7 (female more than male)
agoraphobia with panic disorder	–
social phobia	10–15 (female equal to male)
specific phobia (animals, blood, vomiting, dental phobia)	5–15 (female more than male)
Obsessive-compulsive disorder	1–3 (female slightly more than male)
Generalized anxiety disorder	4–6 (female more than male)
Stress disorders	
acute stress reactions	–
post-traumatic stress disorder	1–3
Anxiety disorders (all)	15–20

SPECIFIC ANXIETY DISORDERS

The specific anxiety disorders for which operational diagnostic criteria exist are described below.

Panic disorder

Panic disorder consists of episodic crescendo anxiety that is recurrent and unpredictable and which occurs in the absence of a stimulus. Each episode is characterized by an abrupt onset of symptoms, which peak within 10 minutes. DSM-IV criteria for panic attack require four of the following symptoms:

- palpitations or accelerated heart rate
- sweating
- trembling/shaking
- feeling of choking
- sensation of shortness of breath
- chest discomfort
- nausea
- dizziness, unsteadiness
- derealization or depersonalization
- fear of losing control or 'going crazy'
- fear of dying
- paresthesia (numbness or tingling sensations)
- chills or hot flushes.

The selection of four symptoms was arbitrary, but was chosen because individuals with panic episodes with four or more symptoms have greater morbidity than individuals with less symptomatic episodes. Secondary anticipatory anxiety and phobic avoidance may also occur. The DSM-IV diagnosis of panic disorder requires a minimum of three attacks within three weeks in the absence of objective danger and without anxiety between attacks (other than anxiety relating to anticipation of panic). Panic disorder and agoraphobia (see below) is up to six times more common in women than in men and lifetime prevalence rates for panic disorder are approximately 1.2%. As noted above, risk is increased up to 20 times in relatives of probands with the disorder.

In DSM-IV, panic attacks are viewed as the core feature of panic disorder. In ICD-10 agoraphobia is viewed as dominant and panic attacks a secondary feature. A cornerstone of the biological theory of panic is the fact that intravenous infusion of lactate 0.5 mmol/l induces panic attacks in many patients with panic disorder (Klein 1964). This response is not exclusive or specific. Possible mechanisms for lactate-induced panic include hypocalcaemia, metabolic alkalosis, catecholamine release (especially noradrenaline), and the effects of rebreathing carbon dioxide. There appears to be a genetic predisposition to the development of panic disorder and agoraphobia with the risk being increased eight-fold in first-degree relatives of

affected individuals. The genetics of anxiety is discussed further in Chapter 3. As precipitating events are commonly reported by affected individuals a diathesis/vulnerability model has been proposed where illness is precipitated in predisposed individuals in adulthood.

The biology of panic is further underpinned by neuroendocrine studies that suggest reduced noradrenergic and serotonergic function (Charney & Henninger 1986a, b). Noradrenergic agents stimulate panic attacks in patients and, as is the case with anxiogenic stimuli, increase the rate of firing of the locus caeruleus. Involvement of serotonin systems is suggested by symptom response to SSRI medications. Cholecystokinin (CCK) and GABA systems may also be involved as CCK agonists and GABA antagonists also precipitate panic attacks in patients. Positron imaging data also indicates decreased benzodiazepine binding in inferior parieto-temporo-occipital cortex in patients. Psychological factors are also important and panic disorder has also been conceptualized as being primarily due to a phobic attitude and predisposing constitutional factors.

Phobic disorders

In contrast to panic disorder, phobic disorders are characterized by anxiety and intense fear induced by stimuli that leads to avoidance. Phobic anxiety differs from normal fear in that it is unreasonable and disproportionate to the stimulus. The one-year prevalence of phobic disorders is between 2% and 7% in most studies. The commonest phobic anxieties in community samples are specific fears relating to illness, injury, storms or animals, or to agoraphobia. In clinical practice, referral patterns mean that the order of frequency is reversed. Thus agoraphobia is the commonest phobia presenting to primary care practitioners.

The aetiology of phobias is unknown. Recovery from childhood fears occurs in 60% of individuals but fears acquired in adulthood are associated with a poor outcome, particularly when left untreated. Agoraphobia, social phobia and the specific phobias are now considered in some detail.

Agoraphobia

Agoraphobia literally means 'fear of the market place'. In clinical practice, agoraphobia involves multiple phobic symptoms, the most marked of which are extreme anxiety in open spaces, in crowds and on public transport. Almost 75% of agoraphobic patients are female, and the age of onset ranges from 15 to 35 years. There do not appear to be any racial, sociodemographic or educational correlates with agoraphobia. Characteristically, agoraphobic symptoms exhibit generalization so that fear in one situation may lead to fear in many other situations. Patients with agoraphobia often experience dizziness, depersonalization and depression, and secondary alcohol and substance misuse may also occur. Agoraphobic symptoms can be precipitated or intensified by major life events, which, may be more common in this group (e.g. agoraphobia is associated with marital and domestic discord). Agoraphobia is more common in individuals with dependent personality traits and the course of illness is characteristically fluctuating and may be prolonged.

Agoraphobic symptoms are induced by stimuli such as shops, crowds or public transport. The anxiety and fear are disproportionate to the objective risks and characteristically lead to avoidance. Agoraphobic symptoms resemble those of panic and the priority of panic disorder over agoraphobia or vice versa remains unclear. Thus in ICD-10 agoraphobia takes precedence over a diagnosis of panic disorder, while in DSM-IV the reverse is true. What is not in dispute is that both disorders are more common in females and that the six-month prevalence rates are about 1% (ECA study). Twenty per cent of patients with agoraphobia have another anxiety disorder, but while identified agoraphobic patients may repeatedly attend health services, community surveys suggest that less than 25% of patients present for treatment (Briggs & Stirton 1993).

Social phobia

Social phobia consists of fear of social interaction in a crowd and fear of appearing ridiculous when observed by others. Patients tend to avoid social interactions and may even seek to avoid the gaze of others. There is little or no avoidance of shops or public transport and, in contrast to agoraphobia, the sex ratio in social phobia is equal. Age of onset ranges from 15 to 35 years. Social phobia is associated with marked anticipatory anxiety. Alcohol and drug misuse are common and secondary depression occurs in up to 40% of patients. It is essential (and difficult) to distinguish social phobia from avoidant personality disorder and paranoia.

The specific phobias

The specific phobias include animal phobias, phobias of blood and vomitus, dental phobia and fear of urinary or faecal incontinence.

Animal phobias are perhaps the most common specific phobias, but they are nonetheless rare in clinical practice. This is because generalization rarely occurs and thus the phobia does not become disabling. Most patients are female (95%) and the premorbid personality is normal.

Dental phobia affects 5% of the population, while phobias of blood or vomitus and the fear of urinary or faecal incontinence are also very common, especially in females. Such phobias may be medically as well as psychiatrically relevant as they may cause individuals to avoid seeking medical or dental treatment. The specific phobias typically exhibit a prolonged course, they rarely generalize and there is a good response to behavioural treatment.

Obsessive-compulsive disorder

Obsessive-compulsive disorder (OCD) is characterized by obsessional thoughts that repeatedly enter consciousness against the patient's will. The thoughts or ruminations are unpleasant, abhorrent or out of keeping with the patient's character (ego-dystonic). Insight is preserved and patients feel compelled to resist or neutralize the unwelcome thoughts at least initially. The commonest obsessions relate to contamination or doubt. Sexual, violent and religious themes are also common. Obsessions may include vivid mental ideas or images involving contamination, sex or violence. Compulsions are repeated, stereotyped actions, carried out in response to obsessional thoughts. They relieve the tension produced by obsessional thoughts and may have a symbolic, magical quality. They are never pleasurable for the patient to perform. Repeating rituals are seen in 50% of patients with OCD but checking, cleaning and counting are also common. Striving for completeness or symmetry also occurs.

The patient with OCD initially resists the compulsion but this resistance fades and may not be present in severely or chronically ill individuals. Furthermore, insight may be incomplete. OCD symptoms may be confined to a particular location, e.g. 30% of patients may experience symptoms in a domestic setting. A minority of OCD patients, perhaps 4% of the total, and usually male, have obsessional slowness.

The ECA study (Robbins et al. 1984) reported a 3% prevalence of OCD in the community but European data continue to suggest that this figure is an overestimate. Nonetheless it is clear that OCD is no longer as rare as was once thought. The female to male ratio is 1.2:1 and the peak incidence is from 24 to 34 years. The mean age of onset of OCD is 20 years but this may be significantly lower in males. There is commonly a delay of up to seven years between disease onset and seeking treatment. The onset may be insidious and is often associated with depression, which is also common during the course of OCD. This course tends to be continuous with exacerbation. In women, premenstrual or postpartum exacerbations are common. Male patients may have a poor prognosis, and more often exhibit a striving for symmetry, or obsessional slowness. Checking and cleaning rituals are more common in female patients. Tics and abnormal involuntary movements may be more common in male patients, especially those who do not respond to treatment. The differential diagnosis for OCD includes depression with obsessional features, obsessional personality disorder, or normal behavioural rituals of childhood. Occasionally, OCD and schizophrenia may be difficult to distinguish.

There is considerable evidence that OCD is responsive to pharmacological agents that are selective for serotonergic systems. Approximately 50% of patients respond to clomipramine and similar efficacy has been reported for the more selective serotonin (5HT) agents such as fluvoxamine and fluoxetine. Such data led to the development of a 5HT hypothesis of OCD and numerous neuroendocrine abnormalities, further suggesting serotonergic dysfunction, have been reported in OCD, while serotonergic agonists such as metachlorophenylpiperizine (mCPP) are reported to induce OCD symptoms. Serotonergically induced hypo-thalamo-pituitary axis hormone responses are reduced in OCD suggesting a $5HT_2$ receptor abnormality. However, many studies have not had either depression or anxiety disorder comparison groups, and the few studies that have, provide evidence that 5HT abnormality is neither specific nor exclusive to OCD (Lucey 1994). Positron emission tomography (PET) in OCD reveals abnormalities in the orbitofrontal cortex and striatum, findings which have been replicated many times. Abnormalities in regional brain metabolism and regional blood flow may respond to effective treatment with either medication or behavioural psychotherapy (Schwartz et al. 1996).

Despite the 5HT hypothesis and resulting research, the aetiology of OCD remains unknown. Learning theory proposes that rituals are circular and mutually reinforcing, while psychoanalytical views implicate early aggressive sexual trauma with maladaptive use of defence mechanisms such as reaction formation and magical undoing. In addition, there are many clinical associations with striatal diseases including Sydenham's chorea and Tourette's syndrome. Twenty per cent of patients with OCD have motor tics. Less than 50% of DSM-IV-diagnosed OCD patients have axis 2 personality disorder and less than 10% have an obsessional personality disorder. These data, together with the growing functional imaging literature, mean that OCD is increasingly recognized as a neuropsychiatric disorder.

Generalized anxiety disorder

Generalized anxiety disorder (GAD) is probably the commonest anxiety disorder. Patients with GAD experience excessive anxiety that is not caused by another anxiety disorder on most days for a period of at least six months. Uncontrolled anxiety and worry impair social and occupational performance because restlessness, fatigue, poor concentration, irritability, muscle tension and sleep disturbance commonly occur. The utility of GAD as a diagnosis has been questioned recently. The typical symptoms must not be caused by any other anxiety disorder such as panic disorder, OCD or a stress disorder. As a result, GAD has largely become a label for non-specific persistent anxiety, diagnosed more by the exclusion of other anxiety disorders than by its own specific features.

Stress disorders

Stress disorders include acute stress reactions and post-traumatic stress disorder (PTSD).

Acute stress reaction (disorder)

Patients develop acute stress reaction (disorder) following exposure to a threatening event such as assault, a major road accident or a natural catastrophe. The threatening event is extreme and involves actual or threatened death or serious injury to self or others (e.g. war, criminal assault or rape). In ICD-10 criteria this can also include a sudden or threatening change to a persons network (e.g. multiple bereavements in an accident). They present within minutes to hours in a dazed and disorientated state with prominent autonomic signs of anxiety. There may be a subjective sense of numbing, detachment or absence of emotional responsiveness, along with derealization, depersonalization or dissociative amnesia. Patients may be agitated, stuporose or in a fugue. They usually have no premorbid psychiatric diagnosis and there is usually complete resolution of the acute stress reaction within a short period of time. In ICD-10, resolution must take place within 2–3 days, while in DSM-IV, acute stress disorder symptoms may persist for up to four weeks. The DSM-IV ASD diagnosis has been criticized on a number of counts. First, the diagnosis may pathologize transient stress reactions. Second, the diagnosis was introduced to predict risk of post-traumatic stress disorder (PTSD), even though the two diagnoses differ primarily on symptom duration and the predictive power of ASD is limited as most cases of ASD resolve without chronic symptoms. Finally, many cases of PTSD are not precipitated by ASD and indeed prospective research indicates that no particular ASD syndrome profile or symptom is predictive of PTSD. The 'normal' response to chronic stress involves a habituation process and development of coping mechanisms. A few studies have reported the effects of chronic exposure to stressors (such as terrorism) and these suggest that exposed individuals do not develop a high level of psychiatric morbidity (Bleich et al. 2003).

Post-traumatic stress disorder (PTSD)

The symptoms of PTSD arise only after an exceptionally threatening event that is outside the normal range of experience, e.g. combat, rape, attempted murder or torture. The traumatic events can be experienced or witnessed and as such are likely to cause distress (fear, helplessness or horror) in almost anyone. The disorder may be especially severe if the trauma is by human design (e.g. rape or torture). The likelihood of developing PTSD increases as the intensity of and physical proximity to the stressor increases. The DSM-IV diagnosis of PTSD also requires that the individual has a subjective response to the situation that includes horror, helplessness or fear (many would argue that numbness should also be included). The onset is delayed in PTSD with a latency of many weeks to several months. Characteristic symptoms include:

- Repeated reliving of trauma as daydreams, intrusive memories, flashbacks or nighmares.
- Persistent numbness or emotional bloating.

- Avoidance of thoughts about, or reminders of, the trauma, which may lead to marked detachment from personal involvement or relationships. This could include avoiding the scene of the event or other people involved with the event. Such avoidance can extend to similar themes in conversation or in media.
- Symbols, anniversaries or similar events often prompt exacerbation of symptoms.
- Marked irritability.
- Hyperarousal.
- Hypervigilance.
- Insomnia.
- Secondary drug and alcohol abuse is common and there may be overlap with generalized anxiety disorder and depression.

The lifetime prevalence of PTSD is estimated at between 1% and 3%, although high-risk groups, such as soldiers, may have much higher rates. Most patients are young adults but children and older adults may develop the disorder. Epidemiological research suggests that most people will experience at least one traumatic event in their lifetime. Although men experience a larger number of traumatic events, women experience more severe events, which may partially explain why women are twice as likely to develop PTSD in response to trauma as men. Three factors predict the onset of PTSD (Van der Kolk 1996):

- the scale of the trauma
- the patient's previous experience of trauma
- the level of social support available.

In studies undertaken to date, industrial or military disasters were common precipitating traumas in men, while assault and rape were common precipitants in women. A substantial proportion of individuals who develop ASD or PTSD symptoms recover without treatment, particularly in the first year following a traumatic event. However, at least a third of individuals who initially develop PTSD stay symptomatic for three years or longer. Clinical experience suggests that the initiating stress affects both acute and chronic adaptation to stress, with long-term consequences for the manner in which an individual copes with subsequent stress. Neuroendocrine research provides evidence that PTSD patients have chronically increased sympathetic activity, while veterans with PTSD have low levels of urinary cortisol, even in the presence of major depression (Yehuda et al. 2001). Several prospective studies indicate that after a traumatic event cortisol levels are lower in individuals who subsequently develop PTSD. Recent magnetic resonance imaging evidence suggests that hippocampal volume is decreased in PTSD, and this and other data support theories associating the development of PTSD with limbic dysregulation and disturbances of memory.

Conditioning theory has been applied to PTSD aetiology: through classic conditioning stimuli present at the time of the trauma become associated with fear and arousal responses. As a result conditioned stimuli trigger similar responses when present on their own. In the aftermath of the trauma a wide variety of stimuli may become triggers by stimulus generalization. Avoidance behaviours are negatively reinforced by reducing PTSD symptoms. Cognitive responses to traumatic events may also be important in the development and maintenance of PTSD. Excessive negative appraisal of the trauma or its sequelae and a disturbance of autobiographical memory may mediate the cognitive response to trauma. In support of this theory, several recent studies indicate that excessively negative or catastrophic appraisals of the trauma within the first three months of the traumatic event predict chronic PTSD. In one study, poor retrieval of specific memories in the acute phase of trauma accounted for 25% of the variance in severity of subsequent PTSD symptoms. This cognitive response is influenced by personality and it has been suggested that certain personality traits such as dependence or obsessionality may increase risk. Pre-existing mental disorder can also have a negative impact on the course of illness.

TREATMENT OF ANXIETY DISORDERS

Few studies compare treatment across the different anxiety disorders and most randomized controlled data relate to the treatment of agoraphobia/panic. However, this is not the problem it might at first seem because in clinical practice, treatments tend to be applied and to be effective across the range of anxiety disorders. The psychological treatments most commonly used include behavioural and cognitive methods, in either individual or group settings. A number of pharmacological treatments are also used.

Psychological treatments

Behavioural therapy/cognitive therapy
Psychological methods offer enduring, non-toxic treatments for many anxiety disorders. These range from non-specific interventions such as relaxation therapies and supportive psychotherapies to more specific therapies that target behavioural and cognitive features of anxiety. Research indicates that specific therapies are more effective, but non-specific interventions may be important in helping individuals cope with distressing symptoms and in motivating/supporting cognitive or behavioural adaptation.

Preventative psychological interventions after traumatic events have been widely practised; only recently have these methods been empirically tested. Psychological debriefing aims to educate trauma survivors about stress reactions, normal post-trauma symptoms and normal coping strategies. Originally a group intervention, but also practiced with individuals, the therapist promotes expression of thoughts and feelings about the event and provides information about possible further interventions. In assessing scientific studies of such interventions it is important to realise that the normal course of psychological response to trauma is poorly understood. Many debriefing studies have even failed to include untreated control populations. A recent systematic review of 11 randomized controlled trials found that a single session of individual debriefing did not reduce stress or prevent PTSD (Rose 2002). Several studies have even indicated negative effects for individual (but not group) debriefing. If psychological debriefing proves to be ineffective are there other psychological interventions for trauma survivors?

An alternative approach is to offer psychological intervention to a subgroup of trauma survivors. This subgroup is offered several sessions of individual cognitive behavioural therapy (CBT). Most studies have included education about psychological effects of trauma, imaginal reliving of the event, cognitive restructuring, and reversal of avoidance behaviours. But which survivors to select? Many studies have identified patients based on early symptoms of PTSD or a diagnosis of ASD, although prospective evidence suggests that these measures have limited predictive value for chronic PTSD symptoms. Longer CBT interventions (5–6 session programme) have demonstrated significant superiority to supportive counselling on measures of post-traumatic symptoms, anxiety and depression both post treatment and at four-year follow-up. However, these studies did not include an untreated control group and the supportive counselling group reported higher levels of symptoms than reported by untreated controls in other studies. A full course of CBT does appear to be an effective intervention for trauma survivors with moderate to high PTSD symptoms in the months after trauma.

Most research relates to behavioural treatments involving exposure and response prevention. Cognitive techniques, which emphasize conceptual adaptation of the mindset, or cognitive restructuring, have also been studied. Some therapies combine behavioural and cognitive approaches, in either individual or group settings.

A recent randomized study compared in vivo exposure alone with cognitive therapy combined with in vivo exposure in two groups of patients with severe agoraphobia. Both groups received eight sessions of in vivo exposure. One group of 12 patients received four sessions of cognitive therapy followed by eight sessions of in vivo exposure, while another 12 patients received four sessions of 'associative therapy', a presumably inert treatment that controlled for therapist attention, followed by eight sessions of in vivo exposure. There were no additional benefits from cognitive therapy in agoraphobia and exposure alone clearly produced significant reduction in phobic avoidance and self-rated anxiety (Van den Haut et al. 1994). However, a randomized controlled study of 156 agoraphobic patients in which cognitive techniques were combined with behavioural methods including exposure (cognitive–behavioural therapy) found a marked superiority of cognitive–behavioural therapy over waiting list management (Telch et al. 1995).

The relative superiority of behavioural psychotherapy over cognitive restructuring for agoraphobia/panic is disputed. Bouchard et al. (1996) studied 26 agoraphobic/panic patients randomly assigned to either exposure or cognitive restructuring. All patients improved and the differences between the two groups at the end of the study were marginal. Nevertheless, behaviour therapists stress the importance of exposure elements to efficacy and claim that the benefits of exposure-based treatments may be longer lasting than those of other treatments. Follow-up of 32 agoraphobic patients for up to 12 months (during which patients continued to apply self-exposure instructions) showed that 66% of patients reached a clinically significant improvement by 15 months. Furthermore, 36% of this benefit was achieved during the follow-up period (Jansson et al. 1986).

It is increasingly recognized that cognitive and behavioural treatments are synergistic. When cognitive techniques were combined with education and exposure in a group setting, 64% of 34 randomly assigned patients benefited significantly, compared to only 9% of untreated patients on a waiting list who served as controls. At six-month follow-up, 63% of treated patients met criteria for recovery (Telch et al. 1993). The Nottingham study of neurotic disorder compared pharmacological and psychological treatments in a large randomized controlled trial of 74 patients with panic disorder. These were compared with 71 outpatients with generalized anxiety disorder and 65 patients with dysthymia. Diagnoses were made according to DSM-III criteria and each subject was randomized to one of five treatments: diazepam ($n = 28$), dothiepin ($n = 28$), placebo ($n = 28$), cognitive–behavioural therapy ($n = 84$), or a self-help treatment programme ($n = 42$). All treatments were administered for six weeks. Blind data analysis revealed no significance outcome differences between the groups. Diazepam was less effective than dothiepin, cognitive–behavioural treatment or self-help, while these latter three treatments had similar efficacy. Patients treated with dothiepin or cognitive–behavioural therapy used the smallest amount of additional psychotropic medication during the trial. Overall, the data from this trial suggested that in the short term, cognitive–behavioural therapy was no more effective than placebo during treatment (Tyrer et al. 1988). The Nottingham group later examined the influence of therapist training and competence on outcome with cognitive–behavioural therapy. The therapists, mainly community psychiatric nurses, of 70 patients with a DSM-III diagnosis of either dysthymia, panic disorder or generalized anxiety disorder, were separated into two groups on the basis of their perceived competence in the eyes of their supervisor. Patients were rated at regular intervals over two years by assessors blind to knowledge of treatment group or therapist. Results revealed patients treated by competent therapists ($n = 30$) showed greater improvements than those allocated to therapists of uncertain competence ($n = 40$). Benefits were greatest with respect to depressive symptoms and persisted for over two years following cessation of cognitive–behavioural therapy (Kingdon et al. 1996). Thus therapist skill appears to be crucial to the efficacy of cognitive psychological treatments in generalized anxiety disorder. This conclusion has obvious and substantial implications for service provision of psychological treatments for patients with anxiety disorder.

Pharmacological treatments

Pharmacological treatments for anxiety disorders include: serotonin reuptake inhibitors, such as fluoxetine or sertraline; azapirones, such as buspirone and gepirone; benzodiazepines, such as diazepam or alprazolam; tricyclic antidepressants, most notably imipramine; monoamine oxidase inhibitors, such as phenelzine sulphate; and reversible inhibitors of monoamine oxidase-A. Simple comparison of these treatments may be misleading because the nature of control groups and the size of the placebo effect vary considerably between studies.

Serotonin reuptake inhibitors

In recent years, great attention has been paid to the efficacy of old and new serotonin reuptake inhibitors in panic/agoraphobia syndrome. Imipramine and clomipramine, tricyclics with potent serotonin reuptake inhibiting properties, were both shown to be effective (Fahy et al. 1992). In 18 patients with panic/agoraphobia previously resistant to in-patient behavioural treatment, significant benefit was observed for clomipramine in a 12-week double-blind placebo-controlled crossover study (Hoffart et al. 1993). A double-blind comparison of clomipramine and fluvoxamine showed that the two drugs were equally potent in reducing anxiety symptoms, while clomipramine 150 mg for six weeks was more potent than fluvoxamine 100 mg daily in ameliorating self-rated depressed mood (Den Boer et al. 1987). In panic disorder patients sensitive to 35% carbon dioxide, treatment with paroxetine for one month was as effective as imipramine in reducing the panic response (Bertani et al. 1995). Recently Boyer (1995) carried out a meta-analysis of 27 studies in panic disorder in which the efficacy of imipramine, alprazolam and the serotonin reuptake inhibitors paroxetine, fluvoxamine, zimelidine and clomipramine were studied. The results demonstrate a significant superiority for serotonin reuptake inhibitors in alleviating panic, and they were superior to both imipramine and alprazolam, even where doses of imipramine or alprazolam were increased (Boyer 1995). The authors conclude that serotonin reuptake inhibitors should be first-line pharmacotherapy for patients with panic disorder (Boyer 1995) for reasons of efficacy as well as safety.

Furthermore, this superior efficacy is not merely a function of antidepressant effect, because benefits are observed even when depression is not a prominent feature. Preliminary evidence indicates that venlafaxine (a serotonin and noradrenaline reuptake inhibitor) is also effective in the treatment of anxiety.

High-potency benzodiazepines

High-potency benzodiazepines such as alprazolam, adinazolam and clonazepam have proven efficacy in placebo-controlled trials of panic disorder, with the further benefit of a rapid onset of action (Beauclaire et al. 1994; Fleishaker et al. 1994; Jonas & Cohon 1993). Unfortunately, these benzodiazepines also have a relatively high potential for abuse and dependence, and their long-term use may be associated with cognitive impairment. Prescribers are advised to consult the BNF guidelines on long-term prescribing of high potency benzodiazepines (see Chapter 38).

Benzodiazepines have demonstrated superiority over placebo in most trials involving panic disorder. Most studies have investigated alprazolam and predictably somatic symptoms appear to respond better to treatment than psychic symptoms (worries, etc.). However, despite this the merits of benzodiazepines in panic disorder/agoraphobia remain disputed. This is primarily in the context of using benzodiazepines in combination with psychological treatments. The most controversial dispute arose from a trial involving a cross-national (London and Toronto) randomized study of alprazolam 5 mg daily in patients with chronic panic disorder and agoraphobia (Marks et al. 1993). The 154 patients in this study received eight weeks' treatment with either alprazolam and behavioural therapy involving exposure, or placebo and exposure, or placebo and relaxation. All four groups of patients improved on clinical measures of panic, but the exposure group had twice the benefit of the alprazolam-treated patients on measures of avoidance and disability. Alprazolam provided slight additional benefit when combined with exposure in effect size, but the authors claimed that long-term outcome was impaired by the addition of alprazolam and placed emphasis clearly on the benefits of exposure treatment (Marks et al. 1993). Further concerns were raised about the risk of aggressive behaviours and impaired memory functions with benzodiazepines and it has been suggested that the attribution of recovery to benzodiazepines is a predictor of relapse. Wardle et al. (1994) have examined the impact of benzodiazepine use in 91 patients with chronic agoraphobia receiving behaviour therapy. Half had received long-term treatment with benzodiazepines and these were compared with patients who had not received benzodiazepines. Both groups responded to a behavioural programme based on exposure, with the only difference being an increased rate of anxiety symptoms in patients subsequently withdrawn from benzodiazepines. Benzodiazepine-treated patients were more likely to abandon behaviour therapy, but there was no evidence that the outcome of exposure was significantly affected by benzodiazepine use (Wardle et al. 1994).

Tricyclic antidepressants

The anxiolytic effect of tricyclic antidepressants has been recognized since the early 1960s (Klein 1964), when it was discovered that imipramine had proven ability to block both spontaneous panic attacks (Klein 1964) and panic precipitated by intravenous sodium lactate. The mechanism by which sodium lactate induces panic is unclear and it is not certain why imipramine is effective in protecting against this effect. However, imipramine potently inhibits the reuptake of both 5HT and NA, and it may be that its anti-panic effects are mediated as much by 5HT as by NA. But whatever the mechanism, numerous studies have confirmed the efficacy of imipramine in the treatment of panic disorder. This effect is not specific to imipramine and research suggests similar efficacy for clomipramine and lofepramine, although withdrawal rates of the order of 30% were reported for clomipramine-treated patients. The side-effects of tricyclics used in the short-term treatment of panic disorder include blurred vision, tachycardia, insomnia, sleep disturbance, excitement, malaise, dizziness, headache and nausea and their onset of action is typically delayed by 2–3 weeks.

Azapirones

The azapirones gepirone and buspirone have both been studied in patients with panic disorder. Gepirone, a potent serotonin $5HT_{1A}$ receptor agonist, was used in doses ranging from 2 mg to 12 mg daily in 21 patients with generalized anxiety or panic disorder/agoraphobia. This six-week study was open and uncontrolled, but significant benefits were apparent within one week of treatment (Pecknold et al. 1993). Buspirone is a partial $5HT_{1A}$ agonist with dopamine antagonist properties. It was studied in a multicentre randomized controlled trial of cognitive therapy with buspirone or placebo in 91 patients with agoraphobia/panic. After an initial 16 weeks of treatment, double-blind status was maintained for a further 52 weeks. Buspirone appeared to enhance the effects of cognitive–behavioural therapy in the short term only, and by week 64 there was no added effect of buspirone (Cottraux et al. 1995).

Monoamine oxidase inhibitors

Monoamine oxidase inhibitors such as phenelzine were studied in the pre-operational diagnostic era and were frequently shown to be superior to imipramine or placebo in the treatment of anxiety disorder. Monoamine oxidase inhibitors may be more effective than tricyclic antidepressants in anxiety disorders when depressed patients have a prominent phobic anxiety component. The use of MAOIs is limited by the dietary restrictions required and the risk of hypertensive crisis. The development of the

reversible monoamine oxidase A inhibitors renewed interest particularly as clinically significant reductions in panic and avoidance were reported in brofaromine treated patients. Unfortunately, development of this agent has been discontinued and results from meclobemide have been less promising.

Other agents

Small studies of other agents appear to provide promising results. Inositol, an intracellular second messenger precursor thought to be an effective antidepressant, was studied in 21 patients with panic disorder. Patients completed a double-blind randomized controlled trial with crossover design. Inositol (12 g/day) for four weeks was significantly more effective than placebo and had relatively few side-effects (Benjamin et al. 1995). Preliminary data also indicates that GABA reuptake inhibitors (e.g. tiagabine) may be effective treatments for PTSD and other anxiety disorders (Taylor 2003).

Combination psychological and pharmacological treatments

The potential benefits of exposure in vivo for panic agoraphobia with the addition to the exposure regimen of fluvoxamine or psychological training (repeated hyperventilation and respiratory training) have also been studied in 96 patients randomly assigned to double-blind placebo-controlled treatment. All treatments involving exposure were equally effective. However, the combination of exposure in vivo with fluvoxamine had twice the effect of the other treatments on agoraphobic avoidance (De Beurs et al. 1995). Thus many clinicians pragmatically combine pharmacological and psychological treatments in the management of patients with anxiety disorders.

Future developments in psychological treatment

One major potential limitation of psychological methods arises from the shortage of trained therapists and the limited ability of severely disabled phobic patients to participate in therapy. A recent study of 42 panic/agoraphobic patients living in remote regions of Ontario, Canada suggests that telephone-administered behaviour therapy for panic disorder with agoraphobia may be effective. Compared to waiting list controls, patients who received an eight-session telephone behaviour programme made substantial gains, with significant time by treatment interactions. Patients originally on the waiting list then received the same form of treatment and made similar gains, and benefits in both groups were maintained at three and six months follow-up. Computer systems of self exposure therapy (such as fear fighter) may be a method of increasing availability of psychological therapies. A recent study of this approach in patients with phobia or panic disorder found comparable improvement and satisfaction in groups where self-exposure therapy was guided by computer or by clinician. Further investigation of this approach is required as the drop-out rate was higher in the computer-guided group (43%) than in the clinician-guided group (24%) (Marks et al, 2004).

FURTHER READING

Allen SN & Bloom SL (1994) Group and family treatment of post-traumatic stress disorder. *Psychiatric Clinics of North America* **17**: 425–37.

Gray AJ (1982) *The Neuropsychology of Anxiety*. Oxford: Oxford University Press.

REFERENCES

American Psychiatric Association (1994) *Diagnostic and Statistical Manual of Mental Disorders*, 4th edn. Washington, DC: APA.

Beard GM (1890) *A Practical Treatise on Nervous Exhaustion (neurasthenia)*, Edited by AD Rockwell. London: HK Lewis.

Beauclair L, Fontaine R, Annable L et al. (1994) Clonazepam in the treatment of panic disorder: double-blind placebo-controlled trial investigating the correlation between clonazepam concentrations in plasma and clinical response. *Journal of Clinical Psychopharmacology* **14**: 111–18.

Benjamin J, Levine J, Fux M et al. (1995) Double-blind placebo-controlled cross-over trial of inositol treatment for panic disorder. *American Journal of Psychiatry* **152**: 1084–6.

Bouchard S, Gauthier J, Laberge B et al. (1996) Exposure versus cognitive restructuring in the treatment of panic disorder with agoraphobia. *Behavioural Research and Therapy* **34**: 213–24.

Boyer W (1995) Serotonin uptake inhibitors are superior to imipramine and alprazolam in alleviating panic attacks: a meta-analysis. *International Clinical Psychopharmacology* **10**: 45–9.

Bremner JD, Randall PR, Scott TM et al. (1995) MRI based measurement of hippocampal volume in post-traumatic stress disorder. *American Journal of Psychiatry* **152**: 973–81.

Briggs AC & Stirton RF (1993) Epidemiology of panic. In: Montgomery SA(ed.) *Psychopharmacology of Panic*, pp. 25–37. Oxford: Oxford University Press.

Burton R (1621 edition 1896) *The Anatomy of Melancholia*, vols 1–111, edited by AR Shillito. London: George Bell.

Charney DS & Deutch A (1996) A functional neuroanatomy of anxiety and fear: implications for the pathophysiology and treatment of anxiety disorders. *Critical Review of Neurobiology* **10**(3–4): 419–46.

Charney DS & Henninger GR (1986a) Serotonin function in panic disorders. *Archives of General Psychiatry* **43**: 1059–65.

Charney DS & Henninger GR (1986b) Abnormal regulation of noradrenergic function in panic disorders. *Archives of General Psychiatry* **43**: 1042–5.

Cottraux J, Note ID, Cungi C et al. (1995) A controlled study of cognitive behavioural therapy with buspirone or placebo in panic disorder with agoraphobia. *British Journal of Psychiatry* **167**: 635–41.

Crowe RR, Noyes R, Paul DL & Slymen D (1983) A family study of panic disorders. *Archives of General Psychiatry* **40**: 1065–6.

Davis M, Walker DL & Lee Y (1997) Roles of the amygdala and bed nucleus of the stria terminalis in fear and anxiety measured with the acoustic startle reflex. Possible relevance to PTSD. *Annals of the New York Academy of Science* **821**: 305–31.

De Beurs E, Van Balkom AJ, Lange A et al. (1995) Treatment of panic disorder with agoraphobia: comparison of fluvoxamine, placebo and psychological panic management, combined with exposure and of exposure in vivo alone. *American Journal of Psychiatry* **152**: 683–91.

Den Boer JA, Westenberg HG, Kamerbeek WD et al. (1987) Effect of serotonin uptake inhibitors in anxiety disorders: a double-blind comparison of clomipramine and fluvoxamine. *International Clinical Psychopharmacology* **2**: 21–32.

Drevets WC, Videen TO, MacLeod AK et al. (1992) PET images of blood flow changes during anxiety: correction. *Science* **256**: 1696.

Fahy TJ, O'Rourke D, Brophy J et al. (1992) The Galway study of panic disorder. 1: clomipramine and lofepramine in DSM III-R panic disorder: a placebo-controlled trial. *Journal of Affective Disorders* **25**: 63–75.

Fleishaker JC, Greist JH, Jefferson JW & Sheridan AQ (1994) Relationship between concentrations of adinazolam and its primary metabolite in plasma and therapeutic untoward effects in the treatment of panic disorder. *Journal of Clinical Psychopharmacology* **14**: 28–35.

Glas G (1996) Concepts of anxiety: a historical reflection on anxiety and related disorders. In: Westenberg HGM, Den Boer JA & Murphy DL (eds). *Advances in the Neurobiology of Anxiety Disorders*, pp. 2–19. Chichester: Wiley.

Hoffart A, Due Madsen J, Lande B et al. (1993) Clomipramine in the treatment of agoraphobic inpatients resistant to behavioural therapy. *Journal of Clinical Psychiatry* **54**: 481–7.

James W (1884) What is an emotion? *Mind* **9**: 188–205.

Jansson L, Jerremaln A & Ost LG (1986) Follow-up of agoraphobia in patients treated with exposure in vivo or applied relaxation. *British Journal of Psychiatry* **149**: 486–90.

Jonas JM & Cohon MS (1993) A comparison of the safety and efficacy of alprazolam versus other agents in the treatment of anxiety, panic, and depression: a review of the literature. *British Journal of Psychiatry* **149**: 486–90.

Kingdon D, Tyrer P, Seivewright N et al. (1996) The Nottingham study of neurotic disorder: influence of cognitive therapists on outcome. *British Journal of Psychiatry* **169**: 93–7.

Klein DF (1964) Delineation of two drug-responsive anxiety syndromes. *Psychopharmacologia* **5**: 397–408.

Kosten TR, Mason JW, Giller EL et al. (1987) Sustained urinary norepinephrine and epinephrine elevation in PTSD. *Psychoneuroendocrinology* **12**: 13–20.

Kramer MS, Cutler NR, Ballenger JC et al. (1995) A placebo-controlled trial of L-365, 260, a CCKB antagonist, in panic disorder. *Biological Psychiatry* **37**: 462–6.

Lucey JV (1994) Towards a neuroendocrinology of obsessive compulsive disorder. *Journal of Psychopharmacology* **8** (4): 250–7.

Marks IM (1987) Physiology of fear. In: Marks IM (ed.) *Fears, Phobias and Rituals, Panic, Anxiety and their Disorders*, pp 177–228. Oxford: Oxford University Press.

Marks IM, Swinson RP, Basoglu M et al. (1993) Alprazolam and exposure alone and combined in panic disorder with agoraphobia. A controlled study in London and Toronto. *British Journal of Psychiatry* **162**: 776–87.

Myers JK et al. (1984) Six month prevalence rates of psychiatric disorders in three communities. *Archives of General Psychiatry* **41**: 959–60.

Pecknold JC, Luthe L, Scott Fleury MH & Jenkins S (1993) Gepirone and the treatment of panic disorder: an open study. *Journal of Clinical Psychopharmacology* **13**: 145–9.

Robbins LN, Helzer JE, Weissman M et al. (1984) Life time prevalence rates of specific psychiatric disorders in three sites. *Archives of General Psychiatry* **41**: 949–58.

Roy-Byrne PP, Lewis N, Villacres E et al. (1989) Preliminary evidence of benzodiazepine subsensitivity in panic disorder. *Biological Psychiatry* **26**: 744–8.

Schwartz JM, Stoessel PW, Baxter LR Jr et al. (1996) Systematic changes in cerebral glucose metabolic rate after successful behaviour modification treatment of obsessive-compulsive disorder. *Archives of General Psychiatry* **53**: 109–13.

Sheehan DV, Ballenger J & Jacobsen G (1980) Treatment of endogenous anxiety with phobic, hysterical, and hypochondriacal symptoms. *Archives of General Psychiatry* **37**: 51–9.

Sheehan DV, Ballenger J & Jacobsen G (1987) Relative efficacy of monoamine oxidase inhibitors and tricyclic antidepressants in the treatment of endogenous anxiety. In: Klein DF & Rabkin J (eds) *Anxiety:New Research and Changing Concepts*, pp. 47–67. New York: Raven Press.

Swinson RP, Fergus KD, Cox BJ & Wickwire K (1995) Efficacy of telephone administered behavioural therapy for panic disorder with agoraphobia. *Behavioural Research and Therapy* 33: 465–9.

Taylor FB (2003). Tiagabine for posttraumatic stress disorder: a case series of 7 women. *Journal of Clinical Psychiatry*; 64; 1421–5.

Telch MJ, Lucas JA, Schmidt NB et al. (1993) Group cognitive behavioural treatment of panic disorder. *Behavioural Research and Therapy* 31: 279–87.

Telch MJ, Schmidt NB, Jaimez TL et al. (1995) Impact of cognitive behavioural treatments on quality of life in panic disorder patients. *Journal of Consultation in Clinical Psychology* 63: 823–30.

Tyrer P, Seivewright N, Murphy S et al. (1988) The Nottingham study of neurotic disorder: comparison of drug and psychological treatments. *Lancet* 2: 235–40.

Tyrer P & Shawcross C (1988) Monoamine oxidase inhibitors in anxiety disorders. *Journal of Psychiatric Research* 22 (suppl. 1): 87–98.

Van den Haut M, Arntz A & Hoekstra R (1994) Exposure reduced agoraphobia but not panic, and cognitive therapy reduced panic but not agoraphobia. *Behavioural Research and Therapy* 32: 447–51.

Van Der Kolk B (1996) The body keeps the score: the evolving psychobiology of post traumatic stress. In: Westenberg HGM, Den Boer JA & Murphy DL (eds) *Advances in the Neurobiology of Anxiety Disorders*, pp. 362–82. Chichester: Wiley.

Van Emmerik AA, Kamphuis JH, Hulbosch AM, Emmelkamp PM (2002). Single session debriefing after psychological trauma: a meta-analysis. *Lancet* 360: 766–71.

Van Vliet IM, Westenberg HG & Den Boer JA (1993) MAO inhibitors in panic disorder. clinical effects of treatment with brofaromine. A double-blind placebo-controlled study. *Psychopharmacology* 112: 483–9.

Wardle J, Hayward P, Higgitt A et al. (1994) Effects of concurrent diazepam treatment on the outcome of exposure therapy in agoraphobia. *Behavioural Research and Therapy* 32: 203–15.

Westphal C (1872) Die Agoraphobie, eine neuropathische erscheinung. *Archiv fur Psychiatrie und Nervenkrankheiten* (Berlin) 3: 138–61.

World Health Organization (1992) The ICD-10 Classification of Mental and Behavioural Disorders: Clinical Descriptions and Diagnostic Guidelines. Geneva: WHO.

Yehuda R (2001) Biology of posttraumatic stress disorder. *Journal of Clinical Psychiatry* 62: 41–46.

Liaison psychiatry and psychosomatic medicine

Louise M Howard and Lisa A Page

WHAT IS LIAISON PSYCHIATRY?

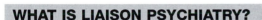

Liaison psychiatry (or consultation-liaison (CL) psychiatry/ general hospital psychiatry) can be defined as a psychiatric subspecialty concerned with the diagnosis, treatment, study and prevention of psychiatric morbidity among physically ill and/or somatizing patients and the provision of psychiatric consultations, liaison and education for non-psychiatrists (Lipowski 1983).

The overlap between medicine and psychiatry in, for example, endocrine problems, HIV, epilepsy, acute confusional states etc. will be covered in other relevant chapters and will not be specifically covered here. However, liaison psychiatrists (and perhaps all psychiatrists) need to have expertise in these areas as they will often encounter such problems in the general medical hospital.

LIAISON PSYCHIATRY IN THE UK

In the 19th century many general medical hospitals had some provision for hysteria and related conditions in addition to organic disorders such as delirium. 'Shellshock' during the First World War led to many physicians emphasizing the importance of psychological care in the 1920s and 1930s. In the 1930s the psychoanalytic movement stimulated interest in the role of psychological factors in medical problems, e.g. Alexander's specificity theory for diseases such as asthma, hypertension, ulcerative colitis. Although research did not support these psychosomatic theories, liaison services grew in the USA.

After 1948, when the National Health Service (NHS) was established in the UK, psychiatrists became increasingly based in general hospitals for outpatient services and provided informal consultations to medical colleagues. In 1961 the Ministry of Health recommended psychiatric assessment of all cases of deliberate self-harm (this is no longer mandatory), which led to more psychiatric input to the general hospital. Piecemeal development of services then continued; some pioneers (e.g. Sir David Hill at the Middlesex Hospital, London) developed liaison attachments with individual medical units, but liaison has often been provided by duty doctors of sector teams. In the last few years there has been a further expansion of services, but some regions still do not have a liaison psychiatrist and numbers still fall short of that recommended by the Royal College of Psychiatrists (Swift & Guthrie 2003).

WHY HAVE A LIAISON SERVICE?
(see Benjamin et al. 1994)

Assessment and management of deliberate self-harm

An average UK health district of 250 000 will have 500 deliberate self-harm (DSH) hospital attendances per year. In 2002 the Department of Health published the National Suicide Prevention Strategy in order to fulfil the Government's pledge to reduce death by suicide in England by 20% between 2002 and 2010. A key component of this strategy is improved management of DSH in general hospitals.

The National Institute for Clinical Excellence has published guidelines for the management of DSH within general hospitals in 2004.

A specific DSH service at the general hospital can:

- see patients more quickly and is more administratively efficient
- provide consistency of approach
- provide specific training and education
- provide brief psychosocial interventions, which can improve social adjustment, depression and hopelessness (there is also some evidence for a trend in reduction in repetition rates) (Townsend et al. 2001).

Assessment/treatment of Accident and Emergency, ward and outpatient referrals

Patients with physical illness have more than twice the rates of psychiatric disorder compared with the general population and 25% of male medical in-patients have a current or previous alcohol problem (Lloyd et al. 1982). Some units have particularly high rates of psychiatric disorder, e.g. neurological in-patients. Psychiatric symptoms can occur in the context of medical disease in the following ways:

- as a direct result of the disease itself, e.g. irritability in hyperthyroidism, depression in Cushing's disease
- as a psychological reaction to the disease, e.g. adjustment disorder in cancer
- the medical disease acts as a precipitant in patients who already have underlying mental illness
- the psychiatric disorder leads to physical problems, e.g. DSH, alcohol misuse
- the psychiatric disorder is mistaken for physical disorder as in somatization.

This comorbidity affects patients' quality of life, reduces the ability to benefit from treatment for medical problems, is associated with poor outcome for the physical problems and increases the cost of medical care. Yet psychiatric problems in the medically ill are underdiagnosed and under-treated. Liaison psychiatrists aim to:

- reduce morbidity, e.g. antidepressants improve depressive symptoms in a range of medical conditions (Gill & Hatcher 2003); cognitive therapy improves quality of life in cancer patients (Greer et al. 1992)
- reduce costs, e.g. by reducing length of hospital stay
- reduce problem-drinking through brief interventions (Bien et al. 1993).

Provision of specialized services—chronic somatization

At some medical clinics, 30–50% of new attendances are due to somatization (Van Hemert et al. 1993). These patients view themselves as more seriously ill than general medical patients and their use of health care services may be as high as nine times that of the general population (Smith 1994). Specialist psychiatric interventions can:

- improve outcome
- provide earlier and better assessment
- reduce inappropriate demand on medical services reduce costs of multiple investigations (which include financial costs, iatrogenic medical problems, delay of appropriate treatment and reinforcement of patients' beliefs in organic pathology)

Education of non-psychiatric staff to identify and manage psychological problems

Liaison psychiatrists cannot see all of the many patients with psychiatric morbidity in the general hospital. It is therefore important to educate hospital staff about how to recognize and manage common psychiatric problems and when and how to refer to liaison psychiatry services. This can be done by:

- including psychiatric teaching within training
- being actively involved in the postgraduate teaching programme of the hospital
- developing close links with staff who are likely to need supervision, e.g. specialist nurses in oncology and transplantation services, midwives, social workers, etc.

Advise on issues of capacity and consent

Although all doctors above pre-registration house officer level are allowed to assess capacity, liaison psychiatrists are often asked to comment on issues of capacity and consent in medical and surgical patients. Likewise, liaison psychiatrists will need to advise on when it is and is not appropriate to use the Mental Health Act in the general hospital setting.

Research in liaison psychiatry

More research is needed into the prevalence of psychological morbidity in the general hospital, the needs of non-psychiatric staff involved in the care of these patients and evaluation of the effectiveness of different psychiatric interventions (Guthrie & Creed 1994). Liaison psychiatrists are well placed to undertake multidisciplinary research in these areas.

RECOMMENDED STRUCTURE OF IDEAL LIAISON SERVICE
(Royal College of Physicians & Royal College of Psychiatrists 2003)

A liaison service should include:

- a service developed in consultation with non-psychiatrists in general hospital and other psychiatrists in district providing catchment area services and specialized services such as substance misuse
- an accessible system for collecting referrals, simple protocols for the detection and management of psychiatric problems by general hospital staff
- a well-organized medical record system, with standardized records of consultations for audit
- private facilities in accident and emergency (A&E), wards and outpatients for interviews
- adequate staff, e.g. for a district general hospital with 600 beds:
  (a) consultant liaison psychiatrist (full time), clinical supervision of DSH service, clinical work and supervision of ward referrals, A&E, administration and organization and outpatient clinic

(b) full-time trainee psychiatrist

(c) five liaison nurses

(d) clinical psychologist and/or physiotherapist, social worker

(e) administrative support.

MODELS OF LIAISON PSYCHIATRY

Consultation model

This refers to individual psychiatrist–patient consultation. The psychiatrist makes a full assessment of the patient's problems and advises a non-psychiatrist on further management. This is the model used by all other medical specialties in secondary care. Problems with this model include:

- it is reactive and not proactive
- it depends on nonpsychiatrists detecting psychiatric morbidity
- it depends on non-psychiatrists' attitudes towards psychiatric referral
- patients may be reluctant to see a psychiatrist
- there are few opportunities to discuss case with referring doctor
- there are few opportunities to exchange ideas on management of patients.

Liaison model

This is a collaborative model where the psychiatrist is a member of the medical/surgical team and is in regular contact, e.g. at ward rounds so that psychiatrist can identify where psychiatric input can be helpful and advise/provide support on staff problems in relationship to their patients and each other. When links are developed with a particular unit the referral rate of patients who can benefit from psychiatric help can increase two- to three-fold (Sensky et al. 1985). The main problems of this model include the following:

- it is time consuming
- it is costly (as it needs higher levels of staffing)
- it may not be wanted by physicians.

Liaison models have also been described as *patient-oriented*, *crisis-oriented* (therapeutic consultations with assessment and a brief psychotherapeutic intervention at the bedside), *consultee-oriented* (where main target is the consultant and his/her main problem with the patient) or *situation-oriented* (focus on interaction between patient and clinical team) consultations (Lipowski 1983).

In practice, most liaison psychiatrists use a combination of models and develop links with units where patients are at particularly high risk of psychiatric problems, e.g. oncology (see below).

(see Guthrie & Creed 1996)

PSYCHIATRIC ASSESSMENT OF PATIENTS WITH PHYSICAL ILLNESS

Conducting the consultation

1. Discuss the case with referrer before seeing the patient to clarify the reason for referral and establish whether patient has been told of the referral.
2. Review the medical notes.
3. Ensure privacy for the interview.
4. Consider gaining informant history from family/general practitioner (GP).
5. Discuss assessment with referrer and establish ongoing medical responsibility.
6. Liaise with nursing staff and GP.

Interviewing skills

1. Address patient's feelings about psychiatric referral.
2. Ask about physical symptoms and general medical history.
3. Ask about psychological symptoms.
4. Be aware of verbal and non-verbal cues of emotional distress and be empathic.
5. Take a comprehensive history and mental state examination.
6. Record consultation in medical notes.

Particular problems

Assessment of depression in the physically ill

Somatic symptoms (e.g. fatigue, weight loss, insomnia, pain) may result from physical illness or depression. Assessment should therefore focus more on affective and cognitive symptoms (diminished interest or pleasure, psychomotor retardation/agitation, irritability, non-reactive mood, suicidal thoughts); depressed mood, morning depression and hopelessness provide good discrimination between depressed and non-depressed medically ill patients.

Assessment of patients with somatization (with or without additional organic pathology)

These patients may be particularly reluctant to see a psychiatrist and feel the referral means their doctors believe there is nothing wrong with them. The psychiatrist should:

- acknowledge the reality of their symptoms, recognize that their symptoms are not imaginary
- explain that all illnesses and their treatments have an emotional component and that treatment needs to focus on both psychological and physical dimension
- acknowledge the fear of labelling and stigma
- take a full history of physical symptoms to allow patient to *feel understood* and to investigate precipitating and

maintaining factors, while establishing a positive collaborative relationship
- ask the patient about their past experience of contact with the medical system.

Engaging the patient may be easier if the first consultation is in the medical clinic, possibly as a joint appointment with the physician, or in a specialized liaison psychiatry clinic.

MEDICALLY UNEXPLAINED SYMPTOMS

Definitions

Many of these terms are used interchangeably:

- *Medically unexplained symptoms* are physical symptoms that are disproportionate to identifiable physical disease.
- *Somatization* is the process by which people with psychological disorders present in non-mental health settings with somatic symptoms which are not due to physical disease.
- *Functional symptoms* imply that there is an abnormality of functioning but no detectable physical pathology.

Other terms include *hysteria*, *somatoform* and *psychosomatic*.

Somatization has been operationally defined in a study of primary care patients by Bridges & Goldberg (1985) as:

- patient seeks help for physical complaints
- these complaints are not attributed to a psychological cause
- psychiatric disorder can be diagnosed
- treatment of psychiatric disorder would improve physical symptoms.

(The last two criteria may not always apply in clinical practice – medically unexplained symptoms can occur in the absence of psychiatric disorder.)

Somatization is common– in Bridges & Goldberg's study up to 1 in 5 new consultations were related to somatic symptoms for which no specific cause could be found.

Other definitions

- *Abnormal illness behaviour* has been defined as 'inappropriate or maladaptive mode of experiencing,

evaluating or acting in relation to one's own state of health, which persists despite the fact that a doctor has offered accurate and reasonable information concerning the person's health status' (Pilowsky 1997).
- *Somatoform disorders* are defined in the ICD-10 (World Health Organization 1992) as 'repeated presentation of physical symptoms, together with persistent requests for medical investigations, in spite of repeated negative findings and reassurances' (Box 16.1)

Somatoform disorders have a confusing terminology with overlapping criteria; in clinical practice it can be difficult to differentiate different disorders but all encompass 'abnormal illness behaviour'. DSM-IV (American Psychiatric Association 1994) includes conversion disorder within somatoform disorders; ICD-10 combines somatoform disorders with conversion disorders, 'stress related' and 'neurotic' disorders and 'neurasthenia'.

The so called *functional somatic syndromes* are not included in ICD-10 (although neurasthenia is included). Examples include chronic fatigue syndrome, irritable bowel syndrome, fibromyalgia, non-cardiac chest pain. They are defined by their symptoms, lack an underlying organic aetiology and have considerable overlap with each other.

Aetiology

Psychiatric disorders (particularly anxiety and depression) can act to predispose, precipitate or perpetuate somatic symptoms. Psychological, physiological and social factors are important.

Predisposing factors:

- personality traits including neuroticism, excessive health consciousness, somatic amplification (tendency to increased awareness of normal bodily sensations)
- early childhood experience – illness beliefs (e.g. from family attitudes to illness), parental lack of care and experience of parental illness as a child
- female gender
- genetic predisposition, e.g. results of some twin studies suggest a genetic influence in the experience of fatigue (Afari & Buchwald 2003).

Precipitating factors:

- physical injury or illness
- life events have been implicated in the onset of medically unexplained symptoms akin to depression (Craig et al. 1994).

Perpetuating factors:

- pathophysiological mechanisms, e.g. autonomic arousal, hyperventilation, sleep disorders, muscle tension (see Sharpe & Bass 1992)
- poor coping techniques such as avoidance (e.g. of physical activity leading to increasing fatigue) and catastrophizing

Box 16.1   ICD-10 somatoform disorders (World Health Organization 1992)
Somatization disorder
Undifferentiated somatoform disorder
Hypochondriacal disorder (includes body dysmorphic disorder)
Somatoform autonomic dysfunction
Persistent somatoform pain disorder

- iatrogenic factors – doctors' fears of missing pathology may lead to inappropriate tests and treatments
- secondary gain – disability benefits are associated with longer duration of disability
- family – can inadvertently reinforce abnormal illness behaviour
- social factors – e.g. media articles on physical causes for functional syndromes (e.g. 'candidiasis', 'total allergy syndrome'), Internet support groups.

Consequences

- Inappropriate and expensive investigations and admissions.
- Prescribed drug misuse.
- Poor doctor–patient relationship.
- Impact on family.
- Disability and loss of employment.
- Potentially harmful and inappropriate treatments.
- 'Addiction' to health care system for social support.

Management

- Make patient feel understood and engaged in treatment (see above).
- Avoid unnecessary investigations and treatment – it may help to negotiate a final test.
- Reassure patient there is no serious organic pathology – to do so it is necessary to know what the patient fears is wrong. May need to reassure that physical rehabilitation is safe.
- Explore possible mechanisms for symptoms (physiological and psychological factors).
- Treat associated psychiatric disorder, e.g. with antidepressants.
- Offer specific psychological therapies shown to be effective in randomized controlled trials:
  (a) cognitive–behavioural therapy (e.g. in chronic fatigue syndrome)
  (b) brief psychodynamic therapy (e.g. in irritable bowel syndrome)
  (c) graded exercise (e.g. in fibromyalgia).

Prognostic factors

Younger age, short duration of symptoms, employment, lack of disability payments and psychological/social attributions are associated with good prognosis.

SPECIFIC SOMATOFORM DISORDERS

Assessment, aetiological factors, general management, etc., discussed above apply here but further details are given for specific disorders.

Somatization disorder (previously known as Briquet's syndrome)

Definition

Patients experience persistent recurrent multiple physical symptoms starting in early adult life (or earlier), with a long history of unhelpful medical and/or surgical investigations and procedures and high rates of disability.

Epidemiology

Studies using DSM-III criteria have found that full somatization disorder (SD) is rare with a prevalence of less than 1%, but SD is present in 8% of new attendees in general medical clinics. 'Abridged SD' is commoner and accounts for one-quarter to one-half of new patients attending medical clinics who do not have an organic explanation for their symptoms and receive a diagnosis of a functional somatic syndrome (e.g. irritable bowel syndrome, fibromyalgia). SD is more common in women and comorbid psychiatric disorders are common, especially anxiety and depressive disorders. Over 70% of SD patients have an associated personality disorder. There is a strong association between the number of somatic symptoms and psychological distress and level of disability.

Somatoform pain disorder and chronic pain

Definition

Persistent, severe and distressing pain not fully explained by a physical disorder (note that the location of pain may not be clearly different in somatoform pain disorder (SPD) and organic disorders). Chronic pain is also often the presenting complaint in somatization disorder, other somatoform disorders and neurasthenia. Comorbid psychiatric disorder is common – depression is found in up to 45% of chronic back pain patients – but frequently unrecognized and/or untreated. Pain can lead to secondary insomnia, inactivity, pain behaviour, depression and cognitive dysfunction – *chronic pain syndrome*.

The *gate control theory of* pain is based on the concept of a 'gate' in the dorsal horn of the spinal cord where effects of afferent nerve impulses are modified by pathways from brain (Melzack & Wall 1965), incorporating the influence of psychological and physical factors.

Treatments

Operant-based behavioural and cognitive treatments (see below) may lead to sustained improvement but there is no clear evidence for long-term superiority of any one specific psychological intervention. Integrated biological and psychosocial treatment approaches are important. Cure of the pain may not be possible but restoration to normal function in spite of pain can be helpful and important to patient.

Multidisciplinary pain clinics

- Many medical specialties (anaesthetists, physicians, psychiatrists), psychologists, nurses, physiotherapists, occupational therapists, social workers, etc.
- Emphasis on reducing disability.
- Eclectic managements including exercise programmes, behavioural principles (goals, hierarchies of activities, consistent, graded exposure to activity), drugs (antidepressants can be useful in chronic pain, e.g. tricyclics for facial pain).

The psychiatrist's role in these clinics is to evaluate emotional factors and diagnose and treat associated psychiatric disorders. Multidisciplinary treatment for chronic back pain has been found to be superior to all types of control procedures (see meta-analysis by Flor et al. 1992).

Hypochondriasis

Definition

Preoccupation with the possibility of one or more serious illnesses, which persists despite medical reassurance. Hypochondriacal ideas can occur secondary to other conditions such as affective disorders and should be distinguished from primary hypochondriasis (see Table 16.1). There is a large overlap with obsessive-compulsive disorder (OCD).

Epidemiology

The prevalence of hypochondriacal concerns in community unknown. The six-month prevalence of DSM-IIIR hypochondriasis in general medical outpatients is 4–6.3% (Barsky et al. 1990).

Cognitive–behavioural model

Central feature is a tendency to misinterpret innocuous physical symptoms as evidence of serious illness with associated anxiety; anxiety leads to reassurance-seeking, avoidance, bodily checking and increased bodily focus, which in turn leads to further misinterpretation of innocuous symptoms. Hypochondriasis is also associated with faulty assumptions about health and illness.

Treatment

Treatment consists of cognitive-behavioural therapy (CBT) (see Warwick et al. 1989), involving:

- explanation of treatment rationale
- self-monitoring of symptoms, anxiety, negative thoughts, illness-related behaviour
- reattribution
- exposure and prevention of reassurance-seeking behaviour
- identification and modification of faulty assumptions.

(CBT for other somatoform disorders involves similar principles tailored for the particular central features of the disorder.)

There is some limited evidence that antidepressants can be helpful in primary hypochondriasis.

Dysmorphophobia (body dysmorphic disorder)

Dysmorphophobia is included under hypochondriacal disorder in ICD-10.

Definitions

Dysmorphophobia is an excessive concern (overvalued idea) about trivial or non-existent physical abnormalities, which are perceived to be deformities. Such concerns can occur as part of other psychiatric disorders, such as OCD, depression or schizophrenia, or may be associated with social phobia or personality disorders. Depression may be secondary to the

---

Table 16.1 Differences in diagnostic criteria and associated features between somatization disorder and hypochondriasis in ICD-10

Somatization disorder	Hypochondriasis
Emphasis is on multiple recurrent physical symptoms	Preoccupation, fear and/or belief concerning serious disease
Persistent refusal to accept advice or reassurance of several doctors that there is no physical explanation for symptoms	Number of symptoms unspecified
Symptoms not due to pathophysiologic mechanisms	Symptoms from normal sensations or minor abnormalities
Chronic (>2 years), onset usually in early adult life	Persistent, can begin at any age; rare to present for first time after 50
Much more common in females	Sex ratio equal
Familial associations reported	No familial associations
Associated with impairment of social and family functioning	Variable associated disability

Adapted from Murphy MR (1990) Classification of the somatoform disorders. In: Bass C (ed.) *Somatization: Physical Symptoms and Psychological Illness*, p. 31. With permission from Blackwell Science Ltd.

dysmorphophobia. Beliefs about deformity which are of delusional intensity are classified with delusional disorders.

Management

Management of dysmorphophobia depends on its underlying cause (see Goodacre & Mayou 1995).

- Treat associated disorder where present; assess for suicidal ideation.
- Good liaison with GP, surgeons, etc., is important to avoid unnecessary and unhelpful surgery; joint appointments may be helpful to ensure consistent advice.
- SSRIs/neuroleptics – no randomized controlled trials – case reports and open trials suggest that drugs may be helpful, particularly when there are clear symptoms of depression/delusional beliefs.
- Exposure therapy.
- Plastic surgery (follow-up studies difficult to interpret due to selection bias, but studies suggest that surgery is not always contraindicated, particularly when psychopathology is not severe and some deformity is present).

Chronic fatigue syndrome (CFS/neurasthenia/ME)

Definition

Symptoms of physical and mental fatigue and significant disability for at least six months, without identifiable organic disease. Various recent operational definitions exist, with the American Center for Disease Control (CDC) definition including the presence of four or more somatic symptoms such as sore throat, painful muscles, lymph nodes and new headaches. Excludes psychotic disorders, eating disorders or organic disorders.

Epidemiology

Fatigue is very common in the community, e.g. substantial fatigue in 38% in one survey; present for >6 months in 18% (Cox et al. 1987). The prevalence of CFS depends on definition – with rates in general adult population ranging from 0.007–2.8% (Afari & Buchwald 2003). CFS is more common in women – the relative risk for women is 1.3–1.7. White, middle-class patients are over represented in clinic samples but not in community samples. About 50–75% of patients have a lifetime history of other psychiatric disorders, particularly anxiety, depression and somatization disorder, with 25% currently fulfilling criteria.

Aetiology
Biological

- Genetic – early twin and family studies indicate a probable genetic influence, larger scale studies are needed.

- Endocrine/neurotransmitter – about one-third of CFS patients are hypocortisolaemic, this is likely to be due to abnormalities of hypothalamic-pituitary axis; the converse is found in depression. It is not clear whether this is a primary or secondary effect. Abnormalities of the serotonin system is also implicated, with CFS patients showing an increase in serum prolactin in response to serotonin agonists.
- Infection – studies to date do not confirm hypothesized link between CFS and specific infective agents. Non-specific immune dysfunction has been found but these do not relate to outcome and there are no diagnostic immunological tests.
- Physical deconditioning leads to an increase in symptoms on mild exertion which, in some, reinforces abnormal illness behaviour.

Psychological

- Illness attributions – CFS patients that believe their illness has a physical cause (e.g. a virus or pollution) have a poorer prognosis.
- Avoidance strategies are associated with a worse prognosis.

Social

- Family attitudes have been shown to reinforce poor functioning.
- Support groups – some studies have shown that membership of CFS support groups to be a poor prognostic sign.

Management

1. Graded exercise – improves fatigue and physiological outcomes in CFS patients without psychiatric disorders.
2. Cognitive–behavioural therapy involving graded exposure to activity, addressing patient's attributions of symptoms to physical disease, negative thinking and patient's unrealistic expectations – improves fatigue and level of disability.
3. Randomized controlled trials of SSRI antidepressants show no evidence of improvement of CFS, but are useful for associated depression. Monoamine oxidase inhibitors such as moclobemide and phenelzine may be more promising.

Conversion disorder

Definition

The classic definition of conversion disorder (CD) is of an alteration or loss of physical functioning suggestive of physical disorder but which is an expression of a psychological conflict or need with primary and secondary gain; symptoms are neither consciously produced nor explained by physical disorder. ICD-10 presumes CDs are 'psychogenic' in origin, but does not include concepts derived from any particular theory (such as unconscious conflicts or secondary gain). Symptoms may have an acute onset after a specific stressor. Typical symptoms are of motor or sensory loss, or 'pseudoseizures' (non-epileptic seizures).

Left-sided symptoms are over-represented, suggesting that there may be a functional disturbance of the non-dominant hemisphere.

Epidemiology

One per cent of all diagnoses in postgraduate psychiatric and neurological centres; the prevalence is higher in developing countries (Toone 1990). It is commoner in women than men. CD can be associated with organic disease. Hysterical personality disorder may be marginally over-represented, but an association between CD and hysterical personality is not inevitable.

Treatment

1. Explain to the patient that the disability is not caused by a physical lesion but that there is a block preventing the messages from the nervous system getting to the affected limb/eye/other body part.
2. Encourage normal behaviour through physiotherapy.
3. Eliminate factors that are reinforcing the symptoms.
4. Help the patient cope with any stresses that may have precipitated the disorder.
5. Treat any associated psychiatric disorder such as depression.
6. Some centres advocate the use of hypnosis as an adjunct to the above.

Prognosis

Disorders of recent onset usually recover quickly; a longer history of symptoms (>1 year) is associated with worse prognosis. Organic disease may be misdiagnosed as hysteria: Slater & Glithero's classic (1965) study found that a third of patients diagnosed with hysteria at a tertiary referral neurological hospital developed an organic illness within 7–11 years and a further third developed depression or schizophrenia. However, a more recent follow-up study of unexplained motor symptoms in the same hospital found a low incidence of physical or psychiatric diagnoses that explained patients' symptoms or disability: only 3 of 64 subjects developed neurological disorders that explained their previous symptoms; however, a high level of psychiatric comorbidity was found (Crimlisk et al. 1998). This may reflect improved diagnostic skills and better investigative techniques.

SPECIAL MEDICAL SERVICES

Specialist units in the general hospital often require specialized psychiatric services. Special links may be made between medical/surgical teams and liaison psychiatrists which help these units provide treatment more effectively. This is illustrated here by describing the role of liaison psychiatry in cancer care. The principles involved can be extended to other services such as neurology, diabetes, intensive care, plastic surgery and transplantation; though each specialty will have particular needs as demonstrated by research (e.g. see Howard & Fahy 1997 for liaison psychiatry and liver transplantation).

Psycho-oncology (see Maguire & Howell 1995)

Epidemiology

Cancer patients have a 3–4 times increased risk of psychiatric problems:

- 25–33% develop a generalized anxiety disorder, major depressive disorder or adjustment disorder within the first 2 years of diagnosis
- up to 25% have body image problems after losing a body part or its function
- 25–33% have sexual problems
- 10–40% have an acute confusional state usually due to hypercalcaemia, brain metastases, drugs or infections

Detection of these disorders is low by all hospital and primary care staff, partly due to patients not disclosing their problems and partly due to medical staff focusing on physical problems and using distancing strategies if patients try to discuss psychological issues.

There is a growing, though controversial, body of evidence that suggests that psychological factors are not only linked to quality of life but may also impact on physical outcomes, e.g. patients who score highly on helplessness and hopelessness and depression measures are more likely to relapse or die from breast cancer (Watson et al. 1999), and social support is associated with lower mortality rates in breast and prostate cancer. This research suggests that psychological coping may be important; patients should therefore be helped to find the optimum coping strategies for them, though they should not be made to feel that their behaviour/personality has contributed to their illness.

Management

Psycho-oncology services can intervene by the following:

1. Seeing referrals causing particular concern (the consultation approach discussed earlier), although relying on referrals will miss most morbidity.
2. Training and supervising specialist nurses in recognition and treatment of psychological disorders using anxiety management and cognitive–behavioural therapy (which can improve quality of life even in advanced cancers).
3. Supervising staff who run patient support groups.

4 Training doctors and nurses in cancer care to upgrade their psychological assessment skills, including breaking bad news effectively (see below).

5 Arranging screening for psychological morbidity using instruments validated in cancer patients such as the Hospital Anxiety and Depression Scale or the Rotterdam Symptom Checklist (though this should only be done where resources are available for further assessment and treatment).

Breaking bad news

Staff need to be aware of the following steps for breaking bad news:

1 Ensure a private consultation in a comfortable area with a relative or friend present.

2 Check what the patient already knows about his/her disease.

3 Find out what the patient wants to know, e.g. by using a hierarchy of terms ('serious', 'tumour', etc.) and judging the patient's response ('you tell me what to do; I'll leave the details to you', indicating patient prefers to leave it to the expert). Patients may want a limited amount of information on the first consultation but staff should state that more information is available to them if and when they want it ('If you want to know more in the future we can discuss it again then').

4 Share the appropriate amount of information with the patient, clarifying and educating without jargon, giving information in small chunks and in writing; allow pauses for assimilation and acknowledge distress, asking for key concerns and discussing them in turn.

5 Plan future consultations with the patient and summarize the present consultation.

Care of the dying and bereaved

Psychological adjustment to dying

There are several competing theories of bereavement (including psychoanalytic, stage, stress and social support theories). The stage theory is characterized as having five stages (Kubler-Ross 1970), though not all patients will pass through each stage. The stages are *denial and isolation*, *anger*, *bargaining*, *depression* and *acceptance*.

Psychiatric aspects of dying

Patients who are close to dying may fear death, though this should not be assumed and fear of becoming a burden or of pain may be more prominent. Regular talks to express fear and grief with a trusted health professional, or a prescription of diazepam to break a cycle of fear can be helpful. Adequate pain relief is also important. Psychiatric disorders such as depression or anxiety should be treated, however 'understandable' they may seem; patients with a terminal illness are at increased risk of suicide. Sedative antidepressants may be particularly helpful in patients with insomnia, and cognitive–behavioural therapy can also improve quality of life (see above under psycho-oncology). Paranoid states can be treated with low dose haloperidol and acute confusional states need assessment and management (see Chapter 26).

The psychiatrist's role is to advise the multidisciplinary team on assessment and management of the patient's and relatives' psychological needs and psychiatric complications, and support the multidisciplinary team who have to cope with their feelings of sadness and anger, which may lead to difficulties in staff interactions.

Support should be available for close relatives, when it is wanted, though the family may not be open to offers of help until after the patient has died.

The 'classic' stages of bereavement are:

- numbness (lack of emotional reactivity)
- acute 'pangs of grief' (anxiety and severe distress)
- chronic background of depressive type symptoms (restlessness, poor concentration, poor memory, loss of appetite, weight and sleep, guilt, pseudohallucinations)
- acceptance.

These stages are normal and the bereaved tend to complain more of physical symptoms than patients with depressive disorders and are less likely to feel suicidal. The professionals involved with the patient who has died should ensure transfer of care for relatives to others outside the hospital/hospice (e.g. GP or local psychiatrist when necessary) so that adjustment can be made to a life without the patient.

Bereavement and physical health

For a fuller review of bereavement see Parkes (1996). Mortality is increased in bereaved relatives, with heart disease as the most frequent cause of death. It is not clear whether this is due to increased smoking or changes in diet or may be due to emotional factors more directly affecting the cardiovascular system. Increased mortality after bereavement is also due to liver cirrhosis, accidents and suicides. Newly bereaved people, particularly those under 65, consult their doctor more frequently than they did previously, for physical and psychological symptoms, possibly due to aggravation of pre-existing conditions.

Bereavement and psychiatric disorder

Bereavement is associated with an increased risk of depression, anxiety disorders, post-traumatic stress disorders after horrific types of bereavement, and a worsening of pre-existing alcohol misuse. Risk factors for these disorders include:

- the nature of the relationship
  (a) spouse, child, loss of parent before age 20
  (b) strength and security of relationship
  (c) intensity of ambivalence

- type of death, e.g. sudden and unexpected, or violent and horrific death
- previous mental illness
- other life events around the time of the bereavement
- lack of social support
- female
- lack of religion or cultural factors influencing expression of grief.

The role of the liaison psychiatrist

1. Training of A&E staff in breaking bad news.
2. Support for staff in frequent contact with the bereaved.
3. Provision of relevant information to those in contact with bereaved, e.g. information on CRUSE (UK bereavement counselling service).
4. Appropriate treatment of patients referred with psychiatric disorder; patients avoiding grieving may benefit from 'guided mourning' (using exposure therapy), patients with chronic prolonged grief may benefit more from problem-focused therapy to promote social reintegration.

SUBSTANCE MISUSE IN THE GENERAL HOSPITAL

A more detailed account of substance misuse is given in Chapters 27 and 28. Substance misuse is included here, however, as it contributes to a large amount of the psychiatric morbidity in the general hospital. Thorough assessment and provision of services (whether advising on management of acute withdrawal, providing brief therapeutic interventions or transferring to specialized services) is a very important part of the liaison psychiatrist's job.

Epidemiology

Twenty-five per cent of male medical admissions are problem drinkers (Lloyd et al. 1982); 18.3% of 1000 attendees at an A&E department were found to have drug-related problems (Ghodse 1981).

Presentation

Alcohol has effects on many body systems. In addition to detection of alcohol misuse in patients presenting with medical problems such as gastrointestinal disorders, liver cirrhosis, etc. Psychiatrists in the general hospital need to be particularly aware of the possibility of alcohol withdrawal symptoms and full-blown delirium tremens in postoperative patients or patients admitted with medical problems a few days previously (see Chapter 26):

- *Delirium tremens* (DTs) can start after 2–3 days of abstinence from alcohol. It presents with tremor, high blood pressure, anxiety, insomnia, mild pyrexia, clouding of consciousness, illusions, hallucinations (typically small 'Lilliputian' visual hallucinations), delusions and convulsions. Cardiac arrhythmias can occur secondary to electrolyte imbalances (of sodium, potassium or magnesium).
- *Wernicke–Korsakov syndrome* is not uncommon in chronically alcohol-dependent patients who are medically unwell or detoxifying. May present with any of the following: confusion, ataxia, opthalmaplegia, nystagmus (see Chapters 26 and 27 for further details).

Management

Doctors often do not take an adequate alcohol history. Liaison psychiatrists are therefore often involved in teaching junior doctors how to take a good alcohol history and in the use of simple tools such as the CAGE screen or the Paddington Alcohol Test. Early recognition of problem drinking, with discussion and simple advice, is effective in reducing alcohol intake (Bien et al. 1993). A brief counselling intervention should therefore be pursued in problem drinkers in the general hospital and can be administered by non-mental health workers. Advice should be offered on how to change habits as well as treatment options. Liaison psychiatrists should be prepared to advise in difficult cases of alcohol withdrawal; likewise in opiate-dependent patients.

Delirium tremens is a potentially life-threatening condition and psychiatrists may be involved in its diagnosis and advice on further management. Patients should be assessed physically and mentally, with daily checks of electrolytes and for signs of associated infection such as pneumonia. It should be treated with reducing doses of benzodiazepines such as chlordiazepoxide or diazepam over a period of approximately seven days. Chlormethiazole should not be used as it can cause respiratory depression and is also more likely to be abused by patients. Withdrawal convulsions may require increases in the dose of benzodiazepine, use of intravenous diazepam and/or the addition of carbamazepine. Patients should be nursed in a well-lit room and need to be assessed for the level of supervision required: a registered mental nurse may be required to provide constant supervision.

Wernicke–Korsakov is under-recognized and under-treated in general hospitals. Parental thiamine (i.e. Pabrinex ampoules) should be used in all inpatient detoxifications and suspected cases of Wernicke's.

PHYSICAL ILLNESS IN SEVERE MENTAL ILLNESS

People with severe mental illness have increased physical morbidity and mortality, for example patients with schizophrenia have a three-fold increase in all cause mortality (Standard Mortality Rate – SMR 298), a 12-fold increase in death by unnatural cause, such as suicide (SMR 1273), and live an average of 9 to 12 years less than the general population (Brown et al. 2000). There are medical, social and behavioural reasons for this excess (Mirza & Phelan 2002):

- lifestyle factors:
  - (a) smoking
  - (b) substance misuse
  - (c) poor diet / lack of exercise
  - (d) antipsychotic medication – can cause weight gain, diabetes, cardiac arrhythmias, dystonias, lowering of seizure threshold
  - (e) risky sexual behaviours
  - (f) self-harm
- social factors:
  - (a) poverty/poor housing
  - (b) stigma.

Patients with severe mental illness often have difficulty accessing appropriate physical health care. This is due to *patient-specific* factors, such as failure to keep outpatient appointments, difficulty spontaneously reporting physical symptoms, high pain threshold, cognitive problems limiting adherence to treatment; and *system-specific* factors, such as insufficient outpatient time, emphasis on mental health problems, inadequate attention to explanation/health education, staff perception that mental health patients are difficult or cannot benefit from intervention. For example, one recent study showed that patients with schizophrenia and other serious mental illnesses were much less likely to be offered revascularization procedures for ischaemic heart disease than the general population (Lawrence et al. 2003).

Liaison psychiatrists are often involved in advising and supporting medical staff when patients with severe mental illness are admitted to hospital. Good communication between all involved teams is required.

FURTHER READING

Benjamin S, House A & Jenkins P (eds) (1994) *Liaison Psychiatry. Defining Needs and Planning Services*. London: Gaskell.
House A, Mayou R & Mallinson C (eds) (1995) *Psychiatric Aspects of Physical Disease*. London: Gaskell.
Guthrie E & Creed F (eds) (1996) *Seminars in Liaison Psychiatry*. London: Gaskell.
Mayou R, Bass C & Sharpe M (eds) (1995) *Treatment of Functional Somatic Symptoms*. Oxford: Oxford University Press
Royal College of Physicians & Royal College of Psychiatrists (2003) *The Psychological Care of Medical Patients. A Practical Guide*, 2nd edn (joint working party report). London: RCP.

REFERENCES

Afari N & Buchwald D (2003) Chronic fatigue syndrome: a review. *American Journal of Psychology* 160: 221–36.
American Psychiatric Association (1994) *Diagnostic and Statistical Manual of Mental Disorders*, 4th edn. Washington, DC: APA.
Barsky A, Wyshak G & Klerman G (1990) The prevalence of hypochondriasis in medical outpatients. *Social Psychiatry and Psychiatric Epidemiology* 25: 89–94.
Benjamin S, House A & Jenkins P (eds) (1994) *Liaison Psychiatry. Defining Needs and Planning Services*. London: Gaskell.
Bien TH, Miller WR & Tonigan JS (1993) Brief interventions for alcohol problems: a review. *Addiction* 88: 315–36.
Brown S, Inskip H & Barraclough B (2000) Causes of the excess mortality of schizophrenia. *British Journal of Psychiatry* 177: 212–17.
Bridges K & Goldberg D (1985) Somatic presentation of DSM–111 psychiatric disorders in primary care. *Journal of Psychosomatic Research* 29: 563–69.
Craig T, Drake H, Mills K & Boardman AP (1994) The South London somatisation study II: influence of stressful life events and secondary gain. *British Journal of Psychiatry* 165: 248–58.
Crimlisk HL, Bhatia K, Cope H et al. (1998) Slater revisited: 6-year follow up study of patients with medically unexplained motor symptoms. *British Medical Journal* 316(7131): 582–5.
Cox B, Blaxter M, Buckle A et al. (1987) *The Health and Lifestyle Survey*. London: Health Promotion Research Trust.
Flor H, Fydrich T & Turk DC (1992) Efficacy of multidisciplinary pain treatment centres: a meta-analytic review. *Pain* 49: 221–30.
Ghodse H (1981) Drug related problems in London accident and emergency departments: a 12-month survey. *Lancet* 1: 859–62.
Gill D & Hatcher S (2003) Antidepressants for depression in medical illness (Cochrane Review). *The Cochrane Library*, issue 3. Oxford: Update Software.
Goodacre TEE & Mayou R (1995) Dysmorphophobia in plastic surgery and its treatment. In: Mayou R, Bass C & Sharpe M (eds) *Treatment of Functional Somatic Symptoms*, pp. 231–51. Oxford: Oxford University Press.
Greer S, Moorey S, Baruch JDR et al. (1992) Adjuvant psychological therapy for patients with cancer: a prospective randomised trial. *British Medical Journal* 304: 675–80.
Guthrie E & Creed F (1994) The relevance of research. In: Benjamin S, House A & Jenkins P (eds) *Liaison Psychiatry. Defining Needs and Planning Services*, pp. 104–13. London: Gaskell.
Howard LM & Fahy T (1997) Liver transplantation for alcoholic liver disease. *British Journal of Psychiatry* 171: 497–500.
Kubler-Ross E (1970) *On Death and Dying*. London: Macmillan.
Lawrence DM, Holman CJ Jablensky AV & Hobbs MST (2003) Death rates from ischaemic heart disease in Western Australia psychiatric patients 1980–1998. *British Journal of Psychiatry* 182: 31–6.
Lipowski ZJ (1983) Current trends in consultation-liaison psychiatry. *Canadian Journal of Psychiatry* 28: 329–37.
Lloyd G, Chick J & Crombie E (1982) Screening for problem drinkers among medical in-patients. *Drug and Alcohol Dependency* 10: 355–9.
Maguire P & Howell A (1995) Improving the psychological care of cancer patients. In: House A, Mayou R & Mallinson C (eds) (1995) *Psychiatric Aspects of Physical Disease*, pp. 41–54. London: Gaskell.
Mirza I & Phelan M (2002) Managing physical illness in people with severe mental illness. *Hospital Medicine* 63: 535–9.
Melzack R & Wall P (1965) Pain mechanisms: a new theory. *Science* 50: 971–9.
Murphy MR (1990) Classification of the somatoform disorders. In: Bass C (ed.) *Somatization: Physical Symptoms and Psychological Illness*, pp. 10–39. Oxford: Blackwell Scientific Publications.
Parkes CM (1996) *Bereavement: Studies of Grief in Adult Life*, 3rd edn. London: Routledge.
Pilowsky I (1997) *Abnormal Illness Behaviour*. Chichester: Wiley.
Royal College of Physicians & Royal College of Psychiatrists (2003) *The Psychological Care of Medical Patients. A Practical Guide*, 2nd edn (joint working party report). London: RCP.
Sensky T, Cundy T, Greer S & Pettingale K (1985) Referrals to psychiatrists in a general hospital: a comparison between two methods of liaison psychiatry. *Journal of the Royal Society of Medicine* 78: 463–8.
Sharpe M & Bass C (1992) Pathophysiological mechanisms in somatisation. *International Review of Psychiatry* 4: 81–97.
Slater E & Glithero E (1965) A follow-up of patients diagnosed as suffering from hysteria. *Journal of Psychosomatic Research* 9: 9–13.
Smith GR Jr (1994) The course of somatisation and its effects on

utilisation of health care resources. *Psychosomatics* **35**: 263–7.

Swift G & Guthrie E (2003) Liaison psychiatry continues to expand: developing services in the British Isles. *Psychological Bulletin* **27**: 339–41.

Toone BK (1990) Disorders of hysterical conversion. In: Bass C (ed.) *Somatization: Physical Symptoms and Psychological Illness*, pp. 207–34. Oxford: Blackwell Scientific Publications.

Townsend E, Hawton K, Altman DG, Arensman E et al. (2001) The efficacy of problem solving treatments after deliberate self-harm: meta-analysis of randomised controlled trials with respect to depression, hopelessness and improvement in problems. *Psychological Medicine* **31**: 979–88.

Van Hemert AM, Hengeveld MW et al. (1993) Psychiatric disorders in relation to medical illness among patients of a general medical out-patient clinic. *Psychological Medicine* **23**: 167–73.

Watson M, Haviland JS, Greer S et al. (1999) Influence of psychological response on survival in breast cancer: a population-based cohort study. *Lancet* **354**: 1331–6.

Warwick H & Salkovskis PM (1989) Hypochondriasis. In: Scott J, Williams J & Beck AT (eds) *Cognitive Therapy: A Clinical Casebook*, pp. 78–102. London: Routledge.

World Health Organization (1992) *The ICD-10 Classification of Mental and Behavioural Disorders: Clinical Descriptions and Diagnostic Guidelines*. Geneva: WHO.

Eating disorders

Sarah H Majid and Janet L Treasure

OVERVIEW

The eating disorders constitute a range of illnesses characterized by abnormal eating behaviour and specific psychopathology (Box 17.1). They typically affect young women in Westernized societies and are a significant source of morbidity and mortality in this population. Approximately 3-5% of young Western women are currently thought to suffer with significant symptoms of eating disorder, and it is the third commonest chronic condition in adolescence. Currently, bulimia nervosa is the most common with around 1% of young Western women fulfilling criteria of both frequent binge eating and purging. The apparent increase in incidence since the late 1950s has been attributed to sociocultural changes in attitudes and behaviour over time. Attention has focused in particular on the media contribution to the idealization and normalization of an underweight female figure. This increase probably represents vulnerable individuals who might have developed other forms of illness such as hysterical conversion or anxiety states in a different cultural context.

ASSESSMENT OF A PATIENT WITH AN EATING DISORDER

History

History of presenting complaint

The patient should be asked about the following:

- Why seek help now and whose idea was it? Do they have misgivings about change – are there things they value about their current state of fear about weight gain?
- Concerns about current well being in following domains physical, psychological, family, social, education, career, spiritual.
- Response to prospect of weight gain.
- Current beliefs about size/shape/weight and ideal weight.

- Current weight control methods.
- Duration of recent weight loss.

The consequences of low weight include the following:

- **Physical**: starvation, tired, feeling cold, difficulty climbing stairs, dry skin, thin hair, increased body hair, oedema, constipation, giddiness, headache, amenorrhoea, reduced fertility (compensatory behaviours: sore mouth, dental erosion, haematemesis, irritable bowel, faintness, dehydration).
- **Psychological**: low mood, irritability, poor concentration, reduced enjoyment, worsening obsessionality, rituals, compulsions and disturbed sleep.
- **Social**: isolation, alienation from friends because of tiredness and avoidance due to food context.
- **Family**: parental concern/conflict/drawing together.
- **Work/school**: unable due to fatigue/poor concentration, job threatened due to time off, advantages (ballerina/model).

Pay attention to positive as well as negative sequelae from the point of view of the patient. This will help engage the patient by acknowledging his/her ambivalence about treatment, while also identifying some potentially motivating factors. It will also help clarify the patient's

Box 17.1   ICD-10 eating disorders F50
Anorexia nervosa Atypical anorexia nervosa
Bulimia nervosa Atypical bulimia nervosa (including normal weight bulimia)
Overeating associated with psychological disturbances (e.g. reaction to bereavement; excluding obesity as a cause of psychological disturbance)
Vomiting associated with psychological disturbances (including psychogenic vomiting, psychogenic hyperemesis gravidarum)
Other eating disorders (including psychogenic loss of appetite) Eating disorder, unspecified

position in the cycle of change (see motivational enhancement therapy below).

Past psychiatric history

The following details should be elicited:

- history of eating disorder
- premorbid fussy 'eating' or robust appetite, special dietary regimens, attributes to weight or size
- onset: age, contextual or precipitating factors (school, family, relationship, work)
- weight: lowest, highest, pattern and rate of fluctuation
- history of weight control methods
- physical complications
- history of comorbid psychiatric disorder such as depression, anxiety, OCD or self-harm
- previous treatments, hospital admissions, detention under mental health legislation.

Background

- Family history of traits of obesity/thinness, psychiatric illness (depression, eating disorder) or personality traits (obsessional, dependent), family dynamics (enmeshment, poor parental relations) and interpersonal style (emotionally inexpressive, critical, isolated).
- Personal history, especially childhood anxiety disorders, personality traits (obsessional, perfectionistic, rigid compliant avoidant), traumatic experiences (loss, separation, abuse), feeding difficulties, special diets.
- Physical illness, comorbidly or as a complication of low weight or weight loss methods.
- Psychosexual history including menstrual history and attitude to this.
- Occupational history: to what extent has eating behaviour interfered with occupation? Does school or sociocultural context (e.g. ballet or fashion school) perpetuate illness?

Psychological assessment instruments

- **EAT** (Eating Attitudes Test): a self-report questionnaire validated in clinical samples, though thought to have poor sensitivity and specificity in community samples (Garner et al. 1983).
- **EDI** (Eating Disorders Investigation): a self-report questionnaire incorporating factors from the EAT in addition to personality dimensions (Garner et al. 1983).
- **BITE** (Bulimic Investigatory Test, Edinburgh): a self-report questionnaire widely used for bulimic features (Henderson & Freeman 1987).
- **EDE** (Eating Disorders Examination): a structured interview to assess the psychopathology of eating disorders (Cooper et al. 1989).
- **Morgan–Russell scales**: measures outcome of anorexia nervosa in terms of physical status (weight,

menstruation) and psychological status (specific psychopathology, attitudes to shape, weight and eating, psychiatric comorbidity, psychosexual adjustment, socioeconomic adjustment and relationships within the family).

Information gathering

It may be possible to gain additional information from the patient's family regarding anorexic behaviours, weight history, premorbid personality and potential psychosocial precipitants or maintaining factors that the patient may not have linked to his or her illness. In addition this will be an important opportunity to engage the family and assess family dynamics and interpersonal style.

The general practitioner (GP) is another essential source of additional information, and is important in the support of longer-term treatment. With younger patients it may also be useful to contact the school if the family are in agreement with this.

Box 17.2   Mental state examination

Appearance: excessive clothing to keep warm or hide body

Behaviour: rapport, cooperativeness with assessment

Speech: spontaneity, rate, fluency, tonal variation

Mood: depression (biological features) anxiety/obsessions/compulsions (include exercising)/routines/rituals. Panic attacks/agraphobia, social phobia, post-traumatic stress disorder

Thought content: overvalued ideas about current body shape/weight; exclude delusions/hallucinations

Insight: attitude to assessment/treatment; recognition of difficulties consequent on low weight; recognition of advantages of low weight (inhibiting change)

Box 17.3   Physical examination

Emaciation or obesity

Skin: general pallor (conjunctiva), Raynaud's phenomena, chilblains, burns, pressure areas, petechial rash, purpura, lanugo hair, calluses on hand, signs of self-mutilation

Mouth and teeth: loss of enamel, caps, abrasions, ulcers, parotitis

Cardiovascular system: look for signs of dehydration or circulatory failure (lying/standing blood pressure, jugular venous pulse bradycardia, arrhythmia)

Neurological system: look for proximal myopathy (ability to rise from a squat) and nasal voice (loss of palatal muscle tone)

Gastrointestinal system: bowel sounds, palpable constipation

Respiratory system: chest infection

Weight (kg) and height (m): calculate body mass index (BMI) (see Table 17.1):

$$BMI = \frac{[weight]kg}{[height]m^2}$$

Table 17.1 Chart of weight thresholds

Height in metres (feet/inches)	Weight (kg)		
	Healthy range BMI 20–25	Diagnosis of anorexia nervosa BMI 17.5	Danger level BMI 13.5
1.50 (4'11")	45.0-56.3	39.4	30.4
1.52 (5'0")	46.2-57.8	40.4	31.2
1.55 (5'1")	48.1-60.1	42.0	32.4
1.57 (5'2")	49.3-61.6	43.1	33.3
1.60 (5'3")	51.2-64.0	44.8	34.6
1.62 (5'4")	52.5-65.6	46.5	35.9
1.65 (5'5")	54.5-68.1	47.6	36.8
1.68 (5'6")	56.5-70.6	49.4	38.1
1.70 (5'7")	57.8-72.3	50.6	39.0
1.73 (5'8")	69.9-74.8	52.4	40.4
1.75 (5'9")	61.3-76.6	53.6	41.3
1.78 (5'10")	63.3-79.2	55.5	42.8
1.80 (5'11")	64.8-81.0	56.7	43.7
1.83 (6'0")	67-83.7	58.6	45.2
1.85 (6'1")	68.5-85.6	59.9	46.2

Investigations

Blood tests:

- haematology/haemoglobin – normochromic normocytic anaemia, reduced white cell count reduced platelets
- erythrocyte sedimentation rate usually normal (an important test to rule out alternative diagnosis)
- urea and electrolytes (important to review regularly with refeeding or if person is in high medical risk category)
  - (a) low – potassium (anorexia nervosa with bingeing and purging behaviour); phosphate; urea (low in anorexia nervosa but raised in anorexia with bingeing and purging and dehydration)
  - (b) raised – bicarbonate; liver enzymes
- protein usually normal (can be low)
- thyroid function tests (as part of differential diagnosis), sex hormones
- urine tests – laxative screen (if required)
- electrocardiogram – if severe vomiting or purging, or if considering drugs with effect QT interval
- bone scan (for osteoporosis if duration >1 year) and relevant for management.

Box 17.4 Key points in assessment

Diagnosis

Engagement primarily with patient but also family

Clarify motivation and resistance to change

Extent of weight loss (BMI)

Physical complications (dehydration, circulatory failure, metabolic abnormalities)

Is admission required urgently for safety of patient? What is medical risk?

Comorbid physical, psychiatric illness or personality traits.

Family history and current dynamics

Psychosocial factors (especially precipitating life events)

Differential diagnosis

MEDICAL COMPLICATIONS OF CHRONIC ANOREXIA NERVOSA OR BULIMIA NERVOSA

- **Musculoskeletal**: stunted growth and osteoporosis with pathological fractures. May be irreversible if onset in early puberty. Proximal myopathy. Skin and bone collagen loss.
- **Dermatological**: dry skin, dorsal finger calluses caused by biting when inducing vomiting (Russell's sign).
- **Dental**: loss of enamel, caries, abscesses. Mainly due to vomiting, exacerbated by acidic or sugary foods grinding and overbrushing.

- **Reproductive**: loss of ovulation and amenorrhoea as a result of reduced gonadotrophin-releasing hormone, leutinizing hormone and follicle-stimulating hormone in most anorexics and 60% of bulimics. Small, multifollicular ovaries (starvation). Polystic ovaries/bulimia nervosa. If women do become pregnant they are at increased risk of miscarriage, poor fetal growth, prematurity, low birthweight and perinatal mortality, and for children, poor growth and eating disorder.
- **Cardiovascular system**: bradycardia (40 bpm). A proportion of mortality from sudden deaths is thought to result from acute dysrhythmias. May be accounted for by prolonged QT interval on ECG as well as electrolyte abnormalities (hypokalaemia, hypomagnesaemia). Suggested increased proportion of mitral valve prolapse. Clinically more common is collapse due to hypovolaemic circulatory failure (as a result of dehydration) and/or reduced sympathetic response (postural hypotension). Idiopathic oedema with refeeding, heart failure as a complication with refeeding syndrome.
- **Central nervous system**: confusion/fits/coma – low glucose or electrolyte especially phosphate abnormality as part of refeeding syndrome. Cognitive deficits in attention, concentration, memory, visuospatial analysis, new learning, judgment and problem solving. Demonstrated neuroimaging abnormalities include widened sulcal spaces, cerebroventricular enlargement and reduced size of pituitary and midbrain. These changes largely improve with weight restoration, although there may be lasting impairment of brain development if onset in adolescence or early adulthood.
- **Gastrointestinal system**: parotid enlargement, oesophagitis, gastric tears (bleeding), delayed gastric emptying, peptic ulcers, gastric dilatation, superior mesenteric artery syndrome (as part of refeeding syndrome), constipation, paralytic ileus, irritable bowel syndrome rectal prolapse.
- **Haematological**: anaemia (30%), leukopenia (30%), thrombocytopenia (rare).
- **Renal function**: prerenal failure, impaired concentrating function, hypokalaemic nephropathy, renal stones.

Important perpetuating complications

Low mood, cognitive deficits and weakness and physical illness increase sense of vulnerability and inadequacy and perpetuate the drive for control through rigorous dieting. Regression of secondary sexual characteristics and loss of libido, sexual thoughts and menstruation perpetuate the illness in cases where sexuality precipitates seemingly insurmountable anxieties. During refeeding, early fluid retention and oedema and delayed gastric emptying exacerbate fear of fatness and a sensation of bloating. Low

dietary tryptophan may alter central 5HT and maintain the illness, low oestrogen may disturb neurotransmitter function.

ANOREXIA NERVOSA

History

The earliest clinical descriptions were by Gull (1874) and Lasegue (1873) who described a disorder characterized by inexplicable severe emaciation and amenorrhoea with associated mental state disturbance that was not clearly defined. It was not until much later that the psychopathology of 'weight phobia' (Crisp 1967) or 'morbid fear of fatness' (Russell 1970) was delineated.

The first widely accepted criteria were by Russell (1970) who emphasized the core characteristic features of *behaviour* to produce weight loss, *fear* of becoming fat and *endocrine* disturbance (Box 17.5). These are reflected in the current ICD and DSM criteria (Box 17.6).

Box 17.5   Key features of anorexia nervosa
Significant weight loss
Self-induced
Fear of fatness
Amenorrhoea

Box 17.6   Diagnostic criteria
ICD-10 F50
Significant weight loss (BMI < 17.5 kg/m) or failure of weight gain
Weight loss *self-induced* by dietary restriction plus one of: vomiting/purging/excessive exercise/appetite suppressants/diuretics
Dread of fatness as an intrusive overvalued idea, and a self-imposed *low weight threshold*
Endocrine disorder with amenorrhoea/loss of sexual interest or potency (males), raised growth hormone and cortisol; reduced thyroid hormone level
DSM-IV
Refusal to maintain body weight over a minimal norm leading to body weight 15% below expected or failure to gain weight during growth
Intense fear of gaining weight or becoming fat
Disturbance in the way in which one's body weight, size or shape is experienced and undue influence of this on self-evaluation, or denial of the seriousness of the current low bodyweight
Absence of three consecutive menstrual cycles (or if periods only occur following hormones)
Restricting type: Binge/purging type: binge eating or vomiting, misuse of laxatives, diuretics, enemas engaged in regularly during this episode

A small proportion of patients deny concerns regarding weight or shape as motivating the behaviour that results in low weight. However a failure to implement weight gain after consultation can be diagnostic in such cases. More recent definitions such as 'self-imposed reduced nutrition in the context of psychosocial stress' where weight loss and self-starvation assume a psychological significance and compulsion through solving an underlying psychological problem (Szmukler & Patton 1995).

This broader definition facilitates historical and cross-cultural comparison, with the current ICD-10 (World Health Organization 1992) and DSM-IV (American Psychiatric Association 1994) diagnostic criteria reflecting the culture-specific presentation in the UK and USA (Box 17.6). For example, the group of Chinese patients described by Lee (1991) complained of abdominal discomfort after eating a small amount of food rather than a desire for thinness. Brumberg (1988) has drawn parallels between a modern anorexic's pursuit of bodily perfection through denial of appetite and self-starvation in pursuit of spiritual perfection practised by religious devotees in earlier centuries.

Research findings differentiate between anorexic patients who purely restrict food and those who engage in bingeing/purging behaviour. This bulimic subtype has a higher prevalence of other impulsive behaviours (stealing, drug abuse, suicide attempts, self-mutilation), premorbid and familial obesity and affective liability. (Such patients are classified as anorexia, binge/purge subtype rather than as bulimia nervosa if the weight loss criteria for anorexia nervosa are met.)

Other psychiatric conditions such as depression, obsessive-compulsive disorder or personality disorder may feature as comorbid or differential diagnoses. It is important to exclude anorexia as a result of delusional beliefs about food or eating occurring in the context of other delusional beliefs or hallucinatory experiences that might suggest a psychotic depression or schizophrenic illness. Somatic causes of weight loss such as Crohn's disease, a malabsorption syndrome, malignancy or other chronic debilitating illness must also be considered, either as differential or coexisting disorders.

Epidemiology

Incidence rates for anorexia nervosa, a predominantly female disorder, vary from 4 to 8 per 100 000 population per year. Prevalence rates among young women in general practice (aged 15–29 years) are approximately 0.15%. Studies focusing on females in their late teens show much higher prevalences of approximately 1%. Specific high-risk groups include dieters, dancers and models, with rates of 6.5–7% in ballet and modelling students (for review see Van Hoecken et al. 2003).

Comorbidity

Depression

Most studies have shown an increased prevalence of depression in patients with anorexia compared to controls, at presentation and at follow-up, with reported rates ranging from 36% to 68%. The diagnosis of depression at presentation is complicated by low mood, lack of energy, poor motivation, reduced enjoyment and other features of depression occurring as a consequence of low weight and improving with weight gain, rather than as an independent diagnosis. In some patients, recurrent depressive episodes can be seen to precede a relapse of anorexic behaviour.

Anxiety disorders

A number of studies suggest a high prevalence of anxiety disorders, in particular, social phobia and obsessive-compulsive disorder. The lifetime prevalence of anxiety disorder is approximately 65% with 26% obsessive-compulsive disorder and 34% social phobia. These are associated with a worse prognosis. It has been suggested that anorexia is a form of obsessive-compulsive disorder, since obsessional traits are common antecedents to illness and obsessive-compulsive disorder is more prevalent in first-degree relatives.

Personality

Cluster C (anxious) disorders are common in restrictive AN. Those with binge/purge AN have cluster B traits.

Aetiology

Genetic factors

There is now a substantial amount of evidence supporting the importance of genetic factors in the development of anorexia nervosa (Box 17.7). Family studies show an increased rate of eating disorder (5–7%) among first-degree relatives of probands with either anorexia nervosa or bulimia nervosa Studies looking at families with multiple cases of anorexia suggest that the genotype can be passed through maternal or paternal lines, that in most cases the phenotype is not expressed and that expression occurs most commonly in women and family members of the same generation, with sisters being most commonly affected. Twin studies have consistently shown a higher level of concordance in identical compared to nonidentical twins. Treasure & Holland (1989) found 66% monozygotic

Box 17.7 Aetiological factors in anorexia nervosa
Genetic (predisposing)
Family environment (maintaining)
Life events (precipitating)
Sociocultural (predisposing/maintaining)

concordance compared to 0% dizygotic concordance in a sample of 62 twins, with estimated heritability of 70%, consistent with earlier studies. This supports the model of a genetic predisposition, with exacerbation within a family environment and illness precipitated by a stressful event. Suggestions as to what might mediate the genetic vulnerability include perfectionist/compulsive personality traits; abnormalities in serotonin (5HT), noradrenaline and corticotrophin-releasing hormone (CRH) function, or a particular physiological response to starvation that maintains illness.

There has been much interest recently in linkage studies, which have found an association with chromosome 1 (Grice et al. 2002). For review of research into genetic factors see Treasure & Holland (1995). It is difficult to interpret findings from association studies with candidate genes most studies have been low-powered and not replicated.

Family factors

Since the earliest accounts of anorexia by Gull (1874) and Lasegue (1873) there has been an attempt to identify aetiological factors in the family background. Though there was early evidence for high social class as an important sociodemographic factor, this has not been supported by more recent community-based studies (Rastam & Gillberg 1991) and may reflect referral patterns to specialist centres.

A number of authors claim to have identified typical features of family functioning or parental personality, mostly based on clinical observation. Attempts to find empirical proof for such hypotheses using self-report questionnaires or observational studies have been largely unsuccessful. There is no evidence to support proposed parental stereotypes of dominant, over-involved but emotionally unavailable mothers and distant, marginal, weak fathers. Where differences between the families of anorexics and those of controls have been identified, it remains unclear whether these differences represent the effect of the illness on the family rather than an aetiological factor. More recently, family theorists have focused on understanding the features of a family as the context within which the illness has arisen and is maintained rather than the cause. This allows a therapeutic focus on identifying the features that make it hard for the anorexic patient and the family to find a solution and move on, rather than the family being a focus of blame for the patient being unwell.

Family systems theorists focus on the family as the context of the illness, and look at the constant interaction between the different components of the family system, and so cause and effect cannot be distinguished and any causality is circular. Most espouse the model of an extremely close family, with blurred intergenerational boundaries where conflict and disagreement are feared and avoided. Selvini-Palazzoli (1974) emphasized the transgenerational conflict of loyalties and the family's need to have a compliant, perfect child. Other models emphasize lack of

facilitation of the adolescent process of individuation and separation (Stierlin et al. 1985). Clinically, illness often occurs at important stages in the lifecycle for individual and family and can be seen as an attempt to negotiate its stresses and conflicts. Illness can be a way of differentiating from the family while at the same time remaining a child within it. There seem to be links in particular between onset of symptoms and lifecycle stages, which revive separation anxieties, such as entrance into secondary school, puberty, leaving home, marriage, divorce, birth and death.

Probably the best-known model is the 'psychosomatic family' developed by Minuchin et al. (1975), which suggested family characteristics of enmeshment, over-protectiveness, rigidity and lack of conflict resolution, with a physiologically vulnerable child. Illness in the child is maintained by its role as part of the family pattern of conflict avoidance (the evidence for these models has been reviewed by Eisler 1995). There is some suggestion from questionnaire-based studies of restricted communication and affective expression within the family and a dissatisfaction with the level of closeness, with feelings of both isolation and constraint. There is some support from observational studies for the importance of the level of expressed emotion in predicting response to treatment, and its change with successful family treatment. Interpersonal factors in particular family patterns may perpetuate the illness and many treatments include elements of this.

Life events

A severe and difficult life event has been reported as directly preceding the onset of illness in 76% of cases (Schmidt et al. 1993, 1997). Adverse events in the family such as death, separation, family break-up and sexual and physical abuse have been particularly investigated. There have been many studies attempting to assess child sexual abuse as a risk factor for anorexia nervosa. The reported rates vary widely and seem to be higher than in the general population, but the same as or lower than in other psychiatric populations, suggesting that this is not a specific risk factor.

Sociocultural factors

The emphasis on pursuit of thinness or dread of fatness in patients is seen as reflecting a sociocultural risk factor of less relevance in AN than BN (Klump 2003), although they may play a role in their mainstream preoccupation with female body ideals emphasizing slimness. This is supported by studies showing an increased incidence of anorexia correlating with changing cultural attitudes and behaviour. These changes have been assessed using studies of models in fashion magazines (Silverstein et al. 1986) and of beauty pageant contestants (Garner et al. 1980). Other writers have emphasized the contradictory roles for women with increasing apparent autonomy in a still patriarchal society, which are seen as underlying the drive to perfection and autonomy (Palazzoli 1974). Bruch (1978) emphasized the greater range of opportunities for young women – in particular, sexual experience – which the illness may be an attempt to manage.

Functional brain scanning has found that food cues produce abnormal activation in the orbifrontal cortex and anterior angulate and that this persists after recovery (Uher et al. 2003).

Biological models

A number of studies have demonstrated abnormalities in the hypothalamo-pituitary-gonadal (HPG) axis and the hypothalamopituitary-adrenal (HPA) axis. People with AN show raised cortisol secretion with loss of diurnal variation and reduced suppression to dexamethasone. They also show raised growth hormone level. Luteinizing hormone (LH), follicle-stimulating hormone (FSH) and oestrogen levels are reduced to infantile or prepubertal levels – reflected in amenorrhoea. Thyroid-stimulating hormone (TSH) and tri-iodothyronine (T$_3$) levels are also reduced, with a blunted TSH response to thyrotrophin-releasing hormone (TRH). These changes were initially thought to indicate primary hypothalamic dysfunction as a model for anorexia nervosa. However, these abnormalities have been replicated in healthy subjects who are starved, and most normalize when anorexic patients gain 10% weight or regain their normal weight as a result of refeeding. They are therefore understood to describe a physiological response to starvation, low bodyweight or reduced caloric intake – which in anorexia is self-induced. Some abnormalities of HPA axis persist after recovery and a neurodevelopmental model which includes abnormality within this system has been developed (Connan et al. 2003)

Similarly, many of the psychological features of AN have been described as a result of experimental semi-starvation, including tiredness, sensitivity to noise, irritability, apathy, loss of concentration, loss of libido, loss of vigilance, emotional instability, depression and reduced motor activity (see Keys et al. 1950). One biological model of anorexia is that there is abnormal regulation of appetite. Some strains of lean animal are prone to stress-related wasting, so it has been suggested that stress may trigger weight loss in those with a specific biological vulnerability. There is also starvation/exercise model of AN (*Handbook of Eating Disorders*, 2nd Edition).

Several groups have suggested that the vulnerability to develop anorexia nervosa is related to abnormal serotonin (5HT) function (Treasure & Campbell 1994). Serotonin is of particular interest because of its role in both physiological and psychological domains. It is involved in appetite and eating behaviour, and implicated in temperamental traits such as impulsivity and emotional reactivity. The 5HT system can be differentiated from a comparison group in both the acute and recovered state. This may be a trait abnormality. Treatments manipulating 5HT are thought to affect obsessionality, psychosexual function and panic symptoms as well as depression. (Bailer & Kaye 2003).

Research on gastric emptying shows that it slows under conditions of dietary restriction, resulting in a sense of fullness and prolonged satiety after only a small quantity of food. This has been postulated as a mechanism that could shift dieters into anorexia after an initial weight loss. There may be genetic variation in the degree of delay. People with anorexia experience prolonged satiety after eating compared to controls, and this seems to persist even when gastric emptying has returned to normal, suggesting a learned cognitive distortion. Those with AN and BN show a high correlation between gastric contents and 'depression' and 'fatness' scales. In addition they show a lack of correlation between 'hunger' or 'urge to eat' and gastric contents, suggesting that these are dissociated.

Components of treatment

Engagement

A stepped care approach may be used (Fig. 17.1).

Psycho-education

Psycho-education for individuals and families can be provided through literature, videos and groups and wider contact with support groups (e.g. Eating Disorders Association in the UK). These can provide important information on the consequences of anorexia, suggest treatment strategies and help reduce the anxiety, isolation and guilt that families often feel.

Medical risk monitoring/weight restoration plan

It is important to try to reach an agreement with patients on regular weight monitoring as a marker of medical risk (often done by a GP surgery practice nurse) (see www.eatingresearch.com). The goal of treatment will be a compromise between a healthy weight (BMI 20–25) and the patient's ideal. Important information to consider in setting the target weight range includes family weights, premorbid weight, weight threshold for amenorrhoea and the presence of complications such as osteoporosis. However, it is unhelpful to have prolonged arguments about weight and the focus should be on nutritional health with clear information available as to the consequences of poor nutrition. This includes a discussion about how the Mental Health Act might need to be used if it is impossible to safeguard health with out-patient care. Gradual, spaced re-feeding with a vitamin and mineral supplement should be negotiated with an explicit, plan for implementation discussed in precise detail (see www.eatingresearch.com for details).

Psychological treatments

Family treatments

Family intervention

There is limited evidence that for adolescents with anorexia nervosa family involvement improves outcome (Dare &

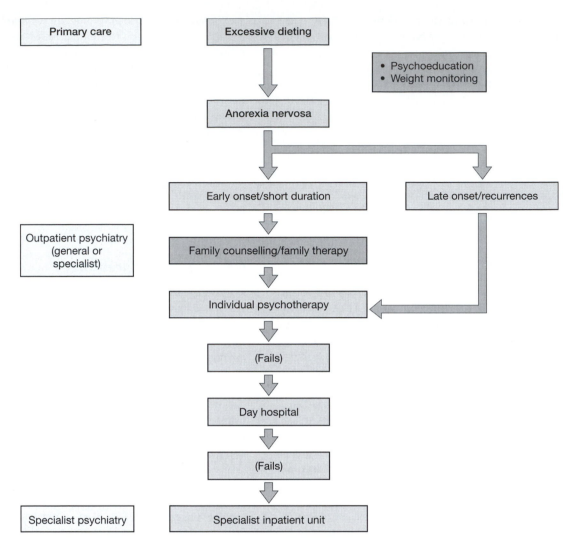

Figure 17.1 Treatment of anorexia nervosa: a stepped care approach.

Eisler 1995). The key to efficacy seems to be for parents to take control of their daughter's eating. It is seen as less important that families change, and unhelpful for families to be seen as the cause of the problem.

The effectiveness of family therapy has been studied systematically in a series of four controlled trials at the Maudsley hospital. The first compares outpatient treatments given *after* an inpatient refeeding programme (Eisler et al. 1997). This study compared one year of outpatient family therapy with one year of individual supportive therapy for 80 consecutive admissions and showed improved outcome with family therapy for patients with early onset (<19 years) and short duration (<3 years). These results at one year were confirmed at five-year follow-up. The second study of 100 severely ill patients with anorexia or bulimia seems to support the finding of a better outcome with family therapy in the early-onset group. The third study compared *family therapy* with *family counselling* for young anorexic patients

and found both interventions to be equally effective by the end of treatment. There is some suggestion that families who expressed high levels of criticism benefited more from family counselling. In family counselling, parents were seen separately. It involved giving information about the condition, problem solving, advising and helping parents to be more confident and direct in their handling of the patient's self-starvation and discussing general issues about the role of parents in relation to the adolescence of their children. This was complemented by individual sessions with the patient. Family therapy involved family systems interventions such as instructions, interpretations and facilitation of negotiations between parents and with children, designed to change aspects of overall family functioning. The interventions are conducted through direct observation of interactional processes and aim to clarify roles, establish age-appropriate hierarchies and boundaries with an adult alliance, and explore the family history to identify specific attitudes and expectations. This would involve identifying the role that the illness had come to play in the pattern of family life and trying to modify patterns that seemed to diminish the capacity of parents to be effective in challenging and restructuring their daughter's eating habits. This was done in addition to giving information and advice on the condition and on parental role, as in family counselling.

Individual therapy

Developing a therapeutic alliance: motivational enhancement therapy

One of the hardest things about working with patients with eating disorders is developing a therapeutic alliance. It is important to avoid confrontation but rather to nurture and mobilize the patient's own motivation to change. Patients often come at the insistence of their families, themselves resisting the suggestion that they have a problem and need to change. Anorexia nervosa is seen as a solution to unhappiness. The rigid adherence to weight loss is defended and attempts to increase weight are resisted as an attack on self. Sympathetic attempts to help can easily degenerate into a stalemate of angry coercion, despair, stubborn refusal or deception.

Motivational interviewing

Attempt to avoid this conflict and build a collaborative therapeutic relationship by exploring ambivalence and considering readiness to change. The therapist gives the patient the opportunity to explore things that concern her with an empathic listener and to focus on costs and benefits of change. Ambivalence is seen as understandable and justifiable and the patient is encouraged to make an informed decision about change. Persuasion and prescription are avoided. It is usually possible to find common ground in medical, social and career concerns.

It is useful to understand the patient's motivational readiness in terms of the transtheoretical model of change developed by Prochaska et al. (1994). Understanding what *stage* the patient is at in the cycle of change helps to clarify which therapeutic techniques (*processes*) will help her move forward and which ones are inappropriate because they will be met with too much resistance.

A patient pressured into treatment by her family may be in *precontemplation*. Emphasis would be on developing a rapport through empathy and reflective listening, eliciting 'good things' and 'less good things' about low weight, and giving additional information about the physical, psychological and social consequences of this if the patient seems receptive.

In *contemplation*, a patient might have a more equal balance of reasons for and against change, e.g. a fear of weight gain but a wish to stop vomiting and secrecy. Balanced feedback of this ambivalence may encourage cognitive reappraisal and a sense of self-efficacy and tip the

decisional balance towards change. It can be helpful to compare the patient's current lifestyle with that hoped for in the future.

A patient in *determination* will need help in planning a course of action to achieve change. This will involve eliciting strategies to address needs; in particular, other ways of obtaining the positive benefits of the eating behaviour. It is useful to try to imagine the future in detail and focus on the things that could get in the way of change.

In the *action* phase, the patient will need help to find specific behavioural strategies to achieve healthy eating, such as avoiding foods that trigger binges, or rewards for regular eating. She will also need to work more generally on improving social support and skills. There will still be areas of ambivalence that need continued exploration. It is useful at this stage to actively consider the worst outcome scenario of not changing.

In *maintenance* it is important to explore the patient's vulnerability to relapse, accept mistakes and minor relapse as a learning opportunity, and continue the development of specific strategies and wider social and occupational skills to prevent relapse.

The motivational approach can be used to facilitate assessment and enhance the therapeutic alliance and effectiveness of other forms of treatment. In our unit it has been formalized into four sessions of *motivational enhancement therapy* with the aid of a workbook to facilitate outpatient and inpatient engagement as a precursor to longer, more intensive forms of psychotherapy (Treasure & Ward 1997a).

Clearly this model deals largely with overt cognitions and behaviour. In some patients, particularly those with chronic illness and personality difficulties, there will be additional resistances to change such as expectations of a care-giving relationship that need to be understood more psychodynamically in terms of relationships to others, including the therapist.

Cognitive–behavioural therapy

A *behavioural* approach is useful in explaining the maintenance of illness in anorexia nervosa. Dieting is understood as a learned behaviour maintained by positive reinforcement of being thin by peers and society and negative reinforcement to avoid disapproval and ridicule of being overweight. There is additional reinforcement through the attention elicited by food-rejecting behaviour, satisfaction of feeling in control and in a conditioned pleasurable response to starvation and having an empty stomach. Slade (1982) proposed a functional analysis looking at antecedents such as difficulties in establishing independence and autonomy, interpersonal anxiety and stressful events such as failure in examinations or interpersonal relationships in the context of a perfectionist personality that needs to feel totally in control and successful in some aspect of life. In this context, a critical comment from peers or family may precipitate dieting behaviour, which is then positively and negatively reinforced and intensified (as above) with additional negative reinforcement through avoidance of the stressors that preceded onset.

The role of *cognitions* has been increasingly emphasized as mediating the external influences that drive and maintain behaviour. Distorted cognitions about bodyweight and shape are characteristic and seem to drive anorexic behaviour. Garner & Bemis (1982) proposed a cognitive–behavioural model analogous to Beck's (1976) model of depression in which the patient with anorexia has a set of underlying dysfunctional cognitions, e.g. 'I am very special if I am thin'; 'The only way I can be in control is through eating'; 'If I am not in complete control I will lose all control'; 'I have gained a pound, I won't be able to wear shorts again'; 'If I enjoy anything it will be taken away'. These are never critically or logically examined and serve to justify self-starvation. As the disorder progresses the patient becomes increasingly isolated and exposed to her own thinking, and this is exacerbated by depression, anxiety and social isolation as a result of starvation, mood-related symptoms and bingeing and vomiting. Fairburn has developed a more specific model in which control plays a key role in maintenance (Fairburn et al.1999).

Cognitive analytic therapy; There has been increasing interest in the use of cognitive analytic therapy (Ryle 1990). This is now the individual psychotherapy used primarily in our treatment centre for adults with anorexia. It shares features with cognitive–behavioural therapy, being time limited (16 or 24 sessions plus follow-up), collaborative, structured and problem orientated; it differs in that it has a greater focus on interpersonal issues. Early sessions are spent identifying *target problems* (low weight, low self-esteem, difficulty in relationships) and *target problem procedures* which maintain these. These are understood as behaviours determined by particular kinds of faulty cognitions. These are *traps* (e.g. trying to please others), *snags* (e.g. sabotaging good things, as if 'I don't deserve them/others may envy me') and *dilemmas* (e.g. either 'I spoil myself and am greedy' or 'I deny myself things and punish myself and feel miserable'; either 'I'm involved and I feel smothered' or 'I stay safely uninvolved but feel lonely and isolated'). The aim is to help the patient to recognize and revise these. They are understood as dysfunctional ways of coping with unmanageable feelings that in fact perpetuate them (*core pain*, e.g. worthlessness, fear), and as having their origins in early experience, particularly in childhood relationships to primary caregivers. These generate a blueprint of relationships to others, conceptualized in terms of *reciprocal roles* and may represent real (e.g. neglecting–neglected, controlling–compliant/ rebellious) or compensatory fantasy (e.g. perfect care–perfectly cared for) interpersonal roles. Promoting recognition and revision of this interpersonal aspect of the patient's difficulties is a crucial aspect of therapy. This includes its manifestation in the patient's relationship with the therapist, an emphasis shared with psychoanalytic psychotherapy

As in cognitive–behavioural therapy, the therapist is collaborative and explicit in his or her understanding of the patient's difficulties and potential strategies to overcome these. To assist in this, great emphasis is placed on the cognitive analytic therapy tools. These include the *reformulation letter* to the patient which communicates the therapist's understanding of target problems and procedures in the context of the patient's own history. This is reinforced by *sequential diagrammatic reformulation*, which emphasizes current procedures and the self-perpetuating way in which unhelpful cognitions are maintained through dysfunctional coping strategies and the experience of painful affect is avoided without being addressed. These underpin the active phase of therapy where a variety of techniques, including diary writing, imagery, role play, reciprocal role interpretations and cognitive–behavioural experiments, are used to promote recognition of target problem procedures and revision of behaviour through the generation of alternatives (exits). At the end of therapy the course of therapy is reviewed explicitly with the exchange of *goodbye letters* focusing on the extent to which target problems have been addressed and the difficulties that remain. In both the course of sessions and in the letters, interpersonal aspects are addressed explicitly in terms of reciprocal roles through reflection on the patient's feelings and behaviour in relation to others, including the here-and-now aspects of the relationship with the therapist (Treasure & Ward 1997b). This approach was more effective than treatment as usual (Dare 2001).

Psychoanalytic psychotherapy

Classic psychoanalysis is not generally considered to be an effective treatment for anorexia nervosa. However, psychoanalytic ideas are useful in making sense of the illness in an individual, and in understanding the difficulties experienced in working therapeutically with this patient group (see Dare & Crowther 1995 for review of psychoanalytic theories in application to eating disorder patients).

In Freudian theory, the refusal of food was understood as a symbolic repudiation of sexuality. This is echoed in more recent formulations by Crisp (1967), who emphasized the effect of starvation on reducing libido and secondary sexual characteristics. Bruch (1978, 1988) is well known for her development and modification of classic technique in extensive psychoanalytic work with eating-disordered patients. She emphasized underlying deficits in sense of self, identity and autonomy. She saw the disturbance in sexual maturation and gender identity as part of a broader maldevelopment. Rather than searching for underlying unconscious conflict, she emphasized the need to reconstruct early development and family interactions, particularly in the pre-illness period. She understood patients as suffering profound deficits in self-concept due to a paucity of consistent and continuing responses to their expression of needs in childhood, or frank disregard of these. In this sense, apparently well cared for and privileged children can be crucially deprived. The absence of regular, consistently appropriate responses to an infant's needs deprives the child of the groundwork for body identity with accurate perceptual and conceptual awareness of own body functions. Such a child grows up with little sense of his/her own needs or feelings, including hunger, and skilled at compliance with parental versions of his/her needs or wants. There has often been little encouragement of independence, so the child has a defective sense of his/her own autonomy or decision-making, tending to be obedient and over-conformist. Often the only sense of love or approval experienced is for being superior or perfect. Perfectionistic behaviour and compliance elicits approval and this pseudo-success for fake behaviour reinforces the child's fear of being spontaneous and interferes with a developing vocabulary or capacity to identify his/her own feelings. This is reassuring during childhood until adolescence, when changes in roles and expectations demand different behaviour and the preoccupation with body and weight usually begins. The increase in urges, in particular sexual, results in an over control of needs, resulting in self-starvation as a concrete solution to the control of impulses more generally. Bruch understands the illness as an attempt at self-cure, seen by the patient as a positive achievement: 'the perfect solution to deep seated unhappiness'. The rigid discipline and over control is an attempt to feel effective, the refusal to eat an attempt to be autonomous, the pursuit of perfection an attempt to mask a deep-seated conviction of worthlessness and helplessness. She sees them as at a Piagetian preconceptual phase, with a concrete expectation that interpersonal effectiveness can be established through bodily discipline.

Thus, the task of psychotherapy is to encourage the patient in her own search for autonomy and self-directed identity through developing an awareness of impulses, feelings and needs that originate from within. This is in the setting of a new interpersonal relationship where what the patient expresses and experiences is closely attended to and a subject of exploration. Resistance is inevitable in view of the denial of illness and family difficulties that defend against a deep sense of worthlessness and failure. Bruch emphasized the need to reconstruct early development, to acknowledge conceptual deficits and distortions, and correct these via a re-evaluation of family interaction. She understood family work as complementary to individual work. It is crucial that the patient be engaged as an active participant in treatment to avoid improvement being a threat to autonomy; receiving interpretations in particular could be experienced as being told what to think or feel,

confirming a sense of inadequacy and lack of trust in the patient's own psychological abilities. Modification of technique seems essential both to engage the patient in therapy and in response to the real physical danger imposed by weight loss.

This model is consistent with object relations theory (Klein 1977) in which the psychology of an individual is dominated by the way the self relates to important people in life. In the infant's earliest experience of a relationship, he/she is undifferentiated from the mother, and swings between two extreme experiences of her; as a loved and completely satisfying source of nourishment (good object) and as attacking, persecutory and hated (bad object). Developmentally, two processes are crucial. Firstly, these split experiences must be integrated so that the infant recognizes that the good mother and bad mother are one. Secondly, the infant must start to differentiate his/her own and the mother's existence as separate. Failure of these processes is associated with a continued longing for completely satisfying care from an ideal, undifferentiated other, at the same time as fearing attack, intrusion and disintegration. Primitive defence mechanisms such as splitting and projection remain prominent. *Splitting* can be seen in the idealization of the anorexic state as the perfect source of complete happiness and goodness in contrast to feared, despised and disgusting fatness. This black-and-white thinking is also evident in relation to others – in particular parents, who may be described as either wonderful and devoted or attacking and neglectful. Similarly a therapist may be idealized, and feel a pressure to collude with the expectation of perfect care from a compliant, childlike patient. This may suddenly switch when (inevitably) the therapist fails and is suddenly experienced as hateful and neglecting. Strong internal feelings of badness are disowned, externalized and attributed to the other (*projection*), who is experienced as cruel and attacking, e.g. in an attempt to feed. Extreme vulnerability and dependency may be completely *denied* with a fantasy of complete self-sufficiency, including survival with no food. Any good that is perceived within another is envied and immediately attacked (spoiling) because needing is experienced so painfully. This is apparent in the continual rejection of food or therapy as not just useless but harmful. Dependency needs may be projected onto parents who are experienced as both demanding and extremely fragile, and about whom there is often excessive concern. This may be reinforced by real parental physical or psychological vulnerabilities. The resistance against food is therefore a struggle against dependency and intrusion and the associated feelings.

These mechanisms are alive in therapeutic work with eating-disordered patients, and may be experienced and acted out in transference and counter transference. Therapists may find themselves trying to collude in the impossible task of providing ideal care. They may experience sudden switches between dealing with a compliant, helpless appealing figure who seems to want and need care and an angry, critical figure who rejects this. They may find themselves feeling helpless, useless, angry or *hungry* – identifying with projected feelings from the patient. They might even act on these feelings, angrily rejecting or coercing a patient who acts out her anger by unexpectedly missing a session or losing weight.

A series of randomized controlled trials at the Maudsley Hospital have compared psychoanalytic psychotherapy (30 individual sessions), individual supportive psychotherapy and family therapy. The most recent of these suggests a significant treatment effect with focal psychoanalytic psychotherapy compared to standard outpatient treatment over one year for adult anorexics (Dare 2001). In focal psychoanalytic psychotherapy (Malan 1979), the therapist explicitly links the patient's relationships to significant people in her past (usually family), the evolving patterns of feelings between the patient and the therapist and the function of symptoms in relationships, particularly symptoms that may help avoid interpersonal feelings and feared risks of being sexual or adult. The symptoms may feel like the only legitimate route to attention and care. The therapist helps the patient to articulate verbally and experience emotionally their bodily communications.

Pharmacological treatments

No primary role has been established for pharmacotherapy in the treatment of anorexia nervosa. Small doses of promethazone are used in patients who continue to show marked anxiety, agitation and inability to eat despite being in a supportive treatment setting. Some centres suggest the use of lorazepam before meals, particularly in the first 2–3 weeks of refeeding, but this is not widely used because of concerns regarding dependence and misuse. Non-pharmacological methods of anxiety reduction are preferable.

There has been much interest and controversy regarding the role of serotonergic-modulating antidepressant medication, since depressive symptoms are so common among anorexics. An open trial suggested that taking fluoxetine helped patients to maintain their weight over the year following admission (Kaye et al. 1997). However, controlled studies of older tricyclic antidepressants (Bierderman et al., 1985; Lacey & Crisp 1980), and more recently of specific serotonin reuptake inhibitors (SSRIs) (Athia et al. 1998), in the acute underweight state have failed to show convincing evidence of efficacy. The risk of side effects is increased due to poor nutritional state, in particular prolongation of the QT interval. Antidepressants may be helpful for patients whose depressive symptoms persist despite weight gain or where recurrent depressive episodes seem to precipitate episodes of anorexia. The requirement of normal circulating levels of oestrogens to prime 5HT

receptor sites has been implicated in this (see Mayer & Walsh 1998 for review).

In-patient treatment

In-patient care is reserved for refeeding and weight restoration in patients with dangerous medical complications or risk of suicide, or where outpatient treatment is not appropriate due to previous failure, social isolation or an intolerable family situation (Box 17.8). Admission may also be used for further assessment where comorbid symptomatology complicates the diagnosis.

A study by Crisp et al. (1991) showed little difference in global measures of improvement between patients randomly allocated to hospital admission, outpatient family and individual therapy, group therapy and a single outpatient assessment. However, the case mix included patients with a good prognosis.

Where admission is required, a specialist unit is preferable. A series of patients at the Maudsley Hospital showed average weight gain of 12.7 kg in a specialist unit, compared with 5.9 kg for the same patients' earlier admission to non-specialist units.

A *specialist nursing team* provides structure and supervision, and aims to maintain a balance between setting clear limits for behaviour and developing patients' autonomy. One of the most difficult tasks is to establish a therapeutic alliance in the face of patients' resistance to treatment and continued attempts to control weight. Primary nursing attempts to develop a trusting relationship and make treatment as collaborative as possible. In our centre motivational enhancement therapy is used to facilitate this. The team creates a ward milieu with a clear structure and rules while maintaining patient individuality. This environment is reinforced by a variety of small and large focused and unstructured groups.

Weight restoration is through regular mealtimes in a controlled environment. One model involves group meals with nurses not only as supervisors but as co-therapists to facilitate exploration of feelings provoked by eating and encourage mutual peer support of eating and challenge of anorexic behaviours. That each patient finishes her meal is seen as a group task. The repeated exposure provides a desensitization to the anxiety that patients associate with

---

Box 17.8 Reasons for admission

Dangerously low weight (BMI < 13.5) or rapid weight loss

Signs of high medical risk

Suicide risk

Failure of outpatient treatment

Comorbid psychiatric/physical illness

Electrolyte imbalance (K^+ < 2.5), hypoglycaemia, severe anaemia or thrombocytopenia, syncope, proximal myopathy

Inadequate support for treatment in community due to social isolation or family features

eating. Weight gain can be positively reinforced through rewards such as an increased range of activities or time off the ward.

Weight gain should be gradual at first and at a controlled rate to reduce patient anxiety and potential physical complications of refeeding. Initially a soft diet is given and is gradually increased in quantity, with the aim of providing 3000 kcal/day and a weight gain of 1–2 kg/week. It is important that patients are aware of the presence of a *target weight range* that their weight will not exceed. This usually encompasses premorbid weight, defined as weight held in late adolescence before onset of illness. If onset preceded this, use BMI 20–22 kg/m². Other important information to consider includes family weights, weight threshold for amenorrhoea and the presence of complications such as osteoporosis. Pelvic ultrasonography is probably the best indicator of weight required for full endocrine recovery (Treasure 1988).

Medical complications associated with refeeding include rebound fluid retention and oedema, especially if the patient has a history of laxative abuse. Limb elevation and salt avoidance may help. Hypophosphataemia may result from a sudden increase in metabolic demands. Rarely there is acute gastric dilatation with vomiting, and abdominal pain and distension (this may progress to perforation).

A *multidisciplinary approach* is essential, with good communication between members of the team to avoid splitting and provide a coherent framework of care. Individual, group and family work may be done by various members of the team. Clinical psychologists may work particularly with patients with marked phobic or obsessive-compulsive symptoms, or features of post-traumatic stress. Occupational therapy is useful to facilitate self-expression and self-awareness (e.g. through projective art), to guide healthy exercise and relaxation, to assist in career planning and retraining and to teach meal planning and cooking. This will complement individual and group work by a dietitian. A social worker is particularly useful in preparing patients for reintegration into the community after discharge (appropriate accommodation, support) and may also do family or individual work that can continue after discharge.

Discharge planning

Relapse after discharge is common, with 48% of patients readmitted at least once in a 5-year follow-up of 112 patients (McKenzie & Joyce 1992). Much of the current emphasis on a collaborative approach to weight gain and engaging the patient and family in treatment is with a view to reducing relapse and sustaining weight gain longer term in the community. It is important to plan discharge in careful coordination with the family GP and community mental health team. This will require continuing psychological support or therapy, an arrangement for regular weight monitoring and a management plan for response to any deterioration in weight or mental state. This is best coordinated through an allocated key worker as part of the *care programme approach*.

Compulsory treatment

Compulsory detention and treatment of anorexia nervosa patients is a controversial area. Coercive treatment practices used in the past have been publicized by patients and their families, and considered both abusive and ineffective. Compulsory measures are not usually necessary, and may be counterproductive to the long-term aim of improving the patient's autonomy. However, it remains appropriate to consider these in cases where physical and psychiatric consequences are life-threatening. They may also be used to prevent irreversible stunting of growth and skeletal development. The decision should be made in close consultation with the family – parents are particularly concerned that their relationship with their daughter will be damaged irrevocably by their agreement. This fear does not seem to be borne out by clinical experience. In our unit approximately 10% of inpatients are detained and treated compulsorily.

For children under the age of 18, parents may provide consent to treatment in opposition to the child's wishes by the execution of parental responsibility as defined in the Children's Act, 1989. For adults, anorexia as a mental disorder defined in ICD-10 falls, in the UK, under the remit of the Mental Health Act, 1983.

Consent to proposed treatment should always be sought. However, it is considered that the capacity to make an informed choice may be compromised by features of the illness, in particular fears of obesity or denial of the consequences of weight loss strategies. This may be the case despite the preserved intellectual capacity to understand the nature, purpose and effect of treatment (Law Commission 1993).

The UK Mental Health Act allows only medical treatment for the mental disorder to be provided compulsorily, and an important issue has been whether this includes compulsory feeding. Following a House of Lords ruling that feeding a patient by artificial means can constitute medical treatment, nasogastric feeding has been accepted by the courts as a medical process, and as forming an integral part of the treatment for anorexia nervosa. Measures to achieve steady weight gain are considered justified as a prerequisite for psychological treatments (see Riverside Health NHS Trust v Fox 1994). However it is important to note that it is unusual to require 'forced' feeding measures. Most patients adhere to the usual therapeutic measures within the group programme.

Compulsory treatment should include exposure to a specialist therapeutic milieu with nursing and rehabilitation under medical supervision. This might include a behavioural programme to help the patient overcome compulsive food refusal. In such an environment less than

1% of patients require tube feeding. (For a more detailed discussion see Mental Health Act Commission 1997; Treasure & Ramsay 1997.)

Prognosis

The Maudsley study followed up patients for 20 years and reported good outcome in 30%, intermediate outcome in 32.5%, and poor outcome in 37.5% and a mortality rate of 17.5% (Ratnasuriya et al. 1991). This supports results of an earlier Swedish study, in which 29% of patients recovered in 3 years, 35% in 3–6 years, and mortality after 33 years (mean) was 18% (Theander 1985).

The standardized mortality rate for anorexics is six times that of the general population and increases dramatically with weight loss (especially if <35 kg). The commonest causes of death are suicide and ventricular arrhythmias (Beaumont et al. 1993). There is a high level of morbidity as a result of weight-related physical complications. In a study of 103 patients over 12 years, 15% died as a result of suicide, infection, gastrointestinal complications and severe emaciation. Of the survivors, 35% had medical complications; the most severe disability was due to osteoporosis with multiple fractures and terminal renal failure (Herzog et al. 1992) (Box 17.9).

Box 17.9 Poor prognostic indicators
Illness-related
Long duration of treatment-resistant illness (>10 years)
Low minimum weight or on admission (<85% ABW)
Late onset (>15 years)
Bulimic behaviour
Premorbid
Personality difficulties
Social or occupational difficulties
Poor relationship with family
Preceding anxiety disorder

BULIMIA NERVOSA

The syndrome of bulimia nervosa was first described by Russell in 1979, as representing a variant of anorexia nervosa (Box 17.10). Subjects are similarly preoccupied with food and a fear of fatness, usually with a sharply defined, abnormally low weight threshold. Bulimia refers to episodes of *uncontrolled excessive eating* or 'binges'. These must be of

Box 17.10 Key features of bulimia nervosa
Binges
Weight control behaviours
Fear of fatness

objectively large amounts (i.e. more than 1000 calories) and occur with a *subjective* sense of *lack of control*. This is accompanied by behaviours to avoid weight gain, similar to those used in anorexia. Subjects are usually of low weight (although severely underweight patients are considered anorexic, if the criteria are met). Patients of normal weight are currently classified in ICD-10 under atypical bulimia nervosa (Box 17.11). Research findings increasingly discriminate between anorexia and bulimia in terms of aetiology, comorbidity and treatment response, so it is increasingly thought of as a separate illness. More recently there has been interest in *binge eating disorder*, which is differentiated from bulimia nervosa by the absence of compensatory behaviours.

Historical accounts of fear of fatness accompanied by alternations between episodic gorging and severe restriction were described earlier this century by Binswanger (1959) and Wulff (1932). Brusset & Jeammet (1971) described bulimic episodes developing later in the course of anorexia. Since the delineation of bulimia nervosa as a clinical category in the late 1970s, there seems to have been a real increase in its incidence, such that cases now exceed those of anorexia in number (Kendler et al. 1991, Lucas & Soundy 1993).

Onset typically occurs following weight loss, usually as a result of strict dieting, though sometimes due to physical illness. One-third of bulimic women have a history of anorexia and another one-third have a history of obesity. Occasionally bulimia nervosa develops in the context of exaggerated fears of food allergies or religious beliefs about the value of fasting.

Self-worth is typically defined in terms of dietary or weight and shape goals. This intense preoccupation may

Box 17.11 Diagnostic criteria for bulimia nervosa
DSM-IV
Recurrent episodes of binge eating (i) large amounts of food in 2 hours (ii) loss of control
Recurrent inappropriate compensatory behaviour
Self-induced vomiting/fasting/excess exercise/misuse of laxatives, enemas or diuretics
Average frequency of binges or compensatory behaviour at least 2 per week for 3 months
Self-evaluation is unduly influenced by body weight or shape
The disturbance does not occur exclusively during episodes of anorexia
Specify type based on current episode: purging/non-purging
ICD-10
Episodes of overeating (large amounts of food consumed in a short period of time) Persistent preoccupation with eating and food craving
Methods to counteract weight gain (at least one of): vomiting/laxatives/fasting/appetite suppressants, metabolic stimulants, diuretics
Morbid fear of fatness with sharply defined abnormally low weight threshold

involve continual calorie counting and frequent weighing throughout the day. Episodes of binge eating are a physiological response to sustained under-eating. Specific binges are often precipitated by feelings of anxiety, loneliness, depression and boredom, or by violations of self-imposed dietary rules. Binges are often experienced as shameful, and kept secret. They exacerbate low self-esteem, self-disgust and self-loathing and reinforce efforts not to eat. Sufferers often find it increasingly hard to eat at all in the presence of others.

The differential diagnosis includes personality disorder, depressive disorder and upper gastrointestinal disorder with recurrent vomiting (characteristic psychopathology absent). These may also coexist.

Epidemiology

Bulimic symptoms are relatively common in the population, and tend to be overrated by self-report questionnaires. Ninety percent of sufferers are female, with similar high-risk groups as for anorexia. Bulimia nervosa tends to have a later age of onset, typically 18 years. The fluctuating course of the illness and varying definitions used in studies make it difficult to achieve a consensus on its incidence and prevalence. Incidence rates of 10–13 per 100 000 per year have been reported in GP settings. The incidence in young women is 52 per 10 000 per year. In the UK the incidence of cases presenting to primary care increased three-fold between 1988 and 1993 (Hoek 1991, Turnbull et al. 1996). The incidence seems to be highest in large cities, intermediate in urbanized areas and lowest in rural areas (Hoek 1995).

The prevalence of bulimia nervosa in Western women is approximately 1–3% (Fairburn & Beglin 1990, Hoek 1991). This rises to over 5% if partial syndromes are included. GPs seem to detect only about 12–15% of cases (Whitehouse et al. 1992). See Van Hoeken et al. 2003 for review of epidemiology.

Comorbidity

Depression is more commonly found in people with bulimia than those with anorexia, with 43% of Russell's original group of 30 meeting criteria. Other studies suggest that at the time of treatment, one-third to one-half will meet criteria for major depression, and one-half to two-thirds will ultimately develop major depression, with lifetime rates reported at 36–70% (Bulik et al. 1996, Herzog et al. 1996). Onset may precede, succeed or be simultaneous, suggesting that neither is purely a secondary phenomenon of the other.

There are also high rates of anxiety disorder (36–64%), in particular, phobia and panic disorder. Post-traumatic stress disorder is common, with a lifetime prevalence rate of 37% reported (Dansky et al. 1997).

Comorbid personality disorder is common (see Herzog et al. 1996 for review). DSM-IV cluster B and cluster C (anxious) disorders have both been reported, with rates of about 30% (Braun et al. 1994).

In some patients, bulimia is one of a variety of impulsive behaviours occurring in association with borderline personality traits or disorder. Deliberate self-harm occurs in a substantial proportion: 18–23% report having taken an overdose and 15–26% report cutting or burning themselves (Favaro & Santonastaso 1997; Welch & Fairburn 1996a). Alcohol and substance misuse seem to be common in clinical samples (42-47%) (Bulik et al. 1997, Lilenfeld et al. 1997), though this is not supported by studies based on community samples (Welch & Fairburn 1996b). Approximately half of clinical samples report stealing. Lacey (1993) has described a subgroup of patients with 'multi-impulsive bulimia nervosa' with high rates of excess alcohol consumption (22%), drug abuse (28%), stealing (21%), overdose (18%), self-cutting (15%) and sexual disinhibition (37%).

Aetiology

Genetic factors

There is an increased rate of eating disorder among the families of patients with both bulimia and anorexia. Bulimia nervosa is more common than anorexia in the families of probands with bulimia, and there are also increased rates of obesity and unspecified eating disorder. Family studies report that first-degree relatives of individuals with bulimia nervosa have a raised lifetime risk of developing an eating disorder (3.4–19.8%), affective disorder (9–37%), substance misuse disorder (8–40%) and DSM-IV cluster B personality disorder (12%) (Lilenfeld et al. 1998). There may be a shared liability with phobia and panic disorder (Kendler et al. 1995). Twin studies show concordance rates that exceed the population risk, supporting the importance of family factors. Linkage of bulimia with chromosome 10 has been implicated (Bulik et al. 2003).

The genetic factors of bulimia may include a shared liability with substance abuse, obesity, anxiety disorders and affective disorder.

Family factors

A family environment where other members diet or make critical comments about weight, shape and eating increases the risk of developing bulimia nervosa. Adverse experiences in childhood (physical and sexual abuse increase the risk). Parental depression and obesity may contribute environmentally as well as genetically. Parents of eating-disordered patients tend to have a history themselves of weight problems or high preoccupation with food (Fairburn et al. 1997).

Life events

Severe life events precipitate the onset of bulimia nervosa in approximately 70% of cases (Schmidt et al. 1997, Welch et al. 1997).

Psychological factors

Childhood risk factors include negative self-evaluation, shyness, absence from school due to anxiety, lack of friends (Fairburn et al. 1997) feelings of helplessness, and pica and problem meals (Marchi & Cohen 1990).

Underlying personality traits thought to increase the risk for the development of bulimia nervosa include perfectionism (Fairburn et al. 1997), impulsivity and mood liability, thrill seeking, excitability and marked dysphoria in response to rejection or non-reward, and a coping style characterized by ruminations.

Specific episodes of bulimic behaviour seem to be associated with negative emotional states and threats to self-esteem. Individuals with bulimia nervosa seem to have an attentional bias towards these. Bingeing, vomiting and purging may reduce awareness of or distract attention from intolerable emotional states.

Sociocultural factors

The high value placed on slimness in Western culture (Keel & Klump 2003; Nasser 1997), reflected in the high prevalence of dieting, is thought to be an important aetiological factor. There is an increased risk in groups under particularly strong pressure to be slim such as female dancers and models (Hamilton et al. 1985) and male performers and sportsmen like jockeys and wrestlers (King & Mezey 1987).

In most cases, dieting precedes bingeing (Bulik et al. 1997) and increases the risk of bulimia nervosa eight-fold (Patton et al. 1999). This may be mediated through cognitive and neurobiological factors.

A number of studies show that bulimia nervosa is more common in immigrant populations living in Westernized society, compared with indigenous populations. Nasser (1986) studied female Arab undergraduates and found increased rates in London compared with those in Cairo. A study of Asian schoolgirls aged 14–16 found a prevalence of 3.4% in Bradford, UK ($n = 204$) compared with 0.6% in the indigenous sample ($n = 355$) (Mumford et al. 1991). This suggests the influence of adopted Western cultural norms either as aetiological factors or as a means of expressing distress. It could also reflect the stress of acculturation increasing psychiatric morbidity more generally (see Mumford 1993 for review).

Biological models

An animal model for BN has been developed by exposing rats to repeated stress and food restriction (Hagan et al. 2003). As for anorexia, neurobiological studies are complicated by the difficulty of assessing which abnormalities predate the symptoms and which are the result of the disorder. Dieting itself may contribute to neurobiological disturbances. Central monoamine pathways, in particular 5HT pathways, have been implicated in the control of feeding behaviour and satiety mechanisms. It has been suggested that 5HT has an inhibitory effect on feeding behaviour and that decreased 5HT function may account for abnormal eating patterns in bulimia nervosa. Several studies show lowered central 5HT in bulimic women (Jimerson et al. 1997). Following recovery there are abnormal levels of 5H2A receptors within the orbito-frontal cortex. It is uncertain whether this is vulnerability trait or a scar from the illness (Kaye et al. 2001). Research has also focused on the role of noradrenaline, endogenous opiates and neuropeptides (such as peptide YY) in the causation or maintenance of bulimia (see Mayer & Walsh 1998 for review).

Peripherally, cholecystokinin is an important satiety signal. In bulimia nervosa, a blunted postprandial cholecystokinin release has been found to lead to impaired satiety, and may maintain the disorder (Devlin et al. 1997).

Neuroimaging studies have shown as in sulcal AN widening and decreased pituitary size. People with BN activate the orbitofrontal cortex when exposed to food cues/similar to people.

Treatment

A stepped care approach may be used as with anorexia:

- *Primary care:*
  (a) self-help manual
  (b) GP/guided selfcare
  (c) psycho-education
- *Outpatient psychiatric treatment:*
- General psychiatry:
  (a) antidepressant medication
  (b) group psychotherapy
- *Specialist unit:*
  (a) individual psychotherapy – motivational enhancement therapy; cognitive–behavioural therapy; interpersonal therapy; cognitive analytic therapy
  (b) group psychotherapy
  (c) daypatient/inpatient care.

Psycho-education

Patients can be provided with information about the following:

- Cultural expectations about food and weight control that affect motivational and behavioural aspects of appetite.
- Biology of weight regulation. Physiological adaptation attempts to maintain weight around a set point. Individual constitutional variability in absolute value of 'healthy weight'.
- Biology and psychology of food intake.
- Weight control methods become perpetuating.
- Strict dieting and starvation leads to preoccupation with food, carbohydrate and strong physiological drive to binge.
- Regular eating will reduce the urge to binge.

- Vomiting reduces tolerance to food in the stomach and reduces the motivation to stop bingeing. Physiological consequences include electrolyte abnormalities, bleeding throat, swollen parotid glands and stomach complications.
- Laxatives and diuretics do not help with weight loss since they alter the body's absorption of water, not food. Physiological consequences such as dehydration, electrolyte abnormalities, bloating and constipation can occur when they are stopped until the digestive system recovers.
- Information on medical consequences of weight loss and weight control methods.

Self-help manuals

Self-help manuals have been shown to be helpful in 20% of patients but may be better with some degree of additional input – for example:

- *Bulimia Nervosa: A Guide to Recovery* (Cooper 1993).
- *Getting Better Bit(e) by Bit(e)* (Schmidt & Treasure 1993).
- *Overcoming Binge Eating* (Fairburn 1995).

Psychological treatments

Individual psychotherapy
Cognitive–behavioural therapy

There has been a growing interest in cognitive–behavioural models of bulimia nervosa, and cognitive–behavioural therapy has been claimed to be the treatment of choice either as an individual or group treatment. Most models emphasize distorted cognitions and dysfunctional assumptions about self-esteem and body shape that predispose to and maintain a cycle of restriction-binge eating-purging behaviour (Fig. 17.2, Box 17.12). Therapy aims to both interrupt the behavioural cycle and help alter the basic assumptions that underlie the body disparagement and need to diet. Therapy is aimed at recognizing the pattern and questioning the validity and inevitability of perpetuating cognitions and behaviours, and encouraging the consideration and practice of alternative ones so that the perpetuating cycle is interrupted. There is some evidence to support predominant cognitive distortions, dysfunctional assumptions and differential processing of information relevant to food and eating in bulimic patients (e.g. they seem to evaluate themselves more negatively following an experience of failure and are more prone to rigid and perfectionistic distortions). There are limitations to the model, in particular in explaining aetiology. However, it is useful in accounting for how proximal factors lead to certain behaviours, how these are maintained and strengthened, and in generating effective strategies of intervention.

Cognitive–behavioural therapy for bulimia nervosa requires adaptation of the standard model by an experienced therapist. A typical treatment will be 20 sessions plus follow-up. The approach is problem orientated and collaborative with explicit questioning and scientific testing of the

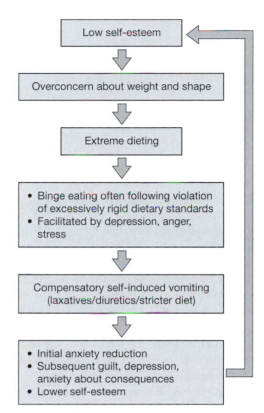

Figure 17.2 Model for bulimia nervosa (from Fairburn C, Cooper Z & Cooper PJ (1986) The clinical features and maintenance of bulimia nervosa. In: Brownell KD & Foreyt J (eds) *Handbook of Eating Disorders. Physiology, Psychology and Treatment*. New York: Basic Books).

Box 17.12 Examples of abnormal cognitions in bulimia nervosa

Selective abstraction: selecting out small parts of a situation while ignoring other evidence, and coming to conclusions on that basis, e.g. 'The only way I can succeed is to control my weight'; 'The only way I can be in control is through eating.'

Dichotomous reasoning: thinking in terms of extremes and absolutes, e.g. 'If I eat any chocolate then I have failed and may as well eat three bars'; 'If I am not in control then I will lose all control'; 'If I put on one pound, I'll go on and put on enormous weight.'

Overgeneralization: deriving a rule from one event and applying it to other situations or events, e.g. 'I was unhappy before I went on a diet'; 'If I stop I will be unhappy again'; 'I failed last night so I'll fail today as well.'

Magnification, e.g. 'I have gained a pound so I won't be able to wear shorts again.'

Superstitious thinking: assuming causal relationships between unrelated things, e.g. 'If I weigh eight stone I am happy. My day is ruined if I weigh eight stone one pound'; 'If I eat this it will be converted into fat immediately.'

Personalization: interpreting events in a self-centred way, e.g. 'What will people think if they see me eating this'; 'They were laughing. I'm sure they were laughing at me.'

patient's beliefs with a view to changing behaviour. There is a large psycho-educational component. CBT produces its effect quickly where as interpersonal therapy takes longer to be effective (Agras 2000).

Breaking the cycle of behaviour involves:

- diary-keeping to facilitate self-monitoring
- recognizing the vicious cycle of dieting and bingeing
- understanding how weight control methods perpetuate this cycle
- steps towards normal controlled eating, aiming at three meals and two snacks per day.

Cognitive restructuring techniques involve explaining and facilitating recognition of automatic thoughts and their effect on mood and behaviour; helping the patient challenge these through socratic questioning of evidence, generation of alternative views, consideration of effects of these, type of thinking error, and potential action to test validity or change situation; and looking for basic assumptions or schemata. These tend to cluster around themes such as control, perfectionism, self-indulgence, weakness and guilt. They are often conditional (because x then y) and may be amenable to evidential challenge or countering by self-coping statements to reduce impact. Deeper schemata may be unconditional and result from maladaptive response patterns learned in early childhood to cope in difficult situations and avoid cognitive dissonance. 'I'm bad, I'm unlovable, I'm a failure.' These will usually require longer-term therapy to address.

Strategies for *relapse prevention* are learned during therapy and may be applied if eating deteriorates or there is risk of relapse due to stress (e.g. diary-keeping, meal planning, planning alternative activities at high-risk times, eating in company, reducing food stocks, reducing excessive weighing, exercising rather than restricting food intake, confiding in others and problem solving), with an emphasis on self-help throughout.

Interpersonal therapy

Interpersonal therapy is a short-term focal psychotherapy, originally developed for treating depression, in which the goal is to help patients identify and modify current interpersonal problems. Treatment is non-interpretive, non-directive, time-limited individual therapy with 15-20 50-minute sessions over 4–5 months. It has been adapted for treatment of bulimia nervosa by Fairburn and colleagues (Fairburn et al. 1993, 1995).

The first stage of treatment consists of *assessment*. It involves explicit discussion of the rationale and method, identification of current interpersonal problems and choosing which to focus on for treatment. Interpersonal problems are understood as predisposing, precipitating and maintaining bulimic behaviour. It is useful to create a life chart integrating the patient's eating and weight history, significant life events, fluctuations in self-esteem and depression and history of interpersonal functioning. Current interpersonal functioning (family, friends, work, partner) and specific precipitants of bulimic episodes are explored. Interpersonal problems are classified into grief, role disputes, role transitions or interpersonal deficits.

The second stage of treatment is largely *patient led*. The therapist is active in encouraging the patient to further explore problem areas and make attempts to change. This helps the patient to remain focused, summarizes and reviews progress and continues to stress the need to change, without making specific recommendations. There is little direct focus on the eating problem – this is seen as a distraction from interpersonal issues. There is rarely any discussion of the patient–therapist relationship.

The third stage involves *review of treatment and progress*, prediction of areas of future difficulty, discussion of how the patient will manage signs of deterioration and discussion of the ending of treatment.

Trials comparing the efficacy of focal interpersonal therapy with cognitive–behavioural therapy and behavioural therapy provide empirical evidence for its usefulness. Improvement is less rapid than with cognitive–behavioural therapy; however, these changes continue after treatment: at 6-year follow-up only 28% of those receiving interpersonal therapy still had an eating disorder, compared with 37% of those receiving cognitive–behavioural therapy and 86% of those receiving behavioural therapy (Fairburn et al. 1986, 1993, 1995). Until further research is available, interpersonal therapy is reserved for use with patients who are unwilling to engage in cognitive–behavioural therapy, or in whom this has been unsuccessful. Further ongoing trials may clarify whether it is preferable to cognitive–behavioural therapy for particular patient groups.

Family therapy

The role of family therapy for people with bulimia is less established than for anorexics. The first Maudsley study showed better outcome at five years in patients who received individual supportive therapy rather than family work, but these results do not seem to be replicated in the second study. There is some suggestion that family therapy is effective for adolescent patients.

Pharmacological treatments

Sedative medication is best avoided due to the high risk of dependency. It is important to help patients find alternative ways of coping with acute anxiety, which may trigger episodes of binge eating or vomiting.

Interest in the use of antidepressant medication has been encouraged by the association with depression both in patients with bulimia nervosa and their families, and by studies implicating 5HT pathways in the control of feeding and satiety. Several trials have demonstrated improvement in the frequency of both binge eating and vomiting with tricyclic antidepressants. However, these have been mainly short-term effects with high rates of relapse after initial improvement and cessation of treatment. This is compounded by poor compliance due to side-effects (weight gain in particular), and high dropout rates.

Mitchell et al. (1990) randomized 171 women and compared treatments with antidepressant alone and combined with group cognitive therapy and placebo. They found a 64% reduction in the frequency of binge eating episodes by imipramine over 12 weeks compared to placebo. However, imipramine did not add to or exceed the marked improvement in response to intensive group therapy, where there was a 90% reduction in binge eating and 51% of patients were free of bulimic symptoms by the end of treatment.

An 8-week trial of 387 women by the Bulimia Nervosa Collaborative Study Group (1992) demonstrated the benefit of fluoxetine in reducing the frequency of binge eating and vomiting and suggested that it was most effective when used in higher doses than for depression (e.g. 60 mg/day). Associated features such as depression, carbohydrate craving and pathological eating attitudes also improved significantly. Predictors of drug response were not identified and in particular, baseline severity of depression was not specifically associated with a response. Unfortunately there are no long-term data available. The high dose should be used with caution due to increased side-effects. Fluoxetine is usually used in patients who have failed to respond to psychotherapy or who are difficult to engage in this, or where there are marked symptoms of anxiety or depression. It should be given for at least eight weeks and usually continued for six months.

Inpatient treatment

This is used rarely, but sometimes indicated in multi-impulsive bulimia nervosa, particularly if there is a risk of self-harm or if outpatient care has failed. A clear contract is needed from the outset, particularly with regard to the management of impulsive behaviours. Some patients, however, may get worse in this setting and a brief admission may be used to gain a thorough assessment and engage in treatment with a view to continuing therapy as an outpatient.

Prognosis

Without treatment the disorder seems to be chronic and fluctuating (Herzog et al. 1991). Of those receiving treatment, 50–70% are symptom-free after 5–10 years while 9–20% still meet criteria for bulimia nervosa and 3–4% develop anorexia nervosa. Approximately 30% will have residual symptoms and may develop milder eating disorders such as binge eating disorder or obesity. Mortality is 0.3–1.1% (Collins & King 1994, Fairburn et al. 1995; Fichter

---

Box 17.13   Poor prognostic indicators in bulimia nervosa
Illness related
Greater severity of bulimic symptoms
Comorbid depression
Multi-impulsive behaviour
Low self-esteem
Premorbid
Personality disorder
Obesity
Discordant family environment

& Quadfleig 1997, Keel & Mitchell 1997) (Box 17.13). Even with successful treatment, one-third of patients experience relapse during the first four years, though the risk of this declines subsequently.

OTHER EATING DISORDERS

Psychogenic vomiting

Psychogenic vomiting consists of chronic and episodic vomiting after meals in the absence of nausea. It occurs more commonly in women in early or middle adult life. In ICD-10 this is classified under vomiting associated with psychological disturbances. Repeated vomiting may also occur in dissociative and hypochondriacal disorders and in pregnancy (psychogenic hyperemesis gravidarum).

Binge eating disorder

This consists of recurrent episodes of binge eating in the absence of the regular inappropriate compensatory behaviours and the over concern about weight and shape that are characteristic of bulimia nervosa. In DSM-IV it is classified under eating disorder not otherwise specified, and in ICD-10, under atypical bulimia nervosa. There has been increasing interest in this as a specific diagnostic category, with criteria proposed by Spitzer et al. (1992). Further empirical evidence is required to establish this. There seems to be an inability to regulate eating both within and between binges, and these are less discreet – for example, lasting all day or occurring towards the end of a regular meal. Most patients are overweight and one-third of patients seeking treatment for obesity have binge eating disorder. Most report intense body disparagement and self-consciousness and want to lose weight, although they seem comfortable with aiming at a roughly average weight and do not seem to have overvalued ideas of thinness. There is a strong association with clinical depression, with over 50% having a lifetime history. There is some evidence that cognitive–behavioural therapy, interpersonal therapy and antidepressants are useful treatments. In addition to modifying maladaptive thoughts about dieting, shape and weight and promoting a normal eating pattern, there is an emphasis on weight loss through exercise and caloric restriction. Patients seem to be helped by weight loss alone. In contrast to bulimia nervosa, this seems to improve binge eating and mood through reinforcing feelings of self-control (Marcus 1997).

Eating disorders in men

Eating disorders in males are not rare, although much less common than in females. There is little research in this area, though it is a growing area of interest. Sex differences in the self-reporting of behaviour and treatment seeking may lead to differential detection of eating disorder. Clinicians may be less likely to consider a diagnosis of eating disorder in men. It has been claimed that 0.2% of all adolescent and young adult males meet stringent criteria for bulimia nervosa, with similar prevalence figures for anorexia. Overall, bulimia nervosa seems to be the more common disorder, and it has been suggested that males account for 10–15% of all cases. In a review of eating-disordered males treated in a district general hospital (Carlat et al. 1997), the most common diagnosis was bulimia nervosa (46%), with 22% meeting criteria for anorexia nervosa and 32% eating disorder not otherwise specified (most commonly binge eating). Males and females with eating disorders seemed to be similar in terms of phenomenological and demographic characteristics such as core weight and body image concerns, comorbid depression, anxiety and personality disorders and age of onset and high-risk occupations. However, male bulimics showed higher rates of parental obesity than female bulimic controls and longer delays between onset of disorder and receiving treatment. This study also suggested increased rates of substance abuse (consistent with increased rates in males) and increased rates of homosexuality/bisexuality compared to females (particularly for bulimic patients and consistent with previous studies). The authors suggested that this reflects an increased emphasis on physical appearance (in relation to self-esteem) in gay culture, such that gay men are under subcultural pressures similar to those experienced by women in the wider culture.

Interestingly, there is increasing evidence that males more generally *are* concerned with physical appearance, and that this has an impact on their self-esteem. However, in contrast to females, males are at least as likely to desire weight *gain* as weight loss, since for men being underweight has a negative impact on self-esteem, body image and social adjustment, in keeping with a sociocultural ideal of a lean but muscular male body. In this context, 'machismo nervosa' has been suggested as a variant of bulimia nervosa in body builders who engage in binge eating, dietary restriction, diuretics, fluid restriction, repeated self-weighing, mirror checking and use of anabolic steroids in an attempt to achieve their ideal shape. They show high levels of body dissatisfaction, perfectionism, ineffectiveness and reduced self-esteem

compared to other athletes, and tend to *underestimate* their size by 15% (Connan 1998).

Eating disorders and chronic physical illness

Medical causes of weight fluctuations due to disease or treatment may be misdiagnosed as an eating disorder. Alternatively they may increase the risk of developing a comorbid eating disorder – especially if occurring in adolescence – and complicate its diagnosis and treatment.

Gastrointestinal pathology, such as Crohn's disease, may present initially with weight loss and amenorrhoea, with relatively minor symptoms of abdominal pain, constipation or diarrhoea (which can occur in anorexia anyway). There may well be anxiety or depressive symptoms, but the characteristic disturbance of body image and intense fear of fatness will be absent. Thorough physical examination (e.g. looking for an abdominal mass or mouth ulcers) and appropriate investigations may clarify the diagnosis (Jenkins et al. 1988). In some cases, however, a comorbid eating disorder may develop as a psychological response to the experience of chronic gastrointestinal illness with pain, operations and a focus on diet. There have been a number of case reports of extreme dieting and preoccupation with weight following the weight gain associated with corticosteroid treatment. Severe restriction may in turn precipitate bingeing and set up a binge–restrict or binge–purge cycle typical of anorexia or bulimia nervosa (Meadows & Treasure 1988). In such cases both diagnoses require consideration and treatment in their own right.

Endocrine causes of weight fluctuation can similarly present as eating disorders or be implicated in their aetiology.

Studies of women with *thyroid disease* show increased prevalence of eating disorders (4%) or an eating disorder not otherwise specified (4%) in thyroid clinic attendees. A significant proportion admits to using thyroxine to manipulate their weight (7%), complicating the management of the condition (Tiller et al. 1994). Hyperthyroid women tend to present for treatment at approximately 84% healthy weight and are restored to 100% weight with treatment, most of the weight gain being in the first three months. Hypothyroid women (who are overweight) initially lose weight with treatment, but this is not usually sustained on treatment alone. Other features such as exophthalmos, goitre or alopecia may exacerbate body image dissatisfaction.

The concurrence of *diabetes* and anorexia nervosa raises particular diagnostic and management concerns. Incidence of eating disorders increased in patients with insulin-dependent diabetes mellitus (IDDM) (see Nielsen & Molback 1998 for meta-analysis). Where IDDM and eating disorder are concurrent, the diabetes usually predates the eating disorder, and interestingly this group shows lower rates of other potential aetiological factors, such as childhood trauma, than non-diabetic eating-disordered controls (Ward et al. 1995). IDDM has been suggested therefore as an aetiological factor when onset is in adolescence and there is a history of obesity. This group seems to have increased psychiatric morbidity more generally (Vila et al. 1995). The focus on body weight and diet, family stress, the stress of a chronic physical illness and weight gain on starting treatment may contribute to the risk. Case studies report patient distress on weight gain, and up to one-third of female diabetics have been reported to misuse insulin by omission or under dosing to achieve weight loss (Peveler 1992). Patients with characteristic psychopathology may be classified as eating disorder not otherwise specified or 'subclinical' bulimia, since insulin misuse may be the only compensatory weight loss strategy for bingeing. Patients may develop more typical anorexia nervosa, with severe dietary restraint in addition to insulin omission. Some alternatively become preoccupied with achieving perfect blood glucose control through dietary restriction. Patients with bulimia may either omit or take insulin after a binge, in an attempt to compensate. Clearly in these patients the diabetes may be 'brittle' or chronically poorly controlled. They are of particular concern because of the high incidence of neurovascular complications at an early age, especially retinopathy, and also nephropathy and neuropathy. They present particular management difficulties since they may default or refuse medical supervision and be secretive about their insulin use, prioritizing desire for thinness over maintaining health and diabetic control. In a psychiatric setting the dietary restrictions associated with diabetes may be used in resistance, and confuse a team attempting to impose a behavioural refeeding regime. Both the eating disorder and the diabetes are therefore harder to treat, and require close liaison between psychiatrist and medical teams. Treatment of the eating disorder may need to be modified, e.g. allowing the patient to retain control of her weight and diet. Rydall et al. (1997) proposed screening of all young IDDM females, and suggested that any eating disturbance be treated to reduce the risk of complications.

REFERENCES

Agras WS, Walsh T, Fairburn CG, Wilson GT & Kraemer HC (2000) A multicenter comparison of cognitive–behavioral therapy and interpersonal psychotherapy for bulimia nervosa. *Archives of General Psychiatry* **57**: 459–66.
American Psychiatric Association (1994) *Diagnostic and Statistical Manual of Mental Disorder*, 4th edn. Washington DC: APA.
Athia E, Haiman C, Walsh BT & Flater SR (1998) Does fluoxetine augment inpatient treatment of anorexia nervosa? *American Journal of Psychiatry* **155**: 546–51.
Bailer UF & Kaye WH (2003) A review of neuropeptide and neuroendocrine dysregulation in anorexia and bulimia nervosa. *Current drug targets. CNS and Neurological Disorders* **2**: 53–9.
Beaumont PFV, Russell JD & Touyz SW (1993) The treatment of anorexia nervosa. *Lancet* **341**: 1635–40.
Beck AT (1976) *Cognitive Therapy and Emotional Disorders*. New York: International Universities Press.
Biederman J, Herzog DB, Rivinus TN et al. (1985) Amitriptyline in the treatment of anorexia nervosa. *Journal of Clinical Psychopharmacology* **49**: 7–9.
Binswanger L (trans. by Mendel WM & Lyons J) (1959) The case of Ellen West. In: May R, Angel E & Ellenberger HF (eds) *Existence: A New Dimension in Psychiatry and Psychology*, pp. 237–364. New York: Basic Books.
Braun DL, Sunday SR & Halmi KA (1994) Psychiatric morbidity in patients with eating disorders. *Psychological Medicine* **24**: 859–67.
Bruch H (1978) *The Golden Cage: The Enigma of Anorexia Nervosa*. England: Open Books.
Bruch H (1988) *Conversations with Anorexics*, edited by Czyzewski D & Suhr MA. London: Aronson.
Brumberg JJ (1988) *Fasting Girls*. Cambridge, MA: Harvard University Press.
Brusset B & Jeammet P (1971). Les periodes boulimiques dans l'evolution de l'anorexie mentale de l'adolescente. *Revue de Neuropsychiatrie Infantile* **19**: 661–90.
Bulik CM, Sullivan PF, Carter FA & Joyce PR (1996) Lifetime anxiety disorders in women with bulimia nervosa. *Comprehensive Psychiatry* **37**: 368–74.
Bulik CM, Sullivan PF, Carter FA & Joyce PR (1997). Lifetime comorbidity of alcohol dependence in women with bulimia nervosa. *Additive Behaviours* **22**: 437–46.
Bulik CM, Devlin B, Bacanu SA, Thornton L, Klump KL, Fichter MM et al. (2003) Significant linkage on chromosome 10p in families with bulimia nervosa. *American Journal of Human Genetics* **72**: 200–7.
Bulimia Nervosa Collaborative Study Group (1992) Fluoxetine in the treatment of bulimia nervosa: a multicentre, placebo-controlled, double-blind trial. *Archives of General Psychiatry* **49**: 139–47.
Bushnell JA, Wells JE & Oakley-Browne MA (1992) Long term effects of intrafamilial sexual abuse in childhood. *Acta Psychiatrica Scandinavica*.
Calam RM & Slade PD (1989) Sexual experience and eating problems in female undergraduate. *International Journal of Eating Disorders* **8**: 391–7.
Carlat DJ, Camargo CA & Herzog DB (1997) Eating disorders in males: a report on 135 patients. *American Journal of Psychiatry* **154**(8): 1127–32.
Carter JC, Olmsted MP, Kaplan AS, McCabe RE, Mills JS & Aime A (2003) Self-help for bulimia nervosa: a randomized controlled trial. *American Journal of Psychiatry* **160**: 973–8.
Collier DA, Arranz MJ, Li T, Mupita D, Brown N & Treanne J (1997) Association between a promoter polymorphism in the 5HT2A gene and anorexia nervosa. *Lancet* **350**: 412.
Collins S & King M (1994) Ten year follow-up study of 50 patients with bulimia nervosa. *British Journal of Psychiatry* **164**: 80–7.
Connan F (1998) Machismo nervosa: an ominous variant of bulimia nervosa? *European Eating Disorders Review* **6**: 154–9.
Connan F, Campbell IC, Katzman M, Lightman SL & Treasure J (2003) A neurodevelopmental model for anorexia nervosa. *Physiological Behaviour* **79**: 13–24.
Connan F & Treasure JL (1998) Stress, eating and neurobiology. In: Hork HW, Treasure TL & Katzman MA (eds) *Neurobiology in the Treatment of Eating Disorder*, pp. 211–36. Chichester: Wiley.
Cooper Z, Coker PJ & Fairburn CG (1989) The validity of the EDE and its subscales. *British Journal of Psychiatry* **154**: 807–12.
Cooper PJ (1993) *Bulimia Nervosa: A Guide to Recovery*. London: Robinson Publishing.
Crisp AH (1967) The possible significance of some behavioural correlates of weight and carbohydrate intake. *Journal of Psychosomatic Research* **11**(1): 117–31.
Crisp AH, Norton KRW, Gower S et al. (1991) A controlled study of the effect of therapies aimed at adolescent and family psychopathology in anorexia nervosa. *British Journal of Psychiatry* **159**: 325–33.
Dansky BS, Brewerton TD, Kilpatrick DG & O'Neil PM (1997) The National Women's Study: relationship of victimization and post-traumatic stress disorder to bulimia nervosa. *International Journal of Eating Disorders* **21**: 213–28.
Dare C & Crowther C (1995) Psychodynamic models of eating disorders. In: Szmukler G, Dare C & Treasure J (eds) *Handbook of Eating Disorders: Theory, Treatment and Research*. Chichester: Wiley.

Dare C & Eisler I (1995) Family therapy. In: Szmukler G, Dare C & Treasure J (eds) *Handbook of Eating Disorders: Theory, Treatment and Research*, pp. 333–49. Chichester: Wiley.

Dare C, Eisler I, Russell G, Treasure J & Dodge L (2001) Psychological therapies for adults with anorexia nervosa: randomised controlled trial of out-patient treatments. *British Journal of Psychiatry* **178**: 216–21.

Devlin MJ, Walsh BT, Guss JL et al. (1997) Postprandial cholecystokinin release and gastric emptying in patients with bulimia nervosa. *American Journal of Clinical Nutrition* **65**: 112–20.

DiNicola VF (1990) Anorexia multiforme: self starvation in historical and cultural context. II. Anorexia nervosa as a culture reactive syndrome. *Transcultural Psychiatric Research Review* **27**: 245–86.

Durand MA & King M (2003) Specialist treatment versus self-help for bulimia nervosa: a randomised controlled trial in general practice. *British Journal of General Practice* **53**: 371–7.

Eisler I (1995) Family models of eating disorders. In: Szmukler G, Dare C & Treasure J (eds) *Handbook of Eating Disorders: Theory, Treatment and Research*, pp. 177–92. Chichester: Wiley.

Eisler I LGD & Asen E (2003) Family interventions. In: Treasure J, Schmidt U & Van Furth E (eds) *Handbook of Eating Disorders*, pp 311–25. Chichester: Wiley.

Eisler I, Dare C, Russell GFM et al. (1997) Family and individual therapy in anorexia nervosa: a 5-year follow up. *Archives of General Psychiatry* **54**: 1025–30.

Ellison ZR & Foong J (1998) Neuroimaging in eating disorders. In: Hoek HW, Treasure JL & Katzman MA (eds) *Neurobiology in the Treatment of Eating Disorder*, pp. 211–36. Chichester: Wiley.

Fairburn CG (1995) *Overcoming Binge Eating*. Lynton: Guildford Press.

Fairburn CG & Beglin SJ (1990) Studies of the epidemiology of bulimia nervosa. *American Journal of Psychiatry* **147**: 401–8.

Fairburn C, Cooper Z & Cooper PJ (1986) The clinical features and maintenance of bulimia nervosa. In: Brownell KD & Foreyt J (eds) *Handbook of Eating Disorders. Physiology, Psychology and Treatment of Eating Disorders*. New York: Basic Books.

Fairburn CG, Jones R, Peveler RC et al. (1993) Psychotherapy and bulimia nervosa: the longer-term effects of interpersonal psychotherapy, behaviour therapy and cognitive behaviour therapy. *Archives of General Psychiatry* **50**: 419–28.

Fairburn CG, Norman PA, Welch SL et al. (1995) A prospective study of outcome in bulimia nervosa and the long term effects of three psychological treatments. *Archives of General Psychiatry* **52**: 304–12.

Fairburn CG, Shafran R & Cooper Z (1999) A cognitive behavioural theory of anorexia nervosa. *Behavioural Research Therapy* **37**: 1–13.

Fairburn CG & Welch SL (1996) Childhood sexual and physical abuse as risk factors for the development of bulimia nervosa: a community based case control study. *Child Abuse and Neglect* **207**: 633–42.

Fairburn CG, Welch SL, Doll HA, Davies BA & O'Connor ME (1997) Risk factors for bulimia nervosa; a community based case control study. *Archives of General Psychiatry* **54**: 509–17.

Favaro A & Santonastaso P (1997) Suicidality in eating disorders: clinical and psychological correlates. *Acta Psychiatrica Scandinavica* **95**: 508–14.

Fichter M, Elton M, Sourdi L et al. (1988) Anorexia nervosa in Greek and Turkish adolescents. *European Archives of Psychiatry and Neurological Sciences* **237**: 200–8.

Fichter M & Noegel R (1990) Concordance for bulimia nervosa in twins. *International Journal of Eating Disorders* **9**: 255–63.

Fichter M & Pirke KM (1986) Effects of experimental and pathological weight loss upon the hypothalamo-pituitary-adrenal axis. *Psychoneuroendocrinology* **11**: 295–305.

Fichter M & Pirke KM (1990) Psychobiology of human starvation in anorexia nervosa. In: Remschmidt H & Schmidt MH (eds) *Anorexia Nervosa*, pp. 15–29. Stuttgart: Hogrefe & Huber.

Fichter M & Quadfleig N (1997) Six-year course of bulimia nervosa. *International Journal of Eating Disorders* **22**: 361–84.

Freeman C (1992) Daypatient treatment for anorexia nervosa. *British Review of Bulimia and Anorexia Nervosa* **6**: 2–8.

Fremouw WJ & Heyneman NE (1983) Cognitive styles in bulimia. *Behaviour Therapist* **6**: 143–4.

Garfinkel PE, Lin E, Goering P et al. (1995) Bulimia nervosa in a Canadian community sample: prevalence and comparison of subgroups. *Journal*.

Garner DM & Bemis KM (1982) A cognitive–behavioural approach to anorexia nervosa. *Cognitive Therapy and Research* **6**: 123–50.

Garner DM & Garfinkel PE (1979) The Eating Attitudes Test: an index of the symptoms of anorexia nervosa. *Psychological Medicine* **9**: 273–9.

Garner DM & Garfinkel PE (1980) Sociocultural factors in the development of anorexia nervosa. *Psychological Medicine* **10**(4): 647–56.

Garner DM, Garfinkel PE, Schwartz D & Thompson M (1980) Cultural expectations of thinness in women. *Psychological Reports* **47**: 483–91.

Garner DM, Olmsted MP & Garfinkel PE (1983) Development and validation of multidimensional eating disorder inventory for anorexia nervosa and bulimia. *International Journal of Eating Disorders* **48**: 173–8.

Garner DM, Vitousek KM & Pike KM (1997) Cognitive–behavioural therapy for anorexia. In: Garner DM & Garfinkel PE (eds) *Handbook of Treatment for Eating Disorders*, pp. 94–144. New York: Guilford.

Grice DE, Halmi KA, Fichter MM, Strober M, Woodside DB, Treasure JT et al. (2002) Evidence for a susceptibility gene for anorexia nervosa on chromosome 1. *American Journal of Human Genetics* **70**.

Gull WW (1874) Anorexia nervosa. *Transactions of the Clinical Society of London* **7**: 2–28.

Hagan MM, Chandler PC, Wauford PK, Rybak RJ & Oswald KD (2003) The role of palatable food and hunger as trigger factors in an animal model of stress induced binge eating. *International Journal of Eating Disorders* **34**:183–97.

Hamilton LH, Brooks-Gunn J & Warren MP (1985) Sociocultural influences on eating disorders in professional female ballet dancers. *International Journal of Eating Disorders* **4**: 465–77.

Hastings T & Kern JM (1994) The relationship between bulimia, childhood sexual abuse and family environment. *International Journal of Eating Disorders* **15**: 103–11.

Henderson M & Freeman CPL (1987) Aself-rating scale for bulimia: 'The Bite'. *British Journal of Psychiatry* **150**: 18–24.

Herzog W, Deter HC, Fiehn W & Petzold W (1997) Medical findings and predictors of long term physical outcome in anorexia nervosa: a prospective, 12-year follow-up study. *Psychological Medicine* **27**: 269–79.

Herzog DB, Keller MB, Lavori PW & Sacks NR (1991) The cause and outcome of bulimia nervosa. *Journal of Clinical Psychiatry* **52**(suppl): 4–8.

Herzog W, Deter HC & Wandereycken W (1992) *The Course of Eating Disorders*. Berlin: Springer.

Herzog W, Nussbaum KM & Marmor AK (1996) Comorbidity and outcome in eating disorders. *Psychiatric Clinics of North America* **19**: 843–59.

Hoek HW (1991) The incidence and prevalence of anorexia nervosa and bulimia nervosa in primary care. *Psychological Medicine* **21**: 455–60.

Hoek HW (1995) Epidemiology of anorexia nervosa and bulimia nervosa in the western world. *CME* **13**: 501–8.

Hsu LKG, Chesler BE & Santhouse R (1990) Bulimia nervosa in eleven sets of twins: a clinical report. *International Journal of Eating Disorders* **9**: 275–82.

Jenkins AP, Treasure J & Thompson RPH (1988) Crohn's disease presenting as anorexia nervosa. *British Medical Journal* **296**: 699–700.

Jimerson DC, Wolfe BE, Metzger ED et al. (1997) Decreased serotonin function in bulimia nervosa. *Archives of General Psychiatry* **54**: 529–34.

Kalucy RS, Crisp AH & Harding B (1977) A study of 56 families with anorexia nervosa. *British Journal of Medical Psychology* **50**: 381–95.

Kaye WH, Gwirstman HE, George DT et al. (1988) CSF 5–HIAA concentrations in anorexia nervosa: reduced values in underweight subjects normalise after weight gain. *Biological Psychiatry* **23**: 102–5.

Kaye WH, Gwirstman HE, George DT & Ebert MH (1991) Altered serotonin activity in anorexia nervosa after long term weight restoration: does elevated cerebrospinal fluid 5-hydroxyindoleacetic acid level correlate with rigid and obsessive behaviour? *Archives of General Psychiatry* **48**: 556–62.

Kaye WH, Weltzin TE, Hsu G et al. (1997) Relapse prevention with fluoxetine in anorexia nervosa: a double-blind placebo-controlled study. 150th APA Meeting, 17 May, p. 178.

Kaye WH, Frank GK, Meltzer CC, Price JC, McConaha CW, Crossan PJ et al. (2001) Altered serotonin 2A receptor activity in women who have recovered from bulimia nervosa. *American Journal of Psychiatry* **158**: 1152–5.

Keel PK & Mitchell JE (1997) Outcome in bulimia nervosa. *American Journal of Psychiatry* **154**: 313–21.

Keel PK & Klump KL (2003) Are eating disorders culture-bound syndromes? Implications for conceptualizing their etiology. *Psychological Bulletin* **129**: 747–69.

Kendler KS, Mclean C, Neale MI et al. (1991) The genetic epidemiology of anorexia nervosa. *American Journal of Psychiatry* **148**: 1627–37.

Kendler KS, Walters EE, Neale MC et al. (1995) The structure of the genetic and environmental risk factors for six major psychiatric disorders in women. *Archives of General Psychiatry* **52**: 374–83.

Kent IS & Copton JR (1992) Bulimic women's perceptions of their family relationships. *Journal of Clinical Psychology* **48**: 281–92.

Keys A, Brozek J, Henschel A et al. (1950) *The Biology of Human Starvation*. Minneapolis: University of Minneapolis Press.

King M & Mezey G (1987) Eating behaviour in male racing jockeys. *Psychological Medicine* **17**: 249–53.

Klein M (1977) *Envy and Gratitude & Other Works* 1946–1963. New York: Delta Books.

Lacey JH (1993) Self-damaging and addictive behaviour in bulimia nervosa. *British Journal of Psychiatry* **163**: 190–4.

Lacey JH & Crisp AH (1980) Hunger, food intake and weight: the impact of clomipramine on a refeeding anorexia nervosa population. *Postgraduate Medical Journal* **56**: 79–85.

Lasegue C (1873) De l'anorexie hysterique. *Archives Generales de Medicine* **21**: 385–403.

Law Commission (1993) Consultation paper no. 129. *Mentally Incapacitated Adults and Decision Making*. Medical Treatment and Research – paragraph 2.18 from Re W (1992) 3 WLR 758. London: HMSO.

Lee S (1991) Anorexia nervosa in Hong Kong: a Chinese perspective.–*Psychological Medicine* **21**: 703–12.

Lilenfeld LR, Kaye WH, Greeno CG et al. (1997) Psychiatric disorders in women with bulimia nervosa and their first degree relatives: effects of comorbid substance dependence. *International Journal of Eating Disorders* **22**(3): 253–64.

Lilenfeld LR, Kaye WH, Greeno CG et al. (1998) A controlled family study of anorexia nervosa and bulimia nervosa. Psychiatric disturbance in first degree relatives and effects of proband comorbidity. *Archives of General Psychiatry* **55**: 603–10.

Lucas AR, Beard C, O'Fallon W & Kurland LT (1991) 50-year trends in the incidence of anorexia nervosa in Rochester, Minn: a population based study. *American Journal of Psychiatry* **148**: 917–22.

Lucas AR & Soundy TL (1993) The rise of bulimia nervosa. Ninth World Congress of Psychiatry, Rio de Janeiro, Brazil, 6–12 June. Abstract 544, p. 139.

Majd SH (in press) *Eating Disorders and Childhood Abuse: Aetiology or Mythology. Advances in Psychiatric Treatment.*

Malan DH (1979) *Individual Psychotherapy and the Science of Psychodynamics*. London: Butterworth.

MalinKrodt B, McCreary BA & Roberson AK (1993) Co-occurrence of eating disorders and incest: the role of attachment, family environment and social competences in incest and eating disorders co-occurrence: family environment and social competences. MalinKrodt B (chair) Symposium presented at the meetings of the American Psychological Association, Toronto.

Marchi M & Cohen P (1990) Early childhood behaviours and adolescent eating disorders. *Journal of the American Academy of Adolescent Psychiatry* **29**: 112–17.

Marcus MD (1997) Adapting treatment for patients with binge-eating disorder. In: Garner DM & Garfinel PE (eds) *Handbook of Treatment for Eating Disorders*, pp. 484–93. New York: Guilford.

Mayer LES & Walsh BT (1998) Pharmocotherapy of eating disorders. In: Hork HW, Treasure JL & Katzman MA (eds) *Neurobiology in the Treatment of Eating Disorder*, pp. 383–405. Chichester: Wiley.

McKenzie JM & Joyce PR (1992) Hospitalization for anorexia nervosa. *International Journal of Eating Disorders* **11**: 235–41.

Meadow G & Treasure J (1988) Bulimia nervosa and Crohn's disease: two case reports. *Acta Psychiatrica Scandinavica* **78**: art. 1174.

Mental Health Act Commission (1997) *Guidance Note 3. Guidance on the Treatment of Anorexia Nervosa under the Mental Health Act 1983.*

Meyer C, Waller G & Waters A (1998) Emotional states and bulimic psychopathology. In: Hoek HW, Treasure JL & Katzman MA (eds) *Neurobiology in the Treatment of Eating Disorder*, pp. 271–89.

Chichester: Wiley.

Miller DAF, McClusky-Fawcett K & Irving LM (1993) The relationship between childhood sexual abuse and subsequent onset of bulimia nervosa. *Child Abuse and Neglect* **17**: 305–14.

Minuchin S, Baker L, Rosman BL et al. (1975) A conceptual model of psychosomatic illness in children. *Archives of General Psychiatry* **32**: 1031–8.

Mitchell JE, Pyle RL, Eckert ED et al. (1990) A comparison study of antidepressants and structured intensive group therapy in the treatment of bulimia nervosa. *Archives of General Psychiatry* **47**: 149–57.

Mumford DB (1993) Eating disorders in different cultures. *International Review of Psychiatry* **5**(1): 109–13.

Mumford DB, Whitehouse AM & Platts M (1991) Sociocultural correlates of eating disorders among Asian schoolgirls. *British Journal of Psychiatry* **158**: 222–8.

Nasser M (1986) Comparison study of the prevalence of abnormal eating attitudes among Arab female students of both London and Cairo universities. *Psychological Medicine* **16**: 621–5.

Nasser M (1997) *Culture and Weight Consciousness*. London: Routledge.

Nielsen S & Molbak AG (1998) Eating disorders and insulin dependent diabetes mellitus – overview and summing-up. *European Eating Disorders Review* **6**: 4–26.

Palazzoli M (1974) *Self-starvation: From Individual to Family Therapy in the Treatment of Anorexia Nervosa*. London: Chaucer.

Patton GC, Selzer R, Coffey C, Carlin JB & Wolfe R (1999) Onset of adolescent eating disorders: population based cohort study over 3 years. *British Medical Journal* **318**: 765–8.

Patton GD, Johnson-Sabine E, Wood K et al. (1990) Abnormal eating attitudes in London schoolgirls – a prospective epidemiological study. *Psychological Medicine* **20**: 282–394.

Peveler RC (1992) Eating disorders in adolescents with IDDM. A controlled study. *Diabetes Care* **15**: 1356–60.

Prochaska JO, Norcross JC & di Clmente CC (1994) *Changing for Good*. New York: William Morrow.

Rastam M (1992) Anorexia nervosa in 51 Swedish adolescents: premorbid problems and comorbidity. *Journal of the American Academy of Child and Adolescent Psychiatry* **31**: 819–29.

Rastam M & Gillberg C (1991) The family background in anorexia nervosa: a population-based study. *Journal of the American Academy of Child and Adolescent Psychiatry* **30**: 283–9.

Ratnasuriya RH, Eisler I, Szmukler GI & Russell GF (1991) Anorexia nervosa: outcome and prognostic factors after 20 years. *British Journal of Psychiatry* **158**: 495–502.

Riverside Health NHS Trust v. Fox (1994) 1 FLR 614–22.

Robinson PH & McHugh PR (1995) A physiology of starvation that sustains eating disorders. In: Szmukler G, Dare C & Treasure J (eds) *Handbook of Eating Disorders: Theory, Treatment and Research*, pp. 109–23. Chichester: Wiley.

Russell GM (1970) Anorexia nervosa: its identity as an illness and its treatment. In: Price JH (ed.) *Modern Trends in Psychological Medicine*, pp. 131–64. London: Butterworth.

Russell GM (1979) Bulimia nervosa: an ominous variant of anorexia nervosa. *Psychological Medicine* **9**: 429–48.

Rydall AC, Rodin GM, Olmstead MP, Deveryi RG & Danam D (1997) Disordered eating behaviour and microvascular complications in young women with insulin dependent diabetes mellitus. *New England Journal of Medicine* **336**: 1905–6.

Ryle A (1990) *Cognitive Analytic Therapy: Active Participation in Change*. Chichester: Wiley.

Schmidt U, Tiller J & Treasure J (1993) Psychosocial factors in the origins of bulimia nervosa. *International Review of Psychiatry* **5**: 51–60.

Schmidt U, Tiller J, Blanchard M et al. (1997) Is there a specific trauma precipitating bulimia nervosa? *Psychological Medicine* **27**(3): 523–30.

Schmidt U & Treasure JL (1993) *Getting Better Bit(e) by Bit(e). A Survival Kit for Sufferers of Bulimia Nervosa and Binge Eating Disorders*. Lawrence Erlbaum Associates.

Selvini-Palazzoli M (1974) *Self-starvation: From the Intrapsychic to the Transpersonal Approach to Anorexia Nervosa*. Hayward's Heath: Chaucer.

Silverstein B, Peterson B & Persue L (1986) Some correlates of the thin standard of bodily attractiveness for women. *International Journal of Eating Disorders* **5**(5): 895–905.

Slade (1982) Towards a functional analysis of anorexia nervosa and bulimia nervosa. *British Journal of Clinical Psychology* **21**: 167–79.

Smolak L, Levine M & Sullins E (1990) Are child sexual experiences related to eating disordered attitudes and behaviours in a college sample? *International Journal of Eating Disorders* **9**: 167–78.

Smoller JW, Wadden TA & Stunkard AJ (1987) Dieting and depression: a critical review. *Journal of Psychosomatic Research* **31**: 429–40.

Spitzer RL, Devlin M, Walsh BT et al. (1992) Binge eating disorder: a multisite field trial of the diagnostic criteria. *International Journal of Eating Disorder* **11**: 191–203.

Steiger H & Zanko M (1990) Sexual traumata among eating disordered, psychiatric, and normal female groups. *Journal of Interpersonal Violence* **5**: 74–86.

Steinhausen HC (2002) The outcome of anorexia nervosa in the 20th century. *American Journal of Psychiatry* **159**: 1284–93.

Stierlin H, Weber G, Schmidt G & Simon F (1985) Why some patients prefer to become manic-depressive rather than schizophrenic. *Journal of Biological Medicine* **58**(3): 255–63.

Szmukler GI (1983) Weight and food preoccupation in a population of English schoolgirls. In: Bargman GI (ed.) *Understanding Anorexia Nervosa and Bulimia.* Report of 4th Ross Conference on Medical Research. pp. 21–27. Columbus, OH: Ross.

Szmukler GI (1985) The epidemiology of anorexia nervosa and bulimia. *Journal of Psychiatric Research* **19**: 143–53.

Szmukler GI, Eisler I, Russell GM & Dare C (1985) Anorexia nervosa, parental 'expressed emotion' and dropping out of treatment. *British Journal of Psychiatry* **147**: 265–71.

Szmukler GI, McCance C, McCrone L & Hunter D (1986) Anorexia nervosa: a psychiatric case register study from Aberdeen. *Psychological Medicine* **16**: 49–58.

Szmukler GI & Patton G (1995) Sociocultural models of eating disorders. In: Szmukler G, Dare C & Treasure J (eds) *Handbook of Eating Disorders: Theory, Treatment and Research*, pp. 177–92. Chichester: Wiley.

Theander S (1985) Outcome and prognosis in anorexia nervosa and bulimia: some results of previous investigations compared with those of a Swedish long-term study. *Journal of Psychiatric Research* **19**: 493–508.

Thiels C, Schmidt U, Treasure JL, Garth R & Troop N (1998) Guided self-change for bulimia nervosa incorporating use of a self-care manual. *American Journal of Psychiatry* **155**: 947–53.

Tiller J, Macrae J, Schmidt U et al. (1994) The prevalence of eating disorders in thyroid disease: a pilot study. *Journal of Psychosomatic Research* **38**(6): 609–16.

Treasure JL (1988) The ultrasonographic features in anorexia nervosa and bulimia nervosa: a simplified method of monitoring hormonal states during weight gain. *Journal of Psychosomatic Research* **32**: 623–34.

Treasure JL & Campbell I (1994) The case for biology in the aetiology of anorexia nervosa. Editorial. *Psychological Medicine* **24**: 3–8.

Treasure J & Holland A (1989) Genetic vulnerability to eating disorders: evidence from twin and family studies. In: Remschmidt H & Schmidt MH (eds) *Anorexia Nervosa*, pp. 59–68. Toronto: Hogrefe & Huber.

Treasure J & Holland A (1995) Genetic factors in eating disorders. In: Szmuklers G, Dare C & Treasure J (eds) *Handbook of Eating Disorders: Theory, Treatment and Research*, pp. 65–81. Chichester:Wiley.

Treasure JL & Ramsay R (1997) Hard to swallow: compulsory treatment in eating disorders. *Maudsley Discussion Paper No. 3.* London: Institute of Psychiatry.

Treasure JL & Ward A (1997a) A practical guide to the use of motivational interviewing in anorexia nervosa. *European Eating Disorder Review* **5**: 102–14.

Treasure JL & Ward A (1997b) Cognitive analytic therapy in the treatment of anorexia nervosa. *Clinical Psychology and Psychotherapy* **4**: 62–71.

Turnbull S, Ward A, Treasure J et al. (1996) The demand for eating disorder care. An epidemiological study using the General Practice Research Database. *British Journal of Psychiatry* **169**: 705–12.

Uher R, Murphy T, Brammer MJ, Dalgleish T, Phillips ML, Ng VW, Andrew CM, Williams SC, Campbell IC & Treasure J (in press) Medial prefrontal cortex activity is associated with symptom provocation in eating disorders. *American Journal of Psychiatry.*

Van Hoeken D, Lucas AR & Hoek HW (1998) Epidemiology. In: Hoek HW, Treasure JL & Katzman MA (eds) *Neurobiology in the Treatment of Eating Disorder*, pp. 97–126. Chichester:Wiley.

Van Hoeken D, Seidell JC & Hoek HW (2003) Epidemiology. In: Treasure J, van Furth EF & Schmidt U (eds) *Handbook of Eating Disorders*, pp 11–34. Chichester: Wiley.

Vila G, Robert J, Nollet-Clemencon C et al. (1995) *European Child and Adolescent Psychiatry* **4**(4): 270–9.

Ward A, Brown N, Campbell I et al. (1998) The neuroendocrine and appetitive effects of d-fenfluramine in recovered anorexia nervosa. *British Journal of Psychiatry.*

Ward A, Troop N, Cachia M et al. (1995) Doubly disabled: diabetes in combination with an eating disorder. *Postgraduate Medical Journal* **71**: 546–50.

Welch SL, Doll HA & Fairburn CG (1997) Life events and the onset of bulimia nervosa. *Psychological Medicine* **27**: 515–22.

Welch SL & Fairburn CG (1996a) Impulsivity or comorbidity in bulimia nervosa. A controlled study of deliberate self harm and alcohol and drug misuse in a community sample. *British Journal of Psychiatry* **169**(4): 451–8.

Welch SL & Fairburn CG (1996b) Childhood sexual and physical abuse as risk factors for the development of bulimia nervosa: a community based case control study. *Child Abuse and Neglect* **20**: 633–42.

Whitehouse AM, Cooper PJ, Vize CV et al. (1992) Prevalence of eating disorders in three Cambridge general practices: hidden and conspicous morbidity. *British Journal of General Practice* **42**: 57–60.

Wilson GT, Fairburn CG & Agras WS (1997) Cognitive–behavioural therapy for bulimia nervosa. In: Garner DM & Garfinkel PE (eds) *Handbook of Treatment for Eating Disorders*, pp. 67–93. New York: Guilford.

Wonderlich SA, Brewerton TD, Jocic Z et al. (1997) Relationship of childhood sexual abuse and eating disorders. *Journal of the American Academy of Child and Adolescent Psychiatry* **36**(8): 1107–15.

Wonderlich SA, Wilsnack RW, Wilsnack SC & Harris TR (1996) The relationship of childhood sexual abuse and bulimic behaviour: results of a US national survey. *American Journal of Public Health* **86**: 1082–106.

World Health Organization (1992) *ICD–10 Classification of Mental and Behavioural Disorders.* Geneva: WHO.

Wulff M (1932) Lieber intersanten ovalen symptomenkomplex und seine bezie hung zur sucht. *Internationale Psychoanalyse Zeitschrift* **18**: 13–16.

Schizophrenia and related disorders

Pádraig Wright

INTRODUCTION

Schizophrenia is probably the single most important cause of chronic psychiatric disability. Fully half the beds in Europe's psychiatric hospitals are occupied by those afflicted with it.

Schizotypal, schizoaffective and persistent delusional disorders represent a heterogeneous group of illnesses that possess many of the features of schizophrenia, may be related to it aetiologically and are frequently difficult to distinguish from it clinically.

SCHIZOPHRENIA

Definition of schizophrenia

In the absence of a biological marker, schizophrenia can only be defined by the nature and persistence of its clinical features (Box 18.1). Indeed, operational diagnostic systems such as the ICD-10 (World Health Organization 1992) or DSM-IV (American Psychiatric Association 1994) require that a number of characteristic symptoms are present for at least one month (see Appendices 1 and 2).

History of the concept of schizophrenia

Epilepsy, mania, dementia and depression are described in ancient writings but there are no unambiguous accounts of schizophrenia. Most physicians thought in terms of a unitary psychosis or *Einheitpsychose*, a type of generic insanity, until well into the first half of the 19th century. Thereafter, the concept of schizophrenia evolved through a number of steps. Partially accurate descriptions were provided by Haslam (1764–1844) and Philippe Pinel (1745–1826) in the 18th century while the description provided by Emil Kraepelin at the end of the 19th century is recognizably similar to the contemporary concept of schizophrenia. It was Eugen Bleuler who first coined the word 'schizophrenia' early in the 20th century while Kurt Schneider delineated the eponymous symptoms of the first rank upon which modern diagnostic criteria depend. The major steps in the development of the concept of schizophrenia are briefly described and their originators listed in Table 18.1.

Emil Kraepelin

Emil Kraepelin (1855–1926) was professor of psychiatry at Heidelburg (1890) and Munich (1903) and was among the first to distinguish between manic-depressive psychosis and the disorder now called schizophrenia. He combined hebephrenia, catatonia, paranoia and later dementia simplex under the rubric of dementia praecox in the fifth edition of his textbook (1896) because he believed that specific symptoms (auditory hallucinations, delusions, autism, abnormal associations of thoughts, affective flattening, impaired insight, stereotypy and negativism) with onset in adolescence and progression to dementia were usual, though not invariable, in all four conditions (1896, translation 1919).

Eugen Bleuler

Eugen Bleuler (1857–1959) was professor of psychiatry at Zurich. He did not consider dementia praecox to be a single diagnostic entity and referred to the four clinical syndromes subsumed within it as 'the group of schizophrenias' (1911). He stated that the primary or fundamental symptoms of schizophrenia were caused by the disease process or its aetiological agent while the clinically more dramatic secondary or accessory symptoms were caused by the primary symptoms (Table 18.1).

Box 18.1 A pragmatic definition of schizophrenia

Schizophrenia usually manifests as a severe psychotic illness with onset in early adulthood, characterized by bizarre delusions, auditory hallucinations, thought disorder, strange behaviour and progressive deterioration in personal, domestic, social and occupational competence, all occurring in clear consciousness.

Table 18.1   The major steps in the development of the concept of schizophrenia and their originators

Historical concept	Description	Originator
Einheitpsychose	Single unitary psychosis	Griesinger and others (to 1850s)
Démence précoce	Mannerisms, intellectual deterioration and personal neglect commencing in adolescence	Morel (1852)
Catatonia	Stereotyped movement, mannerisms, automatic obedience, negativism and stupor	Kahlbaum (1863)
Hebephrenia	Intellectual deterioration and facile behaviour commencing in adolescence	Hecker (1871)
Dementia praecox	Hebephrenia, catatonia and paranoia grouped together as dementia praecox; dementia simplex (simple schizophrenia) subsequently included	Kraepelin (1893)
The schizophrenias	Primary symptoms (abnormal association of thoughts, affective abnormality, ambivalence and autism – the four As) caused by a presumed aetiological agent with secondary symptoms (delusions and hallucinations) caused by primary symptoms	Bleuler (1911)
Non-understandability	The praecox feeling	Jaspers (1913)
Symptoms of the first and second rank	See text and Table 18.2	Schneider (1959)
Biopolitical invention	See text	Szasz, Laing (1960s onwards)
Type 1 and Type 2 schizophrenia	See text and Table 18.4	Crow (1980)
Positive and negative symptoms	See text and Table 18.5	Andreasen (1982)
Three syndromes of chronic schizophrenia	See text	Liddle (1987)
Neurodevelopmental schizophrenia	See text	Murray, Weinberger and others (1990 onwards)
Neuropathological schizophrenia	See text	Numerous (1990 onwards)

Kurt Schneider

The German phenomenologist Kurt Schneider (1887–1967) worked at Munich and Heidelberg. He attempted to operationalize the diagnosis of schizophrenia by describing a number of symptoms that he considered of first-rank importance in differentiating schizophrenia from similar illnesses (1959). He did not believe that any of these symptoms were essential for the diagnosis. Several of Schneider's first-rank symptoms are included among the diagnostic criteria for schizophrenia in both ICD-10 and DSM-IV. Schneider's second-rank symptoms include hallucinations, delusions not already included as first-rank symptoms, and catatonic symptoms. His first-rank symptoms are described below and are listed and further categorized phenomenologically in Table 18.2.

Other German psychiatrists attempted to identify subgroups of patients within the general category of schizophrenia. Thus Leonhard (1957) separated the cycloid psychoses (see below) from schizophrenia, and divided schizophrenia into a progressive or 'systematic' type which included catatonia, hebephrenia and paraphrenia, and a 'non-systematic' type which included periodic catatonia characterized by remitting catatonic symptoms,

schizophasia characterized by severe distortion of speech, and affect-laden paraphrenia characterized by appropriate affective responses to paranoid delusions.

Contemporary authorities

In the recent past, writers such as Thomas Szasz and R.D. Laing of the 'antipsychiatry' school have viewed schizophrenia as the biopolitical invention of psychiatrists, families and society, rather than an understandable reaction on the part of the schizophrenic individual to familial and social pressures (see Chapter 11). Contemporary authorities who have contributed substantially to the development of the concept of schizophrenia include Nancy Andreasen, Tim Crow, Peter Liddle, Robin Murray, Daniel Weinberger and others. Their work and the currently favoured conceptualization of schizophrenia as a neurodevelopmental disorder will be addressed below.

Epidemiology of schizophrenia

General epidemiology

Schizophrenia has been reported in all countries and all cultures (Box 18.2). The lifetime risk is about 1% and the

Table 18.2   A phenomenological classification of Schneider's first-rank symptoms

	Passivity phenomenon	Delusion	Hallucination
Thought insertion	Yes	Yes	
Thought broadcast	Yes	Yes	
Thought withdrawal	Yes	Yes	
Echo de pensée			Yes[1]
Gedankenlautwerden			Yes[1]
Voices arguing (third person)			Yes
Running commentary (third person)			Yes
Made actions	Yes	Yes	
Made impulses	Yes	Yes	
Made feelings	Yes	Yes	
Somatic passivity	Yes	Yes	Yes[2]
Delusional perception		Yes[3]	

[1] Most authorities describe these experiences as auditory hallucinations but some state that the patient's thoughts are repeated in the form of another thought and that *echo de pensée* and *gedankenlautwerden* are not, therefore, auditory hallucinations.
[2] Patients exhibit somatic passivity when they experience a normal perception or a somatic hallucination and attribute their experience to an external force. Somatic hallucination alone is not a first-rank symptom.
[3] The percept in delusional perception is real and is not an hallucination. Delusional perception represents a primary, or autochthonous, delusion.

incidence is about 20 cases (range 7–40) per 100 000 of the population per year. The point prevalence of schizophrenia is between 3 and 5 per 1000 of the population. However, rates as low as 1 per 1000 have been reported in the Hutterite community in the USA while rates of 10 or more per 1000 have been found in parts of Sweden, Ireland and Yugoslavia.

It was recognized almost four decades ago that some of the apparent variations in the prevalence of schizophrenia between countries might be due to differences in diagnostic

Box 18.2   The epidemiology of schizophrenia

Lifetime risk:	1%
Incidence:	20 per 100 000 population per year
Point prevalence:	3–5 per 1000 population
Sex ratio:	males and females affected equally
Age of onset:	male 15–25 years; female 25–35 years
Populations with increased prevalence:	urban populations, lower socio-economic classes, prison populations
Lifetime suicide risk:	10% (see text)
Incidence of suicide: patients per year	147–750 per 100 000 schizophrenic

practice. This led to the initiation of the US–UK Diagnostic Project which found that New York-based psychiatrists – preferring the broader Bleulerian concept – diagnosed schizophrenia more frequently, and affective psychoses less frequently, than their London-based psychiatrists – who preferred the narrower Kraepelinian concept – in newly hospitalized patients (Cooper et al. 1972). However, when these patients were interviewed by psychiatrists associated with the US–UK Diagnostic Project using the Present State Examination, the frequency of schizophrenia was found to be the same in both cities. This result was confirmed by the World Health Organization (WHO) International Pilot Study of Schizophrenia (IPSS) (World Health Organization 1973). However, the World Health Organization ten-country study found that the incidence of broadly defined schizophrenia varied up to four-fold between countries (Jablensky et al. 1992).

There is some evidence that the incidence of schizophrenia has varied over time. Hare (1988) suggested that schizophrenia was uncommon before the 19th century, that its incidence peaked during the rapid industrialization of the 19th and early 20th centuries, and that it is now again becoming uncommon. In keeping with this proposal, decreasing hospital admission rates for schizophrenia have been reported in the UK, Ireland and Australia. Der et al. (1990), for example, examined the Mental Health Enquiry data for England and Wales and reported a 50% decline in first admissions to hospital for schizophrenia over three decades. This apparent reduction in incidence may result from changes in diagnostic practice or in the provision of health services, from improved treatments, or from alterations in background populations. Whether or not schizophrenia exhibits temporal variation remains unknown.

The 'season of birth effect' refers to the well-replicated epidemiological finding that schizophrenic patients are more likely by 7–15% to be born between February and May in the northern hemisphere and between June and October in the southern hemisphere (Mortensen et al. 1999). It has been suggested that prenatal exposure to influenza epidemics may explain this finding (see Wright et al. 1999 for review).

Sex and age

It is generally accepted that schizophrenia is equally common in males and females and Jablensky et al. (1999) reported an equal cumulated risk for the sexes until the sixth decade of life from the IPSS. However, some investigators found an excess of narrowly defined schizophrenia in males (Hafner et al. 1994) and male schizophrenic patients are more likely to experience obstetric complications and to exhibit impaired development during childhood (see below). Male schizophrenic patients are more likely to be hospitalized and are less likely to marry or have children than female patients, although the fertility of female patients is also substantially reduced compared to non-schizophrenic women. These differences may be accounted for by the greater severity of schizophrenia in men and the later onset of illness in women (see below).

Men with schizophrenia are diagnosed most frequently between the ages of 15 and 25 years, while the diagnosis is most likely to be made in women between the ages of 25 and 35 years (Hafner et al. 1994). It is exceedingly rare for schizophrenia to be first diagnosed in men after the age of 45 years, while up to 10% of women are first diagnosed after this age (Goldstein et al. 1989). Some studies report a mean age of onset for schizophrenia of 28 years in men and 32 years in women, but it is likely that diagnosis has been delayed in these individuals and the true age of onset is several years earlier. It is generally accepted that the age of onset in males is 4–5 years earlier than in females.

Social epidemiology

Schizophrenia is commoner in urban areas, in lower socioeconomic groups and in recent immigrants such as the Norwegian immigrants to the United States studied by Ødegaard (1932). These results may be explained by social deprivation and the stresses of immigration increasing the risk of developing schizophrenia. Alternatively, it may be that individuals in the prodromal or prepsychotic phase of a schizophrenic illness are more likely to become socially or financially dependent, and either to migrate to cheap accommodation in urban centres, or to emigrate. This latter hypothesis is supported by reports of schizophrenic patients being financially disadvantaged (McNaught et al. 1997) and by Marshall's (1994) report that up to 40% of men and 65% of women living in hostels or homeless have schizophrenia. Further support for the hypothesis comes from reports of a higher incidence of schizophrenia in Afro-Caribbeans in the

---

Box 18.3 Symptoms of schizophrenia: delusions, hallucinations and formal thought disorders

Delusions	Hallucinations	Formal thought disorders[3]
Delusional mood/Wahnstimmung	Auditory	Overinclusiveness/circumstantiality
Primary (autochthonous)	Somatic[1]	Concrete thinking
Paranoid	Visual[2]	Loosened associations/derailment
Somatic	Tactile[2]	Knight's move/Vorbeireden
Religious	Olfactory[2]	Neologisms
Nihilistic	Gustatory[2]	Word salad/Verbigeration
Grandiose		Tangentiality, illogicality
Complex/fantastic		Thought block
Pseudoscientific		Poverty of thought content
Mystical		

[1]Somatic hallucinations are not unusual in schizophrenia, are often sexual in nature, and are a component of somatic passivity, a Schneiderian first-rank symptom.
[2]Hallucinations other than auditory or somatic should always raise the suspicion of an organic disorder. Olfactory hallucinations in particular suggest a frontal lobe lesion or temporal lobe epilepsy.
[3]Formal thought disorder must, of necessity, be inferred from the patient's speech.

UK than in either the background UK population or in Afro-Caribbeans in Jamaica (Bhugra et al. 1997).

Clinical features of schizophrenia

The clinical features of schizophrenia are myriad (Boxes 18.2, 18.3, 18.4 and 18.5). It is unusual for individual patients to exhibit more than a few of the vast array of schizophrenic

symptoms at any point in time during their illness, and even in the course of a lifetime of schizophrenia it is an exceptional and unfortunate patient who experiences the majority of these symptoms. There is considerable phenomenological overlap in schizophrenic symptoms but they may be conveniently subdivided into delusions, hallucinations, formal thought disorders, passivity phenomena and affective abnormalities, and motor, cognitive and social abnormalities. The individual symptoms within these subdivisions are listed below, and are discussed in more detail in Chapter 6.

Less common features of schizophrenia include obsessive-compulsive symptoms (and indeed obsessive-compulsive disorder is an important differential diagnosis for schizophrenia), violence and aggression, and water intoxication. The latter occurs when patients drink water excessively and develop polyuria and hyponatraemia. Seizures, coma and occasional deaths have been reported. The cause of water intoxication in schizophrenia is not known but may include response to delusions or hallucinations, or involvement of the hypothalamo–pituitary axis or other relevant brain structures in the underlying disease process (see Chapter 26).

The IPSS survey undertaken by the WHO determined the commonest symptoms exhibited by schizophrenic patients (World Health Organization 1973; Table 18.3). These are discussed in Chapter 6 but some of them, along with several other schizophrenic symptoms, warrant detailed discussion, either because they are thought to be of specific importance

Box 18.4   Symptoms of schizophrenia: passivity phenomena and affective abnormalities

Passivity phenomena	Affective abnormalities
Thought insertion	Blunted/flattened affect
Thought broadcast	Incongruous affect
Thought withdrawal	Avolition
Made actions	Autism
Made impulses	Anxiety
Made feelings	Euphoria
Somatic passivity	Depression[1]

[1]Depression is common in schizophrenia either because of comorbidity, side-effects of antipsychotic drugs, response to partial insight into the nature of the illness, or as an intrinsic component of the illness. Depressive symptoms can occur at any time during a schizophrenic illness but are thought to be most prominent in the early years of psychosis and are associated with a poor prognosis, disease relapse and with suicide.

Box 18.5   Symptoms of schizophrenia: motor, cognitive and social abnormalities

Motor abnormalities	Cognitive abnormalities	Social abnormalities
Catatonic stupor	Impaired insight	Impaired social skills
Catatonic excitement	Cognitive impairment	Odd appearance
Posturing		Perplexed facies
Flexibilitas cerea (waxy flexibility)		Impaired self-care
Catalepsy		Hoarding
Negativism		
Echopraxia		
Stereotypy		
Mannerisms		
Schnauzkrampf		
Mitmachen		
Mitgehen		
Forced grasping		
Automatic obedience		

Table 18.3 Frequency of commonest schizophrenia symptoms in patients from nine countries

Symptom	Frequency of symptoms in 306 schizophrenic patients (%)[1]
Lack of insight	97
Auditory hallucinations	74
Ideas of reference	70
Suspiciousness	66
Flatness of affect	66
Second-person hallucinations	65
Delusional mood	64
Delusions of persecution	64
Thought alienation	52
Echo de pensée, Gedankenlautwerden	50

[1] The IPSS studied 1202 patients of whom 306 were diagnosed as schizophrenic both by psychiatrists in their own country and by the Catego Present State Examination computer program.

in making a diagnosis of schizophrenia – Schneider's first rank symptoms – or because they are among the symptoms contributing to specific schizophrenic syndromes such as those described by Crow, Andreasen and Liddle.

Schneider's symptoms of the first rank

Schneider considered the 11 symptoms described below to be of first-rank importance in differentiating schizophrenia from similar illnesses. However, while 58% of patients with a diagnosis of acute schizophrenia in the IPSS study did have one or more first-rank symptom, these symptoms occur in almost 10% of nonschizophrenic patients (World Health Organization 1973), while more than 20% of schizophrenic patients never exhibit even a single first-rank symptom (Mellor 1970). Schneider's symptoms of the first rank are as follows:

- **Thought insertion:** the patient believes that the thoughts he experiences are not the product of his own mind but have been inserted into it by an external agency, e.g. 'Thoughts are put into my mind by radio transmitters'.
- **Thought broadcast:** the patient believes that her private thoughts are readily available to others, e.g. 'My thoughts are also transmitted into other people's minds'.
- **Thought withdrawal:** the patient experiences an interruption in the flow of his thoughts and his mind is left completely blank, e.g. 'My thoughts were completely removed by something. My mind just stopped and was emptied'.

- **Thought echo:** two types of thought echo occur. In *Echo de la penseé* the patient experiences his thoughts after thinking them as if hearing an echo, e.g. 'I think something, and then I hear my mind thinking it again and again'. In *Gedankenlautwerden* the patient experiences his thoughts as if he is hearing them simultaneously to thinking them, e.g. 'I hear myself thinking while I'm doing it'.
- **Delusional perception:** the patient develops a bizarre delusion in response to a real sensory perception, e.g. 'I saw the flower bulbs drop on the steps and immediately knew the manager of the factory was in love with me'.
- **Third-person auditory hallucinations – running commentary:** the patient experiences hallucinatory voices referring to him as 'he', e.g. 'Here he comes. There he goes. He's wearing that old grey coat again'.
- **Third-person auditory hallucinations – voices arguing:** the patient experiences two or more hallucinatory voices referring to her as 'he' in an argumentative manner, e.g. 'She's evil. She's excellent. Evil witch. She's a saint'.
- **Made feelings, impulses and actions:** these three first rank symptoms are experienced as arising without the patient's volition and are outside his control, e.g. 'I don't hate him. They make me hate him', 'The echo-rays make me want to move my arms upwards. They move me like a puppet' and 'Something speaks with my mouth and my lips. It's got my voice but it's not me'.
- **Somatic passivity:** the patient experiences bodily sensations in the absence of a stimulus (somatic hallucinations) and attributes these to an external force. Somatic passivity is also referred to as the experience of bodily influence, e.g. 'The radioactive emissions from Mars cause the muscles in my limbs to turn inside out. I can feel them turning all the time'.

Crow's Type 1 and 2 schizophrenia

Crow concluded in 1980 that the only consistently reported abnormality from postmortem investigations of brain tissue from schizophrenic patients was that of increased numbers of dopamine receptors. On the basis of this and other observations he proposed a division of schizophrenia into a Type 1 and a Type 2 syndrome (Table 18.4). Subsequent research provides evidence that cognitive impairment and tardive dyskinesia occur most commonly in patients with the Type 2 syndrome and are infrequent in those with Type 1 schizophrenia.

Andreasen's positive and negative symptoms of schizophrenia

The division of schizophrenia into two syndromes based on whether symptoms are predominantly positive or negative was originally proposed by Hughlings-Jackson (1931). Andreasen & Olsen (1982) subsequently provided a set of validated diagnostic criteria that facilitated the subdivision of patients into those with positive, negative or mixed

Table 18.4 Crow's Type 1 and 2 schizophrenias

	Type 1	Type 2
Characteristic symptoms	Hallucinations, delusions, thought disorder (positive symptoms)	Affective flattening, poverty of speech, loss of drive (negative symptoms)
Type of illness in which most commonly seen	Acute schizophrenia	Chronic schizophrenia, the 'defect' state
Response to neuroleptics	Good	Poor
Outcome	Reversible	?Irreversible
Intellectual impairment	Absent	Sometimes present
Postulated pathological process	Increased dopamine receptors	Cell loss and structural changes in the brain

schizophrenia (Box 18.6). The positive and negative symptoms they defined are listed below. Mixed schizophrenia is diagnosed when patients do not meet the criteria for either positive or negative schizophrenia, or meet the criteria for both. Patients with positive-symptom schizophrenia exhibit adequate premorbid adjustment and global functioning, normal cognition and no evidence of cerebral atrophy, while patients with negative-symptom schizophrenia typically demonstrate poor premorbid adjustment, poorer global functioning, impaired cognitive function and cerebral atrophy.

Liddle's three syndromes of chronic schizophrenia

Liddle (1987) used factor analysis to segregate schizophrenic symptoms into three syndromes, each associated with a particular performance profile on neuropsychological

Box 18.6 Andreasen's positive and negative symptoms of schizophrenia

Positive symptoms	Negative symptoms
Hallucinations auditory olfactory visual	*Affective flattening/blunting* unchanging facial expression decreased spontaneous movement paucity of expressive gesture poor eye contact affective non-responsivity lack of vocal inflection
Delusions persecutory delusions of jealousy delusions of sin or guilt grandiose religious somatic ideas/delusions of reference delusions of being controlled delusions of mind reading delusions of thought broadcasting delusions of thought insertion delusions of thought withdrawal	*Alogia* poverty of speech poverty of content of speech blocking slow response to questions *Avolition-apathy* poor grooming and hygiene impersistence at work or school physical anergia
Bizarre behaviour clothing/appearance social/sexual aggressive/agitated repetitive/stereotyped	*Anhedonia-asociality* few recreational interests/activities reduced sexual interest/activity inability to experience intimacy or closeness impaired relationships with friends and peers
Positive formal thought disorder derailment (loosened associations) tangentiality incoherence (word salad, schizophasia) illogicality circumstantiality pressure of speech distractible speech clanging	*Attention* social inattentiveness inattentiveness during mental state examination
Inappropriate affect	

Box 18.7 Liddle's three syndromes of chronic schizophrenia		
Psychomotor poverty syndrome	*Disorganization syndrome*	*Reality distortion syndrome*
Poverty of speech	Inappropriate affect	Voices speak to the patient
Decreased spontaneous movement	Poverty of content of speech	Delusions of persecution
Unchanging facial expression	Tangentiality	Delusions of reference
Paucity of expressive gesture	Derailment	
Affective non-response	Pressure of speech	
Lack of vocal inflection	Distractibility	

testing (Box 18.7). These syndromes were subsequently associated with a specific pattern of regional cerebral blood flow on positron emission tomography (PET) (Liddle et al. 1992).

Presentation of schizophrenia

Premorbid schizophrenia

Schizophrenic patients frequently exhibit subtle cognitive, intellectual, linguistic, motor, behavioural and social abnormalities many years before the onset of frank psychosis. Such premorbid dysfunction is often reported retrospectively by parents and teachers as odd or eccentric behaviour, or as social deviance. Jones et al. (1995) prospectively confirmed such subjective reports in their study of almost 5000 individuals born in 1946 and subsequently evaluated on 11 occasions before the age of 16 years, and on nine further occasions before the age of 43 years. This research revealed that the 30 children who ultimately developed schizophrenia were (1) slower in learning to walk; (2) noted by their mothers to prefer solitary play; (3) rated by their teachers as anxious and asocial at the age of 15 years; and (4) rated themselves as lacking social confidence at the age of 13 years.

Poor performance on cognitive tests, especially non-verbal, verbal and mathematical tests, predicted schizophrenia at all evaluation points throughout childhood. This and other studies provide powerful evidence that schizophrenic patients exhibit a range of childhood developmental, cognitive and social impairments when compared to children who either remain healthy or develop non-schizophrenic psychiatric illness. Cannon et al. (2001), for example, found that abnormal suspiciousness or sensitivity and relationship difficulties in childhood were associated with later schizophrenia while hysterical symptoms and disturbances in eating were associated with later affective psychosis.

Patients with schizophrenia may present with an acute florid psychosis which develops over a few days or weeks, or following a more insidious onset of disease over many months or even over years. It is therefore clinically useful to differentiate between acute and chronic schizophrenia.

Acute schizophrenia

This may develop rapidly and de novo but is not infrequently preceded by a prodrome of days or weeks in duration during which delusional mood (see Chapter 6), increasingly bizarre behaviour and progressively more severe abnormalities of speech and affect occur. These may be accompanied by declining personal, domestic, social and occupational competence. These latter characteristics may be evidenced by poor personal hygiene, failure to clean or change clothing, isolation within the family initially followed by increasingly marked loss of contact with family members and peers, homelessness, unacceptable social behaviour, poor work performance and loss of earning capacity.

Acute schizophrenia is characterized by symptoms that may be described as Schneiderian, Type 1 or positive, or that best fit Liddle's reality distortion syndrome. Thus auditory hallucinations, persecutory delusions, passivity phenomena and thought disorder are common. Catatonic features may also occur although these appear to be becoming less common in industrialized countries. Abnormalities of affect such as anxiety, depression or euphoria are common, and there is an increased risk of both violence and suicide. Cognition is generally held to remain normal in acute schizophrenia, but insight is almost always impaired. Few patients realize that they are ill, attribute their experiences to illness or recognize the need for treatment. Patients with acute schizophrenia may require urgent hospitalization in order to prevent danger to themselves or others, to undertake investigations and to initiate treatment.

Chronic schizophrenia

This is characterized by Bleulerian, Type 2, or negative symptoms, and best fits Liddle's psychomotor poverty and disorganization syndromes. Thus avolition, affective abnormality (including depression), autism, and poverty of speech occur. Patients with chronic schizophrenia do not care adequately for themselves and need repeated encouragement to wash, dress and eat. They remain inactive for long periods of time, undertake activities slowly, do not socialize, converse infrequently or are effectively mute, and may be incontinent. Insight is almost always impaired and violence and suicide may occur. Patients with chronic schizophrenia may be unable to live independently and frequently need help in order to ensure basic personal care and to prevent self-neglect.

It is generally accepted that general intellectual function is not compromised in chronic schizophrenia despite the fact that patients perform poorly on almost all cognitive tests. Payne (1973), for example, demonstrated that the mean IQ of 1284 schizophrenic patients was 96 and also provided some evidence of a decline from a normal mean IQ, based on academic and military records. In contrast, Russell et al. (1997) reported no change in mean IQ over 20 years in 34 children initially evaluated for childhood psychiatric disorder who subsequently developed schizophrenia (although these individuals did have below-average IQs when first evaluated as children). These results suggest that IQ is below normal at or before the onset of schizophrenia and does not decline thereafter. This view is supported by a report of similar neuropsychological function in newly diagnosed and previously diagnosed patients, but of impaired function in both groups when compared to healthy subjects (Censits et al. 1997).

Classification and diagnosis

Classification
The number and variety of symptoms and the variable course of schizophrenia has led to repeated attempts to subtype patients. The classic subtypes of schizophrenia – paranoid, hebephrenic and catatonic— are retained in both ICD-10 and DSM-IV (in which hebephrenia is referred to as disorganized schizophrenia) along with undifferentiated schizophrenia and will now be described (see also Appendices 3 and 4).

Paranoid schizophrenia
This is the commonest subtype and is characterized by prominent delusions (which may or may not be persecutory in content) and hallucinations, usually auditory. Thought disorders, affective abnormality and negative symptoms occur but are not prominent, while the course may be episodic, with partial or complete remission, or chronic.

Hebephrenic (disorganized) schizophrenia
This is characterized by affective abnormality, thought disorder, irresponsible and unpredictable behaviour, and mannerisms. Hallucinations and delusions are inconspicuous, avolition and anhedonia common, and the course often one of progressive deterioration.

Catatonic schizophrenia
Psychomotor disturbances ranging from violent excitement to stupor and including posturing, negativism, waxy flexibly, automatic obedience and perseveration characterize this subtype. Visual hallucinations may occur in a dreamlike or oneiroid state.

ICD-10 also includes simple schizophrenia and post-schizophrenic depression as subtypes while both ICD-10 and DSM-IV include residual schizophrenia.

Simple schizophrenia
Negative symptoms develop slowly and progressively and without evidence of delusions or hallucinations. This uncommon subtype is diagnosed very infrequently.

Postschizophrenic depression
This is characterized by the development of depressive symptoms such that antidepressant treatment is warranted and there is an increased risk of suicide in the aftermath of a schizophrenic episode. Schizophrenic symptoms may persist or be absent and postschizophrenic depression may be difficult to differentiate from negative symptoms or the adverse effects of treatment.

Residual schizophrenia
Negative symptoms progressively replace delusions, hallucinations and other positive symptoms and there is no evidence that these are caused by depression, dementia or other disorders.

It should be noted that it is often difficult to subtype schizophrenic patients and indeed the IPSS (World Health Organization 1973) found no evidence that subtypes exist. Because of this and for other reasons, research may be conducted on subgroups of patients defined pragmatically, for example on the basis of whether or not they have a schizophrenic relative, respond to treatment, or have normal cerebral ventricles on neuroimaging.

Disorders similar to schizophrenia
These disorders confound the diagnosis of schizophrenia. They include schizotypal, schizoaffective and persistent delusional disorders, which will be discussed later in this chapter, and several other psychotic disorders that are similar to, but do not meet the diagnostic criteria for, schizophrenia, which will be discussed now (Box 18.8). Discussion of these disorders is complicated by the numerous diagnostic terms available. ICD-10 nosology will therefore be used when possible and equivalent or similar diagnostic terms will be provided as appropriate.

Acute and transient psychotic disorders
These disorders significantly disrupt global functioning and are characterized by:

Box 18.8   Psychiatric and non-psychiatric disorders that may mimic schizophrenia

Psychiatric	Non-psychiatric
Psychotic disorders	*Neurological disorders*
Affective psychoses	Temporal lobe epilepsy
Schizoaffective psychosis	Other epilepsies
Acute and transient psychoses	Cerebral tumours
Persistent delusional disorders	Cerebrovascular accidents
Cycloid psychoses	Huntington's disease
Induced delusional disorders	Dementia
Non-psychotic disorders	*Infectious disorders*
Schizotypal disorder	Neurosyphilis
Personality disorders	Herpes encephalitis
Obsessive-compulsive	HIV
disorder	
Autism/Asperger's syndrome	*Autoimmune disorders*
	Hyperthyroidism
Drug-induced psychosis	Hypothyroidism
Alcoholic hallucinosis	Diabetes mellitus
Lysergic acid diethylamide	Cushing's disease/syndrome
(LSD)	Systemic lupus erythematosus
Amphetamine	
Cocaine	*Systemic disorders*
Cannabis	Metachromatic leucodystrophy
Ecstasy	Fever
Phenylcyclidine (PCP)	Postoperative
Levodopa	Postpartum
Steroids	Wilson's disease
	Traumatic disorder
	Head injury

- an associated acute psychological stress, the putative precipitant
- an abrupt (within 48 hours of the stress) or acute (within two weeks of the stress) onset, and
- variable and rapidly changing (or polymorphic) schizophrenic symptoms, usually including delusions and hallucinations, that resolve rapidly.

Characteristically, the delusions and hallucinations change in content and sensory modality from day to day or even hour to hour, and are associated with a fluctuating affective state. These disorders are thought to be more common in females and immigrants. Schneiderian first-rank symptoms may occur and it is not infrequently difficult to identify a precipitant. Synonyms for acute and transient psychotic disorders include brief psychotic disorders (DSM-IV), psychogenic psychosis, reactive psychosis, acute paranoid psychosis, *bouffee délirante* and cycloid psychoses.

Cycloid psychoses

Leonhard (1957) differentiated between schizophrenia and favourable outcome or cycloid psychoses. These are difficult to distinguish from schizophrenia and are of three types, each characterized by two groups of symptoms between which patients cycle, as follows:

- motility psychosis in which patients cycle between minimal and maximal psychomotor activity
- anxiety-elation psychosis in which patients cycle between anxiety with delusions and hallucinations and elation, and

- confusion psychosis in which patients cycle between overactivity and excitement, often with formal thought disorder, and minimal psychomotor activity.

Induced delusional disorder

These uncommon psychotic disorders consist of delusions, usually persecutory or grandiose, shared by two or more people (*folie à deux*). Delusions are induced in one individual who has as close relationship with and is dependent upon another individual who is psychotic, most often because of schizophrenia. Typically the two individuals are isolated by geography, culture or language, and these factors make for presentation only after prolonged illness. Despite this, induced psychoses usually resolve when the individuals involved are separated.

Gjessing's syndrome

This extremely rare disorder described by Gjessing (1938) consists of episodes of catatonia and altered nitrogen balance, not necessarily in phase, which can be successfully treated with thyroxine.

Diagnosis

There are no diagnostic tests for schizophrenia and the diagnosis must be made on the basis of the presence of typical schizophrenic symptoms for a minimum duration of time and the exclusion of another psychiatric or non-psychiatric cause for the symptoms. Thus both ICD-10 and DSM-IV require that a minimum number of specific symptoms are apparent for at least one month and that there is no evidence of either a psychiatric disorder such as affective psychosis, or the effects of alcohol or psychoactive substances, or a disorder such as Huntington's disease or hypothyroidism (Appendices 1 and 2).

Differential diagnosis

The numerous psychiatric and nonpsychiatric disorders that may mimic schizophrenia are listed in Box 18.8.

The nonpsychiatric disorders can be conveniently classified as neurological, infectious, autoimmune, systemic, traumatic and other, and while these represent uncommon causes of apparent schizophrenia it is important that they are diagnosed when present so that appropriate treatment may be provided and inappropriate treatment avoided. Diagnosis can usually be accomplished on the basis of a careful clinical history and examination supplemented by laboratory and other investigations. It is especially important to consider a nonpsychiatric disorder masquerading as schizophrenia when schizophrenia manifests at the extremes of age, is characterized by abrupt episodes of psychosis, includes atypical symptoms, fails to respond at least partially to adequate treatment, or recurs after prolonged successful treatment.

Psychotic symptoms are associated with temporal lobe epilepsy (see Chapter 26), which accounts for about 50% of all epilepsies and thus represents an important differential diagnosis for schizophrenia. The psychosis of temporal lobe epilepsy generally differs from schizophrenia as follows:

- there is no family history of schizophrenia
- premorbid personality is normal
- the psychosis develops 10–15 years after the onset of epilepsy, and
- affective abnormality is absent.

Temporal lobe epilepsy should be considered particularly in patients who experience recurrent, stereotyped episodes of psychosis associated with possible clouding of consciousness.

Investigations

There are no biological markers for schizophrenia but laboratory and other investigations are essential in order to (1) exclude non-psychiatric disorders presenting as schizophrenia; (2) exclude other non-psychiatric disorders; and (3) establish baseline measures prior to initiation of pharmacotherapy (Box 18.9).

Investigations never preclude the need for careful clinical history taking and a thorough physical, particularly neurological, examination. Schizophrenic patients – especially those who smoke cigarettes, are substance abusing, or are hostel dwelling or homeless – have an increased risk of illness and an increased mortality (Thakore 2004). Their contacts with psychiatric services may present infrequent opportunities to provide medical care and screening.

Every patient in whom schizophrenia is suspected should have the investigations listed in Box 18.9 performed. This battery of investigations will help exclude or confirm substance abuse (urine), anaemia, iron or vitamin deficiency, thyroid dysfunction, diabetes mellitus or syphilis (blood), normal cardiac function (ECG), temporal lobe or other epilepsy (EEG), and cerebral tumours or cerebrovascular

accidents (CT or MRI), and will provide baseline haematology and ECG prior to the initiation of pharmacotherapy. Abnormal CT or MRI results will rarely be reported and some authorities recommend these investigations only in patients over the age of 40 years. However, effective treatments are becoming increasingly available for some previously untreatable neurological disorders and no effort should be spared in excluding neurological pathology. Other investigations may be indicated by the clinical presentation and the results of the tests listed above and may include autoantibody screens, neuroendocrine assessments, measurement of serum caeruloplasmin or viral antibody titres, chest X-ray, lumbar puncture, additional EEG studies, MRI, genetic studies and HIV testing (with consent and appropriate counselling).

The aetiology of schizophrenia

Our current understanding of the pathogenesis and pathophysiology of schizophrenia is that environmental factors (which have been partially identified) interact with predisposing genes (which have been partially identified) to cause neurostructural, neurochemical and neurofunctional brain changes (which have been partially identified) that manifest as the syndrome of schizophrenia.

These environmental factors and predisposing genes, and the neurostructural, neurochemical and neurofunctional brain changes, will now be discussed. The section will conclude with a discussion of the neurodevelopmental hypothesis of schizophrenia, which represents an attempt to include environmental, genetic and neurological data within a single model.

Environmental factors

Temporal and physical factors appear to play a role in the causation of schizophrenia. Psychological and social factors on the other hand appear to trigger acute episodes of schizophrenia rather than play a role in its causation.

Temporal and physical factors

A very modest excess – <10% – of schizophrenic individuals are born during late winter and spring in the northern (February to May) and southern (July to October) hemispheres. The majority of, but by no means all, longitudinal and case-control studies suggest that this excess may be accounted for by exposure to influenza epidemics during the second trimester of fetal life because this is associated with increased risk of schizophrenia in adulthood (see Wright & Murray 1996 for review). Other research provides evidence that schizophrenic patients exposed to influenza during the second trimester of fetal life are at increased risk of obstetric complications (Wright et al. 1995). However, influenza rarely causes a viraemia so if this effect is real, the mechanism must involve genetically determined maternal immune responses (Wright et al. 1996a, 1996b).

Box 18.9 Investigations recommended during the evaluation of possible schizophrenia	
Sample/technique	*Investigation*
Urine	Drugs of abuse
Blood	Haematology Biochemistry Blood glucose Thyroid function tests Serum tests for syphilis
Electrocardiography (ECG)	
Electroencephalography (EEG)	Standard EEG Sleep EEG
Computed tomography (CT) or magnetic resonance imaging (MRI)	Neuroimaging

Obstetric complications such as preterm birth, prolonged labour and neonatal hypoxia are reported more often in the birth records of, and are reported more often by the mothers of, schizophrenic patients than of controls (McNeil et al. 1995). The direction of causation is unclear and it may be that obstetric complications are caused by, rather than cause, the neurodevelopmental anomalies that are presumed to underpin schizophrenia.

The three main neurochemical hypotheses of schizophrenia are supported by the fact that drugs of abuse that enhance dopaminergic and serotonergic, and inhibit excitatory amino acid, neurotransmission cause symptoms that resemble those of schizophrenia (see below). Furthermore, it is generally accepted that cannabis may cause episodes of acute psychosis in patients with psychotic disorders (Dagenhardt 2004) and most psychiatrists advise such individuals against cannabis abuse. More recent evidence suggests that cannabis abuse may cause schizophrenia de novo, presumably only in those who are genetically predisposed given that the overwhelming majority of those who abuse cannabis do not develop psychosis. Thus a recent review (Arseneault et al. 2004) of five well conducted studies involving >55 000 people concluded that:

- for any individual, cannabis abuse doubles the risk of developing schizophrenia, and
- for society, eliminating cannabis abuse would reduce the incidence of schizophrenia by almost 10%.

Psychological factors

Psychodynamic aetiological theories of schizophrenia have been proposed by Freud, who suggested that schizophrenic delusions represented attempts to attach meaning to external objects and by Klein who theorized that failure to resolve the 'paranoid-schizoid position' led to schizophrenia.

Psychological theories of schizophrenia have concentrated largely on describing and explaining schizophrenic symptoms. Thus Cameron suggested that overinclusive thinking consequent upon the loss of conceptual boundaries was a paramount feature of schizophrenia while Goldstein described concrete thinking and the absence of abstract and metaphorical thought. Payne, on the basis of sorting tests, proposed that the failure of a theoretical filter that separates background sensory 'noise' from useful sensory 'signal' allows for the interpretation of excess sensory input as hallucinations, a theory which was elaborated by Frith and others.

The cognitive defect theory proposes that schizophrenia may be caused by an impaired ability to perceive and analyse cognitive input which in turn leads to misinterpretation of conversation and of facial expression. Left-hemisphere dysfunction in schizophrenia is suggested by the excess of left-handed patients and the poor performance of patients on measures of left hemisphere function such as dichotic auditory and tachistoscopic visual tests.

Social factors

Schizophrenia is commoner in members of lower socio-economic groups, in urban dwellers and in immigrants (see above). This led Hollingshead & Redlich (1958), who found an excess of schizophrenia in Chicago's lower socio-economic classes, to suggest that deprivation was causitive. However, Goldberg & Morrison (1963) suggested that schizophrenia was not caused by, but actually led to, social decline because most patients are of lower socio-economic status than their fathers. Schizophrenia is over-represented in the centres of industrialized cities such as Chicago (Faris & Dunham 1939) and Mannheim (Hafner & Reimann 1970). Is this because deprivation causes schizophrenia (the breeder hypothesis) or because schizophrenia causes social decline and drives schizophrenic and preschizophrenic individuals to cheaper inner city accommodation (the drifter hypothesis)? These two theories have been investigated by Lewis et al. (1992), who segregated the 268 of 4900 male Swedish army conscripts who developed schizophrenia by place of rearing and found that the adjusted incidence of the disease per 100 000 person years was 51.4, 43.2, 39.8 and 31.2 in cities, large towns, small towns and rural areas respectively. However, while these results support the breeder hypothesis, the drifter hypothesis continues to enjoy wide acceptance.

The direction of causality between life events and schizophrenia is similarly uncertain – the illness may be either the consequence of or the cause of life events. Brown & Birley (1968) found that schizophrenic patients experienced more life events, including independent life events that could not be caused by schizophrenia or its prodrome, in the three weeks prior to hospitalization when compared to healthy controls, but not when compared to psychiatric controls. Jacobs & Myers (1976) reported an excess of life events preceding first episodes of schizophrenia but Brown and Birley's results are in keeping with the conclusions of Norman & Malla's (1993) review of this literature.

Familial theories have concentrated on aberrant parenting (especially aberrant mothering) and aberrant communication within families. According to Lidz's (Lidz & Lidz 1949) marital skew and schism theory, either a dominant mother and/or a submissive father (skew), or parents who held conflicting views and were hostile to each other (schism) could cause schizophrenia in an offspring. Bateson et al. (1956) proposed a double-bind communication deviance mechanism and suggested that schizophrenia developed when a child received conflicting instructions – one spoken, the other implied by, for example, behaviour or tone of voice – from a parent.

Predisposing genes

Family, twin and adoption studies

Over 80 years ago Rudin (1916) demonstrated that the risk of schizophrenia was greater in siblings of schizophrenic patients than in the general population. It is now accepted that having a schizophrenic relative is the biggest risk factor for schizophrenia and that 70% of the heritibility of schizophrenia is genetic. Gottesman & Bertelsen (1989) graphically illustrated the inherited risk of schizophrenia when they studied the offspring of twins discordant for schizophrenia. They demonstrated that while the risk of schizophrenia was much less in the offspring of unaffected when compared to the offspring of affected dizygotic twins, the risk was similar in the offspring of unaffected when compared to the offspring of affected monozygotic twins. The risk of schizophrenia is greatest when:

- close relatives are affected
- several relatives are affected
- female relatives are affected
- affected relatives have early-onset schizophrenia
- affected relatives have severe schizophrenia, and
- a monozygotic sibling has schizophrenia.

The approximate lifetime risks of schizophrenia for various degrees of genetic relatedness to a schizophrenic individual are shown in Table 18.5 (Gottesman 1991). These data underpin the importance of familial aetiological factors but do not differentiate between genetic and environmental familial effects – environment sharing increases with degree of relatedness, monozygotic twins even sharing the same intrauterine environment!

Adoption studies were performed in order to exclude environmental factors in heritibility. About 10% of the offspring of schizophrenic individuals who are adopted by non-schizophrenic parents develop schizophrenia (Kety 1983) while there is no increase in schizophrenia among the offspring of healthy individuals adopted by schizophrenic parents (Wender et al. 1974). These results clearly favour genetic heritibility of the disease.

Molecular genetics

It is extremely unlikely that a single gene is responsible for schizophrenia because it is impossible to assign a classic Mendelian model of inheritance to a disease with monozygotic twin concordance of less than 100% and in which over 60% of patients do not have an affected relative. Single-gene (monogenic or single major locus) genetic models have therefore given way to polygenic (schizophrenia results from the combined effects of several predisposing genes) or polygenic/multifactorial (schizophrenia results from the combined effects of both several predisposing genes and a number of triggering environmental factors) models. An important implication of the polygenic/multifactorial model is that schizophrenia may result from genes alone, from the interaction of genes and environmental insults such as obstetric complications or head injury, or from environmental insults alone, and the clinical picture may differ in each case (Box 18.10). The polygenic/multifactorial model is currently the subject of international collaborative efforts to identify the responsible genes and environmental factors (see below and Chapter 3).

Chromosome 6p24–22 was the focus of much research when the first edition of this volume was published (Mowry et al. 1995; see Wright et al. 2000 for review). With the publication of the second edition it appears that the years 2002/2003 may yet prove to be pivotal in our understanding

Table 18.5 Lifetime schizophrenia risks for degrees of genetic relatedness to a schizophrenic		
Relative	*Lifetime risk of schizophrenia (%)*	*Degree of genetic relatedness*
(General population)	(1)	(–)
Spouse of patient	2	Unrelated
First cousin of patient	2	Third
Nephew/niece of patient	4	Second
Grandchild of patient	5	Second
Child of patient, other parent healthy	13	First
Child of patient, other parent with schizophrenia	46	First
Sibling of patient	9	First
Sibling of patient, one of patient's parents has schizophrenia	17	First
Dizygotic twin sibling of patient	17	First
Monozygotic twin sibling of patient	48	First
Parent of patient	6	First

Box 18.10 Genetic, genetic/environmental and environmental models of schizophrenia

Genetic
- Patient has close relative(s) with schizophrenia
- Patient inherits sufficient predisposing genes to cause schizophrenia

Genetic/environmental
- Patient may or may not have close relative(s) with schizophrenia
- Patient inherits insufficient predisposing genes to cause schizophrenia
- Patients experience insufficient environmental insults to cause schizophrenia
- The combined effects of insufficient predisposing genes and insufficient environmental insults are sufficient to cause schizophrenia

Environmental
- Patient has no close relative(s) with schizophrenia
- Patient experiences sufficient environmental insults to cause schizophrenia

of the genetics of schizophrenia. Seven pathophysiologically plausible susceptibility genes were reported during this period and several of the reports were replicated. The reported associations are as follows:

- the neuregulin 1 (NRG1) gene at chromosome 8p12–21 in Icelandic (Stefansson et al. 2002), Scottish (Stefansson et al. 2003) and Han Chinese (Li et al. 2004) populations
- the dysbindin (DTNBP1) gene at chromosome 6p22 in Irish (Straub et al. 2002) and German (Schwab et al. 2003) populations
- the novel G 72 gene at chromosome 13q34 in French–Canadian and Russian populations (Chumakov et al. 2002)
- the D-amino acid oxidase (DAAO) gene at chromosome 12q24 in a French–Canadian population (Chumakov et al. 2002)
- the regulator of G protein signalling 4 (RGS4) gene at chromosome 1q21-22 in American and Indian populations (Chowdhari et al. 2002)
- the proline dehydrogenase (PRODH) gene at chromosome 22q11 (Liu et al. 2002) and
- the catechol-o-methyltransferase (COMT) gene at chromosome 22q11 (Shifman et al. 2002).

Implication of the COMT gene is highly plausible given the dopamine hypothesis of schizophrenia and the role of COMT in degrading dopamine. Implication of the other genes listed above is less obvious. However, schizophrenia is thought to be a neurodevelopmental disorder and NRG1, DTNBP1 and RGS4 may play a role in neurodevelopment. Furthermore, the products of all seven of the genes listed modify glutamatergic neurotransmission and thus the findings may support the glutamate hypothesis of schizophrenia (see Harrison & Owen 2003 for review).

Neurostructural, neurochemical and neurofunctional brain changes

Neurostructural brain changes

Neuropathological and neuroimaging studies of schizophrenia have a long history. Alzheimer (1913) described cortical atrophy in the brains of some of Kraepelin's patients after death, Jacobi & Winkler reported enlarged ventricles in schizophrenic patients using pneumoencephalography in 1927 and Ingvar & Franzen demonstrated hypoperfusion of the frontal cortex using a gamma camera and [133]Xenon in 1974. Contemporary research in these fields benefits from both technical innovation and operationalized diagnosis.

The brains of schizophrenic patients weigh slightly less than those of control subjects. Harrison et al. (2003), for example, reported that the mean brain weight of 540 schizophrenia subjects was 2% lighter than that of 794 controls. Structural neuroimaging provides evidence that the brains of schizophrenic patients also have slightly larger third and lateral ventricles than brains from age- and sex-matched controls (Lawrie and Abukmeil 1998). Ventricular enlargement is present at disease onset in patients who have not been treated with antipsychotic drugs (Harrison 1999), does not progress, is commoner in patients without a schizophrenic relative, and only occurs in the affected twins of monozygotic twins discordant for disease (Suddath et al. 1989).

About 15% of schizophrenic patients have widened sulci and narrowed gyri at postmortem examination and reduced numbers of neurons and specific subpopulations of neurons have been reported (Akbarian et al. 1993). Basal ganglia enlargement may be caused by treatment with older antipsychotic drugs because it is reversed by treatment with clozapine and does not appear to occur in patients treated with clozapine from onset of disease (Chakos et al. 1995). Recent evidence suggests that basal ganglia enlargement may be largely confined to male patients (Heitmiller et al. 2004).

Bogerts et al. (1985) reported smaller hippocampi, parahippocampi and amygdalae in some schizophrenic patients at postmortem and these results have been confirmed with MRI (Suddath et al. 1989). Reduced numbers, reduced size and disorientation of the hippocampal pyramidal neurons and heterotopy of parahippocampal pre-alpha cells have also been reported. Recent MRI studies found smaller thalami, hippocampi and superior temporal lobes bilaterally (Flaum et al. 1995) and Pakkenberg (1990) has reported reduced numbers of thalamic neurons. Gliosis, a marker of brain insult, was reported in schizophrenic brains by Alzheimer but has largely not been confirmed by modern studies. The neuropathology of schizophrenia has been extensively reviewed by Harrison (1999, 2003, 2004).

Neurochemical brain changes

Almost every brain chemical has been implicated in an aetiological theory of schizophrenia but only the dopamine, serotonin, excitatory amino acid (EAA) and phospholipid membrane hypotheses merit detailed description. The transmethylation hypothesis warrants brief mention as the first biochemical theory of schizophrenia. It derives from the fact that mescaline, an hallucinogen, is an orthomethylated metabolite of dopamine and proposes that abnormal methylation of brain monoamines produces an endogenous hallucinogen, dimethyl tryptamine. However, while methyl group donors, e.g. methionine, can exacerbate schizophrenia, methyl group acceptors, e.g. nicotinic acid, are not effective antipsychotics.

The dopamine hypothesis   The dopamine hypothesis derives from the data listed in Box 18.11 and states that schizophrenia is caused by excess dopaminergic activity in mesolimbic and cortical brain regions. The research findings listed in Box 18.12 conflict with the dopamine hypothesis. Nonetheless, the fact that every effective antipsychotic drug blocks dopamine D_2 receptors is powerful evidence of the importance of dopamine in the pathogenesis of schizophrenia. Contemporary investigations of the dopamine hypothesis focus on:

- the influence of dopamine receptor subtypes and their genetic variants on response/non-response to treatment via their relative distributions in various brain structures (Sunahara et al. 1993)
- response/non-response to antipsychotic treatment and D_2 receptor occupancy (Pilowsky et al. 1997)
- the role of the D_3 receptor in both the aetiology of schizophrenia and response to antipsychotic drugs (Kerwin & Owen 1999), and
- the fast dissociation hypothesis of atypical antipsychotic efficacy and safety which postulates that while D_2

receptor occupancy is responsible for antipsychotic effect, rapid dissociation from the D_2 receptor (rather than occupancy of $5HT_{2A}$ or other receptors) accounts for extrapyramidal safety (Kapur & Seeman 2001) (see Chapter 38).

The serotonin hypothesis   The serotonin hypothesis states that schizophrenia is caused by excess serotonergic activity in the brain and is based on the two key research findings:

- that lysergic acid diethylamine (LSD) and psilocybin, $5HT_{2A/2C}$ receptor agonists, cause positive symptoms of schizophrenia in non-schizophrenic individuals
- that newer antipsychotics such as clozapine, olanzapine and risperidone are potent $5HT_{2A}$ receptor antagonists.

However, LSD produces visual hallucinations which are uncommon in schizophrenia, older antipsychotics block serotonin receptors and newer antipsychotics are potent D_2 receptor antagonists. Recent investigations suggest that midbrain serotonergic neurons may modulate limbic and cortical dopaminergic systems and several newer antipsychotics have greater affinity at the $5HT_{2A/2C}$ receptor than at the D_2 receptor. Recent investigations of the serotonin hypothesis have concentrated on the influence of serotonin receptor subtypes and their genetic variants on response/non-response to treatment (Arranz et al. 1995) and on functional neuroimaging of these receptors in patients treated with various antipsychotic drugs (Bussato & Kerwin 1997).

The excitatory amino acid hypothesis   The EAAs include glutamate and aspartate and the EAA hypothesis of schizophrenia states that insufficient EAAs or their kainate, quisqualate or N-methyl-D-aspartate (NMDA) receptors are implicated in schizophrenia (see Chapter 38). Low cerebrospinal fluid levels of glutamate were reported by Kim et al. (1980), and Deakin et al. (1989) found reduced numbers of glutamate receptors in temporal cortex from schizophrenic patients. The hypothesis is further supported by the finding that a single dose of phencyclidine (PCP) (a non-competitive NMDA receptor antagonist) can produce

Box 18.11   Research findings supporting the dopamine hypothesis of schizophrenia

Amphetamine releases dopamine at the synapse and causes positive symptoms of schizophrenia in non-schizophrenic individuals

Levodopa increases central dopamine concentrations and causes positive symptoms of schizophrenia in non-schizophrenic individuals

Disulfiram inhibits dopamine metabolism and exacerbates schizophrenia

All effective antipsychotic drugs are dopamine D_2 receptor antagonists

Only the a isomer of flupenthixol is a D_2 receptor antagonist and an effective antipsychotic; the b isomer is not a D_2 antagonist and is clinically inactive (Johnstone et al. 1978)

Antipsychotic efficacy correlates significantly with D_2 receptor occupancy (Sunahara et al. 1993)

Increased (Wong et al. 1986) and asymmetrical (Farde et al. 1990) brain D_2 receptor densities have been reported in living schizophrenic patients, using PET

Increased concentrations of D_2 receptors (Lee & Seeman 1980) and of dopamine (Mackay et al. 1982) have been found in postmortem brain tissue from schizophrenic patients

Box 18.12   Research findings in conflict with the dopamine hypothesis of schizophrenia

Amphetamine, levodopa and disulfiram do not produce negative schizophrenic symptoms

Antipsychotic drugs are not exclusively 'anti-schizophrenic' and are effective in other disorders

Antipsychotic drugs are ineffective in about 30% of patients with schizophrenia

Antipsychotics block D_2 receptors within hours but antipsychotic efficacy is not apparent for days or weeks

Normal concentrations of dopamine and D_2 receptors (Gur & Pearlson 1993) have been found in postmortem brain tissue from schizophrenic patients

Normal brain D_2 receptor densities have been reported in living schizophrenic patients (Farde 1997)

positive and negative schizophrenic symptoms in non-schizophrenic individuals and exacerbations of schizophrenia in stable patients, and that kainate and NMDA receptors are reduced in number in postmortem temporal cortex from schizophrenia patients (Royston & Simpson 1991).

The phospholipid membrane hypotheses The function of neuronal membranes may be modified by alterations in their phospholipid and cholesterol composition. Horrobin et al. (1999) has therefore proposed a phospholipid membrane hypothesis of schizophrenia based on abnormalities of phospholipid metabolism in both brain and red blood cells and clinical trials of omega 3 fatty acids have been undertaken (Emsley et al. 2003).

Neurofunctional brain changes

The frontal hypoperfusion reported by Ingvar & Franzen (1974) was confirmed by contemporary PET studies. Over ten years ago Sedvall (1990) concluded that PET results in schizophrenia demonstrated decreased brain metabolism overall with particularly decreased frontal metabolism, and increased left-hemisphere metabolism with particularly increased left temporal lobe metabolism. These results appear to be independent of treatment. More recently, Erritzo et al. (2003) reviewed PET and single proton emission tomography (SPET) research and concluded that investigations consistently demonstrated increased presynaptic striatal dopaminergic activity and that this was associated with positive symptoms and a good response to antipsychotic drugs.

Magnetic resonance spectroscopy (MRS) has been used in addition to PET and SPET to study brain function in schizophrenia. Most ^{1}H MRS studies have found reduced N-acetyl-aspartate in frontal and temporal cortex (Cecil et al. 1999) while ^{31}P studies have reported reduced phosphomonoesters and increased phosphodiesters (Frangou and Williams 1996). The exact meaning of these findings is unclear at present.

Attempts to correlate symptomatology and functional neuroimaging data have been undertaken. Thus Liddle et al. (1992) reported that each of his three syndromes of chronic schizophrenia was associated with a specific pattern of regional cerebral blood flow (rCBF) while McGuire et al. (1993) demonstrated hyperperfusion of Broca's area in patients experiencing auditory hallucinations. This latter work has been extended by Shergill et al. (2000) who reported that auditory hallucinations were associated with activation in a network of cortical and subcortical areas (inferior frontal/insular, anterior cingulate and temporal cortex bilaterally, right thalamus and inferior colliculus and left hippocampus and parahippocampal cortex) rather than in a single area.

Functional neuroimaging has also demonstrated that schizophrenic patients show impaired activation of the frontal lobes when undertaking tests of frontal lobe function

(Velakoulis and Pantelis 1996) and Rodriguez et al. (1996) demonstrated higher rCBF in the thalamus and left basal ganglia of clozapine-responsive schizophrenic patients compared to clozapine non-responders.

Abnormalities of event-related evoked potentials, skin conductance and smooth pursuit (and other) eye movements have been reported in schizophrenic patients and these abnormalities are being increasingly incorporated into models of the disease, of treatment response and of prognosis. For example:

- Jeon & Polich (2003) undertook a meta-analysis of P300 and schizophrenia and concluded that the P300 effect size was of reduced amplitude and greater latency in schizophrenia than in healthy controls, and that the latency effect increases with disease duration.
- Dawson & Schell (2002) reviewed studies of skin conductance and schizophrenia and concluded that abnormally high electrodermal arousal and reactivity is predictive of poor outcome in at least some patients.
- Lee & Williams (2000) reviewed available studies and concluded that dysfunction of smooth pursuit eye movements was a trait marker for schizophrenia.

The neurodevelopmental hypothesis of schizophrenia

Neurodevelopmental hypotheses of schizophrenia proposed by Weinberger (1987), Murray & Lewis (1987), Murray (1994) and others state that a proportion of schizophrenia commences with impaired fetal or neonatal neuro-development and not with the onset of psychotic symptoms in early adulthood. Support for the neurodevelopmental hypothesis is provided by:

- the excess of structural brain abnormalities and underlying cytoarchitectoral anomalies described in schizophrenia (see above)
- the excess of congenital brain abnormalities reported in schizophrenic patients (Lewis et al. 1988)
- the increased frequency of craniofacial and dermatoglyphic minor physical anonomies reported in schizophrenia, which is significant because both brain and skin develop from primitive neuroectoderm (Griffiths et al. 1988)
- the lower than average IQ and subtle psychomotor, behavioural, personality and social abnormalities described in schizophrenia (see above), and
- the non-specific neurological soft signs that occur in more than 50% of schizophrenic patients, the abnormal smooth pursuit eye movements that occur in patients and their relatives, and the reduced amplitude and greater latency of event-related evoked potentials described in schizophrenic patients.

Environmental factors are implicated in neurodevelopmental schizophrenia because only the schizophrenic members of disease-discordant monozygotic twin pairs exhibit dilated ventricles. Such environmental factors may include obstetric complications, prenatal viral infections and prenatal malnutrition. However, the vast majority of individuals who experience obstetric complications do not develop schizophrenia. The neurodevelopmental hypothesis therefore implicates predisposing genes and states that environmental factors such as obstetric complications and prenatal viral infections cause the neurostructural, neurochemical and neurofunctional brain changes of schizophrenia in genetically predisposed individuals.

The treatment of schizophrenia

The treatment of schizophrenia is largely psychopharmacological. Repeated double-blind trials have demonstrated that antipsychotic drugs both alleviate acute episodes, and prevent recurrences, of schizophrenia more effectively than either placebo or general tranquillizers (Gilbert et al. 1995). More recently, it has been recognized that optimized psychopharmacological treatment also facilitates a range of educational, psychological and social interventions.

General treatment of schizophrenia
Treating acute episodes of schizophrenia
The advantages of hospitalization for many patients with first episodes or any significant relapse of schizophrenia are summarized below (Box 18.13). Antipsychotic treatment with a single antipsychotic drug should be initiated as soon as the diagnosis of schizophrenia is established because there is evidence that the duration of untreated psychotic symptoms determines time to recovery, extent of recovery and risk of relapse (Loebel et al. 1992). Agitated and/or anxious patients may also require oral or parenteral benzodiazepines. Severely ill patients who are agitated and/or unwilling to accept oral antipsychotic therapy may require a parenterally administered antipsychotic drug (see below and Chapters 35 and 38).

Box 18.13   Some advantages of hospitalization in the treatment of schizophrenia

A period of safe, medication-free observation is possible

Thorough investigation and definitive diagnosis are facilitated

Data on personal development, premorbid personality, medical and psychiatric history, education and ocupation may be collected and collated

Social evaluation may be undertaken

Security and safety may be provided

Respite is provided to family/relatives

Antipsychotic treatment may be initiated, dosage titrated and efficacy/safety evaluated, and education of the patient and family/relatives about schizophrenia and its treatment may be undertaken

---

Once antipsychotic treatment has been initiated, patients must be observed for compliance with and response to therapy, and for the development of adverse-effects (see below). An adequate trial of an antipsychotic drug requires compliance with treatment at a suitable dose for a sufficient period of time (perhaps 2-6 weeks). Thus partial or non-response to antipsychotic therapy may indicate:

- misdiagnosis
- comorbiity
- noncompliance
- inadequate dosage
- inadequate duration of treatment
- concurrent use of psychotomimetic drugs, or
- inefficacy.

These problems may be addressed by reassessment of diagnosis and exclusion of comorbidity, by use of liquid or parenteral preparations to enhance compliance, by increasing dosage, by waiting and/or by careful monitoring to exclude abuse of psychotomimetic drugs. An alternative antipsychotic drug should be prescribed if these problems have been addressed and response remains inadequate.

Preventing recurrences of schizophrenia
The relapse rate in antipsychotic-free schizophrenic patients may be as high as 100% over 1–2 years so once an acute episode has resolved virtually all patients should receive maintenance therapy (Davis 1985). It is well established that risk of recurrence never disappears, even after many years of stability, and maintenance therapy will be lifelong for the great majority of patients (Davis et al. 1994). Maintenance antipsychotics may be administered orally or by long acting depot injections (see below).

Benzodiazepines may be a useful adjunct to antipsychotics for some agitated or anxious patients and adjunctive lithium may be beneficial to patients with affective symptoms. Antidepressant treatment including ECT may be appropriate for patients with post-schizophrenic depression, which is associated with an increased risk of suicide and may be difficult to differentiate from extrapyramidal side-effects or from negative symptoms. Once effective maintenance therapy has been established, patients may be discharged from hospital and a range of educational, psychological and social interventions commenced (see below).

Treatment-resistant schizophrenia
The majority of schizophrenic patients respond adequately to antipsychotic treatment. However, it has been estimated that approximately 30% respond inadequately and 10% of patients show no response. Many of these patients fulfill the Kane et al. (1988) criteria for treatment resistance and have functioned poorly for at least five years, have severe psychopathology and have not responded to at least three

periods of treatment with drugs from at least two different classes of antipsychotics in doses equivalent to 1 g of chlorpromazine per day for at least six weeks' duration (assuming compliance).

Apparent treatment resistance may be caused by non-compliance, use of psychotomimetic agents, comorbid illness or disease severity. These causes may be addressed by ensuring compliance (choose drug and dosage that minimizes adverse effects, consider depot formulations), preventing use of psychotomimetic drugs (when possible), treating comorbid psychiatric or nonpsychiatric disease, modifying dosage or changing to another antipsychotic from a different chemical class. However, a proportion of patients will remain severely ill despite these efforts. There is clear evidence that such patients may respond to clozapine (Lieberman et al. 1994). This should be commenced – with appropriate haematological monitoring – as soon as treatment resistance is established because outcome is determined by duration of psychosis before effective treatment is instituted (see above).

Primary treatment resistance in which symptoms have never been adequately controlled must be differentiated from secondary treatment resistance in which previously well controlled symptoms suddenly or gradually re-emerge. In patients with secondary treatment resistance consideration must always be given to comorbid cerebral tumour, dementia or other pathology.

Atypical and typical antipsychotic drugs

Newer or atypical antipsychotic drugs such as olanzapine, quetiapine and risperidone have largely replaced older typical antipsychotic drugs such as haloperidol in the management of schizophrenia in developed countries. The main advantage atypical antipsychotic drugs have over typical antipsychotic drugs is their reduced propensity to cause adverse effects. Thus they:

- are less likely to cause extrapyramidal adverse-effects because they have less affinity for nigrostriatal dopamine D_2 receptors (atypical antipsychotics reduce spontaneous firing in A10 neurons, typical antipsychotics reduce firing in both A9 and A10 neurons)
- are less likely to cause hyperprolactinaemia and associated adverse effects because they have less affinity for tuberoinfundibular dopamine D_2 receptors and
- have relatively high serotonin $5HT_{2A}$ to dopamine D_2 receptor binding ratios.

Atypical and typical antipsychotic drugs are equally effective against positive symptoms but atypical antipsychotic drugs may be somewhat more effective in treating negative and affective symptoms. There is also increasing evidence that olanzapine and possibly risperidone may improve cognitive function in schizophrenia (Bilder et al. 2002). Given these differences, atypical antipsychotic drugs have been recommended as first-line treatment for almost all patients with schizophrenia by the National Institute for Clinical Excellence (NICE) in the UK and other similar authorities (2002; see also Chapter 38). Typical antipsychotics should only be prescribed for patients who have responded to them in the past without developing significant side effects. However, it is recognized that typical antipsychotics will remain in use for the forseeable future in some areas for economic or other reasons.

Rapidly acting intramuscular injections

Patients who are agitated and/or unwilling to accept oral antipsychotic therapy may require a rapidly acting parenterally administered antipsychotic drug. Such a requirement no longer necessitates the use of typical antipsychotic drugs because a rapidly acting intramuscular formulation of olanzapine is now available for the treatment of agitation and disturbed behaviour (Wright et al. 2001). An intramuscular formulation of ziprasidone is also available in a number of countries (Brook 2003). Intramuscular formulations of atypical antipsychotic drugs are much less likely to cause acute dystonia and other extrapyramidal adverse effects. This reduces the distress experienced by patients during what is an already highly distressing period and may facilitate the patient/doctor relationship and long term adherence to prophylactic antipsychotic therapy. NICE have made the following important treatment recommendations about the care of schizophrenic patients who are agitated (2002; see also Chapter 38):

- oral administration of medication is preferred to parenteral administration
- intramuscular administration of medication is preferred to intravenous administration
- the intramuscular drugs recommended are haloperidol, lorazepam and olanzapine
- a single drug is preferred to a combination of drugs whenever possible
- if haloperidol (or another typical antipsychotic drug) is administered intramuscularly, an anticholinergic drug should also be administered in order to reduce the risk of acute dystonia and other extrapyramidal side-effects.

Long acting intramuscular injections

Patients who adhere poorly to long term prophylactic antipsychotic therapy may benefit from a long acting or depot parenterally administered antipsychotic drug. Such a requirement no longer necessitates the use of typical antipsychotic drugs because a depot formulation of risperidone is now available (Hosalli & Davis 2003).

An algorithm for the psychopharmacological treatment of schizophrenia is presented in Figure 18.1. In using this treatment algorithm, the term efficacy refers not only to adequate control of positive symptoms but also to significant alleviation of negative and affective symptoms. Isolated control of positive symptoms may therefore warrant a change of treatment if negative or affective symptoms persist. The psychopharmacology of typical and atypical antipsychotics is discussed further in Chapter 38.

Extrapyramidal side-effects of antipsychotic drugs
The principal adverse-effects of antipsychotic drugs are discussed in Chapter 38. Acute dystonia, parkinsonism, akathisia, tardive dyskinesia and neuroleptic malignant

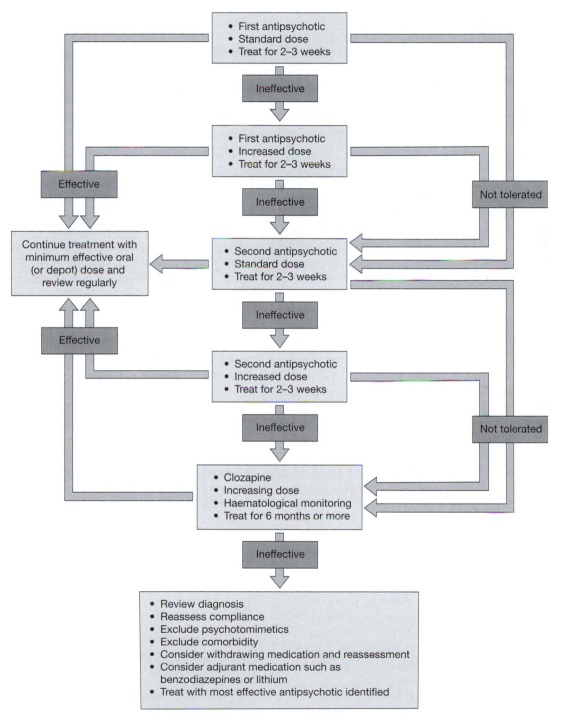

Figure 18.1 Suggested algorithm for the psychopharmacological treatment of schizophrenia. The terms first and second antipsychotic ideally refer to two different atypical antipsychotics (e.g. olanzapine followed by risperidone). In less ideal circumstances, these terms may also refer to a typical and an atypical antipsychotic (e.g. haloperidol followed by olanzapine) or to two typical antipsychotics from two different classes (e.g. chlorpromazine followed by haloperidol). Clozapine should be reserved for treating patients who are treatment resistant or intolerant. The term (or depot) is used because some patients must currently be treated with depot typical antipsychotics and because depot atypical antipsychotics are not widely available.

syndrome may be a component of the schizophrenia syndrome because they were described before the advent of antipsychotic drugs and have been reported in schizophrenic patients who have never been treated with antipsychotic drugs (Waddington 1989). However, typical antipsychotic drugs greatly increase risk for these disorders. Acute dystonia (fixed contortions of the muscles of the head, neck and upper limbs) occurs immediately or within a few days of treatment with an antipsychotic drug, especially in young male patients. Parkinsonism (bradykinesia, mild rigidity and tremor) may only develop after many weeks of treatment and is commonest in older female patients. Both may be treated by anticholinergic/antimuscarinic drugs (which rapidly alleviate acute dystonia if administered parenterally) and/or reducing antipsychotic dosage. Prophylactic anticholinergic treatment should be avoided as it may lead to dependency and may be associated with increased risk of tardive dyskinesia. Akathisia (distressing psychological restlessness and undirected movement) usually develops during the first few days or weeks of treatment.

Tardive dyskinesia is a syndrome of abnormal involuntary movements, typically choreoathetoid and usually complex, rapid and stereotyped. Choreiform lip pursing, tongue protrusion and sucking and chewing movements occur in 80% of cases. Limbs are less often affected and trunk muscles and muscles of respiration only rarely. Patients are often unaware of the movements or are able to suppress them if requested to do so, and are free of them when sleeping. Risk factors for tardive dyskinesia include antisychotic drugs, increasing age, female sex, organic brain damage and diabetes mellitus. The incidence of tardive dyskinesia is about 5% per year, and the prevalence between 20% and 25%, in patients receiving antipsychotic treatment. Aetiological theories, which do not explain the preferential involvement of orofacial muscles, include striatal dopamine receptor supersensitivity (long-term administration of antipychotics causes partial blockade of dopamine receptors which then compensate physiologically by becoming supersensitive to available dopamine), dopaminergic excess/cholinergic deficiency and/or free radical cytotoxicity. There is no effective treatment for tardive dyskinesia and reducing dosage of or discontinuing antipsychotic drugs may exacerbate the disorder. However, the risk of tardive dyskinesia is significantly less with clozapine and transfer of patients from typical antipsychotics to clozapine or another atypical antipsychotic is a useful treatment strategy.

The neuroleptic malignant syndrome consists of extrapyramidal symptoms (rigidity), fluctuating consciousness (delirium, stupor) and autonomic lability (hyperthermia, tachycardia, hypo- or hypertension, sweating, pallor, salivation and urinary incontinence). It is rare, most often develops within a few weeks of initiating or altering antipsychotic therapy, and has a mortality rate of 10–20%. Marked elevation of creatinine phosphokinase occurs and aldolase, liver enzymes and white cells may also be raised. Thromboembolism and renal failure caused by myoglobinuria secondary to muscle necrosis are common and if untreated, death may occur from cardiovascular collapse, respiratory failure or secondary pneumonia (see Chapter 38).

Educational, psychological and social interventions in schizophrenia

Education of patients and their relatives about schizophrenia and its treatment represents good clinical practice and should occur on an ongoing basis. Patients and their relatives should also be advised about and referred to appropriate support organisations.

Cognitive therapy (see Chapter 37) may focus on the alleviation of individual psychotic symptoms or on the global treatment of schizophrenia. The alleviation of auditory hallucinations by treating them as negative automatic thoughts, and of delusions by challenging their inherent illogicality by repeated questioning has been reported (see for example Shergill et al. 1998). Controlled trials of cognitive therapy in the global treatment of schizophrenia have been undertaken by Kemp et al. (1996), who reported improved compliance and global functioning, and by Garety et al. (1994), who reported reduced general symptomatology and improved social functioning in drug-resistant psychosis. It seems likely that as these techniques develop they will be combined with psychopharmacology and that specific patients and/or psychotic symptoms will be targeted.

Brown et al. (1962) found that schizophrenic patients were more likely to relapse if discharged to families exhibiting 'high expressed emotion' (hostility, critical comments and emotional overinvolvement), especially if they were exposed to these families for more than 35 hours per week. Relapse was much less likely in low-expressed emotion families or families that expressed warmth and positive remarks. Leff et al. (1985) demonstrated the interaction between expressed emotion and antipsychotic medication in schizophrenic relapse (Table 18.6), and in a controlled trial, they also showed the effectiveness of family intervention therapy consisting of education about schizophrenia and its treatment, communication training

Table 18.6 The interaction between relapse rates in schizophrenia, exposure to high expressed emotion (EE) for less than or more than 35 hours per week, and treatment with antipsychotic medication

	Low EE	High EE <35 hours	High EE >35 hours
Antipsychotic	12%	15%	53%
No antipsychotic	15%	42%	92%

and support for relatives, in alleviating the effects of high expressed emotion (see also Chapter 7).

Course and outcome in schizophrenia

Course

Perhaps 20% of patients who initially receive a diagnosis of schizophrenia experience a single acute episode, recover fully, and thereafter lead a reasonably fulfilling life. Other patients (particularly males) experiencing a similar acute episode may remain institutionalized and have a life of chronic psychosis punctuated by frequent exacerbations of illness or ended prematurely by suicide. This variability in course and outcome may occur because:

- patients who experienced favourable outcomes were incorrectly diagnosed and did not have schizophrenia
- patients receive different treatments or respond differentially to the treatments they receive
- schizophrenia is a heterogeneous group of psychotic illnesses with variable prognoses, or
- the course and outcome of schizophrenia, in common with many other diseases, is extremely variable.

Irrespective of the cause of these variations, it is generally accepted that schizophrenia follows one of the four courses described by Shepherd et al. (1989) in their report of a 5-year follow-up study of 49 schizophrenic patients (Table 18.7).

Outcome

Schizophrenia is traditionally thought of as a disease characterized by progressive deterioration – the dementia of dementia praecox. However, it may be that this deterioration is caused by institutionalization or medication. Schizophrenic patients scored at least two standard deviations below the mean for a chronically hospitalized physically ill comparison sample on a range of clinical cognitive tests (Owens & Johnstone 1980) and this result has been confirmed in at least 10 further studies (McKenna 1995). Evans et al. (1997) demonstrated that 31 schizophrenic patients performed similarly to 35 brain-injured patients on the behavioural assessment of the Dysexecutive Syndrome test battery. Despite these reports, there is considerable evidence that outcome is not invariably poor and indeed that it may have been improving progressively since schizo-

phrenia was first described over a century ago. Thus while Kraepelin reported that fewer than 1 in 5 of his patients made social recoveries even after many years of illness and treatment, Mayer-Gross, working at the same hospital a decade after Kraepelin, reported social recovery in almost 1 in 3 of his patients over a 16-year interval (1932).

These early reports and subsequent data provide evidence that between 20% and 50% of patients with a diagnosis of schizophrenia make a social recovery, while between 10% and 25% remain substantially disabled. Bleuler, for example, found that 30-40% of 208 schizophrenic patients admitted to hospital in 1942/1943 were socially recovered, 20% were symptomatically recovered and 24% remained severely disabled 22 years later. Bleuler also noted that full recovery usually occurs within 2 years and almost always within 5 years of illness onset, and that further deterioration is rare after 5 years of illness. van Os et al. (1997) have reviewed long-term outcome studies of newly admitted schizophrenic patients reported up to 1990 who met minimum methodological criteria, and concluded that:

- there is significant variability in long-term outcome
- the majority of patients do not recover fully
- there is little evidence that antipsychotic medication has substantially altered the course of illness for the majority of schizophrenic patients, and
- 10–13% of all schizophrenic patients die by suicide.

Outcome following the introduction of atypical antipsychotic drugs The studies cited above were all reported prior to the introduction of atypical antipsychotic drugs. It seems reasonable to assume that the availability of such drugs will improve outcome because they:

- cause fewer adverse effects and thus enhance adherence to treatment and reduce recurrences of illness, and
- alleviate not only positive symptoms but also perhaps negative and affective symptoms and cognitive dysfunction, at least to some extent.

Initial results of controlled trials with these agents are encouraging, Leucht et al. (2003) recently concluding from a meta-analysis of 11 clinical trials involving 1710 patients that compared atypical and typical antipsychotic drugs that '…rates of relapse and overall treatment failure were

Table 18.7 The course of schizophrenia

Course	Symptoms	Interepisodic impairment	% of patients
Course 1	Single episode of acute schizophrenia	No residual impairment	22
Course 2	Recurrent episodes	No or slight impairment	35
Course 3	Recurrent episodes	Significant, non-progressive impairment	8
Course 4	Recurrent episodes	Significant, progressive impairment	35

modestly but significantly lower with the newer drugs'. However, much more research is required before definitive information on the influence of the atypical antipsychotic drugs on disease outcome is available.

Suicide   Suicide rates of between 147 and 750 per 100,000 schizophrenic patients per year have been reported and between 2% and 12% of all individuals dying by suicide have schizophrenia (Heila et al. 1997). It is usually accepted that the risk of suicide is greatest just after schizophrenia is diagnosed, when affective symptoms may be prominent and before insight is lost. In keeping with this view, Mortensen & Juel (1993) found that risk was particularly increased during the first year of follow-up of a Finnish sample of 9156 newly admitted schizophrenic patients, of whom 1100 had died before the study was undertaken. Suicide accounted for 50% of deaths in schizophrenic men and 35% of deaths in schizophrenic women. Heila et al. (1997) reported that 92 schizophrenic patients accounted for 7% of all Finnish suicide victims during a 12-month period, and that 70% of patients had an acute exacerbation of psychosis, depressive symptoms and/or a history of attempted suicide before they died; younger male patients most often used violent suicide methods.

In addition to suicide, schizophrenic patients are at increased risk of death from accidents and from cardiovascular, endocrine, infectious and other diseases. This increased mortality may be caused directly or indirectly by:

- the disease or its treatment
- cigarette smoking, alcohol or other substance abuse and/or obesity which are more prevalent in schizophrenic patients than the general population and
- reduced ability to access health services either because of the effects of schizophrenia or inadequate provision.

Irrespective of cause, schizophrenic patients die on average 10 years earlier than their non-schizophrenic peers (Tsuang et al. 1980).

Predicting outcome for schizophrenia

Factors generally accepted as predictive of favourable and unfavourable outcome in schizophrenia are listed in Table 18.8. The current conceptualization of schizophrenia as a neurodevelopmental disorder implies both a prenatal or early childhood aetiology, and the presence of a prodrome prior to the onset of psychotic symptoms. Features of this prodrome include intellectual impairment, abnormal personality development, poor social skills, and a poor educational and employment record (see above). It is therefore important to realize that some of the apparent predictors of unfavourable outcome listed in Table 18.8 may actually represent aspects of schizophrenia itself. Thus the factors cited in the table may simply be delineating two types of schizophrenia, the neurodevelopmental or less favourable outcome type on the one hand and the non-neurodevelopmental or more favourable outcome type on the other.

Three reports provide evidence that outcome is better in developing than in developed countries:

- Murphy & Raman (1971) reported that schizophrenia had a better prognosis in Mauritius when compared to the UK.
- The WHO (1979) reported that schizophrenia had a better prognosis in India, Columbia and Nigeria when compared to a number of developed countries.

Table 18.8 Predictors of outcome in schizophrenia		
Predictor	Favourable outcome	Unfavourable outcome
Demography	Female Older at onset Higher socioeconomic class Married Living in developing country	Male Younger at onset, especially <15 years Lower socioeconomic class Single Living in developed country
Premorbid status	No family history of schizophrenia No previous psychiatric illness Normal premorbid personality Good educational record Normal social skills Good employment record Normal psychosexual relationships	Schizophrenia in a first-degree relative Previous psychiatric illness Impaired premorbid personality Poor educational record Impaired social skills Broken employment/unemployment Impaired or no psychosexual relationships
Symptomatology	Identifiable precipitant Acute onset Positve and/or affective symptoms Normal brain (neuroimaging) Normal neuropsychology and IQ	No apparent precipitant Insidious onset Negative symptoms Dilated ventricles and/or sulci (neuroimaging) Impaired neuropsychology and IQ <90
Treatment	Brief episode of psychosis Good response to treatment Good compliance	Prolonged psychosis Poor response to treatment Poor compliance

- Sartorius et al. (1986) found that 75% of patients from developing countries had no or minimal social impairment and 45% were clinically recovered at 5-years follow-up, in comparison to 33% and 25% respectively of patients from developed countries.

The cost of schizophrenia

Schizophrenia commences in young adulthood, runs a chronic course, has a relatively low mortality, cannot yet be treated effectively and certainly cannot be cured. It is therefore an emotionally and economically costly disease for individual patients, for their families, and for society.

The financial cost of schizophrenia includes direct and indirect expenditure. Direct expenditure accounts for between 1% and 3% of the national health care budgets of most developed countries. Accommodation and medication account for approximately 75% and 5% of direct expenditure respectively. It has been estimated that about 90% of direct expenditure is utilized in treating patients with chronic schizophrenia (although such patients account for significantly less than 90% of all schizophrenic patients). Patients with chronic schizophrenia are perhaps most likely to benefit from the increased efficacy and safety of newer atypical antipsychotics and there is some evidence that the savings wrought by their improved health may more than offset the cost of these drugs.

Indirect expenditure on schizophrenia is largely accounted for by the loss of productivity experienced by patients and their families. Unemployed patients depend on government funding for accommodation, food and health care and cannot contribute to national wealth by production of goods or services, or by payment of taxes. Such indirect expenditure on schizophrenia may be four times greater that direct expenditure and of the order of £4 billion per year in the UK.

The cost of schizophrenia to the families of patients is both emotional and economic. Emotional costs include worry about their own mental health and that of their relatives, the distress caused by patients' disturbed or embarrassing behaviour or by the attitudes of society to schizophrenic patients, the fear of violence and the relentless stress imposed by living with a dependent, socially withdrawn individual. These emotional costs increase as patients and their parents age. Most schizophrenic patients do not contribute to family finances and the costs of accommodation, medication, repairs to damaged property and transport to and from clinics are not insignificant. There can be little doubt but that the current strategy of caring for schizophrenic patients in (often inadequate) community settings has increased both the emotional and the economic burdens imposed upon patients' families (see Chapter 7 and 11).

Criminality and schizophrenia

Fewer than 1% of all criminally convicted individuals receive a psychiatric disposal and the contribution of psychiatric illness in general, and schizophrenia in particular, to rates of crime is very slight. Aggression and violence are common among schizophrenic patients but are more likely to be self-directed than externally directed. Thus patients may injure themselves, bizarre self-mutilation may occur, and suicide is common. However, externally directed threats or violence represent a significant problem to relatives of patients and to professionals.

There is a small but significant association between fatal externally directed violence and schizophrenia. It has been estimated that 1 out of every 2000 individuals with schizophrenia will commit homicide and that almost 1 in 10 individuals convicted of murder or attempted murder will have schizophrenia (Hafner & Boker 1982). Homicides by schizophrenic patients are generally committed several years after the onset of illness and at an older age than homicides committed by non-schizophrenic individuals. Such crimes may be committed in response to delusions, may appear motiveless and random, often involve victims that are unknown to the patient, and may utilize bizarre methods of killing. There is some evidence that the extremely rare crime of matricide is more likely to be committed by schizophrenic than non-schizophrenic individuals (see also Chapters 30 and 35).

Wallace et al. (2004) recently compared criminal convictions in 2861 people with schizophrenia and an equal number of control subjects over a 25-year period in the Australian state of Victoria. Schizophrenic patients had more criminal convictions overall and were more likely to have been convicted of both any criminal offense (21.6% versus 7.8%) and a violent offense (8.2% versus 1.8%). Furthermore, criminal conviction was more likely in patients with substances abuse problems than in those without (68.1% versus 11.7%).

SCHIZOTYPAL DISORDER

Schizotypal disorder is characterized by eccentric behaviour and unusual thinking and affect. It resembles schizophrenia but characteristic schizophrenic symptoms do not occur. Typical symptoms of schizotypal disorder include eccentricity and aloofness, social withdrawal, paranoid quasi-delusional ideas, magical thinking, obsessive ruminations, depersonalization and derealization, visual and somatic illusions, metaphorical and over-elaborate speech, and transient auditory hallucinations.

Schizotypal disorder is commoner in individuals with a schizophrenic relative and is usually thought of as a schizophrenia spectrum disorder. It behaves like a personality disorder (and indeed is classified as such in DSM-IV) with no clear time of onset, a chronic course with fluctuating intensity of symptoms, and no acute episodes or periods of remission. Schizotypal disorder may occasionally progress to schizophrenia in which case it should probably be retrospectively rediagnosed as prodromal schizophrenia.

SCHIZOAFFECTIVE DISORDER

Differentiating between schizophrenia and affective disorder is often difficult because many symptoms, including Schneiderian first-rank symptoms, are common to both schizophrenia and affective disorder and because depression commonly occurs with schizophrenia. Schizoaffective disorder may be diagnosed when schizophrenic and affective symptoms are episodically, equally and simultaneously prominent. Patients with schizoaffective disorder have an excess of relatives with affective psychosis and the disorder may be thought of as either a schizophrenia spectrum or an affective spectrum disorder.

Schizophrenic symptoms may coexist with manic, depressive or both manic and depressive symptoms in schizoaffective disorder. Schizomanic disorders are associated with a family history of affective disorders, are usually florid with grossly disturbed behaviour, negative symptoms rarely evolve and patients respond to mood-stabilizing drugs and recover rapidly. Schizodepressive disorders are associated with a family history of schizophrenia, are markedly less florid, patients may develop chronic negative symptoms and response to treatment is variable. Mixed schizoaffective disorder is said to be present when schizophrenic, depressive and manic symptoms coexist.

PERSISTENT DELUSIONAL DISORDERS

Persistent delusional disorders may occur in isolation or within the context of a schizophrenic or other psychosis and may be conveniently classified into eponymous and non-eponymous groups (Table 18.9). The eponymous disorders are described in Chapter 22 while the non-eponymous disorders will be discussed here. These disorders are characterized by a persistent, often lifelong, non-bizarre delusion or set of related delusions, most usually arising insidiously in midlife or later. Transient auditory hallucinations may occur but schizophrenic symptoms are incompatible with the pure diagnosis. Affect, thought and behaviour are globally normal but patients' attitudes and actions in response to their delusions are appropriate and may lead to dangerousness in disorders such as Othello syndrome.

Paranoia and paraphrenia are controversial entities that were separated from dementia praecox by Kraepelin, who described paranoia as a persistent systematized delusion arising in later life without evidence of either hallucinations or a deteriorating course, and paraphrenia as an identical syndrome to paranoia but with hallucinations. Kretschmer (1927) considered paranoia a reaction to stress in predisposed individuals (*Der sensitive Beziehungswahn*) while ICD-10 classifies paranoia, (late) paraphrenia and *Der sensitive Beziehungswahn* as persistent delusional disorders that require symptoms of at least three months' duration for their diagnosis.

Delusional dysmorphophobia and paranoia querulans are also included as persistent delusional disorders in ICD-10. Patients with delusional dysmorphophobia are convinced that some physical feature, usually of their head or of a secondary sexual characteristic, is abnormal in shape or size and may repeatedly seek cosmetic surgery to correct the imagined deformity (see Chapter 16). Paranoia querulans is characterized by repeated and prolonged litigation, most often against local or national government authorities, following an imagined or minor event. Some patients in this category undertake elaborate social, religious or political missions and may behave violently towards their imagined opponents.

The treatment of persistent delusional disorders is extremely difficult – patients lack insight and may interpret attempts to help as persecution. Assessment of dangerousness (Chapter 35) is extremely important and compulsory admission may be required. Antipsychotic, anxiolytic and mood-stabilizing drugs may be useful.

Table 18.9 Eponymous and non-eponymous persistent delusional disorders

Eponymous	Non-eponymous
de Clerambault's syndrome (erotomania)	Paranoia
Othello syndrome (morbid jealousy)	(Late) paraphrenia
Capgras syndrome (*l'illusion des sosies*)[1]	*Der sensitive Beziehungswahn*
Ekbom's syndrome (delusion of infestation)	Delusional dysmorphophobia
Fregoli syndrome	Paranoia querulans

[1] Literally 'illusion of doubles'; delusion of doubles is a more accurate phenomenological description

REFERENCES

Akbarian S, Vinuela A & Kim JJ (1993) Distorted distribution of nicotinamide adenine-dinucleotide phosphate diaphorase neurons in temporal lobe of schizophrenics implies anomalous cortical development. *Archives of General Psychiatry* **50**: 178–87.
Alzheimer A (1913) Beitrage zur pathologischen Anatomie der Dementia praecox. *Allgemeine Zeitschift fur Psychiatrie und gerichtliche Medizin* **70**: 810–12.
American Psychiatric Association (1994) *Diagnostic and Statistical Manual of Mental Disorders*, 4th edn. Washington, DC: APA.
Andreasen NC & Olsen S (1982) Negative v positive schizophrenia. *American Journal of Psychiatry* **39**: 789–94.
Arranz M, Collier D & Sodhi M (1995) Association between clozapine response and allelic variation in the 5HT$_{2A}$ receptor gene. *Lancet* **346**: 281–2.
Arseneault L, Cannon M, Witton J & Murray RM (2004) Causal association between cannabis and psychosis: examination of the evidence : 110–17.

Bateson G, Jackson D, Haley J & Weakland J (1956) Towards a theory of schizophrenia. *Behavioural Science* 1: 251–64.

Bhugra D, Leff J, Mallett R et al. (1997) The first contact of patients with schizophrenia with psychiatric services: social factors and pathways to care in a multiethnic population. *Psychol Med* 29: 475–483.

Bilder RM, Goldman RS, Volavka J, Czobor P, Hoptman M, Sheitman B, Lindenmayer JP, Citrome L, McEvoy J, Kunz M, Chakos M, Cooper TB, Horowitz TL & Lieberman JA (2002) Neurocognitive effects of clozapine, olanzapine, risperidone, and haloperidol in patients with chronic schizophrenia or schizoaffective disorder. *American Journal of Psychiatry* 159: 1018–28.

Bleuler E (1911) *Dementia Praecox or the Group of Schizophrenias* (translated edition 1950). New York: International University Press.

Brook S (2003) Intramuscular ziprasidone: moving beyond the conventional in the treatment of acute agitation in schizophrenia. *Journal of Clinical Psychiatry* 64(Suppl 19):13–18.

Brown GW & Birley JLT (1968) Crisis and life change at the onset of schizophrenia. *Journal of Health and Social Behaviour* 9: 203–24.

Brown GW, Monck EM, Carstairs GM & Wing JK (1962) Influence of family life on the cause of schizophrenia. *British Journal of Preventive and Social Medicine* 16: 55–68.

Bussato & Kerwin RW (1997) Perspectives on the role of serotonergic mechanisms in the pharmacology of schizophrenia. *Journal of Psychopharmacology* 11: 3–12.

Cannon M, Walsh E, Hollis C, Kargin M, Taylor E, Murray RM & Jones PB (2001) Predictors of later schizophrenia and affective psychosis among attendees at a child psychiatry department. *British Journal of Psychiatry* 178: 420–6.

Cecil KM, Lenkinski RE, Gur RE & Gur RC (1999) Proton magnetic resonance spectroscopy in the frontal and temporal lobes of neuroleptic naive patients with schizophrenia. *Neuropsychopharmacology* 20(2): 131–40.

Censits DM, Ragland JD, Gur RC & Gur RE (1997) Neuropsychological evidence supporting a neurodevelopmental model of schizophrenia: a longitudinal study. *Schizophrenia Research* 24: 289–98.

Chakos MH, Lieberman JA & Alvir J (1995) Caudate nuclei volumes in schizophrenic patients treated with typical antipsychotics and clozapine. *Lancet* 345: 456–7.

Chowdari KV, Mirnics K, Semwal P et al. (2002) Association and linkage analyses of RGS4 polymorphisms in schizophrenia. *Human Molecular Genetics* 11(12): 1373–80.

Chumakov I, Blumenfeld M, Guerassimenko O et al. (2002) Genetic and physiological data implicating the new human gene G72 and the gene for D-amino acid oxidase in schizophrenia. *Proceedings of the National Academy of Science USA* 99(21): 13675–80.

Cooper JE, Kendell RE, Gurland BJ et al. (1972) *Psychiatric Diagnosis in New York and London*. Maudsley Monograph no. 20. London: Oxford University Press.

Crow TJ (1980) Molecular pathology of schizophrenia: more than one disease process. *British Medical Journal* i: 66–9.

Davis JM (1985) Maintenance therapy and the natural course of schizophrenia. *Journal of Clinical Psychiatry* 46: 18–21.

Davis JM, Metalon L & Watanabe MD (1994) Depot antipsychotic drugs: place in therapy. *Drugs* 47: 741–73.

Dawson ME & Schell AM (2002) What does electrodermal activity tell us about prognosis in the schizophrenia spectrum? *Schizophrenia Research* 54(1–2): 87–93.

Deakin JFW, Slater P & Simpson MDC (1989) Frontal cortical and left temporal glutamatergic dysfunction in schizophrenia. *Journal of Neurochemistry* 52: 1781–6.

Degenhardt L (2000) Cannabis and psychosis. *Australia and New Zealand Journal of Psychiatry* 34: 26–34.

Der G, Gupta S & Murray RM (1990) Is schizophrenia disappearing? *Lancet* 335: 513–16.

Emsley R, Oosthuizen P & van Rensburg SJ (2003) Clinical potential of omega-3 fatty acids in the treatment of schizophrenia. *CNS Drugs* 17(15): 1081–91.

Erritzoe D, Talbot P, Frankle WG & Abi-Dargham A (2003) Positron emission tomography and single photon emission CT molecular imaging in schizophrenia. *Neuroimaging Clinics of North America* 13(4): 817–32.

Evans JJ, Chua SE, McKenna PJ & Wilson BA (1997) Assessment of the dysexecutive syndrome in schizophrenia. *Psychological Medicine* 27: 635–46.

Farde L (1997) Brain imaging of schizophrenia – the dopamine hypothesis. *Schizophrenia Research* 28(2–3): 157–62.

Faris REL & Dunham HW (1939) *Mental Disorders in Urban Areas*. Chicago: Chicago University Press.

Frangous & Williams SCR (1996) Magnetic resonance spectroscopy in psychiatry: basic principles and applications. *British Medical Bulletin* 52: 474–85.

Hollingshead AB & Redlich FC (1958) Social class and mental illness: a community study. *Journal of Psychosomatic Research* 11: 213–18.

Garety PA, Kuipers L, Fowler D et al. (1994) Cognitive behaviour therapy for drug resistant psychosis. *British Journal of Medical Psychology* 67: 259–71.

Gilbert P, Harris MJ, McAdams LA (1995) Neuroleptic withdrawal in schizophrenic patients: a review of the literature. *Arch Gen Psychiatry* 52: 173–188.

Gjessing R (1938) Disturbances of somatic functions in catatonia with a periodic course and their compensation. *Journal of Mental Science* 608–21.

Goldberg EM & Morrison SL (1963) Schizophrenia and social class. *British Journal of Psychiatry* 109: 785–802.

Goldstein JM, Tsuang MT & Farone SV (1989) Gender and schizophrenia: implications for understanding the heterogeneity of the illness. *Psychiatry Research* 28: 243–53.

Gottesman II & Bertelsen A (1989) Confirming unexpressed genotypes for schizophrenia. Risks in the offspring of Fischer's Danish identical and fraternal discordant twins. *Archives of General Psychiatry* 46: 867–72.

Gottesman II (1991) *Schizophrenia Genesis: The Origins of Madness*. New York: Freeman.

Griffiths TD, Sigmundsson T, Takei N et al. (1998) Minor physical anomalies in familial and sporadic schizophrenia: the Maudsley family study. *Journal of Neurology and Psychiatry* 61(1): 56–60.

Hafner H & Boker W (1982) Crimes of violence by mentally abnormal offenders (transl. H Marshall) Cambridge: Cambridge University Press.

Hafner H, Maurer K & Loefler (1994) The epidemiology of early schizophrenia:influence of age and gender on onset and early course. *British Journal of Psychiatry* 164(suppl. 23): 29–38.

Hafner H & Reimann H (1970) Spatial distribution of mental disorders in Mannheim. In: Hare EH & Wing JK (eds) *Psychiatric Epidemiology*. London: Oxford University Press.

Harrison PJ (1999) The neuropathology of schizophrenia. A critical review of the data and their interpretation. *Brain* 122(pt 4): 593–624.

Harrison PJ (2004) The hippocampus in schizophrenia: a review of the neuropathological evidence and its pathophysiological implications. *Psychopharmacology (Berlin)* [published online, accessed 6 March 2004].

Harrison PJ, Freemantle N & Geddes JR (2003) Meta-analysis of brain weight in schizophrenia. *Schizophrenia Research* 64(1): 25–34.

Harrison PJ & Owen MJ (2003) Genes for schizophrenia? Recent findings and their pathophysiological implications. *Lancet* 361(9355): 417–9.

Heila H, Isometsa ET, Henriksson MM et al. (1997) Suicide and schizophrenia: a nationwide psychological autopsy study on age and sex specific clinical characteristics of 92 suicide victims with schizophrenia. *American Journal of Psychiatry* 154: 1235–42.

Heitmiller DR, Nopoulos PC & Andreasen NC (2004) Changes in caudate volume after exposure to atypical neuroleptics in patients with schizophrenia may be sex-dependent. *Schizophrenia Research* 66(2–3): 137–42.

Hollingshead AB & Redlich FC (1958) Social class and mental illness: a community study. *Journal of Psychosomatic Research* 11: 213–18.

Horrobin DF (2002) A new category of psychotropic drugs: neuroactive lipids as exemplified by ethyl eicosapentaenoate (E-E). *Progress in Drug Research* 59: 171–99.

Hosalli P & Davis JM (2003) Depot risperidone for schizophrenia. *Cochrane Database System Review* 4:CD004161.

Ingvar DH & Franzen G (1974) Abnormalities of cerebral blood flow distribution in patients with chronic schizophrenia. *Acta Psychiatrica Scandinavica* 50: 425–62.

Jablensky A, Sartorius N, Ernberg G et al. (1992) Schizophrenia: manifestations, incidence and course in different cultures. A World

Health Organization ten-country study. *Psychological Medicine Monograph Supplement* **20**: 1–97.

Jacobs S & Myers J (1976) Recent life events and acute schizophrenia psychosis: a controlled study. *Journal of Nervous and Mental Diseases* **162**: 75–87.

Jacobi W & Winkler H (1927) Encephalographische Studien auf chronisch Schizophrenen. *Archiv fur Psychiatrie und Nervenkrankheiten* **81**: 299–332.

Jeon YW & Polich J (2003) Meta-analysis of P300 and schizophrenia: patients, paradigms, and practical implications. *Psychophysiology* **40**(5): 684–701.

Jones PB, Murray RM & Rodgers B (1995) Childhood risk factors for adult schizophrenia in a general population birth cohort at age 43 years. In: Mednick SA & Hollister JM (eds) *Neural Development and Schizophrenia*. New York: Plenum Press.

Kane J, Honigfeld G & Singer J (1988) Clozapine for the treatment resistant schizophrenia: a double blind comparison with chlorpromazine. *Archives of General Psychiatry* **45**: 789–96.

Kapur S & Seeman P (2001) Does fast dissociation from the dopamine D_2 receptor explain the action of atypical antipsychotics?: A new hypothesis. *American Journal of Psychiatry* **158**(3): 360–9.

Kemp R, Hayward P, Applewhaite G et al. (1996) Compliance therapy in psychotic patients: randomised controlled trial. *British Medical Journal* **312**: 345–9.

Kerwin R & Owen M (1999) Genetics of novel therapeutic targets in schizophrenia. *British Journal of Psychiatry* Suppl.(38): 1–4.

Kety S (1983) Mental illness in the biological and adoptive relatives of schizophrenic adoptees: findings relevant to genetic and environmental factors in etiology. *American Journal of Psychiatry* **140**: 720–7.

Kim JS, Kornhuber HH, Schmidt-Burgk W & Holzmuler B (1980) Low cerebrospinal fluid glutamate in schizophrenic patients and a new hypothesis of schizophrenia. *Neuroscience Letters* **400**: 330–44.

Kraepelin E (1896) *Psychiatrie. Ein Lehrbuch fur Studierende und Arzte. 5*, Auflage. Leipzig: A. Abel.

Kraepelin E (1919) *Dementia Praecox and Paraphrenia*. Edinburgh: Churchill Livingstone.

Kretschmer E (1927) Der sensitive Beziehungswahn. In: Hirsch SR & Shepherd M (eds) *Themes and Variations in European Psychiatry*. Bristol: Wright.

Lawrie SM & Abukmeil SS (1998) Brain abnormality in schizophrenia. A systematic and quantitative review of volumetric magnetic resonance imaging studies. *British Journal of Psychiatry* **172**: 110–20.

Leff JP, Kuipers L, Berkowitz R & Sturgeon D (1985) A controlled trial of interventions in the families of schizophrenic patients: two-year follow up. *British Journal of Psychiatry* **146**: 594–600.

Lee KH & Williams LM (2000) Eye movement dysfunction as a biological marker of risk for schizophrenia. *Australian and New Zealand Journal of Psychiatry* **34**(Suppl.): S91–100.

Leonhard K (1957) The classification of endogenous psychoses (transl. R Berman). New York: Irvington.

Leucht S, Barnes TR, Kissling W, Engel RR, Correll C & Kane JM (2003) Relapse prevention in schizophrenia with new-generation antipsychotics: a systematic review and exploratory meta-analysis of randomized, controlled trials. *American Journal of Psychiatry* **160**(7): 1209–22.

Lewis SW, Reveley MA & David AS (1988) Agenesis of the corpus callosum and schizophrenia. *Psychological Medicine* **18**: 341–7.

Lewis G, David A, Andreasson S & Allbeck P (1992) Schizophrenia and city life. *Lancet* **340**: 137–40.

Li T, Stefansson H, Gudfinnsson E et al. (2004) Identification of a novel neuregulin 1 at-risk haplotype in Han schizophrenia Chinese patients, but no association with the Icelandic/Scottish risk haplotype. *Molecular Psychiatry* [published online, accessed 6 March 2004].

Lieberman JA, Safferman AZ & Pollack S (1994) Clinical effects of clozapine in chronic schizophrenia: response and predictors of outcome. *American Journal of Psychiatry* **151**: 1744–52.

Liddle PF (1987) The symptoms of chronic schizophrenia. A re-examination of the positive-negative dichotomy. *British Journal of Psychiatry* **151**: 145–51.

Liddle PF, Friston KJ & Frith CD (1992) Patterns of cerebral blood flow in schizophrenia. *British Journal of Psychiatry* **160**: 179–86.

Lidz RW & Lidz T (1949) The family environment of schizophrenic patients. *American Journal of Psychiatry* **106**: 332–45.

Loebel AD, Lieberman JA & Alvir JM (1992) Duration of psychosis and outcome in first episode schizophrenia. *American Journal of Psychiatry* **149**: 1183–6.

Mayer-Gross W (1932) Die Schizophrenie. In: *Bumke's Handbuch der Geisteskrankheiten*, vol. 9. Berlin: Springer.

McGuire PK, Shah GM & Murray RM (1993) Increased blood flow in Broca's area during auditory hallucinations in schizophrenia. *Lancet* **342**: 703–6.

McKenna PJ (1995) General intellectual function in schizophrenia. *Schizophrenia Monitor* **5**: 1–5.

McNaught AS, Jeffreys SE, Harvey CA et al. (1997) The Hampstead schizophrenia survey 1991. 2: Incidence and migration in inner London. *British Journal of Psychiatry* **170**: 307–311.

Mortensen PB & Juel K (1993) Mortality and causes of death in first admitted schizophrenic patients. *British Journal of Psychiatry* **163**: 183–9.

Mortensen PB, Pedersen CB, Westergaard T et al. (1999) Effects of family history and place and season of birth on the risk of schizophrenia. *New England Journal of Medicine* **340**: 603–8.

Murphy HBM & Raman AC (1971) The chronicity of schizophrenia in indigenous tropical people. *British Journal of Psychiatry* **118**: 489–97.

Murray RM (1994) Neurodevelopmental schizophrenia: the rediscovery of dementia praecox. *British Journal of Psychiatry* **165**: 6–12.

Murray RM & Lewis SW (1987) Is schizophrenia a neurodevelopmental disorder? *British Medical Journal* **295**: 681–2.

National Instutute for Clinical Excellence (2002) Schizophrenia: Core Interventions in the Treatment and Management of Schizophrenia in Primary and Secondary Care. Online. Available at: www.nice.org.uk [accessed 26 May 2004].

Norman RM & Malla AK (1993) Stressful life events and schizophrenia: a review of the research. *British Journal of Psychiatry* **162**: 161–6.

Ødegaard Ø (1932) Emigration and insanity. *Acta Psychiatrica Scandinavica* supplement 4.

Owens DGC & Johnstone EC (1980) The disabilities of chronic schizophrenia – their nature and the factors contributing to their development. *British Journal of Psychiatry* **136**: 384–93.

Payne RW (1973) Cognitive abnormalities. In: Eysenck HJ (ed.) *Handbook of Abnormal Psychology*. London: Pitman.

Pilowsky LS, Mulligan RS & Acton PD (1997) Effects of clozapine and typical antipsychotics on striatal and limbic D_2/D_2-like receptors in vivo by ^{123}I epidopride. *Schizophrenia Research* **24**: 181.

Royston MC & Simpson MDC (1991). Post-mortem neurochemistry of schizophrenia. In: Kerwin RW, Dawbarn D, McCulloch J & Tamming A (eds) *Neurobiology and Psychiatry*. Cambridge: Cambridge University Press.

Rudin E (1916) *Studien uber Vererbung und Entstehung geistiger Storungen. I. Zur Vererung und Neuentstehung der Dementia Praecox*. Berlin: Springer.

Russell AJ, Munro JC, Jones PB et al. (1997) Schizophrenia and the myth of intellectual decline. *American Journal of Psychiatry* **154**: 635–9.

Sartorius N, Jablensky A & Korten A (1986) Early manifestations and first contact incidence of schizophrenia in different cultures. A preliminary report on the initial evaluation phase of the WHO collaborative study of determinants of outcome of severe mental disorders. *Psychological Medicine* **16**: 909–28.

Schneider K (1959) *Clinical Psychopathology*. New York: Grune & Stratton.

Schwab SG, Knapp M, Mondabon S et al. (2003) Support for association of schizophrenia with genetic variation in the 6p22.3 gene, dysbindin, in sib-pair families with linkage and in an additional sample of triad families. *American Journal of Human Genetics* **72**(1): 185–90.

Shepherd M, Watt D & Falloon I (1989) The natural history of schizophrenia: a five-year follow up study of outcome and prediction in a representative sample of schizophrenics. *Psychological Medicine Monograph Supplement* **15**: 1–46.

Shergill SS, Murray RM & McGuire PK (1998) Auditory hallucinations: a review of psychological treatments. *Schizophrenia Research* 32: 137–50.

Shergill SS, Brammer MJ, Williams SC, Murray RM & McGuire PK (2000) Mapping auditory hallucinations in schizophrenia using functional magnetic resonance imaging. *Archives of General Psychiatry* **57**(11): 1033–8.

Shifman S, Bronstein M, Sternfeld M et al. (2002) A highly significant association between a COMT haplotype and schizophrenia. *American Journal of Human Genetics* **71**(6): 1296–302.

Stefansson H, Sigurdsson E, Steinthorsdottir V et al. (2002) Neuregulin 1 and susceptibility to schizophrenia. *American Journal of Human Genetics* **71**(4): 877–92.

Stefansson H, Sarginson J, Kong A et al. (2003) Association of neuregulin 1 with schizophrenia confirmed in a Scottish population. *American Journal of Human Genetics* **72**(1): 83–7.

Straub RE, Jiang Y, MacLean CJ et al. (2002) Genetic variation in the 6p22.3 gene DTNBP1, the human ortholog of the mouse dysbindin gene, is associated with schizophrenia. *American Journal of Human Genetics* **71**(2): 337–48.

Suddath RL, Casanova MF & Goldberg TE (1989) Temporal lobe pathology in schizophrenia: a quantitative magnetic resonance imaging study. *American Journal of Psychiatry* **146**: 464–72.

Sunahara RK, Seeman P & van Tol HH (1993) Dopamine receptors and antipsychotic drug response. *British Journal of Psychiatry* **22**: 31–8.

Thakore JH. Metabolic disturbance in first-episode schizophrenia. *British Journal of Psychiatry* **47**(Suppl.): S76–9.

Tsuang MT, Woolsen RF & Fleming JA (1980) Premature deaths in schizophrenia and affective disorders: an analysis of survival curves and variables affecting the shortened survival. *Archives of General Psychiatry* **37**: 979–83.

van Os J, Wright P & Murray RM (1997) Risk factors for emergence and persistence of psychosis. In: van Kammen DP & Welles MPI (eds) *Progress in Clinical Psychiatry 1*, pp. 152–206. London: WB Saunders.

Velakoulis D & Pantelis C (1996) What have we learned from functional imaging studies in schizophrenia? The role of frontal, striatal and temporal areas. *Australian and New Zealand Journal of Psychiatry* **30**(2): 195–209.

Wallace C, Mullen PE & Burgess P (2004) Criminal offending in schizophrenia over a 25-year period marked by deinstitutionalization and increasing prevalence of comorbid substance use disorders. *American Journal of Psychiatry* **161**(4): 716–27.

Waddington JL (1989) Schizophrenia, affective psychosis and other disorders treated with neuroleptic drugs: the enigma of tardive dyskinesia, its neurobiological determinants and the conflict of paradigms. *International Review of Neurobiology* **31**: 297–353.

Weinberger DR (1987) Implications of normal brain development for the pathogenesis of schizophrenia. *Archives of General Psychiatry* **44**: 660–9.

Wender P, Rosenthal D, Kety S et al. (1974) Cross fostering: a research strategy for clarifying the role of genetic and environmental factors in the aetiology of schizophrenia. *Archives of General Psychiatry* **30**: 121–8.

World Health Organization (1973) *Report of the International Pilot Study of Schizophrenia*. Geneva: WHO.

World Health Organization (1979) *Schizophrenia: An Initial Follow Up*. Chichester:Wiley.

World Health Organization (1992) *ICD-10 Classification of Mental and Behavioural Disorders*. Geneva: WHO.

Wright P, Takei N, Rifkin L & Murray RM (1995) Maternal influenza, obstetric complications and schizophrenia. *American Journal of Psychiatry* **152**:1714–20.

Wright P & Murray RM (1996) Prenatal influenza, immunogenes and schizophrenia: a hypothesis and some recent findings. In: Waddington JL & Buckley PF (eds) *The Neurodevelopmental Basis of Schizophrenia*, pp. 43–52. Austin, TX: RG Landes.

Wright P, Sham PC, Gilvarry CM et al. (1996a) Autoimmune disorders in the first degree relatives of schizophrenic and control subjects. *Schizophrenia Research* **20**: 261–7.

Wright P, Donaldson PT, Underhill JA et al. (1996b) Genetic association of the HLA DRB1 gene locus on chromosome 6p21.3 with schizophrenia. *American Journal of Psychiatry* **153**: 1530–3.

Wright P, Takei N, Murray RM & Sham P (1999) Seasonality, prenatal influenza and schizophrenia. In: Susser E & Brown AS (eds) *Prenatal Exposures in Schizophrenia*, pp. 89–112. Washington, DC: American Psychiatric Press Inc.

Wright P, Nimgaonkar VL, Ganguli R & Murray RM (2000) In: Lechler R & Warrens A (eds) *HLA in Health and Disease*. London: Academic Press.

Wright P, Birkett M, David S, Meehan K, Ferchland I, Alaka K, Saunders J, Krueger J, Bradley P, San L, Bernardo M, Reinstein M & Breier A (2001). Double blind, placebo controlled comparison of IM olanzapine and IM haloperidol in the treatment of acute agitation in schizophrenia. *American Journal Psychiatry* **158**: 1149–51.

APPENDIX 1
ICD-10 DIAGNOSTIC CRITERIA FOR SCHIZOPHRENIA (MODIFIED)

The normal requirement for a diagnosis of schizophrenia is that a minimum of one very clear symptom (and usually two or more if less clear-cut) belonging to any one of the groups listed as (a) to (d) below, or symptoms from at least two of the groups referred to as (e) to (h) below, should have been clearly present for most of the time during a period of one month or more. Conditions meeting such symptomatic requirements but of duration less than one month (whether treated or not) should be diagnosed in the first instance as schizophrenia-like psychotic disorder and reclassified as schizophrenia if the symptoms persist for longer periods. Symptom (i) in the list below applies only to a diagnosis of simple schizophrenia and a duration of at least one year is required.

a   Thought echo, thought insertion or withdrawal and thought broadcasting.

b   Delusions of control, influence or passivity clearly referred to body or limb movements or specific thoughts, actions or sensations; delusional perception.

c   Hallucinatory voices giving a running commentary on the patient's behaviour or discussing the patient among themselves, or other types of hallucinatory voices coming from some part of the body.

d   Persistent delusions of other kinds that are culturally inappropriate or completely impossible such as religious or political identity or superhuman powers or abilities (e.g. being able to control the weather, or being in communication with aliens from another world).

e   Persistent hallucinations in any modality when accompanied by either fleeting or half-formed delusions without clear affect content or by persistent overvalued ideas or when occurring every day for weeks or months on end.

f   Breaks or interpolations in the train of thought resulting in incoherence or irrelevant speech or neologisms.

g   Catatonic behaviour such as excitement, posturing or waxy flexibility, negativism, mutism and stupor.

h   'Negative' symptoms such as marked apathy, paucity of speech and blunting or incongruity of emotional responses, usually resulting in social withdrawal and lowering of social performance; it must be clear that these are not due to depression or neuroleptic medication.

i   A significant and consistent change in the overall quality of some aspects of personal behaviour manifest as loss of interest, aimlessness, idleness, a self-absorbed attitude and social withdrawal.

APPENDIX 2
DSM-IV DIAGNOSTIC CRITERIA FOR SCHIZOPHRENIA (MODIFIED)

A. Characteristic symptoms of the active phase

Two (or more) of the following, each present for a significant portion of time during a one-month period (or less if successfully treated).

1   Delusions.
2   Hallucinations.
3   Disorganized speech (e.g. frequent derailment or incoherence).
4   Grossly disorganized or catatonic behaviour.
5   Negative symptoms, i.e. affective flattening, alogia or avolition.

B. Social/occupational dysfunction

For a significant portion of time since the onset of the disturbance one or more major areas of functioning such as work, interpersonal relations or self-care are markedly below the level achieved prior to the onset. (Or, when the onset is in childhood or adolescence, failure to achieve expected level of interpersonal, academic or occupational achievement.)

C. Duration

Continuous signs of the disturbance persist for at least six months. This six-month period must include at least one month of symptoms (or less if successfully treated) that met criterion A (i.e. active phase symptoms) and may include periods of prodromal or residual symptoms. During these prodromal or residual periods the signs of the disturbance may be manifested by only negative symptoms or by two or more symptoms listed in criterion A present in an attenuated form (e.g. odd beliefs, unusual perceptual experiences).

D. Schizoaffective and mood disorder exclusion

Schizoaffective disorder and mood disorder with psychotic features have been ruled out because either (1) no major depressive, manic or mixed episodes have occurred concurrently with the active phase symptoms; or (2) if mood episodes have occurred during active phase symptoms their total duration has been brief relative to the duration of the active and residual periods.

E. Substance/general medical condition exclusion

The disturbance is not due to the direct physiological effects of a substance (e.g. a drug of abuse, a medication) or a general medical condition.

F. Relationship to a pervasive developmental disorder

If there is a history of autistic disorder or another pervasive developmental disorder the additional diagnosis of schizophrenia is made only if prominent delusions or hallucinations are present for at least one month (or less if successfully treated).

APPENDIX 3
ICD-10 DIAGNOSTIC SUBTYPES OF SCHIZOPHRENIA

- paranoid schizophrenia
- hebephrenic schizophrenia (disorganized in DSM-IV)
- catatonic schizophrenia
- undifferentiated schizophrenia

- post-schizophrenic depression
- residual schizophrenia
- simple schizophrenia
- other schizophrenia
- schizophrenia, unspecified.

APPENDIX 4
DSM-IV DIAGNOSTIC SUBTYPES OF SCHIZOPHRENIA

- paranoid schizophrenia
- disorganized schizophrenia (hebephrenic in ICD-10)
- catatonic schizophrenia
- undifferentiated schizophrenia
- residual schizophrenia.

Unipolar depression

Anthony Cleare

INTRODUCTION

Depression represents a considerable public health burden, with a lifetime incidence approaching 20%. There is evidence that the incidence and prevalence of depression have been increasing in recent decades. The WHO estimates that depression is the fourth most important cause of disability worldwide, and that by 2020 it will be the second most important. The phenomenology, epidemiology, aetiology and treatment of depression are described in this chapter.

CLINICAL FEATURES

Phenomenology of depression

The core feature of the clinical syndrome of depression is persistent and pervasive low mood and/or anhedonia. Many other characteristic features make up the full syndrome; they can be divided into behavioural, emotional, cognitive and biological features. Severe cases are associated with the development of psychotic features.

Behavioural features

- Psychomotor retardation or agitation.
- Altered facial expression such as mouth turned down, exaggerated facial lines, lack of facial expressivity.
- Self-neglect and social withdrawal.

Emotional features

- Low mood, distinct from ordinary unhappiness qualitatively (depth and pervasiveness) and quantitatively (DSM-IV requires >2 weeks).
- Tearfulness.
- Loss of interest in activities that would normally have given pleasure.
- Inability to feel pleasure (*anhedonia*).
- Loss of reactivity of mood to external events.
- Irritability.
- Anxiety: psychological and physical components.

Cognitive features
Form of thought:

- Slow speed of thought.
- Reduced speed and latency of speech.
- Reduced volume of speech.
- Reduced tonal modulation and expressivity in speech.
- Subjective impairment in concentration, registration and recall, paralleled by objective impairment in psychometric testing. Memory disturbance may be severe and resemble dementia (*depressive pseudodementia*).

Content of thought:

- Thought content reflects the abnormality in mood, with negative or depressive cognitions: negative views of self (*self-blame*), the world (*negativism*), and the future (*pessimism*).
- Milder forms include a vague pessimistic outlook and a tendency to worry unnecessarily.
- Moderate cases may show hopelessness, worthlessness and excessive guilt. Patients may be unable to distract themselves from these repetitive thoughts (*depressive ruminations*).
- Distorted views of the future may lead to predictions of disaster and *suicidal* thoughts or behaviour.

Biological symptoms

- Diurnal variation of mood (usually, but not always, worse in the morning).
- Sleep disturbance: *early morning waking* (or *late insomnia*) is the classic disturbance, but initial (early) insomnia and restless/disturbed sleep (middle insomnia) are common.
- Loss of appetite.
- Weight loss (DSM-IV specifies 5% as significant).
- Loss of libido.
- Fatigue and generalized lassitude (*anergia*).
- Constipation.
- Amenorrhoea.

Reversed biological features may be present, i.e. hypersomnia (increased sleep), increased appetite and weight gain. *Atypical depression* is a syndrome with reversed biological features, preserved mood reactivity, extreme (leaden) anergia, and interpersonal rejection sensitivity.

Psychotic features

- Delusions: in severe depression, cognitive distortions give way to delusions that are in keeping with the depressed mood (*mood congruent*). Common content involves guilt, poverty and hypochondriasis. The patient may feel he/she is being persecuted, which sometimes, but not always, is viewed as deserved.
- Hallucinations: auditory hallucinations may occur, classically second person accusatory; hallucinations in other sensory modalities can also occur.
- *Cotard's syndrome* characteristically occurs in elderly patients, where severe depression results in nihilistic delusions, often with hypochondriacal content, such as a belief that the bowel has rotted away.

Subtypes and variants of the depressive syndrome

Melancholic depression

While most agree that depression is a heterogeneous condition, there have been innumerable attempts to subdivide depression according to symptom patterns. Most studies of depression have identified a group of patients characterized by certain symptoms: early morning waking, weight loss, poor appetite, anhedonia and agitation. This symptom grouping has been variously labelled as *core*, *endogenous*, *nuclear*, and *melancholic* depression, the latter now being ensconced within DSM-IV. Early conceptualizations of this category noted that patients were said to show a preferential response to antidepressants and ECT, and to show more dysfunction of biological correlates of depression such as the dexamethasone suppression test. Few good studies have made direct comparisons between melancholic depression and other types, preventing firm conclusions from being drawn.

However, this group actually represents the minority of cases of depression. Most patients have milder symptoms, day-to-day fluctuation of mood, initial insomnia and prominent features of anxiety. Results attempting to define these have been conflicting:

- **Newcastle classification:** Roth and colleagues separated out two groups of depressed patients using multiple regression analysis, and argued that the melancholic and neurotic groups were distinct.
- **Kendall's classification:** Kendell was unable to demonstrate that a point of rarity exists between the two forms and proposed that depression represented a continuum with varying degrees of melancholic and neurotic symptoms (Kendell 1976).

- **Paykel's classification:** Paykel (1971) separated four groups of patients using cluster analysis:

  1. psychotic depressives (i.e melancholic)
  2. anxious depressives (middle-aged, moderate depressive symptoms plus anxiety)
  3. hostile depressives (young, hostile)
  4. younger depressives with personality disorders.

More recently, Kendler (1997) used twin pairs to demonstrate that DSM-IV-defined melancholia was associated with an increased genetic loading, as well as increased comorbidity with anxiety disorders (but not alcohol dependence or bulimia), a more severe and recurrent illness course and lower levels of neuroticism. Thus, whilst it represented a valid subtype associated with a particularly high familial liability, the data best supported a quantitative, rather than qualitative, distinction, in keeping with Kendall's description.

DSM-IV depression

Kendler also used this sample to ask whether the DSM-IV criteria represent a truly separate disorder from other depressive disorders, or represent an arbitrary cut off (Kendler & Gardner 1998). Three DSM criteria were studied:

- presence of five out of nine symptoms
- duration of symptoms greater than two weeks
- severity of symptoms or associated functional impairment.

Both severity and number of symptoms in one twin were associated in a linear fashion with risk of depression in the co-twin. This relationship was not found with duration. Using criteria below the threshold for DSM major depression on each of the three measures were all good predictors of future depressive risk, both in individuals and their co-twin. The authors concluded that the DSM-IV criteria are of little use in predicting personal or genetic risk of depression, and that depressive illness is likely to lie on a continuum.

Psychotic depression

The clinical importance of separating out psychotic depression relates primarily to the implications for treatment and prognosis. Some authors have argued that psychotic depression represents a separate and distinct category, based on clinical, genetic, treatment response and biological features. Evidence for this is discussed later in this chapter.

Atypical depression

Atypical depression has been used in the past to mean a number of different conditions, including non-endogenous depression, depression secondary to another condition, depression associated with anxiety or panic, and depression with reversed biological features. However, as the concept has evolved, atypicality has been more tightly defined, and is now included within DSM-IV. It is defined as a subtype of depressive disorder characterized by reversed biological symptoms (e.g. hypersomnia, hyperphagia and variation of mood worse in the evening), preserved mood reactivity, extreme ('leaden') anergia and chronic interpersonal rejection sensitivity. Atypical depression does appear to be a valid concept. Sullivan and colleagues (Sullivan et al. 1998) used data from the large US National Comorbidity Survey, and identified six depressive syndromes, two of which corresponded to mild atypical depression and severe atypical depression respectively. A study of female twin pairs also found an atypical depression syndrome; furthermore, individuals tended to have the same syndrome on each recurrence and the concordance of syndrome type was greater in monozygotic than in dizygotic pairs (Kendler et al. 1996). Importantly, atypical depression probably responds more favourably to monoamine oxidase inhibitors than to tricyclic antidepressants.

Somatization

Epidemiological studies show that physical symptoms are strongly associated with depression; furthermore, patients frequently present with such symptoms rather than emotional symptoms. The physical symptoms may be medically explained, i.e. they represent a comorbid physical illness (physical illness is associated with increased rates of depression). More frequently, they represent medically unexplained, or functional symptoms. Such symptoms may represent the biological disturbance in depression, such as loss of weight or sleep disturbance, or the process of *somatization*. Somatization is a complex phenomenon, dealt with in more detail in Chapter 16, but includes components of heightened symptom production (i.e. via the effects of autonomic arousal), heightened symptom perception (via symptom focusing), abnormal interpretation of symptoms (as representing physical illness), excessive response to symptoms leading to disability (e.g. avoidance behaviour) and seeking medical help. Frequent presentations include fatigue and weakness, headache, gastrointestinal disturbance, chest symptoms, dizziness or pain. Longitudinal studies show that these often precede the emergence of frank affective symptoms. As usual, this process represent a spectrum, and psychiatrists (and other doctors) may need to move gently in the shift of focus from physical to psychological symptoms in order to avoid alienating patients with more extreme tendencies to somatization.

Other descriptors

Impaired social functioning may be the first presentation of depression in the elderly, and has been termed *masked depression*. Such changes should lead to relevant enquiry about the presence of the usual depressive symptoms in order to excluded depression as a cause. Some clinicians separate out *agitated depression* from *retarded depression*, although there is no evidence yet of any great validity to this

distinction, and agitation and retardation can coexist. Also seen is a distinction between primary depression and secondary depression, where the depression can be seen as a response to something else, such as another psychiatric disorder or an obvious cause such as drugs. Clinically, this separation is arbitrary and ignores the usual multifactorial nature of causation.

Comorbidity

Depression is frequently comorbid with other conditions, with, for example, approximately half of all patients having a lifetime history of an anxiety disorder and a quarter with substance misuse (Kessler et al. 2003). Generally, the presence of unaddressed comorbid psychiatric diagnoses will make the depression harder to treat, and vice versa. Depression should therefore always be looked for and treated in other conditions where it occurs commonly. Of particular note is dissociative disorders: patients with various dissociative or conversion disorders are frequently depressed; indeed, this is a relatively good prognostic factor in such cases (Crimlisk et al. 1998).

Abnormal grief reactions

Symptoms of a normal reaction to bereavement are similar to those of depression, although psychomotor retardation and global loss of self-esteem are unusual. Some have characterized distinct stages in a grief reaction; initially there is a stunned phase lasting for a few days, followed by misery and searching behaviour persisting for up to six months (Box 19.1). However, grief reactions merge into depressive illnesses. There is no hard and fast divide as to when grief becomes depression, but, clinically, prolonged reactions, those that markedly interfere with normal function or the presence of symptoms such as suicidality may require intervention.

Murray-Parkes (Murray-Parkes 1998) subdivides abnormal grief into:

- unexpected grief, when the death occurred unexpectedly and often in a horrifying way
- ambivalent grief, occurring after relationships characterized by discord
- chronic grief, which is normal in form, but persistent. It particularly occurs following a dependent relationship with the deceased
- delayed or absent grief, where there is a failure to pass through the normal stages of bereavement.

Box 19.1	Stages of grief
Numbness	
Pining	
Disorganization and despair	
Reorganization	

Other features of abnormal grief reactions include intense anger and feelings of betrayal persisting beyond six weeks. In some cases an anxiety state or psychosis may occur. Features increasing the risk of abnormal grief reactions are listed in Box 19.2.

Box 19.2 Factors associated with abnormal grief reactions
Characteristics of loss
Loss of child
Loss of parent during childhood
Sudden, unexpected death (inc. suicide, murder)
Multiple deaths, e.g. disasters
Attachment of blame to survivor
Characteristics of relationship
Ambivalent relationships
Dependent relationship
Insecure attachment
Characteristics of individual
Previous psychiatric vulnerability
Inability to express grief
Insecurity and low self-esteem
Social circumstances
Social isolation
Absent or unsupportive family

Longitudinal course of depression

Affective disorders may be divided into those which involve only depression (*unipolar* illness) and those in which both episodes of mania and depression occur (*bipolar* illness); the latter are dealt with in Chapter 20. The majority of depressive illnesses are of a recurrent nature, although the frequency of recurrence varies enormously.

Depression with a seasonal recurrence (seasonal affective disorder)

Many subjects describe a seasonal pattern to their illness. The classic presentation is of depression and reversed biological features in winter. There is sometimes evidence of a bipolar course, with mild hypomania in spring or summer. However, many patterns exist. Data from the National Comorbidity Survey suggested that only 1.6% of those with major depression (0.4% of the entire sample) fulfilled the criteria (Blazer et al. 1998). If minor depression was included, this figure rose to 1% of the sample. In those with major depression, a seasonal pattern was higher in male patients and older patients. These prevalence figures are significantly lower than studies of seasonal affective disorder using less stringent criteria.

Postpartum affective disorder

This is discussed elsewhere in this volume (Chapter 23).

Subsyndromal depression

Many people have significant depressive symptoms that fail to meet the usual criteria for a depressive episode. Nevertheless, a significant associated burden of disability has been identified in association with these symptoms. *Dysthymia* describes patients that have depressive symptoms that fail to meet the criteria for severity, but which are of long duration. *Double depression* describes episodes of major depression superimposed on dysthymia: the prognosis and treatment response may be worse. There is some evidence that dysthymia responds to antidepressants, which may need to be given long-term. *Adjustment disorders* describe subsyndromal symptoms that have clearly arisen in response to an identifiable stressor or life change, and which resolve upon alleviation of the stressor or adjustment to new circumstances. *Recurrent brief depression* has been suggested as a descriptor for depressive episodes that reach the criteria for severity, but not duration, of symptoms. It is not yet widely accepted. Treatment response remains unclear.

INTERNATIONAL CLASSIFICATION SYSTEMS

Unipolar depressive disorders are dealt with slightly differently by the two major classification systems (depression as part of bipolar disorder, or bipolar depression, is discussed in Chapter 20).

DSM-IV

Mood disorder is subdivided into Depressive Disorder, Dysthymic Disorder, Adjustment Disorder and Organic Depression in DSM-IV (American Psychiatric Association 1994), as follows:

- Depressive disorders:
  (a) major depressive disorder, single episode
  (b) major depressive disorder, recurrent
  (c) in addition, depressive disorders should be specified with regard to:
    (i) severity (mild, moderate, severe, severe with psychosis)
    (ii) features (melancholic, catatonic, atypical)
    (iii) pattern (post-partum onset, seasonal pattern)
    (iv) course (chronic, with or without full interepisode recovery).
- Dysthymic disorder (two years of depressive symptoms most days insufficient to meet criteria for major depression).
- Adjustment disorder (depressive symptoms insufficient to meet criteria for major depressive disorder and arising in response to an identifiable stressor).
- Organic depression:
  (a) mood disorder due to a general medical condition
  (b) substance-induced mood disorder.

A residual category of depressive disorder not otherwise specified (NOS) includes recurrent brief depressive disorder, premenstrual dysphoric disorder, minor depressive disorder and postpsychotic depression.

ICD-10

Unipolar depression is classified somewhat differently in ICD-10 (World Health Organization 1992) than in DSM-IV, depending on whether they are episodic or persistent, as follows:

- Mood disorders:
  - (a) depressive episode (mild, moderate, severe, severe with psychotic features)
  - (b) recurrent depressive disorder
  - (c) other depressive episodes (including atypical depression and masked depression)
  - (d) other recurrent mood disorders (including recurrent brief depressive disorder).
- Persistent affective states:
  - (a) dysthymia (a chronic syndrome of low mood and associated symptoms never or rarely severe enough to meet criteria for a depressive episode).

Depression is also encountered in other settings, e.g. organic (organic depressive state), other anxiety disorders (mixed anxiety and depressive disorder), or adjustment disorder, which includes brief or prolonged depressive reactions. Postschizophrenic depression is classified under the psychoses.

EPIDEMIOLOGY

Studies of the epidemiology of depression must be seen in the correct perspective, given the large discrepancies often found between them. Important factors include:

- diagnostic schedule (i.e. ICD-10 or DSM-IV)
- screening instrument (self report, lay interview, clinician interview, structured format)
- sample (hospital, primary care, community)
- culture
- era of study (there is evidence of a gradual increase in depression since 1970).

The point prevalence of depressive *illness* varies from 4% to 7%. The point prevalence of depressive *symptoms* is 16–20% in most studies. The National Comorbidity Study in the USA used a representative community sample and administered a structured clinical interview face to face to 8000 individuals (Kessler et al. 1994). Using DSM-IIIR criteria, the 12-month prevalence of depression was 10% (8% in males, 13% in females) and the lifetime prevalence 17% (13% in males, 21% in females). Dysthymia was diagnosable in 6% of the population (5% in males, 8% in females). A recent study,

the NCS-R, using DSM-IV criteria for depression found 12-month rates of 6.6% and lifetime rates of 16.2% (Kessler et al. 2003).

The peak age of onset is 30–40 years for unipolar depression and 50–70 years for psychotic depression. There are some suggestions of a bimodal peak in unipolar depression with the second peak occuring in the 50's (Eaton et al. 1997). There is a female predominance of approximately 2:1 in unipolar depression. The excess of unipolar depression in women decreases with age, particularly in those over 55 years (Bebbington 1998). Using the Present State Examination, 15% of Camberwell (inner city London) women are depressed compared to 8% in the Hebrides (rural Scotland). There is international variation in rates: lifetime rates range from 1.5% in Taiwan to 19% in Beirut, with annual rates ranging from 0.8% in Taiwan to 5.8% in New Zealand (Weissman et al. 1996).

There appears to have been a real rise in both the incidence and prevalence of depression during the last three decades, believed to be a cohort effect (Kessler et al. 2003). This is true for both men and women.

AETIOLOGY

Neurobiological components

Genetics

It has been long been clear that there is a significant genetic component to unipolar depression. Evidence for this comes from studies utilizing a variety of genetic research methodology. Family studies show increased familial risk and the earlier the age of onset, the higher the familial risk. Late onset affective disorder has a lower genetic loading. Twin studies in unipolar depression show concordance rates of approximately 40–50% in monozygotic and 25% in dizygotic twins (McGuffin et al. 1991; Price 1968). The MZ concordance rates seem to be lower for community sampled depression or neurotic depression, suggesting a lesser biological component in these cases (McGuffin et al. 1996). Adoption studies in unipolar depression have found increased rates of illness in biological relatives compared to adopted relatives of probands (Mendlewicz & Rainer 1977).

In terms of the mode of inheritance, there is no compelling evidence of true Mendelian transmission. Although a few studies have reported linkage, none have been adequately replicated. It is probable that there are many genes implicated in mediating differing aspects of the overall genetic predisposition.

How then do these genes confer risk? First of all, there is little support for the suggestion that a higher personal genetic loading leaves an individual needing less environmental stress to become depressed (Tennant 2002). Instead, it is the tendency to become depressed in response to life events that is inherited (Kendler et al. 1995). The situation is further complicated by the recent findings that there is a significant genetic component to life events themselves (Kendler & Karkowski Shuman 1997). Thus, both the tendency to suffer adversity and to respond to it by becoming depressed have genetic components.

However, it has been observed that there is a tendency for each recurrence of depression to be less dependent on precipitating stress, a phenomenon likened to 'kindling' (see later). Kendler and colleagues used a large twin pair sample to discover that genetic risk tended to place people in a 'pre-kindled' state rather than speeding up the process of kindling (Kendler et al. 2001).

It is now clear that there is genetic variation in several biological systems that have important roles in brain homeostasis, linked to the occurrence of polymorphic variation in gene alleles. Various studies have shown that certain polymorphisms at the serotonin (5HT) receptor subtypes (e.g. $5HT_{2C}$ receptor), of tryptophan hydroxylase (the rate limiting enzyme for the synthesis of 5HT) or the 5HT transporter are associated with depression. There is a functional significance of the different alleles: certain polymorphisms are associated with different rates of production of the 5HT receptor or 5HT transporter m-RNA, or differential capacity of the transporter for the reuptake of 5HT into the neuron. Such genetic variation could therefore provide a link between the genetics of depression and the 5HT hypothesis of depression (see later).

Future genetic research may also integrate elements of post-transcriptional changes and modifications, so-called *proteomics* – much of the expression of genetic risk appears to be dependent on what happens during this post-transcriptional period.

Neurochemistry

Brain neurochemistry has long been studied in the search for the biological basis of depression, dating from the original finding that monoamine depletion by the drug reserpine caused depression. The observation that the newly developed antidepressants (monoamine oxidase inhibitors and tricyclic antidepressants) enhanced synaptic mono-amine levels and that there were reduced monoamine breakdown products (5HIAA, HVA and MHPG) in the cerebrospinal fluid (CSF) of depressed subjects led to the monoamine hypothesis of depression. This theory stated that there is a deficiency of noradrenaline (NA) (norepinephrine), dopamine and/or 5HT at monoaminergic synapses. From this original hypothesis, several proposed biological models of depression have developed.

Serotonergic theories

Coppen (1967) originally proposed the 5HT hypothesis of depression, suggesting that 5HT was the specific monoamine involved in depression. Classically, several pieces of evidence are cited to support the theory that many aspects of 5HT physiology may be dysregulated in depression (see Maes & Meltzer [1995] for detailed review). It should be noted that there are at present no ways to measure directly the amount of 5HT present in brain synapses.

First, there is evidence of a reduced availability to the brain of the 5HT precursor tryptophan: there are reduced plasma levels of tryptophan and evidence of an enhanced alternative route of tryptophan catabolism via the kynurenine pathway in the liver.

Second, there are changes in the normal uptake mechanisms for 5HT: evidence for this comes from the finding of a reduced uptake of 5HT into the platelets, which act as a model of the neuronal 5HT transporter system.

Third, there are changes in the status of 5HT receptors in depression. Early work relied on the use of brains obtained from patients who had died by suicide. Several studies found increased $5HT_2$ receptors, which was felt to result from low 5HT synaptic content, and reduced $5HT_{1A}$ hippocampal and amygdala binding. A further approach has been the use of neuropharmacological challenge paradigms to test the integrity of neurotransmitter systems, or receptor sensitivity. Standardized drug challenges are given, ideally centrally acting and selective, and a physiological response is measured, such as hormone release or temperature change. The magnitude of the response is taken as an index of the activity of the system challenged. Many, although by no means all, of these studies have reported impairments in depression. One example is of a blunted prolactin response to fenfluramine, a drug that leads to release of presynaptic 5HT. Other positive examples include a blunted prolactin response to the 5HT precursor L-tryptophan, and a blunted response to the serotonin reuptake inhibitor clomipramine.

Fourth, the technique of tryptophan depletion (TD) suggests that there may be a *causal* relationship between 5HT changes and depression. The TD paradigm involves oral administration of a mixture of amino acids without tryptophan; this leads to a rapid fall in plasma tryptophan since protein synthesis stimulated as a result of the drink utilizes the available tryptophan. This reduction in plasma levels, together with competition from the other ingested amino acids, leads to lowered brain tryptophan entry, and reduced 5HT synthesis. TD in unmedicated depressed subjects has not revealed consistent results, perhaps because the 5HT system is maximally dysregulated (Delgado et al. 1994). On the other hand, TD depletion induces a temporary state of depressive symptomatology in those at increased vulnerability to depression, including patients with a personal (Smith et al. 1997) or family (Benkelfat et al. 1994; Klaassen 1999) history of depression and females (Ellenbogen et al. 1996). This is powerful evidence of a causal link between reduced serotonergic function and depression, rather than merely a cross-sectional association. TD may also be of predictive utility, since the presence of a positive (i.e. mood-lowering) effect of TD in those in remission from depression is associated with a higher rate of relapse in the following 12 months (Moreno et al. 2000). Thus, certain individuals may have a biological vulnerability to short term depressogenic effects of reduced brain 5HT availability, which places them at increased risk of future major depression, possibly as a response to other biological or environmental causes of reduced 5HT availability.

One anomaly in the TD literature is the observation that the mood lowering effect of tryptophan depletion does not occur to a significant degree in remitted depressed patients receiving continuation treatment with desipramine, a noradrenergic specific tricyclic antidepressant (Delgado et al. 1999). They do, however, experience a transient relapse if noradrenaline (norepinephrine) synthesis is inhibited, while, conversely, those who responded to SSRIs are not affected by noradrenaline (norepinephrine) depletion (Delgado et al. 1993).

Fifth, and finally, recent neuroimaging techniques have been utilized to visualize directly brain 5HT changes in depression. PET and SPET imaging can use radiolabelled ligands to measure receptor binding (a product of receptor density and receptor sensitivity) for specific neurochemical targets in the different brain regions.

The status of brain $5HT_2$ receptors has not been clarified by these techniques; receptor binding has been found to be increased, normal or decreased in different studies. The largest study (Yatham et al. 2000) used PET and the $5HT_2$ receptor ligand [18F]septoperone in 20 drug free patients with major depression and 20 matched healthy controls. The main finding was that depressed patients showed a marked global reduction in receptor binding (between 22 and 27% in various regions). Differences from previous studies may have been due to the shorter duration of drug free period in this study (2 weeks). There remains difficulty reconciling the accumulating finding of reduced binding with the fact that effective antidepressant treatments lead to further downregulation of $5HT_2$ receptors (Sheline & Mintun 2002).

The assessment of the status of brain $5HT_{1A}$ receptors in depression was assessed using the PET radioligand [11C] WAY-100635 in a group of 25 depressed patients, 15 of whom were unmedicated, and 10 of whom were rescanned after treatment with a selective serotonin reuptake inhibitor antidepressant (Sargent et al. 2000). There was a generalized reduction in $5HT_{1A}$ receptor binding throughout the cortex. This was also present in the medicated subjects, however, and not altered by prospective treatment with an SSRI. The authors hypothesize a trait reduction in $5HT_{1A}$ receptors that is unaffected by treatment. Results of another study support the reduction in $5HT_{1A}$ binding, particularly in the mesio-temporal cortex (hippocampus–amygdala) and the midbrain (raphe nuclei) (Drevets et al. 1999).

It has been pointed out that measuring receptor numbers may not represent receptor function. A neuroimaging paradigm attempting to assess receptor function extends the neuropharmacological challenge paradigms already described above. Thus, it is possible to measure changes in neural activity in different brain regions using functional imaging with PET or f-MRI after the administration of neuropharmacological challenges. Such serotonergically mediated changes in neural activity after fenfluramine administration are markedly reduced in major depression, suggesting downregulated central 5HT receptors (Mann et al. 1996). However, a study using the more specific d-isomer of fenfluramine could not replicate this finding (Meyer et al. 1998).

One argument against the significance of serotonergic changes in depression comes from observations that either specific behaviours (e.g. suicide) and/or enduring character traits (e.g. impulsivity) may be more closely related to 5HT function. Thus, while initial studies found reduced concentrations of the 5HT breakdown product 5HIAA in CSF from depressed patients, there have been recent suggestions that this is linked more specifically to suicide, impulsivity or aggression (Maes & Meltzer 1995). A further issue is whether or not the serotonergic changes are state or trait related. While the impaired serotonergic responses to neuropharmacological challenge tests usually normalize after successful treatment of depression, the reduced $5HT_{1A}$ receptor binding seen with PET does not (Sargent et al. 2000). This suggests that some of the observed changes in depression may indeed be trait markers, and more closely linked to vulnerability or personality than to depressive state.

Noradrenergic theories

Many effective antidepressants (e.g. desipramine, nortriptyline and reboxetine) are potent inhibitors of the reuptake of noradrenaline (norepinephrine), with little effect on 5HT reuptake. Indeed, several studies found that low urinary levels of the noradrenaline (norepinephrine) metabolite MHPG predict a favourable response to tricyclic antidepressants (Schatzberg & Schildkraut 1995). Neuroendocrine challenge studies have also found evidence of reduced noradrenergic function in depression. For example, reduced GH responses to clonidine (Checkley et al. 1981) and desipramine (Siever 1987) suggest impaired α_2 receptor function, and abnormality that may persist into recovery of depression and thus may represent a trait marker (Siever et al. 1992). Postmortem and platelet studies also provide some support for changes in α and ß adrenergic receptors (Schatzberg et al. 2002). Finally, in a novel, though highly invasive, study, concentration gradients for the main catecholamines and their metabolites were calculated using simultaneous sampling of brachial artery and internal jugular vein blood. In patients with treatment-resistant depression, there was a reduced concentration gradient for norepinephrine and its metabolites and for the dopamine metabolite, homovanillic acid, but no differences in 5HT or its metabolite 5HIAA. These results provide further evidence of reduced noradrenaline (norepinephrine) availability in the brain, particularly in severe, resistant forms of depression (Lambert et al. 2000).

Further support for noradrenergic dysfunction in depression comes from the use of the challenge drug clonidine in combination with PET imaging; this suggests functionally impaired presynaptic α_2 adrenoceptors as well as regionally supersensitive postsynaptic cortical α_2 adrenoceptors (Fu et al. 2001).

Dopaminergic theories

Interest in the dopaminergic system has been stimulated by the introduction of bupropion, an antidepressant that works primarily on dopamine reuptake. There is some evidence of a reduced GH response to the dopamine receptor agonist apomorphine, but results are inconsistent, and there is little other work to date on the dopamine system in unipolar depression (Willner 1995).

Cholinergic theories

Studies have shown an enhanced GH response to the anticholinesterase drug pyridostigmine, a measure of acetyl choline receptor function. Further evidence comes from the observation of reduced rapid eye movement latency and increased REM sleep in depression, effects that may represent increased cholinergic activity. Furthermore, depressed patients show supersensitivity to REM sleep effects of cholinergics. Janowsky proposed the cholinergic-adrenergic balance theory of depression, hypothesizing that increased cholinergic function and reduced noradrenergic function were both important in generating symptoms in depression (Janowsky & Overstreet 1995).

GABA-ergic theories

There is a reduced GH response to baclofen, a GABA-B receptor agonist, suggesting reduced GABA receptor activity in depression (O'Flynn & Dinan 1993). Plasma GABA may also be low (Schatzberg et al. 2002).

Interactions of monoamines

There is now increasing evidence that drugs that affect one neurotransmitter system can also affect another through downstream effects. If one looks simply at 5HT, there are innumerable examples. Thus, $5HT_{1D}$ receptors may act in an inhibitory manner on neurons releasing other neurotransmitters. Similarly, α_1 receptors on serotonergic cell bodies act to increase cell firing and 5HT release, while α_2 receptors are present on serotonergic nerve terminals and are inhibitory to 5HT release. Serotonergic neurones project to other areas of the brain where they can inhibit dopaminergic function (Moghaddan & Bunney 1990). The 5HT transporter protein is thought to interact with the ability of α_2 receptors to inhibit 5HT cell firing (Blier et al. 1990). Finally, noradrenaline (norepinephrine) reuptake inhibition is potentiated in the presence of simultaneous 5HT reuptake inhibition (Engleman et al. 1995).

It is likely that a number of neurotransmitter alterations are present in depression. The clinical relevance of this may be reflected in the finding that drugs that act on both 5HT and noradrenaline (norepinephrine), such as amitriptyline (Barbui & Hotopf 2001) and venlafaxine (Smith et al. 2002), may have slightly enhanced efficacy in the treatment of depression.

Neuroendocrinology

Hypothalamo-pituitary-adrenal axis

The hypothalamo-pituitary or HPA axis (see Fig. 19.1) mediates the response of the body to stress, and has been a focus of biological research into depression, given the close link to stress. Research using 24-hour collections of blood, urine or saliva has clarified that about 50% of depressed patients show a picture of hypercortisolaemia. However, there is considerable variability in these findings: rates are higher in those with features of DSM-IV melancholic depression, strong somatic symptoms or psychosis (Belanoff et al. 2001), while those with predominant features of atypical depression are often found to have the opposite picture, a shift towards hypocortisolaemia (see below).

Assessing the HPA axis is made problematic by the fact that cortisol is a pulsatile hormone with a strong diurnal rhythm, and is released in stressful circumstances, such as blood sampling. This has necessitated more detailed methods of endocrinological assessment. The most widely used in depression research has been the dexamethasone suppression test (DST). Dexamethasone is a synthetic glucocorticoid that suppresses hypothalamic corticotrophin-releasing hormone (CRH) and pituitary corticotrophin

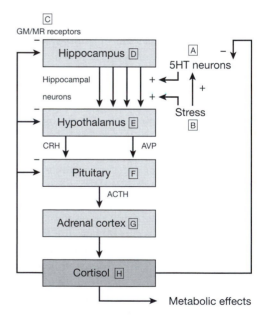

Figure 19.1 Schematic representation of the control of the hypothalamo-pituitary-adrenal (HPA) axis. Abbreviations are: CRH (corticotrophin releasing hormone); ACTH (corticotrophin); AVP (argenine vasopressin); MR (mineralocorticoid receptors); GR (glucocorticoid receptors). Abnormalities in this axis in depression are shown in Box 19.3.

Box 19.3 HPA axis abnormalities in depression (see Fig. 19.1)

A:	decreased 5HT neuronal function
B:	increased incidence of life events
C:	impaired hippocampal fast (rate-sensitive) feedback
D:	shrunken hippocampal structures
E:	raised CRH levels in the cerebrospinal fluid; impaired negative feedback by dexamethasone
F:	impaired pituitary ACTH response to CRH administration; this may represent downregulated CRH receptors or negative feedback from high cortisol levels. Pituitary hypertrophy
G:	hypertrophied adrenal cortices
H:	hypercortisolism

(ACTH) release via its effects on glucocorticoid receptors (see Figure 19.1) and hence suppresses plasma cortisol release. In a proportion of depressed individuals such suppression fails to occur. This observation has lead to the development of the dexamethasone suppression test (DST). There are variants of the test, but the most widely used in depression involves administering dexamethasone 1 mg at 11 p.m., and measuring plasma cortisol measured at 8 a.m., 4 p.m. or 11 p.m. Non-suppression of cortisol below a defined laboratory reference range represents a positive test. Rates of non-suppression vary, but average around 60–70% in melancholic depression and 30–40% in other forms of depression. The test is not specific, however, since non-suppression is also associated with schizophrenia (20%), old age, Alzheimer's disease, weight loss (including anorexia nervosa) and a number of drugs (such as anticonvulsants). Proponents of the test note that it measures the responsiveness of the specific glucocorticoid receptors in the hypothalamus and pituitary glands, and gives an indication of glucocorticoid receptor resistance.

More recently, the combined dexamethasone-CRH test has been developed. The effect of CRH in stimulating ACTH and cortisol release is markedly attenuated after dexamethasone administration in healthy individuals. However, if glucocorticoid receptors are downregulated, the dexamethasone has less effect, and the CRH response is less attenuated. In depression, this test proved more able to distinguish depressed subjects from healthy individuals than the simple DST (Heuser et al. 1994). Box 19.3 outlines the specific findings of various other endocrine tests applied to components of the HPA axis.

These studies show that, in a substantial proportion of depressed patients, there is oversecretion of cortisol and downregulation of glucocorticoid receptors. There are also several reasons for thinking that cortisol hypersecretion could be causally related to depression. Raised cortisol secretion in endogenous Cushing's disease is associated with depression in between 50–85% of cases; this depression usually resolves when cortisol levels decrease after treatment of Cushing's. Even in non-Cushing's depression, reducing the levels or effect of cortisol by administering cortisol synthesis inhibitor drugs such as metyrapone or ketoconazole, using CRH receptor antagonists or using glucocorticoid receptor antagonists can alleviate depression (Murphy 1997). Furthermore, cortisol has been shown to be associated with several other biological changes when present in abnormally high concentrations. For example, cortisol has strong, primarily inhibitory effects on neuronal 5HT neurotransmission; given the links between 5HT neurotransmission and mood changes already discussed, this is a mechanism by which 5HT neurotransmission could become dysregulated. There are also suggestions that prolonged periods of high cortisol can lead to hippocampal atrophy – indeed, in Cushings disease, the decreased hippocampus size can be correlated with plasma cortisol levels and cognitive impairment. Recent studies also suggest hippocampal atrophy in depression (Sheline & Mintun 2002).

Cortisol could also provide links between psychological risk factors for depression and the observed biological changes. For example, since cortisol is the main stress hormone, it is easy to see how it might mediate between life events and biological changes in depression. Similarly, adverse circumstances in childhood, such as losing parents or suffering abuse, are predisposing factors for depression. They are also linked to long-term alterations of the stress response both in childhood (De Bellis et al. 1994) and in later adulthood (Heim et al. 2000) irrespective of the actual presence of depression. Thus, it is also possible to use the HPA axis changes as a biological link between early life stresses and an increased vulnerability to stress and depression.

Others have noted that changes in the HPA axis other than cortisol levels may mediate symptoms. For example, CRH can act as a neurotransmitter, and produces symptoms such as agitation, insomnia and reduced feeding in animals. There is evidence of increased CRH activity in depression: CRH levels in the CSF are increased in depression, and there is more expression of neuronal CRH (and the synergistic ACTH-releaser vasopressin) in depressed suicide victims (Checkley 1996). CRH receptors are consequently downregulated. It is argued that this increased CRH in depression could contribute to some symptoms (Nemeroff 1996).

HPA axis changes in depression are also prognostic indicators. DST non-suppression is associated with a poorer response to placebo and a poorer response to cognitive therapy (Thase et al. 1996). If, despite clinical response to treatment, there is continued non-suppression, the risk of short-term relapse or suicide attempt rises four-fold. DST non-suppression may be the strongest predictor of long term completed suicide, even more so than other factors including past suicide attempts (Coryell & Sehlesser 2001).

Finally, depressed patients may suffer long term effects of raised cortisol such as higher rates of osteoporosis in women (Michelson et al. 1996) and altered body fat distribution in men (Thakore et al. 1997).

In summary, there is no doubt that HPA axis dysfunction is present in a large proportion of depressed patients, particularly those with psychotic or more melancholic symptom patterns. The HPA axis is able to provide a plausible biological mechanism for other known influences on depression; thus, the links between depressive symptoms and stressful life events, chronic social adversity, or traumatic or abusive childhoods could all be explained through the mediating role of the HPA axis.

Hypothalamo-pituitary-thyroid axis

Clinical disorders of thyroid function (both under and overactivity) are known to cause alteration in mood. Classically, patients with hypothyroidism frequently report features similar to depression and, whilst usually more closely linked to feelings of anxiety, depressive reactions are also sometimes seen in hyperthyroid patients.

In depression, several abnormalities in thyroid function have been described (Fig. 19.2 and Box 19.4). The principle findings are:

- The thyroid stimulating hormone (TSH) response to thyrotrophin release hormone (TRH) (*TRH test*) is abnormally blunted in 30% of depressed patients. This may be due to hypersecretion of TRH causing downregulation of TRH receptors on the pituitary (Nemeroff 1989).
- Around 8–17% of depressed patients have subclinical hypothyroidism (high TSH but normal T_4 levels, or an

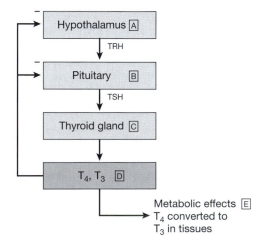

Figure 19.2 Schematic representation of the control of the hypothalamo-pituitary-thyroid (HPT) axis. Abbreviations are: TRH (thyrotrophin releasing hormone); TSH (thyroid stimulating hormone); T_4 (thyroxine); T_3 (tri-iodothyronine). Abnormalities in this axis in depression are shown in Box 19.4.

Box 19.4	Thyroid axis abnormalities in depression (Fig. 19.2)
A:	increased TRH in cerebrospinal fluid
B:	reduced TSH response to TRH administration (30%)
C:	antithyroid antibodies
D:	subclinical hypothyroidism
E:	treatment response to T_3 or T_4 augmentation strategies

enhanced response to the TRH test). This rises to over 50% in those refractory to initial treatment, compared to 5% of the normal population (Howland 1993).
- Antithyroid antibodies (antithyroglobulin and anti-microsomal) are present in 9–20% of cases of depression (Nemeroff et al. 1985). Harris et al. (1992) found that antithyroid antibodies were associated with depressive symptoms post-partum.
- Increased TRH levels in the CSF.

The suggestion that the rate of subclinical hypothyroidism is higher in depression has led to trials of thyroid hormone augmentation therapy. A recent review found six placebo-controlled trials of thyroid hormone supplementation in depression, and concluded that there is evidence that thyroid hormone may potentiate both speed and efficacy of antidepressant medication, although almost all of these studies were undertaken with tricyclic antidepressants (Altshuler et al. 2001). Furthermore, there is also evidence that patients resistant to other treatments may respond to such treatment, although there have been no studies linking pre-treatment subclinical hypothyroidism to this response. There is also some evidence that low T_3 levels are associated with a higher rate of relapse in the long term (Joffe & Marriott 2000).

Dehydroepiandrostenedione (DHEA)

There has been much recent interest in the role of DHEA in depression, particularly as in some aspects DHEA has an anticortisol effect. It has been argued that the 'net' effects of cortisol are enhanced if there is low DHEA, and, conversely, that high levels of cortisol may not be biologically damaging if accompanied by high DHEA levels. For this reason, the cortisol/DHEA ratio may be more relevant to the causation of depression. Initial studies do suggest that this ratio is higher in depression (Young et al. 2002). Small preliminary trials also suggest that DHEA supplementation may be an effective antidepressant, presumably acting by reducing the biological effects of cortisol (Bloch et al. 1999; Wolkowitz et al. 1999).

Cerebral pathophysiology

Recent advances in neuroimaging methodology have allowed researchers to attempt to map the phenomenological abnormalities seen in depression to changes in brain structure and function (Fu & McGuire 1999). Neuroimaging can broadly be broken up into structural and functional techniques.

Structural neuroimaging studies

Evidence is accumulating of changes in brain structure associated with depression. Magnetic resonance imaging has revealed decreased volume in cortical regions, particularly the frontal cortex (see Sheline & Mintun [2002] for review). Several studies also suggest reductions in subcortical structures, such as the hippocampus, amygdala, caudate and putamen, although results are mixed. These findings are supported by postmortem studies finding a loss of both neuronal and glial cells in the orbitofrontal, dorsolateral prefrontal and subgenual prefrontal cortices and hippocampus.

Such findings have been interpreted as having particular relevance to certain symptoms within depression. Thus, the subjective complaints of poor memory in depression are paralleled by objective neuropsychological impairment; hippocampal volume loss has been associated with similar changes such as impaired verbal and declarative memory (Burt et al. 1995).

Early CT studies showed that depression in the elderly was associated with features of cerebral atrophy (sulcal widening and ventricular enlargement) midway between that in depression and dementia, and that patients with pseudodementia have more abnormalities than those without (Jacoby & Levy 1980). More recently, it has been hypothesized that many individuals with late-life depression have 'vascular depression', i.e. underlying cerebrovascular disease affecting areas of the brain important in the control of mood (Alexopoulos et al. 1996). Vascular changes may be obvious, as in post-stroke depression, but there is also an association with the more subtle changes of microvascular disease. For example, the presence of white matter lesions in the MRI scans of 1077, non-demented, elderly adults aged between 60 and 90 was rated in a large cohort study alongside measures of present and past depression (de Groot et al. 2000). Whilst virtually all subjects had some level of white matter lesions, there was a linear relationship between the severity of lesions and measures of depression; those with more severe white matter lesions were up to five times more likely to have depressive symptoms compared to those with only mild white matter lesions. Those with an onset of depression after age 60 had more severe white matter lesions than those with an onset before age 60.

Clinically, depression associated with vascular disease appears to be more resistant to treatment. It is not known whether vascular contributions to late onset depression can be prevented by early monitoring and modification of cardiovascular risk factors.

Functional neuroimaging studies

Functional neuroimaging assesses neural function in different brain region by measuring metabolism (e.g. glucose utilization) or blood flow, both of which are thought to be closely linked to neural activation. The initial wave of investigations in this area concentrated on measuring function in the resting state. Most studies have described hypofrontality, particularly in the dorsolateral prefrontal and anterior cingulate cortices, and some have also described decreased activity in the basal ganglia (Drevets 2001; Fu & McGuire 1999). However, criticisms of these studies include the difficulty in standardizing the 'resting state'; results can be markedly affected by simple design differences such as whether eyes are open or shut (Sheline & Mintun 2002).

An improvement on these designs is to undertake neuroimaging while subjects undertake neuro-psychological tasks. This standardizes what the brain is doing, and also allows specific investigation of particular areas of the brain or particular psychological functions that are thought to be relevant to depression. This approach has consistently found impaired activation in the left anterior cingulate (George et al. 1997), right prefrontal cortex (Elliott et al. 1997), and left caudate (Elliott et al. 1997), while the induction of sadness in healthy individuals leads to similar changes (Mayberg et al. 1999). Depressed subjects also demonstrate an attenuated neural response to neutral or happy objects, but a relatively enhanced one to sad objects, in the same brain regions (Elliott et al. 2002). This may represent a neural substrate underlying the negative cognitive bias in depression.

However, certain neural changes are not specific to depression, and are present in other psychiatric conditions. It has been suggested these abnormalities are more closely related to specific psychological dysfunctions, such as psychomotor retardation (Bench et al. 1993) or depressive pseudodementia (Dolan et al. 1992), rather than diagnosis.

Studies have also been able to show that some pre-treatment abnormalities reverse with treatment. The most consistent finding has been of increased activation of the subgenual prefrontal cortex during an acute depressive state which decreases following successful antidepressant treatment (Mayberg et al. 1999; Mayberg et al. 2000). Other studies have taken a more complex look at dysfunction in the functional connections between brain regions, i.e. brain networks, rather than individual brain areas. Thus, one study revealed a complex picture of cortical and subcortical changes associated with treatment response to fluoxetine, with increases in the dorsal prefrontal cortex but decreases in the hippocampus (Mayberg et al. 2000).

As described earlier, a proportion of subjects with remitted depression relapse after tryptophan depletion. The depressive relapse during tryptophan depletion produces a similar patterns of brain abnormalities as seen in a major depressive episode, both at rest and during a cognitive task

(Bremner et al. 1997; Smith et al. 1999). These studies help link changes in 5HT function with changes in activity in specific brain areas during depressive relapse. Also of note is a study showing that blocking the synthesis of noradrenaline (norepinephrine) can also precipitate a temporary relapse in some recovered depressed patients and that this also results in similar brain changes as in the acute state (Bremner et al. 2003). Thus, different neurochemical mechanisms may be related to common neural changes in depressive relapse.

Cellular factors
Kindling
Neurons show a process of *kindling*, whereby the seizure threshold is gradually lowered when they are repeatedly subjected to convulsions or electrical stimuli; eventually, the cells can become autonomously firing. Post (1992) has suggested that this phenomenon might underlie the tendency for episodes of affective disorder to require fewer provoking life events, or become more refractory, with passing time. He proposes that anticonvulsants prevent this progression by preventing kindling. There is some evidence that this phenomenon occurs in unipolar depression. A study from Virginia (Kendler et al 2000) followed up over 2000 community-based female twin pairs over nine years, and found that each episode of depression was followed by an increased subsequent risk of a further episode of depression. This was an essentially linear relationship up to nine episodes, after which the rate was constant. They also found that the risk that each life event a person experienced would be followed by depression decreased with each successive depressive episode, i.e. each successive episode of depression was less stress-related. These findings are based on a sound methodology and are supportive of the presence of a process similar to kindling. However, the specific mechanisms underlying this effect remain unclear, although investigation into links with the transcription or expression of peptides and neural growth factors is ongoing.

Intracellular signalling
There is evidence that antidepressants are able to modify intracellular signalling, for example by enhancing the cyclic AMP pathway activation occurring after serotonergic receptor stimulation (Duman et al. 1997). It has been hypothesized that G proteins, important signal transducers in the phosphoinositol system, are overactive in depression; they are also potentially important in the mechanism of action of lithium. Several growth factors and neurotrophins are altered in depression, and may be important in neuronal changes seen in depression. Antidepressants also have effects on the expression of these factors. A new cellular model of depression is evolving in which there are felt to be impairments in signaling pathways that regulate neuroplasticity and cell survival (Manji et al. 2001).

Immunology
Psychosocial stress can have an effect on the immune system. Thus, bereavement, marital disturbance and examinations are associated with findings such as reduced natural killer (NK) cell activity, reduced lymphocyte proliferation, and altered white cell counts. While the results in depression are often confusing, given the variety of measures used, in general there is a reduction in indices of immunocompetence as represented by NK cell activity and mitogen-induced lymphocyte proliferation. The degree to which these immunological observations result from other changes in depression, such as the HPA axis and behavioural factors like sleep, remains unclear.

Interferon treatment is strongly associated with the onset of depressive symptoms and illness, and can be a problematic complication in those treated for disorders such as melanoma and hepatitis. The mechanism is unclear, but may be linked to effects on the HPA axis or 5HT metabolism. Treatment with SSRIs can improve symptoms (Musselman et al. 2001).

Sleep studies
Depression is associated with a number of abnormalities of sleep, including reduced REM latency and increased REM sleep (and therefore dreaming/nightmares). These effects may represent increased cholinergic activity. Depressed patients show supersensitivity to REM sleep effects of cholinergics and serotonergics. Antidepressants reduce total REM sleep and reduce REM latency independent of their antidepressant effect.

Neurobiology of atypical depression
In view of the relatively recent addition of atypical depression to the psychiatric nosology, little data exist on the similarities and differences between typical and atypical depression. One of the most frequently observed differences relates to the hypothalamo-pituitary-adrenal axis. While hypercortisolaemia is characteristic of melancholic major depression (see below), several studies have now suggested that atypical depression is associated with hypo-cortisolaemia. Gold and colleagues have suggested that, while typical major depression can be characterized by an excessive activation of both the physiological stress systems, the locus ceruleus-noradrenergic system and the hypothalamo-pituitary-adrenal axis, the opposite changes are present in atypical depression (Gold et al. 1995). Some support for this is provided by studies showing that the control of noradrenergic function is relatively preserved in atypical compared to typical depression (Asnis et al. 1995). Gold and colleagues suggest that it is diminished central corticotrophin-releasing hormone (CRH) activity that is specifically related to the symptoms of hypoarousal of the syndrome (Gold et al. 1995). Support that it is low CRH rather than low cortisol that is related to the atypicality syndrome comes from one detailed study of Cushing's

syndrome, in which cortisol is high and CRH low, where atypical depression was the predominant depressive syndrome (Dorn et al. 1995). Studies of serotonergic function are lacking, though one study suggested that platelet 5HT function is unaltered in atypical depression (Owens & Nemeroff 1994)

Neurobiology of psychotic depression

There is some evidence that there may be biological differences between psychotic depression and non-psychotic depression in terms of a more disturbed HPA axis (see above), increased dopamine turnover (i.e. higher homovanillic acid (HVA) levels in the CSF) and different patterns of disturbance of 5HT pathways (Wheeler Vega et al. 2000). Overall, however, a separation on the basis of neurobiology remains premature.

Psychological components

Psychodynamic

The psychoanalytic view of depression was first developed from the similarities between grief and depression, for example Freud's essay on 'mourning and melancholia'. Thus, the emphasis was on the importance of loss, which may be external (bereavement or separation) or an internally represented loss. Loss of or threat to self-esteem was also emphasized by later writers. Klein suggested that depression was more likely if infants failed successfully to pass through 'the depressive position', when an infant learns to assimilate certain aspects of loss and restitution. Psychoanalytic theory also views depression as a turning inward of aggression and hostility.

Cognitive

The cognitive theory of depression, as first described by Beck (1967), suggests that the cognitive distortions and errors that accompany depression are not just reflections of the lowered mood, but are instrumental in the origin and persistence of the disorder. For example, depressed people have substantial distortions of memory, with access to pleasant memories reduced and to unpleasant memories facilitated. Such distortions serve to amplify low mood. Cognitive theorists identify several specific errors in the thinking of depressed patients, described in Box 19.5.

In addition, Beck theorized that people develop *schema* - characteristic ways of interpreting and looking at the world, based upon development, learning, genetics, etc. These are then instrumental in bringing about cognitive distortions and hence depression.

Behavioural

Seligman (1975) developed a paradigm of chronic stress in animals, and found that some animals lose their capacity to act and avoid the stress. *Learned helplessness* was his term for the situation when reward or punishment is independent of

---

Box 19.5 The cognitive theory of depression

1. Automatic negative thoughts – regarding past, present and future (the cognitive triad: worthlessness, helplessness and hopelessness)

2. Negative expectations

3. Cognitive distortions:
   (i) arbitrary inference – assuming events to have negative implications
   (ii) selective abstraction – concentrating on only the negative aspects of events
   (iii) magnification – attaching undue importance to insignificant matters
   (iv) minimization – underestimating good performance or events
   (v) overgeneralization – extensive conclusions drawn from single incidents
   (vi) personalization

---

any actions of the animal. This is also associated with similar behavioural, endocrine and neurochemical changes to those found in depressed people.

In a cognitive–behavioural formulation, Lewinsohn and colleagues (1970) proposed that a normal mood state depends upon positive behavioural rewards, which may result from job or marital satisfaction, while distressing experiences are associated with negative rewards, and hence depression.

Clinically, behavioural factors may be relevant to understanding the maintenance of some depressive illnesses. Patients may become stuck in a situation of reduced motivation to undertake activities, and hence experience less rewarding experiences. Similarly, there may be other important forces reinforcing unhelpful behaviours such as overprotective or undersupportive partners.

Social components

Predisposing factors (vulnerability)

The study of Brown & Harris (1978) was carried out in two samples of depressed women, one in the community, the other known depressed psychiatric patients. First, they demonstrated the relationship between life events or chronic social stress and depression in both samples (see below). Second, they identified several factors that increased the risk of developing depression after life events (only a minority of life events being followed by depression):

- lack of a confiding relationship
- unemployment
- three or more children under the age of 14 at home
- loss of mother before age of 11.

Others have hypothesized that *low self-esteem* as a result of these factors may be the important mediator of vulnerability. Tennant (2002) and his co-workers suggested it is not the loss of, or separation from, the mother per se that is important, but events consequent on that loss. A further refinement of these links suggests that negative close relationships brought about by many mechanisms confer vulnerability to life events. Death of a parent may lead to a variety of negative experiences and increased likelihood of other stressors.

An important adverse experience that can predispose to depression is a history of an abusive childhood upbringing (see elsewhere in this volume). Many studies show that poor parenting is linked to adult depression irrespective of whether that care was provided by the biological parent. However, the effects of childhood loss, abuse and parenting are not specific for depression. Similar links have been shown for a variety of conditions such as anxiety disorder, schizophrenia, antisocial personality disorder and drug dependence.

Childhood physical ill health, particularly with un-explained physical symptoms such as abdominal pain, is also associated with increased rates of depression in later life, although the mechanism underlying this is unclear (Hotopf et al. 1998).

Bowlby (1980) proposed that people have an innate tendency to seek attachments, and that failure to do so leads to a failure of individual satisfaction (*attachment theory*). Depression is viewed as the end result of disruption of these bonds. *Social isolation* is a powerful predisposing factor for depression, especially in the elderly. It also acts as a strong perpetuating factor.

Precipitating factors (life events)

In the six-month period following a life event, the chance of an episode of depression is increased six-fold (Paykel 1978). The risk of parasuicide is similarly increased. Life events may be *exit events* (e.g. bereavement or separation) or *undesirable events* (e.g. redundancy). Using the concept of *brought-forward time*, Brown et al. (1973) calculated that threatening life events advanced an episode of depression by two years. The measurement of life events is complex, in particular putting a comparative weight upon them, and it seems that individuals have a threshold. The most commonly recorded event in a women's life in the six months prior to onset of depression is marital discord. Recent work suggests that the highest risk is posed by events that involve *loss* or *entrapment*, or are independent of a person's control. Loss events in combination with humiliation (e.g. 'other-initiated separation') are especially depressogenic. Dangerous or threatening events are more associated with the onset of anxiety (Kendler et al. 2003).

People in hospital with a variety of medical illnesses also have an excess of life-events prior to admission. It is possible that life-events are associated with the decision to seek help rather than the actual illness itself. A similar role in the creation of illness behaviour rather than illness has been suggested for early loss of a parent.

A recent review of the literature by Tenant (2002) focused on the literature published between 1980 and 2001 regarding the relationship between stress and depression. A number of findings have emerged, many of which find validity from a clinician's perspective:

- acute stressors are associated with a briefer depressive illness than that occurring without them and have an 'at risk' period of around one month
- chronic stressors lasting six months or more have a much longer at risk period, cause longer depressive episodes and contribute to a greater relapse/recurrence rate
- there is a sensitization effect, in that prior depressive episodes sensitize an individual to develop depression at lower levels of stress in the future; this effect is weaker in those with higher genetic loading for depression
- different characteristics of life events may be associated with producing anxiety or depression
- there is some evidence that some personality variables may increase the risk of stress-induced depression for a given life event
- twin studies have clarified that genetic effects and stressors have approximately equal impact on depression, although, in more clinical samples, genetic factors may be stronger.

However, this relationship is complicated because, as discussed earlier, life events have a genetic component, (subjects tending to select themselves into certain environments) and a tendency to respond to life stress by becoming depressed is also partly genetically determined.

Social networks

Henderson (1982) suggested that depressed persons do not actually lack social networks, but rather that the social bonds within such networks are weaker and provide less support.

Expressed emotions

While most research has been carried out in schizophrenia, there is also evidence that a high expressed emotions environment may increase relapse rates in affective disorders.

Integrative models of the aetiology of depression

The categorization of aetiological factors in depression into biological, psychological and social is convenient, but represents an artificial divide. The various factors are best seen as understanding depression on different levels, but may actually reflect a common substrate. There are many examples of how the biological models of depression can be tied in with other aetiological factors. For example, the predisposition to suffer depression conferred by childhood experiences can be paralleled by the presence of 'endocrine scars'. Acute and chronic stress from the environment can be shown to have profound neurobiological correlates. Artificially induced high cortisol levels are associated with cognitive dysfunction and a tendency to preferentially recall negative experiences. The neural response in depression is selectively larger in response to unhappy stimuli (Elliott et al. 2002). This type of brain dysfunction can be readily linked to the perceptual biases in depression, and also to cognitive theories of depression, without invoking primacy of one level of understanding over another.

Even within the biological factors outlined, it should be remembered that separate systems do not act independently. Just a few examples include the ability of neurochemical systems to modulate the activity of each other, the effect of the HPA axis on neurochemistry, and the effects of both neurochemical and endocrine systems on intracellular pathways.

Understanding the different changes in parallel and on several levels is rarely undertaken, and remains a potent obstacle to a full understanding of the aetiology of depression.

CLINICAL ASSESSMENT

A full assessment of an affective disorder in the clinical setting should aim to obtain a full description of the illness as outlined in Box 19.6. For more complicated cases in specialist care, formal life charting can be useful, for example the method detailed by the NIMH. Also helpful can be the use of structured interviews such as the Schedules for Clinical Assessment in Neuropsychiatry (SCAN, which incorporates the Present State Examination, or PSE) for diagnostically difficult to assess cases.

Rating scales for depression are useful in monitoring severity and response to treatment. The most frequently used interviewer rated tool is the Hamilton Rating Scale for Depression (HAM-D), which has several versions, the 17 and 21 item varieties being in most widespread use. The HAM-D is weighted towards the more biological symptoms of depression, but does include other features. A shorter scale, specifically designed to include those items that are more sensitive to the effects of antidepressant treatment, is the Montgomery–Asberg Depression Rating Scale (MADRS). Other observer rated scales often used include the Bech Melancholia Scale and the Inventory of Depressive Symptoms (IDS), the latter of which is focused on the items of the DSM-IV.

There are also several self-report scales. These have the advantage of being less time consuming for clinicians, but are subject to differing response styles of individual patients. Nevertheless, most have a good cross correlation with the more objective, clinician rated measures. Perhaps the most widely used instrument is the Beck Depressive Inventory. As

might be expected by a scale from Beck, this is heavily weighted towards cognitive features of depression, although it can sometimes pick up longer term difficulties such as low self–esteem as well as more acute changes related to depression. Other widely used scales are the General Health Questionnaire (GHQ) and the Hospital Anxiety and Depression Scale (HADS). The HADS has been designed to be used in those with physical illnesses, while the GHQ is well validated in primary care populations.

Box 19.6   Clinical assessment of depression

Cross-sectional description

Clinical syndrome: features of depressive syndrome

Symptomatic description:
- melancholic (endogenous/biological) features
- psychotic features
- atypical features

Psychiatric comorbidity

Severity: mild, moderate or severe

Behavioural description: retarded, agitated, catatonic

Longitudinal description

Unipolar or bipolar

Degree of recurrence

Seasonal pattern

Responses to treatment in past and present episodes

Aetiological description

Predisposing factors:
- personality
- early life experiences
- family history of depression
- vulnerabilty factors
- chronic social stress

Recent precipitants:
- life-events
- physical illness
- drugs
- childbirth

Perpetuating factors:
- social isolation
- marital relationship
- physical illness
- psychiatric comorbidity
- substance misuse
- ongoing psychosocial stressors
- inactivity and lack of positive events/reinforcement
- adoption of the sick role

Risk Assessment

Suicide

Self-harm

Self-neglect

Harm to others

Thus, choice of scale depends upon the specific purpose required and the time available; however, it is probably true that some degree of objective rating of the effects of treatment is desirable in the management of depression, yet remains rarely implemented by psychiatrists outside of the domains of research.

Differential diagnosis

The main differentials for milder illness are anxiety, dysthymia, OCD or personality disorder. For more severe illnesses, dementing and psychotic illnesses become more important differentials. Organic illness should always be considered in the differential diagnosis.

Normal sadness/bereavement

Normal sadness lacks the other features of the syndrome. Bereavement may have many features of the syndrome, but is regarded as normal unless prolonged (>2 months in DSM-IV) or unusually severe, with features such as profound retardation, suicidal ideas or psychosis. Transient hallucinations of dead person's voice occur normally in about 10% of cases.

Anxiety disorders

It is clear that mild depression shows a large overlap with generalized anxiety disorder. Although in some cases it will be possible to distinguish the two by history (e.g. anxiety only occurring in the setting of a depressive illness) or examination (predominance of one set of symptoms over the other), in many mild cases it is neither practical nor necessary to differentiate between the two; most studies show a good response to antidepressants in both groups. ICD-10 recognized this by including the category of mixed anxiety and depression. Depression is a frequent occurrence in the natural history of agoraphobia, but less so in social and specific phobias.

Obsessive-compulsive disorder

Premorbid obsessional personality traits are a risk factor for depression. Furthermore, obsessional symptoms occur in 20–30% of patients with depression, most of whom do not have premorbid obsessional symptoms. Conversely, 35% of those with obsessive-compulsive disorder will also meet criteria for major depression.

Persistent affective disorders (dysthymia)

The Epidemiological Catchment Area (ECA) study showed that about half of subjects with dysthymia also suffered from recurrent major depression. Dysthymia does not therefore necessarily exclude a past or present diagnosis of depression if the severity criteria are met.

Personality disorder

Although this is a major differential, the presence of a pre-morbid personality disorder does not lessen the likelihood of depression; rather, the opposite is true. Patients with a personality disorder have an increased vulnerability to depression.

Non-affective psychosis

Depressive symptoms are common in schizophrenia. The relative contribution of mood disorder must be determined in anyone presenting with predominantly paranoid features in order not to misdiagnose a psychotic depression. Psychotic features in depression are mood-congruent, i.e. related to themes of punishment, guilt, illness or nihilism. Post-schizophrenic depression is common after the acute psychosis; the best treatment is uncertain at present, but it may respond to antidepressants or antipsychotics.

Organic disorders

Dementia

Depressive pseudodementia may be mild, or severe and difficult to distinguish from organic dementia. Box 19.7 gives the main distinguishing features.

It is likely that there is an overlap in this separation. A large proportion of elderly patients with depression show evidence of cortical atrophy and enlarged ventricles. Thus, even in pseudodementia, there may be a significant organic component; indeed, there is some evidence that patients who develop pseudodementia while depressed have a higher incidence of organic dementia at follow up. If in doubt, the patient should be treated as depressed. A PET study measuring cerebral blood flow showed that depressive pseudodementia showed features distinct from either depression or dementia, namely decreases in the left anterior medial prefrontal cortex and increases in the cerebellar vermis (Dolan et al. 1992).

Others

A variety of medical conditions may be associated with depressive symptoms (see Box 19.8). Similarly, many drugs may produce depressive symptoms (Boxes 19.9 and 19.10). Organic factors must be considered in all cases of depression.

Box 19.7   Distiguishing true and pseudodementia
Illness features that favour a diagnosis of depression or depressive pseudodementia:
<ul><li>rapid onset</li><li>distressed affect</li><li>fluctuating cognitive deficit and patient's complaint of this</li><li>islands of normality, with no dyspraxia or dysphasia</li><li>past or family history of affective disorder</li></ul>
Illness features that favour a diagnosis of dementia:
<ul><li>normal sleep/wake cycle</li><li>no diurnal variation in symptoms</li><li>gradual onset, with prominent memory disturbance, and focal features, such as apraxia, agnosia and dysphasia</li></ul>

Box 19.8   Organic causes of a depressive syndrome

Endocrine: disorders of cortisol, thyroxine or parathormone production; hypopituitarism; hypoglycaemia

Infections: glandular fever, syphilis, AIDS, encephalitis

Neurological: stroke, Parkinson's disease, multiple sclerosis, brain tumours (classically meningioma), trauma, cerebral lupus

Carcinoma: common non-metastatic manifestation, especially pancreatic carcinoma which may otherwise remain occult, and lung carcinoma

Nutritional: deficiencies of folate, nicotinamide (pellagra), vitamins B_{12}, B_1 (thiamine), B_6

Other: cerebral ischaemia, myocardial infarction

Box 19.9   Drugs associated with depressive syndromes

Cardiovascular: methyl-dopa, reserpine, beta-blockers, clonidine, diuretics, digoxin

Endocrine: steroids, oral contraceptive (see text)

Neurological: L-Dopa, bromocriptine

Others: pentazocine, indomethacin, chloroquine, mefloquine

On withdrawal: psychostimulants (e.g. amphetamines, cocaine), benzodiazepines

Alcohol: cause and consequence

Box 19.10   Prevalence of psychiatric side effects of exogenous corticosteroid therapy

Depression	32%
Mania	22%
Mixed affective symptoms	6%
Schizophreniform psychosis/delusional disorder	11%
Delirium	8%

The Royal College of General Practitioners prospective contraception study suggests a small increase in the risk of depression with oestrogen doses greater than 35 micrograms daily (Kay 1984). Kendler's twin study suggested that the tendency to develop depressive symptoms on the oral contraceptive was strongly genetic, but different from the genes controlling baseline susceptibility to depression (Kendler et al. 1988).

MANAGEMENT

General management

The general management of depression must include consideration of the following:

- The need for inpatient or day patient admission:
  - (a) in favour
    - allowing patient and family a breathing space
    - danger of suicide
    - inadequate nutrition and lack of self-care
  - (b) against
    - stigma of hospitalization
    - undermining of ability to cope
    - institutionalization.
- The use of the Mental Health Act.
- Assessment using multidisciplinary team.
- Risk.

Treatments

Pharmacological

Indications, contraindications, side effects, therapeutic effects and drug interactions of the various drugs that may be used in the treatment and prophylaxis of affective disorders are discussed in detail in Chapter 38. The general principles behind drug treatment strategies only are summarized here.

If antidepressant drugs are to be prescribed, the following principles should be observed:

- In view of the risk of overdose, outpatients should be assessed frequently and short supplies of drugs prescribed. Most tricyclic antidepressants are dangerous in overdose, and newer drugs may be preferred where there is concern.
- Patients (and their relatives) should be warned about the delay in treatment response, otherwise they may stop the treatment as ineffective.
- The nature and duration of likely side-effects should be described to aid adherence to treatment as well as to keep patients well-informed. Some patients may prefer some potential side-effect profiles to others. Also, if sedative drugs are to be used, the effects on driving and the sedative interaction with alcohol should be explained. Some measures show amitriptyline to be as cognitively impairing as alcohol above the legal limit.
- The non-addictive nature of antidepressants should be stressed, as patients will frequently harbour a fear of addiction and subsequently not comply.
- Elderly patients may be more prone to develop problematic side-effects on older tricyclics, especially anticholinergic and hypotensive effects, and thus SSRIs or newer agents may be preferred.
- Medically ill: many antidepressants are contra-indicated in heart disease, epilepsy, etc. Also, most SSRIs inhibit some of the cytochrome P450 liver enzymes and may interact with many liver metabolized drugs.
- Occupation: patients who operate machinery or drive should not be given sedative drugs.
- Agitated depression: anxiety or agitation within depression responds to antidepressant treatment. It is not necessary routinely to give sedative drugs in most cases as sedative and anxiolytic effects are pharmacologically distinct.

- Pregnancy: if drugs are necessary, older tricyclics are preferred as there is more experience of their use, although more data and experience is also now emerging with SSRIs.

Physical

Electroconvulsive therapy

ECT is discussed in detail in Chapter 39. Patients with severe depression in whom a rapid response is needed, such as life-threatening states (dehydration, physical complications, stupor or suicidal behaviour) or postpartum, should be considered early for ECT. Otherwise, ECT is reserved for patients resistant to other treatments. Unlike anti-depressants, ECT causes upregulation of postsynaptic $5HT_2$ receptors. Other effects (e.g. normalization of the reduced prolactin response to fenfluramine) are the same. ECT is clearly efficacious for the short term treatment of depression (Geddes 2003). However, the caveats to ECT use include a number of contraindications, side-effects, patient accepta-bility and the tendency to relapse.

Sleep deprivation

Deprivation of sleep, and particular REM sleep, is associated with substantial improvement in mood, although it is not usually a sustained response. Nevertheless, a positive response to sleep deprivation is predictive of future response to other somatic treatments.

Transcranial magnetic stimulation

Transcranial magnetic stimulation uses a strong and rapidly changing magnetic field to stimulate electrical activity in neurons. Early results suggest that it is effective compared to a sham procedure, and induces neurochemical changes similar to ECT, but its role in resistant cases of depression remains unproven.

Vagus nerve stimulation

Vagus nerve stimulation involves surgically attaching an electrode to the vagus nerve in the neck in order to stimulate afferent pathways into the brain. Primarily used as a treatment for refractory epilepsy, it may have some antidepressant properties in resistant cases.

Light therapy

Bright light has been shown to be effective in several placebo-controlled studies of seasonal depression. Morning light is more effective than evening light, and leads to a phase advance of the sleep–wake cycle and dim-light melatonin onset. The exact treatment protocols differ, but those found to be effective include 1.5 hours per day of 6000 lux bright light starting at 6.00 a.m. There is evidence that serotonergic mechanisms may be important in the effectiveness of light treatment (Lam et al. 1996). What remains unclear is the selection of which patients will respond, the regimens which are consistently most effective and the effect size of the treatment in comparison with other potential treatments.

Exercise

Aerobic exercise has beneficial effects on mood, and has been shown in at least one RCT to be of benefit in treating depression.

Neurosurgery

Neurosurgery for mental disorders (NMD, formerly psychosurgery), is described in detail in Chapter 39. This is rarely used, but can be performed for cases of severe, intractable depression using strict controls under the Mental Health Act, including fully informed consent and a second opinion. There are several techniques, including the use of diathermy and radioactive iridium implants in operations such as subcaudate tractotomy. Approximately one-third of patients are reported to gain marked benefit, one-third mild benefit and one-third no benefit. Side-effects can include personality changes of a frontal lobe nature and epilepsy.

Psychological

Behavioural therapy

Behavioural treatments such as problem-solving techniques are effective in mild depression, and supported by several RCTs. Techniques such as behavioural activation and occupational therapy can be very useful adjuncts to treatment, although without clear clinical trial support.

Cognitive therapy

Cognitive therapy aims to alter the disturbed cognitions discussed above. Trials in outpatients have shown it to be as effective for mild to moderate depression in the short-term as antidepressants. Other studies have suggested it may reduce relapse (Blackburn & Moore 1997). Brief versions of cognitive therapy may be effective in primary care (Scott et al. 1997) and postnatally (Appleby et al. 1997).

Psychotherapy

Supportive psychotherapy should be part of the treatment of all depressed patients, with the following aims:

- empathic, supporting relationship
- ventilation of distress
- education about nature of disorder
- general semi-directive counselling.

Brief focused therapies such as described by Malan (1976) may be useful. Dynamic psychotherapy is not a treatment for acute depression, but may help selected patients subject to recurrent depression modify some predisposing factors and develop insight into preventing certain precipitating factors.

Interpersonal therapy

Depression is viewed as a disorder of interpersonal relationships, regardless of aetiology. Therapy aims at symptom relief and a more effective approach to relationships. Reduced frequency therapy is an effective prophylaxis to reduce relapse. There is some evidence that IPT may be effective on a group basis.

Couple therapy

Couple therapy has been shown to be a useful and effective therapy for depression where there is a degree of discord within the relationship, or where aspects of the relationship are felt to be a maintaining factor in a depressive illness.

Social

Effective treatment of depression requires close attention to social factors. Patients may benefit from advice on, or help with, changing adverse social situations such as financial, housing and employment difficulties. Family relationships may need attention and, if indicated, specific family therapy. The meaning of a social situation may be modified by cognitive therapy.

Relative efficacy of treatments

The relative efficacy of treatments is under-researched or suffers from the use of underpowered trials. There is no convincing evidence that any antidepressant or class of antidepressants is more effective than another, although there have been recent meta-analyses suggesting a slightly increased rate of response or remission for the dual 5HT and noradrenergic drugs amitriptyline (Barbui & Hotopf 2001) and venlafaxine (Smith et al. 2002).

A systematic review of RCTS, mostly in secondary care, suggests that cognitive therapy is at least as effective as antidepressant therapy (and behavioural therapies) in mild to moderate depression (Gloaguen et al. 1998). There was also evidence that cognitive therapy was superior to non-directive therapy. The NIMH trial found no clear difference in efficacy between interpersonal psychotherapy and cognitive therapy, although later analyses suggested that there was overlap in the therapies actually received in that study. Several RCTs in primary care suggest that problem solving therapy is as effective as drugs. Evidence regarding the efficacy of nondirective counselling remains poor (Churchill et al. 1999). The combination of antidepressants and cognitive therapy or interpersonal therapy affords a slight benefit over either alone, particularly in more severely ill patients (Thase et al. 1997). A large RCT of a combination of an antidepressant and a form of cognitive therapy in chronic depression (mean duration eight years) showed clear benefits over either therapy alone, in terms both of symptoms and of function (Keller et al. 2000).

Some studies have looked at ways of improving the effectiveness in practice of the various therapies, and have shown that it is possible to improve outcome through means of standardized care pathways (including factors such as improved patient education, telephone follow up and support to the primary care physician).

Illness phase

Treatment of depression is usually thought of as consisting of three overlapping phases:

1. Acute treatment, in which symptoms are alleviated.
2. Continuation treatment, which seeks to prevent relapse of the current episode.
3. Maintenance treatment, which seeks to prevent recurrence of a new episode.

Because of the associated disability, and the higher rates of relapse, current practice is to attempt to treat to remission (e.g. a HAM-D of 7 or less).

Many studies have now demonstrated the necessity for adequate continuation treatment with antidepressants in order to prevent early relapse rates of up to 50%. Current recommendations are for a period of treatment of at least 4–6 months after resolution of the depression, which reduces this early relapse by at least half. A recent systematic review found that continuation treatment after acute response with antidepressants reduced the odds of relapse by 70% (Geddes et al. 2003). The two-thirds reduction in risk of depressive relapse seemed to be largely independent of the underlying risk of relapse, the duration of treatment before randomization, or the duration of the randomly allocated therapy. There did not appear to be a cut-off point for this effect to wear off, and thus continuation therapy merged into maintenance/prophylactic therapy.

Recurrent unipolar depression where there have been three or more episodes, or where episodes have been particularly treatment-resistant or disabling should be considered for long term prophylactic treatment. The issue of full versus reduced dose has not been resolved, though most placebo-controlled evidence for efficacy comes from studies employing full doses of SSRIs or tricyclics.

Other treatment considerations

Treatment-resistant depression

Box 19.11 shows the common causes of treatment resistance. Strategies in treatment resistance are:

- Check for any of the relevant causes and take appropriate action. Compliance can be assessed by asking the patient or an informant, or checking plasma drug levels.
- Pharmacological strategies:
  (a) increase dose
  (b) switch between classes of drug (e.g. tricyclic, SSRI, SSNRI, MAOI)

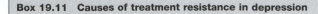

Box 19.11 Causes of treatment resistance in depression

Non-compliance

Inadequate dosage (consider if fast metabolizer of drug)

Insufficient time

Wrong diagnosis (including missed physical illness)

Unaddressed psychiatric comorbidity

Drug interactions

Inadequate account taken of social, family and personal factors

    (c) add lithium (usually has a rapid effect if effective)

    (d) add liothyronine

    (e) other augmentation (e.g. L-tryptophan, olanzapine)

    (f) combination antidepressants (e.g. tricyclic/MAOI).

- Psychological treatments.
- Address modifiable social perpetuating factors (e.g. couple therapy if poor relationship).
- ECT.
- Psychosurgery.

The available treatment options are listed more fully elsewhere (Taylor et al. 2003).

Psychotic depression

The response to tricyclic antidepressants alone in patients with psychotic depression is poorer than in patients with non-psychotic major depression; one meta-analysis found rates to be 35% and 67% respectively (Chan et al. 1987). It is now well-established that the response of psychotic depression to a combination of a typical antipsychotic and a tricyclic antidepressant is superior to either alone, although there are fewer studies of newer antidepressants and atypical antipsychotics (Wheeler Vega et al. 2000). Psychotic depression is an indication for ECT, which is at least as effective as combined antidepressant/antipsychotic therapy (Parker et al. 1992) and may be more effective in psychotic than non-psychotic depression (Petrides et al. 2001).

Residual symptoms of depression

Residual symptoms of depression are common. The presence of residual symptoms predicts early relapse, one study finding rates of early relapse to be 76% in those with residual symptoms and 25% in those without (Paykel et al. 1995), and may herald the beginning of a more severe, relapsing, and chronic future course, even after the first lifetime episode (Judd et al. 2000). For this reason, treatment of depression to remission is preferred.

Cognitive therapy targeted at residual symptoms may be a useful adjunct to modify this high risk of relapse (Paykel et al. 1999). In one study 158 patients with residual symptoms were randomized to receive either routine clinical management or clinical management plus 16 sessions of cognitive therapy over 20 weeks plus two booster sessions. The cumulative relapse rate over 68 weeks was 47% in those receiving clinical management but 29% in those who had cognitive therapy. The mechanism does not seem to be in a marked reduction in depressive symptoms, but rather in improving patients's coping mechanisms to avoid relapse.

Predictors of treatment response

There are no clear predictors of treatment response, most studies claiming to have found such markers not being replicated. However, it is believed that dexamethasone non-suppression and/or shortened REM latency may be associated with response to physical rather than psychological treatments (Thase et al. 1993, 1996). Several studies show that low urinary 3-methoxy-4-hydroxyphenylglycol or MHPG predict response to tricyclic antidepressants, but variability is high, limiting clinical utility (Schatzberg & Schildkraut 1995). Patients with biological features of depression are said to respond more readily to antidepressants than those without.

Biological effects of antidepressant treatment

There are various demonstrations that antidepressants:

- downregulate $5HT_2$ receptors
- up-regulate $5HT_{1A}$ receptors
- downregulate beta adrenergic receptors and presynaptic alpha-2 autoreceptors
- have no effect on clonidine/GH response.

Neuroimaging has been used to investigate brain function during treatment of depression with either psychological therapy or drug therapy. Resting brain glucose metabolism after 12 weeks of treatment with either interpersonal therapy or paroxetine showed similar changes, despite the paroxetine-treated subjects having a greater decrease in depression scores (Brody et al. 2001). Resting brain blood-flow measured before and after six weeks' treatment with either venlafaxine or interpersonal therapy showed a differential change; both treatments caused basal ganglia activation whereas only interpersonal therapy showed limbic blood-flow increase.

OUTCOME AND PROGNOSIS

Data from the original 18-year follow-up study by Lee and Murray (Lee & Murray 1988) showed that psychotic depression responded better in the short term, but worse in the long term with a 75% readmission rate and the majority suffering severe, long-term handicap. In all, 10% of patients with an initial diagnosis of unipolar depression were rediagnosed as suffering with bipolar depression and the suicide rate was 10%. Recovery from melancholic depression (26 weeks) takes longer than other depression (16 weeks).

A meta-analysis of all the older outcome studies of depression (Piccinelli & Wilkinson 1994) showed:

- 50% recover in 6 months
- 25% relapse in 1 year
- 75% relapse in 10 years
- 10% have persistent unresponsive depression.

A more recent 10-year prospective follow-up of major depression found that the diagnosis remained stable in 91% of patients with 6% suffering an episode of mania and 3% developing schizoaffective disorder (Solomon et al. 1997). Between 88% and 92% of subjects recovered at some time, with virtually identical survival curves following recovery from the first five recurrent mood episodes in the 10-year period. The median duration of illness varied from 22 weeks for the first episode to 19 weeks for the fifth episode. There was no difference in rates of recovery or speed of recovery between those with a first-ever onset of depression compared to those with prior episodes of depression. Prospectively, during the first year after onset, approximately 75% of patients recovered. Of those that entered a second year, 38% then recovered. Of those that entered a third year, 27% recovered and of those that entered a fourth year, 16% recovered. Thus, the longer each episode carries on without remission the less likely subsequent recovery will be.

Effect on physical illness

Depression can have a significant effect on the prognosis of concurrent physical illness. All cause mortality (excluding suicide) is raised approximately two-fold or more in depression (Zheng et al. 1997). Specifically, mortality following a myocardial infarction is increased approximately four-fold if a patient suffers from depression during 18 month follow up period (Frasure Smith et al. 1995). Women with recurrent depression (and hence recurrent hypercortisolaemia) have lower bone densities and higher rates of osteoporosis (Michelson et al 1996). Diabetic patients with depression show worse glycaemic control and diabetic complications such as retinopathy (Beardsley & Goldstein 1993). Attempts to modify these increased risks have been less successful than demonstrating that they exist.

REFERENCES

Alexopoulos, GS, Meyers, BS, Young RC et al. (1996) Recovery in geriatric depression. *Archives of General Psychiatry* **53**: 305–12.

Altshuler LL, Bauer M, Frye MA et al. (2001) Does thyroid supplementation accelerate tricyclic antidepressant response? A review and meta-analysis of the literature. *American Journal of Psychiatry* **158**: 1617–22.

American Psychiatric Association (1994) *Diagnostic and Statistical Manual of Mental Disorders*, 4th edition. Washington, DC: APA.

Appleby L, Warner R, Whitton A et al. (1997) A controlled study of fluoxetine and cognitive-behavioural counselling in the treatment of postnatal depression. *British Medical Journal* **314**: 932–6.

Asnis GM, McGinn LK & Sanderson WC (1995) Atypical depression: clinical aspects and noradrenergic function. *American Journal of Psychiatry* **152**: 31–6.

Barbui C & Hotopf M (2001) Amitriptyline v. the rest: still the leading antidepressant after 40 years of randomised controlled trials. *British Journal of Psychiatry* **178**: 129–44.

Beardsley G & Goldstein MG (1993) Psychological factors affecting physical condition. Endocrine disease literature review. *Psychosomatics* **34**: 12–19.

Bebbington PE (1998) Sex and depression. *Psychological Medicine* **28**: 1–8.

Beck A (1967) *Depression: Clinical, Theoretical and Experimental Aspects.* Philadelphia: University of Pennsylvania Press.

Belanoff JK, Kalehzan M, Sund B et al. (2001) Cortisol activity and cognitive changes in psychotic major depression. *American Journal of Psychiatry* **158**: 1612–16.

Bench CJ, Friston KJ, Brown RG et al. (1993) Regional cerebral blood flow in depression measured by positron emission tomography: the relationship with clinical dimensions. *Psychological Medicine* **23**: 579–90.

Benkelfat C, Ellenbogen MA, Dean P et al. (1994) Mood-lowering effect of tryptophan depletion. Enhanced susceptibility in young men at genetic risk for major affective disorders. *Archives of General Psychiatry* **51**: 687–97.

Blackburn IM & Moore RG (1997) Controlled acute and follow-up trial of cognitive therapy and pharmacotherapy in out-patients with recurrent depression. *British Journal of Psychiatry* **171**: 328–34.

Blazer D, Kessler R & Swartz M (1998) Epidemiology of recurrent major and minor depression with a seasonal pattern. The National Comorbidity Survey. *British Journal of Psychiatry* **172**: 164–7.

Blier P, Galsin A-M & Langer SZ (1990) Interaction between serotonin uptake inhibitors and alpha-2 adrenergic heteroceptors in the rat hypothalamus. *Journal of Pharmacology and Experimental Therapeutics* **254**: 236–54.

Bloch M, Schmidt PJ, Danaceau MA, Adams LF & Rubinow DR (1999) Dehydroepiandrosterone treatment in mid-life dysthymia. *Biological Psychiatry* **45**: 1533–41.

Bowlby J (1980) *Attachment and Loss*, volume 3. *Loss Sadness and Depression*. New York: Basic Books.

Bremner JD, Innis RB, Salomen RM et al. (1997) Positron emission tomography measurement of cerebral metabolic correlates of tryptophan depletion-induced relapse. *Archives of General Psychiatry* **54**: 364–74.

Bremner JD, Vythilingam M, Ng CK et al. (2003) Regional brain metabolic correlates of a-methylparatyrosine-induced depressive symptoms: implications for the neural circuitry of depression. *Journal of the American Medical Association* **289**: 3125–34.

Brody AL, Saxena S, Stoessel P et al. (2001) Regional brain metabolic changes in patients with major depression treated with either paroxetine or interpersonal therapy: preliminary findings. *Archives of General Psychiatry* **58**: 631–40.

Brown G & Harris T (1978) *The Social Origins of Depression*. London: Tavistock.

Brown GW, Harris TO & Peto J (1973) Life events and psychiatric disorders: the nature of the causal link. *Psychological Medicine* **11**: 159–76.

Burt DB, Zembar MJ & Niederehe G (1995) Depression and memory impairment: a meta-analysis of the association, its pattern, and specificity. *Psychological Bulletin* **117**: 285–305.

Chan CH, Janicak PG, Davis JM et al. (1987) Response of psychotic and nonpsychotic depressed patients to tricyclic antidepressants. *Journal of Clinical Psychiatry* **48**: 197–200.

Checkley S (1996) The neuroendocrinology of depression and chronic stress. *British Medical Bulletin* **52**: 597–617.

Checkley SA, Slade AP & Shur P (1981) Growth hormone and other responses to clonidine in patients with endogenous depression. *British Journal of Psychiatry* **138**: 51–5.

Churchill R, Dewey M, Gretton V et al. (1999) Should general practitioners refer patients with major depression to counsellors? A review of current published evidence. Nottingham Counselling and Antidepressants in Primary Care (CAPC) Study Group. *British Journal of General Practice* **49**: 738–43.

Coppen A (1967) The biochemistry of affective disorders. *British Journal of Psychiatry* **113**: 1237–64.

Coryell W & Shlesser M (2001) The dexamethasone suppression test in suicide prediction. *American Journal of Psychiatry* **158**: 748–53.

Crimlisk HL, Bhatia K, Cope H et al. (1998) Slater revisited: 6 year follow up study of patients with medically unexplained motor symptoms. *British Medical Journal* **316**: 582–6.

De Bellis M, Chrousos G, Dorn L et al. (1994) Hypothalamic-pituitary-adrenal axis dysregulation in sexually abused girls. *Journal of Clinical Endocrinology and Metabolism* **78**: 249–55.

de Groot JC, de Leeuw F-E, Oudkerk M et al. (2000) Cerebral white matter lesions and depressive symptoms in elderly adults. *Archives of General Psychiatry* **57**: 1071–6.

Delgado PL, Miller HL, Salomon RM et al. (1993) Monoamines and the mechanism of antidepressant action: effects of catecholamine depletion on mood of patients treated with antidepressants. *Psychopharmacology Bulletin* **29**: 389–96.

Delgado PL, Miller HL, Salomon RM, Licinio J, Krystal JH, Moreno FA, Heninger GR, Charney DS (1999) Tryptophan-depletion challenge in depressed patients treated with desipramine or fluoxetine: implications for the role of serotonin in the mechanism of antidepressant action. *Biological Psychiatry* **46**: 212–20.

Delgado PL, Price LH, Miller HL et al. (1994) Serotonin and the neurobiology of depression. Effects of tryptophan depletion in drug-free depressed patients. *Archives of General Psychiatry* **51**: 865–74.

Dolan RJ, Bench CJ, Brown RG et al. (1992) Regional cerebral blood flow abnormalities in depressed patients with cognitive impairment. *Journal of Neurology Neurosurgery and Psychiatry* **55**: 768–73.

Dorn LD, Burgess ES, Dubbert B et al. (1995) Psychopathology in patients with endogenous Cushing's syndrome: 'atypical' or melancholic features. *Clinical Endocrinology* **43**: 433–42.

Drevets WC (2001) Neuroimaging and neuropathological studies of depression: implications for the cognitive-emotional features of mood disorders. *Current Opinion in Neurobiology* **11**: 240–9.

Drevets WC, Frank E, Price JC et al. (1999) PET imaging of serotonin 1A receptor binding in depression. *Biological Psychiatry* **46**: 1375–87.

Duman RS, Heninger GR & Nestler EJ (1997) A molecular and cellular theory of depression. *Archives of General Psychiatry* **54**: 597–606.

Eaton WW, Anthony JC, Gallo J et al. (1997) Natural history of Diagnostic Interview Schedule/DSM-IV major depression. The Baltimore Epidemiologic Catchment Area follow-up. *Archives of General Psychiatry* **54**: 993–9.

Ellenbogen MA, Young SN, Dean P et al. (1996) Mood response to acute tryptophan depletion in healthy volunteers: sex differences and temporal stability. *Neuropsychopharmacology* **15**: 465–74.

Elliott R, Baker SC, Rogers RD et al. (1997) Prefrontal dysfunction in depressed patients performing a complex planning task: a study using positron emission tomography. *Psychological Medicine* **27**: 931–42.

Elliott R, Rubinsztein JS, Sahakian BJ et al. (2002) The neural basis of mood-congruent processing biases in depression. *Archives of General Psychiatry* **59**: 597–604.

Engleman EA, Perry KW, Mayle DA et al. (1995) Simultaneous increases in extracellular monoamines in microdialysates from hypothalamus of conscious rates by duloxetine, a dual serotonin and norepinephrine uptake inhibitor. *Neuropsychopharmacology* **12**: 287–96.

Frasure Smith N, Lesperance F & Talajic M. (1995) Depression and 18–month prognosis after myocardial infarction. *Circulation* **91**: 999–1005.

Fu CH & McGuire PK (1999) Functional neuroimaging in psychiatry. *Philosophical Transactions of the Royal Society of London – Series B: Biological Sciences* **354**: 1359–70.

Fu CH, Reed LJ, Meyer JH, Kennedy S, Houle S, Eisfeld BS, Brown GM (2001) Noradrenergic dysfunction in the prefrontal cortex in depression: an [15O] H2O PET study of the neuromodulatory effects of clonidine. *Biological Psychiatry* **49**: 317–25.

Geddes J (2003) Efficacy and safety of electroconvulsive therapy in depressive disorders: a systematic review and meta-analysis. *Lancet* **361**: 799–808.

Geddes JR, Carney SM, Davies C et al. (2003) Relapse prevention with antidepressant drug treatment in depressive disorders: a systematic review. *Lancet* **361**: 653–61.

George MS, Ketter TA, Parekh PI et al. (1997) Blunted left cingulate activation in mood disorder subjects during a response interference task (the Stroop). *Journal of Neuropsychiatry and Clinical Neurosciences* **9**: 55–63.

Gloaguen V, Cottraux J, Cucherat M et al. (1998) A meta-analysis of the effects of cognitive therapy in depressed patients. *Journal of Affective Disorders* **49**: 59–72.

Gold PW, Licinio J, Wong ML et al. (1995) Corticotropin releasing hormone in the pathophysiology of melancholic and atypical depression and in the mechanism of action of antidepressant drugs. *Annals of the New York Academy of Sciences* **771**: 716–29.

Harris B, Othman S, Davies JA, Weppner GJ, Richards CJ, Newcombe RG, Lazarus JH, Parkes AB, Hall R, Phillips DI (1992) Association between postpartum thyroid dysfunction and thyroid antibodies and depression. *British Medical Jounral* **305**: 152–6.

Heim C, Newport DJ, Heit S et al. (2000) Pituitary-adrenal and autonomic responses to stress in women after sexual and physical abuse in childhood. *Journal of the American Medical Association* **284**: 592–7.

Henderson S, Byrne DG & Duncan-Jones P (1982) *Neurosis and the Social Environment*. London: Academic Press.

Heuser I, Yassouridis A & Holsboer F (1994) The combined dexamethasone/CRH test: a refined laboratory test for psychiatric disorders. *Journal of Psychiatric Research* **28**: 341–56.

Hotopf M, Carr S, Mayou R et al. (1998) Why do children have chronic abdominal pain, and what happens to them when they grow up? *British Medical Journal* **316**: 1196–9.

Howland RH (1993) Thyroid dysfunction in refractory depression: implications for pathophysiology and treatment. *Journal of Clinical Psychiatry* **54**: 47–54.

Jacoby RJ & Levy R (1980) Computerised tomography in the elderly 3: affective disorder. *British Journal of Psychiatry* **136**: 270–5.

Janowsky DS & Overstreet DH (1995) The role of acetylcholine mechanisms in mood disorders. In: Kupfer DJ & Bloom FE (eds) *Psychopharmacology: The Fourth Generation of Progress*, pp. 945–956. New York: Raven Press.

Joffe R & Marriott M (2000) Thyroid hormone levels in recurrence of major depression. *American Journal of Psychiatry* **157**: 1689–91.

Judd LL, Paulus MJ, Schettler PJ et al. (2000) Does incomplete recovery from first lifetime major depressive episode herald a chronic course of illness? *American Journal of Psychiatry* **157**: 1501–4.

Kay CR (1984) The Royal College of General Practitioners' Oral Contraception Study: some recent observations. *Clinical and Obstetric Gynaecology* **11**: 759–86.

Keller MB, McCullough JP, Klein DN et al. (2000) A comparison of nefazodone, the cognitive behavioral-analysis system of psychotherapy, and their combination for the treatment of chronic depression. *New England Journal of Medicine* **342**: 1462–70.

Kendell RE (1976) The classification of depressions: a review of contemporary confusion. *British Journal of Psychiatry* **129**: 15–28.

Kendler KS (1997) The diagnostic validity of melancholic major depression in a population-based sample of female twins. *Archives of General Psychiatry* **54**: 299–304.

Kendler KS, Eaves LJ, Walters EE et al. (1996) The identification and validation of distinct depressive syndromes in a population-based sample of female twins. *Archives of General Psychiatry* 53: 391–399.

Kendler KS, Hettema JM, Butera F, Gardner CO & Prescott CA (2003) Life event dimensions of loss, humiliation, entrapment, and danger in the prediction of onsets of major depression and generalized anxiety. *Archives of General Psychiatry* **60**: 789–96.

Kendler KS & Gardner CO (1998) Boundaries of major depression: an evaluation of DSM-IV criteria. *American Journal of Psychiatry* **155**: 172–7.

Kendler KS & Karkowski Shuman L (1997) Stressful life events and genetic liability to major depression: genetic control of exposure to the environment? *Psychological Medicine* **27**: 539–47.

Kendler KS, Kessler RC, Walters EE et al. (1995) Stressful life events, genetic liability, and onset of an episode of major depression in women. *American Journal of Psychiatry* **152**: 833–42.

Kendler KS, Martin NG, Heath AC et al. (1988) A twin study of the psychiatric side effects of oral contraceptives. *Journal of Nervous and Mental Disease* **176**: 153–60.

Kendler KS, Thornton LM & Gardner CO (2000) Stressful life events and previous episodes in the etiology of major depression in women: an evaluation of the 'kindling' hypothesis. *American Journal of Psychiatry* **157**: 1243–51.

Kendler KS, Thornton LM & Gardner CO (2001) Genetic risk, number of previous depressive episodes, and stressful life events in predicting onset of major depression. *American Journal of Psychiatry*

158: 582–6.

Kessler RC, Berglund P, Demler O et al. (2003) The epidemiology of major depressive disorder: results from the National Comorbidity Survey Replication (NCS-R). *Journal of the American Medical Association* 289: 3095–105.

Kessler RC, McGonagle KA, Zhao S et al. (1994) Lifetime and 12-month prevalence of DSM-III-R psychiatric disorders in the United States. Results from the National Comorbidity Survey. *Archives of General Psychiatry* 51: 8–19.

Klaassen T, Riedel WJ, van Someren A, Deutz NEP, Honig A & van Praag HM (1999) Mood effects of 24-hour tryptophan depletion in healthy first-degree relatives of patients with affective disorders. *Biological Psychiatry* 46: 489–97.

Lam RW, Zis AP, Grewal A, Delgado PL, Charney DS & Krystal JH (1996) Effects of rapid tryptophan depletion in patients with seasonal affective disorder in remission after light therapy. *Archives of General Psychiatry* 53: 41–4.

Lambert G, Johansson M, Ågren H et al. (2000) Reduced brain norepinephrine and dopamine release in treatment-refractory depressive illness: evidence in support of the catecholamine hypothesis of mood disorders. *Archives of General Psychiatry* 57: 787–93.

Lee AS & Murray RM (1988) The long-term outcome of Maudsley depressives. *British Journal of Psychiatry* 153: 741–51.

Lewinsohn PM, Weinstein MS & Alpere TA (1970) A behavioural approach to the group treatment of depressed persons: a methodological contribution. *Journal of Clinical Psychology* 26: 525–32.

Maes M & Meltzer H (1995) The serotonin hypothesis of major depression. In: Bloom FE & Kupfer DJ (eds) *Psychopharmacology. Fourth generation of Progress*, pp. 933–944. New York: Raven Press.

Malan D (1976) *The Frontier of Brief Psychotherapy*. New York: Plenum Medical.

Manji HK, Drevets WC & Charney DS (2001) The cellular neurobiology of depression. *Nature Medicine* 7: 541–7.

Mann JJ, Malone KM, Diehl DJ et al. (1996) Demonstration in vivo of reduced serotonin responsivity in the brain of untreated depressed patients. *American Journal of Psychiatry* 153: 174–82.

Mayberg HS, Brannan SK, Tekell JL et al. (2000) Regional metabolic effects of fluoxetine in major depression: serial changes and relationship to clinical response. *Biological Psychiatry* 48: 830–43.

Mayberg HS, Liotti M, Brannan SK et al. (1999) Reciprocal limbic-cortical function and negative mood: converging PET findings in depression and normal sadness. *American Journal of Psychiatry* 156: 675–82.

McGuffin P, Katz R & Rutherford J (1991) Nature, nurture and depression: a twin study. *Psychological Medicine* 21: 329–35.

McGuffin P, Katz R, Watkins S et al. (1996) A hospital-based twin register of the heritability of DSM-IV unipolar depression. *Archives of General Psychiatry* 53: 129–36.

Mendlewicz J & Rainer JD (1977) Adoption study supporting genetic transmission in manic–depressive illness. *Nature* 268: 327–9.

Meyer JH, Kennedy S & Brown GM (1998) No effect of depression on [(15)O]H2O PET response to intravenous d-fenfluramine. *American Journal of Psychiatry* 155: 1241–6.

Michelson D, Stratakis C, Hill L et al. (1996) Bone mineral density in women with depression. *New England Journal of Medicine* 335: 1176–81.

Moghaddan B & Bunney BS (1990) Acute effects of typical and atypical antipsychotic drugs on the release of dopamine from prefrontal cortex, nucleus accumbens, and striatum of the rat: an in vivo microdialysis study. *Journal of Neurochemistry* 54: 1755–60.

Moreno FA, Heninger GR, McGahueya CA et al. (2000) Tryptophan depletion and risk of depression relapse: a prospective study of tryptophan depletion as a potential predictor of depressive episodes. *Biological Psychiatry* 48: 327–9.

Murphy BE (1997) Antiglucocorticoid therapies in major depression: a review. *Psychoneuroendocrinology* 22: S125–132.

Murray-Parkes C (1998) Coping with loss: bereavement in adult life. *British Medical Journal* 316: 856–9.

Musselman DL, Lawson DH, Gumnick JF et al. (2001) Paroxetine for the prevention of depression induced by high-dose interferon alfa. *New England Journal of Medicine* 344: 961–6.

Nemeroff C (1996) The corticotropin-releasing factor (CRF) hypothesis of depression: new findings and new directions. *Molecular Psychiatry* 1: 336–42.

Nemeroff CB, Simon JS, Haggerty JJ & Evans DL (1985) Antithyroid antibodies in depressed patients. *American Journal of Psychiatry* 150: 1728–30.

O'Flynn K & Dinan TG (1993) Baclofen-induced growth hormone release in major depression: relationship to dexamethasone suppression test result. *American Journal of Psychiatry* 150: 1728–30.

Owens MJ & Nemeroff CB (1994) Role of serotonin in the pathophysiology of depression: focus on the serotonin transporter. *Clinical Chemistry* 40: 288–95.

Parker G, Roy K, Hadzi-Pavlovic D et al. (1992) Psychotic (delusional) depression: a meta-analysis of physical treatments. *Journal of Affective Disorders* 24: 17–24.

Paykel ES (1971) Classification of depressed patients: a cluster analysis derived grouping. *British Journal of Psychiatry* 118: 275–88.

Paykel ES (1978) Contribution of life events to causation of psychiatric illness. *Psychological Medicine* 8: 245–53.

Paykel ES, Ramana R, Cooper Z et al. (1995) Residual symptoms after partial remission: an important outcome in depression. *Psychological Medicine* 25: 1171–80.

Paykel ES, Scott J, Teasdale JD et al. (1999) Prevention of relapse in residual depression by cognitive therapy: a controlled trial. *Archives of General Psychiatry* 56: 829–35.

Petrides G, Fink M, Husain MM et al. (2001) ECT remission rates in psychotic versus nonpsychotic depressed patients: a report from CORE. *Journal of ECT* 17: 244–53.

Piccinelli M & Wilkinson G (1994) Outcome of depression in psychiatric settings. *British Journal of Psychiatry* 164: 297–304.

Post RM (1992) Transduction of psychosocial stress into the neurobiology of recurrent affective disorder. *American Journal of Psychiatry* 149: 999–1010.

Price J (1968) The genetics of depressive behaviour. In: Coppen A & Walk S (eds) *Recent Developments in Affective Disorders*. British Journal of Psychiatry special publications number 2.

Sargent PA, Kjaer KH, Bench CJ et al. (2000) Brain serotonin1A receptor binding measured by positron emission tomography with [11C]WAY-100635: effects of depression and antidepressant treatment. *Archives of General Psychiatry* 57: 174–80.

Schatzberg AF, Garlow SJ & Nemeroff CB (2002) Molecular and cellular mechanisms in depression. In: Davis KL, Charney D, Coyle JT et al. (eds) *Neuropsychopharmacology. The Fifth Generation of Progress*, pp. 1039–50. Philadelphia: Lipincott Williams & Wilkins.

Schatzberg AF & Schildkraut JJ (1995) Recent studies on norepinephrine systems in mood disorders. In: Bloom FE & Kupfer DJ (eds) *Psychopharmacology. Fourth Generation of Progress*, pp. 911–20. New York: Raven Press.

Scott C, Tacchi MJ, Jones R et al. (1997) Acute and one-year outcome of a randomised controlled trial of brief cognitive therapy for major depressive disorder in primary care. *British Journal of Psychiatry* 171: 131–34.

Seligman MEP (1975) *Helplessness: On Depression, Development and Death*. San Francisco, CA: Freeman

Sheline YI & Mintun MA (2002) Structural and functional imaging of affective disorders. In: Davis KL, Charney D, Coyle JT et al. (eds) *Neuropsychopharmacology. The Fifth Generation of Progress*, pp. 1065–80. Philadelphia: Lipincott Williams & Wilkins.

Siever LJ (1987) Role of noradrenergic mechanisms in the etiology of the affective disorders. In: Meltzer HY (ed.) *Psychopharmacology: The Third Generation of Progress*. New York: Raven Press.

Siever LJ, Trestman RL & Coccaro EF (1992) The growth hormone response to clonidine in acute and remitted depressed male patients. *Neuropsychpharmacology* 6: 165–77.

Smith D, Dempster C, Glanville J et al. (2002) Efficacy and tolerability of venlafaxine compared with selective serotonin reuptake inhibitors and other antidepressants: a meta-analysis. *British Journal of Psychiatry* 180: 396–404.

Smith KA, Fairburn CG & Cowen PJ (1997) Relapse of depression after rapid depletion of tryptophan. *Lancet* 349: 915–19.

Smith KA, Morris JS, Friston KJ et al. (1999) Brain mechanisms associated with depressive relapse and associated cognitive impairment following acute tryptophan depletion. *British Journal of Psychiatry* 174: 525–9.

Solomon DA, Keller MB, Leon AC et al. (1997) Recovery from major depression. *Archives of General Psychiatry* **54**: 1001–6.

Sullivan PF, Kessler RC & Kendler KS (1998) Latent class analysis of lifetime depressive symptoms in the national comorbidity survey. *American Journal of Psychiatry* **155**: 1398–406.

Taylor D, Paton C & Kerwin RW (2003) *The South London and Maudsley NHS Trust 2003 Prescribing Guidelines*, 7th edn. London: Martin Dunitz.

Tennant C (2002) Life events, stress and depression: a review of recent findings. *Australian and New Zealand Journal of Psychiatry* **36**: 173–82.

Thakore JH, Richards PJ, Reznek RH et al. (1997) Increased intra-abdominal fat deposition in patients with major depressive illness as measured by computed tomography. *Biological Psychiatry* **41**: 1140–2.

Thase ME, Dube S, Bowler K et al. (1996) Hypothalamic-pituitary-adrenocortical activity and response to cognitive behavior therapy in unmedicated, hospitalized depressed patients. *American Journal of Psychiatry* **153**: 886–91.

Thase ME, Greenhouse J. B, Frank E et al. (1997) Treatment of major depression with psychotherapy or psychotherapy-pharmacotherapy combinations. *Archives of General Psychiatry* **54**: 1009–15.

Thase ME, Simons AD & Reynolds CFD (1993) Psychobiological correlates of poor response to cognitive behavior therapy: potential indications for antidepressant pharmacotherapy. *Psychopharmacology Bulletin* **29**: 293–301.

Weissman MM, Bland RC, Canino GJ et al. (1996) Cross-national epidemiology of major depression and bipolar disorder. *Journal of the American Medical Association* **276**: 293–9.

Wheeler Vega J, Mortimer A & Tyson PJ (2000) Somatic treatment of psychotic depression: review and recommendations for practice. *Journal of Clinical Psychopharmacology* **20**: 504–19.

Wheeler Vega J, Mortimer A & Tyson PJ (2000) Somatic treatment of psychotic depression: review and recommendations for practice. *Journal of Clinical Psychopharmacology* **20**: 504–19.

Willner P (1995) Dopaminergic mechanisms in depression and mania. In: Bloom FE & Kupfer DJ (eds) *Psychopharmacology: The Fourth Generation of Progress*, pp. 921–31. New York: Raven Press.

Wolkowitz OM, Reus VI, Keebler A et al. (1999) Double-blind treatment of major depression with dehydroepiandrosterone. *American Journal of Psychiatry* **156**: 646–9.

World Health Organization (1992) *ICD-10 Classification of Mental and Behavioural Disorders*. Geneva: WHO.

Yatham LE , Liddle PF, Shiah I-S, Scarrow G, Lam RW, Adam MJ, Zis AP & Ruth TJ (2000) Brain serotonin$_2$ receptors in major depression: a positron emission tomography study. *Archives of General Psychiatry* **57**: 850–8.

Young AH, Gallagher P & Porter RJ (2002) Elevation of the cortisol-dehydroepiandrosterone ratio in drug-free depressed patients. *American Journal of Psychiatry* **159**: 1237–9.

Zheng D, Macera CA, Croft JB et al. (1997) Major depression and all-cause mortality among white adults in the United States. *Annals of Epidemiology* **7**: 213–18.

Bipolar disorders

Paul Mackin and Allan Young

INTRODUCTION

Bipolar disorders have until recent times been a relatively neglected area of psychiatry, and our understanding of these disorders remains in its infancy. The fact that this chapter is devoted to bipolar disorders, and that this spectrum of disorders has not subsumed under the heading 'Affective disorders' as in the first edition of this textbook, is testimony to the increasing research interest and activity characterizing the past decade, and to the burgeoning high-quality literature that has been published in recent years. This chapter will consider the historical aspects of bipolar disorders and examine the concept of the 'bipolar spectrum'. The phenomenology, classification, differential diagnosis, epidemiology, aetiology, treatment and outcome of bipolar disorders will also be discussed.

HISTORY OF BIPOLAR DISORDER

Accounts of disturbances of mood, speech and behaviour can be found in ancient Hindu texts, and in the writings of the Babylonians and Mesopotamians dating from 600 BC. Contemporary concepts such as melancholia, mania, schizophrenia, anxiety and hysteria have their origins in the writings of pre-classical Greek philosophers, priests and physicians, although the descriptions of these concepts are in some instances far removed from our current understanding of the terms. The Greek physicians of the classical period were influential in establishing the concept of bipolar disorder(s), and Hippocrates (c460–357 BC), who had a special interest in mental diseases, was the first to describe systematically the syndromes of mania and melancholia. Hippocrates believed diseases to be a result of aberrant physiological processes, or due to environmental influences, rather than the result of intervention by the gods as punishment for some misdemeanour. He formulated the first classification of mental disorders, and described melancholia, mania and paranoia, as well as hypomania and

hyperthymic temperaments. The classic concepts of mania and melancholia are broader than the modern concepts, and although symptoms and patterns of behaviour compatible with contemporary definitions of mania and melancholia were described, also included were other disorders that might now be classified as schizophrenia or organic psychoses. The term mania, in particular, was used to describe a variety of human experiences including rage or anger, 'erotic inspiration', and a divine state, as well as a temperamental subtype and a biologically defined disease.

Mental disorders captivated the interest of many Greek and Roman physicians, but it was Areatus of Cappadocia who described the similarities and connections between the various psychic maladies. Living in the 1st century AD, Areatus was among the most prominent members of the 'Eclectics', while at the same time being strongly influenced by Hippocrates. Eclecticism was not bound by any single theoretical or philosophical perspective but selected ideas from a variety of sources. Areatus described mania and melancholia as a part of the same disease process, and he is credited with establishing the concept of bipolar disorder (Marneros 2001). In his work *On the Aetiology and Symptomology of Chronic Diseases*, descriptions of melancholia are given in Chapter 5 and mania in Chapter 6. He wrote: 'The development of mania is really a worsening of the disease (melancholia) rather than a change into another disease'.

Despite the progress in terms of an understanding of the relevance of biology in the aetiology of mental disorders that emerged during classical Greek and Roman times, the momentum towards further discovery was not maintained in subsequent centuries. The mediaeval period witnessed a resurgence of religious fervour and the soul was seen as a battleground between the Devil and the Holy Ghost. The mentally ill, often judged to be suffering from demoniacal possession, were vilified, imprisoned, tortured and executed. Over 200 000 people, mainly women, were executed during the bloody excesses of witch- and heresy-hunting that eventually culminated in scepticism, expressed by both the public and physicians, about supernatural possession (Porter 2002).

The dark shadow cast over those suffering from mental illness and its causes did not begin to lift until the 19th century. Once again, the oscillations between mood states which characterize bipolar disorders were described by several European psychiatrists including Hienroth who was the first German psychiatrist to be appointed to a university chair in 'Mental Medicine'. The influential German psychiatrist Griesinger (1845) described links between manic and depressive states and their association with seasonality, but it was the coining of the term *folie circulaire* by Falret (1851) which marked the birth of the modern concept of bipolar disorder. This term was later introduced into German psychiatry by Karl Kahlbaum, and quickly gained acceptance across Europe.

Emil Kraepelin (1896), considered by many to be the 'father of modern psychiatry', made significant further contributions to the understanding of manic-depressive illness. He divided 'endogenous' psychoses into *dementia praecox* and *manic-depressive insanity*, and included all affective disorders within the latter category. Strong opposition was mounted to Kraepelin's classification, led by Carl Wernicke and Karl Kleist. Although many of Kraepelin's supporters remained dogmatic in their opinions, Kraepelin was more accommodating of the views of his contemporaries who posited alternative classifications, and he adapted his own works to take account of new insights. Wernicke (1900) attempted to distinguish subtle differences between affective syndromes, and argued that single episodes of mania or melancholia were different from manic-depressive insanity. Kleist differentiated between unipolar and bipolar affective disorders, but his classification was complicated and unwieldy.

Over a half of a century elapsed before the next milestone in understanding of bipolar disorder was reached, when two influential papers by Jules Angst (1966) and Carlo Perris (1966) were published. These studies highlighted the importance of genetics in both bipolar and unipolar affective disorders and the influence of gender. The differences between unipolar depression and bipolar disorder in terms of genetics, gender and illness-course were described and the very strong relationship between 'unipolar mania' and bipolar disorder was emphasized. These landmark studies set the scene for the subsequent four decades of research and the attendant insights into bipolar disorders (Box 20.1).

THE BIPOLAR SPECTRUM

Although current psychiatric classification systems employ operational definitions of syndromes and disorders, the creation of distinct 'entities' may simply be an illusion masking complex and overlapping phenomena, and the status of current research suggests that this may be a particular problem with the bipolar disorders. The concept of a spectrum of bipolar illnesses is not new. Mania, hypomania, drug-induced manic or hypomanic states, cyclothymia, and depression in individuals with a family history of bipolar illness have for many years been considered by some researchers to exist within the bipolar spectrum. Kraepelin, for example, included hyperthymic temperaments within the category of manic-depressive illness, and Angst (1978) developed a continuum of bipolar disorders along which he placed hypomania (m), cyclothymia (md), mania (M), mania with mild depression (Md), mania with major depression (MD), and major depression and hypomania (Dm). More recently Akiskal & Mallya (1987) proposed the 'soft' bipolar spectrum, within which are included those with hyperthymic temperaments who experience recurrent depression without mania or hypomania, but with a family history of bipolar illness (also referred to as pseudo-unipolar disorders) (Akiskal 1996).

The place of personality disorders within the bipolar spectrum has also attracted interest, and evidence supports the inclusion of the 'histrionic-sociopathic' and 'borderline-narcissistic' groups of personality disorders (Akiskal et al. 1977), as well as hyperthymic and cyclothymic temperaments within the modern concept of the bipolar spectrum. Equally, the group of schizoaffective disorders, which have been subcategorized as unipolar and bipolar, may occupy an extreme position along the continuum of bipolarity, but further research is needed to clarify this issue.

CLINICAL FEATURES

Although phenomenologically similar, depressive states in bipolar disorders may differ subtly from those occurring in

Box 20.1 Important dates in the history of bipolar disorders	
Pre-classical era	Origins of the concepts of melancholia, mania, schizophrenia, anxiety and hysteria
c.460–357 BC	Hippocrates systematically described mania and melancholia
1st century AD	Areatus of Cappadocia establishes the concept of bipolar disorder
Mediaeval period	Witch and heresy hunts. The mentally ill were vilified and executed
1845	Griesinger described links between manic and depressive states
1851	Falret coins the term *folie circulaire*
1896	Kraepelin divides the major psychoses into dementia praecox and manic depressive insanity
1966	Influential studies by Angst and Perris marking the 'rebirth' of bipolar disorders

unipolar affective disorder, and subsyndromal depressive symptoms are a common feature of bipolar disorders. The clinical features of depression are described elsewhere in this volume (Chapter 19), and the following account will focus on the phenomenology of hypomanic and manic states, and the salient clinical features of manic stupor, mixed states and cyclothymia.

Mania and hypomania

The manic syndrome is well defined but nevertheless may be mistaken for schizophrenia or a disorder of personality. The core feature of mania is an alteration of mood, but behavioural, emotional and cognitive changes characterize this pathological mood state. Mania is a severe syndrome that causes significant impairment of functioning, and the individual suffering a manic episode often requires treatment in a psychiatric in-patient facility. Hypomania is a term best reserved for less severe mood shifts, and is often only recognized by close family and friends or mental health professionals – function is less impaired, indeed some individuals when hypomanic become more productive, and with early detection and treatment hospitalization can often be avoided. A summary of the clinical features of hypomania and mania is given in Table 20.1.

Appearance

Appearance may be unremarkable in hypomanic states. The outward appearance of an individual experiencing a manic state, however, is often striking. Brightly coloured clothes, inappropriate for the prevailing climate, may be worn and there is often an excessive use of make-up, which may be erratically applied, and jewellery reflecting the current mood state. In more severe states the individual may appear dishevelled and neglected. Shoes may not be worn and it is not uncommon for individuals to walk great distances without footwear, which may result in serious injury and/or infection. The demeanour may be cheerful, but fatigue and tearfulness are often evident.

Behaviour

Disinhibition is characteristic of mania, and is usually first noticed by family or friends. This may have ruinous consequences in terms of personal relationships, occupation and finances. When present it is often evident during the psychiatric interview and the individual may be over-familiar, outspoken or abusive. Overactivity may be mild or severe. In its more severe form, food and fluid intake may be reduced with serious biochemical disturbance, and physical exhaustion may ensue. More typical is inner restlessness and increased motor activity manifested by an inability to remain seated during an interview, pacing around the room or excessive use of gestures. Occasionally increased activity may be productive, but often the individual is unable to complete tasks, and engages in disorganized and purposeless activity, which may occur in response to environmental stimuli.

Table 20.1 Clinical features of hypomania and mania		
	Hypomania	*Mania*
Appearance	May be unremarkable Demeanour may be cheerful	Often striking Clothes may reflect mood state Demeanour may be cheerful Dishevelled and fatigued in severe states
Behaviour	Increased sociability and disinhibition	Overactivity and excitement Social disinhibition
Speech	May be talkative	Often pressured with flight of ideas
Mood	Mild elation or irritability	Elated or irritable Boundless optimism Typically no diurnal pattern May be labile
Vegetative signs	Increased appetite Reduced need for sleep Increased libido	Increased appetite Reduced need for sleep Increased libido
Psychotic symptoms	Not present Thoughts may have an expansive quality	Thoughts may have an expansive quality Delusions and second-person auditory hallucinations may be present often grandiose in nature 10-20% have Schneiderian First Rank symptoms
Cognition	Mild distractibility	Marked distractibility More marked disturbance in severe states
Insight	Usually preserved	Insight often lost, especially in severe states

Speech

Changes to speech may be one of the most striking features of mania or hypomania. Individuals frequently seek out others in order to engage in conversation, which may be excessive and wearing. The quantity and rate of speech are increased, which is a manifestation of the rapid influx of thoughts, and patients give accounts of thoughts flooding the mind. When the individual is difficult to interrupt as a result of an incessant desire to talk and express these thoughts, speech is referred to as *pressured*. A more severe disorder of thinking manifested in speech is *flight of ideas* in which there is a logical connection between two sequential ideas, but the goal of conversation is not maintained and is difficult to follow. Flight of ideas often arises out of an extreme degree of distractibility and inappropriate responses to environmental cues. *Puns* and *clang associations* may also punctuate conversation. Although the form of speech may be disordered, important differences exist which differentiate the patterns of speech characteristic of mania and schizophrenia. In schizophrenia there is often a breakdown in association between ideas such that there appears to be no understandable connection between the chain of thoughts and the listener is often left feeling confused and bewildered.

Mood

An altered mood state is the core feature of mania and hypomania. Classically mood is thought to be elated, but frequently it is irritable. The importance of an awareness of the manifestations of hypomanic and manic mood states cannot be overstated as many individuals presenting with irritability, rather than euphoric mania, are incorrectly diagnosed as suffering from unipolar depression with potentially disastrous consequences if treated only with antidepressant drugs. When elated the individual appears inappropriately cheerful and may experience boundless optimism. Elated mood has an infectious quality, and is often accompanied by religious or metaphysical preoccupations. Irritability, however, may predominate, which is intensely distressing and may result in irascible verbal and/or behavioural outbursts and in extreme cases violence may occur. Although during a manic or hypomanic episode mood may change throughout the day it usually does not show the diurnal pattern characteristic of depression. The mood may, however, be labile and frequently shift between elation and tearful dysphoria or irritability.

Vegetative signs

Appetite is frequently increased during hypomania and mania but this is not invariably accompanied by increased food intake. Indeed the converse may occur resulting in weight loss as a consequence of reduced oral intake and increased motor activity. Sleep disturbance is characteristic, and individuals describe a reduced need for sleep and as such are often resistive to suggestions that they retire to bed.

Initial insomnia occurs and sleep may last for only two or three hours, after which energetic activity is resumed. Libido is often increased and there may be increased sexual interest and activity. Individuals may engage in impulsive and reckless liaisons and disregard issues such as birth control. Counselling and, if appropriate, pregnancy testing or referral to a sexual health clinic, should be offered to individuals if necessary.

Psychotic and related symptoms

Thoughts frequently have an expansive quality, which is congruent with the prevailing mood state, and are often grandiose in nature. These thoughts may be overvalued inasmuch as they preoccupy the individual and are pursued beyond the bounds of reason, but are not held with delusional intensity. When delusional ideas exist they may be of a grandiose or persecutory nature. Common grandiose themes are religious conversion or salvation, personal wealth or influence, and royal descent. Persecutory delusions may arise out of a belief that others are trying to frustrate the individual's plans. The content of the delusional idea(s) is often not stable and changes over a period of days. Delusions of reference and passivity phenomena may also occur, and it is estimated that Schneiderian first rank symptoms occur in 10–20% of manic episodes.

Auditory hallucinations are the most common perceptual disturbance occurring during a manic episode. Generally they are mood congruent and in the second person, such as God addressing the individual and offering instructions for world salvation. Reports exist of visual hallucinations occurring during mania, again typically taking the form of a religious scene, but visual hallucinations should alert the clinician to the possibility of an organic brain syndrome.

Cognition

Marked distractibility is common during mania. The immediate environment may provide a rich source of stimulation, which may frustrate any attempts to interview the individual. Orientation is usually preserved except in the most severe cases, but attention and concentration are often impaired. More subtle cognitive impairments, particularly in the realm of executive functioning, have been identified in recent years, but sophisticated neuropsychological testing is required to identify these abnormalities (see below).

Insight

The degree of impaired insight depends on the severity of the episode. Hypomania is often characterized by relatively preserved insight, and it is not uncommon for individuals to recognize a shift into hypomania and to seek medical intervention. In severe mania, however, insight is lost completely and any intervention is met with disdain and resistance. The use of statutory powers, such as those conferred by the Mental Health Act, are often required in order to offer appropriate treatment in the safest environment.

Manic stupor

Following the advent of effective pharmacological treatment of mania the occurrence of manic stupor is now rare. When it does occur it may follow from a period of manic excitement, or more rarely in the transition between depressive stupor and mania. Characteristically the individual is immobile and mute with a serene facial expression or one suggestive of elation. On recovery the events during the stuperose period are recalled, and descriptions are given of rapid thoughts typical of mania.

Mixed states

Periods of depression and (hypo)mania are the hallmark of bipolar disorders. The switch between depression and mania occurs within a variable time frame with or without an intervening period of euthymia. Symptoms of mania and depression, however, may occur concurrently, and the term 'mixed state' is best reserved for such situations. For example, an individual my appear overactive with pressured speech and flight of ideas, but at the same time be experiencing profoundly negative and morbid thoughts. Females are more frequently represented in the group of mixed states, and using broad definitions, more than two thirds of individuals with bipolar disorder have a mixed state at least once during the course of the illness.

Cyclothymia

Cyclothymia is often referred to as a persistent disorder of mood and is associated with significant distress and/or impairment of functioning. It is characterized by numerous hypomanic episodes and periods of depression that do not meet criteria for a diagnosis of bipolar disorder or recurrent (major) depressive disorder (see below). Mood swings often are not related to life events, and diagnosis can be difficult in the absence of clear and detailed accounts of symptoms and their chronology. The picture is also frequently complicated by substance misuse.

CLASSIFICATION

Box 20.2 shows the classification of bipolar disorders in ICD-10 and DSM-IV. Although the two systems share common features, there are important differences, which are discussed in more detail below.

ICD-10

Full diagnostic criteria are given in Appendix 1 to this chapter.

Hypomania

Hypomania is defined in ICD-10 as elevated or irritable mood that is abnormal for the individual and is sustained for at least four days. Features such as over-familiarity, increased activity or talkativeness, distractibility, or reduced

---

Box 20.2 The classification of bipolar disorders in ICD-10 and DSM-IV

ICD-10	DSM-IV
Mood (affective) disorders Hypomania Mania • without psychotic symptoms • with psychotic symptoms Bipolar affective disorder • current episode hypomanic • current episode manic • current episode depression[A] • current episode mixed ([A]Specified as mild, moderate or severe, with or without psychotic features) **Persistent mood (affective) disorders** Cyclothymia	**Mood disorders** *Mood episodes* Hypomanic episode Manic episode *Bipolar disorders* Bipolar I disorder[C] • single manic episode[A] • most recent episode hypomanic • most recent episode manic[A] • most recent episode mixed[A] • most recent episode depressed[A] Bipolar II disorder[C] • current episode hypomania • current episode depressed[B] Cyclothymic disorder [A]Specified as mild, moderate, severe without psychotic features, severe with psychotic features, in partial remission, in full remission [B]Severity and presence of psychotic features are specified [C]Rapid cycling may be used as a course modifier

sleep should also be present, but these symptoms are not present to the extent that they lead to severe social disruption of work or result in social rejection. Criteria for a manic episode should not be met, nor should hallucinations or delusions be present.

Mania

Mania is defined as elevated, expansive or irritable mood that must be sustained for at least one week. Accompanying symptoms may include increased activity or talkativeness, flight of ideas, disinhibition, reduced sleep, grandiosity or reckless behaviour, which lead to severe interference with personal functioning in daily living. Mania may occur without or with psychotic symptoms, which may be mood-congruent or mood-incongruent. Typical mood-congruent hallucinations would take the form of voices telling the individual that he/she had superhuman powers. Mood-incongruent psychotic symptoms may include voices speaking about affectively neutral topics, or delusions of persecution.

Bipolar affective disorder

The minimum ICD-10 criteria for diagnosing bipolar affective disorder are two separate mood episodes, one of which must be hypomania, mania or a mixed affective state. The current episode must be specified, and may be one of the following: hypomania; mania without psychotic symptoms; mania with psychotic symptoms; mild or moderate depression; severe depression without psychotic symptoms; severe depression with psychotic symptoms; mixed episode; or in remission.

Cyclothymia

In ICD-10 cyclothymia is classified under persistent mood (affective) disorders, and is defined as a persistent instability of mood involving numerous periods of depression and mild elation, none of which is sufficiently severe or prolonged to justify a diagnosis of bipolar affective disorder or recurrent depressive disorder. The period of instability of mood must be of at least two years' duration.

DSM-IV

Full diagnostic criteria are given in Appendix 2 to this chapter.

Hypomania

A hypomanic episode is defined as a distinct period during which there is an abnormally and persistently elevated, expansive, or irritable mood that lasts at least four days. Additional symptoms such as inflated self-esteem, decreased need for sleep, distractibility or increase in goal-directed activity, must be present. The episode should not be severe enough to cause marked impairment in social or occupational functioning, or necessitate hospitalization, nor should there be psychotic features.

Mania

In DSM-IV a manic episode is defined as a distinct period of abnormally and persistently elevated, expansive or irritable mood, lasting one week (or any duration if hospitalization is necessary). Accompanying symptoms may include inflated self-esteem, sleep disturbance, pressure of speech and excessive involvement in pleasurable activities. The mood disturbance is sufficiently severe to cause marked impairment in occupational functioning or in usual social activities or relationships with others, or to necessitate hospitalization to prevent harm to self or others. Psychotic features may be present.

Bipolar disorders

Within the DSM-IV classification, bipolar disorders are subdivided into bipolar I disorder, bipolar II disorder, cyclothymia, and bipolar disorder Not Otherwise Specified (NOS).

Bipolar I disorder

The essential feature of bipolar I disorder is a clinical course characterized by the occurrence of one or more manic episodes, or mixed episodes. Often individuals have also had one or more major depressive episodes. The current episode may be specified as: mild; moderate; severe without psychotic features; severe with psychotic features; in partial remission; in full remission; with catatonic features or with postpartum onset. The type of mood episode (hypomania, mania, depression or mixed) should also be specified.

Bipolar II disorder

The essential feature of bipolar II disorder is a clinical course that is characterized by the occurrence of one or more major depressive episodes accompanied by at least one hypomanic episode. The presence of a manic or a mixed episode precludes the diagnosis of bipolar II disorder. Specifiers for current episodes are similar to those for bipolar I disorder.

Cyclothymic disorder

DSM-IV defines cyclothymic disorder as a chronic, fluctuating mood disturbance involving numerous periods of hypomanic symptoms and numerous periods of depressive symptoms. These symptoms should not meet full criteria for a manic episode or a major depressive episode, and should be present for at least two years (one year in children and adolescents).

DIFFERENTIAL DIAGNOSES

Both depressive and manic disorders include schizophrenic illnesses and organic brain syndromes as possible

Box 20.3   The differential diagnoses of manic states

Cyclothymia

Schizophrenia

Organic brain syndromes
- degenerative conditions
- cerebrovascular disease
- epilepsy
- multiple sclerosis
- brain injury
- space-occupying lesions
- HIV/AIDS
- other cerebral infections
- cerebral inflammatory conditions

Illicit substance and alcohol misuse

Iatrogenic causes
- dopamine agonists
- corticosteroids
- thyroid hormones
- anticholinergics

differential diagnoses. The differential diagnosis of depressive disorders is considered elsewhere in this volume, and the following account highlights the important conditions from which manic disorders must be distinguished.

The differential diagnosis of manic disorders (Box 20.3) include:

- cyclothymia
- schizophrenia
- organic brain syndromes
- illicit substance misuse
- iatrogenic causes.

Cyclothymia

As referred to above, cyclothymia shares many of the characteristics of manic-depressive illness, but the severity and duration of symptoms are not sufficient to make a diagnosis of mania or recurrent depressive disorder. In order to make a diagnosis of cyclothymia careful attention must be given to the history of the mood instability, and a corroborative account from a family member or close friend can assist in distinguishing the two disorders. Notwithstanding, a proportion of individuals with cyclothymia will go on to develop frank bipolar disorder (see below).

Schizophrenia

Differentiating mania from schizophrenia can be a difficult diagnostic problem, particularly in an acute setting with an unfamiliar patient. Both conditions share similar clinical features such as psychomotor disturbance, thought disorder and psychotic phenomena. Schneider's first rank symptoms occur in 10–20% of individuals with mania, and their presence should not necessarily point to a diagnosis of schizophrenia. However, delusional beliefs and auditory hallucinations are typically less stable in manic disorders. A previous history of depression or (hypo)mania, or a family history of bipolar disorder may assist in making the diagnosis.

Organic brain syndromes

The presence of symptoms suggestive of mania, particularly in an older patient without previous affective disturbance, should alert the clinician to the possibility of an organic brain syndrome. Careful examination of the mental state, including thorough cognitive assessment may indicate organic pathology. Frontal lobe pathology, such as fronto-temporal dementia or Pick's disease may manifest as a coarsening of social skills or marked disinhibition that may mimic a manic syndrome. Cerebrovascular insults or head injury resulting in brain damage may produce an organic mood disorder characterized by a change in mood or affect, usually accompanied by a change in the overall level of activity. Space-occupying lesions may cause significant mood disturbance, as well as worsening the course of an already established bipolar illness. The rise in the incidence of HIV infection should prompt careful investigation, particularly in younger individuals who present with atypical features.

Illicit substance misuse

A number of recreational drugs can cause affective and behavioural disturbance, which may mimic mania. A careful history of illicit substance use together with urine drug-screening may be helpful in reaching a diagnosis. Typically, the symptoms associated with drug misuse subside when the substance is withdrawn, unlike manic symptoms which persist. Co-morbid substance misuse is a significant problem for many individuals with established bipolar disorder, and continued use often destabilizes the illness and either prolongs recovery or precipitates relapse.

Iatrogenic causes

Prescribed medication can cause states resembling mania. Corticosteroids, especially in high doses can produce elated mood states as well as depression. Dopamine agonists and L-dopa may also cause pathological mood changes which may be difficult to distinguish from mania.

EPIDEMIOLOGY

The lifetime risk of bipolar disorder depends upon the diagnostic criteria used. The rate is usually quoted as approximately 1%, similar to that of schizophrenia. Lifetime prevalence rates of bipolar I and bipolar II disorders have been estimated at 0.6%, giving a combined prevalence of 1.2%. The combined prevalence of bipolar II, bipolar III ('false unipolar' disorder, or hypomania precipitated by antidepressant treatment) and dysthymic disorders has been estimated at 7.7–12%. A 20-year prospective community cohort study of young adults in Zurich has recently estimated the cumulative prevalence of broadly-defined bipolar II disorder to be 10.9%, and the total prevalence of the 'soft bipolar spectrum' (which includes patients with cyclothymia and hypomanic symptoms not reaching DSM-IV criteria for hypomania) was 23.7% (Angst et al. 2003). The point at which 'soft' bipolar symptoms become pathological, however, has yet to be fully determined.

The six-month prevalence of bipolar disorder is similar to the lifetime prevalence, which emphasizes the chronicity of these disorders. The lifetime prevalence of cyclothymia has been estimated to be between 0.4% and 3.5%. Family studies have indicated an aggregation of cyclothymia with both unipolar and bipolar disorders, and a proportion of these individuals eventually develop a bipolar illness.

The prevalence of bipolar illness and cyclothymia is equal between men and women. Epidemiological data suggest, however, that females form a greater proportion of those individuals with bipolar II disorder, the major burden of which is depression (Box 20.4).

Box 20.4 Epidemiological features of the bipolar disorders
M= F
BPII F > M
Combined prevalence of BPI and BPII ~ 1.2%
Combined prevalence of BPII and BPIII ~ 7.7–12%
Prevalence of broadly defined BPII ~ 10.9%
Prevalence of cyclothmia ~ 0.4–3.5%
Total prevalence of the 'soft' bipolar spectrum ~ 23.7%
BPI= bipolar I disorder; BPII=bipolar II disorder; BPIII=bipolar III disorder (or 'false' unipolar disorder).

AETIOLOGY

The understanding of the aetiology of bipolar disorders is in its infancy, but recent years have witnessed significant progress in the fields of genetic research, neuroendocrine, neuropathological and molecular studies of the causes of this heterogeneous group of disorders. The following section highlights the important aspects of our current understanding of the aetiology of bipolar disorders, and also describes some psychological theories of bipolar illness (see Box 20.5).

Biological

Genetic studies

The influence of genetic factors in the aetiology of bipolar disorder have long been recognized, but until recent years there has been little understanding of the areas of the genome that may confer susceptibility to developing bipolar illness, and the mechanisms of genetic transmission. Advances in technology, in particular in the field of molecular genetics, have led to new insights into these complex areas. Notwithstanding, we still await the discovery of susceptibility genes to further our understanding of the pathophysiology of bipolar disorder. Craddock & Jones (2001) have produced an excellent review of the current status of genetic research (see also Chapter 3).

Box 20.5 Biological and psychological aspects of the aetiology of bipolar disorders
Biological
Genetic studies
Family, twin and adoption studies:
• familial aggregation
• increased risk of affective disorders in first degree relatives
• concordance greater in monozygotic twins
• risk greater in biological relatives than adoptive relatives
Linkage studies:
• ?susceptibility gene on chromosome 12q
Association studies:
• ?COMT gene acts as a course modifier
Neuroendocrine studies
Hypothalamic-pituitary-adrenal axis dysfunction:
• increased plasma cortisol levels
• hypersecretion of CRH
• enlarged pituitary and adrenal glands
• impaired feedback mechanisms
• glucocorticoid receptor abnormalities
Hypothalamic-pituitary-thyroid axis dysfunction:
• subclinical hypothyroidism
• reduced pituitary responsiveness to TRH
• thyroid supplementation enhances antidepressant treatment
Neuropathological studies
Postmortem studies:
• increased brain weight
• abnormalities of parahippocampal cortex
• smaller temporal horns
Cyto-architectural studies:
• malformations in the entorhinal lamination
• reduction in hippocampal non-pyramidal neurons
• anterior cingulate glial cell abnormalities
MRI studies:
• temporal lobe abnormalities
• cerebral white matter lesions
Psychological
Psychodynamic theory:
• importance of loss
• manic defence
• protection against psychic pain

Family, twin and adoption studies

The familial aggregation of a number of psychiatric disorders is well known, and there is overwhelming evidence demonstrating the role of genetic factors in mood disorders. Studies of family pedigrees, however, reveal that the mode of inheritance is complex and does not follow simple Mendelian patterns. Closer examination of these pedigrees also suggests that many psychiatric illnesses do not 'breed true' and that there is a spectrum of illness phenotype within families. Much of the early data highlighting the importance of familial factors in the aetiology of mood disorders were derived from family, twin and adoption studies.

A number of family studies have consistently shown an increased risk of bipolar disorder in first-degree relatives of bipolar probands, which has been estimated to be 5–10 times that of the general population (Craddock & Jones 1999). Moreover, the risk of unipolar depressive disorder is also increased in first-degree relatives of individuals with bipolar illness (8–20% lifetime risk).

Twin studies have provided additional insights into the importance of genetic factors in bipolar disorder. The risk of developing bipolar disorder in a monozygotic co-twin of a proband with bipolar disorder is greatly increased (around 45 to 75 times that of the general population) compared with a dizygotic co-twin. These studies have also revealed that even if the co-twin does not develop bipolar disorder, many will experience some form of affective morbidity, usually severe depression, during their lifetime. A recent twin study has estimated the heritability of bipolar disorder to be in excess of 80%, suggesting that all of the familiality of bipolar disorder could be accounted for by additive genetic effects with no contribution from family environment (McGuffin et al. 2003).

Two small adoption studies have shown that the risk of bipolar disorder is greater in the biological relatives rather than the adoptive relatives of the probands.

Taken together all these data provide robust evidence of the importance of genetic factors in the aetiology of bipolar illness, but nevertheless the discordance between monozygotic twins emphasizes the contribution of non-genetic factors. Even with this persuasive evidence, the mechanism(s) of inheritance continue to elude us. Current research does not favour a single gene model of inheritance, but rather a polygenic model in which several interacting genes confer susceptibility to developing bipolar disorder. The relative contribution of individual genes is unclear, and a considerable number of studies have endeavoured to identify areas of the genome, which may have pathogenetic significance.

Linkage studies

Linkage studies of bipolar disorder recruit families in which more than one family member is affected by the disease, and a number of such studies have been conducted in an attempt to identify candidate genes. An unusual and striking example of the contribution of linkage studies to our understanding of the genetics of bipolar disorder can be found in the identification of a family in which several members had a rare skin disease called Darier's disease (an autosomal dominant condition), together with major affective disorder (bipolar disorder and severe depression). The gene for Darier's disease has been located on chromosome 12q23-q24.1, and the possibility of a susceptibility gene for bipolar disorder existing within the region of the Darier's gene has been raised. A number of researchers have investigated this possibility by conducting linkage studies, and there is some evidence that there may indeed be a bipolar susceptibility gene on chromosome 12q. Other chromosome regions of interest include 4p16, 16p, 21q22 and Xq24-q26.

Association studies

Association studies of bipolar disorder use unrelated affected individuals and appropriate control subjects. A number a candidate gene studies (in which the researcher proposes a specific gene, which may be involved in the pathogenesis of a disease) have been undertaken using the association approach. One such example is a recent study which investigated the relationship between catechol-o-methyl transferase (COMT), an enzyme involved in the breakdown of catecholamines, and rapid cycling bipolar disorder. The results of this work suggested that the COMT gene is not a susceptibility gene as there was very little difference in allele frequency between the bipolar group and controls. However, those individuals within the bipolar group who had the low-activity COMT allele were more likely to have rapid cycling bipolar disorder, and, moreover, there was a dose-dependent relationship between the number of copies of the low-activity allele and rapid cycling. Although these data are preliminary and require replication, the evidence is consistent with COMT acting as a course modifier rather than as a susceptibility gene.

Ethical considerations

The ethical aspects of genetic research are complex and beyond the scope of this chapter. However, this brief survey of the status of genetic research highlights some important areas that are likely to impact on the practice of many mental health professionals:

- The identification of susceptibility genes for bipolar disorder is likely to fundamentally alter the perception of mental illness by patients, the general public and professionals alike.
- A better understanding of the genetics and pathophysiology of bipolar disorder will potentially improve treatment and outcome.
- Developing genetic tests for psychiatric disorders has important implications regarding access to, and use of genetic information.

- Research into psychosocial and ethical aspects of genetic research should exist alongside current pathophysiological and molecular genetic studies.

Neuroendocrine studies

The role of the endocrine system in the pathogenesis of psychiatric disorders has attracted the interest of many researchers over the years, including Kraepelin and Freud, but technical limitations prevented any real understanding of the interaction of endocrine systems with neuronal circuits. More recently, however, advances in technology have resulted in improved methodology, and consequently a clearer understanding of the contribution of endocrine systems to the pathophysiology of mood disorders. Neuroendocrine studies to date have largely focused on the hypothalamic-pituitary-adrenal (HPA) axis, and the thyroid gland.

The hypothalamic-pituitary-adrenal axis

The current state of research regarding the HPA axis, and the implications for future therapeutic targets has been reviewed by McQuade & Young (2000). The HPA axis comprises the tissues of the hypothalamus, pituitary and adrenal cortices, regulatory neuronal inputs, and a variety of releasing factors and hormones (see Figure 20.1). Neurosecretory cells within the paraventricular nucleus of the hypothalamus secrete corticotropin-releasing hormone (CRH) and arganine vasopressin (AVP) into the microportal circulatory system of the pituitary stalk. CRH and AVP cause the release of adrenocorticotropic hormone (ACTH) from the anterior lobe of the pituitary. Cortisol, which may be considered to be the final product of the HPA axis, is released from the adrenal cortex in response to ACTH. Cortisol has a number of central and peripheral effects which are mediated via glucocorticoid receptors.

The activity of the HPA axis is highly regulated. Secretory cells within the paraventricular nucleus receive neuronal inputs from a number of brain regions including the amygdala, hippocampus and nuclei within the midbrain. The HPA axis also has an autoregulatory mechanism mediated by cortisol. Endogenous cortisol binds to glucocorticoid receptors in the HPA axis and acts as a potent negative regulator of HPA activity. These regulatory mechanisms are important in determining basal levels and circadian fluctuations in cortisol levels. Changes in glucocorticoid receptor number or function may be important in altering the homeostatic function of the HPA axis observed in healthy individuals.

Abnormalities of the HPA axis in depression have been well described. Plasma cortisol levels of patients with depression are higher than those of healthy controls. This observation has been consistently replicated, and studies have shown that HPA hyperactivity, as manifested by hypersecretion of CRH, increased cortisol levels in plasma, urine and cerebrospinal fluid, exaggerated cortisol responses to ACTH, and enlarged pituitary and adrenal glands, occurs in individuals suffering from severe mood disorders. Hypersecretion of CRH causing hypercortisolaemia may be a result of impaired feedback mechanisms resulting from glucocorticoid receptor abnormalities. Evidence of glucocorticoid receptor function abnormalities has been demonstrated in postmortem studies of patients with severe mood disorders. Reduced glucocorticoid receptor messenger RNA (mRNA) has been demonstrated in the hippocampi of individuals with unipolar and bipolar affective disorders, and there is accumulating evidence to suggest that antidepressant and mood-stabilizing drugs stimulate glucocorticoid receptor mRNA thus enhancing HPA autoregulation resulting in reduced CRH secretion and cortisol levels. The role of the HPA axis in bipolar disorders, and the place of antiglucocorticoid drugs as therapeutic agents in the management of these disorders are the focus of ongoing research activity (see below).

The hypothalamic-pituitary-thyroid axis

Abnormalities of thyroid function occur in mood disorders. Subclinical hypothyroidism is seen in a significant proportion of depressed patients, and an even higher proportion of those with treatment-resistant depression. T_3 (tri-iodothyronine) and T_4 (thyroxine) supplementation has been shown to enhance the effects of standard antidepressant treatment with regard to response rate and time to recovery, and may be particularly beneficial in those with treatment-resistance.

In mania there are also abnormalities of thyroid function which include subclinical hypothyroidism and reduced pituitary responsiveness to thyrotropin-releasing hormone. Thyroid dysfunction has frequently been implicated in rapid

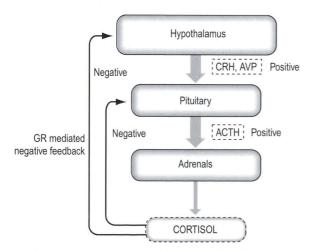

Figure 20.1 The hypothalamic-pituitary-adrenal (HPA) axis. CRH = corticotropin-releasing hormone; AVP = arginine vasopressin; ACTH = adrenocorticotropin hormone; GR = glucocorticoid receptor.

cycling bipolar disorder, and is one of the most consistent findings within this subpopulation of those with bipolar illness. Thyroid supplementation may also be of some benefit in the treatment of rapid cycling.

Neuropathological studies

Studies of neuropathological changes in mood disorders, unlike studies in schizophrenia, are in their infancy. Findings are preliminary, and in many cases, inconsistent. Methodological difficulties with these studies, such as retrospective design, do not allow for straightforward interpretation of the available data, but these early studies have provided an impetus towards further investigation using suitable methodology. We await with interest further insights into the neuropathology of mood disorders, but a number of potentially important preliminary findings are briefly discussed below (Baumann & Bogerts 2001).

Increased brain weight, thicker parahippocampal cortex and smaller temporal horns have been described in a post-mortem study of individuals with affective disorders compared with schizophrenic illnesses. Adding support to the suggestion that patients with mood disorders may have structural abnormalities in the parahippocampal cortex is another postmortem study, which showed a reduction in cortex size in suicide victims compared with non-psychiatric controls. Cyto-architectural studies have also revealed malformations in the entorhinal lamination in patients with bipolar disorder and major depression. Additionally, further evidence of abnormalities of temporal lobe structure in bipolar disorder is provided by the reported reduction of non-pyramidal neurons in the CA2 region of the hippocampus of patients with bipolar disorder and schizophrenia. These studies add weight to the evidence provided by magnetic resonance imaging (MRI) studies, which have suggested temporal lobe pathology to exist not only in schizophrenia, but bipolar disorders, too.

The prefrontal lobe, the medial prefrontal cortex and the anterior cingulate cortex have also attracted attention in attempts to identify neuroanatomical abnormalities in mood disorders. Decreased cortical and laminar thickness have been demonstrated in the dorsolateral prefrontal cortex in patients with bipolar disorder and major depressive disorder, and volume reduction together with fewer glial cells have been observed in the subgenual prefrontal cortex (part of the anterior cingulate cortex) in familial mood disorders.

MRI studies have also identified a variety of other structural brain abnormalities in patients with bipolar disorder. Cerebral white matter lesions, as shown in Figure 20.2, have attracted particular attention, and a recent study has revealed that subcortical white matter lesions are associated with poor outcome in bipolar disorder (Moore et al. 2001). The significance of these lesions in the aetiology of bipolar disorders, or as course modifiers, remains to be elucidated.

Taken together these findings provide convincing evidence that mood disorders are associated with diverse neuroanatomical changes which may be indicative of circumscribed neurodevelopmental disturbances. An excellent review of the neuropathology of mood disorders can is given by Harrison (2002).

Psychological theories

A variety of psychological theories of the aetiology of depression and mania have been posited, and although there is evidence to support the use of some psychological treatments for depression, the aetiological significance of psychological theories of depression, and in particular mania, is controversial.

Loss is central to the psychodynamic view of the precipitant of depression and mania. Freud believed that the loss of an ambivalently loved object resulted in turning against the self. In depression this results in anxiety, guilt and possibly suicidality; in mania the ego is released from oppressive domination by the super-ego. Melanie Kleine proposed the term *manic defence*, which she suggested to be a defence mechanism employed by the ego to protect against the psychic pain of depression and anxiety. Omnipotent control, triumph and contempt result and prevent the process of reparation. Few psychiatrists now attach aetiological significance to these theories, but they may be useful in understanding the content of the ideas that often characterize the manic state.

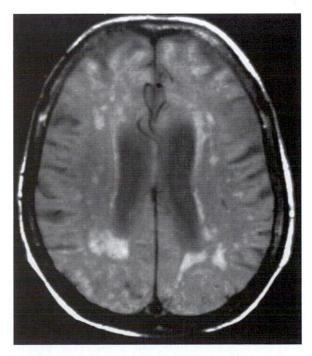

Figure 20.2 MRI scan showing white matter lesions.

COURSE AND OUTCOME

Illness course

Initial presentation
Bipolar illness often becomes clinically manifest in the late teenage years, although a substantial number of individuals are initially misdiagnosed with unipolar depression. Such misdiagnosis may have serious consequences if antidepressant drugs are used without mood-stabilizing agents. The proportion of 'false unipolars' in the diagnosis of unipolar depressive disorder has been estimated to be between 10.7% and 28.4% (Goodwin & Jamison 1990). Patients presenting for the first time with depressive symptoms should be carefully investigated for a history suggestive of (hypo)mania.

There is good agreement in the literature that the peak onset occurs in the 20s (between 25 and 30) (Goodwin & Jamison 1990), and the mean age of first hospitalization is at around the age of 26 years. Frequently there have been previous episodes of affective disturbance that have not required admission to psychiatric in-patient facilities. With the increasing implementation of community-based psychiatric assessment and treatment services that are able to provide intensive home-based treatment and support, some of these admissions may be avoided. Those experiencing severe manic or depressive episodes, with their attendant risks of self-harm and social disruption, are, however, likely to continue to require in-patient care.

In females there is a secondary peak of mania occurring around the age of 45–50 years, which has caused some to speculate about the role of hormonal influences in this group of individuals. First onset of mania in late life is likely to be associated with organic brain disease and is often referred to as 'secondary mania'. Such individuals should be investigated for vascular, infective, inflammatory or degenerative disorders as well as space-occupying lesions and iatrogenic causes.

Number of episodes
Bipolar disorder is a chronic and recurrent condition, and the average number of mood episodes has been estimated to be 10. There is, however, huge variation with many individuals experiencing many more then 10 episodes in their lifetime. There are individuals who experience only one episode in a lifetime, but these are exceptions. The vast majority of patients have numerous mood episodes, but the patterns of mood disturbance in bipolar I and bipolar II disorders are different. Bipolar I disorder, the classic manic-depressive psychosis, is characterized by episodes of frank mania and depression, usually at well-spaced intervals. The defining characteristic of bipolar II disorder is the occurrence of hypomanic, but not manic, episodes. It is now clear that the major burden of illness in bipolar II disorder is depression, rather than hypomania, which has important treatment

implications, particularly with regard to the use of antidepressant medication.

Frequency of episodes and length of cycles
The frequency of episodes can be estimated by evaluating the number and length of cycles. A cycle is defined as the time from one episode to the onset of the next. A variation in cycle length usually reflects variations in the length of intervals between episodes, as the length of episodes within an individual is often relatively stable. Survival analysis has shown that the first cycle is usually longer, and the second cycle shorter than all the others; later episodes usually arise at irregular intervals.

Length of episodes
The duration of depressive episodes in both unipolar and bipolar patients exceeds that of manic episodes. The duration of episodes of mania prior to the advent of effective pharmacological intervention was typically 3–12 months. It appears that duration of episodes is dependent on a number of factors, of which the most important is response to pharmacological treatment. The duration of a full depressive episode is typically 2–5 months, and that of manic episodes is on average two months (Goodwin & Jamison 1990). Within individuals the length of mood episodes is often relatively stable, although as the illness progresses the frequency of episodes may increase and the onset of each episode may be more abrupt.

Precipitants
Some theories on the pathogenesis of affective disorders assign primary causal relevance to the psychosocial environment, but it is now generally accepted that psychosocial or physical events contribute more to the timing of an episode than to causing it. Causality is likely to be largely biological, and especially genetic (Goodwin & Jamison 1990). Precipitating events seem to be important in the onset of the first episode but not in subsequent ones. One study found that approximately 53% of unipolar patients and 47% of bipolar patients had stressful life events prior to the onset of an episode (Marenos et al. 1990). The kind of life event seems to be unspecific, and the only common factor in all life events appears to be sleep reduction.

Rapid cycling
Although the cycling nature of bipolar disorder (*la folie circulaire*) was described by Falret in 1851, it was not until the 1970s that researchers began to identify and investigate the subpopulation of patients with bipolar disorder who experienced a high frequency of mood changes. During the past decade the phenomenon of rapid cycling bipolar disorder has been widely accepted and its significance as a course modifier, particularly with respect to pharmacological intervention, has attracted considerable research interest. 'Normal cycling' in the context of bipolar disorder has not been defined, but the definition of rapid

cycling most frequently cited in the literature is that of Dunner & Fieve (1974): four major depressive, manic, hypomanic or mixed states are required to have occurred within a 12-month period.

Approximately 13–20% of individuals will develop rapid cycling bipolar disorder during the course of their illness. Those who develop rapid cycling are greatly over-represented in the bipolar II group, with a large female preponderance. Hypothyroidism (which is more prevalent in females) and menstrual cycle irregularities have been suggested as causal factors in the switch to rapid cycling. An alternative explanation cites the observation that rapid cycling is greatly over-represented in those individuals with bipolar II disorder, the hallmark of which is depression. The well-documented female predisposition to depressive recurrence may thus account for the unequal sex distribution of rapid cycling.

The differing pharmacological response profile of patients with rapid cycling is intriguing, and raises the question of whether rapid cycling should be classified as a distinct subtype of bipolar illness. Current data do not, however, support this view – to date, studies have recognized few genetic or phenotypic differences between rapid cycling and non-rapid cycling bipolar patients. For example, several family studies have reported a similar family history of bipolar disorder in rapid and non-rapid cycling probands, and suggest that rapid cycling does not breed true. A recent study has investigated the prospective course of illness and potential risk factors for rapid cycling (Kupka et al. 2003). The factors that were most strongly associated with rapid cycling gradually increased with episode frequency, failing to indicate a non-linearity at four episodes per year, or at any other time point. Thus, the concept of rapid cycling as a distinct sub-type of bipolar disorder does not gain support from the literature.

Antidepressant-induced cycling

The role of antidepressant medication in the induction of mania and cycle acceleration is controversial. Historical studies have attempted to correlate switching rate with increasing use of antidepressant drugs. A retrospective study examining mood fluctuation patterns in patients with affective disorders hospitalized over three decades revealed that rapid mood fluctuations were absent among bipolar patients in 1960, but were evident in 1975 and 1985 suggesting an association with prescribing practices (Wolpert et al. 1990). Not all studies, however, support this view.

There is a considerable body of literature that implicates antidepressants in the induction of mania, and a number of studies have shown an association between rapid cycling and antidepressant use. Moreover, certain classes of antidepressants have been suggested to be associated with a higher risk of mania induction and/or cycle acceleration. A meta-analysis by Peet (1994) concluded that a manic switch was less likely to occur with selective serotonin reuptake inhibitors (SSRIs) than with tricyclic antidepressants. A recent study has examined the influence of antidepressant use and gender in the genesis of rapid cycling (Yildiz & Sachs 2003). A significant association was found between rapid cycling and antidepressant use prior to the first episode of (hypo)mania for women, but not for men.

Outcome

Kraepelin's assertion that affective psychoses have a 'good' outcome was over-optimistic. Long-term studies have shown that a significant proportion of patients with affective disorders have an unfavourable outcome, although individuals with affective disorders have a generally more favourable outcome than those with schizophrenic or schizoaffective disorders.

Studies of outcome in affective disorders are limited by heterogeneous definitions of 'unfavourable outcome', and the findings of these studies differ. However, studies focusing on disability and disturbances of social functioning report that approximately one-third of bipolar patients do not have a 'social full remission', and approximately 25% of patients have persisting alterations to psychosocial functioning (Goodwin & Jamison 1990).

Suicide

The problem of suicide in patients with unipolar and bipolar affective disorders is one of the greatest problems in medicine. Patients with unipolar and bipolar disorders are far more likely to commit suicide than individuals in any other psychiatric risk group. The mortality rate for untreated bipolar patients is higher than that of most types of heart disease and many types of cancer (Goodwin & Jamison 1990). Approximately 15% of patients with bipolar disorder will commit suicide, and the rate of suicidal ideas is much greater. The risk of suicide appears to be greater during the first few years after onset of illness, with rates of completed suicide diminishing over time.

Recent evidence has strongly suggested that lithium reduces the rate of suicide among bipolar patients (Baldessarini et al. 1999), and, additionally, lithium has been shown to have antiviral and immunomodulatory action, which may explain the reduction of mortality in bipolar patients, beyond its anti-suicidal and mood-stabilizing effects (Lieb 2002). A recent study has also demonstrated that risk of suicide attempt and completed suicide is lower during treatment with lithium that during treatment with divalproex (Goodwin et al. 2003).

Comorbidity

A large proportion of individuals with bipolar disorder also abuse drugs and alcohol. Around 35% of patients with bipolar disorder may drink alcohol excessively, and studies have found that women with bipolar II disorder are much more likely to abuse alcohol than their bipolar I counterparts, whereas among the men, bipolar I and bipolar II patients were equally likely to drink alcohol excessively (Goodwin & Jamison, 1990).

The data on drug abuse are much less extensive than those on alcohol abuse, but there is convincing data that shows that the rate of misuse of illicit substances such as cocaine and marijuana is greater in bipolar patients than in the general population. These drugs may destabilize the illness and trigger (hypo)mania. Early detection and treatment of drug or alcohol misuse is an essential part of the clinical management of those with bipolar disorders.

Neuropsychology

Kraepelin's proposed separation of the psychoses into dementia praecox and manic-depressive insanity, the latter being characterized by an episodic course and benign prognosis, is further undermined by emerging data revealing cognitive dysfunction not only in acute episodes but also in the euthymic phase of bipolar disorder. This intriguing field of research has recently been reviewed by Chowdhury et al. (2003).

A number of studies have reported a wide spectrum of cognitive impairments in patients with bipolar disorders in both the manic and the depressive phases of the illness. Abnormalities have been found in tests of frontal lobe function, verbal fluency, verbal memory and sustained attention. More recently cognitive assessment of euthymic bipolar patients have been undertaken in order to identify trait-dependent rather than state-dependent neuropsychological deficits. A recent study has demonstrated impairment of executive function, which entails a variety of processes responsible for the control of cognition and the regulation of behaviour and thought, in a cohort of patients prospectively verified as euthymic (Thompson et al. 2003). Other studies have also demonstrated impairment in verbal recall, verbal and visual declarative memory, recognition and general learning in euthymic bipolar patients.

It is currently unclear when, in relation to the natural history of the illness, cognitive deficits develop. Neuropsychological deficits may represent a progressive disease process, possibly mediated by hypercortisolaemia, resulting in hippocampal cell toxicity, decreased glucocorticoid receptors, and eventual cell death. The balance of evidence supports the view that even during periods of euthymia there remain residual, and possibly progressive, cognitive deficits. Long term, prospective studies are awaited to elucidate further the neuropathophysiological relevance of these early findings.

MANAGEMENT

Early identification and relapse signatures

Emerging studies in schizophrenia suggest that early intervention is important in improving outcome.

Accumulating evidence supports the notion that the psychotic process may have a 'toxic' effect upon the brain with long-term sequelae. Such studies are lacking in bipolar disorder, and the neurobiological consequences of delaying detection and diagnosis are currently unknown. It is clear, however, that both the depressive and manic phases of bipolar disorder are characterized by severe disruption to interpersonal, social and occupational functioning, as well as the risks associated with reckless and disinhibited behaviour, and suicidal ideation. In order to minimize impairment of function and risk it is imperative that clinicians are competent in diagnosing these conditions and arranging suitable management.

Patterns of symptoms characterizing a relapse of depression or mania are often stable within individuals, and many patients are able to identify changes in emotional, behavioural or cognitive functioning that herald a relapse. These patterns of symptoms are often referred to as 'relapse signatures'. Family members or close friends may be the first to notice these symptoms, and they should be encouraged to seek appropriate help from relevant professionals.

Appropriate referral and treatment settings

Individuals suspected of suffering from bipolar disorder should be referred to a psychiatrist to clarify the diagnosis, and to commence appropriate treatment. Patients with milder illness may be managed as outpatients, often with support from the community mental health team, family and friends. Those with more severe mania or depression, particularly when associated with aggression, reckless behaviour or suicidal behaviour, may require assessment and treatment in psychiatric in-patient facilities.

Severe mood episodes may be accompanied by a loss of insight, and patients may refuse voluntary admission to hospital. In such situations consideration should be given to the use of statutory powers for compulsory admission. Although involuntary detention may be traumatic for patients and their families and friends, often it is necessary to arrange hospital admission in order to prevent further deterioration and expedite treatment.

Hospital admission

Following admission to hospital all patients should undergo a full physical examination as soon as is practicable. Particular attention should be given to hydration, signs of intercurrent physical illness, and neurological abnormalities. Laboratory investigations should usually include full blood count, baseline urea and electrolytes, tests of thyroid and liver function and urine drug screening. It may be appropriate to request serum drug levels in patients already taking psychotropic medication. An electrocardiogram (ECG) should be considered for all patients on psychotropic medication, particularly high dose regimens, and measurement of metabolic parameters such as fasting blood glucose, triglycerides and cholesterol may be indicated in those on antipsychotic agents. The need for other investigations such as an electroencephalogram (EEG) or neuroimaging will be determined by the history and physical examination.

Manic patients may require individual attention by members of nursing staff, particularly if hyperactive, aggressive or disinhibited. Occasionally it may be necessary to arrange transfer to a locked unit to prevent the individual from leaving. Over-stimulation should be avoided, and restrictions on visiting times or other social activities may need to be implemented. An acutely manic patient can cause considerable disruption to other patients on the ward, and may test limits imposed by ward staff. A firm, non-negotiable approach should be employed by all members of staff in order to minimize disruption and facilitate communication. Behaviour prior to admission may have resulted in alienation from family members or friends, and these issues should be addressed through careful negotiation and education.

Physical treatment

Pharmacological treatment is the cornerstone of the management of bipolar disorders (see also Chapter 38). As a consequence of the relative dearth of high quality research into bipolar disorders, it has been difficult to assert with confidence the optimal treatment for patients suffering from manic-depressive illness. In recent years, however, the pharmacological management of bipolar disorder has attracted considerable research interest and a number of methodologically robust drug trials, combined with ongoing basic science research, have provided important information to guide treatment. As a testimony to recent advances in the treatment of bipolar disorders, the British Association for Psychopharmacology has recently published evidence-based treatment guidelines (Goodwin 2003).

Drugs used in the management of bipolar disorders (Table 20.2)

Mood-stabilizers

A mood-stabilizer can be defined most simply as a drug that improves either depression or mania and does not worsen or precipitate either state. Additional criteria include efficacy in the treatment of both poles of the illness and prevention of recurrence of mood episodes. The most commonly used mood-stabilizing agents prescribed for the treatment of bipolar disorder are lithium and the anti-convulsant drugs sodium valproate and carbamazepine. These drugs are used either alone or in combination.

Lithium

Historically lithium salts were used as salt substitutes in heart disease, but they were banned in the USA in 1949 following several deaths resulting from toxicity. In the same year John Cade investigated the use of lithium in psychosis,

Table 20.2 Commonly used drugs in the management of bipolar disorder

Drug	Uses
Mood stabilizers: Lithium, Sodium valproate, Carbamazepine, Lamotrigine	Acute and maintenance treatment. Depressive and manic phases of the illness may respond preferentially to different agents
Antipsychotics: *Typical agents* Butyrophenones (e.g. haloperidol), Phenothiazines (e.g. chlorpromazine), Thioxanthenes (e.g. zuclopenthixol) *Atypical agents* Amisulpride, Clozapine, Olanzapine, Quetiapine, Risperidone, Zotepine	Acute and maintenance treatment. Acutely disturbed patients may require parenteral administration. Atypical agents may be associated with less long-term side effects, and have recently been shown to have mood-stabilizing properties
Antidepressants: all classes are potentially useful, but some classes (e.g. TCAs) may be associated with cycle acceleration	Treatment of acute depressive episodes. Should not be used 'unopposed' by a mood-stabilizer. May precipitate (hypo)mania
Benzodiazepines	For acute management of hyperactivity or agitation. Use the lowest possible dose for the shortest possible duration

and he found that there was a therapeutic effect in mania. The problems with toxicity remained until the introduction of serum monitoring in the 1960s. Subsequently lithium has been widely prescribed for the treatment of severe affective disorders.

Approximately 50% of manic patients will show a favourable response to lithium, but its full therapeutic effect is usually not evident until about three weeks after initial treatment. Used alone it is often more effective for the management or mild, rather than severe cases of mania. Patients with classic mania and a family history of bipolar disorder tend to respond more favourably than those with a mixed or dysphoric presentation. Lithium tends not to be effective in rapid cycling bipolar disorder, or mania secondary to organic brain disease.

Combinations of lithium and high-dose antipsychotic agents have been associated with neurological complications including irreversible brain damage. Antipsychotic drugs have been shown to increase intracellular lithium levels, and patients on such combinations should be carefully monitored for the development of neurological symptoms.

Side effects of lithium therapy include:

- **Thyroid dysfunction:** hypothyroidism, manifested by raised TSH, weight gain and lethargy, is the most common thyroid abnormality, although cases of hyperthyroidism associated with lithium treatment have been reported.
- **Renal dysfunction:** approximately one-third of patients receiving lithium treatment will experience polyuria and polydipsia. These conditions are usually reversible, and may respond to a reduction in dose.
- **Central nervous system effects:** a fine tremor of the hands may occur in up to a quarter of patients taking lithium. Extra-pyramidal side effects may also be exacerbated in patients who are prescribed antipsychotic drugs.
- **Cognitive side effects:** there is controversy about the effects of lithium therapy on cognitive function, including memory. Some studies have shown evidence of memory impairment in patients on long-term lithium treatment, but this finding has not been replicated in all studies.
- **Skin:** lithium can cause psoriasis and acne, or exacerbate these conditions. Hair loss may also be a problem in a minority of patients.
- **Blood:** lithium may produce reversible leucocytosis.
- **Weight gain:** weight gain may be a significant problem. Lithium is known to cause alterations to glucose tolerance and insulin metabolism, which may be the causal link.
- **Gastrointestinal:** mild abdominal discomfort with loose stools may occur during initial treatment with lithium.

Lithium toxicity is potentially fatal and is manifested by three groups of symptoms: gastrointestinal; motor and cerebral. Toxicity can be classified as mild, moderate or severe:

- **Mild:** nausea and diarrhoea; severe fine tremor; impaired concentration.
- **Moderate:** nausea, vomiting and diarrhoea; coarse tremor, cerebellar ataxia and dysarthria; drowsiness and disorientation.
- **Severe:** vomiting and incontinence; Parkinsonism, myoclonus, cerebellar dysfunction and seizures; apathy and coma.

Signs of toxicity usually develop over a period of days. Patients receiving lithium therapy who are at risk of salt-depletion, are particularly prone to develop lithium toxicity. The onset of diarrhoea, vomiting or excessive sweating should alert the clinician to the possibility of impending toxicity. Glomerular filtration rate in the elderly is reduced and lower doses are required to reach therapeutic serum levels.

Sodium valproate

Sodium valproate is a branched-chain fatty acid and mildly inhibits cytochrome enzymes. It is of use in a proportion of patients with mania, and those who do not respond to lithium or carbamazepine may benefit from valproate either alone or in combination. The time to onset of action is similar to that of lithium. Valproate may also be useful in prophylaxis of bipolar disorder, and it may have a particular role in the management of rapid cycling. A recent Cochrane review examined the role of valproate in the maintenance treatment of bipolar disorder and summarized the efficacy and acceptability of valproate (Macritchie et al. 2002).

Valproate semisodium ('Depakote') is an equimolar combination of sodium valproate and valproic acid, and this formulation has recently been granted a licence in the UK for the treatment of manic episodes associated with bipolar disorder. The National Institute for Clinical Excellence (NICE) has also recently recommended the use of valproate semisodium for the control of the acute symptoms associated with the manic phase of bipolar I disorder (NICE 2003a).

Valproate is generally well tolerated, but side effects include vomiting, tremor, ataxia, weight gain, rash, hair loss, and potentially acute liver damage. In children and patients with a history of liver disease liver function tests should be performed before treatment, and subsequently monitored.

Carbamazepine

Carbamazepine is a dibenzazepine derivative with a tricyclic structure. Trials show that 50–60% of patients with mania show a favourable response to carbamazepine. There is less evidence to support the role of carbamazepine in the prophylaxis of bipolar disorder, and there is a suggestion that despite the initial response rate, its effectiveness may diminish over 2–3 years.

The most common side effects are nausea, dizziness, ataxia and diplopia. Other side effects include headache, drowsiness and nystagmus. Occasionally, serious toxic side effects may develop such as agranulocytosis, aplastic anaemia or Stevens–Johnson syndrome. Leucopenia may develop in 1–2% of patients, and this is most frequently transient occurring at the initiation of treatment.

Other mood stabilizing agents

A number of other anticonvulsant drugs have recently been shown to have efficacy in the management of bipolar disorders. This is unlikely to be a class effect, as not all anticonvulsants have therapeutic effects in the management of depression or mania. Lamotrigine has been shown to have antidepressant effects in bipolar depression, but it appears only to have a weak antimanic effect. It may be particularly useful in the management of bipolar II disorder and rapid cycling bipolar disorder. Gabapentin, used in treatment-resistant temporal lobe epilepsy, may also have a role as adjunctive therapy in bipolar disorder, but recent trials have failed to show any clear benefit in the management of either mania or depression.

Antipsychotics

Antipsychotic drugs are conventionally divided into 'typical' and the newer 'atypical' agents, and both groups have played a role in the management of bipolar disorders. Of the typical antipsychotics, haloperidol (a butyrophenone) is frequently used in the treatment of mania, but phenothiazines and thioxanthenes are also effective. In acutely disturbed patients who refuse oral medication intramuscular preparations may be used. Improvement in manic symptoms usually begins 1–3 days after commencing treatment, and more gradual improvement occurs over the following two weeks. Apart from the drowsiness which is associated with treatment with antipsychotic agents, particularly in high dose, extrapyramidal side effects, particularly acute dystonia, may be troublesome. Anti-parkinsonian medication, such as procyclidine given orally or parenterally, should be used if these side effects emerge. Typical antipsychotic depot preparations currently retain a role in the management of bipolar disorder, but it is possible they will be supplanted by the newer atypical depot agents in the future. More detailed description of the side effects associated with antipsychotic drugs is given elsewhere in Chapter 38.

The currently available atypical agents are amisulpride, clozapine, olanzapine, quetiapine, risperidone and zotepine. Of these, at the time of writing only olanzapine and quetiapine have a licence in the UK for the treatment of manic episodes, and recent NICE guidelines recommend the use of olanzapine for control of the acute symptoms associated with the manic phase of bipolar I disorder (NICE 2003a). Atypical antipsychotics may be better tolerated than the older agents, and extrapyramidal side effects may be less frequent.

The anti-manic effects of antipsychotic drugs are likely to be mediated through blockade of the dopamine (D2) receptor, but other pharmacological mechanisms cannot be excluded.

Antidepressants

The treatment of depression and a description of the various classes of antidepressant drugs are discussed elsewhere in this volume. The management of depression in bipolar disorder can be particularly challenging given the risk of precipitating a switch to (hypo)mania and rapid cycling. As discussed above, tricyclic antidepressants may be associated with a greater risk of destabilizing the illness and causing cycle acceleration.

Benzodiazepines

Benzodiazepines may have a role in the management of acute episodes of affective illness in bipolar disorder, particularly in manic patients who are overactive and require night sedation. The use of benzodiazepines, however, should be limited to the lowest possible dose for the shortest possible time, because of their potential for dependence.

Electroconvulsive therapy (ECT)

ECT is an effective treatment for mood disorders despite the negative public perception. The effectiveness of ECT has recently been demonstrated in a meta-analysis of the efficacy and safety in depressive disorders (UK ECT Review Group 2003). NICE has recently published guidelines on the use of ECT. These recommendations state that ECT should be used only in patients with severe depressive illness, catatonia or a prolonged or severe manic episode, and only then after an adequate trial of other treatment has proven ineffective and/or when the condition is considered to be potentially life-threatening (NICE 2003b).

Treatment of different phases of bipolar illness

The treatment of bipolar disorder can be divided into several phases:

- acute manic or mixed episode
- acute depressive episode
- prophylactic treatment
- treatment in special situations.

Drug management of acute mania or mixed episodes

A summary of the efficacy of commonly used drugs in the treatment of bipolar disorder is given in Table 20.3.

Table 20.3 Summary of the efficacy of commonly used drugs in the treatment of bipolar disorder

	Mania	Depression	Rapid cycling	Prophylaxis
Lithium	+++	+	+	+++
Semisodium valproate	+++	+	++	+
Carbamazepine	+++	+	++	+
Lamotrigine	+	+++	+++	++
Typical antipsychotics	+++	−	+	+
Atypical antipsychotics	+++	+	++	++

+++ = good evidence; ++ = some evidence; + = limited evidence; − = no evidence

For patients not already established on long-term treatment for bipolar disorder, severe manic or mixed states should be treated with an antipsychotic or valproate because of their rapid antimanic effect. Parenteral medication (antipsychotic or benzodiazepine drugs) may be required in the more disturbed patient refusing oral medication. Less severe forms of mania may be treated with lithium or carbamezepine. If the patient is receiving antidepressant medication this should be tapered and stopped.

If the patient is already receiving long-term treatment for bipolar disorder, it is likely that a mood stabilizing agent(s) will have been prescribed. Compliance with prescribed medication should be ascertained, and measuring serum levels of lithium, carbamazepine or valproate may be helpful. If poor compliance is an issue this should prompt a careful enquiry into any side-effects from prescribed medication. Increasing the dose to ensure that the highest well-tolerated dose is offered may control symptoms. If symptoms are inadequately controlled then a combination of lithium or valproate with an antipsychotic should be considered. Clozapine may be considered in refractory illness. Psychotic symptoms during a manic or mixed episode should be treated with an antipsychotic drug, and preferably an atypical agent because of their more favourable side-effect profile.

When full remission of symptoms occurs, drugs used for the treatment of the acute episode may be tapered over a two-week period and discontinued. Drugs which have been shown to be effective in preventing relapse (especially lithium and valproate) may be continued when long-term treatment is planned (see below).

Drug management of acute depression

Antidepressant monotherapy is not recommended for patients with a diagnosis of bipolar disorder. An antidepressant and an antimanic agent (e.g. lithium, valproate or an antipsychotic) should be considered for the treatment of an acute depressive episode. An antipsychotic should be used if there are psychotic symptoms present. If depressive symptoms are less severe then initial treatment with lamotrigine, lithium or valproate may be effective. If the patient fails to respond to these strategies then augmentation or switching the antidepressant drug may be effective. ECT should be considered for patients with high suicidal risk, psychosis or severe depression during pregnancy (see above).

The choice of antidepressant for the treatment of bipolar depression should be guided by the risks of precipitating a switch to (hypo)mania. SSRIs are probably safer than tricyclic antidepressants in this regard, but tricyclics may have a role in treatment-resistant depression.

Episodes of bipolar depression which remit tend to be shorter than unipolar depression, and antidepressant treatment should be tapered and discontinued when symptoms have fully resolved. This may occur after as little as 12 weeks of treatment.

Maintenance treatment

Long-term treatment should be considered in a patient who presents following a single manic episode. Patient education is crucial to inform the individual of the importance of maintenance therapy in reducing the risks or relapse, and to encourage compliance with medication. Even in patients established on long-term treatment who have remained well for a number of years, the risks of relapse remain high following discontinuation of mood-stabilizing agents, and encouragement to remain on treatment indefinitely should be offered.

Lithium monotherapy should be considered initially as it has been shown to have efficacy in preventing both manic and depressive relapse, although it is more effective in preventing mania. Lithium also is associated with a reduced risk of suicide in bipolar illness. If lithium is poorly tolerated or ineffective then valproate, or carbamazepine may be considered. Other options include olanzapine and lamotrigine. Olanzapine has been shown to have mood stabilizing properties and prevents manic more than depressive relapse. Lamotrigine prevents depressive more than manic relapse. If monotherapy fails then a combination of mood-stabilizing agents should be considered. If the main burden of illness is (hypo)mania then two antimanic drugs (lithium, valproate or an antipsychotic) should be considered, and where the burden is depression, lamotrigine or an antidepressant in combination with an antimanic agent may be effective.

Drug treatment of rapid cycling

The treatment of rapid cycling bipolar disorder presents a significant challenge. It is important to identify and treat co-morbid conditions (such as hypothyroidism or substance misuse) that may be contributing to cycling. Antidepressants should be tapered and discontinued. Lithium may not be as effective in treating rapid cycling, but several recent studies have provided compelling evidence to support the use of anticonvulsants, particularly lamotrigine.

Drug treatment during pregnancy

Some psychotropic drugs used in the maintenance phase of bipolar illness have teratogenic potential. The risk does not appear to be as great with antipsychotic agents, lamotrigine and antidepressants. Lithium, carbamazepine and valproate are all associated with higher risk of foetal abnormalities. With regard to breastfeeding, there is no absolute contraindication with any of the drugs used in bipolar disorder, but women taking lithium should be advised not to breast feed.

Experimental drug treatments

Omega-3 fatty acids

The role of omega-3 fatty acids (derived mainly from fish oil) has been investigated in cardiovascular disease with encouraging results, but more recently a link has been suggested between omega-3 fatty acid consumption and depression. One small study has shown that adjunctive eicopantanoic acid (EPA) and docosahexanoic acid supplements, used as maintenance therapy, improve symptoms in patients with bipolar disorder (Stoll et al. 1999). A recent randomized four-month, placebo-controlled trial of EPA in bipolar depression showed significant improvements in 'Global Assessment of Function' and improvement on the 'Inventory of Depressive Symptoms' in patients who remained on treatment for greater than 10 weeks, but no differences between placebo and EPA-treated patients at endpoint (Keck et al. 2003). Additional trials are needed to clarify these findings, and further investigation into their possible mode of action is awaited.

Antiglucocorticoids

As referred to above, abnormalities of HPA axis function characterize both unipolar and bipolar affective disorders, and elevated corticosteroid levels are found. Such abnormalities may cause or exacerbate both neurocognitive and depressive symptoms, and reduction of cortisol levels may have therapeutic value. Preliminary data suggests that cortisol synthesis inhibitors may have antidepressant effects, and the role of glucocorticoid receptor antagonists in affective disorders has attracted recent research interest. At high doses, the progesterone receptor antagonist mifepristone (RU-486) becomes an antagonist of the glucocorticoid receptor subtype of the corticosteroid receptor, and a recent preliminary study in patients with bipolar disorder has shown that treatment with mifepristone resulted in selective improvement in neurocognitive functioning and mood (Young et al. 2004). Further studies are needed to establish the therapeutic value of these agents.

Non-physical management

Although pharmacological treatment is the cornerstone in the management of bipolar disorder, the past several decades have witnessed a growing interest in the role of psychological approaches to alleviate symptoms, restore psychosocial functioning and prevent relapse and recurrence. Some of these developments are considered below.

Psychoeducation

There is a paucity of data on the effects of psychological interventions in bipolar disorder. The psychoeducative approach has been investigated by researchers for many years, but the first studies of its efficacy have only recently been published. Many of the published studies have reported only data on indirect measures of efficacy such as a change in patients' attitudes to medication. The 'Life Goals Programme' is a form of group psychoeducation, which when used as a part of a multimodal programme, has been shown to reduce emergency department use and costs and was one of the first well-structured group interventions specifically designed for bipolar patients.

The first randomized blinded clinical trial comparing the efficacy of group psychoeducation with standard treatment of bipolar I and bipolar II disorder has recently been published (Colom et al. 2003). The treatment tested in this study combined three interventions which have shown some efficacy individually: early detection of relapse signatures, enhancement of treatment compliance, and induction of lifestyle regularity. Group psychoeduction significantly reduced the number of relapsed patients and the number of recurrences per patient, and increased the time to depression, manic, hypomanic, and mixed occurrences. The number and length of hospitalizations per patient were also lower. Although these results are encouraging, the nature of the efficacy of psychoeducation is unknown, and future studies are needed to examine the specific content of the program which is associated with a better outcome.

Interpersonal and social rhythms therapy

Bipolar disorder is associated with persistent deficits in functioning over time, and for many patients psychosocial functioning remains markedly impaired. Until recently psychotherapy was considered to be superfluous in the treatment of this patient group, but within the last decade serious attempts have been made to develop and study manual-based psychological treatments for patients with bipolar I disorder. *Interpersonal and social rhythm therapy* (IPSRT) is a present-focused interpersonal treatment that views the core deficit in bipolar disorder as one of instability and that disturbed biological rhythms may arise from disruptions in social routine. IPSRT appears to be beneficial in terms of reducing the time to recovery from bipolar depressive episodes, but this form of psychotherapy has not proved to be useful in preventing relapse.

Cognitive therapy

The place of cognitive therapy in the management of bipolar disorder has been reviewed by Scott (2001). Beck's original cognitive model of depression and mania has been adapted to provide a framework for understanding the psychopathology of bipolar disorders. Cognitive therapy using this model is designed to facilitate acceptance of the disorder and the need for treatment; to help the individual recognize and manage psychosocial stressors and interpersonal problems; to improve medication adherence; to teach strategies to cope with depression and hypomania; to teach early recognition of relapse signatures; and to identify and modify negative automatic thoughts, and underlying maladaptive assumptions and beliefs.

Preliminary findings indicate that cognitive therapy may be beneficial for patients with bipolar disorder, and may be particularly suitable for patients who wish to take an equal and active role in their therapy. Randomized, controlled trials are needed, however, to establish the short-term and long-term benefits of cognitive therapy in bipolar disorder, and whether any reported health gain exceeds that of standard treatment.

CONCLUSIONS

It is clear that in recent years the concept of bipolar disorder has expanded, and the inclusion of more subtle variations of mood within the bipolar spectrum has challenged the often quoted lifetime incidence rate of ~1%. The increasing recognition of the importance of accurate diagnosis and treatment of individuals with bipolar disorders has significant public health and funding implications. Sadly, compared with schizophrenia, for example, the bipolar disorders remain the poor relation, and it is only in recent years that researchers have turned their attention to the investigation of the pathogenesis and management of these severe mental illnesses. Although still in its infancy, our understanding of these disorders is rapidly increasing. Continued research interest and activity should provide us with further insights into the mechanisms underlying the development of bipolar disorders, which ultimately may have profound consequences for the timing and choice of treatment.

FURTHER READING

Marneros A & Angst J (eds) (2000) *Bipolar Disorders: 100 Years After Manic Depressive Insanity*. Dorddrecht, Boston, London: Kluwer Academic Publishers.
Cookson J, Taylor D, Katona C (2002) *The Use of Drugs in Psychiatry*. London: Gaskell.

REFERENCES

Akiskal HS (1996) The prevalent clinical spectrum of bipolar disorders: beyond DSM-IV. *Journal of Clinical Psychiatry* **17**(suppl 3): 117–22.
Akiskal HS, Djenderedjian AH, Rosenthal RH et al. (1977) Cyclothymic disorder: validating criteria for inclusion in the bipolar affective group. *American Journal of Psychiatry* **134**: 1227–33.
Akiskal HS & Mallya G (1987) Criteria for the 'soft' bipolar spectrum: treatment implications. *Psychopharmacology Bulletin* **23**: 68–73.
Angst J (1966) Zur Ätiologie und Nosologie endogener depressiver Psychosen. Eine genetisch, soziologische und klinische Studie. Berlin, Heidelberg, New York: Springer.
Angst J (1978) The course of affective disorders. II. Typology of bipolar manic-depressive illness. *Archiv für Psychiatrie und Nervenkrankheiten* **226**: 65–73.
Angst J, Gamma A, Benazzi F, Ajdacic V, Eich D & Rossler W (2003). Toward a re-definition of subthreshold bipolarity: epidemiology and proposed criteria for bipolar II, minor bipolar disorders and hypomania. *Journal of Affective Disorders* **73**: 133–46.
Baldessarini RJ, Tondol L & Hennen J (1999) Effects of lithium treatment and its discontinuation on suicidal behaviour in bipolar manic depressive disorders. *Journal of Clinical Psychiatry* **60**(suppl 2): 77–83.
Baumann B & Bogerts B (2001). Neuroanatomical studies on bipolar disorder. *British Journal of Psychiatry* **178**(suppl 41): s142–7.
Chowdhury R, Ferrier IN & Thompson JM (2003) Cognitive dysfunction in bipolar disorder. *Current Opinion in Psychiatry* **16**: 7–12.
Colom F, Vieta E, Martinez-Aran A et al. (2003) A randomized trial on the efficacy of group psychoeducation in the prophylaxis of recurrences in bipolar patients whose disease is in remission. *Archives of General Psychiatry* **60**: 402–7.
Craddock N & Jones I (1999) The genetics of bipolar disorder. *Journal of Medical Genetics* **36**: 585–94.
Craddock N & Jones I (2001) Molecular genetics of biplar disorder. *British Journal of Psychiatry* **178**(suppl 41): s128–33.
Dunner DL & Fieve RR (1974) Clinical factors in lithium carbonate prophylaxis failure. *Archives of General Psychiatry* **30**: 229–233.
Falret JP (1851) De la folie circulaire ou forme de maladie mentale caracterisèe par l'alternative règulière de la manie et de la mèlancolie. *Bulletin of the Academy of Natural Medicine*, Paris.
Goodwin FK & Jamison KR (1990) *Manic Depressive Illness*. New York: Oxford University Press.
Goodwin FK, Fireman B, Simon GE, Hunkeler EM, Lee J & Revicki D (2003) Suicide risk in bipolar disorder during treatment with lithium and divalproex. *Journal of the American Medical Association* **290**: 1467–73.
Goodwin GM (2003) Evidence-based guidelines for treating bipolar disorder: recommendations from the British Association for Psychopharmacology. *Journal of Psychopharmacology* **17**: 149–73.
Griesinger W (1845) *Die Pathologie und Therapie der psychischen Krankheiten für Ärzte und Studierende*. Krabbe, Stuttgart.

Harrison PJ (2002) The neuropathology of primary mood disorder. *Brain* **125**: 1428–1449.

Keck PE, McElroy SL, Freeman MP et al. (2003) Randomized, placebo-controlled trial of eicopentanoic acid in bipolar depression. *Bipolar Disorders* **5**(suppl1): P100.

Kraepelin E (1896) Dementia praecox. In: *The Clinical Roots of the Schizophrenia Concept* (1897), pp15–24. Cambridge: Cambridge University Press.

Kupka R, Luckenbaugh D, Post R, et al. (2003) Rapid and non-rapid cycling bipolar disorder: A comparitive study using daily prospective mood ratings in 539 outpatients. *Bipolar Disorders* **5**(suppl 1): 62.

Lieb J (2002) Lithium and antidepressants: inhibiting eicosanoids, stimulating immunity, and defeating microorganisms. *Medical Hypotheses* **59**: 429–32.

McGuffin P, Rijsdijk F, Andrwe M, Sham P & Cardno A (2003) The heritability of bipolar affective disorder and the genetic relationship to unipolar depression. *Archives of General Psychiatry* **60**: 497–502.

McQuade R & Young AH (2000). Future therapeutic targets in mood disorders: the glucocorticoid receptor. *British Journal of Psychiatry* **177**: 390–5.

Macritchie KAN, Geddes JR, Scott J, Haslam DRS & Goodwin GM (2002) Valproic acid, valproate and divalproex in the maintenance treatment of bipolar disorder. *The Cochrane Database of Systematic Reviews*. Volume 4.

Marenos A, Deister A & Rohde A (1990) The concept of distinct but voluminous bipolar and unipolar diseases. Part III: Unipolar and bipolar comparison. *European Archives in Psychiatry & Clinical Neuroscience* **240**: 90–5.

Marneros A (2001) Expanding the group of bipolar disorders. *Journal of Affective Disorders* **62**: 39–44.

Moore PB, Shepherd DJ, Eccleston D, Macmillan IC, Goswami U, McAllister VL & Ferrier IN (2001) Cerebral white matter lesions in bipolar disorder: relationship to outcome. *British Journal of Psychiatry* **178**: 172–6.

National Institute for Clinical Excellence (2003a) Olanzapine and valproate semisodium in the treatment of acute mania associated with bipolar I disorder. Technology Appraisal No.66. Available at http://www.nice.org.uk [accessed 12/5/04].

National Institute for Clinical Excellence (2003b) Guidance on the use of electroconvulsive therapy. Technology Appraisal No.59. Available at http://www.nice.org.uk [accessed 12/5/04].

Peet M (1994) Induction of mania with selective serotonin reuptake inhibitors and tricyclic antidepressants. *British Journal of Psychiatry* **164**: 549–50.

Perris C (1966) A study of bipolar (manic-depressive) and unipolar recurrent depressive psychoses. *Acta Psychiatrica Scandinavica* **194**(suppl): 1–89.

Porter R (2002) *Madness: A Brief History*. Oxford: Oxford University Press.

Scott J (2001) Cognitive therapy as an adjunct to medication in bipolar disorder. *British Journal of Psychiatry* **178**(suppl 41): s164–8.

Stoll AL, Severus W, Freeman MP et al. (1999) Omega3 fatty acids in bipolar disorder: a preliminary double-blind, placebo-controlled trial. *Archives of General Psychiatry* **56**: 407–12.

Thompson JM, Gray JM, Mackin P, Ferrier IN, Young AH, Hamilton C & Quinn JG (2003). The executive-visuo-spatial sketchpad interface in euthymic bipolar disorder: implications for visuo-spatial working memory architecture. In: Kokinov B & Hirst W (eds).

Constructive Memory. NBU Series in Cognitive Science, pp305–317. Sofia: New Bulgarian University.

UK ECT Review Group (2003) Electroconvulsive therapy – systematic review and meta-analysis of efficacy and safety in depressive disorders. *Lancet* **361**: 799–808.

Wernicke C (1900) *Grundriss der Psychiatrie*. Leipzig: Thième.

Wolpert EA, Goldberg JF & Harrow M (1990) Rapid cycling unipolar and bipolar affective disorders. *American Journal of Psychiatry* **147**: 725–8.

Yildiz A & Sachs GS (2003) Do antidepressants induce rapid cycling? A gender-specific association. *Journal of Clinical Psychiatry* **64**: 814–18.

Young AH, Gallagher P, Watson S, Del-Estal D, Owen B & Ferrier IN (2004) Improvements in neurocognitive function and mood following adjunctive treatment with mifepristone (RU-486) in bipolar disorder. *Neuropsychopharmacology* [In press]

APPENDIX 1
DIAGNOSTIC CRITERIA: ICD-10

Hypomania

a The mood is elevated or irritable to a degree that is definitely abnormal for the individual concerned and sustained for at least four consecutive days.

b At least three of the following signs must be present, leading to some interference with personal functioning in daily living:

1 increased activity or physical restlessness
2 increased talkativeness
3 difficulty in concentration or distractibility
4 decreased need for sleep
5 increased sexual energy
6 mild overspending, or other types of reckless or irresponsible behaviour
7 increased sociability or overfamiliarity.

c The episode does not meet criteria for mania, bipolar affective disorder, depressive episode, cyclothymia or anorexia nervosa.

Mania

a Mood must be predominantly elevated, expansive or irritable, and definitely abnormal for the individual concerned. The mood change must be prominent and sustained for at least one week (unless it is severe enough to require hospital admission).

b At least three of the following signs must be present (four if the mood is merely irritable), leading to severe interference with personal functioning in daily living:

1 increased activity or physical restlessness
2 increased talkativeness ('pressure of speech')
3 flight of ideas or the subjective experience of thoughts racing
4 loss of normal social inhibitions, resulting in a behaviour that is inappropriate to the circumstances
5 decreased need for sleep
6 inflated self-esteem or grandiosity
7 distractibility or constant changes in activity or plans
8 behaviour that is foolhardy or reckless and whose risks the individual does not recognize, e.g. spending sprees, foolish enterprises, reckless driving
9 marked sexual energy or sexual indiscretions.

c There are no hallucinations or delusions, although perceptual disorders may occur (e.g. subjective hyperacusis, appreciation of colours as especially vivid). (If delusions or hallucinations are present then the episode is specified as 'mania with psychotic symptoms'.)

d The episode is not attributable to psychoactive substance use or to any organic mental disorder.

Bipolar affective disorder

a The current episode meets the criteria for hypomania, mania, depression or a mixed state.(If the current episode is classified as mixed then both manic and depressive symptoms must be prominent most of the time during a period of at least two weeks.)

b There has been at least one other affective episode in the past, meeting the criteria for hypomanic or manic episode, depressive episode or mixed affective episode. (If the current episode is classified as depression then there must have been at least one authenticated hypomanic or manic episode or mixed affective episode in the past.)

Cyclothymia

a There must have been a period of at least two years of instability of mood involving several periods of both depression and hypomania, with or without intervening periods of normal mood.

b None of the manifestations of depression or hypomania during such a two-year period should be sufficiently severe or long-lasting to meet the criteria for manic episode or depressive episode (moderate or severe); however, manic or depressive episode(s) may have occurred before, or may develop after, such a period of persistent mood instability.

c During at least some of the periods of depression at least three of the following should be present:

1 reduced energy or activity
2 insomnia
3 loss of self-confidence or feelings of inadequacy
4 difficulty in concentrating
5 social withdrawal
6 loss of interest in or enjoyment of sex and other pleasurable activities
7 reduced talkativeness
8 pessimism about the future or brooding over the past.

d During at least some of the periods of mood elevation at least three of the following should be present:

1 increased energy or activity
2 decreased need for sleep
3 inflated self-esteem
4 sharpened or unusually creative thinking
5 increased gregariousness
6 increased talkativeness or wittiness

7 increased interest and involvement in sexual and other pleasurable activities

8 over-optimism or exaggeration of past achievements.

APPENDIX 2
DIAGNOSTIC CRITERIA: DSM-IV

Hypomania

a A distinct period of persistently elevated, expansive, or irritable mood, lasting throughout at least four days, which is clearly different from the usual non-depressed mood.

b During the period of mood disturbance, three (or more) of the following symptoms have persisted (four if the mood is only irritable) and have been present to a significant degree:

1 inflated self-esteem or grandiosity

2 decreased need for sleep

3 more talkative than usual or pressure to keep talking

4 flight of ideas or subjective experience that thoughts are racing

5 distractibility

6 increase in goal-directed activity

7 excessive involvement in pleasurable activities that have a high potential for painful consequences.

c The episode is associated with an unequivocal change in functioning that is characteristic of the person when not symptomatic.

d The disturbance in mood and the change in functioning are observable by others.

e The episode is not severe enough to cause marked impairment in social or occupational functioning, or to necessitate hospitalization, and there are no psychotic features.

f The symptoms are not due to the direct physiological effects of a substance (e.g. a drug of abuse, a medication, or other treatment) or a general medical condition (e.g. hyperthyroidism).

Mania

a A distinct period of abnormally and persistently elevated, expansive, or irritable mood, lasting throughout at least one week (or any duration if hospitalization is necessary).

b During the period of mood disturbance, three (or more) of the following symptoms have persisted (four if the mood is only irritable) and have been present to a significant degree:

1 inflated self-esteem or grandiosity

2 decreased need for sleep

3 more talkative than usual or pressure to keep talking

4 flight of ideas or subjective experience that thoughts are racing

5 distractibility

6 increase in goal-directed activity

7 excessive involvement in pleasurable activities that have a high potential for painful consequences.

c The symptoms do not meet criteria for a mixed episode.

d The mood disturbance is sufficiently severe to cause marked impairment in occupational functioning or in usual social activities or relationships with others, or to necessitate hospitalization to prevent harm to self or others, or there are psychotic features.

e The symptoms are not due to the direct physiological effects of a substance (e.g. a drug of abuse, a medication, or other treatment) or a general medical condition (e.g. hyperthyroidism).

Bipolar I disorder

Bipolar I disorder, single manic episode

a Presence of only one manic episode and no past major depressive episodes.

b The manic episode is not better accounted for by schizoaffective disorder and is not superimposed on schizophrenia, schizophreniform disorder, delusional disorder, or psychotic disorder not otherwise specified.

Bipolar I disorder, most recent episode hypomanic

a Currently (or most recently) in a hypomanic episode.

b There has previously been at least one manic episode.

c The mood symptoms cause clinically significant distress or impairment in social, occupational, or other important areas of functioning.

d The mood episodes in criteria A and B are not better accounted for by schizoaffective disorder, and are not superimposed on schizophrenia, schizophreniform disorder, delusional disorder, or psychotic disorder not otherwise specified.

Bipolar I disorder, most recent episode manic

a Currently (or most recently) in a manic episode.

b There has previously been at least one major depressive episode, manic episode, or mixed episode.

c The mood episodes in criteria A and B are not better accounted for by schizoaffective disorder, and are not superimposed on schizophrenia, schizophreniform disorder, delusional disorder, or psychotic disorder not otherwise specified.

Bipolar I disorder, most recent episode mixed

a | Currently (or most recently) in a mixed episode.
b | There has previously been at least one major depressive episode, manic episode, or mixed episode.
c | The mood episodes in criteria A and B are not better accounted for by schizoaffective disorder, and are not superimposed on schizophrenia, schizophreniform disorder, delusional disorder, or psychotic disorder not otherwise specified.

Bipolar I disorder, most recent episode depressed

a | Currently (or most recently) in a major depressive episode.
b | There has previously been at least one manic episode or mixed episode.
c | The mood episodes in criteria A and B are not better accounted for by schizoaffective disorder, and are not superimposed on schizophrenia, schizophreniform disorder, delusional disorder, or psychotic disorder not otherwise specified.

Bipolar II disorder

a | Presence (or history) of one or more major depressive episodes.
b | Presence (or history) of at least one hypomanic episode.
c | There has never been a manic episode.
d | The mood episodes in criteria A and B are not better accounted for by schizoaffective disorder, and are not superimposed on schizophrenia, schizophreniform disorder, delusional disorder, or psychotic disorder not otherwise specified.
e | The symptoms cause clinically significant distress or impairment in social, occupational, or other important areas of functioning.

Cyclothymic disorder

a | For at least two years, the presence of numerous periods with hypomanic symptoms and numerous periods with depressive symptoms that do not meet criteria for a major depressive episode. (In children and adolescents, the duration must be at least one year.)
b | During the above two-year period (one year in children and adolescents), the person has not been without the symptoms in criteria A for more than two months at a time.
c | No major depressive episode, manic episode, or mixed episode has been present during the first two years of the disturbance
d | The symptoms in criteria A are not better accounted for by schizoaffective disorder, and are not superimposed on schizophrenia, schizophreniform disorder, delusional disorder, or psychotic disorder not otherwise specified.
e | The symptoms are not due to the direct physiological effects of a substance (e.g. a drug of abuse, a medication, or other treatment) or a general medical condition (e.g. hyperthyroidism).
f | The symptoms cause clinically significant distress or impairment in social, occupational, or other important areas of functioning.

Suicide and deliberate self-harm

Shankarnanarayan Srinath

SUICIDE

Epidemiology

Suicide is recognized as an important public health issue in the UK and the world (Department of Health 1992). According to the World Health Organization, 814 000 killed themselves in the year 2000 (World Health Organization 2001). The suicide rate in the UK is 9.7 per 100 000 population and constitutes nearly 1% of deaths from all causes annually. A total of 10 040 suicides and probable suicides were reported in the two–year period between April 1996 and March 1998. Two-thirds were confirmed by coroners as suicide and a third carried open verdicts or deaths from undetermined causes (Safer Services 1999).

Suicide rates have increased by 60% in some countries in the last 45 years (Bertolote et al. 2003). The rate for young men is starker and is significantly higher in comparison with the older population. In the UK the rate for male adolescents and young men aged 15–24 years is 12.2 per 100 000 (Commonwealth Department of Human Services and Health 1995) and if the age range is narrowed to 15– to 19–year-olds, the rate increases to 13.2 per 100 000 (Shaffer & Piacentini 1994). A recent study of suicides in 15– to 19–year-olds in rural Southern India reported alarming rates of 148 per 100 000 girls and 58 per 100 000 boys (Aaron et al. 2004).

Suicide is rare in children under the age of 14, but it is increasing in the USA in this age group. Shaffer (1974, 1985) found that social isolation, as in adults, was an important factor in child suicide. Large proportions of the suicidal children were school refusers and many of them killed themselves at home while their parents were at work. Shaffer suggests that the protection that family and school provide may account for the low rate of suicide in children. Also children's concept of death is limited by their cognitive immaturity. Children below the age of nine see death as a temporary state (Nagy 1948) and as a reversible, external event – as going away on a journey from which one returns later (Jones 1911; Rochlin 1959; Speece & Brent 1984). Weininger (1979) found that children younger than 4 years did not understand the distinction between animate and inanimate objects and only 20% of children under the age of nine saw death as final.

Statistical data grossly under-represent the true figures for suicide for several reasons:

- A legal verdict of suicide demands evidence of intent. A rigorous application of this definition excludes a large number of deaths from this category where the intent is not clear or the method renders the intent more ambiguous. For example, only 54% of deaths by drowning are deemed to be suicides while 98% of deaths by hanging are recorded as such (Williams & Pollock 1993). Many deaths which may appear as accidents may indeed be suicides, such as those who may be viewed as falling out of windows instead of jumping out, and those who are killed in road accidents when they are drunk (Zilbroog 1937).
- Social, cultural and religious attitudes often inhibit disclosure of deaths by suicide. Suicide has evoked greater primitive fear and censure than murder throughout history (Anderson & Dartington 1998).
- Suicide has been seen as a dishonourable act, a sin or a work of the devil from around 500 BC, an act so terrible that Death would return to haunt the living. Unsuccessful suicides suffered severe retribution. Successful ones were denied a decent burial and their property was confiscated. Their bodies would not be bought out of the house through the door but through a window or hole in the wall. Attempted suicide was indeed a punishable offence in the UK from 1745 until as late as 1961 (Retterstol 1998; 2000).

Suicide rates have fluctuated in the 20th century. The rate declined significantly during the two World Wars. It rose in the 1930s possibly because of the economic depression and again after the Second World War through the 1950s and the early 1960s. It fell in the late 1960s and the early 1970s, but has steadily increased since, especially among young men. The reasons for these changes are not clear.

The most common methods of suicide are hanging, self-poisoning (usually overdoses) and carbon monoxide poisoning through car exhausts. Fifty-four per cent of the sample reported by the recent National Confidential Inquiry (Safer Services 1999) used violent methods such as hanging, jumping from a height or in front of a moving vehicle, accounting for two-thirds of male and two-fifths of female suicides. Men took their lives more commonly by physical methods followed by overdoses; women most frequently resorted to overdoses, followed in frequency by hanging. Occasionally suicide is a result of a suicide pact, a *folie-á-deux*, and sometimes it may follow murder.

The drugs most frequently used in overdoses are prescribed psychotropic drugs. Suicides who have previously harmed themselves are more likely to kill themselves with psychotropic drugs. Paracetamol ingestion surprisingly accounts for only 4% of the suicides by overdose.

Patient characteristics associated with suicide

- The male to female ratio is 3:1. Men outnumber women in all age groups (Arto et al. 1988; Barraclough & Hughes 1987; Safer Services 1999). This may be because women are freer in expressing their feelings (Gould 1965) and the less aggressive methods such as drug overdose that they employ are also less effective. The ratio is higher among teenagers and young people (Burton et al.1990; McClure 1987; Moser et al.1987; Safer Services 1999).
- Nearly half of the suicides will have made an attempt previously (Hawton & Catalan 1987). However, three-fifths of men and two-fifths of women succeed at their first attempt (Isometsa & Lonnqvist 1998).
- Unbearable psychological pain characterizes suicide. Schneidman (1993) terms it as 'psychache'. Feelings of rage, hopelessness and despair predominate. Rage and violence are intimately linked in youth suicide (Hendin 1991). Furman (1984) and Zetzel (1965) highlight the depressed person's incapacity to maintain hope when confronted with loss. Beck and his colleagues (1975) argue that hopelessness is a more accurate indicator of suicide than is depression.
- Severe mental illness is common, especially depression (Arto et al. 1988; Barraclough & Hughes 1987,), and also schizophrenia, personality disorders, drug and alcohol dependence. About a half have comorbid illness (Safer Services 1999). Around 38% abuse alcohol, 23% abuse drugs and 17% misuse both. Drug addicts are at a higher risk and prescribed drugs, particularly antidepressants and methadone, make the risk greater (Oyefeso 1999). Young men are vulnerable in the early phase of a first major depressive episode (Brent et al. 1993). The risk is also pronounced in the phase of recovery from a major depression (Arieti 1959; Kernberg 1984).

- Depression is an important element in those who are suffering from schizophrenia. They more often kill themselves in nonpsychotic periods when they have acquired some insight into the devastating consequence of their illness (Roy 1982).
- Women who suffer from postpartum psychiatric disorders are vulnerable to suicide, particularly in the first year (Appleby et al. 1998).
- Self-harm and violence are significant associations. Of those who kill themselves 63% have a history of self-harm and 19% a history of violence (Safer Services 1999).
- Suicides are associated with bereavement and a failure to mourn. A recent loss such as death of a parent or spouse is significantly more common (Barraclough 1987), particularly in the first year (Bunch 1972; McMahon & Pugh 1971). According to Bunch and Barraclough (1971) suicides tend to take their lives around death anniversaries, especially of parents.
- Suicide is linked with chronic and severe physical illness (Harris & Barraclough 1994), particularly in the elderly (Sainsbury 1962). In the younger age group, suicide is four times more common in those suffering from epilepsy (Barraclough 1987; Sainsbury 1986).
- Suicides are more frequent in the spring and summer. The seasonal variations have however greatly diminished in England and Wales in the last two decades of the 20th century (Yip et al. 2000).

The social characteristics associated with suicide

- Living in over-crowded inner city areas with significant social deprivation and poor economic conditions has a strong association with suicide, especially among young men (Diekstra 1989; Dooley 1989; Platt 1984; Pritchard 1988, 1992,). About two-thirds of suicides are unemployed (Safer Services 1999). The association with unemployment is stronger in the younger age group both among men and women (Gunnell et al. 1999). Poor physical health and reactive depression commonly accompany unemployment.
- Social isolation (Sainsbury 1955) and absence of an intimate relationship are also linked with a higher incidence of suicide. Two-thirds live alone and nearly three-quarters are without a partner (Safer Services 1999). Suicide is thus more common among those who have remained single, are divorced or widowed.
- Suicide is more frequent among prisoners compared with the general population (Gunn & Taylor 1993). Death from abuse of opioids is ten times more common in prisons (Harris & Barraclough 1998, Gore 1999).

The National Confidential Inquiry into Suicide and Homicide, which monitored suicides by people with mental illness over a two–year period between 1996 and 1998 (Safer

Services 1999), while confirming the above patient characteristics, adds:

- The risk is greater in the first year of mental illness, especially after a major affective disorder. Twenty-two per cent of the suicides reported occurred in the first year of illness and 15% had more than five admissions prior to the suicide.
- Four per cent of all suicides were psychiatric in-patients and a third of these killed themselves on the ward, usually by hanging in the evening or at night. Twenty-five per cent of the wards reported that the ward design made it difficult to observe seriously-at-risk patients and another 27% reported nurse shortages at the time of the suicide.
- Three per cent were homeless and these were more often young men with a history of depression, schizophrenia or drug and/or alcohol dependence. Twent-eight per cent of the patients were disengaged with the mental health services, having discharged themselves against medical advice or having been discharged at their own request. They were usually non-compliant with medication.
- Patients who killed themselves were particularly vulnerable in the first few months after discharge. A quarter of post-discharge suicides happened within three months of discharge from the hospital, usually within the first week, more commonly on the day after discharge. About two-fifths of the post-discharge suicides happened before the first follow-up appointment.

Contact with services and communication of risk

The recognition of suicidal thoughts in patients arouses anxiety in the professionals. Doctors often do not recognize the risk and fail to ask suicidal patients about suicide plans or previous suicide attempts (Michel & Valach 1992; Murphy 1975; Richman & Rosenbaum 1970).

Nearly a quarter of all suicides will have been in contact with mental health services in the year before death (Barraclough et al. 1974; Murphy 1975). In the sample monitored by the National Confidential Inquiry, half had been in contact with the mental health services in the week before death and a fifth in the previous 24 hours.

According to the findings of the Inquiry, at final contact, the risk of suicide was estimated to be low or absent in 85% of cases. When the risk was estimated to be moderate or high, the information was not communicated to other members of the mental health team in 14% of cases. When patients were seen by two services prior to suicide, important information known by one service was frequently unknown to the other. Only in just over half the suicides, the mental health services had contact with the family of the deceased.

Characteristics of adolescent suicides

Suicide is the most common cause of death after road traffic accidents among male adolescents. Fifty per cent of adolescents who have attempted suicide before re-attempt (Pfeffer et al. 1994) and 1–11% of these eventually kill themselves. Suicidal male adolescents and young men are less likely than older adults to maintain contact with their GPs or seek alternative help (Vassilas & Morgan 1993). Sexual and physical abuse are frequently associated with adolescents who take their lives (Romans et al. 1995). There is often a history of bullying. Pregnant teenage girls (Gabrielson et al. 1970) and children who have run away from home (Shaffer & Caton 1984) are particularly vulnerable to suicide. Dysfunctional family background, mental illness and/or suicide of a parent and mental illness of a sibling contribute significantly to suicides in young people (Agerbo et al. 2002). Adolescents, depending on their personality, development and family circumstances, may find a melancholic solution (depression, suicidal behaviour) or a manic solution (alcohol, drugs, reckless driving) to their problems (Polmear 2003).

DELIBERATE SELF-HARM

Definitions

Non-fatal self-harm has been defined variously in the last fifty years as 'attempted suicide', 'parasuicide', 'deliberate self-harm' (which is classified further as 'deliberate self-poisoning' and 'deliberate self-injury'), and 'suicidal act'. Stengel (1952) believed that this behaviour, although not fatal, carried a measure of suicidal intent and called it 'attempted suicide'. Kreitman (1977) described it as 'parasuicide', Morgan (1979) as 'deliberate self-harm' suggesting that the actions, although volitional, did not reflect a wish to die. Critics (Asch 1980) argue that the term 'deliberate self-harm' has a punitive connotation and underplays the emotional intensity characterizing the act. The distinction between suicidal behaviour and deliberate self-harm is often a matter of degree. Campbell and Hale (1991), highlighting the ambivalence inherent in the behaviour, propose the term, 'suicidal act', defining it 'as the conscious or unconscious intention at the time of the act to kill the self's body'.

Epidemiology

The prevalence of self-harm has risen significantly in the West since the 1960s (Hawton & Catalan 1987). The rate fell briefly in the 1980s and has returned to its rising trend in the 1990s.

The prevalence of self-harm in the general population is reckoned between 14 and 600 persons per 100 000 population per year in different parts of the world (Soni 1996). It is common in Europe, especially in young people. An estimated 140 000 hospital referrals for deliberate self-harm are made in England and Wales each year (Hawton et al. 1998). The prevelence for self-harm, like the suicide data, is an under-estimation because the source of this information is mainly hospital records, and a large proportion of self-harmers may not report the incident, may only see their family physician or may seek help from an agency that is not linked to a hospital, for example, the Samaritans. Self-destructive behaviour also takes many forms other than overt attacks on the body – for example, addiction, reckless driving, dangerous sexual behaviour, repeated accidents and provoking others to attack. These behaviours are not necessarily conscious and do not fit within the narrow definition of 'deliberate self-harm'.

Overdoses are the most common method of self-harm requiring acute admission to hospital, especially among women. Self-poisoning constitutes 90% of self-harming behaviour, and self-injury, mainly in the form of cutting of forearm and wrist, contributes largely to the rest. Frequently the self-harm includes both cutting and overdose. There is often concomitant heavy drinking and/or drug abuse.

The drugs used for overdoses follow the pattern described with completed suicides and mirror the prevalent prescribing trends and availability of drugs. Psychotropic drugs are more commonly used by those being treated for mental illness, and non-opiate analgesics such as paracetamol and aspirin are more frequently used by young people because of their easy access. The use of minor tranquillizers and sedatives in overdoses has diminished reflecting the changes in prescribing habits (Hawton 1996).

Patient characteristics

- Deliberate self-harm is commoner in women and the female to male ratio is 1.3 : 1. It is more frequent in the younger age group, mainly between the ages of 15 and 24. However, the incidence of self-harm in adolescent boys is low.
- Self-harm is usually impulsive, especially among adolescents. It is frequently accompanied by alcohol and drug abuse, more so in male teenagers (Fombonne 1998).
- Patients who cut habitually may be highly aroused prior to the self-harm and may experience feelings of depersonalization. The cutting may relieve the tension.
- A sense of hopelessness, difficulty in controlling feelings of anger and hostility, and a tendency to aggression are frequently associated with self-harm (Brent 1997). Individuals who harm themselves are self-critical and over-sensitive to criticism. They oscillate between thick-skinned and thin-skinned states of mind, being sometimes inaccessible and defensively aggressive (thick-skinned) and being fragile and vulnerable (thin-skinned) at other times (Bateman 1998; Rosenfeld 1987).

- Patients who self-harm have problems in relationships. A charged incident or event, such as an argument with parents or a break-up of a relationship, may trigger the self-injury.
- There is often a history of loss of a parent in early life either by separation or by death. Emotional neglect, physical and sexual abuse during development are strongly associated with self-injury (Cohen-Sandler et al. 1982, Links 1990; Romans et al. 1995; Shearer et al. 1990). Victims of sexual abuse are most likely to cut themselves. The earlier the origin of such abuse in childhood development, the greater is the propensity to cut and the severity of such behaviour. The families of self-harmers are often dysfunctional with unresolved conflicts and limited support. There is frequently a family history of depression, alcohol and/or drug abuse, violence and life-threatening behaviour. Parents who self-harm have a poor relationship with their children.
- There may be a history of mental illness, most commonly personality disorder or depression, which may of course coexist. Self-injurious behaviour is also seen in other psychiatric conditions such as bipolar affective disorder, schizophrenia (for example, amputation when in a psychotic state), eating disorders, obsessive compulsive disorder, post-traumatic stress disorder, dissociative disorder, and anxiety and panic disorders. Favazza (1987) argues for a separate diagnostic entity called deliberate self-harm syndrome because of the heterogeneity of the condition. About 5–8% of self-harming patients may require hospital admission for treatment of the mental illness (Hawton 1996).
- Chronic physical illness, as with suicide, is associated with self-harm. Men suffering from epilepsy are more prone to harm themselves.

Social characteristics associated with deliberate self-harm

The social characteristics associated with deliberate self-harm are similar to those found with suicides and include poor socio-economic conditions, over-crowded inner city areas with considerable social deprivation, homelessness, unemployment, social isolation, and remaining single or having been divorced. Self-harm is more common in young people who have run away from home (Rotheram-Borus 1993). It is also more frequent in those with a previous criminal record and in those who are held in custody (Feldman 1988, Gunn & Taylor 1993).

THE FAMILY AND THE SUICIDAL PERSON

The family environment is of vital importance in the origin of suicidal behaviour (Marsh 1998). A child's development is influenced by the dynamic organization of the family, how his/her parents assume their responsibilities and relate to each other, and by their responses to his/her development. The process is inevitably affected by traumatic experiences such as loss of a parent or sibling, exposure to violence, seduction and deprivation, and physical and mental illness in the family. How a child is marked by these events will depend on how his/her family reacts to them, the availability of other significant people in the child's life, and his/her age (Ackerman 1958; Schafer 1968).

Suicidal patients have a strong family history of affective disorders, alcohol and drug abuse (Brent et al. 1994). Shaffer (1974) found that 55% of families that had suffered suicides of children had a family member who had consulted a general practitioner or a psychiatrist previously. The families of suicidal individuals also display significant marital conflict, family disharmony, domestic violence and suicidal behaviour. Carroll et al. (1980), note that self-harming patients have a higher family prevalence of separation, violence, physical abuse and sexual abuse compared with other psychiatric populations. A high proportion of suicidal patients report their parents as cold, distant, secretive, resistant to change and intolerant of crisis (Shaffer & Piacentini 1994; Simpson 1976). Early exposure to family violence has been linked with uncontrolled rage and aggression in children who later kill themselves (Hendin 1991). Children of parents who have committed suicide are afraid that they may be overwhelmed by their potential for self-destruction (Schwartz et al. 1974).

Sometimes suicide may be attempted as a solution to a conflict if the family fails to address it for fear of confrontation. Children frequently act as receptacles for family tensions and help to maintain a precarious equilibrium within the family. They become the focus for family hostility and the scapegoating is often a contributory factor in the suicidal behaviour (Sabbath 1969).

Richman and Rosenbaum (1970) found in their family studies that aggression was a striking feature in the behaviour of all family members involved with the suicidal person. The families saw themselves as victims of the suicidal person's difficult behaviour and he/she was frequently the repository of aggression within the family. Families, reacting to their anger, often withdraw from the suicidal or self-mutilating patient.

Suicide is a catastrophic event and may buckle even the most resilient family. It leaves behind many damaged lives and broken relationships. It creates enormous personal suffering and provokes a gamut of feelings: shock, perplexity, anger, despair, blame, guilt, shame and abandonment. The family is seized by a sense of failure that it had not ensured the safety or survival of its family member. The grief may persist for a lifetime. There is also a loss of hope invested by the family in the person who has killed him/herself.

The death may also cause considerable family disruption and shift in responsibilities. For example, children may be forced to assume adult responsibilities in the wake of a parent's suicide. The family may be forced into economic difficulties. The suicide may leave the family with little emotional reserve to comfort each other. Many families disintegrate after a suicide. In Shaffer's study, 25% of families had broken up 1–4 years after a child's suicide.

The impact of suicide on the family members is determined by their roles and responsibilities within the family (for example, of parents, spouses and siblings), their developmental stages (for example, of children) and histories, and the cultural and religious beliefs within the family. The various members of the family mutually affect one another by their reactions to the violent and untimely death.

THE IMPACT OF SUICIDE ON MENTAL HEALTH PROFESSIONALS

The reaction of mental health professionals to the suicide of their patients is not commonly discussed (Gitlin 1999). In a survey of Scottish consultants in psychiatry, a third of them reported depressive symptoms in response to the most distressing suicide of their patients (Alexander et al. 2000). Themes that emerged included guilt, lack of support, feeling blamed and unrealistic expectations from within and outside the profession that the suicide was preventable.

PSYCHOANALYTIC THEORIES OF SUICIDE AND SUICIDAL BEHAVIOUR

Suicide is a tragic end to an inner turmoil. It derives from a complex interplay of internal and external factors determined by the individual's psychic development and his conscious and unconscious attitudes to life and death.

The psychic meaning given to death by suicidal patients can be conceived overall as reactions to separation, loss and abandonment (Hendin 1991). These may be triggered not only by a real person, but also by indignities, disappointments and loss of significant parts of oneself (for example, health). Freud (1917), in his seminal paper, 'Mourning and Melancholia', observed that the ambivalent feelings of love and hatred for what was lost were inherent in pathological depression. Anger and aggression, as reactions to loss, are so unacceptable to the depressed individual that they are repressed and turned upon himself. Indeed the term, 'melancholia' has its roots in the Greek words, 'menos' and 'cholos', meaning black bile or black fury (Rycroft 1968). There is an unconscious feeling of damage and destruction, and to quote Padel (1995), 'Melancholic depression is pathological mourning, not necessarily of a real person, but of an internal object you feel you have destroyed'.

Campbell and Hale (1991), drawing on Freud's formulation, highlight the role that ambivalence and violence play in a suicidal act. They suggest that suicide is a form of 'acting out' whereby the unconscious conflict generating unbearable psychic tension finds relief in the physical action of killing oneself.

Violence in suicide is under-estimated. *The Oxford English Dictionary* defines suicide as an act of taking one's life, a self-murder – a self that submits to murder by itself (derived from Latin *sui* meaning self, *caedere* meaning to kill). Suicide and homicide indeed have a common unconscious origin. The outcome depends on whether the victim is located inside oneself as in suicide or outside as in homicide (Asch 1980). Suicide thus has two components: an aggressive wish to kill and a submissive wish to be killed (Menninger 1933), with an accompanying confusion between the self and the other (Maltsberger 1993; Pollock 1975).

Internal motives and suicide phantasies

Campbell and Hale argue that suicidal behaviour is driven by suicidal phantasies and these are rooted in childhood. Their argument is based on 500 interviews over a four–year period with patients seen within 24 hours of a suicide attempt in the accident and emergency (A&E) department of a large metropolitan hospital and on comments made by suicidal patients in psychoanalytic psychotherapy before and after suicide attempts.

Laplanche and Pontalis (1973) define 'phantasy' as 'an imaginary scene in which the subject is a protagonist, representing the fulfillment of a wish in a manner that is distorted to a greater or lesser extent by defensive processes'. It is distinguished in Britain from the word 'fantasy', which is used in the sense of 'caprice, whim and fanciful invention' (Rycroft 1968). Phantasies are primarily about the body and express the instinctual aims and the defences in relation to people and what they represent (termed 'objects' in psychoanalysis) (Hinshelwood 1989).

A suicide phantasy involves a disturbed relationship between two people (Asch 1980). It carries sets of opposing elements: a passive victim and an intolerable persecutor, an idealized good self and a bad body, a conscious wish to die and a less conscious desire to survive (Campbell & Hale 1991). An alarming state of confusion, chaos and loss of control result when the suicidal patient, who had hitherto kept the conflicting elements apart, is not able to maintain the split. The body is identified with the intolerable persecutor. The patient repudiates the body, and thus attacks the internal persecutor, with the hope that the core part of the self will remain alive – what Campbell and Hale call the 'surviving self' – even when the body is being killed (Maltsberger & Buie 1980).

Several suicide phantasies may be at play. The phantasies are not mutually exclusive, although a particular phantasy may be dominant in a particular individual. The wish to die and the attendant suicidal phantasies may fluctuate in the patient's mind.

The most common suicide phantasy is of merging. The wish to kill oneself may be driven by a desire to reside in a world beyond where all that is lost or denied in this life would be restored. Death may be seen as a return to the heaven where we were born, i.e. to the mother's womb (Jones 1911), to sleep in order to wake up to a better life. The gods of sleep and death in Greek mythology, *Hypnos* and *Thanatos*, are indeed brothers (Friedlander 1940).

The aim of suicide may also be a desire for fusion with another person (Sandler 1960, Meissner 1981). The suicidal person may identify him/herself with a significant other who has died, for example, a parent, a sibling or a partner. He or she may be driven to kill him/herself by a wish to join the dead, thereby regaining in his/her mind the loved person who is lost. The identification is particularly strong if the death has occurred in the person's childhood or adolescence, predisposing him to depression when beset with a loss in later life (Bowlby 1973; Zilbroog 1937). The experience of good family relationships before the loss, the family's ability to mourn and the availability of other carers will of course modify this outcome (Birtchnell 1980).

The act of dying together (e.g. as in a suicide pact) may result from a similar yearning for fusion and a belief in sharing life as well as death. The wish may also find expression in religious beliefs with phantasies of fusion with God (Asch 1966). Suicide in the wake of a murder also may follow such belief, at least in the mind of the murderer-suicide, but is more often a result of extreme jealousy.

Suicide phantasy may also involve the notion of punishment, either as revenge against others or as self-punishment.

The phantasy of revenge is aimed at people who are important to the suicidal person such as parents or other loved ones. The person, seeking retribution for perceived neglect or wrong-doing, is preoccupied with the impact of his or her death on others. The 'surviving self', in the role of the invisible observer, enjoys the anguish, guilt and remorse that would be evoked by his or her death (Campbell & Hale 1991). As Menninger (1933) observes, the greatest hurt a child could inflict on his/her parents is to attack what is most precious to them, i.e. him/herself. 'A rejection of life usually includes a rejection of the parents from whom the life originated' (Hendin 1991).

The wish for self-punishment is driven by a severe sense of guilt. Freud (1916) notes: 'The sense of guilt was present before the misdeed, ... it did not rise from it, but conversely the misdeed arose from the sense of guilt'. The guilt may be associated with unconscious feelings of hostility and forbidden impulses, particularly in adolescents. Freud also links guilt with a sense of failure in matching the expectations of one's ideal self. Sometimes the guilt may be over real events, as observed in combat soldiers. The suicidal person, in his/her desperate attempts to placate the oppressive conscience, may seek punishment by submitting him/herself to dangerous situations or by enlisting others to punish him/her.

Suicide is sometimes impelled by a fear of punishment or retaliation, real or imaginary, especially in children. They may be afraid of being chastised for what they perceive as their transgression of parental rules. Suicide may also be an attempt to escape unbearable feelings of shame, humiliation and loneliness.

Another suicide phantasy is of elimination (Campbell & Hale 1991), which is seen predominantly in adolescents with disturbances of body image. Adolescence demands negotiating bodily changes and developing a sense of ownership of the body. A teenager, who is frightened by his growing body and is unable to master his urges, sees his body as alien and a danger to himself. 'It was as if puberty had suddenly changed the body into an enemy' (Laufer 1968). He is acutely persecuted by his body and wishes to be rid of it in self-defence. The phantasy of elimination may also be dominant in elderly people who are frightened of growing old or of dying badly.

A suicide phantasy may carry an irresistible fascination with death and the act of killing oneself, an addiction to near-death (Joseph 1982). It offers an illusion of mastery over a situation and compensates for feelings of helplessness and loss of control over one's life (Hendin 1991). The phantasy harbours a grandiose wish to triumph over death by actively seeking it. The individual gambles with his/her life and risks his/her body in various ways, such as drink-driving, delinquency and reckless sexual behaviour.

Another phantasy seen in suicidal individuals is the rescue phantasy. The individual sees him/herself as a victim in a submissive relationship with Death. He/she plays a game of Russian roulette with fate as the executioner who will decide if he/she lives or dies, thus expressing his ambivalence about living (Asch 1980). Similarly he forces others, for example, a parent or a wife, by manipulation or blackmail, to be responsible for his survival. The threat of suicide is used to control the behaviour of others by evoking guilt feelings in them (Hendin 1981; Kernberg 1984). Behind the wish to be rescued may also lie a panic that he is no longer safe in his own hands.

BEHAVIOURAL AND COGNITIVE THEORIES

Behavioural and cognitive theories mainly examine processes underlying anxiety and depression. According to learning theories, an individual becomes vulnerable to depression if adequate reinforcements are not available in the environment, either because of changes in the environment or because of the person's limited capacity to generate reinforcers, as for example, when a child loses a parent (Ferster et al. 1997; Shaffer & Piacentini 1994).

Families of suicidal patients have a greater tendency for suicidal behaviour compared with other psychiatric patients (Kreitman et al. 1970; Shaffer & Piacentini 1994). Learning theories posit that such behaviour is a learned currency of communication within this 'subculture'. The self-harm also elicits attention from others and this reinforces the behaviour through operant conditioning. The behaviour may be reinforced through a similar mechanism if the self-harm generates pleasurable sensory stimulation.

The focus of cognitive theories is on thought processes. Ellis (1962) observed that irrational thinking led to emotionally destructive states of mind. Beck (1974) proposed that depression was a result of negative attributions to experience, for example, seeing oneself as wholly responsible for one's misfortunes (internalized attributions), generalizing experiences that were particular (global attributes), and expecting negative experiences to repeat themselves (stable attributes). Beck and his co-workers (1987), differentiating between anxiety and depression, state that a depressed patient 'takes his interpretations and predictions as facts. In anxiety, they are simply possibilities'.

Seligman (1975) introduced the notion of 'learned helplessness'. He and his colleagues, while studying the relationship between fear and learning, found that dogs subjected to electric shocks each time they tried to leave their cage, later made no effort to escape even when it was possible. Brown et al. (1977), extending Seligman's theme, suggest that the loss of a parent in early life sensitized a child, through learned helplessness, to respond to a future loss with depression. Beck (1974, 1975) has argued that hopelessness is a catalyst for suicide and is a more sensitive marker than depression. Fawcett and her associates (1987), followed up 954 patients with major affective disorder in a prospective study over a four–year period and found similarly a strong relationship between hopelessness and suicide in the 25 patients who killed themselves.

Klerman (1986), advocating interpersonal therapy, emphasized the difficulties that a depressed individual encounters in his interactions with others because of conflicts and criticism.

SOCIAL THEORIES

Emile Durkheim, an influential sociologist of the late 19th and early 20th centuries, was concerned with the pathological states of society that provoked individuals to suicide (Harre et al. 1986). He argued that suicide was caused by a breakdown in the relationship between society and the individual, and that it resulted from a failure in man's integration into society and in the regulation of his relationship with it.

Durkheim classified suicide into several types based on the nature of the disturbance between the individual and society. Over-integration into society with an under-developed sense of one's individuality makes man susceptible to an *altruistic* suicide. The socially accepted suicide of early Christians who sought martyrdom to reach God, the immolation of Buddhist priests in protest against social oppression and persecution, and the suicide of whole troops of soldiers in the face of the conquering enemy may be seen as examples of altruistic suicide (Asch 1966). Conversely, under-integration and an overdeveloped sense of individuality impel man to an *egoistic* suicide because of a loss of meaningful life with people and social isolation.

Over-regulation of a man's relationship with society restricts his freedom and may drive him into a *fatalistic* suicide. Under-regulation results in breakdown of social rules of behaviour and leads to a state of hopelessness – *anomie* – and thus provokes an *anomic* suicide. Anomie can be economic or domestic and can take both acute and chronic forms. Acute economic anomie is caused by sudden changes in a person's financial fortunes, either by an economic disaster or a sudden fortune, the individual in either situation failing to adjust to the change. Chronic economic anomie stems from greed and endless pursuit of novelty. Acute domestic anomie follows divorce and in its chronic form is a result of man's marital discontent.

Durkheim's theories have several flaws (Harre et al. 1986). They imply that psychological equilibrium is possible only under certain social conditions. They underplay the individual's psychological structure that contributes to his/her self-destruction. They also ignore the cultural differences in reactions to social situations.

Phillips (1974), elaborating on Durkheim's hypothesis that anomic individuals are vulnerable to suicide, suggests that these individuals are more at risk when the notion of suicide has been heavily publicized. He argues that suggestion, contrary to Durkheim's assertion, has a significant impact on suicide rates through imitation. He calls it the 'Werther Effect' after Goethe's semi-autobiographical novel, *The Sorrows of Young Werther*, describing the suicide of its young grief-stricken hero. The publication of the book in 1774, towards the height of the Romantic Movement, was followed by an alarming swell of suicides in Europe. Phillips found in his study, comparing the numbers of suicides before and after publicized suicides, that national rates increased in the month after a highly publicized suicide. For example, there was a 12% rise in the USA and a 10% rise in the UK following the death of Marilyn Monroe, and a 10% increase in the USA and a 17% increase in the UK after the suicide of Stephen Ward, the osteopath involved in the Profumo affair. Presentations for deliberate self-harm by women rose by 44% in England and Wales in the week after the death of Diana, Princess of Wales, and suicides rose by 17% after the funeral. The latter was particularly marked in women between the ages of 25 and 44 years (Hawton et al. 2000). Phillips suggests that the size of the Werther effect varies with the strength of the publicity and the regional importance of the death.

The adverse media influence on suicidal behaviour, especially of adolescents, through coverage of news and television dramas has been much debated. The studies are beset with methodological problems and the findings are conflicting (Simkin et al. 1995). Schmidtke & Hefner (1988) described a significant rise in suicides in Germany in the wake of a television film depicting a young man's suicide. Platt (1987), investigating the impact of a suicidal attempt in a British soap opera, found the result inconclusive.

Conversely, a more recent study (Salib 2003) argues that a brief but significant reduction in suicides in England and Wales found after the terrorist attacks in America on 11 September 2001, supports Durkheim's theory that periods of external threat create group integration within society and lower the suicide rate through greater social cohesion.

ETHOLOGICAL THEORIES

Jones & Daniel (1996) report that several non-human mammals such as primates (macaques, marmosets, squirrel monkeys), carnivores (leopards, lions, jackals, hyenas), rodents and marsupials (opossums) resort to self-harm when they are in high states of arousal and the usual modes for expression of aggression are denied to them. Self-harming behaviour in animals, according to Chamove et al. (1984), is displaced social aggression. Physical isolation provokes self-directed aggression, as it does in incarcerated human populations. Jones & Daniel suggest that the developmental, biochemical and genetic constituents of such behaviour may be common in man and these animals.

Harlow (1959) found that an infant monkey sought physical contact from its carers. It formed an attachment to a soft fluffy 'mother' in preference to a metal wire 'mother' with a rubber nipple. Anderson & Chamove (1985), in experiments with macaques, found that maternal deprivation and insecure early attachment, for example, separation of the baby from its mother, predispose these primates to self-aggression later in life. Reuniting the baby with its mother, however, may mitigate this behaviour. Rosenblum and his colleagues (1998), in their experimental studies of the macaque's susceptibility to panic, show that insecure social attachments result in inadequate social and cognitive skills to master unexpected triggers and may lead to 'acute endogenous distress' similar to human panic disorder.

SUICIDE BOMBING

A suicide bomber may be defined as a person who kills him/herself deliberately while detonating a bomb. The phrase, 'suicide bomb', was used by the Times newspaper in London in August 1945 to refer to a Japanese kamikaze plane.

Suicide bombing, which has serious social, political and economic consequences, has become common news in the last 20 years. In more modern times it began with the Hezbollah in Lebanon in 1982 and has been used with telling effect by Palestinian organizations in the Middle East, by the Tamil Tigers in Sri Lanka, and more recently in Iraq. The most devastating example is the attack on the World Trade Centre in New York and the Pentagon outside Washington, DC on 11 September 2001, which resulted in nearly 3000 deaths.

Suicide attacks have been common in war throughout history, as a desperate measure to prevent capture, as self-sacrifice and as offensive action. The Japanese used their men as bomb-laden human missiles when they attacked American ships and aircraft carriers from the sky (in the form of kamikaze pilots) and in the water (through midget submarines) in the Second World War. These actions had political and social support, and had precedents in the country's history and culture. Suicide bombings have been targeted not only on military installations, but also on civilian populations in the last decade.

The psychology behind suicide bombing is complex and appears to have its own logic. Nasra Hassan, a Pakistani journalist, interviewed nearly 250 recruit and training bombers in the Middle East and found that they are usually young unmarried men between the ages of 17 and 28 years, educated, religiously devout and fiercely loyal to their group. They are not depressed, nor impulsive, lonely, helpless or driven by economic despair, although the despair of their community may explain the support for them (Margalit 2003).

The motives for suicide bombing are varied. It is sustained by a fiery mixture of nationalism, and religious and revolutionary ideology. It is seen not only as defiance against oppressive occupation, but also as an act of religious martyrdom. The bombers are encouraged by their organizations to 'greet death as an old friend' and not to fear it. Suicide bombing is frequently an act of revenge for a specific event, or for the killing of a close relative or friend.

Suicide bombing evokes visceral fear and horror in the targeted population. It also provokes rage and hatred. The bombers, by making themselves the victims of their own act, also aim to claim the moral ground for their cause.

PHYSICIAN-ASSISTED SUICIDE

In 2001, Diane Pretty, a 43–year-old woman who was paralyzed from motor neuron disease, petitioned to the High Court that she should be allowed to commit suicide with the help of her husband because she suffered from the terminal stage of the illness. The Court, while sympathetic to her cause, refused her request stating that the law had a duty to protect the weak and vulnerable. She appealed to the Law Lords and the European Courts, but they refused to upturn the decision of the High Court.

The case of Diane Pretty rekindled the debate on euthanasia and assisted suicide. It highlighted the legal, moral, ethical and religious dilemmas surrounding the issue.

Ward & Tate (1994) state that nearly 30% of British doctors are confronted with requests for euthanasia by patients with severe disability or terminal illness. Pain, humiliation and futility are cited as the most common reasons (Van der Mass et al. 1991).

A distinction should be made between voluntary and involuntary euthanasia, and assisted suicide. Euthanasia refers to intentional killing or shortening of life of a seriously ill person by an act of omission or commission, seemingly for the benefit of the person. It is voluntary if it is at the individual's request, and involuntary if no request is made or no consent given.

Euthanasia became a public debate for the first time in the late 19th century when it was argued that it was necessary to achieve a good death by allowing the patient to die with less pain. The Nazi regime made euthanasia a pernicious state policy in the 1930s and the 1940s to eliminate the sick, the disabled, the mentally ill and those deemed 'unworthy of life'.

The preoccupation of medicine in the 1950s to the 1970s was to extend life at all costs (Van Delden 1998). However, the twin concept of patient rights and patient autonomy have brought to the forefront the seriously ill person's right to decide how and when he or she should die (Heintz 1994).

Only a handful of states in the world have endorsed the practice of physician-assisted suicide. Switzerland has allowed it with stringent guidelines since 1941. The state of Oregon (USA) made it lawful in 1997, the Netherlands in 2001 and Belgium in 2002. The Northern Territory of Australia legalized it in 1997, but the Federal Parliament repealed it seven months later.

The advocates of assisted suicide contend that if doctors could withdraw life-sustaining treatment to relieve suffering and accelerate death at the request of a mentally competent patient, assisted suicide could be justified on similar moral grounds (Doyal & Doyal 2001).

A moral argument against assisted suicide is the double effect – that an action while arguably good in itself has an unintended but foreseen negative consequence (Jeffrey 1994). Another moral argument against it is 'the slippery slope'. It is feared that regulations cannot be adequately enforced and vulnerable sections of society such as the poor, elderly and mentally ill, may be seen as burdens to society or their families and 'seduced to death' (Hendin 1997). Hendin argues that palliative care has become a casualty of the Dutch euthanasia policies.

FACTORS THAT INCREASE THE RISK OF SUICIDE ATTEMPTS

- The tendency to deal with internal conflict with physical action (Campbell & Hale 1991). Suicidal patients who are withdrawn and manifestly neglectful of their physical state are more likely to act out conflicts with their bodies.

- A suicide plan. A pre-meditated and planned attempt with a suicide note, secrecy, precautions against discovery and preparations in anticipation of death, such as giving away one's possessions and making a will, makes the patient more vulnerable to repetition. (Hawton & Catalan 1987).
- A previous suicide attempt, especially if planned, carries a risk that is 27 times greater than in the general population (Hawton & Fagg 1998). The risk is higher in the first year after an attempt. The use of a dangerous method, such as hanging, jumping from a height or in front of a moving vehicle, shooting and carbon monoxide poisoning in a previous attempt heightens the risk (Brent 1997).
- Young men with a history of several previous narcotic overdoses are also at greater risk. (De Moore & Robertson 1996; Hawton & Fagg 1988; Nordentoft et al. 1993; Suokas & Lonquist 1991).
- A recent experience of failure or of loss through death, separation or divorce.
- Chronic unresolved grief. Patients who have not mourned their losses adequately are particularly at risk especially around death anniversaries.
- Family history of suicide or deliberate self-harm. These patients are twice as likely to attempt suicide as those without the history (Roy 1984).
- A lack of concern in the suicidal patient for him/herself and for others, and in others for him/her (Campbell and Hale 1991). A patient who is cut off from him/herself fails to evoke concern in others. Professionals should be alert to experiences of loss of empathy for an actively suicidal patient.
- Hopelessness, which is a more accurate indicator of suicide than depression (Beck 1975, Fawcett 1984). Patients who feel hopeless are more likely to drop out of treatment (Brent et al. 1995).

Of course, social characteristics such as unemployment, poverty, social isolation and absence of a close relationship, as described earlier, predispose an individual to suicide and self-harm.

MANAGEMENT OF SUICIDAL BEHAVIOUR

Assessment

Assessment should be prompt and should be made before the crisis is dissipated, especially in teenagers. The impetus for assessment and treatment may be lost if the adolescent's family and/or caretakers are not involved from the beginning (Sprague 1997).

The assessment should be detailed and should include interviewing the patient, his partner and family members and other helping agencies involved. The behaviour of the patient should be closely observed. It is important to note that the patient's mental state may be clouded by the drugs used in the overdose and by alcohol. Psychotropic drugs in large doses impair the patient's cognitive ability and make a proper assessment difficult (Sprague 1997).

The assessment should evaluate (Brent 1997):

1. The characteristics of the attempt.
2. The patient's psychopathology and the continuing risk of suicide.
3. The patient's coping resources, and family and social supports (Hawton & Catalan 1987).

The characteristics of the attempt
The gravity of the suicidal intent should be evaluated. Efforts should be made to establish whether the attempt was impulsive or carefully planned, what measures the patient had taken to avoid discovery, and whether or not the suicidal intent was conveyed to others. Patients often appear unusually calm once they have made a firm suicide plan. The suicide plan should be fully unravelled.

Patients often deny dysphoria or a desire to re-attempt perhaps because of a cathartic effect of the suicide attempt (Van Praag & Plutchik 1985).

The seriousness of the suicidal act should be gauged. It should include knowledge of the method employed by the patient to harm him/herself, and whether or not the patient understood the consequences of the method used – for example, the actions and lethal effects of the drug used in an overdose. Beck's suicide intent scale (1974) and Pierce's modified version (1981) have been commonly used to quantitatively assess the suicide risk of patients.

Finally, the current problems of the patient should be appraised. Attempts should be made to trace the event leading up to the suicidal act and to determine its triggers. The trigger may sometimes seem small or trivial to the observer, but its meaning is enormously significant to the suicidal patient.

The patient's psychopathology and the continuing risk of suicide
It is important to establish whether the person continues to entertain suicidal thoughts or maintains a plan to kill him/herself (Lewinson et al. 1994; Pfeffer et al. 1991; Reinherz et al. 1995). The examination of the patient should include a survey of past suicidal behaviour; current abuse of alcohol and drugs; the presence of a serious psychiatric illness such as depression, borderline personality disorder or schizophrenia, and if so, its symptoms and signs, whether it is acute or chronic, whether it is amenable or resistant to treatment; the patient's compliance with medication; and a family history of mental illness, alcohol or substance abuse, violence or suicidal behaviour.

The despair of the patient is often missed in adolescents and psychotic patients because they are likely to be less communicative of their thoughts and feelings. Suicidal young men, particularly university students, may become less accessible by intellectualizing their distress.

The patient's coping resources, and family and social supports

The patient's ability to tolerate anxiety should be assessed. The capacity to endure psychic pain varies between patients. A patient's reactions to previous failures, losses and stressful situations give a measure of his/her coping resources. The availability and the strength of support from family and friends should also be determined.

Counter-transference feelings

All patients evoke emotional responses in the professionals who care for them and these responses, called counter-transference, if recognized and understood, can be helpful in gaining a better understanding of the patient (Heimann 1950).

Winnicott (1949) acknowledges the emotional burden of caring for the mentally ill on doctors and nurses. The suicidal and self-mutilating patient arouses intense and disturbing feelings of anxiety, fear, helplessness, despair and guilt in family members, friends and staff involved in his care. He may refuse offers of help leaving the professional feeling unskilled. He may also provoke strong negative feelings such as manipulation, irritation, dislike, revulsion, anger, and hostility (especially if he injures himself horribly). Winnicott (1949) cautions against ignoring them: 'However much the psychiatrist loves his patients, he cannot avoid hating and fearing them and the better he knows this the less will hate and fear be the motives determining what he does to his patients'.

When a professional is reduced to therapeutic helplessness by a difficult suicidal patient, he/she may become authoritarian and moralistic (Hinshelwood 1999). The patient may be seen as a burden: playing games, wasting valuable clinical time, taking up beds undeservedly. The professional may react by minimizing the seriousness of the suicidal intent, sometimes colluding with the patient; or by taking a 'scientific attitude' and seeing the behaviour as merely a manifestation of an illness (Hinshelwood 1999); or by seeing the patient's action as deliberate and wilful. Alternatively the patient may be treated gingerly if he/she generates anxiety and fear. Suicidal patients sometimes present themselves in ways that provoke rejection, thereby convincing themselves that they are hated and the suicide is justified (Ogden 1979).

Morgan (1979) introduced the term 'malignant alienation' to describe a process whereby there is a gradual erosion of the therapeutic alliance between certain patients and the staff caring for them. These patients may have an intrinsic difficulty in communicating their needs and wishes and may do so in improper ways, thereby eliciting mixed reactions from their carers. Such patients may be perceived as provocative, unreasonable, over-dependent, inaccessible, difficult to engage, demanding, moody, manipulative, self-abusive, unwilling to progress and thus difficult to treat (Watts & Morgan 1994). Such feelings may pervade the whole team or may create splits within the team, and may interact adversely with the staff's aspirations to 'heal all, know all and love all' (Maltsberger & Buie 1974), more so if the staff are inexperienced, poorly supervised and work in a culture less receptive to open discussion of the powerful negative feelings evoked when working with seriously ill patients. The staff, if unaware of these strong feelings, may act them out against the patients. Malignant alienation was a theme in 55% of suicides among psychiatric patients in a study in Bristol (Morgan & Priest 1991).

Wheat (1960), in a retrospective study of 30 patients who killed themselves during or after hospitalization, notes that the professional expects rational behaviour from the suicidal patient far in excess of the patient's capacity at the time and this contributes to the breakdown of communication between them.

Treatment

- The primary aim should be to alleviate the distress. The approach should be non-punitive. A punitive reaction inhibits a patient from returning for help (Sprague 1997).
- Admission to hospital may be necessary. There is frequently a pressure to discharge the patient prematurely and it should be resisted.
- Continuity of care is essential. The family physician should be actively involved in the planning and maintenance of treatment. Similarly the therapist should be involved if the patient is in psychotherapy.
- The underlying mental illness should be treated. Alcohol and drug addiction should be addressed if they are contributing to the problem.
- Appropriate psychological treatment with an experienced therapist should be offered as soon as possible.
- Family support should be mobilized. Communication with people who are significant to the patient such as parents, family and spouse is essential. Family work is important with suicidal adolescents. Conflicts between the adolescent and his parents and other family members should be explored.
- The child or adolescent, if there is on-going sexual or physical abuse, should be moved to a place of safety. It is important to ensure that the patient does not return to the same patterns of relationships and the same abusive environment.
- Links should be made with school or college, if the suicidal individual is a student.

- Drugs with lesser side-effects should be prescribed. The number of tablets or capsules for prescriptions should be limited. Australian studies suggest that the fall in suicide rates in the country in the 1960s and 1970s was strongly influenced by the legal restriction in the number of tablets or capsules for each prescription of sedative and hypnotic drugs (Oliver & Hetzel 1973).

- Measures should be taken to ensure compliance with treatment – medication and follow-up (Brent 1997). Efforts should be made to maintain contact with patients who become disengaged:

  (a) a definite appointment for follow-up should be offered after the assessment, if admission to hospital is not thought to be necessary

  (b) a 24–hour back-up should be available. A study comparing a group with 24–hour availability with another group without such a back-up found fewer incidents of continuing suicidal behaviour in the former (Morgan et al. 1993)

  (c) at-risk patients not attending for follow-up should be pursued with phone calls, letters or visits

  (d) patients should be helped to understand the illness and the need for treatment.

- Staff in the A&E department and on medical wards who encounter suicidal and self-mutilating patients should be supported.

The National Confidential Inquiry (Safer Services 1999) recommends the following:

- administrative aspects of clinical care should be simplified
- information about the risk must be shared by services involved
- mental health services should be more accessible to families of suicidal patients
- ward structure should facilitate good observation of at-risk patients
- in-patient and community care should be better coordinated.
- there should be an active care-programme approach (CPA) with adequate documentation and communication, especially in the first 3 months after discharge, more so with reference to the first week
- good practice should be established in dealing with the aftermath of suicide with a multidisciplinary review of the case
- survivors of suicide should be looked after. These include not only the family, but the professionals involved, such as nurses and doctors
- a comprehensive training should be offered to psychiatric staff in the assessment and management of suicidal behaviour and its risk.

REFERENCES

Aaron R, Joseph A, Abraham S, et al. (2004) Suicides in young people in rural Southern India. *Lancet* **363**: 1117–18.

Ackerman NW (1958) *The Psychodynamics of Family Life*. New York: Basic Books.

Agerbo E, Nordentoft M & Mortensen PB (2002) Familial, psychiatric and socio-economic risk factors in young people: nested case-control study. *British Medical Journal* **125**: 74–7.

Alexander DA, Klein S, Gray NM et al. (2000) Suicide by patients: questionnaire study of its effects on consultant psychiatrists. *British Medical Journal* **320**: 1571–4.

Anderson JR & Chamove AS (1985) Early social experience and the development of self-aggression in monkeys. *Biology of Behaviour* **10**: 147–57.

Anderson R (1998) Suicidal behaviour and its meaning in adolescence. In Anderson R & Dartington (eds) *Facing It Out*, pp. 65–78. Duckworth: Tavistock Clinic Series.

Appleby L (1997) *National Confidential Inquiry into Suicide and Homicide by People with Mental Illness: Progress Report 1997*. London: Department of Health.

Appleby L, Mortensen PB & Faragher EB (1998) Suicide and other causes of mortality after post-partum psychiatric admission. *British Journal of Psychiatry* **173**: 209–12.

Arieti, S (1959) Manic depressive psychosis. In Arieti S (ed.) *American Handbook of Psychiatry I*. New York: Basic Books.

Arto M, Demeter E, Rihmer Z et al. (1988) Retrospective psychiatric assessment of 200 suicides in Budapest. *Acta Psychiatrica Scandinavica* **77**: 454–6.

Asch S (1966) Depression: three clinical variations. *Psychoanalytic Study Child* **21**.

Asch S (1980) Suicide and the hidden executioner. *International Review of Psycho-Analysis* **7**: 51–60.

Barraclough BM (1987) The suicide rate of epilepsy. *Acta Psychiatrica Scandinavica* **76**(4): 339–45.

Barraclough BM, Bunch J, Nelson B et al. (1974) A hundred cases of suicide: clinical aspects. *British Journal of Psychiatry* **125**: 355–73.

Barraclough BM & Hughes J (1987) *Suicide: Clinical and Epidemiological Studies*. Beckenham: Croom Helm.

Bateman A (1998) Narcissism and its relation to violence and suicide. *International Journal of Psycho-Analysis* **79**: 13–25.

Beck AT (1974) The development of depression: a cognitive model. In: Freidman R & Katz M (eds) *The Psychology of Depression – Contemporary Theory and Research*, pp. 3–27. Washington, DC: Winston-Wiley.

Beck AT, Brown G, Steer RA et al. (1987) Differentiating anxiety and depression: a test of cognitive content-specificity hypothesis. *Journal of Abnormal Psychology* **96**(3): 179–83.

Beck AT, Kovacs M & Weissman A (1975) Hopelessness and suicidal behaviour. *Journal of the American Medical Association* **234**: 1146–9.

Beck AT, Weissman A, Lester D & Trexler L (1974) The measurement of pessimism: the hopelessness scale. *Journal of Consulting and Clinical Psychology* **42**: 861–5.

Bertolote JM, Fleischmann A, De Leo D & Wasserman D (2003) Suicide and mental disorders: Do we know enough? *British Journal of Psychiatry* **183**: 382–3.

Birtchnell J (1980) Women whose mothers died in childhood: an outcome study. *Psychological Medicine* **10**: 699–713.

Bowlby J (1973) *Separation: Attachment and Loss*, Volume 2. New York: Basic Books.

Brent DA (1993) Depression and suicide in children and adolescents. *Pediatric Review* **14**(10): 380–88.

Brent DA (1997) The aftercare of adolescents with deliberate self-harm. *Journal of Child Psychology and Psychiatry* **38**(3): 277–86.

Brent DA, Birmaher B, Holder D et al. (1995) A clinical psychotherapy trial for adolescent major depression. Symposium conducted at the 42nd Annual Meeting of the American Academy of Child and Adolescent Psychiatry, October, New Orleans, LA.

Brent DA, Johnson B, Bartle S et al. (1993) Personality disorder, tendency to impulsive violence, and suicidal behaviour in adolescents. *Journal of American Academy of Child and Adolescent Psychiatry* **32**: 69–75.

Brent DA, Perper JA, Moritz G et al. (1994) Suicide in affectively ill adolescents: a case control study. *Journal of Affective Disorders* **31**: 193–202.

Brown G, Harris T & Copeland J (1977) Depression and loss. *British Journal of Psychiatry* **130**: 1–18.

Bunch (1972) Recent Bereavement in relation to suicide. *Journal of Psychosomatic Research* **16**, 316–26.

Bunch J & Barraclough BM (1971) The influence of parental death anniversaries on suicide dates. *British Journal of Psychiatry* **118**: 621–6.

Burton P, Low A, Briggs A (1990) Increasing suicide rates among young men in England and Wales. *British Medical Journal* **300**(6741): 1695–96.

Campbell D & Hale R (1991) Suicidal acts. In: Holmes J (ed.) *Textbook of Psychotherapy in Psychiatric Practice*. London: Churchill Livingstone.

Carroll J, Schaffer CB, Spensley J et al. (1980) Family experiences of self-mutilating patients. *American Journal of Psychiatry* **137**: 852–3.

Chamove AS, Anderson JR & Nash VJ (1984) Social and environmental influences on self-aggression in monkeys. *Primates* **25**: 319–25.

Cohen-Sandler R, Berman AL & King RA (1982) Life stress and symptomatology: determinants of suicidal behavior in children. *Journal of American Academy of Child Psychiatry* **21**(2): 178–86.

Commonwealth Department of Human Services and Health (1995) *Youth Suicide in Australia: A Background Monograph*. Canberra: Australian Government Publishing Service.

De Moore GM & Robertson AR (1996) Suicide in the eighteen years after deliberate self-harm. *British Journal of Psychiatry* **169**: 489–94.

Department of Health (1992) *The Health of the Nation: A Strategy for Health in England*. London: HMSO.

Diekstra RFW (1989) Suicide and attempted suicide: an international perspective. *Acta Psychiatrica Scandinavica* **80**: 1–24.

Dooley D, Catalan R, Rook K et al. (1989) Economic stress and suicide: multi-variate analysis of economic stress and suicidal ideation. Part 2. *Suicide and Life Threatening Behaviour* **19**: 337–51.

Doyal L & Doyal L (2001) Why active euthanasia and physician assisted suicide should be legalised. *British Medical Journal* **323**: 1079–80.

Ellis A (1962) *Reason and Emotion in Psychotherapy*. New York: Lyle Stuart.

Favazza AR (1987) *Bodies Under Siege: Self-mutilation in Culture and Psychiatry*. Baltimore and London: John Hopkins University Press.

Fawcett J, Scheftner WA, Clark D et al. (1987) Clinical predictors of suicide in patients with major affective disorders: a controlled prospective study. *American Journal of Psychiatry* **144**: 35–40.

Feldman MD (1988) The challenge of self-mutilation: a review. *Comprehensive Psychiatry* **29**: 252–69.

Ferster CB, Skinner BF, Cheney CD & Morse WH (1997) Schedules of reinforcement.

Fombonne E (1998) Suicidal behaviours in vulnerable adolescents. *British Journal of Psychiatry* **173**: 154–9.

Freud S (1916) Some character-types met within psycho-analytic work. Standard Edition, 14.

Freud S (1917) Mourning and melancholia. Standard Edition, **14**: 237–258

Friedlander K (1940) On the longing to die. *International Journal of Psycho-Analysis* **21**, 416–26.

Furman E (1984) Some difficulties in assessing depression and suicide in childhood. In: Sudak H, Ford AB & Rushforth B (eds) *Suicide in the Young*, pp. 245–58. Boston: John Wright/PSG Inc.

Gabrielson LW, Gabrielson IW, Klerman LW et al. (1970) Suicide attempts in a population pregnant as teenagers. *American Journal of Public Health* **60**: 2289–301.

Gitlin MJ (1999) A psychiatrist's reaction to a patient's suicide. *American Journal of Psychiatry* **156**: 1630–4.

Gore SM (1999) Suicide in prisons: reflection of the communities served or exacerbated risk? *British Journal of Psychiatry* **175**: 50–5.

Gould RE (1965) Suicide problems in children and adolescents. *American Journal of Psychotherapy* **21**: 228–45.

Gunn J & Taylor PJ (1993) *Forensic Psychiatry*. Oxford: Butterworth-Heinemann.

Gunnell D, Lopatatzidis A, Dorling D et al. (1999) Suicide and unemployment in young people. Analysis of trends in England and Wales, 1921–1995. *British Journal of Psychiatry* **175**, 263–70.

Harlow HF (1959) Love in infant monkeys. *Scientific American* June: 68–74.

Harre R & Lamb R (eds) (1986) *The Dictionary of Personality and Social Change*. London: Blackwell Reference.

Harris EC & Barraclough BM (1994) Suicide as an outcome for medical disorders. *Medicine* **73**: 281–96.

Harris EC & Barraclough BM (1998) Excess mortality of mental disorder. *British Journal of Psychiatry* **173**: 11–53.

Hawton K (1996) Self-poisoning and the general hospital. *Quarterly Journal of Medicine* **89**(12): 879–80.

Hawton KE (1996) Deliberate self-harm. *Medicine*, 77–80.

Hawton KE, Arensman E, Townsend E et al. (1998) Deliberate self-harm: systematic review of efficacy of psychosocial and pharmacological treatments in preventing repetition. *British Medical Journal* **317**: 441–7.

Hawton KE & Catalan J (1987) *Attempted Suicide: A Practical Guide to its Management*, 2nd Edition. Oxford: Oxford University Press.

Hawton KE & Fagg J (1988) Suicide and other causes of death, following attempted suicide. *British Journal of Psychiatry* **152**: 359–66.

Hawton KE, Harriss L, Appleby L et al (2000) Effect of death of Diana, Princess of Wales, on suicide and deliberate self-harm. *British Journal of Psychiatry* **177**: 463–6.

Heimann P (1950) On counter-transference. *International Journal of Psycho-Analysis* **31**: 81–4.

Heintz APM (1994) Euthanasia: can be part of good terminal care. *British Medical Journal* **308**: 1656.

Hendin, H (1991) Psychodynamics of suicide with particular reference to the young. *American Journal of Psychiatry* **148**: 1150–8.

Hendin H (1997) *Seduced by Death: Doctors, Patients, and the Dutch Cure*. Norton.

Hinshelwood RD (1989) *A Dictionary Of Kleinian Thought*. London: Free Association Books.

Hinshelwood RD (1999) The difficult patient: the role of 'scientific psychiatry' in understanding patients with chronic schizophrenia or severe personality disorder. *British Journal of Psychiatry* **174**: 187–90.

Isometsa ET & Lonnqvist JK (1998) Suicide attempts preceding completed suicides. *British Journal of Psychiatry* **173**: 531–5.

Jeffrey D (1994) Active euthanasia: time for a decision. *British Journal of General Practitioners* **44**: 136–8.

Jones E (1911) On dying together. In Jones E, *Essays in Applied Psychoanalysis*, volume I (1951), pp. 9–21. London: Hogarth Press.

Jones IH & Daniels BA (1996) An ethological approach to self-injury. *British Journal of Psychiatry* **169**: 263–7.

Joseph B (1982) Addiction to near-death. *International Journal of Psycho-Analysis* **63**: 449–56.

Kernberg OF (1984) Diagnosis and clinical management of patients with suicide potential. In: Kernberg OF, *Severe Personality Disorders: Psychotherapeutic Strategies*, pp. 254–263. Yale University Press.

Klerman GL (1986) Evidence for increase in rates of depression in North America and Western Europe in recent decades. In: Hippius H et al. (eds) *New Results in Depression Research*. Berlin and Heidelberg: Springer-Verlag.

Kreitman N (1977) *Parasuicide*. London: Wiley.

Kreitman N, Smith P & Tan ES (1970) Attempted suicide as language: an empirical study. *British Journal of Psychiatry* **116**: 465–73.

Laplanche J & Pontalis J-B (1973) *The Language of Psycho-Analysis*. London: The Hogarth Press.

Laufer M (1968) The body image, the function of masturbation and adolescence. *Psychoanalytic Study of Child* **23**: 114–37.

Lewinsohn PM, Rohde P & Seeley JR (1994) Psychosocial risk factors for future adolescent suicide attempts. *Journal of Consulting and Clinical Psychology* **62**: 297–305.

Links PS (1990) *Family Environment and Borderline Personality Disorder*. Washington, DC: American Psychiatric Press.

Maltsberger JT (1993) Confusions of the body, self and others in suicidal states. In: Leenaars A (ed.) *Suicidology: Essays in Honour of Edwin Schneidman*. Northvale, NJ: Jason Aronson.

Maltsberger JT & Buie, Jr DH (1974) Countertransference hate in the treatment of suicidal patients. *Archives of General Psychiatry* **30**: 625–33.

Maltsberger JT & Buie, Jr DH (1980) The devices of suicide: revenge, riddance and rebirth. *International Review of Psycho-Analysis* **7**: 61–72.

Margalit A (2003) The suicide bombers. *The New York Review of Books* **50**(1), 16 January.

Marsh DT (1998) *Serious Mental Illness in the Family*. Chichester: Wiley.

McClure GMS (1987) Suicide in England and Wales. *British Journal of*

Psychiatry **150**, 309–14.

McMahon B & Pugh TF (1971) Suicide in the widowed. *American Journal of Epidemiology* **81**: 23–31.

Meissner WW (1981) *Internalization in Psychoanalysis*. New York: International University Press.

Menninger KA (1933) Psychoanalytic aspects of suicide. *International Journal of Psycho-Analysis* **14**: 376–90.

Menninger K (1938) *Man Against Himself*. New York: Harcourt Brace and World Inc.

Michel K & Valach L (1992) Suicide prevention: spreading the gospel to general practitioners. *British Journal of Psychiatry* **160**: 757–60.

Morgan HG (1979) *Death Wishes: The Understanding and Management of DSH*. Chichester: Wiley.

Morgan HG, Jones EM & Owen JH (1993) Secondary prevention of non-fatal self-harm: The green card study. *British Journal of Psychiatry* **163**: 111–12.

Morgan HG, Pocock H, Pottle S (1975) The urban distribution of non-fatal deliberate self-harm. *British Journal of Psychiatry* **126**: 319–28.

Morgan HG & Priest (1991) Suicide and other unexpected deaths among psychiatric in-patients. The Bristol confidential inquiry. *British Journal of Psychiatry* **158**: 368–74.

Moser KA, Goldblatt PQ, Fox AJ et al. (1987) Unemployment and mortality: comparison of the 1971 and 1981 longitudinal study census samples. British Medical Journal 294: 86–9.

Murphy GE (1975) The physician's responsibility for suicide. II Errors of omission. *Annals of Internal Medicine* **82**(3): 305–9.

Nagy M (1948) The child's theories concerning death. *Journal of Genetic Psychology* **73**: 3–27.

Nordentoft M, Breum L & Munck LK (1993) High mortality by natural and unnatural causes: a 10 year follow-up study of patients admitted to a poisoning treatment centre after suicide attempts. *British Medical Journal* **306**: 1637–41.

Ogden TH (1979) On projective identification. *International Journal of Psycho-Analysis* **60**: 357–73.

Oliver RG & Hetzel BS (1973) An analysis of recent trends in suicide rates in Australia. *International Journal of Epidemiology* **2**(1): 91–101.

Oyefeso A, Ghodse H, Clancy C & Corkery JM (1999) Suicide among drug addicts in the UK. *British Journal of Psychiatry* **175**: 277–82.

Padel R (1995) *Whom Gods Destroy – Elements of Greek and Tragic Madness*. Princeton, NJ: Princeton University Press.

Pfeffer CR, Hurt SW, Kakuma T et al. (1994) Suicidal children grow up: suicidal episodes and effects of treatment during follow-up. *Journal of the American Academy of Child and Adolescent Psychiatry* **33**(2): 225–30.

Pfeffer CR, Klerman GL, Hurt SW et al. (1991) Suicidal children grow up: demographic and clinical risk factors for adolescent suicide attempts. *Journal of the American Academy of Child and Adolescent Psychiatry* **30**(4): 609–16.

Phillips DP (1974) The influence of suggestion on suicide: substantive and theoretical implications of the Werther effect. *American Sociological Review* **39**: 340–54.

Platt S (1984) Unemployment and suicidal behaviour: a review of the literature. *Social Science and Medicine* **19**(2): 93–115.

Platt S (1987) The aftermath of Angie's overdose. Is soap opera damaging your health? *British Medical Journal* **294**: 954–7.

Pollock GH (1975) On mourning, immortality and utopia. *Journal of the American Psychoanalytic Association* **23**: 334–62.

Polmear C (2003) Dying to live: mourning, melancholia and the adolescent process. Unpublished manuscript.

Pritchard C (1988) Suicide, unemployment and gender in the British Isles and European Economic Community (1974–1985). A hidden epidemic? *Social Psychiatry and Psychiatric Epidemiology* **23**(2): 85–9.

Pritchard C (1992) Is there a link between suicide in young men and unemployment? A comparison of the UK with other European Community Countries. *British Journal of Psychiatry* **160**: 750–6.

Reinherz HZ, Giaconia RM, Silverman AB et al. (1995) Early psychosocial risks for adolescent suicidal ideation and attempts. *Journal of the American Academy of Child and Adolescent Psychiatry* **34**(5): 599–611.

Retterstol N (1998) Suicide in a cultural history perspective Part 1. *Suicidologi* **2**.

Retterstol N (2000) Suicide in a cultural history perspective Part 2. *Suicidologi* **3**.

Richman J & RosenbaumM (1970) A clinical study of the role of hostility and death wishes by the family and society in suicide attempts. *Israel Annals of Psychiatry and Related Disciplines* **8**: 213–31.

Rochlin GR (1959) The loss complex: a contribution to the aetiology of depression. *Journal of the American Psychoanalytic Association* **7**: 299–316.

Romans SE, Martin JL, Anderson JC et al. (1995) Sexual abuse in childhood and deliberate self-harm. *American Journal of Psychiatry* **152**: 1336–42.

Rosenblum LA (1998) Experimental studies of susceptibility to panic. NIMH Grant Award MH-42545, New York State Psychiatric Institute, Columbia University, New York.

Rosenfeld H (1987) Afterthought: changing theories and changing techniques in psychoanalysis. In: *Impasse and Interpretation*. London: Tavistock, New Library of Psychoanalysis.

Rotheram-Borus MJ (1993) Suicidal behavior and risk factors among runaway youths. *American Journal of Psychiatry* **150**(1): 103–7.

Roy A (1982) Suicide in chronic schizophrenia. *British Journal of Psychiatry* **141**: 171–7.

Roy A (1984) Family history of suicide. *Archives of General Psychiatry* **40**: 971–4.

Rycroft C (1968) *A Critical Dictionary of Psychoanalysis*. London: Nelson.

Sabbath (1969) The suicidal adolescent – the expendable child. *Journal of the American Academy of Child Psychiatry* **8**:272–289.

Safer Services (1999) *National Confidential Inquiry into Suicide and Homicide by People with Mental Illness, Report 1999*. Department of Health.

Sainsbury P (1955) *Suicide in London*. Maudsley Monograph no 1. London: Chapman and Hall.

Sainsbury P (1962) Suicide in later life. *Gerantologia Clinica* **4**: 161–70.

Sainsbury P (1986) Epidemiology of suicide. In: Roy A (ed.) *Suicide*. Baltimore, MD: Williams and Wilkins.

Salib E (2003) Effect of 11 September 2001 on suicide and homicide in England and Wales. *British Journal of Psychiatry* **183**: 207–12.

Sandler J (1960) On the concept of the super-ego. *The Psychoanalytic Study of the Child* **15**: 128–62.

Schafer R (1968) *Aspects of Internalization*. New York: International University Press.

Schmidtke A & Hafner H (1988) The Werther after television films: new evidence for an old hypothesis. *Psychological Medicine* **18**: 665–76.

Schneidman ES (1993) Suicide as psychache. *Journal of Nervous and Mental Disease* **181**: 147–9.

Schwartz DA, Flinn DE & Slawson PF (1974) Treatment of the suicidal character. *American Journal of Psychotherapy* **28**: 194–207.

Seligman MEP (1975) *Helplessness: On Depression, Development and Death*. San Francisco: WH Freeman.

Shaffer D (1974) Suicide in childhood and early adolescence. *Journal of Child Psychology & Psychiatry* **45**: 406–51.

Shaffer D (1985) Notes on developmental issues in the study of suicide. In Rutter, Izard & Read (eds) *Depression in Childhood: Developmental Issues*. New York: Guildford Press.

Shaffer D & Caton C (1984) *Runaway and Homeless Youth in New York City*. Unpublished manuscript.

Shaffer D & Piacentini (1994) Suicide and attempted suicide. In Rutter, Taylor & Hersov (eds) *Child and Adolescent Psychiatry, Modern Approaches*, pp. 407–24. Oxford: Blackwell.

Shearer SL, Peters CP, Quaytman MS & Ogden RL (1990) Frequency and correlates of childhood sexual and physical abuse histories in adult female borderline inpatients. *American Journal of Psychiatry* **145**: 1424–7.

Simkin S, Hawton K, Whitehead L et al. (1995) Media influence on parasuicide: a study of the effects of a television drama portrayal of paracetamol self-poisoning. *British Journal of Psychiatry* **167**: 754–9.

Simpson MA (1976) Self-mutilation and suicide. In Schneidman ES (ed.) *Suicidology: Contemporary Developments*, pp. 281–315. New York: Grune and Stratton.

Soni RV (1996) Suicide patterns and trends in people of Indian subcontinent and Caribbean origin in England and Wales. *Ethnicity Health* **1**: 55–63.

Soni Raleigh V & Balarajan R (1996) Suicide and self burning among Indians and West Indians in England and Wales. *British Journal of Psychiatry* **161**: 365–8.

Speece MW & Brent SB (1984) Children's understanding of death: a review of three components of a death concept. *Child Development* **55**: 1671–86.

Sprague T (1997) Clinical management of suicidal behaviour in children and adolescents. *Clinical Child Psychology and Psychiatry* **2**(1): 113–23.

Stengel E (1952) Enquiries into attempted suicides. *Proceedings of the Royal Society of Medicine* **45**: 613–20.

Suokas J & Lonnquist J (1991) Outcome of attempted suicide and psychiatric consultation: risk factors and suicide mortality during a five-year follow-up. *Acta Psychiatrica Scandinavica* **84**: 545–9.

Van Delden JM (1998) Review of book: Physician-assisted Suicide. Ed. Robert F Weir. *British Medical Journal* **316**: 1543.

Van der Mass PJ, Van Delden JJM et al. (1991) Euthanasia and other medical decisions concerning the end of life. *Lancet* **338**: 669–74.

Van Praag HM & Plutchik R (1985) An empirical study of the 'cathartic effect' of attempted suicide. *Psychiatry Research* **16**: 123–30.

Vassilas CA & Morgan HG (1993) General practitioners' contact with victims of suicide. *British Medical Journal* **307**: 300–1.

Vassilas CA & Morgan HG (1997) Suicide in Avon. Life stress, alcohol misuse and use of services. *British Journal of Psychiatry* **170**: 453–5.

Ward BJ & Tate BA (1998) Attitudes among NHS doctors to request for euthanasia. *British Medical Journal* **308**: 1332–4.

Watts D & Morgan G (1994) Malignant alienation: dangers for patients who are hard to like. *British Journal of Psychiatry* **164**: 11–15.

Weininger O (1979) Young children's concept of the dying and dead. *Psychological Reports* **44**: 395–407.

Wheat W (1960) Motivational aspects of suicide in patients during and after psychiatric treatment. *Southern Medical Journal* **53**: 273.

Williams & Pollock (1993)***

Winnicott DW (1949) Hate in the countertransference. *International Journal of Psycho-Analysis* **30**: 69–74.

World Health Organization (2001) *World Health Report 2001: Mental health – new understanding, new hope*. Geneva: WHO.

Yip PSF, Chao A & Chiu CWF (2000) Seasonal variation in suicide: diminished or vanished. Experience from England and Wales, 1982–1996. *British Journal of Psychiatry* **177**: 366–9.

Zetzel E (1965) On the incapacity to bear depression. In: Schur M (ed.) *Drives, Affects and Behaviour*, Volume 2. New York: International University Press.

Zilbroog G (1937) Considerations on suicide with particular reference to that of the young. *American Journal of Orthopsychiatry* **7**: 15–31.

Unusual psychiatric syndromes

Sadgun Bhandari

INTRODUCTION

The unusual psychiatric syndromes are a collection of largely eponymous symptom complexes and conditions, which are relatively rare and are unusual in their presentations. The first six syndromes described are delusions or delusional disorders and most may be diagnosed using contemporary classificatory systems. Othello syndrome, De Clerambault's syndrome, Ekbom's syndrome and *folie à deux* are diagnosed as delusional disorders in the ICD-10 (World Health Organization 1992) and DSM-IV (American Psychiatric Association 1994) where they present as pure syndromes. Munchausen syndrome is classified under somatoform disorders as factitious disorder and Munchausen by proxy is a form of child abuse and does not feature in contemporary classifications. The culture-bound syndromes will be discussed separately.

CAPGRAS' SYNDROME

Capgras' syndrome was first described by Capgras and Reboul-Lachoux in 1923. The main characteristic of the syndrome is the delusion that a person, usually a close relative, has been replaced by a double or an imposter (Box 22.1). Christodoulou (1991) suggests that Capgras' syndrome is of a group of four syndromes known collectively as the *delusional misidentification syndromes*:

Box 22.1   Capgras' syndrome
One of the four delusional misidentification syndromes
Characterized by a delusion that another person, usually a close relative, has been replaced by a double
Usually a symptom of either a psychotic disorder (70%), most commonly schizophrenia, or of an organic disorder (30%)
Patients may be violent towards misidentified persons

[1] Capgras' syndrome is the delusional negation of a familiar person (or persons), in which the patient believes that the misidentified and familiar persons are identical physically but different psychologically.

[2] Fregoli syndrome is the delusional identification of a familiar person in strangers. The misidentified and the familiar persons are perceived by the patient as being physically different but psychologically identical.

[3] The syndrome of intermetamorphosis is characterized by the belief that the persons in his environment interchange with each other. The syndrome is similar to Fregoli but the person also believes that there are physical similarities between the misidentified and familiar persons.

[4] Syndrome of subjective doubles is the delusional belief that a stranger has been transformed physically but not psychologically into the patient's own self.

It is suggested that the four syndromes represent variants of the same basic condition and they may often coincide or interchange. A related misidentification syndrome is that of reduplicative paramnesia in which the patients believe that a physical location has been duplicated.

Clinical aspects

Capgras' syndrome is very often a symptom of a recognized psychosis and is rarely thought to occur in its pure form. When it occurs as a symptom, its onset is not dependent on the length of the illness of the condition it accompanies. Usually one person who is very familiar to the patient is persistently misidentified. In most married patients the spouse is the double. In other cases the misidentified persons are usually close relatives. In some cases healthcare staff may also be misidentified.

Diagnostic significance

In 70% of the cases the person suffers from a psychotic disorder, usually schizophrenia, and it has also been described in affective disorders. It is not part of the delusional disorders in either the ICD-10 and DSM-IV classificatory systems.

Capgras' syndrome has been described in a wide variety of organic conditions, (structural brain injury, infection and encephalitis, drug intoxication or withdrawal, endocrine disorders, epilepsy, and AIDS) and can herald the onset of dementia. When it occurs in organic conditions, confusion and cognitive deficits are usually present.

Fleminger & Burns (1993) found that a history of paranoid delusions preceding the onset of the misidentification syndrome was common in non-organic conditions. Also misidentification of place was common in organic conditions and misidentification of person in functional psychoses.

Explanatory theories

Psychodynamic and organic explanations for the syndrome have been proposed. Enoch & Trethowan (1991) consider Capgras' syndrome as a psychological solution to the love–hate conflict. Projection and splitting is used to direct hate towards the bad impostor while the original continues to be ideal. Prosapagnosia (face non-recognition) and right-hemisphere dysfunction have also been put forward as possible explanations.

Management

Since 30% of cases have organic aetiology it is important that patients are fully investigated. As Capgras' syndrome is very often a symptom rather than a syndrome the accompanying condition should be treated.

Dangerousness

Violence against the misidentified persons is possible and is more likely when delusions are well developed. Past history of aggressive behaviour, delusions against a specific person and suspiciousness and hostility contribute towards dangerousness.

DE CLERAMBAULT'S SYNDROME

De Clerambault's syndrome is also known as *psychose passionelle*, erotomania, delusions of love or delusions of passion. De Clerambault first described the syndrome in 1942. He stated that it is characterized by the patient, usually a woman, and referred to as the subject, suddenly developing a delusion that a man or object, with whom she may have had a little or virtually no contact, is in love with her (Box 22.2). The term erotomania is used to designate the delusion that a person of higher social standing loves the patient. There are a number of derivative themes (Signer 1991):

Box 22.2   De Clerambault's syndrome

Characterized by a delusion that a person of a higher social or economic status is in love with the patient
May present as a primary delusional disorder, or a symptom of schizophrenia or affective disorder
May result in stalking behaviour and the risk of violence is high. This may be directed both towards the object of love or those who are thought to be in the way

---

- The object is unable to be happy or to have a sense of self-esteem without the subject.
- The object is unmarried or if married, the marriage is invalid.
- The object attempts to make contact, has indirect conversation with and exerts continuous surveillance or protection of the subject by means of phenomenal resources.
- There is almost universal sympathy or support for the relationship.
- The object shows a paradoxical or contradictory attitude toward the subject. Paradoxical conduct means that the patient interprets all denials of love by the object as being secret affirmations of love or as 'tests' of the strength of their love.

The last theme is given singular importance and is always present.

Clinical aspects

There is considerable debate as to whether a pure form of erotomania exists. The criteria for a primary syndrome include, apart from the themes described above, a sudden onset, the belief that the object is the first to fall in love and make advances, persistence of the same love object, a chronic course, absence of hallucinations and no cognitive deficits. Erotomania is characterized by the subject bombarding the object with letters and telephone calls and also by following them without respite.

Erotomania has also been described in males, although Menzies et al. (1995) suggest that it is uncommon and usually associated with other disorders. Health professionals are recognized as being at high risk of becoming objects (Mullen & Pathe 1994a).

Diagnostic significance

A pure erotomanic delusion should be diagnosed as one of the delusional disorders. When part of another disorder schizophrenia is commonest but erotomania has also been described in patients with affective disorders.

Management

Erotomania is difficult to treat and there are no systematic studies available on the management of erotomania. Hospitalization may be necessary to protect others. Antipsychotics should be prescribed, and Mullen & Pathe (1994b) found antipsychotics in a low to moderate dose to be more effective when coupled with supportive yet gently challenging psychotherapy. If the erotomania is secondary to other psychiatric disorders the primary disorder should be treated.

Dangerousness

The phenomena of stalking has been linked with erotomania and describes a constellation of behaviours in which one individual inflicts on another unwanted intrusions and communications. The intrusions can involve following, loitering nearby, maintaining surveillance and making approaches (Pathe & Mullen, 1997). Harmon et al. (1995) found that stalking tends to occur with disorders other than erotomania, including delusional disorders, and non-erotomanic stalking represents the greater risk. Menzies et al. (1995) suggest that in male erotomanics, predictors of dangerousness include the presence of more than one object and a history of unrelated antisocial behaviour. Violence can be directed towards the love object, as well as rivals or people thought to be in the way of the relationship. It has also been suggested that the risk of violence is low in pure erotomania but high when erotomania is associated with other conditions.

Behaviour similar to erotomania is seen sometimes where there has been a previous relationship that has gone 'sour.' This relationship may be personal, professional or business (Zona 1993).

OTHELLO SYNDROME

Othello syndrome is characterized by the delusion of infidelity of the sexual partner (Box 22.3). Jealousy does not always occur as a delusion and may also manifest as an overvalued idea, depression or an anxiety state. In the majority of patients it is quite clear when malignant jealousy exists, but in borderline cases jealousy of

Box 22.3 Othello syndrome
Characterized by a delusion of infidelity
Can present as a delusional disorder or as a symptom of schizophrenia, affective disorder, organic disorder and alcohol abuse
Dangerousness is significantly high as morbid jealousy contributes to both wife battering and homicide

apparently normal proportions merges imperceptibly into delusional jealousy.

A related syndrome is that of *retrospective ruminative jealousy* in which the patient is preoccupied with the past sexual activity of the sexual partner but without delusions of infidelity.

Clinical aspects

The condition occurs in both sexes but is commoner in males. It usually presents in the fourth decade. Onset is sudden but a history of increasing suspiciousness is often present. The person acts on the delusion by checking for signs of infidelity, such as examining undergarments, going through pockets, watching and spying on the partner, following and interrogating the partner for hours in an attempt to confirm their belief and obtain a confession. Sexual activity may increase as the person demands more sex and in the context of ongoing relationship problems this may cause further difficulties.

Aetiology

Psychodynamic explanations include projection of feelings of unfaithfulness and latent homosexual feelings. Morbid jealousy is frequently associated with sexual disorders especially erectile dysfunction. Partners frequently report sexual difficulties but it is difficult to determine whether the sexual problems are primary or secondary. Feelings of inadequacy are central to the disorder and may arise due to the partner being more sexually attractive.

Diagnostic significance

Delusional jealousy can occur as a monodelusional disorder and is then diagnosed as a delusional disorder. It can also occur as a symptom of other disorders most commonly schizophrenia, alcohol abuse and affective disorders, (especially depression, which may enhance feelings of inadequacy). Alcohol abuse is present in 6% to 20% with morbid jealousy. According to Soyka (1991) this association holds good for male alcoholics only.

Morbid jealousy has also been described in a number of organic conditions including infections, endocrine disorders and dementia.

Enoch & Trethowan (1991) also suggest that psychiatric disorders such as depression are often quite common in relatives of patients suffering from delusional jealousy.

Management

Treatment is primarily with antipsychotics. As with schizophrenia, currently atypical antipsychotics would be an important aspect of pharmacological management. If the delusions are part of another disorder then the underlying disorder should be treated. Compliance with medication may be poor due to the nature of the delusion and in such cases compulsory treatment may be necessary.

Psychotherapy for morbid jealousy has included:

1. behavioural psychotherapy employing treatments for obsessions
2. cognitive behaviour therapy that focuses on addressing factors that precipitate and maintain the jealousy and factors in the individual's personality that predispose to jealousy
3. marital therapy
4. conjoint therapy.

Dangerousness

Delusional jealousy carries a high risk for violence. It is a major contributor to wife battering and is one of the commonest motivations for homicide (Mullen 1990). Delusional jealousy has a high rate of recurrence and can reoccur when a new partner replaces a former partner. Instances of repeat homicides following release from hospital or prison having been reported (Scott 1977). For the safety of partners of patients with morbid jealousy, temporary or permanent separation may be necessary.

FOLIE À DEUX

Folie à deux is also known as communicated insanity, contagious insanity, infectious insanity, psychosis of association, and induced psychosis. In DSM-IV it is called *shared psychotic disorder*. The term was first coined by Lasegue & Falret in 1877. It refers to several syndromes in which mental symptoms, particularly paranoid delusions, are transmitted from one person to one or more others with whom the apparent instigator is in some way intimately associated; thus two or more individuals come to share the same delusional ideas (Enoch & Trethowen 1991) (Box 22.4). In rare cases whole families are affected (*folie à famille*). Various subtypes of this rare syndrome have been described; the commonest is *folie imposée* where the patient who suffers from the primary psychosis is dominant and imposes the delusion on the second individual, who is both submissive and suggestible. Delusions are usually persecutory.

Box 22.4   *Folie à deux*
Characterized by two persons, usually closely related, sharing the same delusion
The dominant partner has the primary illness and induces the delusion in the submissive partner
Separation often resolves the delusion in the secondarily affected person

Clinical aspects

This condition is rare and information is mainly obtained from case reports. Three essential criteria have been proposed for the diagnosis of true *folie à deux* (Dewhurst & Todd 1956):

1. marked similarity in the general and sometimes specific content of the partner's psychosis
2. unequivocal evidence that the partners accept, support and share each other's delusions
3. evidence that the partners have been intimately associated over a long period of time.

About 90% of relationships described are within the nuclear family, sister–sister dyads being the most common.

The duration of association between the two persons is long but the duration of exposure to the psychosis is variable. One of the most consistent findings is that of social isolation; this refers not to physical isolation but the impairment of the extent and/or nature of communication with others.

Explanatory theories

The psychological mechanism of identification is considered to be most important. Hereditary factors have also been postulated as the condition tends to occur in close relatives, although it does occur in husband–wife dyads as well.

Diagnostic significance

In the primarily affected individual, schizophrenia is the commonest diagnosis but delusional disorder and affective disorder can also occur. The cases secondarily affected might also suffer from schizophrenia or other psychiatric disorders.

Management

The first step in treatment is separation of the two persons suffering from the delusions because about 40% of the cases who are secondarily affected respond to this treatment. Primary cases need treatment of the underlying condition, usually schizophrenia, and secondary cases who do not improve with separation may require antipsychotic medication.

To prevent recurrence, social isolation needs to be addressed. Social support is important and family therapy may also be appropriate.

COTARD'S SYNDROME

Cotard's syndrome is characterized by nihilistic delusions which at their most extreme are manifested by the person denying his own existence or that of the external world (Box

Box 22.5   Cotard's syndrome

Characterized by nihilistic delusions ranging from denial of the integrity of body organs to denial of internal and external existence
Syndromal presentation rare, Cotard's syndrome usually accompanies depressive illness

Box 22.6   Ekbom's syndrome

Characterized by a delusion of infestation with small organisms
Condition rarely presents to psychiatrists, more commonly to dermatologists
Can present as a delusional disorder, or as a symptom of schizophrenia or depression, especially in the elderly

22.5). Cotard described his case in 1880 and in 1897 Seglas first used the eponym. It has been suggested that in his original description Cotard had described a syndrome with related symptoms but over time the name applied to nihilistic delusions (Berrios & Luque 1995). There is a considerable amount of debate as to whether Cotard's syndrome is a distinct clinical entity.

Clinical aspects

The condition is characterized by delusions of negation (beliefs that specific body parts do not exist, that the person is dead or that the world does not exist). Accompanying features include delusions of guilt and immortality, anxiety, depression, suicidal behaviour, hypochondriacal delusions, and auditory hallucinations with depressive content. The commonest delusions reported are those involving the body followed by those about existence. Cotard's syndrome occurs more commonly in late middle age.

Diagnostic significance

In their review of 100 cases reported in the literature Berrios & Luque (1995) found comorbid depression reported in 89% of the cases. Cotard's syndrome has also been reported with schizophrenia and organic disorders.

Management

The treatment of Cotard's syndrome is essentially that of the underlying condition, most often depression. Since psychotic symptoms are present, ECT may be indicated. Risk of suicide is high.

EKBOM'S SYNDROME

Synonyms for Ekbom's syndrome include delusions of infestation, delusional parasitosis, and delusional infestation (Box 22.6). Ekbom (1938) described eight patients with the delusional conviction that they were infested with small organisms such as mites or insects, a condition he called *Dermatozoewahn* or 'delusion of animal life in skin'. Patients with this uncommon condition, the subject of sporadic case reports, most often presents to dermatologists.

Clinical aspects

The condition occurs more frequently with advancing age and the female to male ratio is 2:1. Patients tend to delay clinical consultation. Insects such as spiders, dragon flies and fleas are among the commonest complained of and patients may show 'the matchbox sign' by bringing specimens of the alleged organisms. Cleaning rituals are common and patients may fear contaminating others.

Diagnostic significance

Delusional infestation alone is diagnosed as a delusional disorder or *monosymptomatic hypochondriacal psychosis* (Munro 1980). It has been described in association with organic disorders, schizophrenia and affective disorders. Depression is a likely cause in the elderly (Morris & Jolley 1987) and *folie à deux* may be associated in 5–15% of these cases (Enoch & Trethowen 1991). Delusional infestation with tactile hallucinations may occur in cocaine users – 'cocaine bug.'

Management

Whether presenting as a delusional disorder or as a schizophrenic symptom, treatment is with antipsychotics. Pimozide has been often used in the past although there is no conclusive evidence that it is more effective than any other antipsychotic agent and moreover due to cardiac side effects it would be no longer recommended. Recent studies suggest that atypical antipsychotics are more effective (Kiraly et al. 1998).

MUNCHAUSEN'S SYNDROME

Otherwise known as hospital hobos, peregrinating problem patients, hospital addiction syndrome or factitious disorder, this syndrome was first described by Asher in 1951. It is classically characterized by a patient presenting to hospital with dramatic symptoms suggesting a medical emergency, and necessitating investigations and treatment including surgery (Box 22.7). Patients have a history of wandering from one hospital to another with a similar presentation, with no obvious gain. The term may be applied to other presentations, not necessarily dramatic, where physical

Box 22.7   Munchausen syndrome

Characterized by recurrent, feigned dramatic presentation of a medical condition in order to obtain investigations and treatment
Not much is understood about underlying aetiological factors
Management is difficult due to lack of engagement in treatment

signs or abnormal laboratory results are fabricated, all these conditions subsumed under the rubric of factitious disorders. Asher originally described three subtypes (acute abdominal, haemorrhagic and neurological), but over time a much wider variety of presentations have been described. Munchausen has been also used to describe factitious presentations of psychiatric symptoms but diagnostic criteria are not clear (Enoch & Trethowan 1991).

Clinical aspects

The disorder is commoner in males. The patients are well-informed about medical conditions and may be members of the medical or allied professions. A criminal record is common. The course varies from episodic to a chronic unremitting one. Presentation is often late at night or at weekends, patients are demanding and attention-seeking, often 'break the rules', and have no visitors.

Association with a range of physical and psychiatric conditions (eating disorders, depression, borderline personality disorder, diabetes, asthma and brain damage) has been described (Robertson & Hossain 1997).

Explanatory theories

Many psychological mechanisms have been postulated to explain this behaviour but not enough is known about the condition to understand the aetiological factors completely. Sussman et al. (1987) suggest that Munchausen syndrome is a result of complex interaction of personality factors and psychosocial stressors.

Diagnostic significance

The condition must be differentiated from those in which patients adopt a patient role in order to obtain drugs or shelter, or in response to an acute psychosocial crisis. Malingering should be ruled out, although it is unlikely to present recurrently.

Management

Management is difficult as the patients are reluctant to engage in treatment. Early detection is important. Treatment is primarily psychotherapeutic and should aim to promote social integration and reduce inappropriate behaviour

(Robertson & Cervilla 1997). Prognosis is regarded as generally poor.

MUNCHAUSEN SYNDROME BY PROXY

The syndrome was first described by Meadow in 1977 and is also known as Munchausen by proxy syndrome, Meadow's syndrome or Polle syndrome (Box 22.8). Munchausen syndrome by proxy consists of the induction of an appearance, or a state, of physical ill health in a child, by a parent (or someone *in loco parentis*), where the child is subsequently presented to health professionals for diagnosis and/or treatment, usually persistently. The perpetrator denies the aetiology of the child's illness and the acute symptoms and signs of the illness decrease after separation from the perpetrator (Bools et al. 1992). The harm to the child results from the direct production of physical signs and diseases in the child and indirectly through medical intervention.

Box 22.8   Munchausen syndrome by proxy

Characterized by repeated fabrication of an illness in a child, in order to obtain medical intervention for the child, resulting in harm to the child
Almost all cases are perpetrated by the biological mother
Not enough is known about the characteristics of the perpetrators
Requires a high index of suspicion to facilitate early identification and intervention

Clinical aspects

The most common presentations involve seizures, failure to thrive, vomiting and diarrhoea, asthma/allergies and infections. Abuse usually involves young children, starting from the first year of life, with the average age just over three years at diagnosis, and the mortality is estimated at 9% (Rosenberg 1987). Average length of time to establish a diagnosis of Munchausen syndrome by proxy generally exceeds six months, and often there is a history of a sibling having died of undiagnosed causes, suggesting that cases may go undetected (Schreier & Libow 1994).

In nearly every case the perpetrator is the biological mother (Rosenberg 1987). They usually have a health professional background or are medically knowledgeable. They usually appear caring and doctors and other professionals are reluctant to believe that the mothers are responsible for the cruelty to the child (Schreier & Libow 1994). In 30–35% of cases returning home, the fabrication of illness is repeated. The long-term psychological outcome is poor regardless of the child returning home or going into care outside the home (Bools et al. 1993).

Diagnostic significance

Little is known about the relation between psychiatric disorders and Munchausen syndrome by proxy. Depression and personality disorder have been diagnosed in patients assessed by psychiatrists.

Management

The key to management is early identification. Clues include the nature of presentation of the illness and attitude of mother. Covert video surveillance has also been used (Samuels et al. 1992). Once identified, the management is aimed at protecting the child (and other siblings). Treatment of the perpetrator may be through family therapy or psychiatrists.

GANSER'S SYNDROME

This syndrome was first described by Ganser in 1898. It is characterized by a patient giving approximate answers to simple and familiar questions, in a setting of disturbed and clouded consciousness (Box 22.9). The other two features of the complete syndrome include hysterical conversion symptoms and hallucinations. Associated features include psychogenic amnesia. It is thought to be a hysterical dissociative state that occurs as a result of an unconscious effort by the subject to escape from an intolerable situation (Enoch & Trethowan 1991). The symptom that has attracted the most attention is that of approximate answers or talking past the point (*vorbeireden*).

Box 22.9   Ganser's syndrome
A rare syndrome characterized by approximate answers, clouded consciousness, hallucinations and hysterical conversion symptoms
Symptom of approximate answers is more common
Resolution is the likely outcome

The complete syndrome is very rare. Scott (1965) suggested that it is useful to distinguish between the Ganser *symptom* (approximate answers) and Ganser *syndrome*, the symptom being more common. Lishman (1987) discusses the difficulty with the concept of the symptom as it requires an element of subjective interpretation on the part of the examiner and it is unclear how approximate the answer should be before the symptom is considered to be present.

Diagnostic significance

This condition needs to be distinguished from true dementia, pseudodementia (in depression or schizophrenia) and conscious simulation of symptoms (malingering).

Management

Hospitalization may be necessary for investigation and in order to remove the patient from the stressful environment. Underlying depression should be treated. Improvement is the most likely outcome.

CULTURE-BOUND SYNDROMES

The term 'culture-bound syndromes' conjures up images of rare and exotic psychiatric disorders, and indeed many disorders are described as culture-bound syndromes. However, there are difficulties with the term because the disorders it is applied to are often not distinct disease entities and are not strictly culture-bound, occurring in multiple cultures. The culture-bound syndromes therefore include a heterogenous group of phenomena, some of which are true syndromes, some culturally based aetiologic explanations for psychiatric disorders, and others, folk terms for common behaviours or emotions, otherwise known as 'idioms of distress' (Levine & Gaw, 1995). According to Littlewood (1990), the term 'culture-bound' was applied to local patterns of behaviour that did not fit into the Western psychiatric classifications. Littlewood also suggests that the term is redundant because all reactions are to an extent culturally determined. Patterns characteristic of Western societies such as overdoses and anorexia nervosa are as culture-bound as any others.

The following are some of the common conditions described under this heading:

- koro
- amok
- latah
- wihtigo (Windigo)
- possession states
- others.

Koro

This occurs in south-east Asia and affects Chinese people. Patients are usually males, who believe that the penis is withdrawing inside the abdomen. This results in a panic as the person also believes that once the penis has completely retracted he will die. Remedial action is taken by tying the penis with strings and getting help from relatives and friends. It can affect females as well and may occur individually or in epidemics. Koro responds to reassurance and education. In psychiatric terms koro is an anxiety state and is not delusional.

Koro epidemics have been described in other cultures including Thailand (*rok joo*) and Assam in India (*jinjina bemar*).

Koro-like states characterized by fear of the penis shrinking have been described in individuals from outside south-east Asia, but these patients do not show the other features of koro and have a history of psychiatric conditions including anxiety, depression and schizophrenia (Berrios & Morley, 1984).

Amok

This occurs in the Philippines and Malaysia and is confined to males who, after a real or imagined insult, brood for several days and then return in a blind fury during which they attempt to kill everyone encountered. The frenzy is halted only when the person himself is killed or is caught and bound. There is amnesia for the behaviour. The essence of amok is blind, murderous violence arising out of extremely heightened emotions but without other features of psychiatric illness.

Latah

This occurs in Malaysia, affecting the Malay and Iban peoples. It predominantly affects women. Characteristically the sufferers show hypersensitivity to sudden fright or startle, echopraxia, echolalia, automatic responses to commands, and dissociative behaviour. Psychiatrically, latah is similar to the dissociative phenomena.

Similar behaviours have been described in other cultures including Burma (*yuan*), Thailand (*bah-tsche*), Philippines (*mali-mali*), Siberia (*myriachit*), Lapland (Lapp panic), among the Ainu of Japan (*imu*) and the French Canadians of Maine (jumpers) (Simons 1980).

Wihtigo (Windigo)

This occurs in North America and affects the Indians of the Cree, Ojibway, and Salteaux tribes, who experience very severe winters and scarcity of food. Initially sufferers experience a distaste for food, and if this fails to subside anxiety develops, which rapidly reaches a climax. The sufferer then construes the repugnance for food as evidence that he or she is turning into a wihtigo, which is a cannibalistic ice spirit of giant size (Leff 1988). There are doubts about the actual occurrence of cases of wihtigo (Neutra et al. 1977). Phenomenologically, it is an anxiety state.

Possession states

These occur widely across a number of traditional societies and usually affect women, who assert that they are possessed by a spirit, which may be a god or a demon. There is a dramatic change in behaviour and in voice, and unusual desires are expressed. Possession states usually occur in the context of a ritual designed to encourage their induction and

are transient. They are usually not maladaptive but rather help people cope with everyday life and its attendant misfortunes (Jadhav 1995).

Other culture-bound conditions

Apart from the well known entities described earlier there are a number of other conditions:

- Pibloqtoq: occurs among the Arctic and sub-Arctic Eskimos, mainly affects women and is characterized by abrupt episodes of extreme excitement, often followed by apparent seizures and transient coma.
- Susto: seen throughout Latin America where it is believed that a sudden fright will make the soul leave the body making the person vulnerable to a variety of illnesses long after the fright.
- Brain fag: term used in West Africa. The predominant complaint is of fatigue and it occurs mostly in male students in response to the stress of schooling.
- Dhat: it is seen in India where a number of ailments are attributed to semen loss. Similar beliefs prevail in other Asian countries.

REFERENCES

American Psychiatric Association (1994) *Diagnostic and Statistical Manual of Mental Disorders*, 4th edn. Washington, DC: APA.

Asher R (1951) Munchausen's syndrome. *Lancet* **1**: 339–41.

Berrios GE & Luque R (1995) Cotard's syndrome: analysis of 100 cases. *Acta Psychiatrica Scandanavica* **91**: 185–8.

Berrios GE & Morley SJ (1984) Koro-like symptom in a non-Chinese subject. *British Journal of Psychiatry* **145**: 331–4.

Bools CN, Neale BA & Meadow SR (1992) Co-morbidity associated with fabricated illness (Munchausen syndrome by proxy). *Archives of Diseases of Children* **67**: 77–9.

Bools CN, Neale BA & Meadow SR (1993) Follow-up of victims of fabricated illness (Munchausen syndrome by proxy). *Archives of Diseases of Children* **69**: 625–30.

Capgras J & Reboul-Lachaux J (1923) Illusion des sosies dans un delire systematise chronique. *Bulletin de la Societe Clinique de Medecine Mentale* **2**: 6–16.

Christodolou GN (1991) The delusional misidentification syndromes. *The British Journal of Psychiatry* **159**(Suppl 14): 65–9.

Dewhurst K & Todd J (1956) 'The psychosis of association': folie à deux. *Journal of Nervous and Mental Diseases* **124**: 451–8.

De Clerambault GG (1942) *Les Psychoses Passionelles. Oeuvre Psychiatrique*. Paris: Presses Universitaire.

Ekbom K (1938) Praeseniler Dermat-zooenwahn. *Acta Psychiatrica Scandanavica* **13**: 227–59.

Enoch MD & Trethowan W (1991) *Uncommon Psychiatric Syndromes*. Oxford: Butterworth-Heinemann.

Fleminger S & Burns A (1993) The delusional misidentification syndromes in patients with and without evidence of organic cerebral disorder: a structured review of case reports. *Biological Psychiatry* **33**: 22–32.

Ganser SJM (1898) Ueber einen eigenartigen hysterischen Daemmerzustand. *Archiv fur Psychiatrie und Nervenkrankheiten* **30**: 633–40. Transl. by Schorer CE (1965) *British Journal of Criminology* **5**: 120–6.

Harmon RB, Rosner R & Owens H (1995) Obsessional harassment and erotomania in a criminal court population. *Journal of Forensic Sciences* **40**(2): 188–96.

Jadhav S (1995) The ghostbusters of psychiatry. *Lancet* **345**: 808–9.

Jones DPH (1994) The syndrome of Munchausen by proxy. *Child Abuse and Neglect* **18**: 769–71.

Kiraly SJ, Gibson RE, Ancill RJ & Holliday SG (1998) Risperidone: treatment response in adult and geriatric patients. *International Journal of Psychiatry in Medicine* **28**: 255–63.

Lasegue C & Falret J (1877) La folie à deux (ou folie communiquée). *Annales Medico-psycholoques* **18**: 321. Transl. R Michand (1964) *American Journal of Psychiatry* **121**(suppl.): 4.

Leff J (1988) *Psychiatry Around the Globe. A Transcultural View*. London: Gaskell.

Levine RE & Gaw AC (1995) Culture-bound syndromes. *The Psychiatric Clinics of North America* **18**(3): 523–36.

Littlewood R (1990) From categories to contexts: a decade of the 'new cross-cultural psychiatry'. *British Journal of Psychiatry* **156**: 308–27.

Lishman WA (1987) *Organic Psychiatry*. Oxford: Blackwell Scientific.

Meadow R (1977) Munchausen syndrome by proxy: the hinterland of child abuse. *Lancet* **2**: 343–5.

Menzies RPD, Fedroff JP, Green CM & Isaacson K (1995) Prediction of dangerous behaviour in male erotomania. *British Journal of Psychiatry* **166**: 529–36.

Morris M & Jolley D (1987) Delsuisional infestation in late life. *British Journal of Psychiatry* **151**: 272.

Mullen P (1990) Morbid jealousy and the delusions of infidelity. In: Bluglass R & Boweden P (eds) *Principles and Practices of Forensic Psychiatry*. Edinburgh: Churchill Livingstone.

Mullen PE & Pathe M (1994a) Stalking and pathologies of love. *Australian and New Zealand Journal of Psychiatry* **28**: 469–77.

Mullen PE & Pathe M (1994b) The pathological extensions of love. *The British Journal of Psychiatry* **165**: 614–23.

Munro A (1980) Monosymptomatic hypochondraical psychosis. *British Journal of Hospital Medicine* **24**: 34–8.

Neutra R, Kevy JE & Parker D (1977) Cultural expectations versus reality in Navajo seizure patterns and sick roles. *Culture, Medicine and Psychiatry* **1**: 255.

Pathe P & Mullen PE (1997) The impact of stalkers on their victims. *The British Journla of Psychiatry* **170**: 12–17.

Robertson MM & Cervilla JA (1997) Munchausen's syndrome. *British Journal of Hospital Medicine* **58**: 308–12.

Robertson MM & Hossain G (1997) Munchausen's syndrome, co-existing with other disorders. *British Journal of Hospital Medicine* **58**: 154–6.

Rosenberg D (1987) Web of deceit: a literature review of Munchausen syndrome by proxy. *Child Abuse and Neglect* **11**: 547–63.

Samuels MP, McClaughlin W, Jacobson RR, Poets CF & Southall DP (1992) Fourteen cases of imposed upper airway obstruction. *Archives of Childhood Diseases* **67**: 162–70.

Schreier HA & Libow JA (1994) Munhausen by proxy syndrome: a modern pediatric challenge. *Journal of Pediatrics* **125**: 110–15.

Scott PD (1965) The Ganser syndrome. *The British Journal of Criminology* **5**: 127–31.

Scott PD (1977) Assessing dangerousness in criminals. *British Journal of Psychiatry* **131**: 127.

Signer SF (1991) Les Psychoses Passionnelles reconsidered: a review of De Clerambault's cases and syndrome with respect to mood disorders. *Journal of Psychiatry and Neuroscience* **16**(2): 81–90.

Simons RC (1980) The resolution of the Latah paradox. *Journal of Nervous and Mental Disease* **168**: 195–206.

Soyka M, Naber G & Volcker A (1991) Prevalence of delusional jealousy in different psychiatric disorders. *British Journal of Psychiatry* **158**: 549–53.

Sussman N, Borod JC, Cancelmo JA & Braun D (1987) Munchausen's syndrome: a reconceptualisation of the disorder. *Journal of Nervous and Mental Disease* **175**: 692–5.

World Health Organization (1992) *ICD-10 Classification of Mental and Behavioural Disorders*. Geneva: WHO.

Zona MA, Sharma K & Lane J (1993) A comparative study of erotomanic and obsessional subjects in a forensic sample. *Journal of Forensic Sciences* **38**: 894–903.

Psychiatry and women

Shubuladè Smith

INTRODUCTION

Prior to the sixties, women were felt to be the weaker, more emotional, sex, not very mentally robust and thus prone to nervous disorder. After the sexual revolution, feminism stamped out the differences between men and women, insisting that males and females be treated in the same way in all walks of life. This is a far more acceptable state of affairs for most people; yet ignoring differences between individuals may result in inappropriate comparisons being made and less than appropriate treatments being given. This chapter attempts to redress the balance. It should be remembered that women are different to men in certain ways which may have profound effects on the development, course, outcome and treatment of any disorder. In this chapter we look at some of the most important aspects of psychiatry as it pertains to women.

EPIDEMIOLOGY OF PSYCHIATRIC DISORDERS IN WOMEN

The recent National Psychiatric Morbidity Survey (Jenkins et al. 1997) in the UK revealed that women were far more likely than men to suffer with all psychiatric disorders except for functional psychosis, and alcohol and drug dependence (see Table 23.1). The rates of disorder were very similar to those found in the Epidemiologic Catchment Area Study in the US (Weissman et al. 1998). This discrepancy between the sexes has been challenged by some who feel that increased rates of alcohol and substance abuse seen in men might actually be an expression of underlying distress, much the same as that seen in women, women being more likely to report their distress than men (Hohmann 1989).

Treatment settings

Women are more likely to present to primary care services but less likely to be referrred on to secondary care than men.

However, they still make up the majority of the in-patient hospital population, mainly because of elderly women with dementia (Johnson & Busiewicz 1996).

Far fewer women commit crime than men, but when women do come into contact with the criminal justice system, they are more likely to receive a psychiatric disposal (Maden et al. 1994). The marked gender differences in the forensic population, results in poor service provision for mentally ill female offenders, many being placed on units where they are greatly outnumbered by men and therefore at risk from physical and sexual violence. Maden et al. (1994) demonstrated that women prisoners have higher prevalences of some psychiatric disorders than men, yet many prisons are not equipped to provide adequate psychiatric care for such people.

DISORDERS SPECIFICALLY ASSOCIATED WITH BEING FEMALE

Menarche

There are no specific disorders associated with menarche. Theories that early psychological stress results in earlier age of reproductive maturation have not been upheld. Unpreparedness/early menarche tends to be associated with more negative emotional reactions but is not as traumatic an event as portrayed in the literature. Recently, Bisaga et al. (2002) found that adolescent females who had a later onset of menarche were more likely to report depressive symptoms.

The main importance of puberty to psychiatrists is that it heralds the onset of the reproductive period of a woman's life and this coincides with a greater risk of psychiatric illness, particularly depression.

Menstrual cycle

Cyclical changes in mood and other symptoms may be associated with the menstrual cycle. Frank (1931) described premenstrual tension, now commonly called premenstrual syndrome (PMS).

Table 23.1   Prevalence per 1000 of psychiatric disorders in men and women

Diagnosis	Women (95% CI)	Men (95% CI)
Generalized anxiety disorder	51 (45-57)	39 (33–45)
Major depressive disorder	27 (23-31)	18 (14–22)
Phobic disorder[1]	25 (21-29)	12 (8–16)
Panic disorder[1]	15 (11-19)	9 (7–11)
Obsessive-compulsive disorder[1]	20 (16-24)	12 (8–16)
Alcohol abuse/dependence[2]	21(17-25)	75 (65–85)
Drug abuse/dependence[2]	15 (11-19)	29 (23–35)
Schizophrenia[2]	4 (2-6)	4 (2–6)

[1] 1-week prevalence
[2] 1-year prevalence
From: Jenkins R, Lewis G, Bebbington P et al. (1997) *Psychological Medicine* **27**: 775-89 with permission.

Clinical features

- anxiety
- irritability
- depression
- lethargy
- headache
- abdominal distension/bloatedness
- breast swelling and tenderness
- fluid retention and weight gain.

Most women having ovulatory cycles experience some cyclical symptoms, but for some 3%, these symptoms are severe and result in a marked disturbance of their every-day functioning.

In the ICD-10 (World Health Organization 1992), premenstrual symptoms are classified under genitourinary diseases, and in the UK few psychiatrists will be confronted by women complaining specifically of premenstrual syndrome, this being more commonly seen by gynaecologists (Box 23.1). In America, however, the symptoms associated with the premenstrual phase have made their way into DSM-IV (American Psychiatric Assocation 1994) and are classified as a mood disorder, not otherwise specified – premenstrual dysphoric disorder (PMDD). Until now there has been little consensus with regard to diagnosis; there has been frequent use of unstandardized rating scales and retrospective self-reporting. It thus comes as no surprise that the prevalence of the disorder ranges from 3% in some studies to 90% in others. Despite the acceptance of the diagnosis in DSM-IV, there remains controversy regarding the disorder. For a diagnosis of PMDD symptoms should:

- recur cyclically during the luteal phase of the cycle
- remit after the onset of menses and remain absent for at least one week during the follicular phase
- cause marked interference with usual activities of life
- have been documented by prospective daily ratings during at least two consecutive cycles.

Aetiology

PMS is only associated with ovulatory cycles: hysterectomy and ovariectomy eliminate PMS, whereas symptoms persist when hysterectomy is undertaken and the ovaries left, hence the implication that something about ovulation causes profound changes in mood. Progesterone deficiency, progesterone excess, raised prolactin levels, and raised and decreased levels of oestrogen have been postulated as causal, as have changes in oestradiol:progesterone ratio, although no difference in hormonal levels has been found between PMS sufferers and non-sufferers.

Serotonin may play a role as 5HT uptake in platelets and levels of 5HT in whole blood are reduced during the late luteal phase in women with PMS compared to non-suffers. There have also been reports of significant response to SSRIs in women with PMS (Young et al. 1998).

Recently, reduced levels of blood-cell calcium have been found in those with PMS, fuelling speculation that the disorder may be related to a calcium deficiency state or a metabolic defect involving calcium (Shamberger 2003).

Women who report PMS have a higher prevalence of coexisting depressive disorder, anxiety disorder and substance misuse, tend to be unemployed and have poor marital relationships, and are more likely to experience psychological disturbance related to reproductive events. This latter finding may indicate an inherent abnormality of steroidal hormone metabolism/response in these women.

Treatment

- Progesterone vaginal suppositories were found to have no better effect than placebo.
- Oestrogen has had little success, the fears about endometrial hyperplasia severely curtailing widespread use of this method.

Box 23.1   Premenstrual symptoms and psychiatry

Premenstrual syndrome is unlikely to be the sole complaint of a patient attending a psychiatrist. The main importance of PMS to most psychiatrists is that patients with major mental illness such as schizophrenia and bipolar disorder might have premenstrual exacerbations of their illness. This may in part be related to changes in fluid balance, especially for drugs such as lithium. The control of drug levels in certain patients may be extremely difficult at this time. There is also a possibility that there is a change in receptor sensitivity that coincides with the marked hormonal changes that occur particularly in the late luteal phase.

The oral contraceptive pill has not been very effective, its use being implicated in the onset of depression in certain women.

Other treatments range from diet alteration, exercise, vitamin B_6 and evening primrose oil, to more drastic interventions such as GnRH agonists, danazol and even surgical ablation. The SSRIs have been found to significantly relieve symptoms of PMS in women (Young et al. 1998).

DISORDERS ASSOCIATED WITH CHILDBIRTH

Pregnancy

This is generally associated with a decreased rate of major mental illness and suicide, despite pregnancy being a major life event. Studies have described psychiatric disturbance in 5–10% of women attending antenatal clinics (Kumar & Robson 1984). When psychological problems do occur they often take the form of mild anxiety. Depression occurring in late pregnancy may persist as a postnatal depression.

Most at risk are young single mothers with little social support. Psychiatric symptoms when seen tend to occur in the first trimester and are often a reaction to an unplanned pregnancy in the context of a poor marital relationship. These problems are best helped with counselling, education and reassurance. A psychotherapeutic approach addressing the issues of impending motherhood, the meaning of this to the woman and exploration of her own parenting may reveal important concerns about her own ability to mother (Raphael-Leff 1986).

Exceptions to the above are women with a past psychiatric history, who are at much higher risk of breakdown during pregnancy and as such should be monitored closely throughout. This is especially so for those with bipolar illness. Medication may need to be prescribed but care must be taken to minimize the risk of foetal toxicity.

Pregnancy in women with major mental illness

Significant numbers of people with chronic psychosis fail to practise adequate contraceptive strategies (Raja & Azzoni 2003). In particular, women with schizophrenia are likely to have fewer planned pregnancies, more unwanted pregnancies and more abortions than controls (Miller & Finnerty 1996).

The newer atypical antipsychotics are less likely to cause hyperprolactinaemic-induced subfertility, thus patients taking these medications are more likely to get pregnant. Women with a history of psychotic illness, particularly those with schizophrenia, are at increased risk for poor obstetric outcomes, including stillbirth, preterm delivery, low birth weight, neonatal death and neonates who are small for their gestational age (Howard et al. 2003; Patton et al. 2002). However, it is possible for women with severe mental illness to successfully give birth and care for their children. The clinician can facilitate this.

Managing pregnancy in women with severe mental illness

- Inform all women of reproductive age about the risks of pregnancy with unprotected sexual intercourse, especially if they are taking one of the newer prolactin-sparing medications, e.g. olanzapine, quetiapine, ziprasidone or clozapine.
- Encourage female patients to discuss any plans for pregnancy *before* they actually get pregnant and to let their clinician know as soon as they think they might be pregnant.
- Prepregnancy counselling should include discussion of risks of medication versus risks of stopping medication; antenatal care; perinatal psychiatric services (if available); contingency plans in case of relapse; social services involvement/support and breastfeeding.
- Refer patient to specialist perinatal psychiatric services if available.
- Ensure regular liaison with primary care and specialist perinatal/obstetric services.
- Social services should be informed about any woman with a severe mental illness who is due to give birth. They should invite all interested agencies (including family) to a prebirth planning conference at which contingency and crisis plans can be discussed, from no support to full care by social services.
- The role of the psychiatric team is very important to ensure that there is adequate understanding of the woman's illness and capabilities (these can easily be under- or overestimated by other agencies). A significant proportion of women with chronic mental illness are able to care for their children, although they may need support from social services. These supports can be predicted and put in place before the child is actually born.

Pharmacological treatment of pregnant women with severe mental illness

- Avoid polypharmacy.
- Try to avoid medication in the first trimester, however, do not stop medication suddenly, as abrupt cessation may be associated with rebound psychosis (especially with the newer atypical antipsychotics).
- Use the lowest dose possible of the most established medications.
- Withdrawing antipsychotics towards the end of pregnancy may prevent extrapyramidal side effects in the neonate, but may increase risk of relapse in the mother.

- Lithium in the first trimester is particularly associated with Ebstein's anomaly and should be avoided. Likewise, other mood stabilizers such as sodium valproate and carbamazepine are associated with congenital abnormalities, mainly spina bifida. If they have to be continued, patients should be given folic acid supplements.
- Some of the newer antipsychotics are also effective in bipolar illness and there are reports that they have been used during pregnancy with no ill-effects to the foetus (Mendekhar et al. 2002; Ratnayake & Libretto 2002; Taylor et al. 2003).

Disorders associated with the puerperium

Following childbirth, the incidence of psychiatric disorder increases greatly. The disturbances range from the mild postnatal blues to severe disabling psychoses, which frequently require hospital admission and may interfere with mother–infant bonding. Some believe there are distinct aspects to puerperal illness that deserve separate recognition, others feel there is not enough evidence to distinguish puerperal disorders from major psychiatric disorders occurring at any other time. In ICD-10 there is provision for classification of disorders associated with the puerperium (F53), but the recommendation is that this classification should be used only for mental disorders that do not meet the criteria for disorders classified elsewhere and it is felt that most could be classified under the mood (affective) disorders (F30–F39).

Postpartum blues (maternity blues, postnatal blues)

This is a transient mood disturbance occuring 3 to 5 days after childbirth. It occurs in 50-60% of mothers and usually resolves within about 2 days. It is very common but may cause considerable distress to mother and relatives

Clinical features

- crying
- irritability
- depression
- lability of mood
- maximal depression and lability on day 5 postpartum.

The aetiology is unknown. There is no association with changes in levels of oestrogen, progesterone or adrenal steroids. Women with severe postnatal blues are at particular risk of developing a postnatal depression, which implies that their aetiology may be linked (Sutter 1997). The 'blues' might herald the onset of postnatal depression. With the current vogue for early discharge from hospital, severe blues may be missed and thus all those involved in the care of the mother in the community (midwives, GPs and health visitors) should be alert to the diagnosis.

Treatment

- support
- reassurance
- the condition is self-limiting
- observe for development of a major illness, if episode seems prolonged or severe.

Postnatal depression

Postnatal depression (PND) is a common disorder that is often missed by health professionals despite occurring when women are under more scrutiny than at any other time in their lives: 10–15% of mothers become non-psychotically depressed within 6–8 weeks of childbirth. This finding has been replicated in different countries and cultures.

Non-detection of PND occurs for a number of reasons. Symptoms usually manifest after the third day postpartum, but many mothers have been discharged home by this time. Health professionals and family may be more concerned with the mother's physical health than her emotional wellbeing. Those dealing with postnatal care may expect to see the 'blues,' and therefore ascribe any mood disturbance to this self-limiting disorder. Mothers themselves may not report depression as they may not realize what is happening or because of the stigma attached to mental illness, especially at a time when they are meant to be experiencing 'parental bliss.'

Paykel et al. (1980) described risk factors associated with postnatal depression: stressful life events, previous history of psychiatric disorder, younger age, poor marital relationship and absence of social support. More recently it has been found that PND is associated with unplanned pregnancy, not breast-feeding and unemployment. Also, women who were discharged within 72 hours of childbirth were found to have a significantly increased risk of developing PND. It is of note that up to 50% of women who develop postnatal depression report a previous history of sexual abuse.

Clinical features

- tearfulness and profound sadness
- poor concentration and indecisiveness
- irritability and loss of libido
- marked anxiety about the baby's health and fears that it may be deformed
- negative thoughts of failure and inadequacy as a mother
- sleep disturbance
- suicidal ideas and thoughts of harm to the baby.

Aetiology

Depression occurs in much higher rates after childbirth than during pregnancy. However the rates are very similar to those found in non-pregnant, community samples. Nonetheless, researchers have attempted to compare biochemical changes occurring around childbirth with those seen in non-puerperal depression in an effort to elucidate any underlying biological basis to the disorder.

Harris et al. (1992) found that women with positive thyroid antibodies scored significantly higher on depression scores than women who were antibody-negative and concluded that depressive symptoms are associated with positive thyroid antibody status in the puerperium. Ten per cent of women are thyroid antibody-positive and therefore identifying and monitoring these women may help in prevention. Women who experience a more rapid reduction in beta-endorphin at birth are more prone to depression postpartum (Smith et al. 1990). Sichel et al. (1995) hypothesized an 'oestrogen withdrawal state' resulting from the sudden reduction in oestrogen after delivery, after finding that high dose oral oestrogen was effective in preventing relapse in women at high risk of puerperal depression. McIvor et al. (1996) demonstrated that women with a past history of major depression who subsequently relapse after childbirth have significantly greater growth hormone response to apomorphine than those who remain well. Thus the development of increased sensitivity of hypothalamic dopamine D_2 receptors may predict the onset of depressive disorder.

Treatment

The following psychological treatments have been found to improve outcome in the short-term although they are not superior to spontaneous remission in the long-term (Cooper et al. 2003):

- A full psychiatric history should be taken, with particular reference to deliberate self-harm or harm to baby.
- Counselling/psychotherapy/cognitive behaviour therapy.
- Antidepressants can be given even if breastfeeding (see below). Lithium should be avoided when breastfeeding.
- Admit (preferably to specialist mother and baby unit) if illness is severe and risk of deliberate self-harm or harm to baby.

Prevention

- Preventative measures include adequate training especially for midwives and GPs.
- Education antenatally may help mothers distinguish between the blues and more severe mood symptoms that may require professional help.
- Antenatal detection, close follow-up and prophylaxis in high risk patients.
- Early detection – monitor mothers with severe postnatal blues as there is a high risk of depression later.
- Screening, e.g. Edinburgh Postnatal Depression Scale.

Prognosis

Most postnatal depression will have resolved by six months after birth. Unfortunately, the depression may have serious detrimental effects on the marital relationship and mother–infant relationship.

Postnatal depression and child development

Severe mood disturbance during the postnatal period may affect child development by interfering with usual mother–child bonding process. Depressed mothers are more unresponsive to infants, cries, and usually more withdrawn or hostile than non-depressed mothers (Murray et al. 1996). The infant's way of relating to others may be negatively influenced by this early relationship to a depressed mother. Finally, children whose mothers are depressed at three months postpartum have been found to have significantly lower IQ scores, with boys being more negatively affected than girls. These children also have more attentional problems, more difficulty with mathematical reasoning and are more likely to have special educational needs (Hay et al. 2001).

Puerperal (postnatal) psychosis

Epidemiology

These are mainly affective, but can be schizophrenic or organic. They occur after 0.2% of live births. There is a substantial increase in the risk of a mother being admitted to a psychiatric unit within 90 days of parturition. The risk is 2.2/1000 births. In the first 30 days after childbirth, there are seven times as many admissions as in the same group of people as before pregnancy, and for primigravidas, the risk of being admitted to a psychiatric hospital with psychosis within this 30-day period is 35 times higher than before pregnancy (Kendell et al. 1987).

Hippocrates described puerperal psychoses in 5th century BC, thinking they were the result of breast milk erroneously entering the brain. Much later, in 1858, Marcé's study of 310 women with mental illness associated with childbirth seemed to confirm a distinct clinical syndrome consisting of a predominance of delirium and lability of mood occurring 4–5 days postpartum. Today, researchers continue to search for the humoral mechanism that might underlie the aetiology of this disease, but the distinction of postnatal psychosis from other major psychotic illness remains in doubt. This is because the clinical features of puerperal psychoses closely resemble those of psychoses occurring at other times and no differences have been found between the subsequent psychiatric morbidity or hormone levels of psychotic mothers compared with mothers with nonpsychotic illness or mothers who remain well postpartum.

However, the clinical picture shows these women with puerperal psychosis to be more deluded, hallucinated, labile and more likely to be disorientated than in non-puerperal psychosis, and onset is usually within two weeks after delivery, implying that there may be some biological trigger to the disorder.

Aetiology

Kendell et al. (1987) found that there is an increased risk of psychiatric admission if the mother is unmarried, if it is her first baby and if delivery is by Caesarean section, all indicating that psychological stress may be the important factor. However, depressive/manic presentations are commoner: a past history of manic depression or postnatal psychosis leads to a 1 in 5 chance of an affective disorder after childbirth, i.e. much higher risk of relapse, and in high risk women who do relapse after childbirth, it has been shown that the onset of psychotic symptoms is preceded by increased dopamine receptor sensitivity (Wieck et al. 1991). These findings support a biological basis to the illness.

Clinical features

- Severe insomnia in the absence of a crying baby.
- Confusion and memory impairment.
- Markedly changeable behaviour with rapid shifts from elation to profound sadness or rage, from inappropriate laughter to tearfulness.
- Paranoid delusions re: hospital staff or family.
- Thought interference.
- Periods of florid psychosis may be interspersed with intervals of lucidity.
- Marked guilt, depression, anxiety, irritability.
- Suicidal and/or infanticidal thoughts.

Often the initial stages of mood lability may be difficult to distinguish from postnatal blues

Management

In-patient treatment is often needed, preferably with the baby but not if the mother is too disturbed or infanticidal. Mother and baby units are specialist wards where the baby is cared for by nurses and the mother's care of the child can be monitored over time. Midwife and health visitor involvement should be maintained.

The mother should be observed for up to one week prior to discharge to ensure she is coping adequately with the baby. Any coexisting illness should be treated. Don't forget the postnatal examination just because the person is in a psychiatric unit, and don't forget the father. He may be confused, upset and may even be the subject of a delusion. Lovestone & Kumar (1993) found that fathers whose partners become postnatally unwell have much higher rates of psychiatric disorder, compared with fathers whose partners remain well after birth. Information, education and reassurance about his partner's illness, together with involving him in the care of his child, will help to alleviate some of his concerns, at the same time as facilitating the bonding process.

Treatment

- Antipsychotics (choice of drug will depend on whether mother is breastfeeding or not).
- Antidepressants (usually given in conjunction with an antipsychotic as the illnesses are often affective in nature).
- ECT.
- Lithium has been used prophylactically in patients at high risk of relapse, but there are concerns about teratogenicity. Stewart et al. (1991), found that giving lithium late in the third trimester or immediately after delivery was effective in reducing the risk of relapse. However one woman in their sample had an unexplained stillbirth after taking lithium in the third trimester. The changes in fluid balance that occur after birth can make it very difficult to control blood levels of lithium and therefore toxicity is always a risk.
- Lithium should not be given to breastfeeding women.
- Sichel et al. 1995, used prophylactic oral oestrogen to prevent relapse in high risk patients.

Breastfeeding

Many women will wish to breast feed, but psychotropic medications enter the breast milk and may affect the neonate (Burt et al. 2001, Patton et al. 2002). The following points about breastfeeding should be considered (see Chapter 38):

- It is generally advisable to keep doses to a minimum and use shorter-acting drugs if psychotropic medications are given to a breastfeeding woman.
- Time feeds to avoid peak drug levels, e.g. giving the dose after the last breastfeed at night in older infants may help to reduce exposure to the drug.
- The infant should be monitored for adverse drug effects as well as close attention being paid to their feeding, growth and development.

Yoshida et al. (1998), found that breastfed infants whose mothers were given large or multiple doses of antipsychotics showed decline in their developmental scores, but found no acute toxic effects and no evidence of developmental delay in infants breastfed by mothers taking tricyclic antidepressants. Wisner et al. (1996), found that adverse effects in breastfed infants were seen with doxepin and fluoxetine, but not with sertraline, amitriptyline, desipramine, dothiepin or clomipramine. For a review of psychotropic use in breastfeeding see Maudsley Prescribing Guidelines 2003 and Chapter 30.

Prognosis

For the acute illness, the prognosis is very good, but the risk of relapse after further births is very high (up to 50%).

Other disorders associated with childbirth

Phobias, OCD and anxiety states may interfere markedly with childcare. Recently there has been interest in PTSD occurring after traumatic childbirth, Wijma et al. (1997) finding a prevalence of 1.7% in postnatal women.

MENOPAUSE

The menopause is defined as 12 months after the last menses. The average age of menopause in British women is 51 years. This time in a woman's life is associated with many changes, including children leaving home, death of parents and the loss of reproductive capability. The time of menopause calls for a reappraisal of roles, particularly the maternal one.

The menopause is another time in the reproductive cycle that is anecdotally associated with psychiatric symptoms, yet studies have found little evidence for a mood disorder specifically related to the menopause, symptoms being no different from those found with mood disorders occurring at any other time.

There is insufficient evidence to show that menopause causes depression (Box 23.2). Pearce et al. (1995) found that psychological morbidity (not amounting to psychiatric disorder) preceeds natural menopause and follows surgical menopause, but psychosocial factors are more relevant than hormonal factors. Many women developing psychiatric symptoms around the time of the menopause appear to belong to a vulnerable population who are likely to develop symptoms in response to stress. These women were also more likely to attend clinic than matched controls.

The role of hormone replacement therapy

Hormone replacement therapy (HRT) has been said by many women not only to improve their physical symptoms, but also their mood. Evidence of improvement in psychological symptoms has been found only in those women who have undergone surgical menopause. When sexual symptoms are the main complaint, HRT seems to be more effective.

Women presenting with psychological symptoms should be treated with psychological interventions, as the response to HRT has been found to be no better than placebo. More recently there have been concerns about the risk of certain cancers in women taking HRT in the long-term, and therefore, given the lack of evidence for their efficacy in psychiatric disorder, their use for mood improvement is not recommended.

Box 23.2 Menopausal symptoms and psychiatry

No real correlation between any psychiatric illness and the menopause has been found. The main predictors of depression during the menopause are psychosocial and do not differ from those risk factors associated with depression occurring at other times of life, i.e. past history of depression, stressful life events and unemployment (for review see Nicol-Smith 1996).

Hormonal aspects of psychiatric illness

Stewart & Boydell (1993) found that women who suffer from affective disorders following one reproductive event are more vulnerable to recurrences associated with others. A proportion of women may have increased sensitivity or an abnormal response to the neuromodulatory effects of hormones, which result in them being more vulnerable to psychiatric disorder during times of hormonal flux. This would tally with the findings of Bebbington et al. (1998) that the excess of depression in women disappeared in the post-menopausal years, which was not explained in terms of social variables. On the other hand, the later onset of schizophrenia in women may be a result of protective effects of oestrogen.

DISORDERS SHOWING HIGHER PREVALENCE IN WOMEN

Eating disorders, depression, anxiety, agoraphobia, dementia, somatization, borderline personality disorder and parasuicide are all discussed in the relevant chapters in detail, but are briefly mentioned to highlight the gender bias they have in common.

Eating disorders

Anorexia nervosa has a prevalence of 1%; 86% of sufferers are female. Bulimia nervosa is on the increase – it is more culture-bound than anorexia and is associated with other maladaptive behaviours. It has a higher prevalence in ballerinas, models, etc (see Chapter 17).

Depression, anxiety and phobic disorders

Consistently shown to occur almost twice as much in women as men (see Table 23.1 and Chapter 15).

Dementia

Thought to be seen more in women as they live longer. There are possible beneficial effects of oestrogen on cognitive function and HRT may be prophylactic against the development of symptoms (see Chapter 26 and 31).

Somatization disorder

Also known as St Louis hysteria or Briquet's syndrome, this disorder occurs almost exclusively in females. In the Epidemiological Catchment Area study, the prevalence was 0.38% of the general population (see Chapter 15).

Borderline personality disorder

Borderline personality disorder (BRD) is classified in ICD-10 under emotionally unstable personality disorder. There is much controversy over the definition of BPD and therefore statements about the epidemiology of the disorder are difficult to make. It is generally felt to be much more common in women than men, and appears to be associated with a previous history of abuse or neglect (see Chapter 14).

Deliberate self-harm

Deliberate self-harm (DSH) occurs more frequently in women than men, and completed suicide is three times as common in men as women (Charlton et al. 1992). Women use less violent methods than men. People who self-harm are more often female, young adult, in a situational crisis, have no major mental illness. People who commit suicide are more often male, young or middle-aged adult and have a major mental illness such as schizophrenia (see Chapter 21).

Management

- Assess suicide risk; it must be noted that recurrent parasuicide attempts are associated with subsequent completed suicide and this should always be borne in mind when assessing patients who self-harm.
- Try to help the person manage the situation. This may involve couple/family work. Remember that the patient is genuinely distressed and at the time of the attempt may not have been able to think of another solution to the crisis.
- Offer counselling and follow-up but try to avoid making the person a psychiatric patient if there is no mental illness present.
- Some time in sessions should be given to teaching better coping strategies such that should a similar stressful situation arise, the patient will be better able to deal with it.

DISORDERS SHOWING LOWER PREVALENCE IN WOMEN

Alcohol dependency

Alcohol dependency is felt to occur more in men because alcohol is seen as an acceptable coping mechanism. Men are felt to cope with their emotional distress by self-medicating with alcohol rather than seeking support from their GP as women do (Hohmann 1989).

Drug addiction

Drug addiction is also felt to be a maladaptive coping mechanism used by emotionally vulnerable men to overcome their fears.

Violent crime

This is less associated with women than men, but recent years have seen an increase in violent crime by women. This may be a reporting bias due to people being more likely to complain of assault by women or it may reflect a true increase in violence perpetrated by women. d'Orban & Dalton (1980), found that 44% of women committed violent crime during the paramenstrum, although offences were unrelated to symptoms of PMS. The diagnosis of PMS has been accepted as a defence in cases of violent crime (R v Craddock 1982 and R v English 1983). Women who do commit violent crimes are more likely to receive a psychiatric disposal and to have diagnoses of schizophrenia or personality disorder.

DISORDERS PRESENTING DIFFERENTLY IN WOMEN COMPARED TO MEN

Schizophrenia

This disorder has an equal prevalence in males and females but presents differently in men and women. In women it starts later and typically has a less severe course. Women tend to have more affective symptoms and to achieve a higher educational level. Men have a greater vulnerability to negative symptoms. Women may have a better treatment response. Women have a greater prolactin response to antipsychotic medication and appear more prone to tardive dyskinesia. They are possibly less likely to respond to treatment if the disease is chronic than men. Women may be protected by the neuromodulatory effects of oestrogen on dopamine receptors in the brain.

Bipolar Illness

This illness also has an equal prevalence in men and women, but bipolar disorder tends to occur later in women than men. Women experience depressive episodes, mixed mania, and rapid cycling more often than men and more often have a seasonal pattern of mood disturbance. Bipolar II disorder, which is predominated by depressive episodes, also appears to be more common in women than men (Arnold 2003).

TREATING WOMEN WITH PSYCHIATRIC ILLNESS

With female patients, there are a number of factors that can greatly influence treatment and outcome and should be taken into account when treating women.

Pharmacological factors

Throughout Europe and America, women receive twice as many prescriptions for psychotropic medication as men.

These are drugs that in the most part, have been developed from research in young healthy male subjects. Women differ from men in terms of their physiology, and thus differ in the way that they metabolize drugs. Physiological mechanisms showing gender differences include total blood volume, absolute percent body fat, gastric emptying, hepatic metabolism and renal clearance. These all tend towards increased blood levels of a drug after ingestion and decreased renal clearance compared with men. This is especially true for those drugs that are mainly metabolized by the liver, as most psychotropic medications are. These effects are not simply countered by dosing on a mg/kg basis because the effects of gender affect multiple mechanisms underlying the pharmacokinetics. Thus for the same weight, a man will clear a drug quicker and have lower plasma levels than a woman. Women may therefore be more at risk of adverse effects because the drug stays in the body for longer (see chapter 38).

For women there exist particular physiological states which do not occur in men. The menstrual cycle, pregnancy and menopause all represent physiologically normal processes that may affect drug metabolism in women. Menstrual phase changes may affect drug distribution and metabolism, e.g. variable dosing of antidepressants and lithium is needed in some patients to control symptoms during the different stages of the menstrual cycle. The oral contraceptive pill can interact with psychotropic medication, e.g. to decrease clearance of benzodiazepines. In pregnancy, large changes in drug kinetics and dynamics may be expected and in addition there is the presence of the fetus and the added risk of teratogenicity. The risks to the infant of giving psychotropic medications to breastfeeding mothers must also be taken into account.

Women are frequently excluded from drug trials, but there is a growing body of research that indicates the need for specific gender differences to be taken into account when drug research is being done, including:

- cytochrome P450 metabolism (differs in men and women)
- the prolactin response to neuroleptics is increased in women compared to men
- women respond better to smaller doses of neuroleptic than men, but are more likely to get tardive dyskinesia later in life.

Prescribing factors

The psychotropic drugs prescribed in greatest amounts are hypnotics and the highest prescribing is associated with being female aged 65 years and over living in socially deprived areas (Pharoah & Melzer 1995). Women presenting with the same psychiatric complaint as men are significantly more likely to receive prescriptions for anxiolytics and antidepressants (Hohman 1989)

Sexual abuse

This is an extremely relevant risk factor for psychiatric disorder. Women are up to three times more likely to be sexually abused than men. Depending on definition, studies have found that almost 50% of female patients report sexual abuse. Patients who have been sexually abused are more likely to present with maladaptive coping mechanisms and polydiagnosis.

The true extent of the problem is unknown. Reporting bias, and a lack of consensus as to what constitutes sexual abuse (it being partly dependent on the extent of the sexual interaction, and also on the individual's response to the sexual involvement) has resulted in difficulties assessing the prevalence of sexual abuse.

Sexual abuse is particularly associated with low self-esteem, suicidal behaviour, borderline personality disorder, eating disorder, sexual dysfunction, somatization disorder and substance misuse. Severity of abuse is related to the degree of adult psychopathology and psychiatric disorder is more likely to occur in those from disturbed backgrounds (Mullen et al. 1993). Although most reports link childhood sexual abuse with the development of dissociative symptoms, patients with chronic psychosis report significant levels of childhood sexual trauma. Women with severe mental illness experience higher levels of sexual abuse in early life than those without mental illness, and women with schizophrenia are most at risk (Darves-Bornoz et al. 1995; Nettelbladt et al. 1996). Although sexual abuse does not appear to be causally related to the development of psychosis, it appears to worsen outcome in these disorders (Lysaker et al. 2001). Unfortunately, having a severe mental illness appears to put women at much greater risk than the general population of sexual abuse throughout their lives (Darves-Bornoz et al. 1995). This is something that clinicians need to be aware of and alert to.

Physical abuse

Violence towards women frequently occurs in the domestic context. Like sexual abuse, domestic violence is associated with an increased risk of psychiatric disorder. It is particularly associated with depression, anxiety and low self-esteem.

Service provision

Women are major users of psychiatric services, suffering mainly with affective conditions. Current psychiatric services are targeted to psychotic illness and thus some women may be neglected. Services specific to their needs, e.g. crèche facilities, availability of individual/group work for survivors of abuse, should be provided in addition to the usual psychiatric services (see Gadd 1996). If psychiatric services were able to target women more effectively, the benefits would be felt in terms of parenting; family life; costs to the Health Service caused by repeated morbidity and indeed the recovery of working hours lost to psychiatric illness. The return to better functioning of a sizeable group can only be of advantage to society as a whole.

REFERENCES

American Psychiatric Association (1994) *Diagnostic and Statistical Manual of Mental Disorders*, 4th edn. Washington, DC: APA.

Arnold LM (2003) Gender differences in bipolar disorder. *Psychiatric Clinics of North America* **26**(3): 595–620.

Bebbington P, Dunn G, Jenkins R et al. (1998) The influence of age and sex on the prevalence of depressive conditions: report from the National Survey of Psychiatric Morbidity. *Psychological Medicine* **28**(1): 9–19.

Burt VK, Suri R, Altshuler L, Stowe Z, Hendrick VC & Muntean E (2001) The use of psychotropic medications during breast-feeding. *American Journal of Psychiatry* **158**(7): 1001–9.

Charlton J, Kelly S & Dunnell K (1992) Trends in suicide deaths in England and Wales. *Population Trends* **69**: 10–16.

Cooper PJ, Murray L, Wilson A & Romaniuk H (2003) Controlled trial of the short- and long-term effect of psychological treatment of post-partum depression. I. Impact on maternal mood. *British Journal of Psychiatry* **182**: 412–19.

Darves-Bornoz J, Lemperiere T, Degiovanni A et al. (1995) Sexual victimization in women with schizophrenia and bipolar disorder. *Social Psychiatry and Psychiatric Epidemiology* **30**: 78–84.

Frank R (1931) The hormonal causes of premenstrual tension. *Archives of Neurology and Psychiatry* **26**:1053.

Gadd E (1996) Developing psychiatric services for women. In: Abel K, Busiewicz M, Davison S, Johnson S & Staples E (eds) *Planning Community Mental Health Services for Women*, pp. 6–19. London: Routledge.

Harris B, Othman S, Davies J et al. (1992) Association between postpartum thyroid dysfunction and thyroid antibodies and depression. *British Medical Journal* **18**: 305(6846):152–6.

Hay DF, Pawlby S, Sharp D, Asten P, Mills A & Kumar R (2001) Intellectual problems shown by 11-year-old children whose mothers had postnatal depression. *Journal of Child Psychology and Psychiatry* **42**(7): 871–89.

Hohmann A (1989) Gender bias in psychotropic drug prescribing in primary care. *Medical Care* **27**(5): 478–90.

Howard LM, Goss C, Leese M & Thornicroft G (2003) Medical outcome of pregnancy in women with psychotic disorders and their infants in the first year after birth. *British Journal of Psychiatry* **182**: 63–7.

Jenkins R, Lewis G, Bebbington P et al. (1997) The National Psychiatric Morbidity Surveys of Great Britain – initial findings from the Household Survey. *Psychological Medicine* **27**: 775–89.

Johnson S & Busiewicz M (1996) Women's mental health in the UK. In: Abel K, Busiewicz M, Davison S, Johnson S & Staples E (eds) *Planning Community Mental Health Services for Women*, pp. 6–19. London: Routledge.

Kendell R (1985) Emotional and physical factors in the genesis of puerperal mental disorders. *Journal of Psychosomatic Research* **29**: 3–11.

Kendell R, Chalmers J & Platz C (1987) Epidemiology of puerperal psychoses. *British Journal of Psychiatry* **150**: 662–73.

Kumar R & Robson K (1984) A prospective study of emotional disorders in childbearing women. *British Journal of Psychiatry* **144**: 35–47.

Lovestone S & Kumar R (1993) Postnatal psychiatric illness: the impact on partners. *British Journal of Psychiatry* **163**: 210–16.

Lysaker PH, Meyer P, Evans JD et al. (2001) Neurocognitive and symptom correlates of self-reported childhood sexual abuse in schizophrenia spectrum disorders. *Annals of Clinical Psychiatry* **13**: 89–92.

McIvor R, Davies R, Wieck A et al. (1996) The growth hormone response to apomorphine at 4 days postpartum in women with a history of major depression. *Journal of Affective Disorders* **40**(3): 131–6.

Maden T, Swinton M & Gunn J (1994) Psychiatric disorder in women serving a prison sentence. *British Journal of Psychiatry* **164**(1): 44–54.

Mendhekar DN, War L, Sharma JB & Jiloha RC (2002) Olanzapine and pregnancy. Pharmacopsychiatry **35**(3): 122–3.

Miller LJ & Finnerty M (1998) Family planning knowledge, attitudes and practices in women with schizophrenic spectrum disorders. *Journal of Psychosomatics Obstetrics and Gynaecology* **19**: 210–17.

Mullen P, Martin J, Anderson J et al. (1993) Childhood sexual abuse and mental health in adult life. *British Journal of Psychiatry* **163**: 721–32.

Murray L, Fiori-Cowley A, Hooper R & Cooper P (1996) The impact of postnatal depression and associated adversity on early mother–infant interactions and later infant outcome. *Child Development* **67**(50): 2512–26.

Nettelbladt P, Svensson C & Serin U (1996) Background factors in patients with schizoaffective disorder as compared with patients with diabetes and healthy individuals. *European Archives of Psychiatry and Clinical Neuroscience* **246**: 213–18.

Nicol-Smith L (1996) Causality, menopause and depression: a critical review of the literature. *British Medical Journal* **313**: 1229–32.

d'Orban P & Dalton J (1980) Violent crime and the menstrual cycle. *Psychological Medicine* **10**(2): 353–9.

Patton SW, Misri S, Corral MR, Perry KF & Kuan AJ (2002) Antipsychotic medication during pregnancy and lactation in women with schizophrenia: evaluating the risk. *Canadian Journal of Psychiatry* **47**(10): 959–65.

Paykel E, Emms E, Fletcher J & Rassaby E (1980) Life events and social support in puerperal depression. *British Journal of Psychiatry* **136**: 339–46.

Pearce J, Hawton K & Blake F (1995) Psychological and sexual symptoms associated with the menopause and the effects of hormone replacement therapy. *British Journal of Psychiatry* **167**(2): 163–73.

Pharoah P & Melzer D (1995) Variation in prescribing of hypnotics, anxiolytics and antidepressants between 61 general practices. *British Journal of General Practice* **45**(400): 595–9.

Raja M & Azzoni A (2003) Sexual behaviour and sexual problems among patients with severe chronic psychoses. *European Psychiatry* **18**: 70–6.

Raphael-Leff J (1986) Facilitators and Regulators: Conscious and unconscious processes in pregnancy and early motherhood. *British Journal of Medical Psychology* **59**(pt 1): 43–53.

Ratnayake T & Libretto SE (2002) No complications with risperidone treatment before and throughout pregnancy and during the nursing period. *Journal of Clinical Psychiatry* **63**(1): 76–7.

Shamberger RJ (2003) Calcium, magnesium, and other elements in the red blood cells and hair of normals and patients with premenstrual syndrome. *Biological Trace Element Research* **94**(2): 123–9.

Sichel D, Cohen L, Robertson L et al. (1995) Prophylactic oestrogen in recurrent postpartum affective disorder. *Biological Psychiatry* **38**(120): 814–18.

Smith R, Cubis J, Brinsmead M et al. (1990) Mood changes, obstetric experience and alterations in plasma cortisol, beta-endorphin and corticotrophin releasing hormone during pregnancy and the puerperium. *Journal of Psychosomatic Research* **34**(1): 53–69.

Stewart D & Boydell K (1993) Psychological distress during menopause: associations across the reproductive life cycle. *International Journal of Psychiatry in Medicine* **23**(2): 157–62.

Stewart D, Klompenhouwer J, Kendell R & van Hulst A (1991) Prophylactic lithium in puerpural psychosis. The experience of three centres. *British Journal of Psychiatry* **158**: 393–7.

Sutter A, Leroy V, Dallay D et al. (1997) Post-partum blues and mild depressive symptomatology at days three and five after delivery. A French cross sectional study. *Journal of Affective Disorders* **44**(1): 1–4.

Taylor TM, O'Toole MS, Ohlsen RI, Walters J & Pilowsky LS (2003) Safety of quetiapine during pregnancy. *American Journal of Psychiatry* **160**(3): 588–9.

Weissman MM, Leaf PJ, Tisschler GL et al. (1988) Affective disorders in five US communities. *Psychological Medicine* **18**: 141–53.

Weike A, Kumar R, Hirst A et al. (1991) Increased sensitivity of dopamine receptors and recurrence of affective psychosis after childbirth. *British Medical Journal* **303**: 613–16.

Wijma K, Soderquist J & Wijma B (1997) Posttraumatic stress disorder after childbirth: a cross sectional study. *Journal of Anxiety Disorders* **11**(6): 587–97.

Wisner K, Perel J & Findling R (1996) Antidepressant treatment during breast-feeding. *American Journal of Psychology* **153**(9): 1132–7.

World Health Organization (1992) *ICD-10 Classification of Mental and Behavioural Disorders*. Geneva: WHO.

Yoshida K, Smith B, Craggs M & Kumar R (1998) Neuroleptic drugs in breast-milk: a study of pharmacokinetics and of possible adverse effects in breast-fed infants. *Psychological Medicine* **28**(1): 81–91.

Young S, Hurt P, Benedek D & Howard R 1998 Treatment of premenstrual dysphoric disorder with sertraline during the luteal phase: a randomized, double-blind, placebo-controlled crossover trial. *Journal of Clinical Psychiatry* **59**(2): 76–80.

Adult sequelae of childhood sexual abuse

Sue Stuart-Smith

INTRODUCTION

There is substantial evidence that sexual abuse of children is a widespread problem and has adverse consequences for many of those who have been subjected to it. In a considerable proportion it occurs in the context of neglect and other forms of childhood abuse. As a result, it is a complex area to study and research in this field is fraught with methodological difficulties. Mullen et al. (1988, 1993, 1994) have attempted to overcome many of these difficulties by identifying the potentially confounding variables, in what they term 'the matrix of family disadvantage'. By taking into account factors such as concurrent physical abuse and the nature of the child's relationship with the parents, they have been able to calculate what appear to be the direct effects of childhood sexual abuse. Nevertheless, many of these variables may well act in an additive way and a child who has experienced other forms of abuse and neglect may be particularly vulnerable to adverse effects. Not surprisingly, no clear-cut post-abuse syndrome has emerged from this and other research. Rather, what has emerged is a series of significant associations with a number of psychiatric disorders, as well as impairments in sexual, social and interpersonal functioning. This chapter explores these associations and considers implications for treatment.

HISTORY

Children have been sexually abused throughout history; what changes is the extent to which it is acknowledged and the significance that is placed upon it. Aristotle was one of the earliest writers to observe a link between childhood abuse and adult behaviour. Writing in the 4th century BC, in his *Ethics* (transl. Thomson 1976), he discusses the origin of 'perverse pleasures'. He attributes a proportion of cases of male homosexuality to a 'habit acquired in those who have been victimized since childhood'. Just over a century ago, as a result of his work with female hysterics, Freud (1896) proposed that childhood sexual experiences lay at the root of the psychoneuroses. Shortly after this, in 1897, he abandoned his so-called seduction theory in favour of his developing theory of infantile sexuality and the Oedipus complex. He has been accused by some of betraying the reality of childhood abuse, thereby contributing to the denial of the problem in society as a whole. It is important to appreciate, however, that what Freud retracted was not the existence of childhood sexual abuse, but the idea that it was at the root of all psychoneurotic illness. He continued to acknowledge its damaging effects, even if his interests increasingly lay elsewhere: 'the external influences of seduction are capable of provoking interruptions of the latency period or even its cessation...it seems, moreover, that any such premature sexual activity diminishes a child's educability' (Freud 1905).

Nevertheless, the full extent of the problem of childhood sexual abuse only began to be acknowledged in the 1970s, largely as a result of feminist writers who drew attention to the frequency of childhood victimization. Researchers started to try to measure the extent of the problem. Finkelhor's (1979) study of college students revealed that one-fifth of females and one in 11 males had been sexually abused as children. This, and other similar studies, led to a gradual acceptance by health care professionals in the 1980s that childhood sexual abuse was an important and relevant problem. In contrast, the 1990s have witnessed a highly polarized debate, originating in the USA, about the status of memories of sexual abuse, recovered as a consequence of therapy and the plausibility, or not, of the so-called false memory syndrome. There is little doubt that at least some of this has arisen as a consequence of over-zealous therapists, believing that repression of memories of childhood abuse lies at the root of much psychiatric morbidity and seeking to uncover it in therapy. Brandon et al. (1998) review this debate and discuss implications for clinical practice. It would be a pity if these issues were to detract from the progress that has been made in the recognition and treatment of the effects of childhood sexual abuse, when for the majority of sufferers the problem is not difficulty in remembering, but difficulty in forgetting. Childhood sexual abuse remains a highly emotive subject and one on which it can be hard to retain an appropriate perspective without falling into the trap of either over- or underemphasizing its significance.

DEFINITION

There is no universal definition of child sexual abuse, although Schechter & Roberge's (1976) definition is widely accepted. This refers to the sexual exploitation of children as:

> The involvement of dependent, developmentally immature children and adolescents in sexual activities that they do not fully comprehend, are unable to give informed consent to, and that violate the social taboos of family roles.

This is a broad definition. The area can be further conceptualized according to the following description of the acts involved (after Sheldrick 1991):

- **Exposure:** the viewing of sexual acts, pornography and exhibitionism.
- **Molestation:** fondling the genitals of the child or asking the child to touch the adult's genitals.
- **Sexual intercourse:** vaginal, anal or oral intercourse, without use of excessive force.
- **Rape:** strictly speaking, this is vaginal intercourse without consent, but other forms of intercourse may also involve the threat of violence or actual violence.

The term 'child sexual abuse' thus covers a wide range of experiences. In addition, it includes experiences with other children as well as with adults, ranging from strangers to close members of the family. The abuse may take the form of a single incident or, at the other extreme, consist of repeated, sadistic sexual assaults.

'Sadistic sexual abuse involves the terrorization of children, and its aim is total domination of the child. It has much in common with acts of torture. Certain features may alert a clinician that sadistic abuse has been involved, including: descriptions of ritualistic punishments; abuse requiring hospitalization or surgical repair; and bizarre acts including bondage, the use of excreta or the use of confinement or sensory deprivation' (Sinason 1994). Following the allegations of ritualistic abuse on the UK island of Orkney in 1991 there remains controversy about the extent of so-called satanic abuse. In this form of abuse, children may be subject to sexual abuse as part of 'satanic' or 'black magic' ceremonies. To date, seven cases of ritualistic abuse have successfully been brought to prosecution in the UK.

METHODOLOGICAL DIFFICULTIES

Since the early 1980s, the number of research studies being carried out has increased rapidly, so there is now a substantial amount of literature on the psychological sequelae of childhood sexual abuse. However, the quality of these studies is variable and there remain a number of methodological problems to be addressed. The most important of these are outlined below:

1. **Lack of a universally accepted definition:** as a result of this, studies vary in the definitions they use. Some confine themselves to abuse involving physical contact only, while others use a much broader definition. In addition, a number of studies employ a measure of age discrepancy between perpetrator and victim. Where this is applied, an age difference of at least five years is usually required for an experience to count as abuse. Some research is limited solely to abuse within the family, while other research includes any unwanted sexual experiences. There is also a wide variation in the upper age limit applied to victims, ranging from 12 to 18 years. Because of the diverse definitions used, it is hard to make valid comparisons between many of the studies. Furthermore, the range of definitions used has led to a wide variation in estimates of incidence and prevalence (see below).

2. **Retrospective nature of most studies:** the majority of studies that have been carried out are retrospective, cross-sectional and correlational, rather than longitudinal. Subjects of sex abuse research are often questioned simultaneously about abusive events in the past and their current level of psychological functioning. Childhood abuse reports are then treated as independent variables whereas psychological functioning is considered a dependent variable. However, cause and effect may not be so straightforward; for example, it is possible for current psychological distress to influence retrospective reports of abuse. Some subjects may not report abuse that they have experienced for a number of different reasons, including amnesia, distress, embarrassment and a desire to forget (Femina et al. 1990). If these subjects are then included in 'no abuse' comparison groups, the between-group differences will be obscured. It is also possible that some subjects will make false claims of abuse and there is no satisfactory way to ensure the validity of responses. There are a small number of prospective studies (Bagley & McDonald 1995; Banyard & Williams 1996; Noll et al. 2003) that follow up verified cases such as those on social service registers. While this approach has the advantage of externally validated cases, the results may not generalize to all instances of childhood sexual abuse because such a small proportion of cases (about 5%) are reported to the authorities. Such cases are also likely to be more severe in nature and in addition have lost the shroud of secrecy that encompasses most instances of abuse.

3 **Nature of the population studied:** the subjects chosen for many studies include specific 'problem population's, for example, prostitutes, drug addicts and psychiatric patients. While these studies confirm a high prevalence of childhood sexual abuse in these particular populations, it is not clear what percentage of all sexually abused children go on to develop these problems. Many studies have been carried out on college students (e.g. Finkelhor 1979), but this is not a group representative of the general population in terms of intelligence and social class. The majority of studies have also been on Caucasian subjects, but at least one (Russell et al. 1988) has suggested that Afro-American incest victims report greater degrees of trauma than white victims. The majority of studies have looked at effects on female victims. This means that there is a comparative lack of data on the long-term effects of childhood sexual abuse on men. King et al. (2002), have recently published a study of the child and adult sexual molestation of men, in an attempt to redress the balance.

4 **Confounding effects of other forms of abuse:** there has been a tendency for research in this area to examine sexual abuse in relative isolation, in spite of the fact that it frequently occurs in the context of physical and psychological abuse. If other forms of abuse are not taken into account, it is difficult to infer any specific causality to sexual abuse alone. Studies vary in the extent to which they examine other forms of abuse. Briere (1992) suggests that future research should encompass all three forms of abuse and use multivariate procedures in the analysis in order to try to overcome this problem.

5 **Data collection methods:** there are many different methods used to elicit information about sexual abuse, including face-to-face or telephone interviews, symptom rating scales, case note studies and questionnaires. Childhood sexual abuse is a sensitive subject and, not surprisingly, the method used will influence the results obtained. Wyatt & Peters (1986) conclude, for example, that face-to-face interviews yield higher prevalence rates than self-administered questionnaires. It is generally accepted that female interviewers are most appropriate for both female and male victims. A validated, structured sexual trauma interview has been used in many general population studies (Russell 1983), but a number of other studies use measures of unknown reliability.

PREVALENCE

The variation in the definition of sexual abuse has led to wide discrepancies in prevalence rates, which range from less than 10% to over 30%. In addition, many studies focus only on women. The rates depend on whether an age difference between the individuals involved is taken as a defining factor, what the upper age limit is, whether encounters involving no physical contact are included and whether multiple or single episodes are considered. If the most rigorous definition of unwanted sexual assaults involving attempted or actual penetration is applied, then it is estimated that approximately 5–10% of children will have been sexually abused by the age of 16 (Fergusson & Mullen 1999). The majority of abusers of girls are male, but up to 20% of the abusers of boys may be female. Girls are most often abused by a family member and boys by someone outside their immediate family. The risk of abuse by a stepfather is almost five times the risk of abuse by a biological father. According to Bagley & Thurston (1996), the increasing rate of divorce and subsequent formation of reconstituted families may be linked to an increased incidence of sexual abuse in those born after 1950. This increase has mainly been observed in some North American recall studies.

In an important study, Baker & Duncan (1985) interviewed a representative sample of 2000 British men and women. Twelve per cent of the women and nearly 9% of the men reported having been sexually abused before the age of 16 years. Forty-six per cent of the incidents involved physical contact and 5% consisted of full sexual intercourse. The authors estimate that there are 4.5 million adults in the UK who were sexually abused as children. Other findings were that the onset of abuse in girls tends to be at a younger age, with a mean age of 10.7 years compared to 12 years for boys. Forty-nine per cent of the abusers were known to the child, and girls were at greater risk of incestuous abuse. Boys (44%) were more likely than girls (33%) to experience abuse by someone known to them but not related to them. Sixty-three per cent had experienced one incident but 23% were abused repeatedly by one person, and 14% by a number of people. Girls were more likely than boys to experience revictimization. Fifty-four per cent of the sample reported a damaging effect on their lives. This study indicates that social class is not a factor in the risk of abuse, although some North American studies have found an association with lower social class.

Russell (1983) surveyed a community sample of 900 women in San Francisco and found much higher rates, with 28% having been sexually abused before the age of 14 years and 38% before the age of 18 years. Only 2% of the intrafamilial cases and 6% of the extrafamilial cases had been reported to the police. Twenty-three per cent of the intrafamilial abuse was classified as very serious. The data suggest that when stepfathers abuse their stepdaughters, they are much more likely than any other relative to abuse at the most serious level: 47% of all abuse carried out by stepfathers was classified as very serious. In New Zealand, Anderson et al. (1993) found, in a general population study of women, an overall prevalence of abuse before the age of 16 years of 32%. Nearly 20% reported unwanted contact with their genitalia and in 12% the abuse involved attempted or completed intercourse. Clearly, sexual abuse is a significant international problem. There may be many reasons for the variation in prevalence rates between countries, including methodological differences, but equally it is possible that sexual abuse is more common in some countries than in others.

There is generally less information available about the prevalence of sexual abuse of boys. Much of the attention paid to the problem of sexual abuse arose from the activity of the women's movement and many studies have focused only on women. Finkelhor (1984) reviews the literature on sexual abuse in boys and estimates that the prevalence rates for abusive experiences under the age of 13 or before puberty lie between 2.5% and 5%. In 1999, a primary care survey of over 2000 men in England found a prevalence rate of 5% (Coxell et al. 1999). In 81% of these the perpetrator was male and the mean age at the first episode was 11 years.

THE CONSEQUENCES OF CHILDHOOD SEXUAL ABUSE

The initial and short-term effects are reported in a number of studies which are reviewed by Browne & Finkelhor (1986). These include states of fear, anxiety, depression, anger and hostility as well as inappropriate sexual behaviour, somatic symptoms, truancy and delinquency (Box 24.1). It is important to recognize that the short- and long-term effects of sexual abuse may be different. As an abused child matures

into an adult, his or her understanding of what has taken place often changes and powerful emotions such as guilt and shame take effect. The debate about 'recovered memory' aside, clinical experience suggests that it is possible in some cases for memories of sexual abuse to be suppressed, only for them to re-emerge later in life in response to specific triggers.

More common is the phenomenon of so-called sleeper effects, which are silent during childhood but emerge with considerable impact in adulthood. This is particularly the case with sexual dysfunction but applies to other symptoms as well. There are no specific or unique adult outcomes of childhood sexual abuse and not all children subjected to it will go on to develop problems. It is estimated that about one-third of victims report no long-term adverse effects. Some features of sexual abuse are consistently associated with a poor outcome (Box 24.2).

Long-term effects

Emotional/psychological

Mullen et al. (1993) studied the relationship between childhood sexual abuse and mental health in adult life, and found that women who had experienced penetrative abuse were significantly more likely to suffer from eating disorders, anxiety, depression, suicidal behaviour and substance misuse than those who had experienced other forms of abuse. The high rates of psychopathology were associated with psychiatric admission rates between 5 to 16 times the rates in the non-abused control groups. Seriously

Box 24.1 Psychological effects of sexual abuse			
Nature of trauma	*Acute responses*	*Modifiers*	*Outcomes*
Type of abuse	Fear	Family and peer support	*Direct:*
Duration	Anxiety	Temperament	Feelings of guilt, shame, anger and hostility
Frequency	Depression	Attachment	Flashbacks
Relationship to abuser	Anger		Sleep disturbance
Use of force	Hostility		Sexual dysfunction
Age of onset	Sexualization		Dissociation
			Difficulty with close relationships
			Revictimization
			Becoming an abuser
			Indirect:
			Depression and low self-esteem
			Anxiety
			Self-harm and suicidal behaviour
			Eating disorder
			Somatization
			Substance misuse
			Personality disorder, especially borderline states

Box 24.2   Abuse characteristics that predict adverse outcome

Abuse by father or stepfather
Associated violence and/or threats
Penetrative sexual acts
Multiple abusers
Bizarre abuse

---

abused women were significantly more likely to come from families where emotional and/or physical abuse took place. Logistic regression revealed that the impact of sexual abuse was much reduced when the effect of associated risk factors was taken into account, although cases involving intercourse remained statistically significant.

Depression, low self-esteem and suicidal behaviour
Depression is the most commonly reported symptom in women who have been sexually abused as children, and the association has been demonstrated in many studies (Bagley & Ramsay 1986; Hill et al. 2001; Mullen et al. 1988). Childhood abuse and lack of parental care both increase the risk of depression in later life. In a North London community sample, Bifulco et al. (1991) found that 64% of women who had a history of childhood sexual abuse were clinically depressed at some point during their two-year study, compared to 26% of those who had not been sexually abused. The highest rates of depression were seen in those who had experienced intercourse. Lack of parental care, separation from a parent and physical abuse all also had significant links with depression, and these appeared to interact additively. Only 5% of the sample had experienced sexual abuse in isolation from these factors. A wide range of depressive symptoms are reported by women who had been sexually abused, including feelings of guilt, inferiority, low self-esteem and impaired feelings of interrelatedness (Mullen et al. 1993). A recent study has examined the role of adult relationships in moderating the link between childhood abuse, neglect and depression. The authors found that the risk for depression associated with childhood sexual abuse was unaffected by the quality of intimate adult relationships, while the risk associated with poor parental care was substantially altered (Hill et al. 2001).

Another study has attempted to unravel some of the complex interactions between self-esteem in adulthood and childhood adversity (Romans et al. 1996). It was found that women who report childhood sexual abuse have a greater expectation that unpleasant things will happen to them and are less sure that they can affect their own destiny than other women. The abuse only affected self-esteem directly if it had involved attempted or completed intercourse.

Many studies have found a link between past sexual abuse and self-harm (Browne & Finkelhor 1986). Rates of suicide attempts in women with a history of childhood

sexual abuse have been found to be 2–3 times the rates in control groups (Green 1993). Mullen et al. (1993) found very high levels of suicidal behaviour (70 times that in the control group) in a group of women who had been subjected to severe abuse, many of whom had been subjected to physical abuse as well. It may well be that where physical force has been involved in the abuse, victims are at much greater risk of self-harm than was previously thought. Most of the studies in this area have focused on the mental health consequences in women. It has been hypothesized that there may be differences between the sexes, with women more likely to internalize their feelings of anger, which are then expressed in self-destructive behaviours, whereas men are more likely to project their anger outwards (Hilton & Mezey 1996). However, a study by King et al. in 2002 found that men who reported childhood sexual abuse were 2.4 times more likely to report any type of psychological disturbance and 3.7 times more to have self-harmed than those in the comparison group.

Anxiety, post-traumatic stress and dissociation
Anxiety, tension, insomnia and nightmares are all commonly reported by adults who suffered childhood sexual abuse (Bagley & Ramsay 1986, Browne & Finkelhor 1986). It appears that anxiety is most likely to be a consequence where force or threat of force has been used. Some authors regard these symptoms as manifestations of delayed or chronic post-traumatic stress disorder (PTSD). In some cases, symptoms of anxiety and intrusive memories of the trauma do seem to be elicited by exposure to events that evoke memories of the original abuse (Lindberg & Distad 1985). Women who have been sexually abused also report a higher incidence of dissociation experiences than do non-abused comparison groups. It has been hypothesized that dissociation, which has originally been used as a coping mechanism during abuse, later becomes a symptom in its own right (Briere & Runtz 1988).

Eating disorders and somatization
Mullen et al. (1993) found a strong link between a history of childhood sexual abuse and both anorexia and bulimia (Chapter 17). It appears that about 30% of patients with eating disorders have experienced previous sexual abuse. There has been much recent debate about whether childhood sexual abuse is a specific risk factor for eating disorders, and in particular it has been suggested that this may be the case in bulimia nervosa. A community study found a rate of 26% for contact sexual abuse in subjects with bulimia. This rate was significantly higher than the rate in the control group but not significantly higher than figures for patients with other psychiatric diagnoses (Welch & Fairburn 1994). A recent study compared patients with bulimia, depressed patients and a control group and found that childhood sexual abuse appears to be a vulnerability factor for psychiatric disorder in general rather than for

eating disorder in particular. There was some evidence that eating-disordered patients who had been sexually abused were also more likely to have a history of taking overdoses and shoplifting (Vize & Cooper 1995). Another study has confirmed findings of increased comorbidity in similar patients, including an increased risk of suicide attempts and substance abuse (Sullivan et al. 1995).

Patients who suffer from somatization disorder have been shown to be more likely to have been sexually abused than a control group (Morrison 1989). An association has also been shown, in a number of studies, between childhood sexual abuse and gynaecological symptoms, especially unexplained chronic pelvic pain (Lampe et al. 2003). Walker et al. (1988) have shown that the rate of sexual abuse in sufferers of pelvic pain is twice that found in a general population survey. They also found that chronic pelvic pain was strongly associated with a lifetime history of depression. Pelvic pain may be a metaphorical way of describing chronic psychological pain and could also confer secondary gain, such as the avoidance of sexual contact. There is also an association with other forms of abdominal pain, in particular irritable bowel syndrome and functional constipation. The latter may start in childhood when it can present as faecal soiling and in some cases is related to anal sexual abuse. Scarinci et al. (1994) studied women with gastrointestinal disorders and a history of abuse. They found that the women tended to have a lower pain threshold and a tendency to set low standards for judging a stimulus to be noxious. The authors relate this to their history of sexual abuse which is likely to have involved acute pain, and ascribe their current symptoms to a state of hypervigilance.

Borderline personality disorder, multiple personality disorder and psychotic symptoms

The diagnosis of borderline personality disorder and its differentiation from other personality disorders is highly variable in clinical practice. The diagnosis of multiple personality disorder is even more controversial and it is one that is rarely made outside North America. It has been renamed dissociative identity disorder in DSM-IV. A number of studies have detected high rates of childhood sexual abuse in patients with borderline personality disorder. Figures range from 40% up to 80%. Herman et al. (1989) regard borderline personality disorder as a complicated form of PTSD, in which the trauma becomes integrated into the total personality organization. They also relate the higher rate of this diagnosis in women to the increased incidence of childhood sexual abuse in girls. Certain features of borderline personality disorder, such as suicidal or self-harming behaviour, affective instability and depression, have all been established independently as typical sequelae in adult survivors of sexual abuse. It seems likely that a borderline personality organization results from aspects of severe childhood sexual abuse. Figueroa & Silk (1997) have found that patients diagnosed with borderline personality

disorder are less likely to give a history of mild or transient abuse and more likely to give a history of severe and/or long-lasting abuse than patients in other diagnostic groups.

A number of studies have linked multiple personality disorder with a history of childhood sexual abuse, generally finding rates of 70–90% (Ross et al. 1990). Many of the studies are flawed by the small number of patients involved and the lack of standardized criteria for the diagnosis.

Few studies have looked at the association of childhood sexual abuse with psychotic illnesses, and studies that do exist have tended not to differentiate between physical and sexual abuse. Dissociative symptoms may overlap with psychotic symptoms and contribute to an atypical presentation (Goff et al. 1991). A study of first-episode psychosis found a prevalence rate of childhood abuse (both physical and sexual or combined) of 53% (Greenfield et al. 1994).

Learning disability

Until recently, the association between sexual abuse, metal health and behavioural problems in people with learning disabilities had not been examined in a controlled study (Sequeira et al. 2003). This study found that sexual abuse was associated with increased rates of mental illness, behavioural problems and post-traumatic stress. Psychological reactions to abuse were similar to those observed in the general population but with the addition of stereotypical behaviours.

Sexual adjustment

Almost all clinically based studies found problems of later sexual adjustment in women who had been sexually abused as children (Browne & Finkelhor 1986). This is hardly surprising, given that sexual abuse gives rise to an experience in which sex is contaminated by exploitation, coercion and guilt. Mullen et al. (1994) found that those who had been sexually abused as children were just as likely to be sexually active as controls, but were far more likely to express dissatisfaction with their sex lives and to experience difficulties with their own sexuality. It is not uncommon for sexual experiences to trigger flashbacks to the abuse and even where this is not the case many women suffer from difficulties such as anorgasmia or vaginismus. A recent prospective study has found that sexually abused participants were more preoccupied with sex and tended to be younger at first consensual intercourse as well as more likely to have a teenage pregnancy than the comparison group women (Noll et al. 2003). This study supports the notion that sexual abuse may be a risk factor for early and risky sexual activity.

Much less is known about the long-term effects in male victims. In boys, the type of abuse experienced is less likely to be one of chronic abuse and more likely to be a homosexual encounter with someone outside the home.

Dhaliwal et al. (1996) review the literature, and while it seems that a range of sexual problems, including avoidance, compulsivity and erectile difficulties, may be related to childhood sexual abuse, the evidence is far from clear. The relationship of childhood sexual abuse to adult homosexual orientation remains controversial. Finkelhor (1979) reported that men who had been sexually abused before the age of 13 years were four times more likely to define themselves as homosexual than controls. However, subsequent studies have failed to confirm this scale of effect. Likewise, in women there appears to be a small but significantly increased rate of later homosexuality (Beitchman et al. 1992).

Interpersonal relationships

The effect of childhood sexual abuse on interpersonal relationships is often profound and far-reaching. It can lead to difficulties in relating to parents, peers, partners and the victim's own children. Hostile feelings towards the mother for failing to protect the victim are common and may be stronger than hostile feelings towards the abuser (Browne & Finkelhor 1986). Incest victims are more likely to have difficulties with close relationships where there has been a history of poor attachment to the mother.

Child sexual abuse is known to be associated with insecure and disorganized attachments (Alexander 1993), as well as with physical abuse. Given that each of these in its own right will exert a considerable influence on interpersonal functioning, there is a need to try to disentangle the effects of sexual abuse from the general effect of the context within which it so often occurs. Mullen et al. (1994) have attempted to do this by taking into account these potentially confounding variables. They found that those reporting childhood sexual abuse were more likely to show a general instability in their close relationships, with a marked tendency to evaluate their current partner negatively. Twenty-three per cent of those sexually abused and 36% of the most severely abused went so far as to say that they had no meaningful communication with their partner on an intimate level; this compared with 6% in the control group. When considering sexual abuse as a single variable, they found that it exerted a greater effect than any of the other variables studied, accounting for 3–6% of the variance in interpersonal and sexual difficulties.

Women who have been sexually abused as children are vulnerable to revictimization in later life. Russell (1986) found that 30-60% of sexual abuse victims were subsequently raped, compared with 17% of a control group. In addition, they are more likely to enter into a relationship with a man who is violent towards them (Coid et al. 2001). Revictimization is more likely to occur in children from families where the sexual abuse coexisted with emotional and/or physical abuse or alcoholism or mental illness in a parent (Bagley & Thurston 1996).

Social functioning

The difficulties with both academic performance and behaviour that sexually abused children experience in the school environment are well recognized. It would not be surprising, therefore, if their later educational and employment prospects were impaired. Few studies have looked at this. Mullen et al. (1994) have shown that women who have been sexually abused are more likely to engage in unskilled work than a control group, even where they have higher educational qualifications.

Prostitution

The prevalence of reported childhood sexual abuse among both male and female prostitutes is extremely high, generally reported as between 45% and 70%. Bagley & Young (1995) found that the earlier the age of entry into prostitution, the more likely a history of childhood sexual abuse. Some in this sample had entered prostitution as young as 12 or 13 years old. Sometimes the entry into prostitution seems to be a direct route following on from sexual abuse. In other cases it appears to be a process of drift in young people attempting to escape from abusive homes, who find themselves trying to survive on the streets.

Drug and alcohol abuse

Between 20% and 30% of adults who have been sexually abused as children will give a history of substance abuse (Browne & Finkelhor 1986; Mullen et al. 1993). A study of patients with alcohol problems (Moncrieff et al. 1996) found that sexually abused subjects had higher alcohol problem scores than non-abused subjects. They also started their drinking careers at an earlier age than their non-abused counterparts and were at greater risk of comorbid psychiatric disorders.

Sexual offending and victim to abuser cycles: male and female perpetrators

While the majority of children who have been sexually abused do not become adult perpetrators, a high proportion of child sex abusers give a history of sexual abuse themselves, although the figures vary. Green (1993) found that 50–80% of convicted rapists and child molesters reported having been sexually abused as children. Other studies suggest lower figures, for example Glasser et al. (2001) found that 35% of perpetrators gave a history of having been a victim themselves. Ninety per cent of child abusers are men. Many have a personality disorder that interferes with their capacity to form intimate relationships. There is increasing recognition that the incest offender may also abuse children outside the home and that paedophilic and incestuous abuse represent more of a continuum than was previously thought. Because only a minority of victims of sexual abuse will become adult perpetrators, factors other than sexual abuse alone must account for the victim to abuser cycle. Watkins & Bentovim (1992) have identified risk factors likely to be associated with becoming an abuser (Box 24.3) and Finkelhor (1984) has proposed four preconditions for sexual abuse to take place (Box 24.4).

Until recently, the fact that 10% of the perpetrators of child sexual abuse are female has largely been ignored. This neglect parallels the relative neglect of male victims in prevalence and outcome research. Both are the result of cultural stereotypes which promote women as victims and men as abusers. At the start of the 1990s, a telephone helpline for abused children called Childline was set up in the UK. Nine per cent of callers reporting abuse reported that the perpetrator was a woman (Rosen 1996). From this and other sources in the literature, it is estimated that in 30% of these cases, the female abuser is the mother. Finkelhor & Russell (1984) estimate that 14% of perpetrators against boys and 6% of perpetrators against girls are female. The implication of these findings is that women actually abuse girls more frequently than boys because the overall number of girls who are abused is so much greater. The few existing studies of female sexual offenders indicate that 50–95% of them have been sexually abused during childhood. Welldon (1996) presents an account of female perversions in which the aim of the perversion is the woman's own body or that of her babies or children. Within this framework female perversions include attacks on the body such as bulimia, anorexia and self-harm as well as the sexual and physical abuse of children. Self-abuse and sadomasochistic relationships often precede the abuse of children in such women.

Factors that influence outcome

About one-third of adults who have been sexually abused as children consistently report no long-term effects. The impact of the abuse will vary according not only to the severity of the abuse but also to the phase of the child's development when it occurs, the resilience and temperament of the individual child and the nature of the family environment. The damaging effect of early abuse reflects not just the increased vulnerability of young children but also the fact that perpetrators of such abuse are generally more disturbed.

It has been hypothesized that individual differences in resilience and temperament may partly explain the variation in outcome. Binder et al. (1996) have studied a group of women who were functioning well following experiences of childhood sexual abuse. While the severity of the abuse explained this to some extent, lower levels of symptomatology were also seen in women who had special talents or abilities and who had not felt responsible for the abuse. Having a supportive relative in the background had also helped a number of them.

The child's family environment is extremely important. In particular, a good relationship with the mother can protect a child from the more severe consequences of the abuse. Peters (1988) found that lack of maternal warmth was the strongest predictor of difficulties in adulthood. If a child discloses sexual abuse, the support of other family members is essential for a benign outcome. If the child is not supported but is disbelieved or blamed for breaking up the family, then an adverse outcome is much more likely. Only about 5% of children disclose their sexual abuse during childhood. Some only disclose as adults because they fear that a younger relative may be at risk from the same perpetrator. This latter situation can place clinicians in a difficult position with the issue of confidentiality, on the one hand, and the requirement to report to social services any child who is currently at

---

Box 24.3 Watkins & Bentovim's (1992) factors influencing the development of sexually abusive behaviour

Gender
Male (linked to temperamental factors)

Abuse
Male
Close relative
Multiple perpetrators

Type of abuse
Repeated
Long duration
Greater severity

Age of child
Impact is greater with younger children

Effects
Anxious sexualization as a result of own victimization
Externalizing coping adaptation (influenced by concurrent physical abuse)
Sexual identity confusion
Identification with the aggressor

Diagnosis
Conduct disorder
Post-traumatic stress disorder
Attention deficit disorder
Learning difficulty
General immature functioning

Box 24.4 Finkelhor's (1984) four preconditions for sexual abuse

Emotional congruence: a fit between the adult's and the child's emotional needs

Sexual arousal: by children

Blockage: inability to fulfil sexual and emotional needs in relationship to adults

Disinhibition: includes factors such as poor impulse control and alcohol consumption

significant risk of abuse, on the other. See Crowe & Dare (1998) for a discussion of this predicament.

Recently, attachment theory has been applied to the study of outcome. Many of the family dynamics associated with childhood sexual abuse, such as role reversal and rejection, are consistent with a model of insecure attachments. Alexander (1993) has studied the differential effects of abuse characteristics and attachment as predictors of the long-term effects of childhood sexual abuse. This work suggests that symptoms such as depression, distress, intrusive thoughts and avoidance are best predicted by characteristics of abuse severity. Personality functioning such as borderline and avoidant personality disorders appear to be better predicted by attachment measures. The weakness of this work is that it is retrospective in nature, and there is a real need for prospective studies in this area.

Factors outside the family may also be important in determining outcome. Russell et al. (1988) showed that Afro-American incest victims suffered from worse sequelae than white American victims. This was partly explained by their being subject to more severe abuse, but this did not account for all of the variance. The authors suggest that being raised as an Afro-American female in a racist and sexist society may compound the effects of abuse.

CHILDREN MOST AT RISK

Emotional and physical abuse and disorders of family interaction often precede and accompany child sexual abuse and exacerbate its effects. Growing up in a dysfunctional family increases the risk, not only of intrafamilial sexual abuse, but also of extrafamilial sexual abuse. Children who are neglected and unloved are more vulnerable to approaches from those with paedophilic intentions. Certain family characteristics are linked to an increased risk of child sexual abuse (Box 24.5).

THEORIES OF CHILDHOOD SEX ABUSE EFFECTS

Post-traumatic stress disorder

Researchers in the area of child sexual abuse have noted that the constellation of symptoms described by many adult childhood abuse victims resembles the diagnostic criteria for PTSD (Herman 1994) (Chapter 15). In this model, psychological trauma occurs when human coping mechanisms are overwhelmed by a force in the face of which the individual is powerless. This leads to symptoms such as anxiety, sleep disorders, hypervigilance, intrusive memories or flashbacks and dissociative reactions. While many victims of childhood sexual abuse continue to describe such symptoms long after the abuse took place, this model is

limited in that it does not take into account the wider interpersonal and social problems that many victims experience. In addition, it focuses on force and powerlessness as the main threat to the child, which is not always the case. In the more seductive forms of abuse, there may not be much force involved and the child may even enjoy some aspects of the attention at the time, only realizing later the significance of what happened to him or her. Guilt, shame and feelings of being responsible for the abuse are common consequences of childhood sexual abuse. It can damage a child's developing capacity for trust, intimacy, sexuality and self-esteem, and these are not readily accounted for in the PTSD model.

Finkelhor's traumagenic factors

Finkelhor & Browne (1986) have proposed an alternative model of four traumagenic dynamics (Box 24.6). This model encompasses many features of PTSD but also goes beyond it and allows sexual abuse to be conceptualized as a situation or a process rather than an event.

Box 24.5   Factors placing a child at risk of sexual abuse (Finkelhor 1984)

Having a stepfather

Having lived without the mother

Not being close to the mother

Mother never having finished secondary school

Having a mother who is punitive about sexual matters (e.g. masturbation)

No physical affection from the mother

Low family income

Having two friends or fewer in childhood

'Box 24.6   Finkelhor & Browne's (1986) 'traumagenic' factors

Traumatic sexualization

This results from reinforcement of the childs sexual responses, such that the child learns to use sexual behaviour to gratify non-sexual needs. Gives rise to inappropriate and premature sexual activity, confused sexual identity, and aversion to sex and intimacy, as well as deviant patterns of sexual arousal.

Stigmatization

The child's sense of being damaged by and blamed for the abuse. This may be reinforced by the abuser, by peers or other family members. Leads to shame, guilt and low self-esteem

Betrayal

The child's well-being is disregarded and the abuser exploits the child's trust and vulnerability. Leads to depression, mistrust, anger and fear of intimate relationship

Powerlessness

The child is unable to protect him- or herself. Leads to anxiety, fear, perception of self as victim and identification with the aggressor

---

Psychodynamics and attachment theory

Childhood sexual abuse often takes place in the context of emotional neglect and in some cases physical abuse as well, and tends to occur in families that are characterized by insecure and disorganized patterns of attachment. Within such environments, many features that are known to facilitate healthy psychological development may be lacking. The central focus of the psychodynamic view of early infant development is the attachment to the mother. This two-person stage of development involves the formation of 'affectional bonds' (Bowlby 1988). A nurturing and secure base is established from which the infant is able to explore both the inner and outer worlds. An infant needs to be helped to deal with separations and other painful and threatening experiences as well as with the powerful internal feelings that these give rise to. If the parent feels threatened by the infant's protests and is unable to help the infant to contain his or her feelings, then the infant has no model on which to base the regulation of his or her own affect. Instability of affect, an unstable sense of the self and a view of intimate relationships as threatening may all result. The importance of the early environment is borne out in research that indicates that an adverse outcome is much more likely where there is a disturbed relationship with the mother. In many families, childhood sexual abuse takes place as a result of a 'cycle of deprivation', in which one or both parents experienced some form of abuse as a child.

Following on from the two-person stage of development is the three-person or 'Oedipal' stage of development. A normal child is able to play with the 'fantasy' of marrying his or her opposite-sex parent and learns that this wish cannot be fulfilled in reality. However, in incest, the child actually takes the place of the mother or father. This rupture of the normal barrier between fantasy and reality is both traumatic and psychologically damaging. The childs ability to fantasize and deal with internal and external reality in a symbolic way is jeopardized. See Garland (1991) for further discussion of this theory of trauma.

Another important contribution of psychodynamic theory to the understanding of childhood sexual abuse is the concept of unconscious defence mechanisms. Powerful intrapsychic defence mechanisms may come into play in order to help the child to survive the trauma. These in turn can contribute to later psychopathology. If emotions are too painful to be borne, the victim may resort to using earlier, infantile defence mechanisms such as splitting, projection and denial. The split-off and denied experience is then not integrated with the rest of the victims internal world. Other unconscious defence mechanisms that are often seen in sexually abused patients include: the compulsion to repeat the trauma; turning passive into active; somatization; and identification with the aggressor (Rosen 1996). All these can contribute to personality disorders and distorted object relations.

THERAPEUTIC APPROACHES

(Therapeutic approaches are discussed in greater detail in Chapters 36 and 37.) When taking a history from a patient, it is important that a history of childhood sexual abuse is inquired about in a sensitive way. Many psychiatric patients who have been abused do not spontaneously give a history of sexual abuse and may not be aware of its relevance to their symptoms. Jacobson & Herald (1990) studied psychiatric in-patients and found that 44% of them had experienced serious sexual abuse which had not, until then, been disclosed to any of their therapists or doctors. Their study suggests that this important aspect of the history is often neglected. It is up to clinicians to routinely ask about sexual abuse in a manner that is not intrusive and which respects the patient's threshold for discussing aspects of the abuse further. Without awareness of the underlying trauma, sexually abused patients suffering from depression, substance abuse, eating disorders and so on, can come to be regarded as 'treatment-resistant' patients.

The selection of psychotherapy for patients who have experienced childhood sexual abuse must be guided above all by what the patient feels able to cope with. It is also important to assess what areas of healthy functioning the patient possesses and the degree of familial and social support he or she has access to. The therapeutic process can be disturbing and distressing for a patient who has been sexually abused, and it may well have an impact on his or her family as well. Some patients will need supportive therapy over a considerable period of time before being able to acknowledge their traumatized feelings. Many patients will prefer to see a female therapist.

The initial task in any of the therapeutic approaches described below is to develop a sense of trust between the patient and the therapist. If this is established, the patient may idealize the therapist as a longed-for, caring parent and may find separations such as the therapist's holidays difficult to cope with, necessitating additional arrangements at these times. Equally, the dynamic of abuser and abused will almost inevitably enter the therapeutic relationship at some stage and the therapist should be alert for this in the transference. It is important that the abuse itself is not focused on exclusively, as this may reinforce a patient's self-image as a victim. The whole person needs to be taken into account and, given the disturbed and deprived family backgrounds that often accompany sexual abuse, there are inevitably significant other dimensions to the therapy. Work with patients who have been severely sexually abused often needs to be long-term in nature. Where resources exist, the various modes of therapy can offer victims of childhood sexual abuse different therapeutic opportunities, and it is not uncommon for patients to move from one type of treatment to another, e.g. individual therapy may precede group treatments.

Cognitive and solution-focused therapy

This type of therapy aims to identify and modify the patient's cognitive distortions. Many victims of sexual abuse believe that they are bad themselves and were responsible for the abuse. An attributional style of self-blame is often combined with low self-esteem and feelings of powerlessness in intimate relationships. Distorted beliefs are challenged in the therapy with more accurate alternatives. Jehu (1988) gives a detailed account of cognitive therapy with childhood sexual abuse victims.

Psychodynamic therapy

This focuses on enabling patients to work through, or psychologically process, the complex mixture of feelings that inevitably arise from sexual abuse. The therapist needs to help patients to foster a more positive sense of self, while creating an environment in which the patient feels safe enough to disclose the most painful aspects of their experience. Initially a patient may fear that the therapist will not be able to bear hearing about the worst aspects of the abuse. These patients often need to explore feelings of intense anger, not only towards the abuser but also towards those who failed to protect them. There may be disturbing fantasies of revenge as well as shame and guilt. The patient will unconsciously transfer onto the therapist expectations of seduction, exploitation, abandonment or neglect. The therapist's focus on the patient's internal world may at times be felt to be intrusive and even abusive. As with all psychodynamic therapy, the working through of the transference forms the cornerstone of the work. See Grant (1991) for a case study and discussion of long-term, individual psychotherapy with a childhood sexual abuse survivor.

Couple therapy

The relationships of previously sexually abused men and women are often characterized by discord, overdependence, dissatisfaction and distress. It is not uncommon for sexual abuse to be disclosed in the context of a relationship problem or in the treatment of sexual difficulties. Sometimes a combination of couple therapy and individual therapy for the victim is required (Douglas et al. 1989). Jehu (1988) gives an account of couple therapy and treatment for sexual dysfunction.

Family therapy

Family therapy is more often used in the treatment of children and their families, but it can have a place in the treatment of adolescents or adults within the family context. In particular, family therapy is useful for focusing on the role reversals and the loss of boundaries that tend to occur in abusive and dysfunctional families. The collusion of the non-abusing parent and the secondary gain achieved by scapegoating the victim will often need to be addressed. Bentovim et al. (1988) give a full account of assessment and treatment using family therapy.

Group therapy

The treatment of childhood sex abuse survivors in therapeutic groups can be particularly effective at reducing the sense of isolation that many victims suffer from (Chapter 36). Discovering that others have also been abused can help patients to talk about experiences that they have not previously been able to share. A sense of trust develops such that feelings of hostility, shame and guilt can be worked through. In a group environment, the secrecy that has surrounded the abuse is inevitably challenged and this in itself can be therapeutic. Patients vary in their capacity to make use of groups and careful assessment of this is needed. Possible group treatments include long-term, analytic group therapy, either in a group of childhood sexual abuse survivors or in a heterogeneous group. A more informal setting may be provided by self-help groups in the community, who aim to offer support. Welldon (1998) gives an account of group therapy within a specialist forensic psychotherapy service. In this service, perpetrators and victims of incestuous sexual abuse (not previously known to each other) are treated together, in the same group. She argues that this is a powerful therapeutic milieu in which the intergenerational nature of the abuse can be addressed and in which perpetrators have to face the damage they have inflicted. She also highlights the careful assessment process required in considering treatments for both victims and perpetrators.

CONCLUSION

Psychotherapy is an important part of treatment for survivors of childhood sexual abuse, but their other treatment needs should not be overlooked. Depression, eating disorders, substance abuse and other comorbid psychiatric disorders will often require treatment in their own right. In this respect, the treatment of childhood sexual abuse victims is similar to that of other patients suffering from these disorders.

REFERENCES

Alexander PC (1993) The differential effects of abuse characteristics and attachment in the prediction of long-term effects of sexual abuse. *Journal of Interpersonal Violence* 8(3): 346–62.

Anderson J, Martin J, Mullen P et al. (1993) Prevalence of childhood sexual abuse experiences in a community sample of women. *Journal of the American Academy of Child and Adolescent Psychiatry* 32: 911–19.

Aristotle (1976) *Ethics* (transl. by JAK Thomson). London: Penguin.

Bagley C & McDonald M (1995) Adult mental health sequels of child sexual abuse, physical abuse and neglect in maternally separated children. In: Bagley C (ed.) *Child Sexual Abuse and Mental Health in Adolescents and Adults*, pp. 15–28. Aldershot: Avebury.

Bagley C & Ramsay R (1986) Sexual abuse in childhood: psychosocial outcomes and implications for social work practice. *Journal of Social Work and Human Sexuality* **4**: 33–47.

Bagley C & Thurston WE (1996) *Understanding and Preventing Child Sexual Abuse*, vol. 2. Aldershot: Arena.

Bagley C & Young L (1995) Juvenile prostitution and child sexual abuse: a controlled study. In: Bagley C (ed.) *Child Sexual Abuse and Mental Health in Adolescents and Adults*, pp. 70–76. Aldershot: Avebury.

Baker AW & Duncan SP (1985) Child sexual abuse: a study of prevalence in Great Britain. *Child Abuse and Neglect* **9**: 457–67.

Banyard VL & Williams LM (1996) Characteristics of child sexual abuse as correlates of women's adjustment: a prospective study. *Journal of Marriage and the Family* **58**: 853–65.

Beitchman JH, Zucker KJ, Hood JE et al. (1992) A review of the long term effects of child sexual abuse. *Child Abuse and Neglect* **16**: 101–18.

Bentovim A, Elton A, Hildebrand J et al. (eds) (1988) *Sexual Abuse in the Family: Assessment and Treatment*. London: Wright.

Bifulco A, Brown G & Adler Z (1991) Early sexual abuse and clinical depression in adult life. *British Journal of Psychiatry* **159**: 115–22.

Binder RL, McNiel DE & Goldstone RL (1996) Is adaptive coping possible for adult survivors of childhood sexual abuse? *Psychiatric Services* **47**: 186–8.

Bowlby J (1988) *A Secure Base: Clinical Applications of Attachment Theory*. London: Routledge.

Brandon S, Boakes J, Glaser D & Green R (1998) Recovered memories of childhood sexual abuse. Implications for clinical practice. *British Journal of Psychiatry* **172**: 296–307.

Briere J (1992) Methodological issues in the study of sexual abuse effects. *Journal of Consulting and Clinical Psychology* **60**(2): 196–203.

Briere J & Runtz M (1988) Post sex abuse trauma. In: Wyatt G & Powell G (eds) *Lasting Effects of Child Sexual Abuse*, pp. 85–99. Newbury Park: Sage.

Browne A & Finkelhor D (1986) Initial and long-term effects: a review of the research. In: Finkelhor D (ed.) *A Sourcebook on Child Sexual Abuse*, pp. 143–79. Newbury Park: Sage.

Coid J, Petruckevitch A, Feder G, Chung W, Richardson J & Moorey S (2001) Relation between childhood sexual and physical abuse and risk of revictimisation in women: a cross-sectional survey. *Lancet* **358**: 450–4.

Coxell A, King M, Mezey G & Gordon D (1999) Lifetime prevalence, characteristics, and associated problems of non-consensual sex in men: cross sectional survey. *British Medical Journal* **318**: 846–50.

Crowe M & Dare C (1998) Survivors of childhood sexual abuse: approaches to therapy. *Advances in Psychiatric Treatment* **4**: 96–100.

Dhaliwal GK, Gauzas L, Antonowicz DH & Ross RR (1996) Adult male survivors of childhood sexual abuse; prevalence sexual abuse characteristics and long term effects. *Clinical Psychology Review* **16**(7): 619–39.

Douglas A, Matson IC & Hunter S (1989) Sex therapy for women incestuously abused as children. *Sexual and Marital Therapy* **4**: 143–60.

Femina DD, Yeager CA & Lewis DO (1990) Child Abuse: adolescent records vs. adult recall. *Child Abuse and Neglect* **14**: 227–31.

Fergusson DM and Mullen PE (1999) *Childhood Sexual Abuse: An Evidence Based Perspective*. Thousand Oaks: Sage.

Figueroa E & Silk KR (1997) Biological implications of childhood sexual abuse in borderline personality disorder. *Journal of Personality Disorders* **11**(1): 71–92.

Finkelhor D (1979) *Sexually Victimized Children*. New York: Free Press.

Finkelhor D (1984) *Child Sex Abuse: New Theory and Research*. New York: Free Press.

Finkelhor D & Browne A (1986) Initial and long term effects: a conceptual framework. In: Finkelhor D (ed.) *A Sourcebook on Child Sexual Abuse*, pp. 180–98. Newbury Park: Sage.

Finkelhor D & Russell D (1984) Women as perpetrators: review of the evidence. In: Finkelhor D (ed.) *Child Sex Abuse: New Theory and Research*, pp. 171–87. New York: Free Press.

Freud S (1896) *The Aetiology of Hysteria*, standard edition, vol. 3. London: Hogarth.

Freud S (1905) *Three Essays on the Theory of Sexuality*, standard edition, vol. 7. London: Hogarth.

Garland CB (1991) External disasters and the internal world: an approach to psychotherapeutic understanding of survivors. In: Holmes J (ed.) *Textbook of Psychotherapy in Psychiatric Practice*, pp. 507–32. London: Churchill Livingstone.

Glasser M, Kolvin I, Campbell D, Glasser A, Leitch I & Farrely S (2001) Cycle of child sexual abuse: links between being a victim and becoming a perpetrator. *British Journal of Psychiatry* **179**: 482–94.

Goff DC, Brotman AW, Kindlon D et al. (1991) Self-reports of childhood abuse in chronically psychotic patients. *Psychiatry Research* **37**: 73–80.

Grant S (1991) Psychotherapy with people who have been sexually abused. In: Holmes J (ed.) *Textbook of Psychotherapy in Psychiatric Practice*, pp. 489–505. London: Churchill Livingstone.

Green AH (1993) Child Sexual abuse: immediate and long term effects and intervention. *Journal of the American Academy of Child and Adolescent Psychiatry* **32**(5): 890–902.

Greenfield SF, Strakowski SM, Tohen M et al. (1994) Child abuse in first episode psychosis. *British Journal of Psychiatry* **164**: 831–4.

Herman JL (1994) Anew discovery. In: Herman JL (ed.) *Trauma and Recovery*, pp. 115–29. London: Pandora.

Herman JL, Perry JC & van der Kolk BA (1989) Childhood trauma in borderline personality disorder. *American Journal of Psychiatry* **146**: 490–5.

Hill J, Pickles A, Burnside E, Byatt M, Rollinson L, Davis R & Harvey K (2001). *British Journal of Psychiatry* **179**: 104–9.

Hilton MR & Mezey GC (1996) Victims and perpetrators of child sexual abuse. *British Journal of Psychiatry* **169**: 408–15.

Jacobson MD & Herald C (1990) The relevance of childhood sexual abuse to adult psychiatric inpatient care. *Hospital and Community Psychiatry* **41**: 154–8.

Jehu D (1988) *Beyond Sexual Abuse. Therapy with Women who were Childhood Victims*. Bath: Wiley.

King M, Coxell A & Mezey G (2002) Sexual molestation of males: association with psychological disturbance. *British Journal of Psychiatry* **181**: 153–7.

Lampe A, Doering S, Rumpold G, Soelder E, Krism M, Kantner-Rumplmair W, Schubert C & Soellner W (2003) Chronic pain syndromes and their relation to childhood abuse and stressful life events. *Journal of psychosomatic Research* **54**(4): 361–7.

Lindberg FH & Distad LJ (1985) Post-traumatic stress disorders in women who have experienced childhood incest. *Child Abuse and Neglect* **9**: 329–34.

Moncrieff DC, Drummond B, Candy K et al. (1996) Sexual abuse in people with alcohol problems. A study of the prevalence of sexual abuse and its relationship to drinking behaviour. *British Journal of Psychiatry* **169**: 355–60.

Morrison J (1989) Childhood sexual histories of women with somatization disorder. *American Journal of Psychiatry* **146**: 239–41.

Mullen PE, Martin JL, Anderson JC (1993) Childhood sexual abuse and mental health in adult life. *British Journal of Psychiatry* **163**: 721–32.

Mullen PE, Martin JL, Anderson JC et al. (1994) The effect of child sexual abuse on social, interpersonal and sexual function in adult life. *British Journal of Psychiatry* **165**: 35–47.

Mullen P, Romans-Clarkson S, Walton V & Herbison G (1988) Impact of sexual and physical abuse on womens mental health. *Lancet* **1**: 841–5.

Noll JG, Trickett PK & Putnam FW (2003) A prospective investigation of the impact of childhood sexual abuse on the development of sexuality. *Journal of Counselling and Clinical Psychology* **71**(3): 575–86.

Peters SD (1988) Child sex abuse and later psychological problems. In: Wyatt GE & Powell GJ (eds) *Lasting Effects of Child Sexual Abuse*, pp. 101–18. Newbury Park: Sage.

Romans SE, Martin J & Mullen P (1996) Women's self-esteem: a community study of women who report and do not report childhood sexual abuse. *British Journal of Psychiatry* **169**: 696–704.

Rosen I (1996) The adult sequelae of childhood sexual abuse. In: Rosen I (ed.) *Sexual Deviation*, 3rd edn, pp. 361–81. Oxford: Oxford University Press.

Ross CA, Miller SD, Reager P et al. (1990) Structured interview data on 102 cases of multiple personality disorder from four centres. *American Journal of Psychiatry* **147**: 596–601.

Russell DEH (1983) The incidence and prevalence of intrafamilial and extrafamilial sexual abuse of female children. *Child Abuse and Neglect* **7**: 133–46.

Russell DEH, Schurman RA & Trocki K (1988) The long term effects of incestuous abuse: a comparison of Afro-American and white American victims. In: Wyatt GE & Powell GJ (eds) *Lasting Effects of Child Sexual Abuse*, pp. 119–34. Newbury Park: Sage.

Scarinci IC, McDonald-Haile J, Bradley LA & Richter JE (1994) Altered pain perception and psychosocial features among women with gastrointestinal disorders and history of abuse: a preliminary model. *American Journal of Medicine* **97**: 108–18.

Schechter MD & Roberge L (1976) Sexual exploitation. In: Helfer RE & Kempe CH (eds) *Child Abuse and Neglect: The Family and the Community*, pp. 127–42. Cambridge, MA: Ballinger.

Sequeira H, Howlin P & Hollins S (2003) Psychological disturbance associated with sexual abuse in people with learning disabilities. Case-control study. *British Journal of Psychiatry* **183**: 451–6.

Sheldrick C (1991) Adult sequelae of child sexual abuse. *British Journal of Psychiatry* **158**(suppl 10): 55–62.

Sinason V (1994) *Treating Survivors of Satanist Abuse*. London: Routledge.

Sullivan PF, Bullick CM, Carter FA & Joyce PR (1995) The significance of a history of childhood sexual abuse in bulimia nervosa. *British Journal of Psychiatry* **167**: 679–82.

Vize CM & Cooper PJ (1995) Sexual abuse in patients with eating disorder, patients with depression and normal controls. *British Journal of Psychiatry* **167**: 80–5.

Walker E, Katon W, Harrop-Griffiths J et al. (1988) Relationship of chronic pelvic pain to psychiatric diagnoses and childhood sexual abuse. *American Journal of Psychiatry* **145**: 75–80.

Watkins B & Bentovim A (1992) The sexual abuse of male children and adolescents: a review of the research literature. *Journal of Child Psychology and Psychiatry* **33**: 197–248.

Welch SL & Fairburn CG (1994) Sexual abuse and bulimia nervosa: three integrated case control comparisons. *American Journal of Psychiatry* **151**: 402–7.

Welldon E (1996) Women as abusers. In: Abel K, Buszewicz M, Davison S et al. (eds) *Planning Community Mental Health Services for Women*, pp. 176–89. London: Routledge.

Welldon E (1998) Group therapy for victims and perpetrators of incest. *Advances in Psychiatric Treatment* **4**: 82–8.

Wyatt GE & Peters SD (1986) Methodological considerations in research on the prevalence of child sexual abuse. *Child Abuse and Neglect* **10**: 241–51.

Sexual disorders

Mark Jones

INTRODUCTION

Sexual disorders have been recognized for generations. One of the first 'behavioural treatments' for a sexual disorder (paradoxical intervention) was described in the 18th century as follows:

> ... go to bed with this woman, but first promise to himself that he would not have any connection with her for six nights, let his inclinations and powers be what they would; which he engaged to do; and also to let me know the result. After about a fortnight he told me his resolution had produced such a total alteration in the state of his mind, that the powers soon took place, for instead of going to bed with the fears that he should be possessed with too much desire, too much power, so as to become uneasy to him, which really happened.
> John Hunter 1786

Today, however, sexual or psychosexual medicine is a neglected and misunderstood but important discipline. Sexual medicine is a biopsychosocial discipline. Sexual dysfunction is common at any age. Sexual disorders are characterized by disturbance in sexual desire and drive, and the psychophysiological changes that characterize the sexual response cycle can cause marked distress and interpersonal difficulties. The terms 'disorder' and 'dysfunction' are interchangeable and reflect the complex interaction of psychic and often unclear biological determinants of the presenting complaint, as well as the dynamic interpersonal relationships between sexual partners. Dissatisfaction, the failure to satisfy one's own or one's partner's sexual needs (either stated or unstated), is a frequent cause of referral to sexual, marital or couple therapy clinics, and may in part have sexual dysfunction at its core.

One-fifth to one-third of the general population complain of sexual dysfunction or dissatisfaction at some time (Saunders 1985, 1987). Many clinicians are unaware of the scale of the problem and psychosexual services have arisen in response to the increased awareness of the numbers being referred to specialities, most commonly urology, gynaecology and psychiatry. Yet many patients do not reach secondary care services, instead using self-help literature or being contained in general practice and family planning services. Such different approaches, which are inherently a part of the practice of specialists, are divisive while the all too rare multidisciplinary approach can yield a holistic result that does not ignore any one part of the complex interplay of factors resulting in sexual dysfunction.

A HISTORY OF SEXUAL DISORDERS

- Havelock Ellis began a scientific enquiry into sexuality in 1910.
- Up until the 1940s only psychoanalysts discussed sex as the central pivot in the neurotic conflict.
- Kinsey et al. (1948, 1953) published two books leading to a wider appreciation of sexual relationships and their problems. Due to non-random sampling, and the over-representation of American white, middle-class sex offenders and criminals in the sample their studies are flawed. However, they remain a cornerstone of the literature and have been widely generalized to the population.
- Between 1940 and 1970 specific behavioural techniques were proposed for premature ejaculation (stop–start technique, Semans 1956), vaginismus and anorgasmia (self-stimulation, attributed to Hastings).

In 1970 Masters & Johnson published *Human Sexual Inadequacy*, which became the template for the development of modern approaches to sexual therapy. It emphasizes the importance of the relationship as an integral part of the sexual problem, predicting outcome. Therapy targeted the 'marital unit' and behavioural techniques were superimposed. Masters & Johnson's published work has never been replicated in subsequent studies (Hawton 1986).

- AIDS/HIV infection was first described in 1981 and it has since transpired that it is associated with significant psychological morbidity, as are all chronic medical conditions (Jones et al. 1994).

In 1992 the British government made sexual health (and psychiatric well-being) a priority in the Health of the Nation strategy (Department of Health 1994). With the establishment of the Faculty of Family Planning and Reproductive Health Care of the Royal College of Obstetricians and Gynaecologists in 1993, they supported both closer links and liaison between family planning and genitourinary medicine with input from psychiatric and psychological services (Royal College of Obstetricians and Gynaecologists 1993). The government has proposed a module as part of higher specialist training, which expects trainees to acquire skills in reproductive medicine and the ability to recognize and refer patients with psychosexual problems. The expectations of the Royal College of Psychiatrists are that training schemes give the opportunity to experience psychosexual and marital therapy. Some physicians are clearly concerned at the lack of expertise for such a large problem, and have suggested that genito-urinary clinics are the obvious place to develop integrated services. Yet specialist clinics are not generalized or well-established within the National Health Service (NHS) in the UK and many individuals feel uncomfortable about discussing their sexual health needs with their general practitioners (GPs).

In 1994, Johnson et al. published a major survey of British sexual attitudes, the most comprehensive to date. For a summary see Puri & Hall (1998).

THE EPIDEMIOLOGY OF SEXUAL DISORDERS

The most common sexual problems reported are loss of sexual drive and erectile failure (which increases markedly with age: 0.8% at age 30, 6.7% at age 50 and 55% at age 74), but less is known about the specific prevalence of other disorders. Premature ejaculation has been reported as occurring in at least 20% of married men, and anorgasmia during intercourse in 42% of women. Up to 38% of women report anxiety and inhibition during sexual activity and 16% complain of lack of pleasure (Rosen et al. 1993). Although the dysfunction may be purely organic or psychological, it is usually a mixture of both (Crowe & Jones 1992).

THE CLASSIFICATION OF SEXUAL DISORDERS

The general classification of sexual disorders

Kaplan (1974) and Hawton (1986) both arrived at the following distinctions, essentially growing out of the work of Masters & Johnson: sexual problems can be broadly divided into problems of motivation (sexual desire), problems of arousal (erection, lubrication and penetration) and problems of orgasm (see Table 25.1).

Masters & Johnson found the subcategories of *primary vs secondary* and *total vs situational* useful in assessment. Primary dysfunction is present since the first attempt at intercourse, and secondary follows a period of successful function, whereas total dysfunction is present under all circumstances, compared with situational which appears only under certain circumstances.

Clearly in many cases there are combinations of problems; for example, a male partner may experience both impotence and impaired sexual interest, while premature ejaculation in a man may be associated with lack of interest on the woman's side. The other frequently quoted, but less helpful, classification is that of *functional vs organic*. Using the example of impotence caused in part by diabetic neuropathy, a man may experience *performance anxiety* leading to an expectation that he will fail to achieve an erection. Equally, where no specific physical cause can be found for impotence in an ageing male, there may be some, as yet, undiscovered physical change occurring; the frequency of this problem throws doubt on the *psychogenic* label.

There are a range of behaviours not yet discussed but which were described as far back as 1877 by Lasegue, who

Table 25.1 Categories of sexual dysfunction		
Aspect of sexuality affected	*Women*	*Men*
Interest	Impaired sexual interest	Impaired sexual interest
Arousal	Impaired sexual arousal or poor lubrication	Erectile dysfunction (impotence)
Orgasm	Orgasmic dysfunction	Premature ejaculation Delayed ejaculation Ejaculatory pain
Other types of dysfunction	Vaginismus Dyspareunia (pain during intercourse) Sexual phobias	Dyspareunia Sexual phobias

coined the term *l'exhibitionisme* (exhibitionism). Such behaviours are often linked with other similar behaviours, and the term *paraphilias* or *parasexual* has been assigned to them. Some have suggested that they be labelled *antisocial sexual behaviours*. The risk here is that we are approaching the interface with legal aspects of sexuality, and society's general misinterpretation of sexual orientation or preference and gender identity. The question of deviation often comes to light because of distress caused to others, such as partners or the general public, and public disorder offences, and only rarely by self-referral (see Chapter 30).

ICD-10 and DSM-IV classification of sexual disorders

Both ICD-10 (World Health Organization 1992) and DSM-IV (American Psyhciatric Association 1994) provide operational systems for the diagnosis and classification of sexual disorders. The following disorders are recognized within a single section of ICD-10:

- lack or loss of sexual desire
- sexual aversion and lack of sexual enjoyment
- failure of genital response
- orgasmic dysfunction
- premature ejaculation
- non-organic vaginismus
- non-organic dyspareunia
- excessive sexual drive
- other sexual dysfunction, not caused by organic disorder or disease
- unspecified sexual dysfunction, not caused by organic disorder or disease.

In addition to the above sexual disorders, gender identity disorders, disorders of sexual preference (paraphilias), and psychological and behavioural disorders associated with sexual development (sexual maturation disorder, egodystonic sexual orientation, sexual relationship disorder, and unspecified others) are recognized within other sections of ICD-10.

In contrast to ICD-10, DSM-IV includes all sexual disorders within one section entitled, 'Sexual and Gender Identity Disorders'. Thus the sexual dysfunctions as listed in ICD-10 are coupled with:

- Sexual dysfunction due to a general medical condition: characterized by a disturbance in the processes that

characterize the sexual response cycle (Box 25.1) or by pain associated with sexual intercourse.
- Substance-induced sexual dysfunction: characterized by disturbance in sexual desire and in the psychophysiological changes that characterize the sexual response cycle and causes marked distress and interpersonal difficulty.
- Paraphilias: characterized by recurrent, intense sexual urges, fantasies, or behaviours that involve unusual objects, activities or situations and cause significant distress or impairment in social, occupational, or other important areas of functioning. The paraphilias include:
  (a) exhibitionism
  (b) fetishism
  (c) frotterism
  (d) paedophilia
  (e) sexual masochism
  (f) sexual sadism
  (g) transvestic fetishism
  (h) voyeurism
  (i) paraphilia not otherwise specified (e.g. telephone scatology).
- Gender identity disorders: characterized by a strong and persistent cross-gender identification accompanied by persistent discomfort with one's biologically assigned sex.
- Sexual disorder not otherwise specified: one's personal judgements must also take into account society's notions of deviance and concepts of gender role, with some (accepted) activities varying from culture to culture.

At the turn of the 21st century, reproductive endocrinologists and neuro-anatomists began to question the whole psychological emphasis that had been placed on sexual disorders and dysfunction, suggesting through experimental work with rats that there was a much greater role than previously thought for central and peripheral neurotransmitters at each stage of the sexual cycle. The advent of first-generation phosphodiesterase type 5 (PDE-5) inhibitors and the success of sildenafil in male erectile dysfunction has fuelled interest in pharmacological treatment of female sexual dysfunction. The emphasis has changed (much to the dismay of many sex therapists) from the psychosocial to the organic with the possibility that these partially effective treatments might soon allow a greater organic understanding and therefore potential for pharmacological solutions.

Particular attention has been paid to the (i) amygdala, periventricular nucleus of the hypothalamus and median preoptic area centrally and peripherally (ii) the effects of dopamine, noradrenaline and acetylcholine (iii) vasoactive intestinal peptide responses mediated by parasympathetic fibres and (iv) sympathetic and parasympathetic spinal cord chain and nuclei responses.

Firstly, although psychological and physical factors interact in sexual dysfunction, the experimental evidence so

---

Box 25.1 Normal sexual response cycle

Desire
Arousal, mediated by parasympathetic and central nervous system
Plateau
Orgasm, mediated by sympathetic and central nervous system
Resolution, longer in men and increases with age

far indicates that *female sexual arousal* is a neuromuscular and vasocongestive event controlled by parasympathetic and *inhibitory* sympathetic inputs. Autonomic preganglionic parasympathetic and inhibitory sympathetic fibres to the vagina and clitoris originate in the spinal cord in the sacral parasympathetic nucleus at the sacral level and in the dorsal gray commissure/intermediolateral cell column at the thoracolumbar level respectively (see Chapter 2).

Parasympathetic fibres are conveyed by the pelvic nerve and sympathetic fibres by the hypogastric nerve and the paravertebral sympathetic chain. The activity of these spinal nuclei is controlled by descending projections from the brain and sensory afferents (conveyed in the pudendal, pelvic and vagus nerves) *from* the genitalia.

A key but unresolved issue concerns the neuro-transmitters involved in the control of vaginal smooth muscle contractions. It appears that vasoactive intestinal peptide and nitric oxide may be responsible for the increase in vaginal blood flow during sexual arousal, whereas noradrenaline is inhibitory. Acetylcholine, previously thought to be crucial, now appears to play only a minor role compared to noradrenaline and acetylcholine in the regulation of vaginal blood flow.

Within the central nervous system, serotonergic projections from the brain to the spinal cord are inhibitory to the induction of genital arousal via a spinal reflex. Dopamine seems the most likely candidate (with as yet other unidentified transmitters) regulating the display of sexual behaviour. Anatomists and electrophysiologists point to a contribution from the paraventricular nucleus of the hypothalamus and the median preoptic area, respectively, as key elements in genital arousal. These recent animal models should assist in deciphering the neurochemical pathways controlling vaginal sexual arousal and the development of suitable pharmacological treatments for female sexual dysfunctions.

As an elaboration on DSM-IV and ICD-10, one paper in particular merits a re-examination of long-held beliefs relating to the physiology of erectile function and dysfunction (Sachs 2000), including the idea that there is a *singular physiology of erection*. Sachs claims that there appear to be pleural neural, neurochemical and endocrine mechanisms at work on which erectile function depends. He argues for a behavioural context in which erection occurs founded on a context-dependent physiology researched using laboratory rats. The medial amygdala is essential for *non-contact* erection in response to inaccessible oestrous females, but not for erection during copulation. Even the specific dopamine receptors important to erection may differ, depending on context. It follows that if there is not a singular physiology of erectile dysfunction, the general physiology of erectile dysfunction may vary from context to context. Thus, some disorders of the central nervous system may not be manifested in sleep related erection and consequently labelled 'psychogenic' erectile dysfunction.

Like Freud and later Francis Crick (The Amazing Hypothesis) this concept supports the axiom that all psychological processes have a somatic basis and therefore there can be no psychogenic dysfunction that does not involve organic processes, which may respond to drug treatment.

A revised classification is suggested for erectile dysfunction based on this idea and a closer attention should be paid to male sexual arousal and its relationship to sexual motivation. Indeed the former term has so many meanings in the literature that it is impeding research into the physiology of sexual arousal, where so much depends upon comparisons between animals and humans. It is a logical progression of this research that attention should now be paid to two variables: whether or not erection occurs and whether the context is sexual. Currently the occurrence of penile erection *within* a sexual context is viewed as the only case in which sexual arousal may be inferred unambiguously.

SEX THERAPY

There are three steps in the provision of sex therapy: referral, assessment and treatment.

Referral

The 'ticket' of entry to the GP can be a casual, incidental or disguised problem. Identification can be problematic, since with the time constraints of an average GP, once the patient's history has been taken and a physical examination performed, more time is needed for further listening, non-judgemental reassurance, and possibly counselling. The neutrality of a GP is not felt by all attenders, but talking about a sexual problem can dispel fears and reduce anxiety. Simple behavioural techniques (stop–start for premature ejaculation or a sensate focus approach – see below) are rarely beyond most practitioners' abilities, yet their lack of basic training makes many feel disempowered to offer straightforward, sensible advice. Referral often ensues, despite the fact that primary care will remain the first point of contact for many patients and successful treatment can be effected in the community.

In Canada in 1985, Maurice called for sexual medicine to be advanced as a new medical subspeciality. The development to date has been fragmented and haphazard. Joint clinics providing collaborative academic and clinical integration is the probable way forward, attractive to providers and purchasers alike. The training opportunities that should be available to all higher trainees will then be more widespread in availability. At present, joint multidisciplinary clinics are a rarity. Where a GP refers a patient to, will depend upon local relationships with providers of secondary care and knowledge of specialist services. At present specialized services exist because of the dedication of a few consultant psychiatrists, urologists and gynaecologists, who frequently work without extra staff or resources. The family GP is often consulted for help and this trend will probably continue as trusts squeeze this perceived patient luxury out of their service.

Assessment

The components of the assessment of patients and couples referred for sex therapy are as follows:

1. Assessment: history from both partners, separately and together. Remember to ask about:
   (a) physical pathologies, especially diabetes, hypertension, neurological disorders (especially multiple sclerosis) and endocrine disorders (e.g. hypogonadism, hyperprolactinaemia)
   (b) sexually transmitted diseases, including HIV serostatus
   (c) alcohol and illicit drug use
   (d) prescribed medications and contraception if appropriate
   (e) physical disabilities
   (f) genital deformities
   (g) marital disharmony/relationship difficulties
   (h) stress or problems in other areas of the patient's lives, e.g. financial worries
   (i) psychiatric morbidity, especially anxiety and depression, psychoses
   (j) sexual preferences.
2. Physical examination: coupled with reassurance.
3. Education: explain simple functional anatomy and physiology to develop common ground for discussion. Allow free expression of language and identify areas of confusion.
4. Screening: routine haematological and biochemical screening, and proceed to hormonal studies if indicated.

Taking the history alone can take two or three sessions, and it is useful to send the patient/couple a self-assessment questionnaire prior to their initial visit. Patients sometimes find it easier to write down their problems and return them so that an appropriate member of the multidisciplinary team can do an initial assessment based on the answers received. It may be that what transpires at interview is very different from what the patient(s) initially identified as the problem, in which case feedback and discussion can be very helpful in formulating a management plan, which may involve a number of health professionals.

Treatment

Sex therapy draws its treatment options from several areas of psychological and physical medicine. Techniques include:

- counselling with or without behavioural programmes (e.g. Masters & Johnson 1970)
- cognitive therapy (Beck et al. 1979)
- psychodynamic psychotherapy
- systemic couple therapy (Crowe & Ridley 1990)
- hypnosis (Fromm et al. 1970)
- drug treatments, e.g. sildenafil, yohimbine, anti-androgens and hormonal replacement
- a combination of psychodynamic and behavioural techniques (Kaplan 1974)
- mechanical sex aids, e.g. vibrators, dilators and vacuum tumescence pumps with penile ring constriction
- local drug treatments, e.g. intracavernosal injections of papaverine, phentolamine and prostaglandins (Virag 1982a)
- vascular surgery for correction of a venous 'leak' and proximal vessel reconstruction for arteriosclerosis (usually unsuccessful because distal disease usually coexists) (Virag 1982b)
- penile prosthetic implants (Loeffler 1960).

Practitioners vary considerably in the emphasis they place on physical, psychological and relationship factors in sex therapy. However, it is preferable, and the general consensus is moving in this direction, to treat sexual disorders as far as possible in the context of a relationship, married or unmarried, heterosexual or homosexual. Extremely sensitive individuals can be treated alone, at least initially, and if a patient has no partner, therapy along individual lines is still possible.

Whatever the outcome of the assessment, psychological factors are most likely to be responsible for sexual dysfunction unless a patient is clearly physically ill and a treatable organic cause is present. Psychological/behavioural techniques should generally be tried first, and only if these fail or the patient refuses to engage after persistent encouragement to do so, should pharmacological or surgical solutions be resorted to. Psychological/behavioural techniques, relationship issues and their impact on sexuality and mechanical and pharmacological treatments are now discussed.

Psychological/behavioural techniques

The Masters & Johnson (1970) *sensate focus approach* aims to reduce anxiety and improve non-verbal, tactile communication between partners. Essentially, it is a set of homework exercises designed to help couples become more comfortable with physical contact and closeness. Patients are encouraged to communicate using touching, although speaking is not forbidden. However, this is a graded approach to re-establishing a sexual dialogue, and initially breast and genital touching is not allowed; this has two purposes:

- reduces anxiety
- can liberate sexual urges.

Some couples 'break' the ban and have intercourse, but the therapist does not sanction this, predicting failure if they break the ban again.

If sensate focus proves successful, the therapist instructs the couple that it will enhance other aspects of their relationship.

The non-genital sensate focus stage (Box 25.2) may be followed after 1–2 weeks by the genital sensate focus stage (Box 25.3).

The therapist discusses any problem encountered, such as guilt, anxiety and resistance to tasks as they arise. Couples with particular dysfunctions are introduced to the next stage of treatment, which precedes intercourse. The application of psychological/behavioural techniques to each specific sexual disorder is now discussed.

Premature ejaculation

Premature ejaculation is usually treated using Semans' *stop–start technique* (1956). A behavioural treatment, the man masturbates to the point of 'ejaculatory inevitability' (just before ejaculation) and then stops touching himself and allows the urge to abate. The 'squeeze technique' can be used to prevent ejaculation by squeezing the tip of the penis to help control the ejaculatory urge. The penis becomes unresponsive and subsequent vigorous stimulation does not cause ejaculation. The same technique is repeated for 15 minutes, and the exercise repeated with the man using body oil on his hand to make control more difficult. The man's partner then stimulates his penis, first with a dry hand and

---

Box 25.2 Non-genital sensate focus approach to sexual problems

Instruct the couple to find a warm and comfortable place to practise

Tell the couple to undress and, having carried out some relaxation exercises, stroke and caress each other's bodies in turn, using oil or lotion on their hands

The emphasis should be on physical communication through the hands of the active partner and the body of the recipient

Tell the couple they can talk, but only to describe their emotional responses to being touched and to request other types of touching

---

Box 25.3   Genital sensate focus approach

Touching of the breasts and genital areas is allowed, but intercourse is still banned

Encourage the couple not to try to maintain an erection or achieve arousal in the woman. Instruct them to use the 'teasing technique', with pauses between periods of genital contact to allow the excitement to abate

The couple may be encouraged to use a vibrator or spray from a shower head to stimulate each other. Oral genital stimulation, which provides a good transition between manual stimulation and full intercourse, can be useful for some couples at this stage

---

then with body oil. This process is repeated, gaining control first with oral sex and then intravaginally until control in full intercourse is achieved. Paroxetine has also been used to treat primary premature ejaculation with some success (Waldinger et al. 1994).

Delayed or absent ejaculation

A penile superstimulation technique is used in mutual masturbation. The man is instructed to rub his penis vigorously with body oil on his hand. This may lead to orgasm. If so, on another occasion his partner is asked to masturbate his penis until ejaculation occurs. Full intercourse is then later attempted. Should the masturbation technique described not produce an orgasm, a penile superstimulation technique using a high-frequency vibrator applied to the end of the man's penis can sometimes encourage orgasm. The technique is then incorporated into sexual foreplay, leading to intercourse.

Vaginismus

Vaginismus is caused by spasm of the lavator ani muscle, which encircles the lower third of the vagina. Spasm can totally occlude the vaginal introitus. Before concluding that vaginismus is a purely psychological condition, dyspareunia of non-organic origin should be excluded (Bancroft 1989). A woman with vaginismus can be examined using one finger. After the therapist has done this the partner is then encouraged to examine her. In taking the patient's history consider that the male partner may be contributing to this condition, for example, through impotence and associated female anxiety or phobia of penetration. Graded vaginal trainers (smooth, tapered tubes of different sizes) or fingers can be used to 'train' the vaginal wall to accept penetration.

Encourage the couple to do homework exercises involving gradual dilation of the vagina using graded trainers or one, two and then three fingers, over several weeks. Once this has been achieved the couple are instructed to have careful penetration with the erect penis, with the woman on top.

Female anorgasmia

The couple are encouraged to practise clitoral stimulation using fingers, water spray or a vibrator. Given that around 40% of women do not experience orgasm during intercourse, it is often easier to achieve orgasm in this way than in intercourse, but once achieved the couple can introduce such techniques into their foreplay and intercourse.

Erectile dysfunction or impotence

The term 'impotence' is no longer popular among practitioners, who prefer more general terms like dysfunction, disorder or difficulty. However, impotence is a commonly used and understood term in medicine and is retained here. Masters & Johnson advocate gradual introduction of the penis into the vagina, with the woman on top or the couple side by side, after a sensate focus session. The man is told to concentrate on the erotic sensations, and to relax and enjoy the experience. This behavioural technique is only applicable to those individuals who have a purely 'psychogenic' cause for their impotence (see later).

Masters & Johnson's (1970) studies of 500 couples reported high rates of treatment success: 50% in primary and 70–80% in secondary impotence; 98% in premature ejaculation; and 100% in vaginismus. These rates have never been replicated. Hawton (1986) showed a 60% improvement rate for premature ejaculation and less than 50% for impotence, with both conditions having a significant relapse rate. Vaginismus appears to be the only sexual disorder with a 100% success rate providing follow-up sessions are used by the couple as required.

RELATIONSHIP ISSUES AND THEIR IMPACT ON SEXUALITY

Discord within relationships is the most frequent cause of sexual dysfunction (Hawton 1986) and resentment underlies the cause of sexual dysfunction in many cases. It is perhaps more accurate to say that relationships are the area in which sexual dysfunctions emerge, but relationship problems in themselves are rarely seen by doctors. From an object relations viewpoint, the unconscious partner choice means we choose others who allow us to re-enact earlier developmental dilemmas in the unconscious hope of repairing previous damage. Disappointment occurs when a re-creation of earlier conflicts occurs and impairs sexual responsiveness. Relationships then act to *maintain* the problem, and must therefore become the focus of treatment.

The sexual relationship is central to many intimate relationships and misunderstandings are common when physical and emotional aspects of sexual arousal are out of phase. Sex is often part of the initial attraction and the sexual urge may remain a cohesive force. When things go wrong in a relationship, sex can put things right, albeit temporarily. Good sex, however, does depend upon the quality of the relationship overall, and many relationship problems (including lack of trust, resentment and anger) can lead to tension and sexual dissatisfaction. Untested assumptions about a partner's attitude to sex, partly fuelled by media impressions, create vicious circles of sexual difficulties. Communication between partners breaks down and avoidance of the subject ensues.

Behavioural marital therapies

Clear communication
Accurate empathy on the part of the therapist is important in couple therapy. At the most basic level, it involves encouraging the partners to sit opposite each other and talk together, with the therapist to one side. Checking meaning and understanding using short sentences, taking each other's requests seriously, avoiding making assumptions (mind reading) and making welcoming and constructive comments can be translated into homework exercises lasting 15 minutes each evening.

Negotiation of problems
Hawton (1986) has advocated *reciprocity negotiation* to reduce resentment as the underlying cause of reluctance for sex in many cases. The therapy encourages couples to carry out mutually rewarding behaviour to overcome the problem of complaint and counter-complaint. Sexual intercourse itself can be one of the rewarding behaviours. The tasks are usually reciprocal, arising from complaints or requests and are kept as mundane as possible, e.g. housework.

Arguments and assertiveness
Where relationships have an imbalance of power, there may also exist sexual conflict. The therapist encourages the quieter partner to assert him- or herself, and does not allow withdrawal or deviation from the topic until it has been resolved or fully discussed. Many couples find the exercise liberating and their relationship and sex life improve as a result.

The negotiated timetable
Introduced by Crowe & Ridley (1986), this is a useful approach to marital conflict where the woman is reluctant for sex, while the man has a high drive and presses her for frequent intercourse. The couple are asked to plan their sexual activities for certain days of the week, with a ban on sex on other days. The timetable takes the heat out of the sexual conflict and allows the couple to deal with issues that may underlie it. The timetable is less useful where it is the male partner who is reluctant for sex. A sensate focus timetable may be more useful here, or inducing trivial arguments in therapy sessions, where the man is encouraged to 'keep his end up'. A reversal of overt power may result in a re-established sexual relationship.

MECHANICAL AND PHARMACOLOGICAL TREATMENTS

Of the many commercially available mechanical devices used to augment the sexual response, the vibrator is the most frequently used. In the context of sex therapy it is primarily used to induce orgasm in anorgasmic women, as it is a powerful orgasmic stimulus when applied to the clitoris. It also has a place in inducing ejaculation and orgasm in men with delayed or absent ejaculatory responses.

Other devices used in the treatment of erectile impotence are the penile ring and the vacuum pump. Both of these have a place in the treatment of total erectile failure, but if used alone without any concurrent psychological or pharmacological interventions they are only successful in men who can sustain a partial erection.

The remaining physical treatments of significance are all directed at the treatment of erectile impotence, and fall into four main categories (Box 25.4).

Box 25.4   Categories of erectile impotence treatment
Intracavernosal injections α_1 adrenoreceptor antagonists (phenoxybenzamine and phentolamine) Smooth muscle relaxants (papaverine) Prostaglandins
Orally administered drugs Sildenafil citrate (Viagra) Second generation PDE-5 inhibitors–tadalfil (Cialis), verdenafil (Levitra) α_2 adrenoreceptor antagonists (yohimbine)
Sex hormones Testosterone Luteinizing hormone-releasing hormone Bromocriptine
Surgical Penile prostheses Vascular surgery

ERECTILE DYSFUNCTION (FAILURE OF GENITAL RESPONSE)

Erectile dysfunction (ED) has multiple causes and accounts for around 50% of all men attending psychosexual clinics. Erection is a neurovascular phenomenon which can be interfered with at the conscious/unconscious interface with its cognitive accompaniments, e.g. negative self-image and depression. Fears and phobias, non-sexual stress, and the state of the patient's relationship can contribute to erectile dysfunction.

Normal erection is dependent upon an intact arterial supply and is mediated via the autonomic nervous system via S2, 3 and 4, and intact venous valves. Centrally mediated α_2 effects have been noted by Wagner & Brindley (1980) using the α_2 antagonist, idazoxan, which is similar to yohimbine, administered orally. It is known that there is an age-related increase in impotence that is in part a result of unknown physiological/anatomical changes occurring. The contribution of androgens is uncertain, but they do affect nocturnal erections via the limbic system. Two types of erection are known: *psychic* (mediated via thoracic sympathetic outflow) and *reflex* (mediated via sacral parasympathetic outflow). Clearly, anatomical defects may

interfere with erections, but endocrine, neurological and vascular pathologies are the most prevalent and important causes of impotence:

- **Endocrine:** diabetes via arteriopathy and neuropathy; hypothalamic–pituitary dysfunction (hyerprolactinaemia – phenothiazines and alcohol); hypogonadism (reported in HIV infection); endorphins – naltrexone improves impotence in apparent 'psychogenic' impotence.
- **Neurological:** peripheral and autonomic neuropathy, pelvic surgery/irradiation and multiple sclerosis.
- **Vascular:** arteriopathy of pelvic vascular bed and proximal supply. Incompetent venous valves.

Management

Advanced investigations

The patient's history is elicited as previously mentioned. Investigations in addition to laboratory blood tests can include:

- Nocturnal penile tumescence: indicates the presence of nocturnal erections and may distinguish 'organic' from 'functional' causes. Total absence of early morning and nocturnal erections is strongly suggestive of an organic cause for the impotence.
- Dynamic cavernometry: detects venous incompetence by infusing normal saline into the corpus cavernosum.
- Penile-brachial penile pressure index: indicates local arterial disease to penis. Proceed to angiography if necessary.
- Diagnostic intracavernosal injection of papaverine or phentolamine: indicates 'capacity' for erection (if successful, arterial disease less likely).

Management

Treatment options

Phosphodiesterase-5 inhibitors

A number of chemical pathways are implicated in the erectile response. The most important mechanism involves cyclic guanosine monophosphate (GMP), the formation of which is mediated by nitric oxide. Sildenafil inhibits phosphodiesterase (PDE), increases levels of cyclic guanosine monophosphate (GMP), and thus relaxes smooth muscle in the penis and effects erection. The drug acts through neural mechanisms to restore erectile function in response to sexual stimulation. It is not an aphrodisiac. The dose is 25–100 mg and it has been proven to be effective in patients with depression, diabetes, spinal cord injury, hypertension, and neural damage due to surgery. It is safe for use in patients over the age of 65, but is contraindicated with concomitant use of nitrates. It is fast-acting, with an efficacy window of 25 minutes to 4 hours. The most common adverse events in clinical studies were headache, flushing and dyspepsia – these were usually transient and mild.

Discontinuation due to adverse events was shown to be 2.5% in flexible-dose studies (compared with 2.3% on placebo).

The cascade of neurotransmitter and physiological events that leads to the production of the chemical messenger cyclic guanosine monophosphate (cGMP) causes the blood vessels in the penis to relax, thus increasing blood flow. The enzyme PDE-5 breaks down cGMP, reducing blood flow, which in turn reduces the erection. There are 11 isoforms of PDE, but in the penis the predominant isoform is number 5. The PDE-5 inhibitors reinforce the erectile process and help maintain erections. In addition to sildenafil and the newer tadalafil there is another compound not available in the UK, vardenafil. All three have a similar chemical structure with three to five benzene rings and various side chains of methane, hydrogen and oxygen. Tadalafil is a reversible, potent and efficacious inhibitor of PDE-5. Furthermore, tadalafil's 36 hour duration of action (longer half-life) and faster onset coupled with its low side-effect profile compared to its competitors suggests that it has the edge over them. It is solely excreted by the liver, but alcohol and food have no influence over this drug's pharmacokinetics (see Chapter 38).

Some PDE inhibitors appear to be less effective in patients with diabetes mellitus types 1 and 2. Sildenafil potentiates the potency of organic nitrates and is associated with significant reductions in blood pressure; there have been case reports of both infarction and ischaemia associated with the use of sildenafil. The use of this drug in patients with pre-existing cardiac disease and those using organic phosphates is discouraged if not contraindicated. In randomized controlled trials with 80 healthy volunteers tadalafil produced no statistically significant differences in blood pressure or heart rate compared with placebo. The incidence of myocardial infarction and cardiac death was the same as placebo. Furthermore, tadalafil has been used safely in over 1300 men with stable cardiovascular conditions complicated by hypertension, diabetes mellitus and hyperlipidaemia.

All drugs have side-effects related to the distribution of the drug and the mode of action. PDE-5 is located in neurons and the gut, so the commonest side-effects are headache, back pain and dyspepsia, with nasal congestion, myalgia and flushing being less prominent. Yet only around 2.1% of patients in trials discontinued the drug because of these effects. As with most medication continued usage reduces side-effects over time.

Intracavernosal injections
Pharmacologically induced penile erection (PIPE) was pioneered by Wagner & Brindley (1980) using α_1 adrenoreceptor blocking drugs. Virag (1982a) used the smooth muscle relaxant papaverine to similar effect. A combination of papaverine and phentolamine, or papaverine alone, can be injected into the base of the corpora cavernosa to produce an erection for intercourse. The dose is usually 120 mg, and the patient or his partner are taught to inject using a sterile technique. An optimal dose produces an erection for between 30 minutes and 2 hours. Although early results showed an impressive response, it is not a treatment acceptable to all (Hollander & Diokno 1984), and is not without risk of priapism or penile fibrosis. Injections should not be used more than twice weekly. Erections that last longer than six hours are potentially dangerous and can cause necrosis; the treatment is to withdraw around 60 ml of blood from the penis and inject phenylephrine 1–5 mg (an α adrenergic agonist), which will allow the erection to subside. Patients must be advised of the risks and given written instructions about what to do if an emergency arises.

Yohimbine
This orally administered drug remains popular with many therapists. Having been available for more than 30 years, its use is on the increase. Being a derivative of the yohimbine tree, it has a mixed pharmacological identity, but the main component is an α_2 adrenoreceptor antagonist with central neural effects, whose main therapeutic influence has been on the 'psychogenic' impotent male. Yohimbine has also been used to treat the anorgasmic male – 20–40 mg 45 minutes prior to applying an erotic stimulus (usually a vibrator), which increases the likelihood of orgasm.

Hormonal treatment
Testosterone plays a small part in the erectile mechanism, being more important for sexual interest and drive. However, lowered testosterone levels can produce impaired sexual interest and ejaculatory failure. Replacement using testosterone or bromocriptine can resolve this, but since testosterone is extensively metabolized by the liver, parenterally administered testosterone esters are preferred. Negative feedback mechanisms do unfortunately produce diminished effects after prolonged usage.

Luteinizing hormone releasing hormone is given to men with hypogonadism, and some women with post-menopausal atrophic vaginitis benefit from the rejuvenating effects of hormone replacement therapy.

Surgical treatments
Surgery does have a place in the treatment of erectile failure of organic origin and psychogenic impotence resistant to other forms of treatment. Loeffler (1960) first described the use of implanted surgical plastic splints into the penis. Since then, flexible/hinged and inflatable implants have been developed. Both types are inserted into the corpora cavernosa bilaterally, but this is a complicated procedure often complicated by technical failure, local infection and wound dehiscence and an unaesthetic outcome. Although they have a place in the treatment of impotence, counselling of both partners should precede the treatment, and in particular it should be made clear to the couple that the procedure is irreversible.

Revascularization of the larger arteries supplying the penile vascular bed affected by peripheral vascular disease is sometimes attempted, but the distal vessels are usually also affected and the results variable and short-lived. Surgical plugging of dysfunctional venous valves within the penis has been successful in some cases.

FUTURE DEVELOPMENTS IN TREATMENT

The future of the treatment of sexual disorders lies partly with the psychosexual behavioural programmes, which remain the best option for female problems, premature ejaculation and motivational difficulties, coupled with pharmacological treatments for impotence unresponsive to first-line therapies. Pharmacological treatments for both erectile dysfunction and female anorgasmia are likely to become increasingly available. The problem to date is the lack of dedicated centres offering a comprehensive service with an eclectic approach to assessment and treatment. With the extent of the problem now more widely acknowledged by various professionals and the public it must be hoped that trainees will gain greater exposure to departments that offer a valuable and rewarding resource.

REFERENCES

American Psychiatric Association (1994) Diagnostic and Statistical Manual of Mental Disorders, 4th edn. Washington, DC: APA.

Bancroft J (1989) Human Sexuality and its Problems. Edinburgh: Churchill Livingstone.

Beck AT, Rush AJ, Shaw BF & Emery G (1979) Cognitive Theory of Depression. A Treatment Manual. New York: Guilford.

Crowe M & Jones M (1992) Sex therapy: the successes, the failures, the future. British Journal of Hospital Medicine 48(8): 474–82.

Crowe M & Ridley J (1986) The negotiated timetable: a new approach to marital conflicts involving male demands and female reluctance for sex. Sexual and Marital Therapy 1: 157–73.

Crowe M & Ridley J (1990) Therapy with Couples. A Behavioural-Systems Approach to Marital and Sexual Problems. Oxford: Blackwell Scientific.

Department of Health (1994) Health of the Nation. HMSO.

Fromm E, Oberlander MI & Gruenwald D (1970) Perceptual and cognitive process in different states of consciousness: the waking state and hypnosis. Journal of Projective Techniques and Personality Assessment 34: 375–87.

Hawton K (1986) Sex Therapy: A Practical Guide. Oxford: Oxford University Press.

Hollander JB & Diokno AC (1984) Successes with penile prostheses from patients' viewpoint. Urology 23: 141.

Johnson AM, Wadsworth J, Wellings K et al. (1994) Sexual Attitudes and Lifestyles. Oxford: Blackwell Scientific.

Jones MB, Klimes I & Catalan J (1994) Psychosexual problems in people with HIV infection: controlled study of gay men and men with haemophilia. Aids Care 6(5): 587–93.

Kaplan H (1974) The New Sex Therapy. New York: Brunner/Mazel.

Kinsey AC, Pomeroy WB & Martin CF (1948) Sexual Behaviour in the Human Male. Philadelphia: Saunders.

Kinsey AC, Pomeroy WB, Martin CF & Gebhard PH (1953) Sexual Behaviour in the Human Female. Philadelphia: Saunders.

Loeffler RA (1960) Perforated acrylic implant in the management of organic impotence. Journal of Urology 97: 716.

Masters WH & Johnson VE (1970) Human Sexual Inadequacy. London: Churchill.

Maurice WL (1985) Sexual medicine. Journal of the Canadian Medical Association 132: 1123–5.

Puri BK & Hall AD (1998) Revision Notes in Psychiatry. London: Arnold.

Rosen RC, Taylor JF, Leiblum SR & Bachmann GA (1993) Prevalence of sexual dysfunction in women: results of a survey study of 329 women in an out-patient gynaecological clinic. Journal of Sex and Marital Therapy 19: 171–88.

Royal College of Obstetricians and Gynaecologists (1993) Report of the RCOG Working Party on Structured Training. London: Chameleon Press.

Sachs BD (2000) Contextual approaches to the physiology and classification of erectile function, erectile dysfunction, and sexual arousal. Neuroscience & Behavioural Reviews 24(5): 541–60.

Saunders D (1985) The Woman Book of Love and Sex. London: Sphere.

Saunders D (1987) The Woman Report on Men. London: Sphere.

Semans S (1956) Premature ejaculation: a new approach. Southern Medical Journal 49: 3–8.

Virag R (1982a) Intracavernous injection of papaverine for erectile failure. Lancet ii: 938.

Virag R (1982b) Revascularisation of the penis. In: Bennet A (ed.) Management of Male Impotence, pp. 219–33. Baltimore: Williams & Wilkins.

Wagner G & Brindley GS (1980) The effect of atropine and alpha blockers on human penile erection. In: Zorgniotti AW & Rossi G (eds) Vasculitic Impotence, pp. 77–81. Springfield: CC Thomas.

Waldinger MD, Hengeveld MW & Zwinderman AH (1994) Paroxetine: treatment of premature ejaculation – a double-blind, randomised, placebo controlled study. American Journal of Psychiatry 151: 1377–9.

World Health Organization (1992) ICD-10 Classification of Mental and Behavioural Disorders. Geneva: WHO.

Organic psychiatry and epilepsy

Pádraig Wright and Thordur Sigmundsson

INTRODUCTION

Contemporary psychiatric research provides ever increasing evidence that many psychiatric disorders have a biological origin. However, with few exceptions, it is not yet possible to classify psychiatric disorders on this basis. These exceptions include a number of amnestic disorders, the dementias, several specific movement disorders, epilepsy, sleep disorders or parasomnias and the psychiatric sequelae of cerebral insult, whether focal or generalized. This chapter discusses the psychiatric aspects of these various disorders. The reader is referred to a textbook of medicine or neurology for a more general account of each disorder and its treatment.

ORGANIC PSYCHIATRY – GENERAL CONSIDERATIONS

An understanding of the individual organic psychiatric syndromes depends on the appreciation that organic psychiatric syndromes have temporal and geographic dimensions. Therefore they may be acute or chronic in onset and/or course, and may cause either a focal brain deficit or a more generalized impairment of intellectual function.

Thus delirium, for example, represents an acute disorder that causes generalized intellectual impairment, dementia represents a chronic disorder that causes generalized intellectual impairment, and head injury represents an acute disorder that often causes focal intellectual impairment. The clinical evaluation of patients with organic psychiatric syndromes is largely directed at differentiating between acute and chronic disorders on the one hand, and between focal and generalized disorders on the other.

Acute and chronic organic psychiatric syndromes

The clinical differentiation of acute (delirium) from chronic (dementia) organic psychiatric syndromes is of paramount importance, as the former represent a medical emergency and patients suffering with them require urgent assessment and treatment. The diagnosis is usually apparent from the history and presentation but it may be difficult on occasion and only become apparent after careful observation. Diagnosis is further complicated by the fact that it is not uncommon for patients to present with an acute organic reaction superimposed upon a heretofore undiagnosed dementia. Such patients may be thought of as having a reduced 'mental reserve' such that even minor physical illnesses can provoke an acute organic reaction that unmasks their dementia. Table 26.1 summarizes the clinical features that may be helpful in differentiating between acute/delirium and chronic/dementia organic psychiatric syndromes.

Focal and generalized organic psychiatric syndromes

Disturbances of brain function may affect either one neuropsychological domain or several. Thus both acute and chronic organic psychiatric syndromes cause generalized intellectual impairment and are characterized by multiple neuropsychological deficits. Focal brain lesions, on the other hand, are more likely to cause one or a few neuro-psychological deficits such as aphasia, an amnestic disorder or frontal lobe syndrome. However, the distinction between focal and generalized dysfunction is not always clear and it is not uncommon for focal deficits to become apparent only after resolution of generalized intellectual impairment. For example, the specific memory disorder associated with Korsakoff's syndrome may only become apparent when the generalized intellectual impairment of Wernicke's encephalopathy has been successfully treated.

Clinical evaluation of patients with organic psychiatric syndromes

The appropriate clinical assessment is determined to some extent by the mode of presentation and the treatment setting

Table 26.1 Clinical features that help differentiate between acute (delirium) and chronic (dementia) organic psychiatric syndromes

Clinical feature	Delirium	Dementia
Onset	Acute or subacute	Usually insidious
Course	Transient and fluctuating	Persistent
Duration	Short, hours to days	Long, months to years
Attention	Impaired	Usually intact initially
Consciousness	Often drowsy	Usually alert
Mood	Agitation, fear, perplexity	Flat, unreactive, apathetic
Thinking	Disorganized, delusions (fleeting and persecutory)	Impoverished
Illusions and hallucinations	Common	Uncommon
Association with physical illness, drugs or alcohol	Common	Uncommon

(see Chapter 32). Thus the emergency assessment of an acutely disturbed patient will be brief and focused and largely based on careful observation of the patient and any further information that is available. The primary objective is to distinguish between psychotic illness, behavioural disturbance caused by a chronic organic illness, personality disorder and acute organic reaction. Patients presenting with a more insidious onset of illness require a more detailed clinical assessment, including a thorough psychiatric history, a physical examination and a detailed neurological examination. The general clinical examination of psychiatric patients is described in Chapter 32, while a schema for cognitive assessment – adapted from Lishman (1997) – is presented below.

Standard cognitive examination in all psychiatric patients

Bedside clinical tests to assess cognitive function are invaluable for screening patients and psychiatrists should familiarize themselves with a small battery of tests for use in routine practice.

Orientation:

- for time (date: day of week, month and year)
- for place (name of present whereabouts and own address)
- for person (own name).

Attention and concentration (record qualitative observations if difficulties are encountered):

- ask patient to name the days of week or months of year backwards
- ask patient to subtract serial 7s from 100
- ask patient to repeat increasing numbers of digits forwards and backwards.

Memory (assess general information and recent and remote personal information):

- reproduction of sentence with immediate and delayed (3-5 minutes) retrieval
- reproduction of name and address (e.g. Mr John Brown, 32 Church Street, Bristol, B8) with immediate and delayed (3-5 minutes) retrieval.

Intelligence:

- a rough estimate of intelligence may be formed from educational and occupational achievements and from interests and leisure activities.

Cognitive examination in psychiatric patients with suspected organic psychiatric syndromes

In addition to the above, patients with suspected organic psychiatric syndromes should be further assessed as follows:

- assess level of cooperation
- assess level of consciousness
- determine if language functions are intact
- test spatial and constructional ability.

Neuropsychological evaluation of patients with organic psychiatric syndromes

Box 26.1 briefly describes some of the tests commonly used by neuropsychologists in the detailed evaluation of cognitive function. Tests of frontal lobe function are also referred to as tests of executive function and although many are sensitive to frontal lobe dysfunction they are not specific. It is increasingly recognized that results depend on intact neural networks, so damage other than to the frontal lobe may impair executive function.

Box 26.1 Tests commonly used by neuropsychologists in the detailed evaluation of cognitive function

Measurement of IQ

The Wechsler Adult Intelligent Scale – Revised (WAIS R) measures general IQ

The National Adult Reading Test (NART) measures premorbid IQ

Progressive Matrices measure non-verbal intelligence

Tests of language functions

The Boston Naming Test

The token test

Tests of memory function

The Rivermead Behavioural Memory Test (RBMT)

The California Verbal Memory Test (CVMT)

The Ray-Osterich Complex Figure Test

Tests of executive function

The Wisconsin Card Sorting Test (WCST)

The Tower of London Test

The Stroop Test

The Controlled Word Association Test or FAS – Verbal fluency test

Scales used to assess the severity of cognitive impairment

The Mini-Mental State Examination (MMSE)

The CAMDEX

The Newcastle Dementia Scale

Investigation of patients with organic psychiatric syndromes

Haematology and biochemistry

Haematological tests including white and red blood cell indices and erythrocyte sedimentation rate should be performed and serum electrolytes, liver function enzymes and tests of renal function evaluated. Other tests may be indicated by the clinical picture including thyroid function tests, fasting blood glucose, calcium, iron, folic acid and vitamin B_{12} levels, serum tests for syphilis, HIV serology, plasma levels of therapeutic drugs and tests for illicit drugs. Further tests may be appropriate to rule out specific illnesses.

Electroencephalography

An electroencephalogram (EEG) is regarded as a routine investigation in patients with neuropsychiatric disorders is certainly indicated if epilepsy is suspected. A standard EEG or sleep EEG may suffice, or an EEG with additional electrodes (in the foramen ovale, nasopharynx and intracranially, for example) may be appropriate if there is high suspicion of epilepsy. A 24-hour EEG recording is also helpful in diagnosing epilepsy and in evaluating possible non-epileptic seizures (see below and Chapter 34).

Neuroimaging

The skull X-ray is occasionally useful but has largely been replaced by computed tomography (CT), which effectively visualizes space-occupying brain lesions, infarcts and white matter lesions, shows brain atrophy and allows for visualization of the ventricular system. Magnetic resonance imaging (MRI) is increasingly replacing CT because it is more effective in detecting abnormalities near the base of the skull and its resolution is higher. Positron emission tomography (PET), single photon emission computed tomography (SPECT) and functional magnetic resonance imaging (fMRI) are increasingly used in clinical practice while the value of magnetic resonance spectroscopy (MRS) is predominantly in research (see Chapter 34).

FOCAL ORGANIC PSYCHIATRIC SYNDROMES

The psychiatric syndromes associated with lesions of specific cortical lobes will now be described (see also Chapter 2).

Lesions of the frontal lobe

The frontal lobe is conventionally divided into the motor cortex anterior to the central sulcus and the prefrontal cortex anterior to the motor cortex. Lesions in the motor area of the frontal cortex may cause Broca's aphasia if the dominant hemisphere is involved and executive aprosodia (difficulty recognizing emotional content and expression of speech) if the non-dominant hemisphere is involved.

The prefrontal cortex represents approximately 30% of the total human cortex. Despite this, it has been called 'the silent region, because even relatively large lesions may not produce significant neurological signs or cognitive impairment. In contrast, however, modest lesions may cause marked change in personality, cognition and behaviour. These are often so stereotyped that the term frontal lobe syndrome has been applied. The clinical features of the frontal lobe syndrome are as follows:

Personality changes

Disinhibition with overfamiliarity, tactlessness, over-talkativeness and sometimes childish excitement. Lack of concern for the future and the consequences of actions. Lack of social and ethical control. Lack of judgement and insight. Irritability and aggression or indifference and apathy. Lack of motivation and initiative with slowing of thought and motor activity.

Cognitive dysfunction

Deficits in sequencing or temporal ordering of behaviour, with difficulties in problem solving, planning and mental flexibility. Memory dysfunction with poor recall and recognition.

Behavioural changes

Three relatively distinct behavioural syndromes may occur depending on the cortical region damaged as follows:

- dorsolateral prefrontal region – executive dysfunction, loss of initiative, slowing of thought and behaviour, perseveration, poor memory recall (as evidenced by poor verbal fluency) and changes in mood – especially depression – commonly follow dorsolateral prefrontal lesions
- medial frontal region – disinhibition, impulsiveness, distractibility, loss of emotional and social control, lability and irritability commonly follow orbitofrontal lesions
- orbitofrontal region – apathy and poor performance on tasks that require suppression of inappropriate responses follows medial frontal lobe lesions.

These behavioural syndromes rarely occur in isolation in clinical practice, but because the dorsolateral prefrontal, medial frontal and orbitofrontal regions are components of specific frontal-subcortical-thalamic circuits (Cummings 1993), lesions (especially bilateral lesions) of the striatum may produce frontal lobe syndrome by disruption of such circuits. It is also worth noting that there is emerging evidence of lateralization of function in the frontal lobe – visuospatial function is more affected by right side lesions and linguistic function by left side lesions.

Lesions of the temporal lobe

The major symptoms of temporal lobe damage are disorders of memory and language. It is important to realize that both of these functions depend on brain regions other than the temporal lobe, most notably the frontal lobe.

Disorders of memory (the amnestic syndrome)

The amnestic syndrome is present when organic memory impairment is out of proportion to other cognitive impairments. It is caused by bilateral damage to medial temporal lobe (hippocampus, amygdala and fornix) and certain mid-line structures (mammillary bodies and medial parts of thalamus). Major causes of the amnestic syndrome are as follows:

- Wernicke's encephalopathy – the clinical picture is usually of an acute onset of clouding of consciousness/delirium with nystagmus, external rectus paralysis, paralysis of conjugate gaze, ataxia and peripheral polyneuropathy.
- Wernicke–Korsakoff syndrome – the delirium of Wernicke's encephalopathy resolves and is followed by anterograde memory disturbance in the presence of intact short-term or working memory. A retrograde

amnesia of a variable degree is also common, as is confabulation (Kopelman 1995). Wernicke–Korsakoff syndrome is caused by thiamine deficiency, which in turn is usually caused by malnutrition in chronic alcohol dependence (see Chapter 2) but may also be caused by malabsorption syndromes associated with carcinoma of the stomach or by hyperemesis gravidarum.

- Head injuries (see below).
- Herpes simplex encephalitis (see below).
- Infarction in posterior cerebral arteries.
- Hypoxia (see below).

Amnesia is also a feature of the Kluver–Bucy syndrome (hyperorality, overattention to external stimuli, agnosia, hypersexuality and loss of fear) which is caused by bilateral damage to the medial temporal lobe as a result of tumour or infection, most commonly herpes simplex encephalitis.

Transient global amnesia consists of attacks of sudden global amnesia lasting several hours and followed by complete recovery. Patients are typically men in their middle years, attacks are sudden and there is usually no clouding of consciousness. Anterograde memory loss is profound but short-term memory remains intact. There is complete amnesia for the attack on recovery. The aetiology of transient global amnesia is unclear but transient ischaemic attacks, epilepsy and migraine have been implicated. The differential diagnosis includes dissociative disorders, hypoglycaemia and temporal lobe epilepsy (Hodges 1994).

Disorders of language

Technical terms used in describing disorders of language include:

- aphasia or dysphasia (impaired ability to formulate and/or comprehend speech)
- dysarthria (impaired ability to articulate words caused by inadequate control of the muscles necessary for speech)
- mutism (failure to produce any speech or sounds)
- alexia (loss of the ability to read)
- agraphia (loss of the ability to write).

The structures subserving speech are largely located in the left hemisphere and include the anterior or Broca's area in the frontal lobe and the posterior or Wernicke's auditory association area in the posteriosuperior temporal lobe. The most important aphasias may be differentiated on the basis of patients' abilities to comprehend speech (including reading and writing), speak fluently and repeat words or phrases as follows:

- Comprehension resides in Wernicke's area and lesions there produce sensory (or receptive or anterior) aphasia in which comprehension and the ability to repeat words is greatly impaired but speech is fluent albeit with paraphasias, jargon and neologisms.

- Lesions involving Broca's area produce expressive (or motor or posterior) aphasia in which comprehension is intact but speech is non-fluent or telegraphic and the ability to repeat words is impaired.
- Lesions involving the arcuate fasciculus which connects Wernicke's and Broca's areas produce conductive aphasias with intact comprehension and fluent speech but with a strikingly impaired ability to repeat words.
- Global aphasia, the most common and severe aphasia, is characterized by an almost complete absence of both speech and comprehension. It is usually caused by large lesions of both Wernicke's and Broca's areas, often following occlusion of the left internal carotid or middle cerebral artery, and almost always accompanied by a right hemiplegia.

Lesions of the parietal and occipital lobes

Lesions of the parietal and occipital lobes may cause a wide variety of symptoms including visuospatial difficulties, dyspraxias, agnosias, disturbances of body image and a specific syndrome, Gerstmann's syndrome. These are described in detail in Chapter 2.

Lesions of the diencephalon and other brain regions

Lesions of the deep midline structures may cause disorders of memory and hypersomnia while lesions involving the hypothalamus commonly cause hyperphagia (although anorexia nervosa has also been described). Tumours in this region can cause an obstructive hydrocephalus with diffuse cognitive impairment.

Lesions of the basal ganglia may be associated with a wide variety of psychiatric symptoms in addition to motor abnormalities. Bilateral lesions of the putamen and caudate, for example, can cause a syndrome identical to frontal lobe syndrome, symptoms identical to the negative symptoms of schizophrenia and obsessive compulsive symptoms (Laplane et al. 1989). Lesions of the basal ganglia can also produce an atypical aphasia, dysarthria and aprosodia.

Thalamic lesions may cause language disorders and executive dysfunction in addition to a disturbance in memory if the dorsomedial nuclei are involved.

GENERALIZED ORGANIC PSYCHIATRIC SYNDROMES

Both acute and chronic organic psychiatric syndromes – delirium and dementia (which will be discussed separately below) respectively – cause generalized neuropsychological deficits.

Delirium

Delirium is also called acute organic reaction, acute confusional state, acute brain syndrome, organic psychosis and ICU psychosis. Impairment of consciousness ranging from mild impairment in concentration and attention to deep coma, and typically worsening at night, is the universal feature of delirium but disturbances of perception, thinking and psychomotor behaviour are also common. Delirium has been defined as impaired consciousness with intrusive abnormalities of perception and affect (Lishman 1987), causes significant morbidity and mortality and is probably the commonest psychiatric syndrome. One study found that 13.5% of patients admitted to a general medical ward had delirium when hospitalized, while a further 3% became delirious during hospitalization (Cameron et al. 1987).

The following terms have been used to describe the various impairments of consciousness observed in patients with delirium:

- clouding of consciousness – the mildest stage of impairment characterized by slight deterioration in thinking, attention, perception and memory
- drowsiness – the patient falls asleep in the absence of sensory stimulation and exhibits slowness of action, slurred speech, reduced muscle tone and reduced reflexes
- sopor – the patient is unconscious but can regain consciousness if strongly stimulated (this term is rarely used in clinical practice)
- coma – the patient is deeply unconscious and cannot be roused
- confusion – an imprecise term is usually referring to unclear and incoherent thought processes that is best avoided
- twilight state – this term is used to describe an organic condition usually associated with epilepsy and characterized by abrupt onset/termination, variable duration and unexpected violent acts or emotional outbursts during otherwise apparently normal behaviour
- oneroid state (dream-like state) – the patient appears disorganized and confused and often experiences elaborate visual hallucinations. Oneroid states are not clearly differentiated from delirium and may be associated with dissociative disorders.

There are many causes of delirium (Box 26.2) but the clinical picture is remarkably similar in all cases (see Box 26.3 for ICD-10 diagnostic criteria). Patients exhibit clouding of consciousness, disturbances of memory (poor registration, retention and recall and amnesia for the duration of the delirium), distractibility, slowed thinking and impaired reasoning progressing to disorganization and fragmentation of thought and ultimately to incoherence. Illusions are frequent and vivid visual hallucinations are common (visual

Box 26.2   Common causes of delirium

Infections
Systemic
Intracranial

Cardiovascular disorders
Intracranial bleeding
Subdural haematoma
Myocardial infarction
Pulmonary embolism
Heart failure

Endocrine disorders
Diabetes
Hypothyroidism
Hyperthyroidism

Gastrointestinal disorders
Hepatic failure
Pancreatitis

Genitourinary disorders
Renal failure
Urinary tract infection

Intoxications
Alcohol
Prescribed and illicit drugs
Carbon monoxide poisoning

Neurological disorders
Head injury
Meningitis
Encephalitis
Tumours

Box 26.3   The ICD-10 diagnostic criteria for delirium not induced by alcohol or other psychoactive substances

Symptoms should be present from each of the following areas for a definite diagnosis:
Impairment of consciousness and attention
Global disturbance of cognition
Psychomotor disturbance
Emotional disturbances, e.g. depression, anxiety or fear, irritability, euphoria, apathy or wondering perplexity

hallucinations indicate an organic lesion until proven otherwise). Delusions – often fleeting and persecutory in content – are also common. Initial fear and anxiety is eventually replaced by apathy and indifference while arousal, agitation and hypervigilance are followed by listlessness and hypoactivity (fluctuation between hyperactivity and hypoactivity is frequent). Disorientation in time and in place is common. Apraxia, dysnomia and dysgraphia are common but are not specific to delirium and

also occur in dementia. The individual clinical picture is coloured by the patient's premorbid personality and the primary illness.

Delirium has a high mortality, 19 of 77 patients (25%) dying within six months in one investigation (Trzepacz et al. 1985). Early diagnosis and aggressive investigation is therefore essential in order to determine the primary cause and initiate appropriate treatment. Delirium associated with alcohol withdrawal is usually treated with reducing doses of benzodiazepines (although these should be used with caution, especially in elderly patients, because they may cause confusion) (see Chapter 16). Small doses of antipsychotics are also useful (although antipsychotics with anticholinergic properties are best avoided because they may worsen delirium). Delirium and its treatment have recently been reviewed by Meagher (2001).

The dementias

The diagnosis of dementia is clinical and requires the presence of acquired, persisting, usually progressive, global impairments of multiple higher cortical functions (especially memory and intellect) and of personality (emotional lability, socially inappropriate behaviour, impaired judgement and avolition) in clear consciousness. Functional impairment is a necessary prerequisite for the clinical diagnosis of dementia, which may be further supported by neuroimaging. While the clinical diagnosis of dementia depends on psychiatric, neuropsychological and neuroimaging evaluations, a precise neuropathological diagnosis can only be made postmortem. The traditional classification of dementia into presenile (onset before the age of 65 years) and senile (onset after that age), or cortical (Alzheimer's, vascular, Lewy body, Pick's, frontal lobe and alcoholic dementias and Creutzfeldt–Jakob and new variant Creutzfeldt-Jakob diseases) and subcortical (Parkinson's disease, Huntington's disease, progressive supranuclear palsy, dementia associated with the acquired immune deficiency syndrome, dementia associated with multiple lacunar infarcts and Binswanger's disease) is referred to in this discussion but is gradually falling into disuse.

Alzheimer's disease

The clinical features, pathology and treatment of Alzheimer's disease are described in Chapter 31. It is important for the psychiatrist to realize that Alzheimer's disease is not a disorder of specific brain regions or of specific neurotransmitter systems. Thus while senile plaques and neurofibrillary tangles are characteristically accompanied by loss of neurons in frontal and temporal cortex and of cholinergic neurons in the nucleus of Meynert and other basal nuclei, neuronal loss and neurotransmitter dysfunction occurs throughout the brain. Neurotransmitter abnormalities are thought to follow neuronal loss and may be summarized as follows:

- **Acetylcholine:** cholinergic neuronal loss occurs in the nucleus of Meynert, the largest cholinergic nucleus, and other basal nuclei. This is associated with reduced choline acetyltransferase activity which correlates with both cognitive impairment and neuropathological findings. Treatments directed at improving cholinergic function may reduce cognitive impairment in some patients with Alzheimer's disease (see Chapter 38). It is also worth noting that oestrogens modulate hippocampal choline acetyltransferase activity and that oestrogen replacement therapy delays the onset of Alzheimers disease. Thus women's increased vulnerability to Alzheimer's disease may be attributable to post-menopausal hypo-oestrogenaemia.
- **Serotonin:** cortical and hippocampal concentrations of serotonin and its metabolites are reduced, as are numbers of serotonin $5HT_2$ receptors.
- **Dopamine:** cortical and basal ganglia concentrations of dopamine are reduced, and the latter is probably responsible for the parkinsonism that patients with Alzheimer's disease may experience.
- **Noradrenaline (norepinephrine):** cortical concentrations of dopamine hydroxylase and subsequently of noradrenaline (norepinephrine) are reduced.
- **Excitatory and inhibitory amino acids:** concentrations of the excitatory amino acid glutamate, and of its N-methyl-D-aspartate receptors, are reduced, as are cortical levels of inhibitory gamma-aminobutyric acid and glutamic acid decarboxylase.

Patients with Alzheimer's disease almost always suffer from weight loss. It is unclear whether this is because they are unable to care for themselves and become malnourished, or because Alzheimer's disease is a systemic disorder and not central nervous system-specific. It is also unclear whether incontinence is secondary to cognitive impairment or follows neuronal deterioration. Alzheimer's disease is inevitably fatal and patients with it have a mortality rate several-fold greater than that of age-matched controls. Death occurs earlier in male patients and in those with a younger age of onset (Burns et al. 1991) and is more frequently due to bronchopneumonia than any other cause.

Vascular dementia and Binswanger's disease

The clinical features, pathology and treatment of vascular dementia – this term is preferred to multi-infarct dementia – are described in Chapter 31. Cerebrovascular disease is the second leading cause of dementia after Alzheimer's disease. It is commoner in men than women and hypertension is the most significant risk factor. The clinical course is often stepwise, with sudden cognitive decline and/or focal signs (primitive reflexes, dysphasias and amnesias, for example) and syndromes (Gerstmann's syndrome, for example) developing after cerebral infarcts or haemorrhages. Postmortem research provides evidence that at least 50 ml of cerebral cortex must be damaged before cognitive impairment develops and that the extent of cortical damage correlates with cognitive impairment (Tomlinson et al. 1970). Treatment directed at hypertension and at the prevention of cerebrovascular disease may slow the progress of vascular dementia. Patients with vascular dementia have a mortality rate two- or three-fold greater than that of age-matched controls, and if Alzheimer's disease coexists, the mortality rate is further increased.

Binswanger's disease causes subcortical dementia (see below) and is a severe form of subcortical cerebrovascular disease (sometimes referred to as progressive subcortical arteriosclerotic – or vascular – encephalopathy) with periventricular white matter demyelination that may occur in patients as young as 50 years of age. It is associated with systemic vascular disease and hypertension and symptoms may include motor and sensor deficits, dementia and pseudobulbar palsy.

Lewy body dementia

The clinical features, pathology and treatment of this dementia – named after the intracytolasmic inclusion bodies, or Lewy bodies, that occur especially in the temporal and cingulate cortex of patients – are described in Chapter 31. Lewy bodies also occur in Parkinson's disease but are not as common as in Lewy body dementia. Conversely, loss of nigrostriatal neurons occurs in Lewy body dementia, but is not as marked as in Parkinson's disease. Senile plaques and increased risk with the apolipoprotein ε4 allele also occur with Lewy body dementia. Thus it may be thought of as a variant of either Alzheimer's or Parkinson's disease. Patients with Lewy body dementia are especially sensitive to antipsychotic drugs, frequently developing extrapyramidal side-effects and even neuroleptic malignant syndrome (see Chapters 18 and 38). The treatment of the disturbed behaviour and hallucinations that are common symptoms of this disorder are therefore difficult, and atypical antipsychotics are preferred to older drugs.

Pick's disease and dementia of frontal lobe type

About 10% of patients with dementia prove to have predominantly frontal or frontotemporal lobe atrophy at autopsy. This dementia has been referred to as Pick's disease since it was first described by Pick in 1892. More recently, Brun (1987), while confirming that 1 in 10 demented patients do have frontal or frontotemporal atrophy, also reported that only 25% of these have classic Pick's disease. The remainder are now usually described as having dementia of frontal lobe type. It is unclear if there is any relationship between Pick's disease and dementia of frontal lobe type.

Pick's disease

The aetiology of Pick's disease is unknown. However, it appears to be inherited as an autosomal dominant disorder in at least some pedigrees and at least 50% of Brun's sample (see above) had an affected first degree relative. The classic pathological features of Pick's disease are as follows:

- asymmetrical 'knife-blade atrophy of the frontal or frontotemporal lobes with absent or modest generalized cortical atrophy
- Pick's bodies, or argentophilic inclusions, in the outer cortical layers, and
- Pick's cells, or chromatophilic neurons, in the outer cortical layers.

Onset is usually in the sixth decade and women are affected twice as frequently as men. The clinical features resemble those of Alzheimer's disease, although frontal lobe symptoms may be more prominent, and intellectual impairment less prominent, at least initially. Thus patients may exhibit disinhibition, lability of mood, impaired judgement and coarsened social behaviour. A Kluver–Bucy-like syndrome with hyperorality, hypersexuality and visual agnosia may also occur, as may extrapyramidal and parietal lobe symptoms. Urinary incontinence occurs early but deterioration, and especially intellectual deterioration, is otherwise relatively slow, the patients described by Brun surviving over 10 years from the time of diagnosis.

Dementia of frontal lobe type

As mentioned above, about 75% of patients with apparent frontal lobe dementia do not have Pick's disease and are now usually described as having dementia of frontal lobe type. The aetiology of dementia of frontal lobe type is unknown but up to 50% of patients have an affected first degree relative. The pathology consists of neuronal loss, gliosis and spongiosis in the frontal lobes while the clinical picture is one of onset in the sixth decade, personality change and progressive dementia with relative preservation of memory.

Dementia associated with alcohol

Dementia caused by the direct neurotoxic effects of alcohol is commoner than Wernicke's encephalopathy or Korsakoff's psychosis (see above and below). Risk factors for alcoholic dementia include female sex, age (older patients are more susceptible than younger patients with a similar history of alcohol misuse) and continuous drinking without periods of abstinence. The disorder is slowly progressive and clinical features include severe cognitive impairment, delusions and hallucinations (see Chapter 27).

Structural neuroimaging provides evidence of cortical atrophy, dilated ventricles and atrophy of the cerebellar vermis in up to 50% of alcohol-dependent patients. These abnormalities may remit with abstinence in some individuals, while they persist despite abstinence in others (Besson 1993). The relationship between these findings and alcoholic dementia is unclear.

Prion protein dementias (spongiform encephalopathies)

The prion protein dementias or spongiform encephalopathies are a group of rare disorders that affect animals and humans and are invariably fatal. Prion protein is a normal cellular constituent that in certain circumstances may undergo a post-translational conformational change such that it acquires a high beta-sheet content, becomes insoluble and accumulates in brain tissue (Fleminger & Curtis 1997, Prusiner 1998). This results in neuronal vacuolation, astrogliosis and amyloid deposition with degeneration of the pyramidal and extrapyramidal systems.

The human prion protein dementias are caused by transmission of prion protein from infected to healthy individuals via neurosurgical instruments, corneal grafts, cadaveric human growth hormone, contact with infected tissue and cannibalism (kuru), and are analogous to bovine spongiform encephalopathy (BSE) in cattle and to scrapie in sheep and goats. About 10% of human prion protein dementias are inherited in an autosomal dominant fashion (familial Creutzfeldt–Jakob disease, Gerstmann–Straussler–Scheinker syndrome and fatal familial insomnia) and are caused by mutations in the prion protein gene on the short arm of chromosome 20 at 20p12-ter.

Kuru

Kuru was reported among the Fore tribe of Papua New Guinea but is now virtually eradicated. It is thought to have been transmitted by ritual cannibalism and largely affected women because they preferentially ate human brain tissue. Symptoms included personality and behavioural disturbances, progressive cerebellar ataxia, dementia and death.

Creutzfeldt–Jakob disease

Creutzfeldt–Jakob disease is the commonest prion protein dementia, affecting 1 in every 3 million people per year. It typically presents in the sixth or seventh decade of life, with personality change followed by a rapidly progressive dementia and accompanied by myoclonus, parkinsonian and choreoathetoid movements, spasticity, dysarthria and dysphagia. Cerebellar ataxia, cortical blindness and seizures may also occur. Akinetic mutism and coma ultimately develop and death is usual within two years of diagnosis. The EEG of up to 90% of patients shows a reduced background rhythm with characteristic triphasic sharp wave complexes at 1–2 Hz (these changes may not be present initially and repeated recordings are necessary). Structural neuroimaging may reveal cerebral atrophy. Treatment is symptomatic and care should be taken to prevent cross contamination.

Gerstmann–Straussler–Scheinker syndrome

This familial disorder is characterized by progressive cerebellar ataxia and dementia. The EEG changes described above have not been reported in Gerstmann–Straussler–Scheinker syndrome. Treatment is symptomatic and death is usual within five years of diagnosis.

Fatal familial insomnia

This disorder may present from the third decade onwards and consists of progressive cerebellar ataxia and dementia, accompanied by intractable insomnia and/or autonomic dysfunction with weight loss. Death is usual within one to two years of diagnosis.

New variant Creutzfeldt–Jakob disease

A new variant of Creutzfeldt–Jakob (vCJD) disease was first described by Will et al. (1996), who reported 10 cases that differed from classic Creutzfeldt–Jakob disease in that psychiatric symptoms dominated the clinical presentation, non-classic EEG changes were present, all patients were less than 40 years old and none had apparent risk factors for Creutzfeldt–Jakob disease. Spongiform encephalopathy was identified postmortem in the brains of all patients.

At the time of writing, 141 deaths from definite or probable vCJD had been reported in the UK by the National Creutzfeldt–Jakob Disease Surveillance Unit (www.cjd.ed.ac.uk) with the highest ever reported annual death rate of 28 being noted in the year 2000. Globally, 153 people have died from vCJD. Authorities disagree on the final number of deaths that are likely, some taking the view that the epidemic has peaked and is in decline while others believe that many thousands are yet to die given that the incubation period may be as long as 15 years. UK researchers recently found three tonsils or appendix samples to harbour vCJD from a total of 12 674 samples removed surgically from patients and stored between 1995 and 1999 but whether all individuals harbouring vCJD prions develop vCJD is not known (Hilton et al. 2004).

It is now apparent that vCJD occurs almost exclusively in the UK, where the first patient was noted 10 years after the identification of bovine spongiform encephalopathy (BSE) in cattle, and where almost 200 000 cases of BSE were reported prior to measures designed to prevent transmission being introduced. Current evidence strongly suggests a causal link between BSE and vCJD, and it is probable that the causative prion was transmitted via contaminated sheep offal which was fed to cattle and thus passed into the human food chain. Collinge et al. (1996) have provided molecular support for this hypothesis by demonstrating that the prion proteins implicated in vCJD and bovine spongiform encephalopathy are identical.

The neuropathological features of vCJD allow differentiation from sporadic, familial and iatrogenic Creutzfeldt–Jakob disease and are as follows:

- spongiform change most marked in the basal ganglia
- deposition of pericellular disease-associated prion protein in the cerebrum and cerebellum

- multiple plaques in the cerebral and cerebellar cortices
- severe gliosis in the thalamus.

The clinical features of the first 35 cases of vCJD disease have been summarized by Will et al. (2000) as follows:

- males and females were approximately equally affected
- the median illness duration was 14 months (range, 8–38 months)
- the median age at death was 29 years (range, 18–53 years).

The clinical features included initial psychiatric symptoms, subsequent ataxia and later involuntary movements and cognitive impairment. Electroencephalograms did not show the classic periodic triphasic sharp wave complexes found in sporadic Creutzfeldt–Jakob disease. Over 70% of patients had bilateral pulvinar high signal on magnetic resonance brain imaging and all were homozygous for methionine at codon 129 of chromosome 20p12-ter on genetic analysis (as indeed are 40% of the general population of the UK). Diagnostic criteria for vCJD have been formulated, which have a high sensitivity and specificity.

The treatment of vCJD involves prevention and symptomatic treatment.

Prevention Measures designed to prevent the spread of BSE within herds of cattle and from cattle to humans involve destruction of herds found to contain infected animals, a permanent ban on the feeding of animal derived foodstuffs to cattle, a temporary ban on the export of animals from the UK and the removal of brain, spinal cord and offal and of older cattle from the human food chain. As with sporadic, familial and iatrogenic Creutzfeldt–Jakob disease, cross contamination is a risk and cases have been reported of transmission of vCJD via surgical instruments, blood and blood products.

Symptomatic treatment There is no effective treatment yet available for vCJD although quinicrine and pentosan polysulphate are being investigated. Advice on symptomatic treatment is available from the National Creutzfeldt–Jakob Disease Surveillance Unit (www.cjd.ed.ac.uk). Bearing in mind the typical presentation, psychiatrists should exercise a high degree of vigilance for new variant Creutzfeldt–Jakob disease.

Subcortical dementias

Subcortical dementias are said to differ from cortical dementias in that psychomotor retardation and depression are prominent, memory may be improved by effort, and apraxia, agnosia and aphasia are mild or absent. However, recent neuropathological investigations which reveal neuronal loss in subcortical regions in Alzheimer's disease and in the cortex in Parkinson's disease cast doubt upon the existence of subcortical dementia as a separate clinicopathological entity. The subcortical dementia associated with multiple lacunar infarcts has many symptoms in common with the subcortical dementias described below and will not be discussed further.

Parkinson's disease

Parkinson's disease affects at least 1% of people over the age of 70 years. The dominant symptoms of akinesia, tremor and rigidity are caused by neuronal loss in the substantia nigra and related brainstem nucleii which in turn causes almost complete dopamine depletion in the striatum, nucleus accumbens, hippocampus and frontal cortex. Treatment is with dopaminergic and/or antimuscarinic/anticholinergic drugs (see Chapter 38).

Depression occurs in almost 50% of patients with Parkinson's disease and psychotic symptoms secondary to dopaminergic medication are not uncommon. However, the relationship between dementia and Parkinson's disease is unclear. Symptoms of dementia in patients with Parkinson's disease, most of whom are elderly, may be caused by:

- difficulties in undertaking cognitive evaluations in patients with bradykinesia and other motor symptoms
- cognitive impairment associated with antiparkinsonian medications
- cognitive impairment associated with normal ageing concurrent Alzheimer's or other dementia.

However, even when all of these potential causes are controlled for, up to 20% of patients with Parkinson's disease have an unexplained dementia which most often manifests late in the course of the illness (Biggins et al. 1992). It is generally accepted that this is an intrinsic part of Parkinson's disease, although reports of reduced choline acetyltransferase activity and of cortical Lewy bodies in the brains of patients with Parkinson's disease raise other possibilities.

Dementia in patients with Parkinson's disease should be treated in the same manner as any other dementia but caution should be exercised when prescribing anticholinergic/antimuscarinic and dopaminergic medications, the former of which may impair cognition and both of which may cause confusion. The treatment of psychosis caused by dopaminergic medication presents clinicians with a problem – reducing the dosage of dopaminergic medication risks losing control of the Parkinson's disease while antipsychotic medication may cause extrapyramidal symptoms.

Huntington's disease

Huntington's disease was first described by George Huntington in New England in 1872. It is now known to affect about 5 per 100 000 of the world's population, males and females equally.

Aetiology Huntington's disease exhibits anticipation (see Chapter 3) and is inherited in an autosomal dominant manner with complete penetrance. The gene was located to the short arm of chromosome 4 in 1983 and was fully identified 10 years later (Huntington's Disease Collaborative

Research Group 1993). It is now known that Huntington's disease is caused by expansion of a CAG trinucleotide repeat beyond 35 repeats. However, the precise pathophysiology is not yet understood (see Chapter 3). There is some evidence of increased risk of schizophrenia in the first-degree relatives of patients with Huntington's disease.

Pathology Huntington's disease is characterized by marked neuronal loss and gliosis in the striatum, particularly the head of the caudate nucleus, and in the frontal lobes. This is accompanied by a reduced concentration of gamma aminobutyric acid in the striatum and an increased concentration of dopamine and somatostatin in other components of the basal ganglia.

Clinical aspects and outcome Onset is usually in the fifth decade of life but may be as early as 10 years of age. Clumsiness is usually the first symptom, followed by uncontrollable twitching of the face, shoulders and fingers. Patients often try to conceal these movements by pretending that they are voluntary, for example by scratching the head following an uncontrolled upward movement of the arm. Symptoms progress to generalized chorea with ataxia, dysarthria, difficulty in swallowing and, ultimately, gross writhing and seizures.

Personality changes predate the onset of chorea by several years in about 40% of patients and range from moodiness and irritability to violence and criminal behaviour. Depression is the commonest psychiatric disorder but affective and paranoid psychosis are not uncommon. A subcortical dementia, often characterized by a prolonged course with relative sparing of memory and insight, may precede the onset of chorea.

The diagnosis of Huntington's disease depended on clinical evaluation, EEG and neuroimaging prior to the development of genetic testing. The EEG reveals low amplitude waves while CT and MRI show caudate, and perhaps frontal, atrophy, Reduced basal ganglia metabolism may be evident on functional neuroimaging prior to the onset of chorea.

The treatment of patients with Huntington's disease is symptomatic. Thus the dementia should be treated as with any other dementia, psychiatric disorder should be treated as appropriate and consideration should be given to treatment of chorea with antipsychotic medication. Planning for the long-term care of an increasingly dependent individual is extremely important. Death typically occurs 10–15 years after diagnosis. Patients with Huntington's disease, and their relatives, have an increased risk of suicide.

Genetic testing for Huntington's disease It is possible to confirm the diagnosis of Huntington's disease in patients, to identify the gene in relatives of patients, and to undertake prenatal testing. Such testing is associated with significant ethical implications and should only be undertaken at appropriate centres and by experienced individuals.

Perhaps somewhat surprisingly, a Canadian study of almost 150 asymptomatic individuals found that testing enhanced psychological wellbeing irrespective of whether results indicated the presence or absence of the gene for Huntington's disease (Wiggins et al. 1992).

Progressive supranuclear palsy
Progressive supranuclear palsy or Steele–Richardson syndrome is a subcortical dementia caused by neuronal loss and gliosis in the brainstem, cerebellum and basal ganglia. Onset is commonest in the sixth decade and the clinical features include paralysis of the extraocular muscles, dysarthria, cervical and truncal dystonia and ataxia. There is no effective treatment.

Human immunodeficiency virus-associated dementia
Minor degrees of cognitive impairment are common in patients with the human immunodeficiency virus (HIV) and 15–30% of such patients develop dementia (Adamson et al. 1999). The prevalence of HIV-associated dementia will increase as a consequence of increased life expectancy in patients who are HIV positive or have developed acquired immunodeficiency syndrome (AIDS). HIV-associated dementia will therefore represent an increasing cause of personal morbidity and mortality and of public health care resource utilization in the future.

Neuropathology It is thought that HIV-infected peripheral macrophages carry the HIV virus into the brain where it damages neurons indirectly, disease onset and progression depending on:

- viral properties (high levels of immunological nitric oxide synthase and of the gp41 protein are particularly associated with severe and/or rapidly progressive dementia)
- host properties (extensive immune activation is associated with severe and/or rapidly progressive dementia)
- concurrent non-HIV infection (cytomegalovirus and other infections are associated with severe and/or rapidly progressive dementia) (Adamson et al. 1999).

Clinical features, treatment and outcome About 10% of all HIV positive patients who develop AIDS present with dementia. The onset is generally insidious, but once established disease progression may be either rapid or modest, death occurring in weeks or years respectively. Clinical features include cognitive impairment, psychomotor retardation, tremor, ataxia, dysarthria and incontinence. Death is usually caused by concurrent opportunistic infection and may be preceded by akinetic mutism and seizures. Mean survival from diagnosis of HIV-associated dementia is about six months (McGuire 1996).

The treatment of HIV-associated dementia is largely symptomatic. However, there is some evidence that high doses of nucleoside reverse transcriptase inhibitors or combination therapy with these and protease inhibitors may delay cognitive decline. It is important to exclude reversible causes of dementia which in patients with AIDS will include concurrent infection and side-effects of anti-HIV and other treatments in addition to those discussed below.

Other dementias
Patients with a number of other relatively rare dementias may occasionally present to the psychiatrist. The causes of these dementias include the leucodystrophies, the commonest of which are metachromatic and adrenocortical leucodystrophy, and Gaucher's and Kuf's diseases.

Metachromatic leucodystrophy
The term leucodystrophy refers to abnormality of the cerebral white matter. Metachromatic leucodystrophy is an autosomal recessive disease that is caused by deficiency of aryl sulphatase A which results in deposition of sphingolipid in neurons and their demyelination (sphingolipid is also deposited in other cells). The activity of aryl sulphatase A may be measured in leukocytes. Infantile and adult forms occur, the latter characterized by psychiatric (personality change, behavioural disturbance, psychosis and dementia) and neurological (cerebellar and pyramidal symptoms, rigidity and seizures) symptoms. Treatment is symptomatic.

Adrenocortical leucodystrophy
The precise pathophysiology of this X-linked disorder is unknown. Symptoms include personality change, dementia, pyramidal features, aphasia, apraxia, dysarthria and blindness. Subclinical or clinical adrenal insufficiency is invariably present.

Gaucher's disease
Gaucher's disease (cerebroside lipoidosis or gluco-cerebrosidase deficiency) is an autosomal recessive, inborn error of metabolism in which glucocerebroside is deposited in the brain and reticuloendothelial system, and Gaucher's cells are present in bone marrow. The infant form causes impaired neurodevelopment while the juvenile form is characterized by systemic manifestations (splenomegaly, hepatomegaly and erosion of limb and pelvic bones) with relative sparing of the brain. These latter features also occur in the adult form and may be accompanied by dementia, psychosis, behavioural disturbance, ataxia, anaemia and jaundice.

Enzyme replacement therapy for Gaucher's disease with alglucerase (a placental preparation of glucocerebrosidase) or imiglucerase (a recombinant enzyme preparation) is efficacious, well-tolerated and safe. Enzyme replacement improves hematological abnormalities, reduces hepato-splenomegaly and increases quality of life in a few months.

Kuf's disease
Kuf's disease is the juvenile or adult form of cerebral sphingolipidosis. Lipofuscin is deposited in the brain and causes dementia, ataxia and myoclonus.

Box 26.4   Causes of potentially reversible dementia

Psychiatric causes (pseudodementia)
Depressive pseudodementia
Schizophrenic pseudodementia
Dissociative pseudodementia

Systemic causes
Drug toxicity
Electrolyte imbalance
Infection (including concurrent infection in patients with AIDS)
Hypoxia
Poisoning
Hypothyroidism
Hypoglycaemia
Vitamin deficiency
Alcohol
Renal failure and dialysis dementia
Hepatic failure including Wilson's disease

Intracranial causes
Normal pressure hydrocephalus
Subdural haematoma
Tumours
Neurosyphilis

Potentially reversible dementias and pseudodementia

Dementia is potentially reversible in a small proportion of patients. Psychiatrists should be aware of the causes of such apparent dementias (Box 26.4) and should undertake suitable investigations and initiate appropriate treatment when applicable. Of the many causes of potentially reversible dementia, normal pressure hydrocephalus and pseudodementia are discussed further below.

Normal pressure hydrocephalus

Normal pressure or obstructive-communicating hydro-cephalus is caused by obstruction within the subarachnoid space rather than within the ventricular system and is therefore potentially reversible. It may be associated with subarachnoid haemorrhage, Alzheimer's disease, head injury, posterior fossa tumour or meningitis. The clinical features include dementia, psychomotor retardation, ataxic gait and urinary incontinence which, in contrast to Alzheimer's disease, occurs early in the course of illness. Psychotic symptoms rarely occur. Neuroimaging reveals dilated ventricles with little or no evidence of cortical atrophy while cerebrospinal fluid (CSF) pressure is normal or low at lumbar puncture.

Treatment most commonly requires the insertion of a shunt between the lateral ventricles and the inferior vena cava and it is important to realize that this may effectively alleviate even severe degrees of dementia (Bekkelund et al. 1999). However, even with a high level of suspicion, early detection and immediate treatment, outcome is uncertain and the dementia often progresses.

Pseudodementia

Pseudodementia may be defined as dementia diagnosed in patients who have psychiatric disorders that are associated with apparent cognitive decline. Depression in elderly patients is especially associated with such cognitive decline, but it may also be present in patients with schizophrenia or with dissociative disorders. A diagnosis of pseudodementia is suggested by the following findings:

- a family history of depression or schizophrenia
- a personal history of depression, schizophrenia or dissociative disorder
- other depressive, schizophrenic or dissociative symptoms are present
- depressive, schizophrenic or dissociative symptoms precede cognitive impairment
- acute onset of cognitive impairment
- retention of normal cognitive function in some domains (patients may be able to learn new information, for example)
- cognitive impairment may be reversed by effort or by taking more time than is usual to complete a task
- cognitive impairment may be reversed by treatment of the underlying depression, schizophrenia or dissociative disorder.

A trial of treatment – usually antidepressant medication or electroconvulsive therapy – is appropriate if there is any doubt about the diagnosis of dementia.

SPECIFIC MOVEMENT DISORDERS

The term specific movement disorders is used to signify a group of syndromes that primarily fall within the clinical practice of neurology, but which may either initially present with psychiatric symptoms, or which are frequently associated with significant psychiatric morbidity. These disorders, which must be considered in the psychiatric differential diagnosis, may be conveniently classified as eponymous and non-eponymous specific movement disorders (Parkinson's and Huntington's diseases have been described above).

Eponymous specific movement disorders

Friedreich's ataxia

Friedreich's ataxia is an inherited spinocerebellar degeneration caused by an expanded triplet repeat (Chapter 3). Sclerosis of the dorsal and lateral columns of the spinal cord causes clumsiness, nystagmus, ataxia, dysarthria, dysphagia, scoliosis, unusual swaying and irregular movements, paralysis of the muscles of the lower limbs and impaired proprioception. Disease onset is usually during adolescence. Many patients develop cardiomyopathy, arrhythmia and/or diabetes mellitus. Dementia does not occur but depression is common and a small proportion of patients have learning disability.

Sydenham's chorea

Sydenham's chorea is an autoimmune disorder of the basal ganglia that follows rheumatic fever. Psychiatric symptoms including irritability, obsessions, compulsions, tics and psychosis accompany the chorea in most patients. Penicillin prevents further attacks while valproate and antipsychotic drugs provide symptomatic treatment. There is some evidence that chorea gravidarum, some cases of obsessive-compulsive disorder and Tourette's syndrome and possibly some cases of schizophrenia represent adult neuro-psychiatric sequelae of Sydenham's chorea.

Gilles de la Tourette's syndrome

Gilles de la Tourette's (1885) eponymous syndrome affects 1 per 2000 of the population and consists of multiple tics (rapidly repeated involuntary muscle movements such as grimacing or blinking) with onset before 16 years and which precede vocal tics, coprolalia, echolalia and echopraxia. Associated features include attention deficit hyperactivity disorder, learning difficulty and obsessive-compulsive disorder. In one study, generalized tics affecting the entire body were found in 64% of patients, coprolalia in 50%, obsessive-compulsive symptoms in 63%, and attention deficit hyperactivity disorder in 17% of patients (Kano et al. 1998).

Concordance for Gilles de la Tourette's syndrome in monozygotic twins is 53% (Pauls and Leckman 1988) and both the syndrome and its associated features are commoner in the first degree relatives of patients. The partial efficacy of dopamine receptor antagonists implicates dopaminergic dysfunction in this disorder, while Anderson et al. (1992) have reported reduced serotonin levels in postmortem brain tissue. Treatment with haloperidol (or pimozide or clonidine less often) is effective in about 50% of patients.

Wilson's disease

Wilson's disease (hepatolenticular degeneration) is a rare, recessively inherited defect in a copper transporter protein which causes defective incorporation of copper into apo-caeruloplasmin and failure to excrete copper in bile. Copper is deposited in the liver (jaundice, cirrhosis, hepato-splenomegaly, ascites and oesophageal varices), basal ganglia (tremor, rigidity, athetosis and dystonia), cerebral cortex (personality change, behavioural disorder, psychosis with delusions and hallucinations, clouding of consciousness, epilepsy and dementia; bulbar symptoms may also occur) and eye (brown/green Kayser–Fleischer rings at the corneal edge). Up to 66% of patients first present to a psychiatrist while 50% have psychiatric symptoms and

receive treatment, including hospitalization, for schizophrenia, depression and anxiety before final diagnosis (Rathbun 1996).

Investigations reveal low serum caeruloplasmin and copper, and high urinary copper. Structural neuroimaging may show basal ganglia cavitation and cortical atrophy. Neurological features are more responsive than hepatic or psychiatric symptoms to treatment with chelating agents such as D-penicillamine.

Non-eponymous specific movement disorders

Benign essential tremor

Benign essential tremor is a fine to moderate, slowly progressive tremor affecting the hands, head and voice. This disorder is dominantly inherited in some patients, is exacerbated by movement or anxiety and alleviated by alcohol, and may be associated with social phobia (George & Lydiard 1994). Propranolol is an effective treatment.

Focal dystonias

Focal dystonias consist of tonic spasm of localized (hence focal) muscle groups. The cause of these disorders is unknown (and patients may present to neurologists or psychiatrists) but they cause significant disability and include:

- blepharospasm (tonic spasm of the orbicularis oculi muscles producing closure of the eye and preventing vision)
- oromandibular dystonia (tonic spasm of the muscles around the mouth preventing speech)
- spasmodic torticollis (tonic spasm of the sternocleidomastoid muscle producing flexion of the neck and rotating the head to the contralateral side)
- writer's cramp (tonic spasm of the muscles of the hand and forearm such that a pen is held and applied to paper with excessive force, preventing writing).

Anxiety exacerbates these disorders and comorbid depression is common. Botulinum toxin injected into the affected orbicularis oculi provides prolonged relief from blepharospasm, while oromandibular dystonia may respond to anticholinergic/antimuscarinic drugs. Spasmodic torticollis generally resolves with time but nerve transection may occasionally be necessary. Writer's cramp may be relieved by altering the way a pen is held (pencil grips designed for children may be useful).

EPILEPSY

Definition

Epilepsy may be defined simply as a tendency to suffer recurrent seizures or more comprehensively as a recurrent abnormality of the electrical activity of the brain, which causes changes in motor, sensory or autonomic function and/or in behaviour or consciousness. A practical clinical definition of epilepsy is of two or more seizures occurring within a year of each other.

Classification

Epilepsy may be classified by clinical description of the seizures (petit mal, grand mal, or tonic–clonic seizures, for example) or by specification of the anatomical location of the epileptic focus (frontal or temporal lobe epilepsy, for example). The most widely used classification is that of the International League Against Epilepsy (ILAE), which relies on both the anatomical location of the epileptic focus and its effect on consciousness and which is currently being revised (Commission on Classification and Terminology of the International League Against Epilepsy 1989; see also www.ilae-epilepsy.org). Thus generalized epilepsy implies impairment of consciousness while partial (focal) epilepsy may occur with (temporal lobe epilepsy, for example) or without (Jacksonian seizures, for example) alteration of consciousness. Partial epilepsy may become generalized (secondary generalization) in which case consciousness becomes impaired. A modified ILAE classification of epilepsy is presented in Table 26.2.

Aetiology

Aetiology of epilepsy

The cause of more than 70% of epilepsy is unknown, while 30% is secondary to trauma, febrile convulsions (unilateral convulsions and/or convulsions that last longer than 10 minutes) or cerebrovascular events. Drugs may cause epilepsy directly (phenothiazines, clozapine and tricyclic antidepressants, for example) or upon withdrawal (alcohol, benzodiazepines and barbiturates, for example). A small but significant proportion of epilepsy is genetic in origin, including juvenile myoclonic epilepsy (gene mapped to the short arm of chromosome 6), benign familial neonatal convulsions (genes mapped to the long arms of chromosomes 8 and 20) and progressive myoclonic epilepsy (gene mapped to the long arm of chromosome 21).

Aetiology of seizures

Seizures are ultimately caused by increased neuronal excitability. The cause of this is unknown but the two most prominent theories are:

- The excitatory/inhibitory neurotransmitter imbalance theory, which postulates that an imbalance exists between excitatory and inhibitory neurotransmitters that allows spontaneous excessive electrical activity in the brain which manifests as a seizure. This hypothesis is based on the probable mechanism of action of antiepileptic drugs (AEDs), many of which inhibit glutamate release or gamma aminobutyric acid (GABA) metabolism, or stimulate GABA receptors.

- The 'kindling' theory, which is based on the finding that the repeated application of a subconvulsive electrical stimulus to the brain will eventually cause a seizure at that or a lower level of electrical stimulation. In patients with epilepsy, it is thought that recurrent discharges which do not cause a seizure, 'kindle' the brain such that a subsequent discharge does cause a seizure.

Epidemiology

The epidemiology of epilepsy is uncertain because of differences in diagnostic and treatment practices between physicians and countries, and because of the stigma that is still attached to the diagnosis. The general epidemiology of epilepsy is summarized in Box 26.5. Patients with complex partial seizures, especially those of frontal lobe origin (Williamson & Spencer 1986), are especially likely to experience psychiatric symptoms and to be misdiagnosed.

The diagnosis of epilepsy

The diagnosis of epilepsy is clinical and relies on a careful history, a thorough neurological and cognitive examination, the evaluation of reports from relatives, teachers and nurses, and on observation of the almost always stereotyped

---

Table 26.2   Classification of epilepsies (modified)

	ILAE	Older terms
Generalized	Tonic-clonic Absence Atonic	Grand mal, major Petit mal, minor Akinetic, drop attacks
Partial (focal)	Simple (consciousness not impaired)	Focal, Jacksonian
	Complex (consciousness impaired)	Temporal lobe, frontal, psychomotor

---

Box 26.5   Epidemiology of epilepsy

Epilepsy in the general population

2% of the general population have one seizure during their lives

0.5% of the general population have epilepsy

Epilepsy is commoner in males, the prison population (0.8%), and mentally handicapped individuals (30% of autistic and 50% of severely intellectually impaired children have epilepsy)

The onset of epilepsy is before the age of 20 years in 60% of epileptic patients (with peaks during both childhood and adolescence) with another peak in onset after the age of 65 years.

Epilepsy in the epileptic population

70% of patients with epilepsy have partial epilepsy (of whom 70% have complex partial seizures, accounting for 50% of all epilepsy)

30% of patients with epilepsy have generalized epilepsy

seizures. It should be remembered that seizures are a symptom of epilepsy and of several non-epileptic disorders. A diagnosis of epilepsy should never be made on the basis of an EEG, but EEG recordings can support a clinical diagnosis of epilepsy. The classic symptoms of the aura of temporal lobe complex partial seizures are:

- nausea
- epigastric burning sensation radiating to throat
- dizziness
- olfactory, gustatory, visual or auditory hallucinations
- palpitations
- macropsia
- micropsia
- altered thought
- panoramic memory
- elation, depression, ecstasy
- dread
- *déjà vu*.

Investigations

The EEG in epilepsy is discussed in Chapter 34. CT and MRI can identify tumours or define mesial temporal sclerosis, and telemetry (simultaneous EEG and closed-circuit television monitoring) can facilitate the correlation of behavioural and EEG changes, especially if a diagnosis of non-epileptic seizures is being considered (see below). Serial serum prolactin measurements may be useful, although generalized seizures are but one cause of transient hyperprolactinaemia.

Epilepsy and psychiatry

Patients with epilepsy may consult psychiatrists because of comorbidity – the occurrence of psychiatric illness largely independent of their epilepsy or its treatment – or because of ictal (during seizures) or interictal (between seizures) psychiatric illness associated with epilepsy or its treatment. Psychiatrists play important roles in the social treatment of patients with epilepsy and in diagnosing non-epileptic seizures, and may be asked to determine if criminal behaviour is a manifestation of epilepsy.

Comorbid psychiatric illness and epilepsy

Epilepsy and psychiatric illness are both common and thus many patients with epilepsy require psychiatric treatment. In addition, both disorders may have common aetiologies such as head injury, tumours, alcohol, drugs (illicit and prescribed) and dementias. There is some evidence that epilepsy increases risk for psychiatric illness although this is less evident in patients with well controlled epilepsy. The treatment of psychiatric patients with epilepsy is the same as that of patients who do not have epilepsy, but the following important aspects must also be considered (see also Chapter 38):

- antipsychotic and antidepressant drugs may lower the seizure threshold and cause seizures
- antiepileptic (AEDs) may cause depression, cognitive impairment or other psychiatric symptoms
- AED-psychotropic drug interactions may occur
- AEDs and psychotropic drugs present potential for accidental or deliberate overdose.

Thus depression in patients with epilepsy is best treated with serotonin reuptake inhibitors or electroconvulsive therapy, and psychosis with atypical antipsychotics other than clozapine. Lower doses of antipsychotics may be effective, and oral rather than depot preparations are probably safer in patients subject to recurrent seizures or status epilepticus. Acute agitation may be treated with parenteral or oral benzodiazepines, and bipolar illness with lithium and/or carbamazepine.

Peri-ictal psychiatric illness

Seizures, especially complex partial seizures, may be preceded by hours, or occasionally days, of a prodrome during which fear, irritability, insomnia or depression occur. Patients may present to psychiatrists with these symptoms and may sometimes be taught to recognize them and to take prophylactic AEDs.

Auras are particularly common in temporal lobe complex partial epilepsy, generally last only a few seconds, and may consist of depersonalization, derealization, or affective change, or any of the symptoms listed above. Unlike a prodrome, an aura is a partial seizure.

Automatisms consist of relatively brief periods of clouding of consciousness during which the patient retains posture and tone and exhibits stereotyped simple behaviours (chewing, lip-smacking, hand movements). Less often, prolonged automatisms or fugue states associated with complex behaviour (wandering, indiscretion or crime) may occur. Automatisms occur during or immediately following an epileptic seizure. Patients cannot recall an automatism but they often have full recall up to its onset and their behaviour may help in localizing the epileptic focus. Automatisms are associated with initial unilateral low voltage θ and subsequent bilateral δ waves on the EEG. Prolonged twilight states during which patients experience intense hallucinations and bizarre thoughts may also occur.

Post-ictally, patients may be extremely agitated and combative (furor), or experience automatisms or twilight states as described above. Auras, automatisms, fugue states and twilight states may be incorrectly diagnosed as psychotic illness in patients who do not experience obvious seizures unless impairment of consciousness is noted.

Interictal psychiatric illness

It was formerly believed that epilepsy was associated with a specific personality type described as pedantic, egocentric, religiose and 'socially adhesive', and patients with complex partial epilepsy have been described as dependent, circumstantial and excessively metaphysical (Tizard 1962). Recent research does not support these reports and there is no evidence of an association between epilepsy and violence (Treiman 1993). The effects of the social, domestic, occupational and treatment implications of epilepsy on patient's lives and behaviour are clearly very significant.

Slater et al. (1963) described a schizophreniform psychosis in patients with epilepsy, almost all of whom had temporal lobe complex partial epilepsy, which differed from schizophrenia as follows:

- the premorbid personality was usually normal
- there was usually no family history of schizophrenia
- there was preservation of affective response
- the psychosis began 10–15 years after the onset of the epilepsy.

Flor Henry (1969) found that this syndrome was commoner in temporal lobe complex partial epilepsy, especially when the focus was in the dominant hemisphere. Whether this psychosis and epilepsy have a common cause or the epileptic discharges cause the schizophreniform symptoms is unclear.

Neuroses and sexual dysfunction are commoner in patients with epilepsy and may be related to the disease and the limitations it imposes, and to the side-effects of AEDs. Depression, deliberate self-harm and suicide also occur more frequently than in the general population.

The episodic dyscontrol syndrome is a somewhat controversial clinical syndrome consisting of unprovoked and senseless violence, personality disorder and EEG abnormalities mapped to the temporal lobes. It may develop following head injury and carbamazepine may be an effective treatment.

The treatment of epilepsy

Medical treatment

The treatment of epilepsy is almost always symptomatic, but if a cause is apparent, for example a tumour, this should be removed. The goal of AED treatment should be monotherapy, and if a second or third AED provides control, the withdrawal of previously added AEDs should be considered. Barbiturates should be avoided in contemporary AED treatment.

A summary of the AED treatment of epilepsy is provided in Table 26.3. However, the treatment of epilepsy is advancing rapidly – eight new AEDs have become available since 1990 (Sander 1998) – and the reader is referred to an appropriate source, for example the British National Formulary in the UK, for the most recent advice (see also Chapter 38).

The plasma levels of AEDs should be monitored (especially with combination therapy, because of the risk of AED–AED interactions such as valproate or phenytoin

induction of enzymes that metabolize carbamazepine) but the 'rule' is that the patient, not the laboratory value, should be treated. Thus if seizures are controlled and the patient is not experiencing side-effects, AED levels above the advised range can probably be ignored. Conversely, if levels are within the advised range but seizures continue, dosage may be increased until effective or until side-effects occur. Equally, the dosage should not be increased if it is effective, despite AED levels below the advised range. In addition to monitoring AED plasma levels, regular full blood counts and evaluations of thyroid, renal and hepatic function are advised with some AEDs (see Chapter 38).

AEDs induce the metabolism of ethinyloestradiol and a dosage of 50 μg is necessary if the contraceptive pill is prescribed. Women with epilepsy should plan their pregnancies and should consider withdrawing AEDs before conception and during pregnancy, although it is almost certainly safer to take AEDs than to have seizures while pregnant. If these occur, patients can be reassured that seizures that do not lead to cyanosis probably do not affect the foetus. Carbamazepine is the least teratogenic AED. Folate supplements are advised for women taking AEDs (and are now advised for all women) before and during pregnancy, and vitamin K supplements are advised for pregnant women taking carbamazepine or phenytoin.

Status epilepticus consists of recurrent seizures without recovery of consciousness between them. Treatment requires immediate intravenous lorazepam, diazepam, midazolam or

Table 26.3 A summary of the AED treatment of epilepsy		
	First line treatment	*Second line treatment*
Generalized		
Tonic–clonic	Carbamazepine Lamotrigine Phenytoin Valproate[1]	Clobazam
Absence	Ethosuximide Valproate[1]	Clonazepam Clobazam Ethosuximide Acetozolamide
Partial (focal)		
	Carbamazepine[2] Lamotrigine[2] Phenytoin[2] Valproate[2]	Clonazepam[3] Clobazam[3] Acetozolamide[3] Gabapentin Tiagabine Topiramate Vigabatrin

[1] Valproate is also effective in patients who experience both tonic/clonic and absence seizures.
[2] If none of these AEDs are effective two of them may be prescribed in combination.
[3] One or other of these AEDs may be added to the most effective monotherapy identified.

clonazepam. This should be followed by an intravenous loading dose of phenytoin and a subsequent phenytoin infusion. Patients with status epilepticus should be transferred immediately to an intensive care unit.

Patients who have not had seizures for a prolonged period may wish to consider AED withdrawal. This must be an individualized decision based on:

- the length of time the patient has been seizure-free (a 2-year minimum is recommended)
- the normality of the EEG with current AED treatment (it would be unwise to withdraw treatment from a patient whose EEG exhibits significant epileptic activity)
- the side-effects of current AEDs
- social factors such as the patient's work, hobbies and need for a driving licence.

If AEDs are to be withdrawn, a careful record of seizure type and frequency must be made and an EEG recorded before reducing dosage, again when dosage is reduced to half the initial dosage, and finally when AEDs are stopped. Any increase in seizure frequency or severity, or deterioration in the EEG, should lead to the planned withdrawal being reconsidered or abandoned or deferred.

Surgical treatment

The surgical treatment of epilepsy has advanced significantly in recent years and is directed at either removal of the cause of the epilepsy (for example a tumour or sclerotic temporal lobe) or prevention of seizure spread by tractotomy, callosotomy or sub-pial resection. Pre-operatively, AED treatment must be optimized, the epileptic focus must be defined (scalp and depth EEG, CT and MRI) and the risk and/or extent of postoperative cognitive and/or motor impairment evaluated. Outcome is best in younger patients, but overall about 50% of patients become seizure-free (most continue to require AEDs). Mortality is less than 1% and morbidity between 5% and 20%, depending on the neurosurgical centre and the site of the lesion.

Legal aspects of epilepsy

All countries impose driving restrictions on people with epilepsy. In the UK, for example, a driving licence may only be obtained if a patient has had no seizures while awake during the previous year, or has had seizures only when asleep during the previous three years.

Aggressive behaviour is probably no more common in patients with epilepsy than in the general population and is usually related to peri-ictal confusion when it does occur. Violence due directly to epilepsy is extremely rare, and is characterized by being unprovoked, sudden, short-lived, undirected, purposeless, and associated with evidence of a seizure such as confusion and absence of recall (Gunn & Fenton 1971). UK law enshrines the concept of *mens rea* or guilty mind. The mind is said to be absent during ictal or peri-ictal automatisms, and thus *mens rea* is not possible. In law, automatisms may be sane and due to an external factor such as head injury, or insane and due to an internal factor such as epilepsy. In general, if found not guilty due to sane automatism, the accused goes free; if found not guilty due to insane automatism the accused is detained in a secure hospital (although judges now have discretion in sentencing). Epileptic automatism is a difficult defence to use and is only likely to succeed when:

- epilepsy has been diagnosed prior to the offence
- there was no evidence of premeditation
- there was no attempt to conceal the crime or escape (which would imply awareness)
- the accused was objectively confused
- there is no evidence of recall of the offence.

NON-EPILEPTIC SEIZURES

Non-epileptic seizures (NES) are also referred to as pseudoseizures, a term best avoided, and as non-epileptic attack disorder. NES is a dissociative disorder which may be defined as a tendency to suffer recurrent seizures which cannot be diagnosed as epilepsy and which occur in association with psychologically stressful events.

It is thought that deep psychological conflicts are responsible for NES but previous learning plays a role. NES is commoner in patients with personality disorder and among health professionals and the relatives of epileptic patients. A significant proportion of patients with NES also have epilepsy (Wada 1985) and research evidence suggests that many patients with NES have been abused during childhood (Betts 1990). Some of the features that help to differentiate between NES and epilepsy are listed in Table 26.4 and EEG telemetry is also helpful in making the diagnosis.

Once diagnosed, behaviour therapy aimed at rewarding seizure-free peroids and not rewarding seizures is effective in about 50% of patients. It is absolutely essential that this is accompanied by psychological support and instruction in appropriate functional behaviour (Betts 1998). Many patients with NES take AEDs because of comorbid epilepsy or through misdiagnosis. AEDs should be discontinued in the latter group, both because of their side-effects and because they may disinhibit the patient and promote NES. However, this is not always possible.

SLEEP DISORDERS (PARASOMNIAS)

Sleep is a recurrent behaviour consisting of inactivity and loss of awareness and of responsivity. Sleep differs from coma in that a sleeping individual either awakens spontaneously or can be roused. The physiology of sleep and

Table 26. 4   Differences between epileptic and non-epileptic seizures (NES)

	NES	Epilepsy
Location	In safety, rarely in public	Anywhere
Seizure type	Asymmetrical, non-stereotyped, prolonged, frequent	Symmetrical, stereotyped, brief, infrequent
Consciousness	Normal	Impaired
Response to stimulus	Present, e.g. resists attempts to open eyes	Absent
Corneal reflex	Normal	May be absent
Plantar reflex	Normal	May be extensor
Injury	Rare	Frequent
Incontinence	Usually absent	May be present
Precipitant	Usually present	Usually absent
EEG/telemetry	Usually normal	Usually abnormal
Prolactin	Usually normal	May be elevated

the EEG changes associated with it are described in Chapter 34, while disorders associated with sleep (parasomnias) and their evaluation and treatment are discussed here.

Insomnia

Insomnia is subjective dissatisfaction with the quantity or quality of sleep. It is commoner with increasing age and may be primary or secondary. Primary insomnia requires training in sleep hygiene (avoid drinks and stimulants for up to six hours before retiring, retire at the same time each night to a comfortable bed in a warm dark room, remain in bed whether sleeping or not, set alarm for the same time each day and always get up at that time, avoid sleeping when not in bed) but a brief period of treatment with hypnotics is sometimes reasonable (see Chapter 38 for further advice). Secondary insomnia usually resolves when the cause is treated.

Nightmares and night terrors

Nightmares, unpleasant dreams that awaken the individual from rapid eye movement (REM) sleep, are very common during childhood but decrease in frequency thereafter. Night terrors are uncommon and familial, occur almost exclusively during childhood, and are unpleasant dreams occurring during non-REM (stages III and IV) sleep, which awaken the child. Although initially terrified, the child usually returns to sleep and has little subsequent recall of the episode. Training in sleep hygiene is helpful and night terrors almost always resolve with age.

Sleep walking, sleep paralysis and Kleine-Levin syndrome

Sleep walking (somnambulism) is a common familial disorder that occurs during non-REM (stages III and IV) sleep and is largely confined to childhood. More or less purposeful actions may be carried out but the patient has no recall of these when awakened. Sleep walkers may harm themselves and should be protected from stairs, windows, knives and machinery. Sleep walking is an automatism and has been used as a defence against criminal prosecution.

Sleep paralysis affects approximately 10% of the population (Penn et al. 1981) and causes patients to awaken while paralysed during REM sleep. Training in sleep hygiene is helpful.

The Kleine–Levin syndrome is rare and consists of periods of compulsive eating, clouded consciousness, visual or auditory hallucinations, and hypersomnia. These last up to 72 hours and are accompanied by bursts of high-voltage δ waves on the EEG.

Narcolepsy

The cardinal symptom of narcolepsy (the narcoleptic syndrome) is excessive daytime drowsiness with the sudden onset of REM sleep, often in unusual circumstances. This must be accompanied by either cataplexy (sudden atonia with resultant collapse, often triggered by an emotional event such as laughter) or frequent (several times per year) sleep paralysis. No consistent neuropathological features have been found. Narcolepsy is virtually always familial and 99.5% of patients have the HLA antigen DR2 (DR15/DQ6), making narcolepsy the disease that most strongly exhibits HLA association and implying a susceptibility gene on the short arm of chromosome 6. Hypnagogic and hypnopompic hallucinations occur in about 25% of narcoleptic patients. The hypersomnia of narcolepsy may be treated with mazindol, dexamphetamine or methylphenidate. Cataplexy responds to selective serotonin reuptake inhibitors, which have fewer side-effects than older treatments such as clomipramine or imipramine.

SEQUELAE OF CEREBRAL INSULTS

The sequelae of cerebral insults may be minimal and short-lived or severe and permanent. Their extent depends on whether the insult is focal or generalized, as well as on its severity and duration. Focal and generalized cerebral insults will now be discussed.

Focal cerebral insult

Focal cerebral insults are the result of intracranial or pericranial pathologies affecting a specific region of the brain.

Head injury

Any trauma to the head that is associated with a skull fracture, loss of consciousness, amnesia and/or headache (as distinct from local pain from the injury) with vomiting constitutes a head injury (HI). About 3 per 100 population suffer HIs each year in developed countries and up to 30% of these HIs are moderate or severe (Powell 1994). At least 50% of all HIs are caused by road accidents in most countries, the remainder being caused by other accidents (30%), sporting injuries (10%) and assaults (10%). Young adults and elderly individuals are at greatest risk of HI and the risk for males is three times that for females.

Classification and pathophysiology
Open HI in which the skull is fractured and the brain injured directly is relatively rare and follows road and other accidents and blunt instrument or gunshot assaults. Closed HIs are commoner and follow similar events which cause brain injury at the site of trauma (coup) and directly opposite it (contrecoup). The frontal, anterior temporal and occipital poles are more susceptible to contrecoup injury because the brain is more mobile in the anteroposterior than in the transverse plane. At a microscopic level, HI causes shearing of nerve fibres, nerve tracts and blood vessels.

General clinical features
Textbooks of neurology or neurosurgery should be consulted for details of the general effects of HI. However, it is important to remember that while HI has obvious direct effects such as skull fracture and loss of consciousness, these

are exacerbated by associated events including the following:

- alcohol and drugs, to which HI is very often related
- raised intracranial pressure caused by bleeding and/or cerebral oedema
- cardiovascular and/or metabolic imbalance following damage to vital centres
- epileptic seizures
- secondary infections
- iatrogenic effects of treatment.

Psychiatric features
Whether or not psychiatric sequelae follow HI depends on pre-HI, peri-HI and post-HI factors as presented in Box 26.6. HI can cause almost any psychiatric disorder and many post-HI patients will suffer more than one disorder, the disabling effects of which are frequently additive. The commonest sequelae of HIs that are of interest to the psychiatrist are the following:

- post-concussional syndrome
- personality disorder
- cognitive disorder
- anxiety disorder
- affective disorder
- psychotic disorder
- epilepsy.

Post-concussional syndrome This is the commonest psychiatric disorder following HI. It develops in up to 20% of patients following severe HI and in a significant

---

Box 26.6 The psychiatric sequelae of HI: pre-, peri- and post-HI aetiological factors

Pre-HI factors

Premorbid personality

Personal history of psychiatric illness, especially alcohol dependence

Family history of psychiatric illness

Peri-HI factors

Site of brain injury (temporal lobe injury is especially likely to cause psychiatric sequelae)

Extent of injury (risk of psychiatric sequelae increases as extent of brain injury increases)

Post-HI factors

Development of epilepsy (psychiatric sequelae are commoner in patients who develop post-HI epilepsy)

Emotional response to the HI, its cause and where responsibility lies (the emotional response to HI sustained in a road accident for which the patient was responsible may differ to that following a serious assault by a stranger, for example)

Marital, domestic, financial, social and occupational consequences of HI and its physical and psychiatric sequelae

Medicolegal issues

proportion following less severe HI. Its aetiology is much debated. An organic genesis with psychologically driven persistence was proposed by Lishman (1988) but it has recently been suggested that psychosocial, cognitive-behavioural and coping factors may greatly influence post-concussional symptoms, especially during their late phase (Jacobson 1995). Such symptoms include headache, fatigue, dizziness, increased sensitivity to noise, sexual dysfunction, mild cognitive impairment, sleep disturbance and alterations in mood (irritability, anxiety and depression).

Post-concussional symptoms generally resolve following mild or moderate HI (although they frequently last many months and often require specific treatment such as antidepressant drugs, in which context it is worth noting that post-HI patients are especially sensitive to such medications) but persist indefinitely in up to 20% of patients following severe HI.

Personality disorder   Post-concussional syndrome is the commonest psychiatric disorder following HI, but it is likely that personality disorder causes the greatest amount of distress to patients and their relatives following HI. Almost all patients who suffer severe HI, especially to the frontal lobes, will develop personality disorder, as will a considerable proportion of patients following less-severe HI. Two changes in personality have been described following HI (and there is some evidence that these may represent the release of previously controlled premorbid personality characteristics):

- emotional blunting accompanied by avolition, apathy and indifference, which make rehabilitation extremely difficult
- emotional irritability accompanied by impaired judgement, egocentric behaviour, rage, verbal and physical aggression and sexual disinhibition, all of which may predispose to criminal behaviour.

Post-HI personality disorder is frequently accompanied by post-HI cognitive disorder, which further compounds the difficulties experienced by patients and those caring for them.

Cognitive disorder   Cognitive disorder develops in a very significant proportion of patients following HI. Risk increases with increasing post-traumatic amnesia (PTA) (almost all patients with PTA of 24 hours or more develop significant cognitive impairment – see below), left-sided HI, penetrating HI and increasing age. Patients suffer a reduction in IQ (typically affecting performance IQ more than verbal IQ), marked short-term memory impairment, and dysphasias (fluent, non-fluent and nominal) and their disability is often compounded by associated neurological dysfunction.

Cognitive improvement continues for up to one year following HI and failure to improve to some extent, or further decline, require that subdural haematoma, hydrocephalus or coincident dementia be excluded.

Anxiety disorder   Anxiety disorder occurs in up to 20% of patients following severe HI. Any anxiety symptom or disorder may develop but dissociative/conversion syndromes (pain, neurological deficits, amnesia, non-epileptic seizures and fugue states), obsessional behaviour (ranging from extreme orderliness which may facilitate coping with cognitive impairment to obsessive-compulsive disorder) and post-traumatic stress disorder (depending on the causative trauma and whether or not this is remembered) are perhaps the most common. Great caution should be exercised in diagnosing post-HI anxiety disorder because the symptoms may well be caused directly by brain injury.

Affective disorder   Depression or mania develop in up to 25% of patients following severe HI, often appearing only many months after the initial injury. The aetiololgy of post-HI affective disorders is uncertain but it is probably best to assume that multiple factors both predispose to them and ensure their persistence. The severity of these disorders contributes to an increased risk of suicide in this group of patients and often warrants psychopharmacological treatment, although it has been suggested that such intervention may impair recovery (Goldstein 1993). Eames (1997) has recently described pathological laughing and crying or dysprosopeia following HI and suggested that this further disables patients by reducing both their social skills and their social acceptability.

Psychotic disorder   Psychotic disorder following HI is relatively uncommon but develops in up to 10% of patients following severe HI, especially those who have suffered temporal lobe injury. Symptoms include poorly formed persecutory delusions, but hallucinations are less common than in schizophrenia. Antipsychotic medication is frequently warranted.

Epilepsy   Epilepsy develops in up to 50% of patients following open HI and in 5% of patients following closed HI. At least 30% of patients who have seizures in the seven days immediately following HI develop epilepsy and require life-long anticonvulsant treatment.

Psychiatric treatment of head-injured patients

This involves care of the patient, care of the patient's family and consideration of medicolegal issues. Care of the patient may involve the management of acute organic reaction and/or aggression in the immediate aftermath of HI and the psychopharmacological, cognitive or behavioural treatment of specific psychiatric disorders subsequently. Occasionally, patients with severely disturbed behaviour following HI may require prolonged institutional psychiatric care.

It is often extremely difficult for patients and their families to adjust following HI. Patients may have significant physical, cognitive and psychiatric disability, and personality changes mean that relatives frequently complain that the patient is not the person they knew before the HI.

Patients and their families need help in coping with changes in family dynamics, occupation, finances and care of children, and with ongoing medicolegal issues. Emotional and sexual dissatisfaction is common in the spouses of individuals that have suffered HI and, accompanied by financial and other stresses, frequently leads to divorce.

Psychiatrists are frequently asked to provide medicolegal reports about post-HI patients who are pursuing claims for compensation. Such reports must provide information about:

- the premorbid personality and any premorbid psychiatric illness
- the current personality and any current psychiatric illness
- the likelihood that the HI was partly or fully responsible for any change in personality or any new psychiatric illness
- the impact of any change in personality or any new psychiatric illness upon the patients personal, domestic, social and occupational functioning
- the likelihood of full or partial recovery with treatment or the passage of time.

There is evidence that ongoing claims for compensation serve to maintain psychiatric illness following HI. In an ideal world such claims would be resolved quickly but unfortunately, and perhaps understandably given the enormous sums that may be paid in compensation, many claims continue for several years.

Outcome

Severity of HI predicts outcome. It has long been known that this is most usefully assessed by the duration of anterograde or post-traumatic amnesia (PTA) (Russell 1932) as presented in Table 26.5, which also describes general outcome in terms of the Glasgow Outcomes Scale (GOS) devised by Jennett and Bond (1975). It will be evident from Table 26.5 that, in general, PTA of <24 hours' duration indicates that future independence is probable, while PTA of >24 hours' duration indicates that future independence is extremely improbable.

The GOS also includes outcome categories of persistent vegetative state (coma with maintenance of vital functions by the brainstem in the absence of cortical activity) and death, which generally follows severe or very severe HI. Retrograde (pre-traumatic) amnesia following HI is a poor predictor of outcome, is usually less extensive than PTA and is characterized by initial loss of most recent memories followed by loss of increasingly distant memories (Ribot's law) with recovery of memory following the reverse sequence.

Neuropsychiatric recovery from HI continues for at least six months and probably for as long as 12 months after the causative trauma following which further improvement is unusual. However, although formal neuropsychiatric improvement may not occur, patients continue to adapt to their disabilities and functional improvement continues for many years. Indeed promoting such functional improvement is the goal of much rehabilitative medicine.

Sequelae of head injuries associated with boxing and other sports

Multiple recurrent HI such as occurs in boxing (and perhaps from repeated heading of the ball in football) has been associated with a subcortical dementia (boxer's encephalopathy or dementia pugilistica) associated with prominent Parkinsonian and cerebellar symptoms, irritability, explosive behaviour, morbid jealousy, pathological intoxication, paranoia and personality change.

Neuropathological changes include cortical atrophy, neuronal loss, neurofibrillary tangles and perforation of the septum pellucidum. Recent evidence suggests that boxers who have an apolipoprotein ε4 allele may be at increased risk of chronic neurological deficits (Jordan et al. 1997).

Cerebrovascular disease

The commonest cerebrovascular diseases that cause psychiatric sequelae are cerebrovascular accident, subarachnoid haemorrhage, intracranial haematoma, cranial arteritis and Binswanger's disease (see above).

Cerebrovascular accident

A cerebrovascular accident or stroke consists of neurological disorder caused by cerebrovascular disease and lasting for

Table 26.5 The association between severity of HI, duration of PTA and eventual outcome		
Severity of HI	Duration of PTA	Outcome (GOS)
Mild	Less than 1 hour	Good recovery (minimal cognitive impairment may persist but there is return to premorbid status with full independence and retention of previous employment)
Moderate	1–4 hours	Moderate disability (moderate cognitive, behavioural and physical impairment persists and global function is considerably worse than premorbidly, but independence is possible)
Severe	1–7 days	Severe disability (severe cognitive, behavioural and physical impairment persists, global function is dramatically worse than premorbidly, and independence is impossible)
Very severe	> 7 days	

more than 24 hours (similar symptoms lasting less than 24 hours are termed transient ischaemic attacks). Stroke is suffered by 2 people per 1000 per year, and is responsible for almost 15% of annual deaths in developed countries. Cerebral infarction is responsible for up to 80% of stroke, cerebral haemorrhage causing the remainder. Stroke may be associated with almost any psychiatric disorder but the commonest are as follows:

- depression
- cognitive impairment
- personality change
- anxiety
- adjustment reactions to post-stroke disabilities and loss of independence
- post-stroke changes in domestic, familial, marital, occupational and social functioning.

Depression affects at least 1 in every 3 patients during the year following a stroke, especially patients who have suffered left frontal lobe damage and/or cognitive impairment (Starkstein & Robinson 1993). Emotional lability may also occur following left frontal lobe damage and in patients who develop pseudobulbar syndromes.

Stroke causes significant cognitive impairment and its non-cognitive effects complicate cognitive evaluation. Focal cortical syndromes are particularly common post-stroke (see above and Chapter 2).

Personality changes following stroke are similar to those following HI and range from apathy, disinterestedness and emotional flattening to increased irritability and obsessionality (a possible compensation for cognitive decline), the latter of which may manifest as a catastrophic reaction with rage, aggression and despair in the face of modest stress. As with patients following HI, spouses frequently complain that their partner post-stroke is not the person they married.

Post-stroke anxiety disorders are myriad but hypochondriasis, especially concerns about further strokes, are very common.

The psychiatric care of post-stroke patients involves their rehabilitation, support for them and their families, and the specific treatment of psychiatric disorders. Antidepressant medication is frequently required although there is some evidence that patients who develop depression post-stroke are relatively resistant to treatment. Further recovery of function is unlikely once 12 months have elapsed after a stroke and at least 50% of post-stroke patients never regain full independence. About 50% of post-stroke patients are destined to suffer a further stroke.

Subarachnoid haemorrhage

A significant proportion of the 50% of patients who survive a subarachnoid haemorrhage develop psychiatric disorders. These frequently warrant treatment and include the following:

- acute organic reaction in the immediate post-haemorrhage period
- personality change (this occurs in 20% of patients, a frontal syndrome frequently following anterior communicating artery haemorrhage)
- cognitive impairment (most often follows middle cerebral artery haemorrhage and frequently associated with neurological deficits)
- anxiety (especially concerns about further subarachnoid haemorrhages)
- minor mood changes (including improvements in mood)
- psychiatric syndromes associated with hydrocephalus and which may not manifest for months or years following the haemorrhage.

Intracranial haematoma

Relatively trivial HI (such as striking the head on overhead cupboards or when getting into a car) may cause acute intracranial haematomas which are usually subdural in elderly and extradural in younger patients. Up to 50% of patients with intracranial haematoma are alcohol dependent. Onset is insidious – often over several months – and clinical features include headache, cognitive impairment, dementia, hyperreflexia, extensor plantar reflexes, pupillary dilation and ptosis (indicating tentorial herniation of the temporal lobe, or coning), hemiparesis, clouding of consciousness and coma. Psychiatrists should maintain a high level of suspicion for intracranial haematoma in elderly and/or alcohol-dependent patients. CT is usually diagnostic and surgical evacuation gives excellent results in at least 50% of patients.

Infection

Most infections that cause significant fever may be associated with delirium, especially in very young or elderly patients. In addition, a considerable number of infectious diseases are associated with intracranial infection and cause illness ranging in severity from headache and anxiety through delirium to dementia and death. A list of the more common infectious processes that are associated with psychiatric symptoms is presented in Box 26.7 and they will be discussed below. The infections listed may exert their effect directly, indirectly via toxins or immunologically via the host's immune response to the infectious organism.

Encephalitis

Encephalitis, or inflammation of the brain, is generally thought to have a viral origin, although it is rarely possible to demonstrate the causative virus. Lyme disease is caused by a bacterium and the cause of encephalitis lethargica is unknown.

The neuropsychiatric features of encephalitis include headache, photophobia, impaired consciousness ranging from clouding to coma, focal neurological signs, seizures, postencephalitic amnesia and death. Symptoms may be subtle and the diagnosis of encephalitis should be considered in all patients with confusion or dementia. Investigations are often inconclusive apart from diffuse slow waves on the EEG, but protein and white cells may be increased in CSF, antibody titres may increase in blood, and structural neuroimaging may reveal areas of necrosis.

The commonest causes of viral encephalitis are listed in Box 26.7. The following infections deserve mention:

- herpes simplex is the commonest cause of clinically significant encephalitis in Europe and warrants aggressive investigation because antiviral medication may attenuate the effects of infection which include psychiatric symptoms and postencephalitic amnesia
- subacute sclerosing panencephalitis is caused by the measles virus, affects adolescents and is associated with myoclonus, epilepsy, dementia and death within a few years of diagnosis
- papovavirus causes progressive multifocal leucoencephalopathy leading to paresis, aphasia, dementia and death in immunocompromised patients
- rabies is associated with an acute organic reaction, psychomotor arousal and seizures
- arthropod-borne viruses (especially *Ixodes* and *Culex* species) are responsible for several epidemic encephalitides such as Russian endemic encephalitis, Semliki forest encephalitis and West Nile encephalitis.

First described in a patient from Lyme, Connecticut, USA, Lyme disease is an arthropod-borne encephalitis caused by the spirochaete *Borrelia burgdorferi*. A small proportion of patients, especially those with CSF antibody to *B. burgdorferi*,

develop fatigue, depression, amnesia and sleep disorders months or years after the primary infection (Kaplan et al. 1999). Treatment is with penicillin (erythromycin or tetracycline if penicillin-allergic).

Encephalitis lethargica (von Economos encephalitis) is an epidemic encephalitis that was reported from a number of countries during the early decades of this century. Patients experienced increasing lethargy and ophthalmoplegia initially, followed by parkinsonism, dystonia, oculogyric crisis, tics, personality change, schizophreniform psychosis and marked apathy.

Meningitis
Viral meningitis rarely causes significant psychiatric morbidity. Bacterial meningitis was once a common cause of neuropsychiatric sequelae but modern antibiotic therapy means that it is now rarely encountered. Tubercular meningitis usually involves the basal meninges and is relatively uncommon. Psychiatric features include irritability, apathy and personality disturbance. Tubercular meningitis is exceedingly difficult to diagnose because physical symptoms including pyrexia, neck stiffness and impaired consciousness appear late. A high level of suspiciousness should therefore be exercised when evaluating high-risk patients with a history of tuberculosis or who are immunocompromised by disease or treatment with psychiatric symptoms. Fungal meningitis is also increasingly common in this group of patients and is clinically similar to tubercular meningitis.

Neurosyphilis
Caused by the spirochaete *Treponema pallidum*, neurosyphilis is now rare in developed countries. However, it was once a major cause of neuropsychiatric illness and remains so in developing countries. About 50% of patients with neurosyphilis develop general paresis of the insane (GPI) while 25% develop tabes dorsalis and a further 25% develop meningovascular neurosyphilis. Cerebral gummata may also occur. The clinical presentation of patients with these syndromes will now be described.

Patients with GPI may present with classic grandiose delusions but depression, psychosis or dementia are more common. Untreated GPI is fatal. Antibiotic therapy prevents disease progression and allows recovery in about 10% of patients. Fleminger (1992) has provided the following useful mnemonic to assist recall of the clinical features of GPI:

P personality (irritability, impaired judgement)
A affect (depression, elation)
R reflexes (increased, extensor plantar reflex)
E eye (Argyll Robertson pupil, which reacts to accommodation but not to light)
S sensorium (clouding of consciousness, dementia, seizures)
I intellectual deterioration
S speech (aphasia) and sensory abnormalities.

Box 26.7 Infectious processes and their causative organisms that are associated with psychiatric symptoms

Encephalitis
Viral encephalitis caused by herpes simplex, influenza, polio, mumps, measles (including subacute sclerosing panencephalitis), rubella, papovavirus (progressive multifocal leucoencephalopathy), rabies and several other viruses, many of which are transmitted by arthropods
Bacterial encephalitis caused by *Borrelia burgdorferi* (Lyme disease)
Encephalitis lethargica (von Economos encephalitis)

Meningitis
Viral meningitis
Bacterial including tubercular meningitis
Fungal meningitis

Neurosyphilis

Cerebral abscess
Bacterial (including tubercular) abscess
Fungal abscess
Parasitic abscess

Malaria

Acquired immune deficiency syndrome

Patients with tabes dorsalis present with pain, ataxia, Charcot's joints (painless, swollen, abnormally mobile joints damaged by excessive movement caused by loss of proprioception and sensation), tabetic facies, urinary incontinence and impotence.

Patients with meningovascular neurosyphilis present with headache, insomnia, lassitude, confusion and seizures, and with focal signs and symptoms (aphasia, monoplegia, hemiplegia, cranial nerve palsies and bulbar symptoms) caused by endarteritis obliterans (inflammation of the superficial vessels of the brain and spinal cord). Response to antibiotic therapy is excellent but relapse may occur.

If suspected, the diagnosis of syphilis should be pursued aggressively. Most psychiatric inpatients have serum tests for syphilis such as the Venereal Disease Research Laboratory (VDRL) and *T. pallidum* haemagglutination (TPHA) tests. The fluorescent treponemal antibody absorption (FTA-ABS) test is more specific and is useful to confirm the diagnosis and exclude false positive results. CSF tests for syphilis are positive in almost all patients with neurosyphilis.

Neurosyphilis is treated with intramuscular procaine penicillin (tetracycline, doxycycline or erythromycin if allergic to penicillin) for 10–21 days. The CSF must be examined regularly for at least five years. The psychiatric manifestations of neurosyphilis should be treated symptomatically.

Cerebral abscess

The signs and symptoms of cerebral abscess are those of a space-occupying lesion (see cerebral tumours below). The onset is usually rapid (evidence of raised intracranial pressure, focal neurological signs and seizures), in which case diagnosis is relatively straightforward. Abscesses of insidious onset are more often confused with psychiatric disorders and the diagnosis should be considered in psychiatric patients with impaired consciousness and/or fever. Neurological signs may be absent or few and early neuroimaging is warranted. Bacteria derived from the middle ear, mastoid or nasal sinuses, systemic infection or head injury are the commonest cause, but tubercular and fungal abscesses may occur in immunocompromised patients. The treatment of cerebral abscess depends on the causative organism.

Malaria

Malaria caused by *Plasmodium falciparum* is a relatively common cause of neuropsychiatric disorder in malarious regions and may occur in travellers returning from such regions. Symptoms include headache, depression and fever, while drowsiness or an acute organic reaction may herald cerebral malaria, which may be fatal or have lasting neuropsychiatric sequelae such as personality change, depression and partial seizures (Varney et al. 1997). Acute organic reactions are less common in patients with *P. vivax*

malaria. Chronic malaria may be accompanied by headache, lethargy, anorexia, fatigue and depression. The diagnosis of malaria relies on demonstrating the parasite in a blood film. Treatment depends on the causative organism and requires expert advice because antimalarial-resistant parasites are increasingly common.

Acquired immune deficiency syndrome

HIV-associated dementia is discussed above. HIV-positive patients are frequently anxious or depressed and have an increased risk of suicide. These and other psychiatric symptoms may be caused by reaction to the diagnosis, infection of the brain by HIV or opportunistic pathogens, treatment with anti-HIV and other drugs, and tumours.

Cerebral tumours

Cerebral tumours cause symptoms common to all space-occupying brain lesions and consequent upon raised intracranial pressure (headache, apathy, emotional blunting, impaired cognition, altered consciousness and brain herniation syndromes) and focal effects (see above), the latter including seizures and depending on the site of the tumour. The absolute size of the tumour and its rate of growth also influence its clinical effects. Thus a small, rapidly growing tumour such as an astrocytoma may cause dramatic symptoms while a slow-growing tumour such as a frontal meningioma may silently reach a very considerable size. A patient's premorbid personality is a further and important determinant of the psychiatric sequelae of cerebral tumours. Cerebral metastases cause symptoms and signs similar to those of primary tumours.

At least 50% of patients with cerebral tumours have psychiatric symptoms (Lishman 1987) and perhaps as many as 1 in every 5 patients with such tumours, especially if malignant, first present to a psychiatrist. Cerebral tumours are found in 4% of psychiatric patients at autopsy in comparison to 2% of the general population. Psychiatrists should therefore be alert to this diagnosis, especially in patients with atypical or treatment-refractory illness. The neuropsychiatric features of patients with cerebral tumours should be treated symptomatically and, if possible, the tumour should be treated specifically.

Generalized cerebral insult

While focal cerebral insults directly affect a specific region of the brain, generalized cerebral insults are the result of pathologies – often extracranial and also affecting the complete organism – that affect the whole brain.

Metabolic disorders

Almost all metabolic disorders can impair the function of the brain, especially if severe or long-lasting. The most important of these are now discussed.

Hypoxia

The effects of hypoxia depend on its severity, rate of onset and duration. Mild acute hypoxia is readily compensated for by increased respirations and pulse. Moderate acute hypoxia causes apprehension and restlessness (air hunger), followed by clouding of consciousness. Seizures, coma and death occur if it becomes severe or persists for too long. Patients who survive moderate or severe hypoxia may suffer chronic amnesia, temporal lobe epilepsy or dementia, caused by the sensitivity of the hippocampus and temporal lobe specifically, and the brain in general, to low levels of oxygen.

Mild to moderate chronic hypoxia is initially compensated for by increased respirations and pulse, increased haemoglobin concentration and reduced activity. Chronic hypoxia of increasing severity is initially associated with fatigue, impaired concentration and judgement, irritability and memory disturbance. Personality change and dementia occur if it increases in severity and/or persists.

Electrolyte imbalance

The neuropsychiatric effects of electrolyte imbalance depend on the ions involved, the severity of the disturbance and the underlying cause. Extreme imbalance may cause an acute organic reaction, seizures or coma, and may ultimately prove fatal. Less severe disturbances are associated with the following psychiatric presentations:

- **Acidosis:** clouding of consciousness gradually progressing to coma; papilloedema may be evident.
- **Alkalosis:** clouding of consciousness, impaired memory, confusion and tetany (overbreathing in patients with anxiety may cause these features as well as perioral and peripheral paraesthesia).
- **Hypocalcaemia and hypercalcaemia:** discussed with parathyroid disorders (see below).
- **Hypokalaemia:** confusion, apathy and lethargy with a flaccid limb paralysis which may be mistaken for a conversion symptom.
- **Hypomagnesaemia:** disorientation, depression, acute organic reaction and coma.
- **Hyponatraemia:** irritability, apathy and clouding of consciousness progressing to coma.

Uraemia and renal dialysis

Uraemia rarely occurs in isolation, and electrolyte imbalance, the causative disease and its treatment will modify the clinical picture. The commonest psychiatric features of moderate uraemia include apathy, fatigue, impaired cognition and drowsiness, while uraemic encephalopathy classically fluctuates, is associated with impaired cognition and may progress to acute organic reaction, convulsions and coma (Burn & Bates 1998). Chronic uraemia is associated with depression which responds to antidepressant therapy.

End-stage renal failure and renal dialysis impose great demands on patients (reduced energy and work capacity, impaired concentration, psychosexual difficulties, side-effects of dialysis and immunosuppressive or other treatments, and fear of organ rejection or death), their relatives (anxiety, financial and marital problems) and renal unit personnel. Because of this, it is increasingly common for a liaison psychiatrist to work with patients, their relatives and personnel in renal units. Quality of life for patients depends on treatment – transplant patients fare better than patients treated with continuous ambulatory peritoneal dialysis who in turn fare better than haemodialysis patients.

Patients undergoing haemodialysis commonly experience anxiety, lethargy, depression and psychosexual difficulties and may experience psychiatric symptoms consequent upon uraemia and electrolyte imbalance (see above). Two specific neuropsychiatric syndromes have also been described:

- **Dialysis dementia:** progressive dementia and seizures probably caused by the accumulation of aluminium from perfusion fluids in the brain. This has become uncommon since the introduction of aluminium-free dialysates.
- **Dialysis disequilibrium:** confusion, acute organic reaction, seizures or coma probably caused by cerebral oedema following excessively rapid haemodialysis.

Hepatic failure

A fluctuating chronic organic state has been described in which psychiatric (drowsiness, confusion, personality change, visual hallucinations, mania and delirium) and physical (motor retardation, flapping tremor of hands, grimacing, ataxia, hyperreflexia, clonus and coma) symptoms wax and wane in unison. This disorder improves with a low-protein diet.

Neuropsychological findings in patients with cirrhosis include selective deficits in attention and fine motor skills with preservation of general intellect, memory, language and visuospatial perception, suggesting a subcortical – possibly basal ganglia – pathophysiology (McCrea et al. 1996).

Polydipsia

Polydipsia may be caused by diabetes insipidus or be associated with schizophrenia or another psychiatric disorder, or its treatment. Diabetes insipidus may be cranial (reduced secretion of antidiuretic hormone or ADH) or nephrogenic (renal insensitivity to ADH, which may be caused by lithium carbonate). Psychogenic polydipsia causes polyuria, which may lead to hyponatraemia (see above). Polydipsia occurs in at least 10% of institutionalized psychiatric patients and may respond to atypical antipsychotics or behaviour therapy (Buckley 1998, Tohen & Grundy 1998).

Porphyria

Three of the six porphyrias may cause psychiatric symptoms. The commonest, acute intermittent porphyria (AIP), may be pecipitated by alcohol, drugs (combined oral contraceptives, barbiturates, sulphonamides, methyldopa and griseofulvin), infection or fasting, and may cause anxiety, irritability, confusion, severe depression, a paranoid psychosis with hallucinations and an acute organic reaction and coma. The 'madness' of King George III has been attributed to AIP. Variegate porphyria and coproporphyria are rare causes of psychiatric symptoms.

Carcinoma (non-metastatic psychiatric effects)

The effects of primary and metastatic cerebral tumours have been described above. Cancers, especially bronchogenic carcinoma, may also cause non-metastatic neuropsychiatric syndromes, the psychiatric symptoms of which include anxiety, depression, acute organic reactions, schizophrenia and dementia (limbic encephalopathy). Three may occur independently of neurological symptoms. Furthermore, psychiatric symptoms may precede physical symptoms in pancreatic (McGee et al. 1994) and perhaps other cancers. Occult cancer is thus a differential diagnosis in patients with treatment-resistant psychiatric illness or dementia. Hormone secretion by tumours may be responsible for these syndromes and many patients have cortical neuronal loss and gliosis.

Carcinoid syndrome

Carcinoid syndrome is caused by metastatic tumours that secrete vasoactive substances such as serotonin and histamine. The majority of patients with this syndrome experience psychiatric symptoms including anxiety, depression, insomnia and confusion.

Vitamin deficiencies

The psychiatric sequelae of vitamin deficiency have been described in prisoners of war, in individuals from developing countries where famine occurs and in those who are elderly, alcoholic, mentally ill or have gastrointestinal disease. Studies have also been undertaken in volunteers. While panvitamin deficiency causes apathy and impaired cognition and may lead to psychosis, specific symptoms are associated with deficiencies of individual vitamins.

Thiamine (B_1) deficiency (cerebral beri-beri) Acute thiamine depletion causes Wernicke's encephalopathy and Korsakoff's psychosis. Replacement therapy generally reverses the confusion, clouding of consciousness and neurological symptoms of the former and will also reverse or reduce memory disturbance in a proportion of patients with the latter, if commenced promptly. Chronic thiamine deficiency causes apathy, fatigue, irritability, depression and cognitive impairment prior to the development of classic beri-beri.

Nicotinic acid (B_3) deficiency (pellagra) Acute nicotinic acid depletion causes encephalopathy with an acute organic reaction, parkinsonism and primitive reflexes. Chronic deficiency causes apathy and lassitude initially, with confusion, depression, paranoid psychosis with hallucinations and occasional violence as the disease progresses. Established pellagra is characterized by the triad of dermatitis, diarrhoea and dementia. Replacement therapy is generally effective at all stages of disease.

Pyridoxine (B_6) deficiency Pyridoxine deficiency may cause depression and, much less frequently, an acute organic reaction.

Cyanocobalamin (B_{12}) deficiency (pernicious anaemia) Anxiety, depression, psychosis, acute organic reaction and dementia have been attributed to vitamin B_{12} deficiency (in addition to subacute combined degeneration of the spinal cord) and are said to respond to replacement therapy (Shulman 1967).

Folate deficiency (folate dementia) Folate deficiency is common and may be associated with lassitude, impaired cognition, depression and dementia. However, it is probable that these symptoms occur only following severe, prolonged deficiency.

Endocrine disorders

Psychiatric symptoms occur in a large proportion of patients with a range of different endocrine diseases, may lead to incorrect psychiatric diagnoses (Box 26.8) and may have medicolegal significance. Such symptoms usually resolve upon treatment of the primary endocrine disease.

Psychiatric treatment may be required if acute organic reactions occur or if treatment of the primary disease is prolonged or impossible.

Hypopituitarism Hypopituitarism may follow pituitary tumours or hypophysectomy. Weight- and hair-loss and impotence or amenorrhoea develop in addition to the psychiatric symptoms seen in Addison's disease – including cognitive impairment – and hypothyroidism. An acute organic reaction leading to coma may occur during pituitary crises.

Replacement therapy for the underlying disease usually ensures resolution of psychiatric symptoms (McGauley 1989) but symptomatic psychotropic treatment may be required in the short term.

Acromegaly Fatigue, avolition, emotional lability and apathy may occur and occasionally are so severe as to resemble depression.

Hyperprolactinaemia Psychotic symptoms have been described in association with hyperprolactinemia.

Treatment is problematic because antipsychotic drugs, being dopamine D_2 receptor antagonists, may worsen the non-psychiatric symptoms of hyperprolactinemia, while bromocriptine, a dopamine D_2 receptor agonist, may worsen psychosis. There is some evidence that atypical anti-

Box 26.8   Endocrine disorders and the psychiatric diagnoses they may be mistaken for

Hypothyroidism
Dementia
Depression
Psychosis

Hyperthyroidism
Anxiety disorder
Depression (agitated)

Addison's disease
Dementia
Depression
Psychosis

Cushing's syndrome
Depression
Psychosis
(Mania with corticosteroid therapy – see below)
Anxiety

Hypopituitarism
Dementia
Depression
Anorexia nervosa
Psychosis

Acromegaly
Depression

Hypoparathyroidism
Anxiety disorder
Depression

Hyperparathyroidism
Depression
Dementia

Phaeochromocytoma
Anxiety disorder
Panic disorder

Diabetes mellitus
(see text)

Hypoglycaemia (insulinoma)
Anxiety
Intoxication
Personality disorder
Automatism
Temporal lobe epilepsy

psychotic drugs maybe effective in combination with bromocriptine (Soygur et al. 1997).

Hypothyroidism Hypothyroidism is caused by low plasma thyroxine (or tri-iodothyronine) caused by thyroid disease, thyroidectomy or drugs.

Symptoms develop insidiously and include impaired concentration, psychomotor retardation, depression, dementia and 'myxoedematous madness', a paranoid psychosis with hallucinations and delusions first described by Asher (1949). Acute organic reaction, seizures and coma may occur.

Myxoedema has been used successfully as a defence against homicide (Easson 1980).

Psychiatric symptoms usually resolve with thyroxine replacement therapy but symptomatic psychotropic treatment may be required in the short term. Depression associated with hypothyroidism is relatively treatment-resistant (Denicoff et al. 1990) and patients with dementia of more than two years' duration do not always recover.

Hyperthyroidism The psychiatric symptoms of hyperthyroidism include overactivity and irritability resembling anxiety, depression, mild to moderate cognitive impairment and acute organic reaction during thyroid crises. Affective or schizophreniform psychosis occurs occasionally.

Psychiatric symptoms almost invariably resolve with treatment of the thyroid disorder.

Hypoparathyroidism The psychiatric features of hypoparathyroidism, which most commonly develops following thyroidectomy, include anxiety, depression, irritability, epilepsy, acute organic reaction and cognitive impairment (if untreated). Psychosis is probably no more common than in the general population.

Psychiatric symptoms increase as hypocalcaemia worsens, but they respond rapidly to treatment with vitamin D.

Hyperparathyroidism Hyperparathyroidism is usually caused by a parathyroid adenoma and is frequently associated with depression, anergia and irritability. About 1 in 3 patients receive a psychiatric diagnosis prior to the definitive diagnosis being made. Cognitive impairment occurs in a large proportion of patients, as does acute organic reaction during parathyroid crisis.

Psychiatric symptoms are related to plasma calcium and respond to removal of the causative adenoma.

Diabetes mellitus There are four psychiatric syndromes associated with diabetes mellitus, as follows:

* Psychological reactions to a lifelong disease that requires treatment with daily injections, imposes limitations on lifestyle and increases risk for disabling (blindness or impotence, for example) and fatal (myocardial infarction or stroke, for example) diseases such as anxiety, hypochondriasis and depression.
* Psychiatric symptoms caused by metabolic imbalance (hyperglycaemia/ketoacidosis, lactic acidosis and hypoglycaemia) such as anxiety, irritability, aggression, confusion and acute organic reaction.
* Psychiatric symptoms associated with the long-term effects of diabetes mellitus including cerebrovascular disease – which may account for the cognitive

impairment and dementia described in some diabetic patients (Perlmutter et al. 1984) – impaired vision and renal failure.

- Comorbid psychiatric illness in diabetic patients that is unrelated to their diabetes mellitus.

Thus a proportion of diabetic patients may require general psychiatric treatment (because of their reaction to the diagnosis and treatment of diabetes mellitus or because of comorbidity) while some will require specific treatment such as antidepressant therapy for pain associated with diabetic neuropathy, psychological and pharmacological treatment of sexual dysfunction and psychoeducation directed towards improved compliance with diabetic treatment regimens.

There is considerable evidence that major depression occurs in at least 20% of diabetic patients and that it is both poorly recognized and poorly treated (Lustman et al. 1997).

Hypoglycaemia Hypoglycaemia may be caused by excess insulin administration, insulinoma, liver disease or alcohol.

Psychiatric symptoms include anxiety, aggression, behavioural disturbance, mood disorder, clouding of consciousness, amnesia and coma. Automatisms may occur and hypoglycaemic automatism has been used as a defence against criminal conviction. Episodic hypoglycaemia may occur with insulinoma and may present as psychiatric disorder while chronic hypoglycaemia has been associated with dementia.

Addison's disease Addison's disease is caused by adrenal failure and is associated with weakness, apathy, fatigue, depression, irritability and weight-loss.

Marked cognitive impairment may occur (and may lead to a diagnosis of dementia) as may an acute organic reaction during Addisonian crises. Psychosis occurs infrequently. Psychiatric symptoms almost always resolve with replacement therapy for the underlying disease but symptomatic psychotropic treatment may be required in the short term.

Cushing's syndrome Corticosteroid treatment is the commonest cause of Cushing's syndrome, with adrenocorticotrophin secreted by pituitary adenomas (Cushing's disease) and other tumours accounting for the remainder.

At least 50% of patients develop psychiatric symptoms which include depression (which is less common with corticosteroid treatment - see below) during which biological and psychotic symptoms may occur and, less often, psychosis, mania, anxiety and cognitive impairment. Impotence and amenorrhoea are common.

Psychiatric symptoms usually resolve with treatment of the underlying disease but psychotropic treatment may be required in the short term.

Phaeochromocytoma Phaeochromocytomas are usually benign (90%) tumours of the adrenal (90%) or sympathetic chain chromaffin cells that secrete adrenaline and noradrenaline and, often in response to emotion or excitement, cause episodes of severe panic with palpitations, sweating, tremor, headache, tachycardia, hypertension, pallor and intense fear. Confusion and excitement may also occur. Catecholamines and their metabolites are increased in blood and urine and the tumour may be detected by MRI.

Psychiatric symptoms may suggest a diagnosis of anxiety or panic disorder but they invariably respond to surgical treatment of the tumour.

Poisoning

Poisoning with carbon monoxide, prescribed and illicit drugs, and toluene is relatively common, while poisoning with heavy metals is relatively rare.

Carbon monoxide poisoning

The hippocampus and basal ganglia are particularly sensitive to carbon monoxide (CO) poisoning (and concurrent hypoxia), which most often occurs during suicide attempts with car exhaust fumes. The neuropsychiatric effects of CO poisoning depend on the concentration of the gas and the duration of exposure:

- **Mild CO poisoning:** an acute organic reaction with amnesia and extrapyramidal symptoms is usual upon recovery of consciousness. These features resolve over days or weeks leaving minimal or no long-term sequelae.
- **Moderate CO poisoning:** a prolonged acute organic reaction with severe amnesia and extrapyramidal symptoms is usual upon recovery of consciousness. These features resolve over weeks or months but relapse often occurs a few weeks after an apparently complete recovery. A small proportion of patients die at this stage while persistent severe extrapyramidal symptoms or dementia develops in some survivors.
- **Severe CO poisoning:** persisting coma leading to death.

Follow-up studies suggest that more than 50% of patients suffer permanent personality change or cognitive deficit while 2% develop permanent extrapyramidal disorders or dementia. It has been suggested that a law requiring catalyst vehicle exhaust systems and automatic idling stop, and exhaust tubes that are incompatible with vacuum cleaner tubes (the commonest means by which CO is transferred from the exhaust pipe to the car interior) would reduce suicides from CO poisoning (Ostrom et al. 1996).

Poisoning with drugs

Many drugs, whether available over the counter, by prescription or illicitly, can alter brain function and cause psychiatric symptoms. Indeed it is largely because of this effect that illicit drugs are abused (see Chapter 28). The psychiatric side-effects of commonly prescribed drugs will now be discussed.

Antibacterial and antituberculous drugs Intramuscular procaine penicillin may cause anxiety and hallucinations, while a large number of antibiotics including chloramphenicol, cefalexin, gentamycin, nitrofurantoin and the sulphonamides have been reported to cause acute organic reactions.

Isoniazid may cause prolonged psychosis and cycloserine has been associated with confusion, depression and schizophreniform psychosis in patients receiving antituberculous therapy.

Anticholinergic/antimuscarinic and dopaminergic drugs Anticholinergic/antimuscarinic drugs may cause confusion, excitement and visual hallucinations, especially in elderly patients, while dopaminergic drugs cause acute organic reactions, affective disorders and psychosis. These side-effects are commoner in patients with a history of psychiatric illness (see Chapter 38).

Anticonvulsant drugs Psychiatric side-effects from AEDs may arise directly or may be mediated indirectly by sedation and disinhibition. Carbamazepine, lamotrigine and topiramate are associated with confusion, depression and agitation (especially in elderly patients). Lamotrigine may also cause irritability and aggression. Most other AEDs cause similar side-effects while psychosis may occur with both vigabatrin and topiramate (see Chapter 38).

Barbiturates, benzodiazepines and related drugs Barbiturates, prescribed infrequently now in comparison to a few decades ago, may cause euphoria and irritability. In addition to dependency, these drugs and benzodiazepines may cause drowsiness, lethargy, ataxia and depression on the one hand, and disinhibition with excitement and aggression on the other. Elderly patients may become very confused. Withdrawal effects from barbiturates are similar to those of alcohol and delirium and seizures may occur (see Chapter 38).

Cardiovascular drugs The neuropsychiatric side-effects of digitalis, the older antihypertensive drugs and diuretics are well recognized, and more recently, similar side-effects have been described for newer cardioactive drugs. Digitalis toxicity is often associated with confusion, disorientation and hallucinations, and depression and excitement have also been reported. Depression or euphoria may be caused by beta-blocking, diuretic, ganglion-blocking (trimetaphan), calcium channel blocking and centrally acting (rauwolfia, methyldopa, clonidine and moxonidine) antihypertensive drugs, and by antihypertensive drugs that affect the renin-angiotensin system. Vasodilator and adrenergic-blocking antihypertensive drugs appear less likely to cause such side-effects.

Corticosteroid drugs It has long been recognized that corticosteroid drugs may cause psychosis with paranoia and auditory hallucinations, mild elation or depression in the short term, and mania or more severe depression with an increased risk of suicide in the longer term. The latter may be associated with an acute organic reaction and may persist for

several weeks. These side-effects are more common with higher dosages and in patients with a history of psychiatric illness. Recovery is usual upon withdrawal of corticosteroid therapy but prolonged psychotropic treatment – including treatment with antipsychotic drugs or lithium if appropriate – may be required if corticosteroid withdrawal is impossible. Acute organic reaction may be precipitated by rapid corticosteroid withdrawal.

Contraceptive drugs Hormonal contraceptive drugs, both combined and progesterone-only formulations, may cause depression. This may resolve with the addition of pyridoxine but if not, discontinuation of hormonal (and initiation of non-hormonal) contraception may be necessary.

Cytotoxic drugs Vinca alkaloid and platinum drugs are neurotoxic, but while they may cause neurological disorders including encephalopathy, pure psychiatric symptoms are relatively uncommon. Confusion has been reported with α and β interferons, and affective and sleep disorders with gonadorelin analogues. Cytotoxic antibiotics and antimetabolites are relatively free from neuropsychiatric side-effects.

Opiate drugs Although widely abused because they induce mild euphoria and drowsiness, opiates are relatively free from significant psychiatric side-effects. Sedation and depression may occur, especially in elderly patients.

Toluene poisoning

The inhalation of toluene in adhesives ('glue-sniffing) produces dizziness and euphoria in the very short term. Hallucinations, seizures and coma may occasionally evolve. In the longer term, a chronic paranoid psychosis, temporal lobe epilepsy and intellectual impairment have been described (Byrne et al. 1991). Suggestions that cortical atrophy may occur are unproven.

Heavy metal poisoning

All heavy metals may cause acute and chronic organic reactions and this and the relative rarity of heavy metal poisoning makes the diagnosis extremely difficult unless a clear account of exposure can be obtained.

Lead poisoning in children causes an encephalopathy that may be associated with permanent intellectual impairment. Adults exhibit anorexia and colic with cognitive impairment and, infrequently and only with chronic exposure, psychosis. Cerebral and cerebellar calcification may occur.

Mercury poisoning causes depression and mild cognitive impairment more frequently than the more famous 'erythism' or Mad Hatter's disease (poor attention and concentration with severe anxiety and agitation), and while there have been suggestions that mercury from dental amalgam may have these effects, there is no evidence that this is the case (Foerster & Breyer-Plaff 1996).

Thallium poisoning almost always follows accidental or intentional ingestion of rat poison. Clinical features include severe peripheral neuropathy, abdominal pain, nausea, vomiting, alopecia and acute organic reaction. The vast majority of patients make a complete recovery.

Arsenic poisoning most often occurs during industrial exposure. Psychiatric symptoms include mild impairment of new learning, recent memory and concentration. This may only manifest a few years after exposure. Recovery is usual on cessation of exposure.

Autoimmune and other disorders

Psychiatric symptoms occur in patients with several autoimmune disorders and may be aggravated by treatment with steroids. Autoimmune disorders therefore deserve consideration in the psychiatric differential diagnosis.

Amyotrophic lateral sclerosis (motor neuron disease)

Amyotrophic lateral sclerosis (ALS) develops from the fifth decade of life onwards. Patients initially present with weakness and atrophy of the muscles of the hands. This progresses proximally and some patients have cranial nerve/craniobulbar muscle weakness which may impair breathing, swallowing and speech, and may be associated with pseudobulbar emotional lability. Many patients with ALS are depressed and have chronic pain and there is evidence that these symptoms are frequently unrecognized and untreated (Ganzini et al. 1999).

Cerebral sarcoidosis

Neurosarcoidosis usually presents with meningo-encephalitis or cranial nerve palsies caused by cerebral sarcoid granulomata. Less frequently, patients present with clouding of consciousness, hallucinations and aphasia (Hayashi et al. 1995). Treatment should be directed at the control of symptoms and at the underlying sarcoidosis.

Systemic lupus erythematosus

Psychiatric symptoms, including anxiety, major depression, affective and schizophreniform psychoses, acute organic reactions and dementia with personality change and emotional lability, occur in at least one-third of patients (Rubio et al. 1998) with systemic lupus erythematosus (SLE) and may occasionally be the presenting symptom. These symptoms are usually short-lived and are best treated symptomatically and by controlling the underlying SLE. Cerebral SLE detected by structural and functional neuroimaging is as common in patients without psychiatric symptoms as in those with such symptoms (Sabbadini et al. 1999).

Multiple sclerosis

A proportion of patients with multiple sclerosis (MS) present to psychiatrists and may receive diagnoses of conversion disorder before MS is identified. Depression is the commonest psychiatric symptom in patients with MS and there is an increased risk of suicide. Patients with bilateral bulbar lesions may exhibit emotional incontinence. Euphoria occurs in less than 10% of patients, being commonest in those with cognitive impairment. Cognitive impairment occurs in 50% of patients and is closely related to the number of cerebral lesions. Dementia may occur. There is some evidence that emotional incontinence is particularly responsive to selective serotonin reuptake inhibitors (Nahas et al. 1998). Otherwise, psychiatric illness in patients with MS should be treated symptomatically.

Myasthenia gravis

A proportion of patients with myasthenia gravis (MG) are referred to psychiatrists with fatigue and muscle weakness and may receive a diagnosis of conversion disorder. Patients with MG may suffer from depression and anxiety and there is some evidence that such symptoms exacerbate the MG.

REFERENCES

Adamson DC, McArthur JC, Dawson TM & Dawson VL (1999) Rate and severity of HIV-associated dementia (HAD): correlations with Gp41 and iNOS. *Molecular Medicine* **5**(2): 98–109.

Anderson GM, Pollak ES, Chatterjee D et al. (1992) Postmortem analysis of subcortical monoamines and amino acids in Tourette syndrome. In: Chase TN, Friedhoff AJ & Cohen DJ (eds) *Tourette Syndrome: Genetics, Neurobiology and Treatment Advances in Neurology*, pp. 123–33. New York: Raven Press.

Asher R (1949) Myxoedematous madness. *British Medical Journal* **ii**: 555–62.

Bekkelund SI, Marthinsen TA & Harr T (1999) Reversible dementia in idiopathic normal pressure hydrocephalus. A case report. *Scandinavian Journal of Primary Health Care* **17**(1): 22–4.

Besson JAO (1993) Structural and functional brain imaging in alcoholism and drug misuse. *Current Opinion in Psychiatry* **6**: 403–10.

Betts T (1990) Pseudoseizures: seizures that are not epilepsy. *Lancet* **ii**: 9–10.

Betts T (1998) *Epilepsy, Psychiatry and Learning Difficulty*. Martin Dunitz: London.

Biggins CA, Boyd JL, Harrop FM et al. (1992) A controlled longitudinal study of dementia in Parkinsons disease. *Journal of Neurology, Neurosurgery and Psychiatry* **55**: 566–71.

Brun A (1987) Frontal lobe degeneration of the non-Alzheimer type 1 – neuropathology. *Archives of Gerontology and Geriatrics* **6**: 193–208.

Burn DJ & Bates DJ (1998) Neurology and the kidney. *Journal of Neurology, Neurosurgery and Psychiatry* **65**(6): 810–21.

Burns A, Lewis G, Jacoby R & Levy R (1991) Survival in Alzheimer's disease. *Psychological Medicine* **21**: 363–70.

Byrne A, Kirby B, Zibin T & Ensminger S (1991) Psychiatric and neurological effects of chronic solvent abuse. *Canadian Journal of Psychiatry* **36**(10): 735–8.

Cameron D, Thomas R, Mulvihill M et al. (1987) Delirium: a test of the Diagnostic and Statistical Manual III criteria on medical inpatients. *Journal of the American Geriatric Society* **35**: 1007–10.

Collinge J, Beck J, Campbell T et al. (1996) Prion protein gene analysis in new variant cases of Creutzfeldt-Jacob disease. *Lancet* **348**: 56.

Commission on Classification and Terminology of the International League Against Epilepsy 1989). Proposal for revised classification of epilepsies and epileptic syndromes. *Epilepsia* **30**:389–399.

Cummings JL (1993) Frontal-subcortical circuits and human behaviour. *Archives of Neurology* **50**(8): 873–8.

Denicoff KD, Joffe RT, Lakshman MC et al. (1990) Neuropsychiatric manifestations of altered thyroid state. *American Journal of Psychiatry* **147**: 94–9.

Dreifuss FE, Bancaud J, Henricksen O et al. (1981) Proposal for a revised clinical and electroencephalographic classification of epileptic seizures. *Epilepsia* **22**: 489–503.

Easson WM (1980) Myxedema psychosis – insanity defense in homicide. *Journal of Clinical Psychiatry* **41**(9): 316–18.

Fleminger S (1992) Organic psychiatry. In: Appleby & Foreshaw DM (eds) *Postgraduate Psychiatry, Clinical and Scientific Foundations*. Oxford: Butterworth-Heinemann.

Fleminger S & Curtis D (1997) Prion diseases. *British Journal of Psychiatry* **170**: 103–5.

Flor Henry P (1969) Psychosis and temporal lobe epilepsy: a controlled investigation. *Epilepsia* **10**: 363–95.

Foerster K & Breyer-Plaff U (1996) Amalgam – 'etiology of psychiatric disorders? *Versicherungsmedizin* **48**(2): 62–4.

Ganzini L, Johnston WS & Hoffman WF (1999) Correlates of suffering in amyotrophic lateral sclerosis. *Neurology* **52**(7): 1434–40.

George MS & Lydiard RB (1994) Social phobia secondary to physical disability. A review of benign essential tremor (BET) and stuttering. *Psychosomatics* **35**(6): 520–3.

Gunn J & Fenton GW (1971) Epilepsy, automatism and crime. *Lancet* **i**: 1173–6.

Hayashi T, Onodera J, Nagata T, Mochizuki H & Itoyama Y (1995) A case of biopsy-proven sarcoid meningoencephalitis presented with hallucination, nominal aphasia and dementia. *Rinsho Shinkeigaku* **35**: 1008–11.

Hodges JR (1994) *Cognitive Assessment for Clinicians*. Oxford: Oxford University Press.

Jacobson RR (1995) The post-concussional syndrome: physiogenesis, psychogenesis and malingering. An integrative model. *Journal of Psychosomatic Research* **39**: 675–93.

Jennett B & Bond MR (1975) Assessment of outcome after severe brain injury: a practical guide. *Lancet* **i**: 480–4.

Jordan BD, Relkin NR, Ravdin LD et al. (1997) Apolipoprotein e4 associated with chronic traumatic brain injury in boxing. *Journal of the American Medical Association* **278**: 136–40.Kano Y,

Laplane D, Levasseur M, Pillon B et al. (1989) Obsessive-compulsive and other behavioural changes with bilateral basal ganglia lesions. A neuropsychological, magnetic resonance imaging and positron tomography study. *Brain* **112**: 699–725.

Lishman WA (1987) *Organic Psychiatry – the Psychological Consequences of Cerebral Disorder*, 2nd edn. Oxford: Blackwell Science.

Lishman WA (1988) Physiogenesis and psychogenesis in the 'post-concussional syndrome'. *British Journal of Psychiatry* **153**: 460–9.

Lishman WA(1997) *Organic Psychiatry*, 3rd edn. Oxford: Blackwell Science.

Lustman PJ, Griffith LS & Clouse RE (1997) Depression in adults with diabetes. *Seminars in Clinical Neuropsychiatry* **2**: 15–23.

McCrea M, Cordoba J, Vessey G, Blei AT & Randolph C (1996) Neuropsychological characterization and detection of subclinical hepatic encephalopathy. *Archives of Neurology* **53**: 758–63.

McGee R, Williams S & Elwood M (1994) Depression and the development of cancer: a meta-analysis. *Social Sciences and Medicine* **38**: 187–92.

McGuire D (1996) Neurological aspects of AIS. *Medicine* 24: 131–3.

Meagher D (2001) Delirium: optimizing management. *British Medical Journal* **322**: 144–9.

Nahas Z, Arlinghaus KA, Kotrla KM, Clearman RR & George MS (1998) Rapid response of emotional incontinence to selective serotonin reuptake inhibitors. *Journal of Neuropsychiatry and Clinical Neurosciences* **10**(4): 453–5.

Ohta M & Nagai Y (1998) Clinical characteristics of Tourette syndrome. *Psychiatry and Clinical Neurosciences* **52**: 51–5.

Ostrom M, Thorson J & Eriksson A (1996) Carbon monoxide suicide from car exhausts. *Social Sciences and Medicine* **42**: 447–51.

Pauls D & Leckman J (1988) The genetics of Tourette syndrome. In: Cohen D, Brun R & Leckman J (eds) *Tourettes syndrome and Tic Disorders: Clinical Understanding and Treatment*, pp. 91–102. New York: Wiley.

Penn NE, Dripke DF, Scharff J (1981) Sleep paralysis among medical students. *Journal of Psychology* **107**: 247–252.

Perlmutter LC, Harami MR, Hodgeson-Harrington C et al. (1984) Decreased cognitive functioning in ageing non-insulin dependent diabetic patients. *American Journal of Medicine* **77**: 1043–8.

Powell T (1994) *Head injury: A Practical Guide*. Bicester: Winslow Press.

Prusiner SB (1998) Prions. *Proceedings of the National Academy of Sciences USA* **95**: 13363–83.

Rathbun JK (1996) Neuropsychological aspects of Wilson's disease. *International Journal of Neuroscience* **85**: 221–9.

Rubio Valladolid G, Gil Aguado A, Balsa Criado A et al. (1998) Prevalence of psychiatric disturbances and psychopathologic status in patients with systemic lupus erythematosus. *Revista Clinica Espanola* **198**: 61–5.

Russell WR (1932) Discussion on the diagnosis and treatment of acute head injuries. *Proceedings of the Royal Society of Medicine* **25**: 751–7.

Sabbadini MG, Manfredi AA, Bozzolo E et al. (1999) Central nervous system involvement in systemic lupus erythematosus patients without overt neuropsychiatric manifestations. *Lupus* 8: 11–19.

Shulman R (1967) Vitamin B_{12} deficiency and psychiatric illness. *British Journal of Psychiatry* **113**: 252–6.

Slater E, Beard AW & Glithero E (1963) The schizophrenia like psychoses of epilepsy. *British Journal of Psychiatry* **109**: 95–105.

Soygur H, Palaoglu O, Altinors N, Corapcioglu D, Erdogan G & Ayhan IH (1997) Melperone treatment in an organic delusional syndrome induced by hyperprolactinemia: a case report. *European Neuropsychopharmacology* **7**(2): 161–3.

Tizard B (1962) The personality of epileptics. *Psychological Bulletin* **59**: 196–210.

Tomlinson BE, Blessed G & Roth M (1970) Observations on the brains of demented old people. *Journal of the Neurological Sciences* **11**: 205–42.

Treiman DM (1993) Epilepsy and the law. In: Laidlaw A, Richens A & Chadwick D (eds) *A Textbook of Epilepsy*. Edinburgh: Churchill Livingstone.

Trzepacz P, Teague G & Lipowski Z (1985) Delirium and other organic mental disorders in a general hospital. *General Hospital Psychiatry* **7**: 101–6.

Wada JA (1985) Differential diagnosis of epilepsy. In: Gotman J, Ives JR & Gloor P (eds) *Longterm Monitoring of Epilepsy*. Amsterdam: Elsevier.

Wiggins S, Whyte P, Huggins M et al. (1992) The psychological consequences of predictive testing for Huntington's disease. *New England Journal of Medicine* **327**: 1401–5.

Will RG, Ironside JN, Zeidler M et al. (1996) A new variant of Creutzfeldt–Jakob disease in the UK. *Lancet* **347**: 921–5.

Will RG, Zeidler M, Stewart GE, Macleod MA, Ironside JW, Cousens SN, Mackenzie J, Estibeiro K, Green AJ & Knight RS (2000) Diagnosis of new variant Creutzfeldt–Jakob disease *Annals of Neurology* **47**(5): 575–82.

Alcohol misuse

Adam Winstock

INTRODUCTION
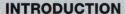

Alcohol is the most commonly used mood altering substance in Western society, with over 90% of the UK population drinking at some time. Although the psychiatrist will usually be concerned with the dependent drinker who is at greatest risk of drink related complications, the cost to society is in fact more related to the lower incidence of problems in the far more numerous *normal drinking* population. This has been termed the 'prevention paradox', since reducing alcohol consumption in that large number who drink just in excess of recommended levels, through public education and brief interventions, may be a more cost- and health-effective option, than the treatment of the smaller number of dependent users whose consumption of resources on an individual basis is enormous. At present, the maximum recommended levels of consumption are 21 units for man and 14 for a woman, although about 30% of the working population drink more than this. A *unit of alcohol* is equivalent to 10 ml or 8 g of absolute alcohol (approximately half a pint (284 ml) of normal strength lager, a glass (125 ml) of average strength wine or a single measure (25 ml) of spirits).

Metabolism

Alcohol is hydrophilic and rapid absorption occurs from all parts of the gastrointestinal tract with peak levels being reached 30–60 minutes after ingestion. This is enhanced by the absence of food in the stomach or the presence of carbon dioxide bubbles (note the effect of Champagne and 'Tequila slammers'). The primary route of metabolism (see Fig. 27.1) is hepatic oxidation by the rate limiting enzyme alcohol dehydrogenase (ADH) to acetaldehyde, which is subsequently oxidized by aldehyde dehydrogenase (ALDH). There is a racial distribution of ALDH2 (responsible for most of the second oxidative process), with the almost complete absence of activity in Orientals being responsible for the 'flushing reaction' (tachycardia, hypertension, a facial flush and weakness) they experience on ingestion of small amounts of alcohol. Such a deficit is seen in half of 'normal' Chinese and Japanese subjects but in only 2% of Japanese alcoholics. With increased consumption of alcohol the cytochrome P450 system starts contributing to alcohol metabolism, enhancing activity of the microsomal ethanol-oxidising system and contributing to the tolerance seen with chronic consumption.

Dependency

The disease concept of alcoholism originated with the writings of Benjamin Rush in the U.S and Thomas Totter who viewed alcoholism as 'a disease of the will'. The clinical syndrome, described by Edwards & Gross (1976), forms the basis for most modern day operationalized definitions of dependence syndromes (see Box 27.1).

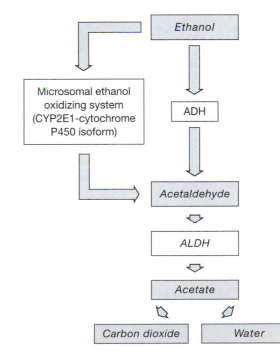

Figure 27.1 Metabolism of ethanol.

413

Box 27.1   Edwards & Gross alcohol dependency syndrome

Narrowing of drinking repertoire (loss of variation in pattern of intake)

Salience (primacy) of drink seeking behaviour

Increased tolerance to alcohol

Repeated attempts at withdrawal from alcohol

Relief or avoidance of withdrawal symptoms by further drinking

Reinstatement of dependent drinking after a period of abstinence

Subjective awareness of compulsion to drink

Identification and assessment

Effective secondary prevention can only be implemented through brief intervention and advice, if harmful drinking levels are detected. Several questionnaires have been developed, such as the 25-item MAST (Michegan Alcohol Screening Test) and the 4-item CAGE questions (Cutdown, Angry, Guilt and Eye opener). These tend to identify those with severe alcohol problems and tend to miss those with hazardous patterns of consumption. More recently WHO have developed the 10-item AUDIT (Alcohol Use Disorders Identification Test) for use by primary care workers. It detects 92% of harmful drinkers and 94% of those who drink above recommended levels. A five-item version of the AUDIT is reproduced in Box 27.2. The use of screening instruments in primary care can markedly improve identification of alcohol problems (Wallace & Haines 1985). Useful measures of alcohol related problems (which correlate with severity of dependence) include self-reporting

---

Box 27.2   Five item AUDIT questionnaire (Piccinelli et al. 1997)

How often do you have a drink containing alcohol?

0 = Never; 1 = Monthly or less; 2 = 2-4 times/month; 3 = 2-3 times/week; 4 = 4 or more times/week

How many drinks containing alcohol do you have on a typical day when you are drinking?

0 = 1 or 2; 1 = 3 or 4; 2 = 5 or 6; 3 = 7-9; 4 = 10 or more

How often during the past year have you found that you were not able to stop drinking once you started?

0 = Never; 1 = Less than monthly; 2 = Monthly; 3 = Weekly; 4 = Daily or almost daily

How often during the past year have you failed to do what was expected of you because of drinking?

0 = Never; 1 = Less than monthly; 2 = Monthly; 3 = Weekly; 4 = Daily or almost daily

Has a relative or friend or doctor or other health worker been concerned about your drinking or suggested you cut down?

0 = No; 1 = Yes, but not in the past year; 4 = Yes, during the past year

A score of 5 or more indicates harmful drinking
From Piccinelli M, Tessari E, Bortolomasi M et al. (1997) Efficacy of the alcohol use disorders identification test as a screening tool for hazardous alcohol intake and related disorders in primary care: A validity study. British Medical Journal 314: 420-4.

Alcohol Problems Questionnaire (APQ) and the Severity of Alcohol Dependence (SADQ).

Other means of identification include physical examination and the use of laboratory investigations. Blood alcohol concentration may also sometimes be a useful instrument in the workplace or in primary care. Biochemical (for a review see Haber & Conigrave 2003). investigations include:

- LFTs especially gamma GT (sensitivity 20–90%, specificity 55–90%). Levels fall quickly with abstinence, with moderate levels (300–500 mmol per litre) returning to normal within a month or two of abstinence
- MCV (sensitivity 20–50%, specificity 55–100%)
- carbohydrate deficient transferrin (an iron transport protein variant) has been used with a sensitivity for heavy drinking of 60–70% and a specificity of 95%.

EPIDEMIOLOGY OF ALCOHOL USE

Prevalence

The average UK per capita level of consumption is just over 10 units a week, with peak mean consumption occurring in males between 25–44 being 18 units/week, with that of women showing a 30% increase over the last decade to over a mean of 8 units/week (UK National Household Survey 2001). Recent national UK studies using the AUDIT screen identify about a third of those aged 16–35 years drinking at hazardous level (50% of M, 25% of F), with half of males between 16–35 years of age drinking at harmful levels. Rates of high risk drinking (defined as equal to or more than 51 units/week in males, 35 in females) are highest in those aged 20–24 years with 13% of males and 6% of females considered to be drinking at high risk. Mean drinking levels are highest in the North and lowest in the West Midlands and London (which has the most dependent drinkers, about 400 000). Prevalence studies in the UK give dependence rates in the last 12 months as 7.5% for men and 2% for women (4.7% overall) (Office of Population, Census and Statistics 1996). Lifetime rates of experiencing alcohol use disorders are higher, with approximately a quarter of men being classified as problem drinkers at some time in their lives (Institute of Alcohol Studies 2004). The Epidemiological and Catchment Area (ECA) study in the US reported a 14% lifetime prevalence of alcohol dependency with a male to female ratio of 2:1 (Reiger et al. 1991). On the basis of available data, there are in excess of three million adults (2.5 million men, 600 000 women) who are to varying degrees dependent on alcohol in the UK.

Patterns of use

In vino cultural countries 80% of alcohol is consumed at moderate levels with food on a daily basis. In the UK, food related consumption is 50%, with a significant proportion consumed during binge drinking episodes. Binge drinking is variously defined as consumption of half or more of the recommended maximum weekly amount during a single session or the consumption of more than six units for women and eight for men during a drinking session. The motive for such consumption patterns is clearly drunkenness. Binge drinking is a normal mode of alcohol consumption among 18- to 24-year-olds (40% of men and 22% of women report binge consumption in the last year). People in the UK binge-drink more than any other Western countries, except for Germany and Finland. Recent proposals to change opening hours in the UK are aimed at reducing the necessity for and frequency of such drinking patterns.

Age

Adults drink less with advancing age. The heaviest drinking occurs in the late teens and early twenties when the sex differences in consumption are least evident. Some groups may be particularly at risk of high risk drinking, such as 'clubbers' where the risk may be compounded by concurrent use of illicit drugs. Marketing of flavoured alcoholic beverages ('alcopops') to young consumers although worrying, must be viewed in light of the fact that the vast majority of alcohol consumed by this age group is in the form of traditional alcoholic beverages. The peak age for dependence is between 30–44 years.

Gender

Men drink about three times as much as women in the UK, and experience the onset of dependency at a earlier age. In Asian and Hispanic cultures the male/female ratio of consumption is nearer 10. Recent studies from many countries suggest that young women are now drinking at levels comparable to young men, with binge consumption posing a significant risk for health and wellbeing.

Harmful patterns of alcohol consumption in women are often compounded by other risky behaviours such as unprotected sex and illicit drug use. Women appear more sensitive to the harmful effects of alcohol as well as experiencing a greater degree of intoxication for a given amount of alcohol. Reasons for this increased vulnerability include having a higher proportion of body fat, lower body mass and smaller livers. Excessive consumption carries both short term risks such as accidents as well as longer term ones including cirrhosis and breast cancer. Women are more likely to have comorbid affective disorder (anxiety, depression and eating disorders) and to develop drinking problems more rapidly once they start. A high proportion of female alcoholics will have experienced physical and/or sexual abuse as adults with a third having been victims of childhood sexual abuse. This increased vulnerability to alcohol-related harm is compounded by the stigma associated with female drunkenness and dependence. Alcohol problems among women are often less visible than those in men, whilst access to acceptable and appropriate treatment services is often inadequate. The majority of trials on both psychological and pharmacological treatments for alcohol-related problems involve male only samples.

Beverage type

Wine is more commonly consumed by social classes 1 and 2, beer among socioeconomic classes 4 and 5, with heavy spirit consumption most common among the higher classes. There is also variation depending on country with France being a 'vino-cultural' country (and also having the world's highest cirrhosis rate).

Religion and culture

Among some religions such as the Islamic faiths, alcohol is prohibited, where among others there is a more permissive stance. The role of culture and religion upon consumption is complex, with highly prohibitive rules perhaps making binge drinking more likely. However, the effect of global marketing and homogenization of social behaviours may diminish the effects of such variables in years to come. More drinkers live in cities than in rural regions and small towns.

Occupation

Jobs permitting access to cheap, easily available sources of alcohol, in unsupervised jobs or those where consumption is regularly seen as 'part of the job', increase the risk of drinking. Other factors include unsociable hours, shift work or time away from the family. Unskilled manual occupations, publicans, traveling salesmen, journalists, dentists and doctors are at particular risk.

Marital status

Heavy drinkers are more likely to be divorced, separated or never married.

Socioeconomic class

In the Whitehall II study the most striking difference between the classes was the increasing prevalence of non-drinkers with progressively lower grade. The lowest mean consumers of alcohol are those classified under 'routine and manual' with a mean of 10.9 units/week and highest are those classified under 'managerial and professional' at 12.4 units/week.

Economic cost

The financial cost of alcohol use is significant. Treating alcohol-related illness and injuries costs the NHS up £1.7 billion/year. More broadly the cost of lost years, sickness, absenteeism, crime and human suffering associated with the consumption of alcohol is estimated as being over £20 billion/year in the UK (three times that gained from alcohol taxation).

Comorbitity

The most likely comorbid diagnosis in someone with alcohol dependency is dependence upon another substance. The combination of diagnoses increases the likelihood of violence and suicide (see below).

Taking a drinking history

The assessment of a patient suspected of having an alcohol use disorder should include the onset, development, pattern and consequences of drinking.

Box 27.3 shows a suggested scheme of enquiry and presentation that permits both diagnosis of harmful use/ dependence. The information gained from enquiring about a typical day from waking to sleep and the role alcohol plays is a useful starting point.

AETIOLOGY

As with most mental health disorders the aetiology is multifactorial with both constitutional and environmental factors playing a role.

Box 27.3 Scheme of enquiry for diagnosis of harmful alcohol use dependence

Current level of intake: volume, type(s) (% alcohol), days per week, duration at this level.

Typical day: time from waking to the onset of symptoms of withdrawal (in severely dependent drinkers these may be experienced on waking), time to first drink and its function (relief of withdrawal symptoms in the alcohol dependent person) social, e.g. familial, occupational and nutritional activities. Place of drinking and antisocial behaviours. Note evidence that suggests primacy and neglect of other interests. Sleep is often disturbed and may be cited as a primary reason for continued drinking.

Drinking history: age first used alcohol. Age first consumed at regular level (note quantities to assess development of tolerance and types of beverage consumed with passing years to demonstrate narrowing of repertoire). Age at which daily drinking started, age first experienced withdrawal and age at which institution of relief drinking began. Note the changing social circumstances especially with respect to family, social and employment.

Alcohol related problems (psycho-socio-biological): enquire about GI symptoms, withdrawal fits, DTs, amnestic blackouts. Continued consumption of alcohol despite problems is another diagnostic criteria.

Previous treatments: (e.g. in and out patient detoxes, AA and length and pattern of abstinent periods). Enquire specifically about the relationship between abstinent periods and the treatment of comorbid psychiatric disorders.

Circumstances surrounding relapse: internal cues (such as positive and negative mood) and external triggers including people, places and things.

Family history: of substance abuse in both immediate and extended family. Also enquire about history of other mental illness, criminality and violence.

Biological

Genetic

Twin studies give higher MZ:DZ concordance rates in male rather than female twins, with figures of 70%:43% for men (Pickens et al. 1991) and 47%:32% for women (Kendler et al. 1992), with the incidence in first degree relatives being raised by about 2.5 times. The evidence for a genetic contribution in women is less consistent than in men. *Adoption studies* demonstrate a four-fold increase in the incidence of alcoholism among male adoptees adopted away from their alcoholic parent(s) (Goodwin et al. 1973).

Biological markers suggest that the genetic contribution is mediated at a number of levels (see Table 27.1). For example, those with a family history of alcohol dependence experience less subjective intoxication with a given dose of alcohol than those with no family history. The apparent corrective effect of alcohol on the baseline low levels of EEG alpha activity seen in alcoholics suggest that in some alcohol may be self-medicating a neurophysiological deficit. Acetaldehyde may also combine with neurotransmitters to form *tetrahydroisoquinolines,* substances with opiate-like qualities, explaining the occasional beneficial impact of naloxone on severe alcohol intoxication. Genetic effects also determine the susceptibility to *alcohol associated physical damage,* for example in the development of cirrhosis, psychosis, haemachromatosis and brain damage (Hrubec & Omenn 1981) and probably the age of the *onset of dependence* (Blum et al. 1990).

Cloniger hypothesizes two types of genetic transmission broadly differentiating between familial and non-familial alcoholism with the former having a younger age of onset, more severe dependency and antisocial personality (Cloniger et al. 1981) (see Table 27.1).

Biological markers

The growth of molecular genetics in the last decade has heralded the possibility of identifying genetic loci that may confer a predisposition to the development of alcohol dependence (see Box 27.4).

Biochemical

Like all drugs of dependence the ventral tegmental dopaminergic reward pathway (see below) probably

---

Box 27.4 Biological markers for alcoholism

Increased static ataxia in first degree relatives

Lower alpha activity on the EEG

Blunted prolactin response to ethanol challenge

Reduced platelet MAO activity

Decreased subjective intoxication

Autonomic stress response increased

Transketolase Km higher

Reduced amplitude and increased latency of the P300 (not specific)

Blunted cortisol response to ACTH especially in family positive

---

Table 27.1 Cloniger subtypes of alcoholism

	Type 1 (milieu limited)	Type 2 (male limited)
Drinking pattern	Loss of control with high psychological dependency and guilt	Less likely to achieve abstinence
Sex	M and F	M
Family history	Parents mild/non abusers	High genetic component for alcohol and antisocial behaviour
Age of onset	Usually >25 years old	Usually <25 years old
Violence and crime	No association	Increased
Personality	Passive dependent traits with high degrees of harm avoidance and reward dependence, low levels of novelty seeking	Impulsive and antisocial traits

underlies the development of dependence (alcohol releases DA in the nucleus accumbens).

Psychological

Psychoanalytic theory

These tend to explain drinking as a result of usually traumatic early life experience, the need for oral gratification and concepts such as the death wish explaining the self-destructive consumptive process.

Conditioning theory

Classic and operant learning theories with relief drinking and cued response/relapse are two commonly cited mechanisms. The two main dimensions of the condition within this framework are seen as withdrawal avoidance and reward, with the latter seemingly the more important. Such explanations have an important role in directing some therapeutic interventions such as relapse prevention. Modelling (vicarious learning) and social learning theory also propose aetiological theories.

Personality traits

Half a century of research has failed to identify the alcoholic or addictive personality, however attractive the idea may sound. Several personality traits have been shown to have an association with alcoholism (see Box 27.5) but only dissocial ones are consistent.

Box 27.5 Predisposing personality traits and alcoholism

Childhood: aggression, inattention, hyperactivity, antisocial behaviours

Locus of control: external

Emotional: dependency, anxiety and alexithymia. Higher neuroticism scores on Eysenck Personality Questionnaire

Life events and stress

The 'tension reduction' hypothesis views alcohol's anxiolytic effects as primary, while other studies show an increased frequency of life events preceding the onset of alcohol misuse.

Sociological

The wider sociocultural context determines both the availability of alcohol and the attitude to drinking and intoxication. Price and other legislative controls have a significant impact on per capita consumption.

NEUROBIOLOGY OF ETHANOL, TOLERANCE, DEPENDENCE AND WITHDRAWAL (Littleton & Little 1994)

Alcohol's psychoactive effects are mediated through modulation at a number of neurotransmitters systems with most attention focused upon glutamate and GABA receptor-gated channels to which alchohol binds directly.

Its anxiolytic activity is probably mediated through the acute potentiation of the inhibitory neurotransmitters including GABA at GABA-A receptors and taurine. Alcohol also inhibits the function of the receptor for excitatory neurotransmitters such as glutamate and aspartate. The attenuating effect of alcohol on the N-methyl-D-aspartate (NMDA) glutamate receptor is thought to contribute to intoxication as well as impaired cognition and blackouts. Chronic alcohol consumption results in up-regulation of the NMDA-type glutamate receptor. Acute withdrawal of ethanol leads to increased glutamate synaptic release with the excitotoxic effects resulting in neuronal cell death (e.g. cerebellar degeneration), seizures and cognitive dysfunction (blackouts) (see Figure 27.2).

So alcohol, an agonist at neuroinhibitory GABA receptors and an antagonist at neuroexcitatory glutamate/NMDA

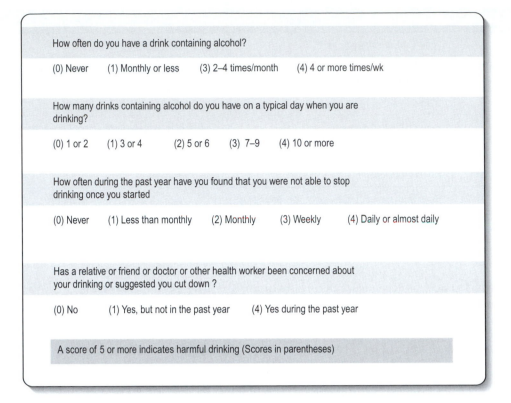

How often do you have a drink containing alcohol?

(0) Never   (1) Monthly or less   (3) 2–4 times/month   (4) 4 or more times/wk

How many drinks containing alcohol do you have on a typical day when you are drinking?

(0) 1 or 2   (1) 3 or 4   (2) 5 or 6   (3) 7–9   (4) 10 or more

How often during the past year have you found that you were not able to stop drinking once you started

(0) Never   (1) Less than monthly   (2) Monthly   (3) Weekly   (4) Daily or almost daily

Has a relative or friend or doctor or other health worker been concerned about your drinking or suggested you cut down ?

(0) No   (1) Yes, but not in the past year   (4) Yes during the past year

A score of 5 or more indicates harmful drinking (Scores in parentheses)

Figure 27.2 Acute and chronic effects of alcohol on GABA and glutamate activity. The neurochemical basis for withdrawal phenomena is thought to be unopposed GABA and NMDA activity, reflecting the general increase in neuronal excitability that is seen on withdrawal. This explains the rational for using benzodiazepines in the management of alcohol withdrawal.

receptors, causes GABA receptor down regulation `and glutamate/NMDA receptor upregulaton with long term use. Alcohol cessation permits unopposed and excessive neuroexcitation mediated by upregulated glutamate/NMDA receptors (Fig. 27.2) Benzodiazepines are effective in treating the symptoms of alcohol withdrawal as a result of the cross-tolerance they demonstrate with alcohol at the GABA-A. It is likely that carbamazepine, also effective in withdrawal, acts through this mechanism. Future pharmacological interventions may focus on NMDA antagonism as a means of reducing both withdrawal and the neuronal toxicity associated with exposure to repeated episodes of withdrawal. The management of alcohol withdrawal is discussed more fully later in this chapter.

Other effects

As with other drugs of dependence, alcohol also releases dopamine from the nucleus accumbens within the limbic VTA DA system as well as impacting on serotonin pathways thought be involved in priming and reinforcing effects. Alcohol also results in increased endogenous opioids which contribute to the euphoria associated with its consumption ands also explains why naltrexone is effective in maintaining abstinence in some dependent drinkers.

In addition to these primarily sedative effects, it must be noted that alcohol may cause stimulation and euphoria most notably when there is a rapid increase in blood alcohol levels and these effects may also be highly reinforcing.

ALCOHOL-RELATED PHYSICAL PROBLEMS

Moderate alcohol consumption of alcohol (1–3 units/day) is associated with reduced mortality compared to either life-long abstention or heavy use (J-shaped curve) with effects most clearly seen in reduced rates of coronary heart disease (mediated through increased levels of HDL). With excessive consumption (>50 units/day) damage may be seen in every physiological system, most commonly the gastrointestinal and nervous systems. Vulnerability to the toxic effects increase with age, female sex, total consumption and pattern of use (constant heavy drinking > binge drinking).

Gastrointestinal tract

- oesophagitis and reflux
- gastritis and ulceration anywhere in tract
- Mallory–Weiss tears

- oesphageal varices
- pancreatitis
- portal hypertension
- carcinoma of tongue, pharynx, larynx, esophagus, rectum and liver.

Liver

- alcoholic hepatitis. Acute inflammation consequent upon heavy drinking. Reversible with abstinence. Mortality of 10%.
- fatty liver. Fatty infiltration which disappears on stopping alcohol.
- alcoholic hepatitis. Here there is hepatocellular necrosis. With continued alcohol consumption, this will frequently lead to cirrhosis.
- alcoholic cirrhosis (in 10-20%).
- haemachromatosis in those with genetic susceptibility.
- hepatic encephalopathy.

Cardiovascular

- arrhythmias – atrial fibrillation and ventricular extrasystoles
- dilated cardiomyopathy, beri-beri with high output failure
- coronary and cerebrovascular disease
- hypertension, important especially in young males.

Metabolic

- hypoglycaemia–fasting or reactive
- ketoacidoisis
- hypertriglyceridaemia with obesity
- hypomagnesaemia
- hyperuricaemia.

Endocrine and reproductive

- hypercortisolaemia with non suppression on the DST. A 'Pseudocushings' picture may be seen usually resolving on abstinence
- hypogonadism with testicular atrophy
- infertility
- decreased libido and impotence.

Musculoskeletal

- proximal myopathy with or without myositis
- Dupytren's contracture (not important in diagnosis of dependency
- gout.

Bone

- avascular necrosis
- osteoporosis
- healed rib fractures on X-ray are a marker for alcoholism.

Haematological

- anaemia-iron, B_{12} or folate
- thrombocytopenia
- disordered clotting.

Respiratory

- tuberculosis
- pneumonia
- bronchiectasis.

Dermatological

- spider naevi
- palmar erythema
- acne rosacea
- discoid eczema and worsening of psoriasis.

NEUROLOGICAL PROBLEMS

Acute intoxication

Initially associated with an elevation in pulse and blood pressure and reduced social inhibition. Increasing doses lead to slurring of speech, ataxia, and sedation with risk of accidental injury. These effects form the basis of roadside sobriety tests, which focus on coordination, balance and attention. Horizontal nystagmus is also a sensitive marker of acute intoxication with alcohol. Poisoning is rare and tends to occur in compromised individuals or those who have taken other substances concurrently.

Pathological drunkenness (*manie a potu*)

The existence or otherwise of this syndrome is much debated and it is not coded for in ICD-10. It is said to be induced by minute quantities of alcohol and is characterized by a rapid and marked behavioural disinhibition often associated with explosive violence.

Methanol poisoning

Although consumption is rare and associated with home production, methanol poisoning has a mortality rate of 20% mediated through it's metabolites, formaldehyde and formate. It causes confusion, ataxia, visual disturbance, optic atrophy and necrosis of the putamen. Ethyl alcohol is used therapeutically in the management of methanol poisoning, by competing for the enzyme ALDH, preventing the build-up of toxic metabolites such as formate.

Amnestic (Korsakoff's) syndrome and Wernike–Korsakoff psychosis

This is characterized by persistent, prominent impairment of recent memory and thus new learning (may also affect remote recall). Immediate recall and procedural memory are preserved. Disturbances in time sense and ordering are common though other cognitive functions are unimpaired. The main feature is that memory loss is out of all proportion to cognitive loss, and new learning is impaired (see Chapter 26).

Aetiology

Alcohol reduces the absorption of thiamine and the activity of the enzyme that activates it. For causes of Korsakoff's syndrome see Box 27.6. Neurological damage is focused in the brain stem, wall of the third ventricle and floor of the fourth ventricle, periaqeductal grey matter, part of the thalamus, the mammillary bodies, the terminal portion of the fornices, anterior lobe and superior vermis of the cerebellum. Myelinated fibres are affected more than neurons while petechial hemorrhages, with astrocytic and histiocytic proliferation dominate the microscopic picture. For the clinical features of Wernike's encephalopathy see Box 27.7.

Korsakoff's syndrome may be defined as 'an abnormal mental state in which memory and learning are affected out of all proportion to other cognitive functions, in an otherwise alert and responsive subject'. Such a picture is differentiated from that seen with bilateral temporal lobe excision by the emotional and intellectual decline and absence of disturbed social behaviour that characterizes Korsakoff's (see Box 27.8).

Confabulation is the *falsification of memory in clear consciousness*. Fragments of genuine memory are dislocated in time resulting in inappropriate recall of 'old recollections with present impressions'. It occurs more commonly in the early stages of Korsakoff's, often setting in as the Wernicke's subsides. Two sorts are described, 'momentary' which relates to the recent past and the rarer but more famous 'fantastic' type in which bizarre autobiographical recollections are prominent with the content often relating to latent wish fulfillment. Confabulation does not occur with bilateral hippocampal destruction.

Neuroimaging of Korsakoff's patients using computed tomography (CT) show frontal lobe atrophy in one third and convolutional atrophy in a quarter, while the EEG shows diffuse slowing (in contrast to delirium tremens).

Prognosis

In Victor's classic 1971 study of 245 patients (Victor et al. 1971) the following conclusions were reached:

- 17% died in the acute phase
- 16% presented with Korsakoff's
- sixth nerve palsies always recovered
- 66% had residual horizontal nystagmus
- of the 186 who were followed up, 84% developed Korsakoff's psychosis; a quarter of these had complete recovery, half had partial recovery and a quarter had no recovery.

Women have a better prognosis than men.

Box 27.7   Clinical features of Wernicke's encephalopathy

Acute onset (may be over days)
Prodromal nausea, anorexia, vomiting
Nystagmus
Abducens and conjugate gaze palsies (90%)
Ataxia of gait (90%)
Peripheral neuropathy (80%)
Clouding of consciousness with disorientation
Lethargy and hypotension
Misidentification
Decreased spontaneous activity and speech
Memory problems (confabulation usually occurs later)
Emotional lability
Anxiety, insomnia
Fear of the dark, apprehension
Signs of malnutrition: angular stomatitis, glossitis, dry skin, etc.
Increased serum pyruvate levels
Cerebrospinal fluid: mild rise in protein
EEG shows diffuse slowing
Abstinence syndrome occurs in 15% with fits and DTs

Box 27.6   Causes of Korsakoff's syndrome

Cancer of the upper GI tract
Malabsorbtion or malnutrition
Heavy metal poisoning
Carbon monoxide poisoning
Tumours of the third ventricle
Head injury
Bilateral hippocampal destruction
Anaesthetic agents

Box 27.8   Clinical features of Korsakoff's psychosis

Apathy and reduced initiative
Loss of interest in alcohol
Thinking is stereotyped, perseverative and facile
Reduced ability to categorize and form concepts
Visuospatial impairment is common
Underestimate age and time in hospital
Reduced insight and confabulation
Impairment of new learning
Variable retrograde amnesia
Procedural memory and digit span are left intact

Other neurological consequences of alcohol

Cerebellar degeneration
The anterior lobe and superior vermis demonstrate Purkinje cell loss leading to ataxia of stance and gait.

Amblyopia
With an onset over a matter of weeks, this retrobulbar neuritis rarely leads to blindness. However, it is associated with loss of central vision, especially in the red/green bands and is associated with peripheral neuropathy.

Marchiafava Bignami syndrome
This is characterized by ataxia, epilepsy, dysarthria and severely impaired consciousness. A slowly progressive form with dementia and spastic paresis also occurs. The neuropathology is demyelination of the corpus callosum, optic tract and cerebellar peduncles.

Central pontine myelinosis
Acutely there may be nausea, vomiting, confusion and coma. Pseudobulbar palsy, quadriplegia and loss of pain sensation in the limbs and trunk may occur. Neuropathologically there is demyelination of pyramidal neurons in the pons.

Epilepsy
There can be a lowering of the seizure threshold in those prone to developing epilepsy. Occurrence of seizures may also arise consequent upon head injury, hypoglycaemia, subdural haematoma or from direct neurotoxicity, as alcohol is epileptogenic.

Dementia
Mild to moderate cognitive deficits are common in alcoholics, particularly visuospatial, frontal (impulse control) and memory impairment. Damage may be due to direct neurotoxicity, head trauma or nutritional deficiency and it would appear that women are more susceptible than men. CT and MRI studies demonstrate ventricular enlargement (Besson 1993) and cortical atrophy (Harper et al. 1985) in about two-thirds of alcoholics with atrophy of the cerebellar vermis seen in about 30%. Functional imaging shows decreased glucose metabolism and blood flow in cortical areas. Abstinence may be associated with some reversibility in these structural cerebral changes, especially in younger drinkers and women (see chapter 26).

Amnesia
Alcoholic blackouts are periods of retrograde amnesia arising during a period of intoxication while fully conscious. Occurring more commonly in the binge drinker, blackouts are not a defence nor reason for being unfit to plead in court.

Fetal alcohol syndome
Alcohol has been implicated as a causative factor in fetal damage for 30 years. First described in the English scientific literature in 1973 by Jones & Smith, fetal alcohol syndrome (FAS) is characterized by pre- and postnatal growth retardation, CNS involvement with developmental delay and a characteristic pattern of craniofacial dysmorphism, with the degree of dymorphism correlating with the decrement in IQ (Steinhausen et al. 1993). Alcohol consumption during pregnancy has been associated with low birthweight and an increased rate of stillbirths (Kaminski et al. 1976). Its incidence is between 0.5–2/1000 live births, though since FAS is a spectrum disorder, there may be many babies with the incomplete syndrome who are overlooked. Alcohol use may also lead to inadequate bonding and parenting (Blume 1986). The threshold 'safe level' of consumption through pregnancy probably lies in the region of 1 standard unit of alcohol/day though even light consumers may demonstrate some decrement in developmental delay compared to abstainers. Alcohol related brain infant neurotoxicity is the most preventable form of intellectual retardation in children. It is in theory 100% preventable.

Features of fetal alcohol syndrome are:

- intrauterine growth retardation
- failure to thrive
- short stature
- developmental delay
- micro-opthalmia
- short palpebral fissure
- short nasal bridge
- microcephaly with prominent forehead
- thin upper lip
- small philtrum
- cleft palate
- maxillary hypoplasia
- gait abnormailties
- irritable, mood disorder and hyeractivity
- cardiac abnormalities
- some show persistent cognitive impairment.

ALCOHOL-RELATED PSYCHOLOGICAL DISORDERS

The comorbidity of alcohol misuse and other psychiatric syndromes is common, present in over two-thirds of alcohol dependants. For a recent review of comorbidity and substance abuse see Hall & Farrell 1997.

Alcoholic hallucinosis
The psychopathology of alcoholic hallucinosis is characterized by auditory hallucinations, paranoid symptoms and

fear. Hallucinations are characteristically third person auditory hallucinations, often derogatory or command, which occur in clear consciousness. They may also take the form of fragments of conversation or music and there may be secondary delusions or perseveration. The symptoms may be highly distressing and may result in violent suicide. The onset is often associated with a reduction in dose or the precipitation of withdrawal and hallucinosis must be differentiated from delirium tremens, though they may appear as a continuation of hallucinations first experienced during this state. They may however arise in the current drinker. Assessment for the presence of other psychotic symptoms is mandatory to exclude other possible functional and organic pathologies, especially Wernicke's encephalopathy. Visual hallucinations, although not typical, may occur. The prognosis is usually good especially in abstinent drinkers, though in some 10–20% hallucinosis becomes chronic persisting for more than six months. The reinstatement of drinking often results in a recrudescence of symptoms. Hospitalization and treatment with antipsychotic medication may be required. Five to twenty per cent of these patients subsequently develop schizophrenia, and have an increased family history of psychosis.

Psychiatric comorbidity

The ECA study reported that having a psychiatric diagnosis triples the likelihood of an individual having a lifetime alcohol disorder. The most common comorbid conditions are drug-use disorders, mood and anxiety disorders, and dissocial PD (for a recent review see Kranzler & Rosenthal 2003). In community-based studies, people dependent on alcohol were seven times more likely to have a drug disorder and two to three times more likely to have a mental disorder compared to others in the community. Rates tend to be higher in clinical samples reflecting the increased rates of treatment-seeking by dual disorder patients (Berkson's bias). Alcohol dependence is also associated with heavy smoking. Relatives of alcoholic probands have higher rates of depression and drug abuse than controls (Winokur 1979). Common or closely linked genes may produce a general increase in vulnerability to both mental and substance misuse disorders consistent with the hypothesis of pleiotrophy. Shared environmental factors such as poverty or childhood abuse may also jointly predispose. High rates of comorbid psychiatric disorders have a detrimental impact on prognosis. Identifying the temporal onset of comorbid disorders is important when planning treatment and considering prognosis, with the primary illness steering the clinical picture.

Affective disorder

Up to 70% of alcoholics complain of dysphoria during heavy drinking. Immediately after detoxification the rate of depression is 50%, and after a month between 15–20%. In the ECA study, 13.4% of alcoholics reported a mood disorder, whilst conversely 22% of those with mood disorder reported alcohol use disorder. Rates of comorbidity are even higher in those with bipolar disorder (>40%), where the result is higher rates of hospitalizations, shorter remissions, more dysphoria and a poorer clinical outcome. During manic episodes alcohol consumption can be very high, and contribute to increased risks.

Twenty years ago, 80–90% of depression in heavy drinkers was assumed to be secondary to alcohol use, but recent large epidemiological studies suggests that a diagnosis of alcohol misuse is as likely to pre- as post-date the onset of affective disorders (Merikangas et al. 1996). The temporal association of drinking and psychiatric disorders does however vary between genders. In women major depression tends to precede drinking, while in men depression follows on from drinking. Similarly, anxiety disorders tend to precede the onset of alcohol-use disorders more commonly in women than men. Certainly the incidence of depressive symptoms falls with abstinence, but careful assessment is required and treatment must be instituted if a primary diagnosis of depression is made, since untreated, it may precipitate relapse. Traditional antidepressant medications are effective in treating major depression in those with alcohol dependence, with the safety profile of the SSRIs making them preferable to TCAs. Dysphoria in the weeks following withdrawal is common and it takes time for appetite and sleep especially to return to normal. Alcohol may interfere with treatment efficacy and compliance with other psychotropic medication and may lead to a pharmacological nihilism in some current drinkers who are upset at remaining depressed while taking their medication. The commencement of their prescription can be contingent upon achieving a period of abstinence to permit accurate assessment and diagnosis, which can form part of a motivational contract.

The degree to which the comorbidity of affective disorders and alcohol dependence is genetically mediated is unclear and may vary with gender. The US National Comorbidity Study (Kessler et al. 1997) reported that among women with alcohol dependence 86% and 72% had a comorbid lifetime psychiatric or drug use disorder respectively, compared to 78% and 57% respectively for men. Recent twin studies assessing comorbidity between major depression and alcoholism in women suggest that the co-occurrence of the disorders may be largely genetic (Kendler et al. 1993), though in men the nature of the association is less clear. Such gender differences also exist in the relative prevalence of different disorders. For example, in men drug disorders and dissocial psychological disorder are the most comorbid conditions compared to mood and anxiety among women. Depression may also occur as a direct result of the pharmacological effects of alcohol as well as in response to the complications of alcohol use. Other explanations for the association may include shared family environment, poverty, social isolation and unemployment, or both conditions may develop as secondary features of other disorders such as personality disorder, polysubstance abuse and Briquet's syndrome.

Suicide

About a quarter of people dependent on alcohol attempt suicide, and lifetime risk of suicide is estimated at 3–4% (Edwards et al 1997). Depression is implicated in at least half of the suicides and the attempt is often preceded by an increase in very heavy drinking.

Risk factors for suicide in alcoholics include:

- male
- divorced
- personality disorder
- increasing age
- other drug use
- physical complications
- unemployed
- psychiatric disorder
- history of deliberate self-harm (DSH).

Dissocial personality disorder

In keeping with the Cloniger subtyping of alcohol dependence, those with dissocial personality disorder have an earlier onset of alcohol use disorders, higher rates of drug use and poorer treatment retention and outcome. Risk assessment and a forensic history should routinely be sought.

Pathological jealousy (Othello syndrome)

This is characterized by the abnormal belief (delusion or overvalued idea) of infidelity of the sexual partner though the actual fact of infidelity may or may not be true. In those with alcohol problems the male:female ratio is 2:1. The predominant characteristic is the abnormal quality of the belief and the accompanying behavioural constellation such as the inspection of underwear or sheets for staining, searching of clothes, diaries etc. in an attempt to prove the infidelity. Repetitive demand for proof may lead to severe aggression and murder and therefore specific enquiry into past and threatened violence is mandatory and the partner should be advised of any risk. In one study conducted at a high-security hospital, 14% of convicted murderers were given this diagnosis (Mowatt 1966). The syndrome is not unique to alcohol, with other causes including organic disorders, paranoid personality and the bipolar and schizophrenic psychoses. Abstinence and possibly hospitalization with treatment with antipsychotics may be indicated. In some however, geographical separation is the only effective means of intervention. For a classic review see Shepherd (1961) (see Chapter 18 and 22).

Anxiety states

According to the 'anxiety reduction' theory, alcoholics self-medicate what otherwise might be disabling anxiety. Although a review by Cook concludes 'anxiety traits do not appear to be an *important* (my italics) causal factor in alcoholism', in combination with learning theory it may be regarded as one route to alcohol abuse. Conflicting evidence demonstrating that alcohol may increase, decrease or not effect anxiety levels further complicates the picture. However, clinical studies (Allan 1995) consistently report an association between alcohol problems with rates of comorbidity of between 20–30%. The most common anxiety state is panic disorder (3F:M), followed by obsessive-compulsive disorder (OCD) and phobias. Social phobia tends to precede drinking problems, the later presumably self-medicating anxiety. The relative risk for alcohol disorders among those with social phobia is about twice that of the general population (Marshall 1994). There is evidence that buspirone may be helpful in managing persistent anxiety and may increase retention in treatment.

PTSD

Alcohol use disorder is the most common comorbid diagnosis of men with PTSD, though PTSD is more common in women (25% versus 10%). CNS depressants are a means of dampening the pathological state of hyperarousal associated with PTSD. It has been suggested that the sympathetic hyperactivity that occurs on withdrawal from alcohol can precipitate symptoms of PTSD and thus act as a negative reinforcer for continued consumption.

Eating disorders

Up to 30% of young women with a serious drinking problem have a significant eating disorder (most commonly bulimia) at some time (Lascey & Moureli 1986), and prevalence rates of alcohol misuse in people with bulimia are between 9 and 49% (Goldbloom 1993).

Other drug use

Dependence upon another drug is the most frequent comorbid disorder in someone with an existing dependence syndrome; most commonly used are sedatives, such as benzodiazepines and chlormethiazole.

SOCIAL CONSEQUENCES OF EXCESSIVE ALCOHOL USE

Employment

Turning up late for work may be the first indicator of an alcohol problem. Acute and chronic consumption is associated with both accidental injury and reduced productivity. Alcohol has been implicated in 40% of fatal industrial accidents and 35% of non-fatal work-related accidents.

Family

Heavy drinking imposes considerable strain on finances and is associated with increased rates of physical and sexual abuse. Children are at increased risk of conduct disorder and juvenile delinquency as well as developing alcohol misuse themselves. Children of problem drinkers have been called the 'forgotten children' and have to contend not only with the disruption to their own lives but often also having to care for their parents.

Crime and violence

About 66% of male and 15% of female prisoners have serious drinking problems, with higher rates for illicit drug use. Alcohol is common in episodes of domestic violence as well as being a common cause of public affray and violence. Approximately 10% of assault injuries are sustained from bar glass injuries, with three quarters of these resulting in trauma to the face (Shepherd 1998). A Scottish study (Gillies 1976) of 400 people accused of murder showed over half were intoxicated at the time of the alleged attack (as were a third of their victims). Alcohol is also associated with rape (40–70%) and paedophile offences. Among the young there is also a positive association between drinking and violent offending (Ferguson et al. 1996).

Drinking and driving

The peak age for drink-driving convictions is 21, with a third of convictions arising in those aged 25 or under. Over three-quarters of fatal road traffic accidents involve alcohol, and alcohol-related road traffic accidents are more severe than those in which alcohol does not play a role. About one-third of pedestrians killed by day and 70% killed at night have measurable blood alcohol levels. The legal limit is 80mg alcohol per 100 ml blood ([urinary concentration] = $1.3 \times$ [blood]).

Alcohol withdrawal

On the cessation of alcohol, the previously adaptive changes in neurotransmitter function that contribute (along with hepatic metabolic changes) to the development of tolerance become maladaptive, resulting in an excitatory state arising from unopposed glutaminergic activity. It exists in a spectrum of severity, onset and duration and outcomes.

Withdrawal often commences before the blood alcohol levels reaches zero following cessation (or marked reduction) of use in the dependant drinker. Symptoms usually commence 6–24 hours after last use, peaking at day 2–3 with the highest risk of fits in the first 24–36 hours. Some dependent drinkers may experience no or only minimal withdrawal, manifesting as a few days of insomnia and irritability coming on a couple of days after their last drink. More severely dependent drinkers are woken by withdrawal symptoms within a few hours of their last drink as blood plasma levels fall, necessitating the immediate consumption of alcohol to relive the symptoms (the can by the bed).

Repeated alcohol withdrawal episodes may be associated with a kindling effect, such that subsequent episodes of withdrawal become more severe. Other factors implicated in the severity of withdrawal include amount and duration of drinking, the use of other sedative drugs such as benzodiazepines and intercurrent medical illnesses.

Alcohol withdrawal features

- **Early (12–24 hours):** sweating, tachycardia, increased blood pressure, tremor, nausea, anorexia and vomiting, agitation, anxiety and panic, insomnia and restlessness, transient auditory hallucinations.
- **Middle (24–72 hours):** temperature elevation, dehydration, grand mal seizures (associated with low K^+ and Mg^{++}), delirium tremens with misperception, loss of insight and visual and/or auditory hallucinations. Tactile disturbances such as pins and needles, burning, crawling and numbness, 'electric flea' tactile hallucinations.
- **Late (72+ hours):** persistent insomnia and nightmares, tremor and confusion, hallucinosis.

DETOXIFICATION AND WITHDRAWAL MANAGEMENT

Medically assisted detoxification is not a stand-alone treatment. Its function lies on a spectrum from an elective admission as part of a planned attempt at abstinence with well considered aftercare plans to a crisis harm-reduction admission, prompted by a severe withdrawal or physical frailty. Detoxification should ideally only be undertaken after a full assessment with a treatment plan that outlines not only immediate treatment but also considers broader psychosocial issues that may be risk factors for relapse on discharge. The relapse rate following treatment is high, with about 60% returning to problem drinking within a year. Incomplete attempts at detoxification can lead to nihilism in the patient. Liaison between referrer, general practitioner (GP), specialist, after-care providers and client should begin before treatment and continue after detoxification.

In most cases withdrawal can be safely managed in the community with the support of a GP or community drug team. Stable accommodation and the commitment of a responsible carer are essential components for any community-based detoxification attempt. In the absence of such supports or in the presence of contraindications to out-patient detoxification, such as a history of delirium tremens (see Box 27.9) the patient should be admitted to hospital.

Treatment regime for medically assisted withdrawal from alcohol

After a full history and examination, treatment of withdrawal should be implemented at the earliest point to minimize the risk of fits. Benzodiazepines with intermediate half-lives and rapid onset of action such as chlordiazepoxide (Librium) and diazepam (Valium) are preferable. Chlormethiazole (Heminevrin) should be avoided because of the risk of severe interactions (respiratory depression in overdose) and risk of abuse. Carbmazepine and barbiturates are also effective detoxification agents, but are rarely used. Although not licensed for use in the UK, GHB (gamma hydroxybutyrate) is an effective agent for alcohol withdrawal and is used widely in parts of Europe.

Medication forms only one part of a medically assisted detoxification. Explanation of symptoms, their progress and how medication helps should be given to all clients preferably before the commencement of detox. Clients will often be agitated throughout withdrawal and explanations and information may need to be repeated.

A starting dose of 40 mg chlordiazepoxide 6-hourly or equivalent acting benzodiazepine such as diazepam 10–20 mg qid and oxazepam 15–30 mg qid in combination with close physical monitoring allows for titration of dosage. Doses may need to be as high as 300 mg chlordiazepoxide a day but undertreatment of withdrawal is potentially more problematic than oversedation. Those with comorbid benzodiazepine dependence may require higher doses. Reduction in dose over 5–10 days is usually sufficient. Adjunctive treatments such as clonidine may be useful in reducing autonomic hyperactivity.

The use of withdrawal scales such as the CIWA-AR (Clinical Institute Withdrawal Assessment for Alcohol Revised) or the AWS (Alcohol Withdrawal Scale) are useful in guiding treatment. Administered three times a day, the CIMA-AR is a 10-item scale scored out of 67. Scores above 10 indicate the patient is at risk of withdrawal complications if treatment is not given.

The concurrent administration of anticonvulsants in those prone to fits (history of epilepsy, withdrawal seizures,

head injury) is used in some units though drugs such as carbamazepine are unlikely to reach therapeutic levels during the peak time for fits. Optimal treatment in such cases includes close monitoring with a withdrawal rating scale and administration of benzodiazepines preferably using a loading dose regime ensuring suppression of withdrawal. Shorter-acting drugs such as lorazepam may be helpful. If the patient experiences recurrent fits they should be investigated to exclude other responsible pathologies such as epilepsy. Valproate may have some role but phenytoin should be avoided. All patients should be given an intramuscular multivitamin preparation on admission and oral supplements, especially of the B group. Daily doses of administered thiamine should not exceed 50–100mg since the absorption is saturable and no benefit is gained from higher doses. Observation for intercurrent infection, dehydration and suicidal behaviour are important especially in those with who experience delirium tremens.

Delirium tremens

Delirium tremens (DTs) is a short-lived toxic, confusional state with somatic disturbance, usually arising as a consequence of absolute or relative withdrawal of alcohol in severely dependent individuals. Disorientation and confusion are the hallmarks of the syndrome accompanied by vivid (usually visual) hallucinations, the risk of seizures and evidence of autonomic overactivity. Occurring in less than 5% of withdrawals, delirium tremens remains potentially fatal, although actual mortality rates are unclear. Reports indicate that of those 5% experiencing DTs, it may be fatal in up to 10%. Historically known as 'the horrors', the DTs peak on day 3–4 (though may occur up to a week after stopping drinking) of withdrawal and are characterized by a dramatic and rapidly changing picture, with a characteristic triad of clouding of consciousness, sensory distortion and tremor. It frequently has its onset at night heralded by a prodrome of agitation, insomnia and fear (see Box 27.10).

Past withdrawal complicated by seizures or DTs is the best predictor of future alcohol withdrawal complications. Management includes aggressive reduction in autonomic arousal and a reduction in seizure risk with benzo-diazepines, which in the highly agitated patient may be more effectively administered intravenously.

Patients should be nursed where possible in a side room, with low but adequate levels of stimulation with frequent review. Neuroleptics may be required in extreme cases especially where hallucinations are not controlled with high dose benzodiazepines. Drugs such as haloperidol should be used cautiously and in low doses (2.5–5 mg) since they may lower an already compromised seizure threshold. Predisposing factors include medical illness and older age, with a physical examination and routine bloods being mandatory to exclude precipitating factors such as dehydration, metabolic disturbance and intercurrent infection, all of which must be treated aggressively if present.

Post detoxification-relapse prevention

Pharmacotherapy

Maintaining abstinence after detoxification is difficult. Approaches include both psychosocial interventions such as AA and CBT as well as drug treatments (Marlatt & Gordon 1985).

Disulfiram

This is an inhibitor of aldehyde dehydrogenase that causes a 'flushing' reaction by blocking further ethanol metabolism at the acetaldehyde level. Its effects may be explained by both classic and operant learning theories as well as cue exposure with response prevention. It is intended to prevent impulsive resumption of drinking in response to craving or other cues (see Chapter 38).

Starting with 3 or 4 days' loading dose of about 600–800 mg per day the usual maintenance dose is 200–400 mg. Consumption of alcohol by the patient will lead to the disulfiram-ethanol reaction, with flushing, tachycardia, dyspnoea, headaches, nausea and vomiting with symptoms due to the accumulation of acetaldehyde. Provided consumption ceases these symptoms will abate, continued consumption may however lead to hypotensive episodes and even myocardial infarction. All patients should carry an Antabuse treatment card. Contraindications to use include cardiac failure, significantly deranged LFTs, breastfeeding, psychosis and severe personality disorder. Those with disordered liver function need regular monitoring since disulfiram may cause hepatic dysfunction.

Consumption should not be unsupervised and regular review in clinic is mandatory to assess progress and occurrence of side effects. It is generally most useful in highly motivated groups and where a wife or friend may provide supervised administration. Community reinforcement programmes have proven highly effective in enhancing the efficacy of disulfiram. The most favorable outcome is seen in those who are male, older, have severe dependence, have fewer psychological problems and stable social support (Miller 1992).

Naltrexone and acamprosate

These improve treatment outcomes in those with alcohol dependence who are motivated and comply with treatment. The effect of both is significantly enhanced when they are delivered as part of a comprehensive psychosocial treatment programme.

Naltrexone is an opiate receptor antagonist, which reduces the positive reinforcing effects of alcohol and opiates in man and is thought to negate the euphoria and reinforcement associated with alcohol and to reduce craving. It reduces the risk of a lapse becoming a relapse. It has been shown to be more effective than placebo (and in a head-to-head trial more effective than acamprosate) and increases the time to first drink, days of abstinence and amount consumed on days when drinking. It should be avoided in those with significant hepatic dysfunction or who are receiving opiates. It is contraindicated during pregnancy and lactation. Side effects include gastrointestinal disturbance, insomnia, drowsiness and blurred vision. The dose is 50 mg daily. Baseline LFTs and biochemical monitoring is advisable.

Acamprosate (calcium bisacetyl homotaurine) is a synthetic GABA analogue. It is thought to reduce craving by reducing glutamate activity and stimulating inhibitory GABA transmission. Trials suggest a positive effect on outcome, with evidence of a dose-related response (Paille et al. 1995) with a post-drug therapy effect. It has a good side-effect profile, no abuse potential and like naltrexone is a non-aversive therapy. There is some evidence that combinations of anticraving pharmacotherapies are more effective that when used alone (Keifer & Wiedman 2002).

Other promising pharmacotherapies include the newer drugs gabapentin and ondansetron. There is little evidence for the SSRIs, bromocriptine or buspirone in the treatment of alcoholism.

Psychological interventions

There is strong clinical evidence from numerous studies supporting the efficacy of CBT in relapse prevention and in treating alcohol dependence. Other effective interventions include cue-exposure with response prevention, contingency management, social skills training and relaxation techniques. Family therapy can be useful especially in the supervision of drug administration. It may be the case that single-sex groups are more beneficial for women in recovery while for men mixed groups are preferable (Hodgins et al. 1997).

Psychosocial relapse prevention strategies

Relapse prevention (RP) describes a range of strategies aimed at identifying, addressing and minimizing risk factors for a return to substance abuse as outlined by Marlatt & Gordon (1985). It supports the individual in maintaining abstinence or moderating consumption patterns. The evidence for psychosocial relapse prevention strategies being effective in reducing alcohol intake, reducing the severity of relapse and improving psychosocial outcomes is strong (Dimeff & Marlett 1994). These are best delivered after acute withdrawal symptoms have subsided and should take into account current coping and social skills, comorbid illnesses, other substance abuse and cognitive impairment. They are composed of a series of cognitive and behavioural strategies which cope with the spectrum from lapse (an initial return to use) to relapse (reinstatement of dependent use). At its core are the identification of triggers for relapse (negative and positive emotional states, poor coping skills, social isolation, craving, family and beliefs) and the development of global self-management strategies (Dimeff & Marlett 1994). Questionnaires such as the Situational Confidence Questionnaire may be helpful in identifying high-risk situations. The three main components of RP are cognitive restructuring, skills training and lifestyle balancing.

Motivational interviewing

Motivational interviewing (MI) or motivational enhancement therapy (MET) describes a means of communication that facilitates a client's readiness to change by addressing ambivalence and moving clients through a cycle of change from precontemplation to action. First described by the American psychologist Bill Miller (Miller et al. 1991), motivational interviewing is based on five key principles that have utility both within the fields of addiction and eating disorders but may also be used in any aspect of the doctor–patient relationship where the patient is ambivalent about implementing a potentially beneficial change. The five tenets are: express empathy; help client to see discrepancies in their behaviours; avoid argument; roll with resistance; support patient's sense of self efficacy. The central issue to appreciate is that people are only motivated to change a behaviour when they 'mind about it', not when the doctor does. This is very different from the usual paternalistic and authoritarian approach on which doctors are reared. It is not enough to expect a patient to do something we tell them to do; people change their behaviours when they perceive that they are able to and that they will be better for it. The results of the Project MATCH study in America showed little difference in outcome between MET, CBT and 12-Step Facilitation psychological treatments and suggested little was gained from matching patient attributes to therapies (Project Match Research Group 1997).

Brief interventions

Consisting of an assessment of alcohol intake, information on harmful drinking and clear advice for the individual, brief interventions have consistently been shown to reduce intake by about 25% (*Effective Healthcare* 1997). Further evidence suggests that brief interventions are as effective as more expensive specialist treatments. Chick (1988) demonstrated no difference in abstinence rates at two years between groups receiving minimal intervention and those receiving more costly intensive therapies. Tiered care delivery with the sequential delivery of increasingly intensive care is an appropriate treatment pathway for many, while attempts at remaining in contact with clients through extended case monitoring can also be useful.

Alcoholics Anonymous

Founded by recovering alcoholics 'Dr Bob' and 'Bill W' in 1935, AA now represents the largest self-help group in the world, with 5–10% of treatment enlisted alcoholics attending. For some it is a panacea, for others another failed therapy. Based on 12 steps, the premise is that alcoholism is a disease without cure that can only be held at bay a day at a time. The fellowship provides friendship, advice and support and takes place at meetings with both diverse clientele and location. Clients admit their powerlessness over the disease and look to a higher power to return their sanity. AA remains a cheap, widely available form of support and all alcoholics should be encouraged to attend at least a dozen or so different meetings to see if the format suits them. Al-Anon and Al-Teen provide support for family members of alcohol dependent individuals.

Residential rehabilitation

These houses are a popular though expensive means of consolidating upon initial abstinence. Often based on the 'Minnesota model' (first five steps of the 12 AA steps), additional interventions include social skills training, relaxation techniques, and structured relapse prevention programmes. They vary greatly in outcome but can be incredibly effective for some clients at a particular stage in their drinking careers.

Provision of service

Primary care is a highly suitable environment for the early detection and treatment of alcohol disorders. Support from specialist services should extend to general hospital services, especially emergency departments and trauma wards. Community alcohol teams should liaise between hospital and GP-based services and where possible support treatment within the community. Specialized assessments may be needed for pregnant women and those being considered for liver transplant.

PROGNOSIS

Outcome is not unitary and recovery is a process not an event. Therefore many dimensions can be assessed for outcome measures, not just alcohol but psychosocial functioning and health. Further, outcome can only be considered at that point in time at which it is assessed, since the course of drinking problems is rarely stable with the majority flitting between points on the abstinent–troubled drinking axis. A poor prognosis is associated with alcoholic brain damage, comorbid psychiatric disorder, divorced status, criminal record, low IQ, poor support and motivation.

The Rand report (Amor et al. 1976), a multicentre trial with an 18-month follow-up, showed only a quarter of patients remained abstinent for six months, with less than 10% at 18 months. However, there were persistent reductions in levels of consumption in over 70% at follow-up.

Edwards' follow-up of alcoholics over 10 years found that 25% had continued troubled drinking and 12% were abstinent (Edwards et al. 1988) The remainder had a patchwork of abstinence and troubled drinking.

A 60-year follow up of two American groups of socially divergent drinkers (Harvard graduates and socially disadvantaged Boston adolescents) demonstrates the varied outcomes of those with drinking problems (Valient 2003). At some point, about a quarter of both groups met the criteria for alcohol abuse. In general, the death rate among those with an alcohol dependence is two to three times higher than the normal population, with the excess deaths attributable to cirrhosis, unnatural causes, lung and oropharyngeal cancers, and cardiovascular disease. The increase in mortality was twice as great for those under 60 than over 60; indeed alcohol dependence was rare after 70 (half had died and a fifth had achieved long term abstinence). Other than severity of dependence, the predictors of a positive outcome were (1) finding a non-pharmacological substitute for alcohol, (2) new relationships, and (3) compulsory contingency supervision (immediate adverse consequence on consumption) or membership of a spiritual group. Men who achieved abstinence had attended on average 20 times more AA meetings than men who continued to drink. Finally, the study suggested that those severely dependent drinkers, with early onset and genetic loading for dependence from socially disadvantaged backgrounds were more likely to achieve stable abstinence than other men. In summary Valiant suggests, '... the most and the least severe alcoholics appeared to enjoy the best, long term chance of remission'.

FURTHER READING

Kendler KS, Heath AC, Neale MC et al. (1992) A twin-family study of alcoholism in women. *American Journal of Psychiatry* **151**: 707–15.
Victor M, Adams RD & Collins GH (1971) *Wernicke-Korsakoff Syndrome.* Philadelphia: FA Davis Company.

REFERENCES

Allan CA (1995) Alcohol problems and anxiety disorders: a critical review. *Alcohol and Alcoholism* **30**: 145–51.
Armor DJ, Polich JM & Stambul HB (1976) *Alcoholism and Treatment.* Santa Monica: Rand Corporation and Interscience.
Bearn J, Gossop M & Strang J (1996) Randomised double blind comparison of lofexidine and methadone in the outpatient treatment of opiate withdrawal. *Drug and Alcohol Dependence.*
Besson JAO (1993) Structural and functional brain imaging in alcoholism and drug use. *Current Opinion in Psychiatry* **6**: 403–10.
Blume SB (1986) *Women and Alcohol Problems: Public Policy Issues. NIAA Research Monograph No 16*, pp. 294–311. Washington: DHHS Publication.
Chick J, Ritson B, Connaughton J et al. (1988) Advice versus extended treatments for alcoholism: a controlled study. *British Journal of Addiction* **290**: 965–7.
Cloniger CR, Bohman M & Sigvardsson S (1981) Inheritance of alcohol abuse cross fostering: analysis of adopted men. *Archives of General Psychiatry* **38**: 861–8.
Davis KM & Wu JY (2000) Role of glutaminergic and GABAergic systems in alcoholism. *Journal of Biomedical Science* **8**: 7–19.
Dimeff L & Marlatt G. (1995) Relapse precention. In: *The Handbook of Alcoholism Treatment Approaches: Effective Alternatives*, pp. 174–96. Massachusetts: Allyn & Bacon.
Edwards G, Brown D, Oppenheimer E, Sheehan M & Taylor C (1988) Long term outcome for patients with alcohol problems: the search for predictors. *British Journal of Addiction* **82**: 801–11.
Edwards G, Marshall EJ & Cook CC (1997) *The Treatment of Drinking Problems: A Guide for the Helping Professions*, p. 95. Cambridge: Cambridge University Press. *Effective Healthcare.* Brief Interventions and Alcohol Use. November 1993, No 7.
Ferguson DM, Lynskey MT & Horwood LJ (1996) Alcohol misuse and juvenile offending in adolescence. *Addiction* **9**: 483–4.
Gillies H (1976) Homicide in the west of Scotland. *British Journal of Psychiatry.* **128**: 105–27.
Goldbloom DS (1993) Alcohol misuse and eating disorders: aspects of an association. *Alcohol and Alcoholism* **28**: 375–81.
Goodwin DW, Hermansen L, Guze SB et al. (1973) Alcohol problems in adoptees raised apart from alcoholic biological parents. *Archives of General Psychiatry* **28**: 238–43.
Hall W & Farrell M (1997) Comorbidity of mental disorders with substance misuse. *British Journal of Psychiatry* **171**: 4–5.
Harper CG, Kril JJ & Hollowat RL (1985) Brain shrinkage in chronic alcoholics: a pathological study. *British Medical Journal* **290**: 501–4.
Hodgins DC, Nady el-Guebaly & Addington J (1997) Treatment of substance abusers: single or mixed gender programmes? *Addiction* **92**: 805–12.
Hrubec Z & Omenn GS (1981) Evidence of genetic predisposition to alcoholic psychosis and cirrhosis: twin concordances for alcoholism and its biological end points by zygosity among male veterans. *Alcoholism, Clinical and Experimental Research* **5**: 207–15.
Institute of Alcohol studies (2004) *Excessive and problem drinking in Great Britain.* Online. Available at: www.ias.org.uk
Jones KL & Smith DW (1973) Recognition of the fetal alcohol syndrome in infancy. *Lancet* **ii**: 999–1001.
Kaminski M, Rumeau-Rouquette C & Schwartz D (1976) Consommation d'alcohol chez les femmes enceintes et isue de la grossesse. *Revue d'Epidemiologie et Sante Publique.* **24**: 27–40.
Keifer F & Wiedman K (2002)
Kendler KS, Heath AC, Neale MC et al. (1992) A population based twin study of alcoholism.
Kendler KS, Heath AC, Neale MC, Kessler RC & Eaves LJ (1993) Alcoholism and major depression in women: a twin study of the causes of comorbidity. *Archives of General Psychiatry* **50**: 690–8.
Kessler RC, Crum RM, Warner LA & Nelson CB (1997) et al. Lifetime co-occurrence of DSM-IIIR alcohol abuse and dependence with other psychiatric disorders in the National Comorbidity Study. *Archives of General Psychology* **54**: 313–21.
Kranzler HR & Rosenthal RN (2003) Dual diagnosis: alcoholism and co-morbid psychiatric disorders. *American Journal of Addiction* **12**: S26–S40.
Lacey JH & Moureli E (1986) Bulimic alcoholics: some features of a clinical sub-group. *British Journal of Addiction* **81**: 389–93.
Littleton J & Little H (1994) Current concepts of ethanol dependence. *Addiction* **89**: 1397–412.
Marlatt G & Gordon J (1985) *Relapse Prevention: Maintainance Strategies in the Treatment of Addictive Behaviours.* New York: The Guildford Press.
Marshall JR (1994) The diagnosis and treatment of social phobia and alcohol abuse. *Bulletin of the Menninger Clinic.* **58**: 58–66.
Merikangas KR, Angst J, Eaton W et al. (1996) Comorbidity and boundaries of affective disorders with anxiety disorders and

substance misuse; results of an international task force. *British Journal of Psychiatry* **168** (June suppl): 58–67.

Miller WR & Rollnick S (1991) *Motivational interviewing: Preparing People to Change Addictive Behaviour*. New York: Guilford Press.

Miller WR (1992) Effectiveness of treatment for substance abuse: reasons for optimism. *Journal of Substance Abuse Treatment* **9**: 93–102.

Mowat RR (1966) *Morbid Jealousy and Murder*. London: Tavistock Publications.

Office of Population, Census and Statistics (1996) report. Her Majesty's Stationary Office.

Paille FM, Guelfi JD, Perkins AC et al. (1995) Double blind multicentre trial of acamprosate in maintaining abstinence from alcohol. *Alcohol and Alcoholism* **30**: 239–47.

Pickens RW, Svikis DS, McGue M et al. (1991) Heterogeneity in the inheritance of alcoholism: A study of male and female twins. *Archives of General Psychiatry* **48**: 19–28.

Project MATCH Research Group (1997) Matching alcoholism treatments to client heterogeneity post-treatment outcomes. *Journal of Studies on Alcoholism*, Jan.

Reiger DA, Farmer ME, Rae DS et al. (1991) Comorbidity of mental disorders with alcohol and other drug abuse results from the epidemiological and catchment area (ECA) study. *Journal of the American Medical Association* **264**: 2511.

Shepherd J (1998) The circumstances and prevention of bar glass injury. *Addiction* **93**: 5–8.

Shepherd M (1961) Morbid jealousy: some clinical and social aspects of a psychiatric symptom. *Journal of Mental Science* **107**: 687–753.

Steinhausen HC, Willms J & Spohr H-L (1993) Correlates of psychopathology and intelligence in children with Fetal Alcohol Syndrome. *Journal of Clinical Psychiatry 1994* **35**: 323–31.

Valiant GE (2003) A 60 year follow up of alcoholic men. *Addiction* **98**: 1043–51.

Victor M, Adams Rd & Collins GH (1971) *Wernike–Korsakoff Syndrome*. Philadelphia: FA Davis Company.

Wallace P & Haines A (1985) The use of a questionnaire in general practice to increase the recognition of patients with excessive alcohol use. *British Medical Journal* **290**: 1949–53.

Winokur G (1979) Alcoholism and depression in the same family. In: Goodwin DW & Erikson CK (eds) *Alcoholism and Affective Disorders: Clinical, Genetic, and Biochemical Studies*, pp. 49–56. New York: SP Medical and Scientific Books.

Psychoactive drug misuse

Adam Winstock

INTRODUCTION

The last 40 years has seen a rapid expansion in the availability, range and popularity of psychoactive drugs with lifetime experience of their use almost normalized as behaviour. A recent study of 3000 second year University students in the UK reported that over 50% reported lifetime use of cannabis, with a third having used other drugs such as LSD or ecstasy (Webb et al. 1996). Although historically demonized by society, the true image of the average consumer of illicit substances is more benign. Drug policies driven by political will and social expectancies have compounded significantly the harm associated with their use.

The harm related to most drugs is more often related to the behaviours and patterns of drug use than to the toxic effects of the drug *per se*. There is a spectrum of drug use within society (see Figure 28.1) and treatment services must respond to both the small number with dependence as well as the far greater proportion of non-dependent users who experience problems related to their use. A more pragmatic view of drug use and societal responses is encompassed in the philosophy of harm reduction, which underpins drug treatment services in most parts of the Western world. Harm reduction accepts that use of drugs will occur and advocates providing the safest environment for consumption combined with education and access to treatment, thereby protecting both the individual and their community. In recent years the opening of supervised injecting rooms, where drug users are able to inject in a safe, sterile and monitored environment, have demonstrated that such approaches save lives, reduce risk and facilitate access to treatment.

DEFINITIONS

Problems associated with substance abuse are categorized in ICD-10 under the heading 'Mental and behavioural

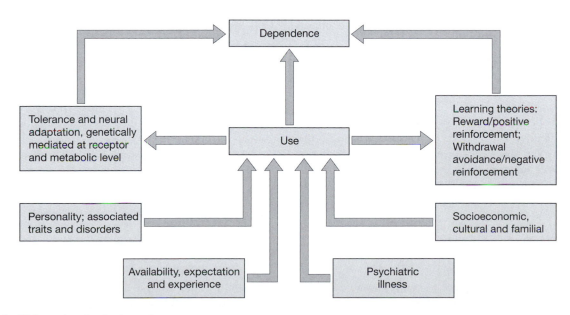

Figure 28.1 Risks and routes to dependence.

disorders due to psychoactive substance abuse' (F10–F19). The available codes denote both substance type and pattern of use as well as the particular disorder consequent upon that type of use. Categories include acute intoxication, psychotic state, amnestic syndrome and withdrawal among others. Some of the ICD definitions are given below.

ICD and DSM definitions are broadly similar. Both are largely based on Gross & Edwards' 1976 definition of alcohol dependency with the main difference between the two being that ICD has a separate item for craving or compulsion to use. Both allow classification of the current status of the user and neither tolerance nor dependence are essential diagnostic criteria in either. Thus contrary to popular belief, a withdrawal syndrome is neither a necessary nor sufficient symptom for the diagnosis. Furthermore, both classification systems recognize dependence as a condition that can exhibit a spectrum of severity. According to ICD-10, dependence may be regarded as 'a cluster of physiological, behavioural and cognitive phenomena in which the use of a substance or a class of substances takes on a much higher priority for a given individual than other behaviours that once had greater value'.

ICD-10 diagnostic guidelines suggest that at least three or more of the following have to have been present together at some time during the previous year:

- a strong desire or sense of compulsion to take the substance
- difficulties in controlling substance-taking behaviour in terms of its onset, termination, or levels of use
- a physiological withdrawal state
- evidence of tolerance
- progressive neglect of alternative interests or pleasures
- persisting with substance abuse despite clear evidence of overtly harmful consequences.

Despite operational criteria allowing uniform diagnosis, dependence is not an all-or-nothing concept. Like other illnesses, it exists as a spectrum, measured not only by the degree of neurophysiological adaptation and loss of control over use but also by the degree of social, physical and psychological harm that has arisen as a result of continued substance use.

Both DSM-IV and ICD-10 also allow for a more general diagnostic category of problem or harmful use. ICD-10 carries a broad definition of harmful use defined as 'pattern of psychoactive substance use that is causing damage to health, physical or mental'. The DSM-IV concept of 'abuse' is perhaps more controversial. Abuse is defined by scoring 1 or more on the following items:

1. Use leading to neglect of personal, social, occupational roles.
2. Use in an unsafe or dangerous situation.
3. Use leading to repeated problems with the law.
4. Continued use despite relationship, domestic, occupation or educational problems.

Reward

Drugs are likeable or reinforcing. All drugs of dependence release DA within the mesolimbic (ventrotegmental 'VTA') DA system, with significant increases in the nucleus accumbens and this is thought to mediate the rewarding effects of drugs. This so-called 'reward or pleasure pathway' underlies most driven human passions, be they food, sex, thirst or chocolate! Drugs of dependence seem to 'highjack' the body's natural rewards pathway such that, after chronic administration, the brain learns to preferentially derive pleasure from drug reinforcers. The reinforcement of drugs differ between individuals with one study showing cocaine to be likeable in those subjects with low D2 receptor levels and associated with unpleasant effects in those with high receptor levels (see Lingford-Hughes & Nutt 2003 for a review of the neurobiology of addiction).

Tolerance and neuroadaptation

The concepts of tolerance, withdrawal and relapse are now beginning to be understood not only at a psycho-behavioural level but also a neurochemical one. Continued administration of a psychoactive drug may lead to adaptive changes at three main levels: *receptor* (up or down regulation through decreased expression, affinity or coupling to secondary messengers); *transmitter* (increased or decreased release or production); and *metabolism* (e.g. enzyme induction or inhibition). The first two types of change may be regarded as neuroadaptation, resulting in the development of *tolerance*. Tolerance may be seen as a homeostatic adaptation to chronic administration of a drug, to ameliorate longer-term toxicity and to allow the organism to continue functioning while chronically intoxicated. Pharmodynamic tolerance is present when higher doses of the drug are needed to produce a given response. Metabolic tolerance is the increased capacity to metabolize a drug. Cross-tolerance occurs when tolerance to a drug is accompanied by tolerance to those of a different chemical group (e.g. alcohol and benzodiazepines at the GABA-A receptor). It should be noted that there are non-biological mechanisms of tolerance which play an important role in the development of dependence, such as behavioural tolerance, which involve associative (classical and operant conditioning) and non associative (habituation) mechanisms (Goudie & Emmett-Oglesby 1989).

Withdrawal

The adaptive mechanisms responsible for the emergence of tolerance are 'adaptive' only in the presence of continued drug administration. When drug administration ceases after a period of chronic use, these adaptive changes are unopposed and become maladaptive and the syndrome of withdrawal ensues (see Chapter 27). Withdrawal may be defined as a characteristic pattern of signs and symptoms (psycho-behavioural and physical) that occur when a drug is stopped after a period of chronic administration or an antagonist is given. The experience is unpleasant, occasionally life-threatening and alleviation of withdrawal distress through use of the drug is often cited as a reason for continued use. Neuroimaging studies in dependent users of heroin, cocaine and alcohol have demonstrated reduced levels of D2 receptors, which may recover to some extent but often last for months (Volkow et al. 1999). Hypodopaminergic function is also believed to underlie some of the common symptoms of drug withdrawal, namely craving, drug seeking, and dysphoria.

Dependence

The reinforcing properties of most drugs of dependence and abuse are mediated through the mesolimbic dopaminergic pathway, which projects to the ventral striatum, with the nucleus accumbens as pivotal (Altman et al. 1996). Although dopamine is thought to be the central neurotransmitter in this process it is becoming clear that many others such as glutamate, 5HT and GABA have major but as yet unclear roles.

The reinforcing properties or the use/abuse liabilities of substances differ between drug classes but can also be impacted significantly by a number of other factors, namely the 'effect profile' (intensity of the effect, the speed of onset and duration of action), which is impacted upon by the dose, preparation, purity and route of administration. The effect profile and its relationship to abuse liability can be broadly expressed in an equation:

$$\text{Abuse liability} = \frac{\text{intensity of effect}}{\text{speed of onset} \times \text{duration of action}}$$

Thus higher potency preparations of a substance are more reinforcing than less potent ones (e.g. cocaine powder versus coca leaves) often because they are associated with a more intense effect, which in turn is often related to the alternative routes of administration that purified products permit. Generally the quicker the onset (smoking and injecting), the shorter the high (crack) and the more intense the high (crack) the more reinforcing the substance and the more frequent the desire and/or need for administrations. For example, cigarettes act as a highly reinforcing nicotine delivery system that requires smokers to light up hourly as plasma levels drop to the point where craving begins. An understanding of the interplay between route and duration of action helps explain why slower delivery systems such as patches are used to wean smokers off nicotine since longer-acting less intense effects are less reinforcing and easier to refrain from. A similar explanation in part helps us understand why oral methadone is preferred in treatment to injectables in many clients seeking abstinence.

THE EFFECT OF DRUGS

The effect of a drug will depend upon the interplay of cognitive 'set' (mood state the person was in at the time of drug consumption), environmental 'setting' (social situation – including the mood of those one is with – in which the drug was taken) as well as the dose, type and purity of drug. As the dose of a drug increases, the role of the environment in drug effect becomes less noticeable while the pharmacologically mediated ones of arousal or sedation become more marked.

PREVALENCE OF SUBSTANCE ABUSE

Almost two-thirds of those aged 16–24 years have taken an illicit drug in the last year. Cannabis is the mostly widely used drug with almost three million users last year (11% of those aged 16–59 years). Class A drug use has remained stable with about 8% having used in the last year. The only drug that appears to be increasing in popularity is cocaine. Levels of drug use are highest in those aged 20–24 years. The 1996 OPCS survey of psychiatric morbidity in the UK population showed the prevalence of substance abuse to be 4.7% for alcohol dependence and 2.2% for drug dependence (Office of Population, Census and Statistics 1996). The American 1991 ECA study (Reiger et al. 1990) reported even higher figures, with lifetime prevalence of 13.5% alcohol abuse, 6.1% substance abuse disorder, 3.2% comorbid substance abuse and other mental disorder, with male:female ratios of 2:1 for alcohol and 4:1 for substance use disorders.

AETIOLOGY (see Figure 28.1)

Constitutional, environmental and childhood factors contribute the majority of risk for developing substance use disorders. Often there is an interplay of various risk factors, each compounding the other, giving rise to an 'interactive web of causation'. Risk factors such as positive family histories, childhood abuse, disorganized neighbourhoods, poor academic attainment, limited opportunity and expectation for success, conduct disorder, attention deficit hyperactivity disorder (ADHD), depression, post-traumatic shock disorder (PTSD), often exist in a matrix devoid of protective factors such as love, achievement, family and religion. Some of the most important aetiological factors are briefly covered below.

Individual factors

Genetics

Overall the heritability of dependence (not use or abuse) is thought be around 30%. It has been suggested that certain

D2 polymorphisms coding for the dopamine receptor may underlie vulnerability to substance dependence through coding for personality traits (Blum et al. 1990). Similarly the DA D4 polymorphism, associated with the behavioural trait of thrill seeking and attention deficit disorder is considered by some to be an indirect risk factor for substance abuse

Personality

Despite 100 years of searching, the Holy Grail of the addictive personality remains elusive. What has become recognized are a number of personality traits that may predispose to or otherwise associate with drug use. For example, both dissocial personality disorder and emotionally unstable 'impulsive' (borderline) personality disorder are associated with substance use, with early antisocial behaviour being one of the best predictors of later drug dependence. Both novelty seeking and low impulse control are also associated, with Cloniger (1994) suggesting that those who are high in novelty seeking and low in harm avoidance may be more prone to substance misuse.

Psychological models

See section on alcohol aetiology in Chapter 27.

Social

Social deprivation, dysfunctional neighbourhoods, childhood abuses, peer group selection and influence, familial drug use, cultural attitudes and drug availability all contribute to the social matrix that the individual's drug use is placed within. Demographic variables such as unemployment, gender, and age are obviously also important.

Dual diagnosis

Given the ubiquitous presence of drug misuse across social classes and races, the likelihood of psychiatric patients presenting with problems related to their use is commonplace. Consequently the dual diagnosis patient (one with a severe mental illness and comorbid problematic use of substances (not just dependence), is becoming the rule and not the exception in many inner cities and now represent perhaps the most needy, but most poorly resourced, group in the whole of psychiatry (Hall & Farrell 1997).

Two recent community studies demonstrate the high rates of coexistence of these disorders. A Camberwell study (Johnson 1997) reported about one third of patients attached to a community mental health team had concurrent alcohol or substance misuse problems. A more recent four-city study of community mental health attendees suggested even higher figures with 44% reporting past year harmful use of alcohol and or problem drug use. Conversely three quarters of drug service and over 80% of alcohol service clients reported past year psychiatric disorder (Weaver et al. 2003).

Cannabis was the drug most frequently reported by problems drug users, although a quarter also reported drinking at harmful levels with 10% experiencing severe alcohol problems.

The comorbidity of substance use and mental illness results in uniformly poor prognosis (see Box 28.1).

Compliance by patients with psychiatric/medications is often poor. It is even worse among those who use substances. For example, Owen et al. (1996) looked at compliance among 161 patients with Schizophrenia and found that they were eight times more likely to be noncompliant with their medication that those who did not abuse substances and this was associated with worst symptoms at six months. Explanations for poorer compliance may include a poorer understating of the nature of the illness and benefits of medication, more difficulty in engagement and retention in treatment contact outside the hospital setting, less family support and possibly higher rates of side-effects due to higher dose of medication. Higher dose may be needed because of drug-exacerbated positive symptoms as well as direct antagonism of neuroleptics (e.g. cannabis). Compliance therapy based on motivational interviewing is useful in improving compliance and treatment outcome.

Possible explanations for the high rates of comorbidity (other than a common environmental or genetic predisposition) include:

- Substance use may lead to psychological problems as a direct result of toxicity or indirectly as a consequence of the psychosocial consequences of drug use (Meyer 1986). Frequently, substance use will aggravate a pre-existing psychiatric condition (see Box 28.2).
- Psychiatric illness may lead to self-medication with psychoactive substances in an attempt to relieve the distress of the illness or the side-effects of treatment they are prescribed, e.g. fatigue, mental sluggishness with neuroleptics.
- A shared common environment characterized by other factors such as socio-economic disadvantage, emotional deprivation, social disorganization, childhood abuse, genetic loading and adult trauma.

Box 28.1   Associations of comorbidity
Increased rates of psychiatric admission – longer admissions, shorter remissions, higher rates of sectioning
Increased rates of violence
Increased rates of suicidal behaviour
Increased rates of health service utilization
Increased rates of non compliance with treatment
Increased rates of depot and high dose neuroleptic treatment
Increased rates of homelessness, unemployment and imprisonment
Poorer treatment access and efficacy
Poorer treatment outcomes in both substance use and psychiatric treatment populations

Box 28.2 How drugs exacerbate mental illness through their pharmacological effects

Compound pre-existing 'cognitive set', e.g. anxiety, paranoia

Direct pharmacological effects, e.g. positive symptoms with stimulants

Antagonize medication effect centrally, e.g. cannabis on neuroleptic medication

Metabolic interactions, e.g. cytochrome P450 induction/inhibition

Impair already compromised information processing system reducing efficacy of psychological/cognitive therapies

Since high rates of comorbidity initially found in clinical settings were replicated in the community it is unlikely that the association is solely attributable to the over-representation of comorbid cases in treatment settings (because those persons with a psychiatric disorder and a substance abuse problem are more likely to encounter in treatment services a bias known as Berkson's paradox. (Hall 1996).

MANAGEMENT

Current issues in service delivery to this group include polarization of specialities and the complexity and severity of the client group. In addition, specialist addiction services focus on alcohol and opiate dependence, while the most problematic and frequent substance use patterns for those in mental health are those of non-dependent use of cannabis, stimulants and alcohol. Harm reduction interventions should be a primary consideration since this group are at higher than normal risk for BBV transmission, and sexually transmitted diseases. Engagement with support focusing on the client's priorities such as housing and welfare then permit the opportunity for introducing other effective interventions such as cognitive-behavioural therapy, motivational interviewing and appropriate pharmacotherapies. Those receiving supervised methadone or buprenorphine may usefully have their other psychotropic medication dispensed at the same time to enhance compliance. Unfortunately they are a difficult group to engage and maintain contact with and in the US and UK this has prompted the development of small caseload, assertive outreach, dual diagnosis teams. There is little evidence so far to support any particular model for dual diagnosis care and it is likely that only when systemic changes occur in training and resourcing will this group be adequately catered for.

TAKING A DRUG HISTORY

- In order to provide the most optimal treatment current drug use is required.

- What drugs they are currently using (last three days' use is a good guide based on recent recall by the client).
- Quantity (weight, money spent, number of pills etc.).
- Frequency (times per day, days in the last month).
- Route of administration.
- Explain to the client that you need to understand the impact their drug use has on their day-to-day activities.
- Ask at what time they wake up and why. People may wake earlier than they would wish because of an alarm clock, other noise (traffic, baby), depression or withdrawals.
- Ask then how they feel when they wake up. Those dependent on drugs often report feeling 'sick' or unwell. If they report the latter, ask them to describe their symptoms of withdrawal. It may also be useful to ask those who do not wake because of withdrawal, how long after waking do they experience withdrawals or first use.
- Ask where and when the first use takes place. Do they leave enough drugs at bedtime to have something to alleviate withdrawal in the morning or do they need to obtain drugs after waking? This may identify risky behaviours (e.g. sex work, criminal activity) or other priorities such as child care or work commitments.
- Ask them how their days start. Do they shower? Do they have breakfast? (Lack of nutrition is common in this group.) Ask how they spend their day. Who do they see? Where do they go? This may identify high risk behaviours (e.g. sharing of injecting equipment) as well as evidence suggesting prioritizing drug-seeking and drug-using behaviour over other activities. It is also possible to ask whether their days were always spent like this or whether they used to get pleasure from other hobbies and interests. What if anything do they do anymore? This may allow the client to reflect positively on non-drug-using periods.
- Ask about their social networks.
- Ask them about evening activities. What do they enjoy? Do they find it easy to get off to sleep? Do they lie awake, do they sleep straight through? Many drug users sleep badly and may chase sleep with a cocktail of depressant drugs, which represent increased risk to the person.
- Their drug use history. The age of their first use, regular use, onset of tolerance and withdrawals, the transition from smoking to injecting.
- Past treatments, e.g. counselling, AA, pharmacotherapies, detoxification, maintenance, in- versus outpatient. Duration and number of abstinent periods. Circumstances of relapse.
- Complications of drug use: psychological, social and physical.

INVESTIGATIONS

Substance misuse must always be considered in young people presenting with psychological problems. A full physical examination may reveal stigmata of substance use (for example, recent injection sites, old tracks, venous scarring, 'puffy hand syndrome', abscesses) and evidence of malnutrition or undetected infection. Laboratory confirmation of self-reported use should be sought, most commonly with urinanalyis, though false negatives can arise through dilution or contamination of samples. In most treatment settings self-report is fairly reliable. Urine tests and their results should not result in punitive consequences for the client (e.g. being discharged from the programme) but should be used in discussion about changes in treatment approach. The provision of takeaway doses of methadone contingent upon clean urines may be a motivator for positive behavioural change as may the risk of losing this option if drug use is detected. Urine tests can tell you if a drug has been used recently but not how much. Serial dilutions of sequential urine samples can however detect reductions in cannabis levels with abstinence. The time windows for detection after last use of commonly used illicit substances are given in Table 28.1.

More recently, hair analysis has been used to retrospectively detect drug use, with most illicit drugs becoming incorporated into the hair follicle 7–10 days after ingestion. Other samples that are being developed to enhance the utility of biological indicators for drug detection include sweat, saliva, finger nails, buccal scrapings and blood.

Viral screens

HIV and AIDS

Among injecting drug users, the risk of viral transmission is high and routine testing should be available with counselling to those at risk. Rates among users show wide geographic variation reflecting differing injecting patterns. Rates of HIV have fallen since the mid 1980s with recent studies suggesting rates of less than 1% among the UK injecting population (Crawford 1997). Much of this reduction in prevalence has been due to the widespread availability of 'needle exchange' services and provision of services focused towards 'harm minimization'. Rates elsewhere in countries without such access are much higher for example in Eastern Europe and parts of South-east Asia. Although opiate users represent the largest group of injecting drug users, some evidence suggests that rates among those who inject stimulant drugs are even higher, (Hunter et al. 1995). One reason may be the higher daily rates of administration and socializing effects of stimulant drugs. Other groups that are at high risk are prison populations, where injecting is more likely to involve sharing of needles, syringes and related paraphernalia without the precaution of adequate cleaning of used equipment.

Hepatitis B and C

Rates of 70% for hepatitis C and 20–40% for hepatitis B infection are found among injecting drug users. The higher virulence and hardiness of hepatitis C explains the rates of infectivity and the need to advise users that risks of sharing extend beyond needles and syringes to include spoons, filters, tourniquets, water, etc. High levels of alcohol consumption, common in many methadone maintenance clients, worsens prognosis significantly. Education and harm reduction provision must therefore continue in order to bring about reductions in prevalence that has been achieved with regard to HIV. Hepatitis C-positive injecting drug users should not be denied antiviral treatment but should be supported to stop injecting and adopt healthier life styles.

Biochemical and viral screens as well as vaccination should be taken opportunistically with pre and post-test counselling and accessible treatment services.

DRUGS OF ABUSE

These are covered individually below. See Tables 28.2 and 28.3 for an overview of drug classification and clinical signs suggestive of use.

Opiates: opium, heroin, methadone and buprenorphine

Opium is derived from the ripe seed capsule of the poppy, *Papaver somniferum*. The extract contains morphine and codeine, alkaloid opiate analgesics. Heroin (diamorphine), and dihydrocodeine are semisynthetic congeners of morphine, while pethidine and methadone are non-opiate morphine-like analgesics. The street purity of heroin varies widely (usually 30–60%) and cost is £30–70/g depending on type, quality, amount purchased, relationship to dealer, availability, and geographical location. Daily consumption is commonly in the region of 0.5–1 g but may be more than 2 g.

Table 28.1 Detection of drug use through urinalysis	
Drug	*Detection window[1]*
Cannabis	3 days–6 weeks
Heroin	2–3 days
Methadone	7–9 days
LSD (photolabile–store away from light)	1 day
Stimulants	1–3 days
[1] Detection window – length of time urine remains positive after last use	

Table 28.2 Drug terminology and classification, cost

Drug type	Example	Slang	Cost
CNS depressants	Heroin, benzodiazepines, alcohol, barbiturates, GHB	Smack, gear, brown, H, jellies, mazzies, barbs, GBH, liquid E	Heroin: £35–70/g (£10 bag = 0.1 g)
CNS stimulants	Cocaine, amphetamine, ecstasy, methamphetamine	Blow, Charlie, whiz, E pills, ice pills, crystal	Cocaine: £40–70/g Crack: £10 rock = 0.1–0.25 g E: £3–10
Cannabis	Herbal marijuana, hashish resin, hash oil	Hash, weed, puff, spliff, skunk, black	Hash: £15 per 1/8 oz Skunk grass: £25 per 1/8 oz (3.5 g)
Hallucinogens	LSD, psilocybin, mescaline, DMT, ketamine, PCP	Tabs, trips, blotters, K	LSD: £2.50–5/tab
Solvents, volatile substances	Toluene, butane, N20 nitrates, solvents, glue	Whippets, gas, tins	£3 for a lighter refill, £4.50 for small pot of glue

Table 28.3 Sign of drug intoxication

	Eyes	Pulse, blood pressure	Speech	Coordination	Arousal
Alcohol	Bloodshot, nystagmus	Reduced	Slurred/slow	Impaired	High/low
Opiates	Pinpoint pupils, shut	Reduced	Slurred/slow	Impaired	Low
Stimulants	Saucer pupil, open	Increased	Fast rubbish	May improve	High
Cannabis	Red eye Shut	Increased	Slow rubbish	Impaired	High/low
Hallucinogens	Dinner plate pupils Shut	Increased	All of the above	Impaired	High

Heroin has been described, as 'the ultimate antidepressant' and 'like being wrapped up in emotional cotton wool'. Such descriptions are better understood if you consider the many dependent users who cite histories of childhood abuses or adult trauma and use opiates for their 'narcotic comfort'. So effective and reinforcing is its effect in some that it has been postulated that if heroin was trialled as a treatment for post-traumatic stress disorder it might look quite promising. Iatrogenic dependence through the injudicious and prolonged use of opiates for an initially painful condition, although rare, is a particular problem in those with past substance use.

Mode of action and neurobiology

Opiate drugs exert their effects by binding to the same receptor sites as endogenous opiates such as the enkephalins and endorphins (see Chapter 38). The highest concentration of these peptide receptors opiate receptors are in the limbic system (particularly the amygdala and periaquductal grey), hypothalamus and sensory systems. They are also found in the gastrointestinal tract.

Of the four main opiate receptor subtypes, the μ (mu) and κ (kappa) receptors are the most important in relation to abuse liability and dependence. Opiates facilitate inhibitory transmission and are coupled to G proteins, which regulate transmembrane transmission and secondary messenger systems. Acutely the administration of opiates leads to the inhibition of adenylate cyclase with reduced conversion of ATP to cAMP. Neuroadaptation to chronic opiate administration includes uncoupling of the receptor from secondary messenger systems and compensatory down-regulation of the opiate μ receptors leading to increased levels of adenylate cyclase, returning cAMP levels to baseline. On cessation of use (or following the administration of opiate receptor antagonism) withdrawal ensues. The symptoms of opiate withdrawal are secondary to a massive surge in noradrenaline (norepinephrine) release (termed the 'noradrenergic' storm) primarily from the locus coerulus. This explains the efficacy of the presynaptic α_2 agonists clonidine and lofexidine in the treatment of the symptoms of acute heroin withdrawal (see Chaper 38).

Route of administration

Heroin is effectively administered through smoking ('chasing the dragon'), intranasal snorting or via injection (IV, IM, SC). While many users may start off smoking heroin, once tolerance develops, the economic consequences and limited bioavailability offered by smoking combined by a desire for an intense effect, leads many users to start intravenous injecting.

Heroin metabolism

Diamorphine (half-life 2min) is really a pro-drug crossing the blood–brain barrier quicker than morphine before being rapidly metabolized to the psychoactive intermediate, 6 mono-acetylmorphine by blood esterases prior to conversion to morphine (half-life 3 hours). Morphine is then metabolized by the cytochrome P450 system (Cyp2D6) in the liver to codeine which undergoes conjugation before excretion in the urine. In most people about 10% of consumed codeine is converted into morphine (having the potential to give a false-positive urine test result for heroin/morphine) (Wolff et al. 1999).

Patterns of use

The majority of heroin users who engage with treatment services are dependent users, who as a result of duration, intensity and pattern of use are the group at risk of the greatest opiate-related harm. Most dependent heroin injectors will inject 2–6 times/day to avoid the onset of withdrawal, though some with low levels of dependence may only need to inject once. Not all people who try heroin become dependent and although rare, so called recreational use of heroin does exist (Blackwell 1983; Zinberg 1984).

Epidemiology

In 1997 when the UK Home Office Addicts Index closed there were 40 000 notified opiate addicts in the UK. This register has since been replaced with regional drug misuse databases. Over the last decade, the number has continued to increase by 10–20% per annum. Its use though is uncommon compared to other class A drugs such as cocaine (5%), with only 0.3% reporting use in the last month in the 2002/3 BCS. The current prevalence of heroin use in the UK is thought to be less than 1% (3M:F), with most new addicts seeking treatment being in their twenties.

The effects of opiates

The physiological effects of opiate drugs are as follows:

- pupillary constriction
- respiratory depression
- decreased sympathetic outflow (bradycardia and hypotension)
- sedation/sleep ('gouching out', 'on the nod')
- cough reflex suppression
- nausea and vomiting
- mood change – euphoria/intense pleasure
- lowering of body temperature
- analgesia.

The acute psychoactive effects vary on dose and route but include euphoria, sedation, emotional numbing, analgesia, and induction of a dream-like state.

Heroin withdrawal

Once dependence and neuroadaptation has been established, abrupt cessation or a marked reduction in dose will result in a withdrawal syndrome. The classic withdrawal syndrome for heroin appears within 6–12 hours after the last dose, peaking at 48–72 hours and subsiding by the end of 7–10 days. There is often a prodromal period before the onset of frank withdrawal symptoms during which time the addict becomes agitated and anxious. Characteristic withdrawal symptoms include aching muscles and joints, dysphoria, insomnia, agitation, lacrimation, dilated pupils, increased sweating with goosefleshing of the skin (hence 'cold turkey ' or 'clucking'), diarrhoea, shivering, yawning and fatigue. Opiate withdrawal is not usually considered to be life threatening although complications may arise from significant dehydration or dysphoria.

Physical complications

Harms from drugs are related to route, dose, purity and environment in which the drugs are used. Two-thirds of the deaths occurring in drug addicts are related to drug use, with the annual mortality for opiate dependent users being between 1–2%, mostly from overdose. Potential complications of opiate use are outlined in Table 28.4 (Hunter et al. 1995; Power et al.1992).

Opiate overdose

Most opiate addicts in treatment have experienced an overdose and/or witnessed it in others (Powis et al. 1999). Those who inject are far more likely to overdose than those who smoke (Gossop et al. 1996). Other risk factors include consumption of other CNS depressants such as benzodiazepines, heroin or alcohol, physical/psychiatric illness, longer duration of injecting career and high risk times when tolerance is low (e.g. after detox or rehab, release from prison etc.). The signs of opiate overdose include:

- in an adult, respiratory arrest with a pulse is almost pathagnmonic of opiate overdose
- pinpoint pupils unreactive to light
- snoring giving way to shallow respirations (rate < 8/min)
- bradycardic and hypotensive
- varying degree of reduced consciousness/coma.

Treatment should be supportive with standard cardio-pulmonary resuscitation and intravenous naloxone (opiate antagonist). However in some users intravenous access may be problematic in which case it may be quicker to give it subcutaneously or intramuscularly. Admission to hospital should always be recommended, since the plasma half-life of naloxone is 45 minutes compared to 4–6 hours for the physiological effects of heroin and 24–36 hours for methadone.

Table 28.4 Complications of opiate use

Infections	Cardiorespiratory	Renal	Neurological
Hepatitis and HIV	Pulmonary oedema Pulmonary emboli	Rhabdomyolysis	Peripheral neuropathy
Bacterial endocarditis, septicaemia	Aspiration pneumonia Needle emboli	Membranous nephropathy Nephrotic syndrome	Transverse myelitis
Pneumonia and TB	Pneumothorax	Necrotizing angiitis	Brain abscesses
Skin abscesses, cellulitis, phlebitis osteomyelitis, necrotizing fasciitis	Cardiac arrythmias Respiratory depression	Secondary amyloidosis	Myopathy, local nerve damage – direct trauma and compression

Psychiatric comorbidity

Seventy per cent of those dependent on heroin meet diagnostic criteria for a current psychiatric disorder, most commonly depression, anxiety, dissocial personality, post-traumatic stress disorder and alcohol dependency. Up to a third of all deaths among intravenous drug users are due to suicide (Frischer et al. 1993). There is high incidence of childhood behavioural problems such as conduct disorder and attention deficit hyperactivity disorder. Recent studies suggest that truanting and juvenile offending are markers for subsequent problematic use. Comorbid psychiatric disorders that may be important in maintaining opiate use should be treated appropriately (Hall & Farrell 1997).

Treatment options

Treatment options for opiate dependence can broadly be divided into maintenance treatment (substitution therapy) or detoxification. Methadone and buprenorphine ('Subutex') are effective and licensed in the UK for both options. Methadone gives a different urine drug screen test result from heroin with both immunoassay and chromatographic drug screening thereby allowing non-prescribed opiate use to be identified. Buprenorphine is not identified on routine drug screens.

Methadone

A synthetic, orally effective, opiate developed by the Nazis in the 1940s as their access to opium became obstructed. Methadone is a long acting μ receptor agonist that is the most widely evaluated treatment for opiate dependence being in use since the 1960s. It is most often prescribed long term with the aim of achieving stable (non injecting) opiate dependence or can be prescribed in the short term to aid withdrawal on a methadone mixture (usually linctus) over 10–21 days. Between 30–40 mg of 1 mg/ml mixture is approximately equivalent to 1/2 g of street heroin.

Methadone has a long half-life (24–48 hours) and a steady state plasma level is thus reached within 5–7 days. Although most symptoms of withdrawal are eased in most users at doses of 30 mg/day, doses above 80 mg/day are claimed to provide a reasonable level of opiate receptor blockade (through the induction of tolerance), such that euphoria from illicit opiates 'used on top' is diminished. Care is required during the induction of patients onto methadone. Because of rising plasma levels over the 4 or 5 days of use (note there is also auto-induction of its metabolism), patients should be monitored before receiving their daily dose and preferably 2–4 hours after the first dose. First doses should not usually exceed 30 mg, with subsequent increments of 5–10 mg every 4–7 days occurring until withdrawal is abolished, craving reduced and tolerance to opiate significantly increased (>60 mg/day). There have been deaths recorded during unsafe and unmonitored induction onto methadone (Caplehorn & Drummer, 1999), usually in opioid naïve persons or those using other depressant drugs such as alcohol and benzodiazepines. Confirmation of the patient's dependent status is therefore paramount, assessed by a careful and comprehensive assessment, observation, examination and where appropriate, objective confirmation by repeat urine drug screens and by direct observation of the patient while withdrawing and assessing the effect of an administered dose of methadone on site.

Buprenorphine (Subutex, Temgesic)

Buprenorphine is a partial μ receptor agonist. This means that it has a ceiling effect on respiratory depression and is thus safer in overdose than methadone. It has recently become an acceptable and effective alternative to methadone (Kosten, 2003). Taken sublingually (it undergoes extensive first pass metabolism thus oral bioavailability is poor), it has a higher affinity for the m opioid receptor than pure agonists like heroin and methadone, but lower intrinsic activity. This results in precipitated withdrawal if it is taken within 6–12 hours of heroin or 24–48 hours of methadone (never give buprenorphine to a patient who has 'pinned pupils'). It is effective as a stabilization agent (where safe induction is faster than that usually achieved with methadone) with maintenance doses of 8–24 mg/day being typical. The maximum dose of buprenorphine to be given on any one day is 32 mg. Because of its high affinity and slow dissolution from the receptor means that at higher doses the duration action extends to 2–3 days. This permits for alternate day or three times a week dosing.

Like methadone (which may be regurgitated or secreted in a bottle), Subutex can be diverted and injected. Supervised consumption is recommended for both methadone and buprenorphine, for at least the first three months of treatment. Careful observation initially at public clinics then at community pharmacies is required to ensure that potentially abusable and lethal drugs are not diverted to the street drug market.

Levo-alpha acetylmethadol (LAAM)

This long-acting (48–72 hours) μ receptor agonist has been used in the treatment of heroin dependence since the 1960s. Although studies have demonstrated equivalence with other substitute therapies it is not licensed for use in the UK because of concerns over the prolongation of the QT interval seen in some persons.

Management of opiate dependence

On a population and individual level the most cost-effective way to reduce drug-related problems is to provide good treatment. Treatment for heroin users must address multiple psychosocial and physical problems. Service provision aims to reduce harm through promoting safer practices and encouraging positive behavioural changes such as entering a treatment programme. Engaging a marginalized group who are involved in an illegal activity is difficult with the assurance of confidentially and trust being essential components of a positive treatment alliance.

The major treatment modalities for heroin dependence are substitution therapy; detoxification and psychological therapies such as cognitive–behavioural therapy, motivational interviewing, social skills training, family therapy and self-help groups.

Pharmacological interventions for opiate users: maintenance and withdrawal

Oral methadone is the mostly evaluated and cost-effective treatment for opiate dependence. Methadone is both an effective treatment for the alleviation of withdrawal as well as in higher blockade doses (>60–80 mg) effective in reducing the craving for heroin and increasing the tolerance to other opiate drugs (protecting against overdose and reducing their reinforcement). Although the recommended dose range for effective maintenance is recommended as 60–80 mg/day, the mean dose prescribed as treatment for opiate dependence in the UK is less than 40 mg! Some patients will require higher does of methadone (up to 200 mg/day), though such clients should have their safety and tolerance continually assessed and in some cases have peak and trough plasma levels checked. Similar findings have been demonstrated (although with less evidence) with buprenorphine, although it may be associated with slightly lower retention within present treatment frameworks.

The National Treatment Outcome Research Study (NTORS) used a 5-year longitudinal, prospective cohort design to follow the outcomes of 650 persons admitted to opiate treatment services (community methadone and residential rehabilitation units) in 1995 (Gossop et al. 1997). About a quarter of those on methadone had become abstinent compared to 38% of those attending rehabilitation. Among those still in treatment heroin use was about half of its entry levels of use and there were also significant reductions in use of benzodiazepines and illicit methadone. Most of the improvement seems to have been achieved within a year, with levels sustained beyond this initial stage. Unfortunately there was little positive impact on use of crack cocaine or alcohol. Both substances, with their different mechanisms of actions, are probably perceived to be a more cost effective intoxicant compared to heroin as the levels of opiate blockade increases. Results from the same group suggest that for every extra £1 spent on treatment, there is a return of more than £3 in cost savings associated with lower levels of victim costs of crime and reduced demands upon the criminal justice system. The benefits of opiate replacement therapy include:

- reduced rates of injecting drugs
- reduced rates of other illicit drug use
- reduction in suicide/overdose
- reduced rates of HIV and viral hepatitis
- reduced rates of criminal activity
- improvement in psychosocial and physical wellbeing.

Other opiate pharmacotherapies: naltrexone and 'Suboxone'

The long-acting orally active opiate receptor antagonist naltrexone can be used in the maintenance of abstinence of opiate dependents. Compliance with treatment is generally poor (and hence ineffective) unless supervised and part of wider treatment programmes. It is also associated with an increase in receptor sensitivity that means following the cessation of its use, people are particularly sensitive to the risk of overdose should they relapse. Recently, naltrexone implants have been trialled and it may be that in certain populations, this way of enhancing compliance may be useful.

Suboxone is buprenorphine combined with naloxone in a ratio of 4:1. Taken as directed sublingually, there is very poor bioavailablity of naloxone compared to buprenorphine, thus the drug works similarly to buprenorphine. However when injected the naloxone now is 100% bioavailable and depending on the current state of intoxication of the user may precipitate withdrawal or at least be less reinforcing than buprenorphine alone. Whether such a combination preparation is significantly less abusable and divertable that the single product is as yet unclear. It is not yet licensed for use in the UK.

Detoxification (see Chapter 27 on alcohol)

Opiate withdrawal is not life-threatening and can be managed safely in the community in the majority of cases. There are three common modes of detoxification used in the UK for the management of opiate withdrawal.

The α_2 agonists, clonidine and lofexidine, may be used in the management of opiate withdrawal to alleviate the withdrawal distress associated with the central noradrenergic hyperactivity that is responsible for many of the symptoms of opiate withdrawal. The dose of α_2 agonists should be titrated against the symptoms and signs of withdrawal, while being careful to avoid hypotensive episodes (less common with lofexidine) and can be used both within outpatient and in-patient settings. Their ability to mange the symptoms of withdrawal is similarly as effective in opiate withdrawal as methadone (Bearn et al. 1996). They are often used in conjunction with other medications such as benzodiazepines for sleep, muscular cramps and agitation; quinine for muscle cramps, and hyoscine for abdominal cramps; NSAIDs and paracetamol for pain and anti emetics such as promethazine or metoclopramide. Methadone dose may be reduced gradually (e.g. 5 mg every 1–2 weeks) though below 35 mg there appears to be little difference between a gradual taper and abrupt cessation and symptomatic treatment. (Kosten 2003).

Buprenorphine can also be very effectively used in the management of detoxification, especially as an outpatient, over 5–10 days, where it is probably superior to symptomatic relief with α_2 agonists (though the two can also be usefully combined).

Withdrawal may also be hastened by administering the long-acting opiate antagonist naltrexone, which 'kicks' the addict into intense but shorter-lived withdrawal, during which time symptomatic relief may be given with clonidine and benzodiazepines. In others this precipitant withdrawal is speeded up even further, with the detoxification procedure being completed under general anaesthetic in about 24 hours, though this is not without risk.

Prescribing drugs to opiate addicts

In the UK all doctors may prescribe methadone for the treatment of dependence and other opiates for analgesia or other clinical indications except dependence. Only doctors in possession of a Home Office license are able to prescribe heroin for the treatment of dependence. At present there are approximately 500 clients receiving heroin from a total of 100 or so prescribers. With recent international evidence (Swiss, Dutch, Australian) mounting to support the provision of 'supervised injecting rooms' and prescription of injectable opiates for dependence, the UK's response to explore the development of prescribed heroin-injecting clinics may increase the expansion of this treatment option. Doctors should be wary of behaviours that are suggestive of possible 'abuse' of prescribed opiates. These include using the script up early, losing the script, asking for escalating doses and attending multiple prescribers. Although the attribution may be incorrect and there may be genuine reasons for the requests, it is the doctor's responsibility to ensure that the drugs are being used as directed.

Other treatment interventions

Psychological

There are numerous psychological approaches that are currently used to assist those with substance related problems, reduce their use of drugs and the harm associated with them, including cognitive–behavioural therapy (CBT), relapse prevention (RP) and psychotherapy (individual, family and group). The most influential approach in recent years has been the relapse prevention mode (Marlatt 1999), which includes the identification of cues or triggers for craving (often people, places or paraphernalia or a certain mood state such as boredom or stress) and the learning of techniques (distraction, relaxation, imagery) to handle high-risk situations in which relapse is more likely. Recently, motivational interviewing based on the work of Bill Miller in the US has become increasingly popular. It aims to move the client along a 'cycle of change' (Miller & Rollnick 1991; Prochaska and di Clemente) (see Chapter 27). Involvement with Narcotics Anonymous and support groups such as Mainliners should be encouraged.

Physical

High levels of physical and psychiatric morbidity are compounded by poor nutrition, homelessness, financial hardship and poor access to primary care. Dentition is often particularly bad. Although methadone reduces salivary flow, poor nutrition, dental hygiene and the masking of dental pain probably contribute more significantly. Efforts at reducing injecting and related risk behaviours are a priority. Safer injecting techniques, sharps boxes, needles and syringe outlets and disposal bins should be combined with advice on safer sex, contraception and general health care. Models of shared care (between GP, specialist services, pharmacists and clients and specialized primary care health teams) have been successful in proactively engaging clients and service providers to effect the delivery of care to this multiply-disadvantaged high risk group. Special attention should be focused on provision of hepatitis testing and vaccination to all users.

Social and educational

High rates of early school drop-out and lower levels of employment skills hamper efforts at reintegration into the community as a non-drug user. All available potential supports should be considered including family, friends, social services or voluntary sector supports, user advocate groups, religious communities and spiritual support groups such as Narcotics Anonymous. Providing credible accessible accurate health information as part of harm prevention initiatives foster a positive alliance with using communities and assist in promoting safer drug using practices with consequent benefit to the individual and society. Therapeutic communities and 'concept houses' based on a religious or abstinent theme offer longer-term care.

Pregnancy

The maternal use of opiates has consequences for both mother and child with increased rates of stillbirth, prematurity, low birthweight, IUGR and vertical HBV/HIV transmission risk. This group should be given priority access to coordinated treatment services with effective liaison between patient, family, antenatal, drug and social support services. In general the aim of treatment should be to engage the mother and reduce risk-taking behaviours, e.g. injecting, and stabilize on methadone (buprenorphine is not yet licensed for use in pregnancy or breastfeeding). Liaison with antenatal and primary care and social services through a multidisciplinary programme ensures the wellbeing of the mother and her environment. Pregnancy should be regarded as a window of opportunity in the drug user.

If considering detoxification, this should be done in the middle trimester. However, the risk of relapse and loss of engagement with services means that many specialists recommend that a woman remains on methadone. Although some women can mange a slow reduction through pregnancy, many may require an increase in dose in the last trimester. The experience of withdrawal by the mother should be avoided at all costs since it risks premature labour. Both benzodiazepines and opiates are slowly metabolized by the newborn infant, so that peri-delivery administration may result in hypotonia and respiratory depression. Both opiates and benzodiazepine dependence in the mother may be associated with protracted withdrawal syndromes in the baby. The neonatal abstinence syndrome seen in babies born to opiate-using mothers is characterized by signs and symptoms in the gastrointestinal tract, respiratory system and autonomic nervous system, with failure to thrive and the risk of seizures. Withdrawal incidence and severity is poorly correlated with dose of methadone, but may be prolonged, requiring hospitalization. Management is with morphine and occasionally barbiturates.

Criminal justice system

Prisoners

About one-third of remand prisoners have a substance abuse dependency problem, most commonly alcohol and opiates. Access to illicit substances is not prevented by imprisonment, indeed some users may first 'pick up heroin' or increase their 'habit' while in prison. Education and good primary health care are vital. Recent interest in the Drug Treatment and Testing Orders may allow those dependent users who are convicted of crimes associated with acquisitive offending to receive a Treatment Order as opposed to a custodial sentence. It is of practical importance that the rate of fatal overdose is increased 50-fold in the week after released from prison.

HIV-positive

Reducing high-risk behaviours by those with HIV is important to limit the spread of the disease. Stabilization on methadone with abstinence from injecting, sharing and unprotected sex should be encouraged. Liaison with medical and psychiatric services is important.

Outcome

Not surprisingly, those persons with multiple comorbid diagnoses and severe dependence psychopathology have the poorest outcomes. Among the strongest correlates of mortality in this group are level of disablity, heavy alcohol use, heavy criminal involvement and tobacco use. Longer treatment contacts tend to be associated with better outcomes (Simpson et al. 1997). Annual mortality rates are between 1–2%, with between a third and a half accounted for by suicide and accidental overdose (an excess mortality ratio of 12).

Stimulants: amphetamines, cocaine and MDMA ('ecstasy')

Amphetamine sulphate-type stimulants ('speed', 'whizz', methamphetamine)

Structurally similar to dopamine, amphetamines are synthetic *sympathomimetic drugs*. Stimulant amphetamines such as D-amphetamine and methyl amphetamine act through inhibition of central presynaptic reuptake of catecholamines (DA<NA) as well as indirect sympathomimetic effects secondary to disruption of vesicular storage of monoamines and inhibition of their breakdown by monoamine oxidates.

Illicit amphetamine is often of very low purity (5%) and costs approx £10–15/g. It can be taken orally, intra-nasally or injected. More recently higher purity preparations (up to 40%), known as 'base' or 'paste', are becoming available and may result in a higher abuse potential of the drug. A more potent, harmful and easily smokeable form of methamphetamine is becoming an increasing problem in South-east Asia and Australasia. Prescribable stimulants such as methylphenindate (Ritalin) and diethylpropion (Tenuate) are also open to abuse.

Pattern of use

Users may be classified as recreational, functional or dependent. People who use amphetamine-type stimulants regularly, in high doses and/or by injection or smoking, develop tolerance rapidly and risk becoming dependent upon it. However, unlike other drugs of dependence such as alcohol and heroin, daily use among users of amphetamine is uncommon since chronic use leads to exhaustion and aversive symptoms becoming more pronounced. A more common pattern of heavy use is in binges, in which high doses of amphetamine are administered repeatedly over a period of days until either the supply or the user is exhausted. This period of intense use is then followed by a period of abstinence in which depressant drugs may be used to help the user 'come down' and get some sleep.

Heavy users may inject >5 g of amphetamine sulphate a day and increase their number of injections to more than 20/day. Recreational users may use the drug sporadically, using considerably less (in the region of 0.5–2 g in a night often taken orally or snorted, often in conjunction with other 'dance drugs'). Functional users include students and long-distance lorry drivers, who use the drug to enhance performance and stamina. Some (particularly women) may also use the drug to control weight.

Effects

Amphetamines elevate mood, induce euphoria and feelings of wellbeing, increase alertness, energy, self-confidence and motor activity, reduce inhibitions, fatigue and appetite, and improve task performance that has been impaired by fatigue or boredom (hence their use by radar operators and bomber pilots in the Second World War).

Sympathetic arousal induced by methamphetamine produces rapid and sometimes irregular heartbeat, sweating, pupillary dilation, hypertension, dry mouth, tremor and blurred vision and increased body temperature. However, unpleasant symptoms such as anxiety and irritability, paranoia and panic often develop. Such a picture could be confused with that of opiate withdrawal.

There have been about 300 amphetamine-related deaths (mostly ecstasy) over the last 10 years – mainly from accidents, hyperthermia, cerebrovascular complications (intracranial bleeds and emboli) and cardiac arrhythmias.

Tolerance

Tolerance does develop and there is now a recognized withdrawal syndrome following cessation of chronic use, characterized by depression, psychomotor agitation, sleep disturbance (rebound REM with disturbing vivid dreams) and fatigue accompanied by dysphoria, irritability, anhedonia, anxiety, hyperphagia and craving. In some respects it resembles an atypical depression. While the withdrawal was previously divided into 'crash', 'withdrawal' and 'extinction', more recent studies suggest a more gradual improvement in mood and functioning over a 3–4 week period. Management of withdrawal is largely supportive and with a safe, well-supported home environment in-patient admission is rarely required. The patient should be placed in quiet surroundings for several days and allowed to sleep and eat as much as is needed. Benzodiazepines may be prescribed on a short-term basis for agitation. If the patient is markedly despondent, a suicide assessment may be necessary. Severe and persistent depression may require antidepressants. Antidepressants are not effective in reducing amphetamine use itself, but can be effective in the management of major depressive episodes associated with their use.

Treatment

The best evidence is for CBT and motivational interviewing, if users are ambivalent. Manualized outpatient and residential services are appropriate delivery sites for these types of treatment and can be usefully enhanced in some instances by the use of contingency management approaches (for a review see Baker & Lee 2003).

Although substitution treatment has been the most effective management approach for opiate dependence, the use of maintenance stimulant treatments is less supported. Concerns focus around the possibility of increasing dependence through daily-dosing individuals who may have previously taken the drug in a binge fashion, with additional concerns over cardiovascular and longer-term neurotoxicity, mood and behavioural problems. Episodes of psychosis may be precipitated in some and there is the risk of drug diversion. There may be a role for carefully monitored oral substitute amphetamine prescribing in some injectors as an interim manoeuvre to reduce intravenous use or to stabilize use before commencing a reduction in dose (Fleming & Roberts 1994). Recent trials from Australia (Shearer & Wodak 2003) and elsewhere also support this approach and it may be that substitute prescribing of dexamphetamine or methylphenidate in some treatment regimens becomes a more widespread harm reduction practice for stimulant users.

At present there is no evidence based effective treatment for amphetamine dependence though there have been a multitude of trialled medications. Underlying attention deficit hyperactivity disorder and other comorbidities should be sought for during abstinence and treated.

Psychiatric morbidity is the most common harm associated with amphetamine use. High proportions of users report symptoms such as anxiety, depression, paranoia, mental confusion and panic attacks.

The use of high doses of amphetamine and methamphetamine may lead to the induction of a temporary psychotic state that may be clinically indistinguishable from paranoid schizophrenia. These often-florid psychoses usually remit within a few days and the user returns to normal functioning, although some retain a vulnerability to such episodes, especially on re-use of the drug. Treatment with sedatives and antipsychotic medication may hasten the resolution of the acute symptoms, but care should be taken with close follow up, and observation of the client medication-free will assist in the correct diagnosis (usually either drug-induced psychosis, schizophrenia, bipolar disorder, exacerbation of an underlying psychotic illness, withdrawal, or a de novo condition) and prevent an erroneous diagnosis of schizophrenia being made.

Cocaine ('charlie', 'coke', 'snow', 'crack')

In a 1980 American textbook of psychiatry, cocaine was described as having little abuse potential. This is now seen as misguided and akin to suggesting that the voting system of Florida has low abuse potential! Cocaine is the major alkaloid constituent of the Andean bush *Erythroxylon coca*. It was chewed by the indigenous people who thought it was a gift from God. It gave them stamina when on hunting parties, and dealt with mountain sickness, all the while keeping their appetites at bay.

Mechanism of action

Cocaine is an indirect sympathomimetic agent that causes an acute but transient blockade of the dopamine transporter (DAT) causing an acute elevation of DA levels, resulting in the experienced pleasure burst. There is also release of DA in the VTA (nucleus accumbens) and perhaps 'highjacks the reward pathway' 'better' than any other drug. Chronic cocaine administration leads to a compensatory increase in DAT levels, such as that with abstinence, and these increased transporter levels lead to a relative reduction in levels of DA outside nerve cells. Acute withdrawal probably reflects decreased dopaminergic activity in the brain, resulting in the symptoms of withdrawal, dysphoria, craving, anergia, sleep and appetite disturbance (usually increased). There is evidence that after chronic cocaine consumption there is persistent reorganization of reward pathways, which subsequently are preferentially reinforced by cocaine. Its half-life is about 50 minutes.

Route of administration

Intranasal use is probably still the major route of administration. Intravenous use either alone or in combination with heroin ('speedball') has a high associated mortality. Smoking the free alkaloid base as 'crack' is becoming increasingly common in some inner-cities in the UK.

Patterns of use

Many people may use powdered cocaine in a recreational fashion for many years before insidiously developing a problem with increasingly regular use. Frequently seen as a way of enhancing confidence and performance, attempts at reducing use are frequently accompanied by a rebound fall in self-esteem, energy and the development of depression. Because of its rapid onset of action and intense but very short-lived euphoria, crack cocaine (also known as 'rocks' or 'stones') frequently lends itself to compulsive, repetitive use with users consuming hundreds of pounds worth of the drug during a session. It is of note that crack is sold in small unit cost deals (£10–20) compared to the dealing unit of cocaine (1 g for £50–80). It may be that there are groups of 'functional' occasional users of crack, but in those with substance use disorders, the pattern of use is often uncontrolled and leads to significant harm.

Toxicity

These are similar to those seen with amphetamines and include signs of sympathetic overdrive (tachycardia, hypertension and severe agitation, hyperthermia, seizures) and severe cardiac problems such as congestive failure, arrhythmias, ischaemia and myocarditis. Cocaine, when consumed with alcohol, results in the formation of the less anxiogenic but more reinforcing and longer lasting, cocaethylene. Concurrent consumption of alcohol and then cocaine, leads to a 30% increase in peak plasma cocaine levels, which may increase the risk of sudden death in a vulnerable minority. Chronic use has more recently been associated with accelerated cerebrovascular ischaemia and strokes in young users.

Psychiatric comorbidity with cocaine dependence is high. About 50% experience alcohol-use disorders, and rates of depression are much higher that of the general population. Depression predicts poorer outcome in cocaine dependence.

Management of dependence and cocaine-use is unclear, though some recent small studies suggest venlafaxine or other antidepressants may have a role in a subgroup of patients (McDowell et al. 2000). Paranoia, panic and irritability are commonly seen acutely, although, perhaps because of its shorter half-life, paranoid psychotic episodes (seen with amphetamine) are less common. Acute adverse effects are seen with crack, because of its greater intensity of effect and dose of drug consumed. A progressive fibrotic condition of the lung associated with smoking crack cocaine, 'crack lung', may be seen in heavy users.

Treatment

Withdrawal management is broadly the same for amphetamine, both having symptoms peaking on days 2–4. Hospital admission for withdrawal may be necessary in some clients, such as those with unstable living conditions, comorbid mental heath or severe physical illness, polydrug dependence, or in whom severe withdrawal has been experienced and attempts of outpatient detoxification have proved ineffective. Symptomatic relief with low dose benzodiazepines (e.g. diazepam 5 mg tds) may be helpful.

Beyond detoxification (as with other stimulant drugs) there is little evidence to support the routine use of any specific pharmacotherapy in either the management of cocaine withdrawal or in maintaining abstinence from it. The evidence suggests the most effective interventions are based on CBT.

At the time of writing there is still interest in the possible role of antibodies being used to bind cocaine and prevent it reaching receptor sites. Efficacy, ethics immunogenicity, and a host of other hurdles make it unlikely that the war on drugs will extend to antibody production any time soon in the UK.

MDMA ('ecstasy')

3,4 Methylenedioxymethamphetamine (MDMA), is a hallucinogenic amphetamine, being a member of the largest family of hallucinogens, the substitute derivatives of mescaline phenyl isopropylamine. Often incorrectly termed a designer drug (one whose molecular structure has been altered to retain its psychoactive properties but no longer be classified as a restricted substance), it was explored as an appetite suppressant and was patented by Merck Chemical Company in 1914. Apart from American Army experiments in the 1950s, the drug remained beneath the radar until the 1970s, when doctors, therapists and hippies rediscovered its unusual empathogenic effects. By the mid-1980s, ecstacy had become mainstream and has continued to be part of the 'recreational drug scene' ever since. Recent studies suggest its use may have peaked with slight falls noted in 2001/2.

Mechanism of action

Taken up into 5HT neurons by a fluoxetine sensitive carrier transporter, MDMA acts as an indirect 5HT agonist (blocks reuptake and causes direct Na^+ dependent release). Acutely, this release of 5HT results in euphoria (maximal 1–4 hours), followed by acute depletion of central nervous system brain 5HT (associated with decreases in 5HT, 5HIAA and tryptophan hydroxylase activity). To a lesser degree, MDMA also blocks DA re-uptake, which is thought important in cognition, movement and reward.

This leads to sympathomimetic effects, not unlike that seen with amphetamine and cocaine, including marked mydriasis, piloerection, hypertension, hyperthermia and increase in locomotor activity. Physical effects of MDMA in man include:

- tachycadia, increased blood pressure
- increased respiratory rate
- increased temperature, increased sweating, sweaty palms, hot and cold flushes
- dilated pupils, tremor, dry mouth
- teeth grinding, jaw tightening (bruxism)
- anorexia, dehydration
- increased motor activity, agitation.

Metabolism

MDMA is primarily metabolized by demethylation by the enzyme CYP 2D6, of which two phenotypes predominate in the population, with 9% being 'poor metabolizers'. There is no evidence as yet to support the notion that this group may be at greater risk of fatalities associated with its use.

Neurotoxicity

There is evidence of selective 5HT neurotoxicity from both animal and human studies. They suggest a dose-related reduction in 5HT activity following chronic exposure, with abnormal axonal regrowth seen with time in rats. Key risk factors in animal models for increasing neurotoxicity are increased temperature, dehydration and dose. The effect of MDMA on thermal regulation is dependent upon the ambient temperature, causing hypothermia in cooler conditions and hyperthermia in hotter ones. PET studies in humans suggest that there may be structural damage to the serotinergic nerve terminal (McCann et al. 1998). The functional significance of this is unclear, and it is probable that whether an individual goes on to develop longer term problematic psychological or behavioural problems following use of MDMA will depend upon the amount consumed, any genetic loading for psychopathology, their baseline balance and level of 5HT activity, and any neuroplasticity that may compensate for any neuronal dysfunction. Theoretically, any vulnerability to mental disorders will be become more evident with time as the generation who first popularized ecstasy start losing functional neurons through the ageing process. Any loss that occurred from MDMA use may lead to early decompensation and functional loss.

Route of administration

MDMA may be injected, snorted or used rectally ('E by bum'), but is most commonly taken orally, with an onset of action after 30–60 minutes. The effects peak at between 90–120 minutes with significant effects persisting for a further 3–6 hours followed by a gradual 'come down'. Tolerance however does occur and the duration and intensity of effect may be reduced. The price of 'pills' has fallen to £5 in many places, making them a cost-effective alternative or additive to alcohol consumption.

Effects

Periodic intense 'rushes' have been described, in combination with a feeling of closeness to others, increased sensuality and being filled with energy. *Adverse symptoms* such as anxiety, panic and paranoia often develop, and a range of psychiatric disorders from psychosis to neuroses and affective disorders have been described following its use. Often there is also nausea, reduced appetite and insomnia. Both auditory and visual hallucinations have been described as have delusions and suicidal feelings while intoxicated.

Psychiatric and cognitive comorbidity and MDMA

It has been difficult to assess the MDMA attributable fraction of depression and other psychopathology in the community. Ecstasy users typically consume a wide variety of substances and baseline levels of depression and other factors contributing to premorbid risk are not readily assessed by retrospective examination. Despite these factors, studies of ecstasy using populations consistently report higher depression ratings on clinical scales than non-using controls. There appears to be a dose effect, with psychobiologic deficits more marked in heavy users. Women appear more sensitive to both acute short effects (midweek blues and hallucinations at higher doses) but also possibly the longer term neurotoxic ones (Maxwell 2003). Despite its prevalence over the years, the number of actual case reports of psychiatric conditions associated with the use of MDMA is rather small, with less than 100 published. Those reported include; depression, anxiety, panic, social phobia, bulimia, sleep disorders, paranoia, cognitive disorders, prolonged depersonalization/derealization, suicide, psychotic episodes, flashbacks and increased impulsivity. Factors that appear to increase susceptibility to psychiatric disorders with MDMA include female sex, dose, frequency and duration of use, polydrug use, and constitutional vulnerability. There is no specificity to the disorders that have been reported with MDMA, indeed those reported are those common in the general population. The direction of causality of drug use and mental disorder is further confused by evidence that poor premorbid adjustment is itself associated with drug use.

Psychosis among club drug users, although rare, may present to the general psychiatrist. Most often following high-dose amphetamine use, especially injected, clients can present floridly, often initially psychopathologically indistinguishable from schizophrenia. Psychopathology is often grandiose/persecutory with multimodality. There may also be evidence of stereotypical behaviours.

Differentiating between drug-induced/drug-precipitated/drug-exacerbated psychosis can be difficult. Drug-induced psychosis tends to occur in premorbidly stable individuals with no prodromal symptoms, while hallucinations are commonly visual (although auditory and tactile do occur). Most importantly, in cases of isolated drug-induced psychosis there is resolution within days or a few weeks at most with abstinence. Management should focus on confirmation of substance use (urine/hair) and observation with symptomatic relief using benzodiazepines or neuroleptics. Continuation of treatment needs to be considered on an individual basis, though the patient should be advised to maintain abstinence and be provided with appropriate follow-up to support non-use and monitor their mental state for any evidence of ongoing symptomatology that may suggest other diagnoses.

Whether there are specific cognitive deficits specifically associated with MDMA continues to be a contentious issue. Research suggests that heavy users have subtle cognitive deficits in working memory and recall, but the role of confounding drug use, especially cannabis, makes it difficult to assess the degree of association (Morgan 2000). These deficits both in cognition and mood are thought to reflect the underlying 5HT neurotoxicity that first became a public concern 20 years ago. The UK will need to monitor the relationship between and MDMA for another 20 years until the nature of the association can be more accurately assessed.

Dependence

Given the prevalence of MDMA use and the reported patterns of use, the possibility of a dependence syndrome similar to that seen with other stimulant drugs remains.

Since the dopaminergic system is also influenced by MDMA, it is likely that the ventral tegmental dopaminergic reward pathway underlies much of the reinforcement of MDMA. Users do report tolerance, loss of control and behavioural and lifestyle changes supportive of a dependence syndrome (Winstock et al. 2001). However, no withdrawal has been reported and there is no specific pharmacological intervention in the management of its use. MAOIs and selective serotonin reuptake inhibitors (SSRIs) should be used with caution since concurrent consumption may place the person at risk of the 5HT syndrome, its reinforcing potential and as such the possibility for the development of a dependence syndrome remains.

There have been several hundred deaths associated with MDMA use over the last two decades. Reported causes include hyperthermia, liver failure, cardiac dysfunction, water intoxication, strokes, haemorrhage, seizures, road accidents and violence (Milroy et al. 1996). Suggested safety measures include the provision of information, air conditioning and free water. Interestingly, dose does not seem to be a major factor, suggesting individual constitutional vulnerabilities.

Gamma hydroxybutyrate (GHB, GBH, liquid ecstasy) (Rodgers et al. 2004)

GHB is an endogenous short-chain fatty acid found in the central nervous system (hippocampus, hypothalamus, cerebellum), kidney, heart, skeletal muscle and brown fat. It is probably derived from GABA (transamination to succinate aldehyde, reduced to GHB). A putative neurotransmitter, its role is unclear though specific binding sites have been identified in the hippocampus, which are linked to DA neurons. It was originally developed as an IV anaesthetic induction agent in 1964. It wasn't very successful, causing unacceptably high levels of vomiting, and tonic–clonic jerks of hand and face at anaesthetic doses. Since the 1980s, it has been used as a supplement by body builders, as a sleep agent, a detox agent and most recently as a dance drug. Usually used in the form of a liquid (also available as capsules, powder or crystals), it is colourless and odourless, with a slightly salty, acidic taste. Until a few years ago the end product and the key ingredients were widely available on the net. However, recent legislations have significantly reduced access to it and its procompounds GBL (gamma butyl-lactone) and 1,4 butanediol.

Although probably derived from GABA, it has little effect on GABA-A or -B receptors at submillimolar concentrations. It does, however, readily cross the blood–brain barrier. Acutely it leads to a transient decrease followed by increase in dopamine levels (accompanied by increase in endogenous opioid release). Increases in Ach, GABA, 5HT are also seen. It exhibits some partial GABA-B activity at high levels (epileptogenic).

Easily prepared at home (mix sodium hydroxide and butyrol lactate and distilled water), incorrect manufacture may lead to caustic formulation with GHB and NaOH (emetic, coma induction and caustic stomach contents).

Taken orally the drug has a rapid onset of action (<15min) and a half-life of 27 min, being broken down to CO_2 and H_2O. It exhibits peak effects after 60 minutes with the total duration of action being 2–4 hours.

Clinically, GHB use should be suspected in particular groups such as clubbers and body builders who present with nystagmus, ataxia, nausea, vomiting, bradycardia and hypotension.

Most recently, GHB has been used by those involved in the dance music scene. Referred to by some as 'poor man's coke', GHB can at low doses induce euphoria, stimulation and arousal. Effects are dose related, however, and there is a steep dose–response curve with a narrow margin between untroubled and unconscious. Overdose risk is compounded by combined use with other depressants (especially alcohol) as well as wide fluctuation in purity, tolerance, context and other drugs consumed. The drug can also be associated with agitation, anxiety, aggressive behaviour, confusion, transient delirium and amnesia. Psychotic episodes have been reported when GHB is combined with stimulant drugs (massive increase in dopamine).

Other problems include increased vomiting, aspiration, weakness, sedation, coma, amnesia and collapse. There has also been a single case report of Wernike–Korsakoff syndrome.

There has been recent concern that GHB is a common date rape drug. Theoretically it may be an efficient 'Micky Fin' since it leads to the onset of rapid coma and amnesia, but the evidence suggests that alcohol alone is by far the most common 'date rape' drug.

GHB dependence is probably a reality and there are reports of chronic users consuming doses of 2–20 g/day. Withdrawal may occur and presents as rapid onset, prolonged alcohol withdrawal picture, with less autonomic arousal and risk of seizures but marked confusion, delirium and, hallucinations which may require enormous doses of benzodiazepines over a waxing and waning two-week period.

Hallucinogens (lysergic acid diethylamide (LSD), ketamine and psilocybin – mushrooms)

Lysergic acid diethylchloride (LSD)
Leaving his lab one day in 1943, the Swiss chemist Hoffman forgot to wash his hands, and accidentally discovered what a little bit of acid could do. Popular in the 1960s, LSD has now found a new audience with the rave drug scene. The drug may be absorbed transdermally, but is usually taken orally after absorption onto a piece of blotting paper, or a gelatine square (window panes) or on a sugar cube. Since the small squares of blotting paper (called 'tabs') are cut from a sheet that has been dipped in LSD and hung out to dry, the variation in strength between 'tabs' taken from the top and bottom corners can vary greatly, making accurate dosing almost impossible. One smuggler claims a bottle smashed while in his suitcase and for years he was selling bits of a suit! Doses as low as 20–50 micrograms cause marked perceptual distortion with visual illusions and hallucinations, without any associated lowering of consciousness. Effects start after 30–90 minutes and may last 3–12 or more hours. The half-life is 3 hours.

Mechanism of action
LSD is an indoleamine hallucinogen and binds to $5HT_1$, $5HT_2$, $5HT_5$ and $5HT_7$ receptors. Hallucinogenic potency in man is closely related to $5HT_2$ binding affinity in animals (Titeler 1988). Further evidence for the major role of 5HT comes from recent human trials, demonstrating that the hallucinogenic effects of psilocybin can be attenuated by pre-treatment with the $5HT_2$ receptor antagonist ketanserin or the atypical antipsychotic risperidone, but not haloperidol (Vollenweider et al 1998), with hallucinogenic effects probably mediated by the agonist action at the $5HT_2$ receptor. However, LSD also has significant stimulant effects mediated through the release of dopamine. Tolerance occurs rapidly due to receptor desensitization, which is evident after 3 or 4 days consecutive use, explaining the absence of a dependence syndrome.

Clinical features
Marked perceptual changes, with an alteration in state of awareness and euphoria are common. Visual (and less commonly auditory and other modality) hallucinations and distortions are frequently reported as is the phenomenon of 'synaesthesia' with loss of the normal boundaries between sensory modalities (e.g sounds are 'seen', colours are 'heard'). At higher doses its sympathomimetic effects become evident including hyper-reflexia and hyperthermia. Sympathetic overactivity may also help explain adverse symptoms such as anxiety and panic (the so called 'bad trip'). As with other psychoactive drugs, use may precipitate a severe mental illness in some vulnerable individuals. Approximately 15% of users report 'flashbacks', a recurrence of experiences previously associated with LSD use, while the individual is drug free.

Treatment
The 'bad trip' usually responds to a supportive and reassuring environment (so called 'talking down'), but if appropriate, benzodiazepines or low dose neuroleptics may be used.

Flashbacks may be associated with an underlying disorder such as anxiety and may be brought on by other drugs such as cannabis. Usually remitting with time they may remain distressing for a minority. Thus problems with LSD and other hallucinogens such as mushrooms are usually self-limiting, though persistent symptomatology may arise in those with a predisposition of psychosis.

Ketamine

Ketamine is a non-competitive antagonist at NMDA receptors. It is similar in action to PCP (but shorter acting), with binding to the cation channel of NMDA receptor being responsible for its analgesic/dissociative and purported neuroprotective effects. It also enhances monoamine transmission resulting in significant symphomimetic properties. It also has analgesic opioid receptor mediated effects. The induction of an anesthetic state and subsequent hallucinations are thought to be due to inhibition of central and peripheral cholinergic transmission.

Ketamine shows marked first pass metabolism and is fairly ineffective when taken orally. More commonly and efficiently ketamine is snorted or injected. It exhibits dose-related psychedelic effects, which show a linear relationship at low doses. Effects are highly sensitive to age, dose, route, sex and setting, and include:

- rapid onset, short duration of action (one hour), wide safety margin
- dissociative anaesthesia 'somatosensory blockade' (analgesia without anaesthesia) – analgesia
- perceptual distortion/hallucinations/near death
- out-of-body experience
- sympathetic stimulation
- emergence phenomena
- cognitive impairment
- though disorder/synaethesia
- little effect on cough reflex
- hypersalivation.

At low doses, sought-after experiences are primarily stimulant and elevation of mood. Psychedelic effects commence at higher doses. The Harvard academic, Timothy Leary, described it as 'the ultimate psychedelic journey'. Users describe entering the 'K hole' where they experience visits to God, aliens, their birth, past lives and the 'experiences of evolution' (Dillon et al. 2003).

Detection by clinical examination relies on identifying mydriasis, tachycardia, elevated blood pressure, slurred speech, blunted affect, ataxia, delirium, nystagmus (not always, < PCP). Urine drug screens do not routinely detect it.

Adverse effects are short-lived (<5 hours) and include frightening hallucinations/out of body experiences, thought disorder, confusion, dissociation, chest pain, palpitations and tachycardia, nausea, vomiting, difficulty breathing, ataxia, temporary paralysis/inability to speak, blurred vision, no awareness of pain, derealization/depersonalization and amnesia. A psychotic picture that can briefly mimic schizophrenia can also be seen.

Management is by supportive monitoring (CVS) in a quiet, low-stimulation room with symptomatic treatment with benzodiazepines if needed. CVS excitation can sometimes be helped by using propranolol. Death is rare and usually only occurs when used in combination with alcohol and other respiratory depressants. Prolonged periods of immobility and unconsciousness may result in rhabdomyolysis. Chlorpromazine should be avoided (because of anticholinergic effects) and haloperidol is largely ineffective. One volunteer study found benefit from using lamotrigine.

Ketamine dependence has been described, with compulsive use a primary symptom. Although tolerance develops there is no evidence for a withdrawal syndrome. Other risks associated with its use include accidents, trauma, risky sexual behaviour and cognitive impairment that appears to be persistent in heavy users (Curran et al. 2001).

'Magic mushrooms'

This is the street name for a variety of hallucinogenic fungi that contain the naturally occurring substituted tryptamines, psilocybin and psilocin. Taken orally (either raw or cooked) mushrooms produce a variable but dose-related psychedelic effect that comes on 30–60 minutes after consumption and lasts for 4–8 hours. Hallucinogenic potency in man is closely related to $5HT_2$-binding affinity in animals.

Although psilocybin causes mydriasis, unlike other psychedelics its autonomic activity is modest with no significant increases in pulse or blood pressure after oral doses.

As with other hallucinogens such as LSD, rapid tolerance develops after repeated use over a few days, which explains why most users report weeks or months between uses. A withdrawal has not been described, although cross tolerance with other psychedelic drugs such as LSD and mescaline is thought to occur.

A broad range of acute psychopathology is seen with psilocybin, though typically a psychotic syndrome is seen with changes in sensory perception and cognition, affective functioning and loosened associations. The pattern of thought and ego disturbance seen with psilocybin resembles an acute schizophrenic episode. Other acute adverse symptomatology include acute toxic stuporous states, amnesia and acute panic reactions.

Apart from the acute risk of significant adverse psychological effects and precipitation and exacerbation of mental health problems, physically use is generally safe, with fewer than half a dozen fatalities reported (Karch 2003). Before the commercialization of mushrooms, one of the greatest risks would have been the ingestion by mistake of a similar looking fungus. Uneventful recovery is the rule for most presenting with 'magic mushroom' poisoning.

Psychiatrists should consider mushroom or other psychedelic intoxication in young people, and be prompted in their suspicion by a clinical examination revealing dilated pupils and behavioural disturbance, in the absence of significant sympathetic stimulation. A urine specimen should be taken and if possible a sample of the consumed fungus obtained.

General sedatives: benzodiazepines and barbiturates

Benzodiazepines

Chlordiazepoxide was the first benzodiazepine to be made available, two years before diazepam in 1962. At their peak, up to one in six of the adult population in many European countries had used a benzodiazepine in the preceding year, though since the mid-1980s this has fallen to approximately one in ten (Hallstrom 1993). National guidelines and education have led to changes in prescribing patterns over the last 20 years with a fall in the prescription of benzodiazepines as hypnotics by a third, though levels of anxiolytic prescribing remain fairly level. This has been mirrored by a move away from longer-acting compounds to shorter-acting benzodiazepines.

Mechanism of action

Acting on a specific receptor site on the GABA-A receptor benzodiazepines enhance the response of the GABA-A receptor to GABA. This leads to hyperpolarization by increasing the frequency of opening of the chloride channel.

Metabolism

Bioavailability following oral administration is almost complete, with peak plasma concentrations being reached after 30–90 minutes. Being highly lipid-soluble and highly bound to albumin, drugs such a diazepam have a wide volume of distribution and diffuse rapidly across the blood–brain barrier and the placenta and appear in breast milk. They may also be given intravenously or intramuscularly, though this latter method may lead to unpredictable rates of absorption as well as local tissue damage. Benzodiazepines undergo significant hepatic degradation with many compounds having active metabolites, whose half-lives exceed that of the parent compound (see Chapter 38).

Tolerance

Tolerance to the different effects of benzodiazepines occurs at different rates. For example, rapid tolerance to the anticonvulsant effects explains why these drugs are not used as prophylaxis in the treatment of epilepsy. Tolerance to the sedative effects begin after 2 or 3 days and are marked by 2–3 weeks. Tacyphylaxis has also been reported. The mechanisms underlying the development of tolerance are:

- changes in receptor numbers/binding
- changes in receptor coupling to effector mechanisms
- secondary changes in neural systems that are affected subsequent to the primary action of the drug.

Tolerance to benzodiazepine use is most likely to be mediated by changes at the receptor level, either down regulation or uncoupling of the links between the receptor and ligand.

Withdrawal

More commonly seen with short-acting, high-potency preparations, benzodiazepine dependence and withdrawal was first highlighted by Petursson & Lader in 1981 (Box 28.3). It is probably the decreased functioning of the GABA-BDZ complex (and its knock-on effects on other neurotransmitters) that is responsible for most of the withdrawal syndrome. There do appear to be prolonged changes in GABA release following withdrawal and this may underlie protracted symptoms some patients experience.

Onset occurs 2–3 days after stopping, being maximum on days 7–10, usually abating by the end of the second week. Withdrawal symptoms may be confused with an unmasking of the original problem or with rebound anxiety. Differentiation should be based on the time sequence of its development and symptoms of sensory disturbance such as hyperacusis, photosensitivity, abnormal perceptual body sway, and flu-like symptoms. Withdrawal is time-limited and duration will be determined by particular pharmacokinetics of the benzodiazepine. Relapse tends to emerge slowly as the dose is reduced and persists well beyond discontinuation. Rebound symptoms of anxiety are more severe than prior to treatment.

Box 28.3 Symptoms of benzodiazepine withdrawal		
Physical	*Psychological*	*Perceptual*
Nausea, anorexia, sweating	Anxiety, dysphoria	Hyperacuity to sound, light and smell
Flu-like symptoms, weight loss	Insomnia with rebound REM (nightmares)	Abnormal sense of body sway
Muscle tension, twitching, increased reflexes and fasciculation	Depersonalization and derealization Hallucinosis and paranoia	Metallic taste in mouth Tinnitus
Tremor, palpitations	Rarely psychosis and delirium	Visual disturbance and hallucinations including formication
Convulsions may occur (day 5–7)	Restless, irritable with poor concentration	Other abnormal bodily sensations

Dependence and management of withdrawal
Those who become dependent upon benzodiazepines can be broadly divided into two groups. The first includes the iatrogenic user who, having had the drug prescribed, shows no escalation of dose and tends to achieve the benefits of improved psychosocial functioning. The other group members often use the benzodiazepine as part of a polysubstance abuse pattern and this is characterized by increased doses, a desire for euphoria and consequent psychosocial problems. Withdrawal attentuation is usually achieved by the careful, flexible, tapered withdrawal of the drug. Generally there is a trade-off between a rapid withdrawal with a more intense but relatively short duration of symptoms and a slower withdrawal period with protracted but less intense symptoms. Studies suggest that a slower withdrawal period is better, with most clinicians switching to a longer-acting compound, though the impact of this is less marked the longer the taper period is. For example, in one study using a 2–4 month taper of benzodiazepine dose 7% reported mild withdrawal and there were no cases of rebound compared to a 2–4 week taper where 35% reported mild withdrawal and 35% rebound anxiety (Pecknold et al. 1988).

Adjunctive therapies seem to have little to offer, although high-dose SSRIs may have some role and in some cases propranolol may be useful in reducing the autonomic features of anxiety.

The percentage of users who become dependent is a function of dose, type and duration of use with longer use being more likely to lead to dependence. Estimates suggest that very few will become dependent with periods of use of less than three months. Between 3–12 months of use 10–20% will become dependant, rising to 20–45% after periods longer than a year. Some patients will be more prone to developing dependence than others. Risk factors for developing dependence on benzodiazepines include:

- high doses for long periods, shorter half-life drugs
- previous history of substance dependence
- those with chronic dysphoria, insomnia and vivid dreams
- cognitive style – low self-esteem, tendency to catastrophize
- those who have psychiatric causes for insomnia
- passive dependent personalities
- female sex.

Dependence on benzodiazepines may thus be prevented by using alternative interventions such as psychological treatments or other pharmacotherapies. Benzodiazepine prescribing should be avoided in high risk, dependence prone groups and should be limited where possible to no more than two weeks.

Barbiturates
Forerunners to benzodiazepines, these drugs have greater abuse potential and overdose toxicity than their successors.

Once popular drugs of abuse, their intravenous usage was noted for its high associated mortality, particularly through respiratory depression. Preparations include phenobarbitone, amylobarbitone and secobarbital. They act by binding to specific receptor sites (distinct from the benzodiazepine site) on the GABA-A receptor.

Clinical features
Use leads to marked CNS depression, especially in the reticular system and the cerebral cortex, manifest by reduced anxiety dysphoria and impaired concentration. Increased doses lead to a cerebellar picture, with dysarthria and ataxia and eventually respiratory depression and death. Chronic use may result in labile affect, poor concentration and incoordination.

Tolerance
Tolerance arises through enzymatic auto-induction and there is therefore cross-tolerance to alcohol with a withdrawal syndrome not dissimilar to alcohol. Withdrawal commences 16–72 hours after drug cessation, with onset dependent upon the elimination half-life. Symptoms of barbiturate withdrawal include:

- nausea, anorexia and vomiting
- anxiety, insomnia (marked REM rebound) and tremulousness
- sweating and hypotension
- tendon hyper-reflexia, excessive sensitivity to light and sound
- hyperpyrexia, convulsions (3–7 days after stopping) and electrolyte imbalance may occur
- delirium, cardiovascular collapse and death have also been reported.

Treatment
Withdrawal should involve a tapering off of the drug by 10% daily decrements. This may be done as an in- or outpatient depending on risk of severe withdrawal and fits, which is increased the greater the daily dependent dose.

Cannabis

Ubiquitous in its use across cultures, the preparations of cannabis, from resin to oil to herbal hybrids, represent the most commonly used illicit psychoactive drug in the Western world. Its psychic effects have been recorded in the literature for centuries with the writings of Baudelaire and Dumas recording the experiences at 'Le Club des Haschischins' in Paris in the mid-1800s. Although difficult to classify because of its wide range of subtle psychoactive effects, most would consider cannabis to be a mild sedative with some hallucinogenic activity at higher doses.

Structure and mechanism of action

Of the several hundred substances within the *Cannabis sativa* and *C. indica* plant extracts, δ-9 tetrahydrocannabinol (THC) represents the major psychoactive constituent, though there are more than 60 cannabinoids in marijuana. Recently identified endogenous receptors stimulated by THC are found not only in the cerebral cortex but also in the hippocampus and brainstem. Like other drugs it causes the release of dopamine within the VTA.

Preparations

Preparations vary in form and potency. Cannabis resin has a THC content of about 2–6% and is commonly smoked in a 'joint' with tobacco. Herbal preparations (marijuana) vary widely in THC content with a new hybrid breed of high potency 'skunk grass' (THC = 10–20%) becoming increasingly available. Hash oil is an ether- and charcoal-released potent extraction from hashish with levels of THC exceeding 50%.

Route of administration

It may be smoked, often with tobacco, or taken orally with food or as a herbal infusion ('ganja tea').

Effects

Effects occur rapidly after inhalation and last from 1–6 hours. Physically it results in conjunctival injection and suffusion, tachycadia and a rise in blood pressure. It may cause brochodilation, though with chronic use the irritant qualities of smoke lead to spasm and parenchymal damage. Increased appetite, relaxation and sedation are common along with enhanced perceptual awareness and mild sensory distortion. Excessive use in non-tolerant users or use in combination with alcohol can lead to a 'whitey' where the users (often a novice) feels nauseous, dizzy and faint. Oral consumption of hash cookies is unpredictable and can result in intense prolonged effects due to a bimodal kinetic profile and metabolic breakdown products.

Physical complications

One joint (cannabis cigarette) is thought to be equivalent to about three cigarettes. Cannabis contains as many carcinogens as tobacco, deposits a third more tar and is a probable risk factor for oropharyngeal and lung cancer as well as coronary heart disease. Pulmonary damage is enhanced not only because joints do not have a particulate filter, but because users tend to inhale more deeply and keep the smoke in their lungs for longer. In fact most of the THC is absorbed in the upper airways so that deep inhalation is neither necessary nor the safest mode of inhalation. Short, brief inhalations of a pure joint is thought to be the safest way of smoking cannabis, with bongs and water pipes actually leading to greater tar deposition and inefficient extraction. The introduction of 'vaporizers' may reduce the pulmonary risk of cannabis inhalation since the cannabis is not combusted.

It is probable that the pulmonary damage caused by cannabis is at least as great as that caused by tobacco (Hall 1998) and since many consume the two substances mixed together they are exposing themselves to an enhanced pathogenic load.

Psychological complications

Panic attacks, paranoia, depersonalization, derealization, hallucinations and psychotic episodes have all been reported with acute intoxication, though the current view is that there is no distinct psychopathological entity as 'cannabis psychosis' (see Thornicroft 1990). The role of cannabis in the aetiology of schizophrenia has long been debated (for a recent review see Aresenault et al. 2004 and Chapter 18). The often-cited Swedish male conscript study by Andressan et al. (1987) showed a marked and linear association with use and risk of later developing schizophrenia (a six-fold increased risk for those having used cannabis more than 50 times). Recent analyses suggest that, even accounting for a wide number of confounders, the risk remains, though at lower levels (2.3 times the risk). Similar findings from a Dutch study also suggest that cannabis use is an independent risk factor for the emergence of psychosis. It would appear that overall cannabis use doubles the risk of developing schizophrenia, but the overall population contribution of cannabis to the incidence of schizophrenia is low. What appears critical is the early onset of use (under 15 years of age) in individuals prone to psychosis. The Dunedin and Christchurch studies reported that the earlier the onset of cannabis use and dependence the greater the increase in rates of psychosis, with an approximately three-fold increase in the incidence of schizophrenia in those who first used cannabis before the age of 15 years. Interestingly, cannabis use at 15 years did not predict depression later in life. The best predictor of that was smoking tobacco.

The association between cannabis and depression is also not as significant as widely thought. A review by Degenehart et al. (2003) suggests that although heavy cannabis use may increase depressive symptoms among some users, it is too early to determine if this association is causal.

Detection

Inactive fat soluble metabolites of cannabis (THC-11-oic acid) are detectable for considerable periods of time after last consumption, ranging from a week for the casual user to eight or more weeks for the heavy chronic user depending on the cut off point for detection. Saliva, buccal scrapings, and clothes sprays are all being investigated as methods to enhance acute identification of cannabis intoxication.

Dependence

Dependence on cannabis is the most common, but most under-recognized consequence of regular cannabis use, with

Hall suggesting that around 1 in 10 people who ever smoke cannabis will become dependent upon it (Hall et al. 1994). Effective treatments include CBT and RP. Concurrent tobacco smoking, which is prevalent in cannabis smokers, is a predictor of poor outcome, so NRT should be encouraged. There is no role for any specific pharmacotherapy to assist in the maintenance of abstinence from cannabis.

Volatile substances

The inhalation of volatile substances is commonly known as 'glue sniffing'. Cheap, easily and widely available, volatile substance abuse (VSA) continues to be common among UK teenagers. The range of abused compounds and the variety of preparations is vast (see Table 28.5). It is responsible for about 100 deaths each year with a modal age of 15 years.

Epidemiology

Studies suggest a prevalence of between 5–10% among secondary school children, with higher rates associated with poverty and deprivation. Though prevalence studies suggest equal sex distribution, deaths are far more likely in males, probably due to a different pattern of use. Most commonly a group activity, more popular after school or during school holidays, only 2–5% will persist with solitary use.

Mechanism of action

These substances are diverse in chemical structure but all probably act through a similar mechanism of alteration of the lipid-rich neuroglial membrane. Metabolism mainly occurs in the liver and kidney. Animal studies confirm their reinforcing nature (for example, rats will self-administer toluene) and although tolerance does develop fairly quickly, there is no evidence of a withdrawal syndrome.

Method of administration

Most commonly the substance will be placed in a bag, where the fumes are allowed to gather, before inhalation. Other solvents (trichloroethane) may be absorbed onto material such as clothing and inhaled. Aerosols may be inhaled directly or through rebreathing with a bag.

Table 28.5 Abused volatile substances	
Type of product	Volatile constituent
Adhesives	Toluene
Aerosols	Propellant 11 and 12
Cleaning solvent products	Tetrachloroethylene
Fuel gases	n-butane, isobutane and propane
Inhalational anaesthetics	Halothane and nitrous oxide

Effects

The inhalation of these substances causes a rapid onset of emotional, perceptual and cognitive change lasting about 30 minutes, with hallucinations, a euphoric mood and an altered state of awareness. At higher doses ataxia, nystagmus, frightening hallucinations and confusion may occur with the associated risks of accidental injury.

Complications

Adverse psychological reactions and accidents due to intoxication may occur. A study of 605 deaths from VSA (Esmail et al. 1993) showed a male:female ratio of 5:1, with 70% of deaths in those under 18, occuring in the 14–16 age range. At the age of 15 years 10% of all deaths and 20% of accident/violent related deaths are due to VSA. Death may result from arrthymias, respiratory depression, inhalation of vomitus, laryngeal spasm with cardiac arrest secondary to vagal stimulation.

Chronic use

Chronic use has been associated with a cerebellar syndrome, while inhalation of lead-containing petrol has been linked with cognitive decline. Liver damage and peripheral neuropathies have also been reported.

Recognition

A high level of awareness and education among parents, teachers and children is needed in order to detect and avert future use in children. Markers of solvent abuse include:

- apparent intoxication with giggling and confusion
- smell of glue or perioral dermatitis
- decline in academic performance or attendance
- erratic, irritable behaviour
- glue stains on clothing.

Stricter controls, limiting the variety and access to VSA by age-limits in combination with high-profile education of relevant parties are required to impact on a vulnerable group

Areca (betel) nut

Use of betel nut (areca nut) and its products is widespread, particularly in the Indo-Chinese continents, being the fourth most widely used substance after tobacco, alcohol and caffeine, affecting approximately 20% of the world's population. There is some evidence of a dependence syndrome, though the greatest risk is oral submucous fibrosis and malignancy. Betel nut, with or without admixed tobacco, is widely used amongst UK Indo-Asian immigrants particularly Gujurate speakers. The chemical composition of the nut is varied containing a number of psychoactive alkaloids, with arecoline being the one present in the greatest quantity. Arecoline may act as a GABA uptake inhibitor as well as a sympathetic stimulant. Anecdotally the nut and arecoline have significant medicinal properties ranging from an anti-helminthic and astringent to an aphrodisiac, digestive enhancement and psychomotor stimulant.

REFERENCES

Altman J, Everitt BJ, Glantier S et al. (1996). The biological, social and clinical basis of drug addiction: commentary and debate. *Psychopharmacology* **125**: 285–345.

Andreasson S, Allebeck P, Engstrom A et al. (1987) Cannabis and schizophrenia: a longitudinal study of Swedish conscripts. *Lancet* **2**: 1483–6.

Aresenault L, Cannon M, Whitton J & Murray J (2004) Causal association between cannabis and psychosis: examination of the evdience. *British Journal of Psychology* **184**: 110–17.

Baker A & Lee N (2003) A review of psychosocial interventions for amphetamine use. *Drug and Alcohol Review* September 22, 323–35.

Bearn J, Gossop M & Strang J (1996) Randomised double blind comparison of lofexidine and methadone in the outpatient treatment of opiate withdrawal. *Drug and Alcohol Dependence*.

Blackwell 1983

Blum K, Noble EP, Sheridan PJ et al. (1990) Allelic association of human dopamine D_2 receptor gene in alcoholism. *Journal of the American Medical Association* **263**: 2055–60.

Caplehorn JR, Drummer OH. (1999) Mortality associated with New South Wales methadone programs in 1994: lives lost and saved. *Med. J Aust* **170**: 104–9.

Cloniger CR (1994) Temperament and personality. *Current Opinion in Neurobiology* **4**: 266–73.

Crawford V (1997) Injecting drug use. *Current Opinion in Psychiatry* **10**: 215–19.

Degenhart L, Hall W, Lynskey M (2003) Exploring te association between canabis use and depression. *Addiction* **98**: 1493–503.

Dillon P, Copeland J, Janen K (2003) Patterns of use and harms associated with non-medical ketamine use. *Drugs and alcohol Dependence* **69**: 23–8.

Esmail A, Meyer L, Pettier A, Wright S (1993) Deaths from volatile substance abuse in those under 18 years: results from a national epidemiological study. *Archives of Disease in Childhood* **69**(3): 356–60.

Fleming PM & Roberts D (1994) Is the prescription of amphetamine justified as a harm reduction measure? *Journal of the Royal Society of Health* **114**: 127–31.

Frischer M, Bloor M, Goldberg D et al. (1993) Mortality among injecting drug users: a critical reappraisal. *Journal of Epidemiology and Community Health* **47**: 59–63.

Gossop M, Griffiths P, Powis B, Williamson S & Strang J (1996) Frequency of non-fatal heroin overdose. *British Medical Journal* **313**: 402.

Gossop M, Marsden J, Stewart D et al. (1997) The NTORS in the UK. Six month follow up outcomes. *Psychology of Addictive Behaviours* **11**: 324–37.

Goudie AJ & Emmett-Oglesby MW (eds) (1989) *Psychoactive Drugs: Tolerance and Sensitisation*. New Jersey: Humana Press.

Hall W (1996) What have population surveys revealed about substance use disorders and their co-morbidity with other mental disorders? *Drug and Alcohol Review* **15**: 157–70.

Hall W (1998) The respiratory risks of cannabis smoking. *Addiction* **93**: 1461–3.

Hall W & Farrell M (1997) Comorbidity of mental disorders with substance misuse. *British Journal of Psychiatry* **171**: 4–5.

Hall W, Solowij N & Lemon J (1994) The Health and Psychological Consequences of Cannabis Use, National Drug Strategy Monograph Series No 25 (Canberra, Australia Government Publishing Service).

Hallstrom C (1993) *Benzodiazepine Dependence*. Oxford: Oxford Medical Publications.

Harper CG, Kril JJ & Hollowat RL (1985) Brain shrinkage in chronic alcoholics: a pathological study. *British Medical Journal* **290**: 501–4.

Hunter GM, Donoghue MC & Stimpson GV (1995) Crack use and injection on the increase among injecting drug users in London.

Addiction **90**: 1397–400.

Johnson S (1997) Dual diagnosis of severe mental illness and substance misuse: a case for specialist services? *British Journal of Psychiatry* **171**: 205–8.

Kosten TR (2003) Buprenorphine for opoid detoxification. *Addictive Disorders and their Treatment*, vol. 2, No. 4.

Lingford-Hughes A & Nutt D (2003) Neurobiology of addiction and implications for treatment. *British Journal of Psychology* **182**: 92–100.

Marlatt

Maxwell JC (2003) The response to club drugs. *Current Opinion in Psychiatry* **16**: 279–89.

McCann UD, Szabo Z, Scheffel U, Dannals RF& Ricaurte GA(1998) Positron emission tomographic evidence of toxic effect of MDMA ('Ecstasy') on brain serotonin neurones in human beings. *Lancet* **352**: 1433–7.

McDowell et al. (2000) Am J D+A Abuse

Meyer RE (1986) How to understand the relationship between psychopathology and the addictive behaviours: another example of the chicken and the egg. In: Meyer RE (ed.) *Psychopathology and Addictive Disorders*, pp. 3–16. New York: Guilford Press.

Miller WR & Rollnick S (1991) *Motivational interviewing: Preparing People to Change Addictive Behaviour*. New York: Guilford Press.

Milroy CM, Clark JC & Forrst AR (1996) Pathology of deaths associated with 'ecstasy' and 'eve' misuse. *Clinical Pathology* **49**: 149–53.

Morgan M (2000) Ecstasy (MDMA): a review of its possible persistent psychological effects. *Psychopharmacology (Berlin)* **152**: 230–48 (Review).

Office of Population, Census and Statistics (1996) report. Her Majesty's Stationary Office.

Owen RR, Fischer EP, Booth BM et al. (1996) Medication non compliance and substance abuse among patients with schizophjrenia. *Psychiatric Services* **47**: 853–8.

Pecknold JC, Swinson RP, Kuch K & Lewis CP (1988) Alprazolam in panic disorder and agoraphobia: discontinuation effects. *Archives of General Psychiatry* **45**: 429–36.

Petursson H & Lader M (1984) *Dependence on tranquillizers*. Oxford: Oxford University Press.

Power KG, Markova I, Rowlands A, McKee KJ, Anslow PJ & Kilfedder C (1992) Intravenous drug use and HIV transmission amongst inmates in Scottish prisons. *British Journal of Addictions* **87**(1): 35–45.

Powis B, Strang J, Griffiths P, taylor C, Williamson S, Fountain J & Gossop M (1999) Self reported overdose among injecting drug users in London: extent and nature of the problem. *Addiction* **94**(4): 471–8.

Reiger DA, Farmer ME, Rae DS et al. (1990) Comorbidity of mental disorders with alcohol and other drug abuse: results from the Epidemiological Catchment Area (ECA) Study. *Journal of the American Medical Association* **264**: 2511–18.

Rodgers J, Ashton H, Gilvarry E & Young AH (2004) Liquid ecstasy on the dance floor. *British Journal of Psychology* **184**: 104–6.

Simpson D, Joe G & Brown B (1997) Treatment retention and follow up outcomes in the drug abuse treatment outcomes study (DATOS). *Psychology of Addictive Behaviours* **11**: 294–307.

Thornicroft G (1990) Cannabis and psychosis. Is there epidemiological evidence for an association? *British Journal of Psychiatry* **157**: 25–33. Published erratum appears in *British Journal of Psychiatry* (1990) **157**: 460.

Volkow ND, Fowler JS & Wang GJ (1999) Imaging studies on the role of dopamine in cocvaine reinforcment and addiction in humans. *Journal of Psychopharmacology* **13**: 337–45.

Weaver T, Madden P, Charles G et al. (2003) Comorbidity of substance misuse and mental illness in community mental and substance misuse services. *British Journal of Psychology* **183**: 304–13.

Webb E, Ashton CH, Kelly P & Kamali F (1996) Alcohol and drug misuse in UK university students. *Lancet* **348**: 922–5.

Winstock AR, Griffiths P & Stewart D (2001) Drugs and the dance music scene: a survey of current drug use patterns among a sample of dance music enthusiasts in the UK. *Drug and Alcohol Dependency* **64**(1): 9–17.

Wolff K, Farrell M, Marsden J, Monteiro MG, Ali R, Welch S & Strang J (1999) A review of biological indicators of illicit drug use, practical considerations and clinical usefulness. *Addiction* **94**(6).

Community psychiatry

Michael Phelan

INTRODUCTION

During the second half of the 20th century there were widespread closures of long stay mental hospitals, throughout the industrialized world. The advent of 'community care' has varied in pace and style, but it is now generally accepted as the optimum approach for caring for people with mental illness. Definitions of community care and community psychiatry are numerous, conflicting and, at times, confusing. Fundamentally, it is concerned with providing mental health services to local populations, on the basis of need. Opinions differ on precisely how best to do this, but there is a reasonable agreement about the principles that must underpin mental health services (Box 29.1).

In the asylum era, patients were frequently housed and treated many miles from their families and homes, in isolated and restricted environments. In contrast, it is fundamental to community psychiatry that services should be provided as close as possible to where people live, and in the least restrictive environment possible. At times services should be provided in people's homes, so that family support is not lost, and that disruption to someone's life is kept to a minimum. The development of local mental health services must be dictated by the needs of the population, not by past service provision, which may have grown up in a haphazard way. Services should be focused on those in most need, rather than just on responding to demand. This

---

Box 29.1 The principles of a community psychiatric service

Local and accessible

Responsible for a defined population

Needs-led rather than service-led

Proactive rather than reactive

Multidisciplinary

Involves users

Emphasizes the needs of carers

Seamless and flexible

Responds to special needs

---

requires a proactive response from staff. The needs of people with mental illness are often numerous and complex; frequently including social as well as health needs. No single professional group can hope to meet this diverse range of needs, and multidisciplinary teams are required. The providers of services must never lose sight of who they are trying to help, and they should be involved in a regular dialogue with service users, who should be actively involved at all levels of service planning and development. The demanding and vital role of carers is often under-recognized. They also need a voice in the development of services, as well as individual assessment and support. Service users need different types and intensities of help at different times, and must be easily able to access all elements of a service. Ethnic and other minority groups are especially vulnerable to mental illness and services should be able to respond to special needs, for instance by having easy access to interpreting services. Finally, services should be constantly evaluated and able to change in response to the changing needs of the population, while providing the best evidence-based treatments.

This chapter describes the legislative and policy framework that has grown up to support and guide the development of effective mental health services, and outlines some of the key working practices that appear to be necessary for services to flourish and be effective. Some of the specific components of a comprehensive service are then described. Much of this chapter primarily relates to the provision of adult services, but the principles apply as much to services for children and older people.

HISTORICAL AND LEGISLATIVE BACKGROUND

Prior to the closure of the large psychiatric asylums there were isolated attempts to provide psychiatric care outside of hospital. For instance an Anglican clergyman, Warren, established a telephone service to try and prevent suicides in New York at the beginning of the 20th century, and during the 1930s a mobile psychiatric team worked in Amsterdam to try and prevent hospitalization. Emptying of asylums, so called deinstituitionalization, gathered pace from the mid-1950s. There were various influences behind this policy. The discovery of effective psychotropic drugs began to bring hope that many patients could be treated outside hospital.

At the same time there was an increasing awareness that asylum care could not only fail to improve patients' functioning, but for some was detrimental. Ernest Goffman (1961) described American State hospitals as 'total institutions', with regimes that were authoritarian, impersonal and inflexible. He described the great divide

Box 29.2   Significant UK government legislation and policy
White Paper 'Better Services for the Mentally Ill' (1975) Set a target of 47 900 in-patient psychiatric beds
Mental Health Act (1983) **Audit Commission 'Making a Reality of Community Care' (1986)** 'The one option that is not tenable is to do nothing about present financial, organizational and staffing arrangements'
The White Paper 'Caring for People' (1990) Introduced distinction between health and social care Gave local authorities lead responsibility for the provision of community care Social service authorities to act as 'arrangers and purchasers of care services rather than monopolistic providers', and as gatekeepers to social care. Local authorities to assume responsibility 'in collaboration with health care professionals for assessing the needs of new applicants for public support to residential or nursing home care'
The NHA and Community Care Act (1990) Incorporated the recommendations from the White Paper
The Care Programme Approach Introduced in 1992 to provide 'a network of care in the community'
The Health of the Nation (1992) Highlighted mental health as one of five priority areas Established three targets: (i)   to improve significantly the health and social functioning of mentally ill people (ii) to reduce the suicide rate by at least 15% by the year 2000 from 1990 levels of 11 per 100 000 (iii) to reduce the lifetime suicide rate of severely mentally ill people by at least 33% by the year 2000
The Ritchie Report on the Care of Christopher Clunnis (1994) Made numerous recommendations including that 'no patient should be discharged from hospital unless those taking the decisions are satisfied that he or she can live safely in the community, and that proper supervision and care are available'
Supervision Registers (1994) All mental health units required to establish lists of the most vulnerable patients. Compliance was always patchy, and policy was subsequently disbanded
The Mental Health Act (Patients in the Community) (1996) Introduced supervised discharge; uptake has always been limited and inconsistent
National Framework for Mental Health in England (1999) Provided a blueprint for services and established seven national standards
Effective Care Coordination in Mental Health Services: Modernising the Care Programme Approach (2000) A policy document from the Department of Health that helped simplify aspects of the care programme approach; changes included the introduction of two levels of CPA (standard and enhanced) and the abolition of supervision registers
Mental Health Policy Implementation Guide (2001) Provided guidelines and targets for the development of specific teams for assertive outreach, crisis resolution, and early intervention in psychosis
Draft Mental Health Bill (2002) Proposed changes include the introduction of compulsory assessment and treatment in the community, and removing the need for 'treatability' when detaining people who pose a significant risk Proposals have received considerable opposition, and have yet to become law

between staff and patients (binary living), and how patients were treated as groups rather than individuals (batch living). An English psychiatrist Barton coined the phrase 'institutional neurosis', to describe how the effects of long term hospitalization could exacerbate the disabilities of mental illness. This view was supported by Brown & Wing (1970), who highlighted the link between poor social environment and patient disability. But hospital closure does not appear to have been driven solely, or even primarily, by scientific evidence. The ever rising costs of asylum care was a major factor; along with an increasing number of critical inquiry reports highlighting cruel and degrading treatment received by some patients. It is also suggested that psychiatrists were keen to leave the isolated asylums, and join their more powerful medical colleagues in the general hospitals

The impact of hospital closure was extensively examined by the Team for the Assessment of Psychiatric Services (TAPS) project (Leff et al. 1993). Researchers demonstrated that there was little change in the mental state or social functioning of patients after they left hospital, but that non-hospital care was preferred. Few patients became homeless, and there was no increase in mortality or crime rate.

In the UK, the government has attempted to support and influence the development of community services with a range of policies, initiatives and legislation, which are summarized in Box 29.2. The trend for mental health legislation to become more liberal is now in reverse. Supervized Discharge Orders were introduced in 1996, giving staff the power to bring people back to hospital if they do not comply with specific conditions, such as attending for daycare and living in supported accommodation. Recent proposals to reform the 1983 Mental Health Act are likely to result in further restrictions, and to extend the boundaries of psychiatric legislation (see Chapter 40).

KEY WORKING PRACTICES

Over the last 30 years various work patterns and approaches have evolved within community psychiatric teams, and there is now a degree of consensus on the key constituents of successful services.

Case management

The terms case management, care management and key working cause confusion. They are often used interchangeably, and are frequently used to describe different things by different people. Burns & Leibowitz (1997) have distinguished between 'brokerage case management', 'clinical case management' and 'key working'. The first of these terms describes the practice of obtaining services for patients. This originates from the US

where it was often the role of non-clinicians to ensure that patients discharged from long stay hospitals were receiving appropriate care. The case manager would have little or no direct contact with the patient, and would not personally provide services. This model is similar to the envisaged role for British social workers, originally referred to as case management, but subsequently renamed care management. In practice, most social workers have significant direct contact as well as a brokerage role in the care of people with severe mental illness.

Clinical case managers are directly involved in the care of patients. They have a wide remit, which extends beyond the traditional roles of specific professions. A case manager is expected to have regular contact with their patient or client, be aware of their current needs, and when possible help them meet these needs. This may involve help with simple household tasks, monitoring of medication or going to a cafe for a chat. At times the case manager will identify needs that he or she cannot meet, and will therefore arrange for another professional to be involved. For instance, the case manager may escort someone to his or her GP for a physical problem, or to a benefits agency to assess his or her entitlement for welfare benefits. This approach has been extensively researched with assertive outreach teams and crisis resolution teams (see Box 29.3), and found to be popular with patients and cost-effective. To be successful, case managers must be well supported by a multidisciplinary team, and prepared to extend their professional role. Smaller case loads do not necessarily bring about any significant improvement in outcome for patients (Burns et al. 1999).

The care programme approach

In the UK, the Care Programme Approach (CPA) introduced the principles of case management into routine mental health practice (Box 29.4). The objectives of the CPA are to promote interprofessional communication and co-ordination of care amongst specialist mental health services, and thus reduce the likelihood of people with severe mental illness falling through the safety net of care. Since its introduction, failure to implement the CPA has frequently been blamed on lack of mental health resources. It has also been hampered by staff having inadequate training and supervision and being reluctant to extend their specialist roles. However,

Box 29.3 Key elements of case management
Treatment is offered in the community
Continuity of care
Patients followed up assertively and engaged
Help patient function independently
Assist in basic needs and daily living activities
Care plan for each patient
Goals are negotiated with patients and carers

> **Box 29.4   The basic requirements of the CPA**
>
> 1. *Needs assessment:* a systematic and comprehensive assessment of the social and health needs of any person who appears to require community services
>
> 2. *Care plan:* decided upon in conjunction with the service user and carers. It should list identified health and social needs, and planned interventions. Crisis and contingency plans must be included, as well as a risk assessment and risk management plan. Unmet needs should also be included (e.g. when someone refuses a service), and the plan should be flexible and adaptable to change as the service user's needs change. Care plans must take into consideration cultural needs
>
> 3. *Care coordinator:* a member of staff is assigned as the focal point of contact for the service user and his or her carers. The care coordinator is responsible for keeping in close contact with them, and for monitoring and coordinating care
>
> 4. *Reviews:* care plans are reviewed regularly, and changed when appropriate. Sometimes this will require a multidisciplinary meeting, but reviews can take place with just the care coordinator and service user. Dates for future reviews must be agreed and recorded

perseverance has produced results and the CPA is now the bedrock of community services in the UK. Recent changes have helped to reduce the bureaucracy of the system (Department of Health 1999).

Sectorization

To enable community based services to provide effective care they are usually organized around specific sectors. This model of care is now widespread in the UK and other European countries (Johnson & Thornicroft 1993). Sectors are usually based on geographical areas, although in Britain services are increasingly determined by primary care registration.

Sectorization has a number of potential benefits:

- higher rates of patient identification and follow-up
- development of close working relationships with a range of local services
- greater knowledge and use of community resources by staff
- facilitates home visiting and treatment
- defined responsibility
- greater budgetary control.

In Nottingham, sectorization resulted in a fall in the number and duration of hospital admissions (Tyrer et al. 1989), but there is little other research comparing sectorized and non-sectorized services. Critics of sectorization point out that it reduces choice for referrers and patients, and results in poor continuity when patients move accommodation (a particular problem in inner city areas). It is also impractical to provide 24-hour crisis services to small sectors, and so these, and other more specialized services, have to be centralized.

The focus point of a sectorized service will usually be a community mental health team (CMHT), situated some

distance away from the hospital in-patient unit. This allows greater access for patients coming to see staff, and encourages staff to visit patients at home.

Needs assessment

Community services should be dictated by the needs of the people served. A need can best be defined as 'what people benefit from', and can be distinguished from demand (what people ask for) and supply (what is provided). An assessment of need will be dependent on who is making the assessment. Need as assessed by a professional, is termed 'normative need', and will often differ from the perceived needs of the patient. For instance, staff may well believe that a man needs to be in supported accommodation, while he feels that he needs a flat of his own.

Individual needs assessment

Although there is agreement that the assessment of need of individuals should be conducted and be the basis of subsequent care, there is less agreement on exactly how needs should be assessed. If a care plan is to be agreed with a patient then clearly the initial assessment of need should incorporate the views of the patient (and possibly the carer) as well as the staff. Any assessment must cover a wide range of health, social and basic needs. Box 29.5 lists the areas of

> **Box 29.5   Areas of potential need included in the CAN**
>
> **Basic needs**
> Accommodation
> Food
> Occupation
>
> **Health needs:**
> Physical health
> Psychotic and neurotic symptoms
> Drugs and alcohol
> Safety to self and others
>
> **Social needs**
> Company
> Intimate relationship
> Sexual expression
>
> **Functioning**
> Household skills
> Self-care and child care
> Basic education
> Budgeting
>
> **Service receipt**
> Information
> Telephone
> Transport
> Welfare benefits

need included in the Camberwell Assessment of Need (CAN), a rating scale designed to quantify need in people with severe mental illness (Phelan et al. 1995). Such an approach has uses in routine clinical work as well as research and evaluation.

Population needs assessment

The ideal way to plan local services would be to assess the needs of all people identified as mentally ill in the area, aggregate the data, and base local service provision on this information. Unfortunately, such detailed information is rarely available. Service planners therefore use a range of proxy measures which are known to give some approximation of the level of need in a population. These measures include sociodemographic information (e.g. proportion of people from an ethnic minority), previous service utilization, and estimates of the prevalence of specific mental disorders. Such assessments are used to decide on the distribution of mental health resource in different areas. It is hoped that the recent emphasis on needs assessment in health care will result in a more equitable distribution of resources, and the provision of more appropriate and targeted help to individuals.

Targeting

The Audit Commission (1994) demonstrated that the proportion of CMHT clients with a psychotic disorder ranged from 25–75% at different sites around the UK. As mental health services become more visible and accessible there is a risk that they become congested with people with less severe mental disorders, while the people with the more severe disorders are neglected. This scenario is encouraged by the increasing accessibility and acceptability of community based mental health services, and the greater recognition of common mental disorders, at a time when more patients with psychotic and major mood disorders are dependent on community services, rather than hospitals, for the bulk of their care. Those with the most severe problems are usually also those who are least able to access and demand services, and at times may not understand that they need help.

In an attempt to tackle this problem numerous definitions of severe mental illness (SMI) have been produced, and used in different settings (see Box 29.6). Such definitions are usually of a dichotomous type, i.e. SMI or not, and are increasingly used as gateways to services. There is wide variation in the extent to which objective and reliable (but not necessarily valid) measures are included e.g. number of admissions, compared to more subjective measures such as psychological distress. There is no consensus on either the dimensions that should be included, or the thresholds that should trigger care (Slade et al. 1996). When used in routine practice such definitions can be unreliable, and should not

be used indiscriminately to determine access to services (Phelan et al. 2001).

Multidisciplinary working

A prominent characteristic of modern community psychiatric practice is multidisciplinary team (MDT) working. This requires close working links across professions, and some loosening of interprofessional links. For instance, a community psychiatric nurse (CPN) needs to identify him- or herself with a community team composed of different professions, rather than the CPN department. In multidisciplinary teams there is a risk that staff will feel isolated, and be concerned that their core professional skills are not recognized or valued. There is an inevitable tension between the need for team management and the necessity for staff to be supervised by someone from their own profession. Successful teams are those that possess a strong sense of team cohesion, and where individual members are clear about their roles.

Multidisciplinary working has led to the use of terms that are acceptable to different professionals, and reflect the multiprofessional input, e.g. mental health services rather than psychiatric services, client rather than patient.

Box 29.6   Definitions of severe mental illness

Goldman (1981)

Diagnosis: patients diagnosed according to DSM IIIR criteria with one of the following:

   schizophrenia and schizoaffective disorder
   bipolar disorder and major depression
   delusional (paranoid) disorder

Duration: at least one year since onset of disorder

Disability: serious impairment of role functioning in at least one of the following:

   occupation
   family responsibilities
   accommodation

McLean & Liebowitz (1989)

At least one of the following must be present:

   Two or more years of contact with services
   depot prescribed
   ICD9, diagnostic code 295 or 297
   three or more in-patient admissions in the last three years
   three or more day-patient episodes in the last two years
   DSMIII-R highest level of adaptive functioning in the past year, five or less

Derived from Patmore & Weaver (1990)

Psychotic diagnosis, organic illness or injury AND previous compulsory admission OR aggregate one year stay in hospital in past five years OR three or more admissions in past five years

Psychotic diagnosis, organic illness or injury OR any previous admissions in past five years

No record of hospital admissions AND no recorded psychotic diagnosis, organic illness or injury

Research has highlighted the high levels of stress amongst community mental health workers. Prosser et al. (1996) found staff to have higher levels of depression and anxiety, and to be more 'emotionally exhausted' than hospital in-patient, day care or out-patient staff. Job satisfaction amongst staff appears to be related to having team role clarity, and identification with the team. The success and sustainability of community care is dependent on reducing burnout and stress amongst staff.

Advocacy and user involvement

A common problem for people in contact with mental health services is to get staff to understand what they want, and to obtain information about their condition, treatment, and rights. This is especially important for those who are compulsorily detained, or who are newly diagnosed with a mental illness. Advocacy and the promotion of user empowerment has been initiated and supported by voluntary organizations such as MIND, Rethink (formerly the National Schizophrenia Fellowship), and UKAN (United Kingdom Advocacy Network (see Chapter 11)). These, and other organizations vary in their membership and views, but together have been instrumental in giving patients, and their carers, a voice in how mental health services are organized, as well as providing support and information to patients and their families. When consulted about local service developments, common priorities among users include (Pigrim 1998):

- advocacy services
- out of hours services
- improved communication and information from professionals
- quality of care in residential settings
- destigmatization.

The importance of user involvement in the development of health services has been widely recognized by the British government, and is demonstrated by the increasing prominence given to user views and satisfaction in recent policy and legislation. The Royal College of Psychiatrists has a patients' and carers' liaison group that helps shape college policy. Members of this group have emphasized the importance of users and carers being involved in the teaching and training of psychiatrists.

SPECIFIC SERVICE ELEMENTS

Community mental health teams

Community Mental Health Teams (CMHTs) are usually the central point of any local mental health service. Although more specialist community teams are being established in many localities (see below), CMHTs are likely to continue to be the main point of contact for most service users. The two main functions of a CMHT are to provide assessment and short term treatment for less severe and time limited disorders, and provide on-going care for people with severe mental health illness, especially those who have complex needs and where there are significant risk factors. CMHT staff must work closely with colleagues in other parts of the service, such as the in-patient unit and assertive outreach team, and have effective links with a wide range of services in the community. For instance, a CMHT should have regular contact with the local police, housing department, welfare benefits advisor and local day care providers. It is also essential that there are excellent links with local primary care teams; this can be encouraged by teams accepting referrals from specific GPs, rather than from a fixed geographical area.

In-patient care

The number of psychiatric hospital beds in England & Wales has fallen by around 75% over the last 50 years, and similar reductions have occurred in most industrialized countries (Japan being the exception where hospital beds have increased three-fold). It is now unlikely that there will be further bed reductions, as it is widely accepted that the need for hospital beds can never be entirely replaced by community services. The atmosphere and functions of in-patient units have changed markedly as the numbers of beds have fallen. Admissions are now much shorter, patients are more ill, and ward environments are more disturbing. With so much emphasis on the provision of effective community services, and alternatives to admission, research and policy into how in-patient units can best be managed has lagged behind. There has, however, been consistent criticism and dissatisfaction about current standards of care, and steps are under way to try and improve provision (Department of Health 2002).

Crisis care

Caring for people in crisis is a core function for community mental health services, but emergency services often receive the fiercest criticism from service users. The provision of crisis services poses some specific problems. There is the broad spectrum of problems that present to emergency mental health services, ranging from acute psychosocial crises through to possible organic confusional states. Services need to be provided on a 24-hour basis, and this will usually require a degree of centralization, and subsequent difficulties in communication with sectorized daytime services. Staff working in emergency services have to cope with frequent intense encounters with distressed and at times aggressive and violent patients. The pressures on staff are compounded by the need to make rapid management decisions based on limited information.

Crisis resolution teams

Numerous studies have compared the outcome of acutely ill people managed by a team providing intensive multi-disciplinary home support, compared to hospital treatment (e.g.Hoult 1986; Muijen et al.; Stein & Test 1980 1992). These studies varied in terms of the patients accepted, the characteristics of the local population, and the intensity of care provided. However, they all reached broadly similar conclusions: many acutely ill patients can be managed effectively and safely outside hospital; such care does not result in significant differences in clinical or social outcome compared to hospital treatment but is usually more popular with patients; and the costs of community treatment are the same as, or less, than hospital care.

Crisis Resolution Teams (CRTs) are now being incorporated routinely into many local mental health services throughout the UK. They offer a 24-hour, 7-day-a-week rapid response service, which can provide an alternative to hospital admission for patients with acute and severe mental health problems. Staff focus on administering medication, providing practical help with the basics of daily living, and working closely with the client's normal support network, which may include family, friends and neighbours. Teams usually consist of around 15 staff members, and have between 20–30 clients on their case load. Contact is intense, but time-limited. Clients may be visited several times a day if necessary, but contact will usually be limited to a few days, or at the most a few weeks. If CRTs are not able to transfer clients rapidly to local community mental health teams they quickly become swamped and ineffective.

Acute day hospital care

Day hospitals have traditionally been used to support and rehabilitate people with long term illnesses, and are perceived as not having a significant role in crisis care. However, this view has been challenged, and research has indicated that many acutely ill people can be effectively and safely managed in a day hospital setting (Creed et al. 1991). This is dependent on having adequate staff, however, including medical staff in a day hospital, and on patients having a supportive and secure home to return to at night.

Non-hospital residential care

Crisis respite care outside a hospital is often asked for by service users, but rarely provided by statutory services. There are difficulties in providing a safe level of staffing in small residential units, and there can be opposition to opening such units in residential areas. Successful schemes have been described, however, and may offer substantial benefits compared to hospital care (Sledge et al. 1995).

A&E departments

The first point of contact for many people with a mental health crisis is the accident and emergency (A&E) department of a general hospital (Johnson & Baderman

1995). The attitudes of A&E staff towards psychiatric patients can be dismissive and hostile. Junior psychiatrists may have to conduct assessments in noisy and unsafe rooms that lack privacy. The appointment of specific mental health liaison nurses can help to improve communication with other agencies, and tackle negative attitudes among other staff.

Assertive outreach teams

There is some research demonstrating that some mentally ill people benefit from long-term community follow-up that is more intensive and assertive than that provided by community mental health teams. In particular it appears that the amount of time that people spend in hospital can be reduced (Mueser et al. 1998). Assertive Outreach Teams (AOTs) are being introduced into mainstream mental health services in the UK. They provide care for people with a severe mental illness, who have a past history of heavy hospital use, difficulty in maintaining contact with standard services, and who have multiple and complex needs. AOTs will usually have a total caseload of around 90 clients, and individual staff will have caseloads of 12 or less. Teams operate seven days a week, and often work extended hours. There is a strong emphasis on team working, with all staff having some knowledge of all the clients, and teams will persevere for months or even years to develop meaningful engagement with reluctant clients, with the aim of promoting recovery.

Early intervention teams

There is a strong belief that early treatment in psychosis is crucial. The hope is that early treatment will help to improve long term outcomes. Currently there is often a significant period between the onset of symptoms and diagnosis and treatment (Birchwood et al. 1997). Early Intervention Teams (EITs) provide a service for young people (usually 14–35 years) presenting with psychotic symptoms for the first time, and aim to reduce the duration of untreated psychosis (DUP). Such teams concentrate on administering the best possible pharmacological treatments and specialist psychological treatments, while focusing on the needs of the young person, such as their education and employment. As the incidence of schizophrenia and psychosis is low, EITs usually cover a population of up to 1 million, and expect to see around 150 new cases a year. There are some excellent examples of successful services, but it is not yet clear whether they will become an established part of mainstream mental health services.

Primary care

The World Health Organization (1973) declared that 'the primary care physicians should form the cornerstone of community psychiatry' as they 'are best placed to provide long-term follow-up and be available for successive periods of illness'. In the UK there is a unique and extensive network of primary care, which makes this declaration feasible. About 98% of the population are registered with a general practitioner (GP), and 60% consult at least once each year. Shepherd et al. (1966) first established the high rates of mental disorders amongst patients attending GPs, and since then several studies have confirmed that 25–30% of patients attending primary care services have a significant psychiatric disorder, of which approximately half is 'hidden' or unrecognized by the GP (Goldberg & Blackwell 1970). Each GP will have on average around seven people with a severe and enduring mental illness on the list, and between 300-600 people with depression and anxiety. Although some patients with a severe mental illness have little or no contact with a GP, the majority have frequent contact and the GP has an opportunity to monitor their mental state and drug treatment, as well has their physical health. Approximately one quarter of people with schizophrenia, have no contact with specialist services, and only see their GP (Johnson et al. 1991).

Deinstituitionalization and short in-patient stays have had an inevitable impact on primary care workload. It is essential for specialist mental health services to work in close collaboration with primary care services, to ensure that the relatively small number of people with severe mental illness receive the necessary physical care, and that GPs are fully supported in caring for the far larger numbers of people with less severe disorders. In south London, Strathdee (1990) found that from the GP's perspective important aspects of the local mental health service included the provision of immediate access to a specialist opinion, personal contact with a senior psychiatrist, and the assessment of patients in their own homes.

It is now common for a variety of mental health workers to be attached to GP surgeries. In recent years there has been a rapid growth in the number of practices with counsellors, and now about 50% of all practices have counsellors, and there is increasing evidence that they are effective in helping people with common mental health disorders, while specialist services increasingly focus on those with severe disorders. Having attached psychiatrists allows the GPs easy access to expert advice, and for patients to be seen in a less stigmatizing environment, compared to mental health facilities. However link workers may drift towards seeing those with less severe disorders, and often the smaller practices do not have the necessary space to accommodate them. In the UK there are plans to introduce new primary care mental health workers. It is envisaged that they will be involved in assessing patients with common mental health disorders, but have other roles such as helping establish mental health case registers in general practice and liaise with local mental health services and with other statutory and non-statutory services providers, such as the housing and welfare benefits departments.

Day care and occupation

As long-stay patients were discharged from asylums, day hospitals and sheltered workshops were the main providers of rehabilitation and day care. Although providing a useful service they were increasingly perceived as being another form of institution, and perpetuating segregation from the wider community. As a result, a wide range of different models of day care and vocational programmes have developed, but in the UK provision remains patchy, and for many service users the options are still limited. There needs to be strong user involvement in any occupational programme to ensure that it is meeting the needs of those that it serves. Most importantly, real jobs for real pay should be available for as many as possible, through supported employment schemes.

Housing

No chapter on community psychiatry would be complete without at least a mention of the importance of housing. If vulnerable mentally ill people are to survive out of hospital it is essential that they are provided with adequate and secure accommodation, with the appropriate level of support. No amount of nursing or other input will compensate for poor housing. The range of accommodation required in any area to cater for different patients will include 24-hour staffed hostels, daytime staffed hostels, group homes with staff visiting and supported flats. Community mental health teams need to develop cooperative links with local housing workers, who are often the first to notice that a tenant is not well when they stop paying rent or fail to look after their property.

There are high rates of mental illness amongst the homeless, and providing psychiatric services to them requires expertise and hard work. To be successful, services must first address the priorities of the homeless person, such as food and shelter, as well as trying to treat specific psychiatric disorders. Specialist multidisciplinary teams need to balance offering a flexible non-coercive approach, with a therapeutic focus and emphasis on the patient's right to receive treatment (Craig 1998) (see Chapter 7).

CONCLUSIONS

Community services can improve the quality of life of many of the most disabled patients in our society. However, providing comprehensive and effective services outside hospital is difficult, and currently the support and treatment they receive is all too often inadequate. Progress has been made, but further improvements will largely be dependent on the willingness of governments to invest sufficient resources into mental health services.

FURTHER READING

Thornicroft G & Szmukler G (eds) (2001) *Textbook of Community Psychiatry*. Oxford: Oxford University Press.

REFERENCES

Audit Commission (1994) Finding a Place: A Review of Mental Health Services for Adults. London: HMSO.

Birchwood M, McGorry P & Jackson H (1997) Early intervention in schizophrenia. *British Journal of Psychiatry* 170: 2–5.

Brown GW & Wing J (1960) Social treatment of chronic schizophrenia: a comparative survey of three mental hospitals. *Journal of Mental Science* 107: 847–61.

Burns T & Leibowitz J (1997) The Care Programme Approach: time for frank talking. *Psychiatric Bulletin* 21: 426–9.

Burns T, Creed F, Fahy T, Thompson S, Tyrer P, & White I (1999) Intensive versus standard case management for severe mental psychotic illness: a randomised trial. *Lancet* 353: 2185–9.

Craig T (1998) Homelessness and mental health. *Psychiatric Bulletin* 22: 195–7.

Creed FH, Black D, Anthony P et al. (1991) Randomised controlled trial of day and in-patient psychiatric treatment. 2. Comparison of two hospitals. *British Journal of Psychiatry* 158: 183–9.

Department of Health (1999) Effective Care Co-ordination in Mental Health Services: Modernising the Care Programme Approach: A Policy Booklet. London: DOH.

Department of Health (2002) Mental Health Policy Implementation Guide: Inpatient Care Provision. London: DOH.

Goffman E (1961) Asylums. New York: Doubleday Anchor.

Goldberg D & Blackwell B (1970) Psychiatric illness in general practice: a detailed study using a new method of case identification. *British Medical Journal* 2: 439–43.

Goldman H (1981) Defining and counting the chronically mentally ill. *Hospital and Community Psychiatry* 32: 21–7.

Hoult J (1986) Community care of the acutely mentally ill. *British Journal of Psychiatry* 149: 137–44.

Johnson E.C (1991) Disabilities and circumstances of schizophrenic patients – a follow-up study. *British Journal of Psychiatry* 159(Suppl. 13).

Johnson S & Baderman H (1995) Psychiatric emergencies in the casualty department. In: Phelan M, Strathdee G & Thornicroft G (eds) *Emergency Mental Health Services in the Community*. Cambridge: Cambridge University Press.

Johnson EC, Owens DGC & Leary J. (1991) Disabilities and circumstances of schizophrenic patients – a follow-up study. VI. Comparsion of the 1975–85 cohort with the 1970–75 cohort. *British Journal of Psychiatry* 159(Suppl. 13): 34–6.

Johnson S & Thornicroft G (1993) The sectorisation of psychiatric services in England and Wales. *Social Psychiatry and Psychiatric Epidemiology* 28: 45–7.

Leff J. (1993) Evaluating the transfer of care from psychiatric hospitals to district-base services. *British Journal of Psychiatry* 162(Suppl. 19): 6.

McLean E & Liebowitz J (1989) Towards a working definition of the long term mentally ill. *Psychiatric Bulletin* 13: 251–2.

Mueser KT, Bond GR, Drake RE, & Resnick SG (1998) Models of community care for severe mental illness: a review of research on case management. *Schizophrenia Bulletin* 24: 37–74.

Muijen M, Marks I, Connolly J, & Audini B (1992) Home based care for patients with severe mental illness. *British Medical Journal* 304: 749–54.

Patmore E.C & Weaver J (1990) *A Survey of Community Mental Health Centres*. London: Good Practices in Mental Health.

Phelan M, Seller J & Leese M (2001) The routine assessment of severity amongst people with mental illness. *Social Psychiatry and Psychiatric Epidemiology* 36: 2000–6.

Phelan M, Slade M, Thornicroft G. et al. (1995) The Camberwell Assessment of Need (CAN): the validity and reliability of an instrument to assess the needs of people with severe mental illness. *British Journal of Psychiatry* 167: 589–95.

Prosser D, Johnson S, Kuipers E, Szmuckler G. Bebbington P & Thornicroft G (1996) Mental health, 'burn-out' and job satisfaction among hospital and community-based staff. *British Journal of Psychiatry* 169: 334–7.

Shepherd M, Cooper B, Brown, A & Kalton, G (1966) *Psychiatric Illness in General Practice*. Oxford: Oxford University Press.

Slade, M, Powell, R. and Strathdee, G (1996) Current approaches to identifying the severely mentally ill. Social Psychiatry, *Psychiatry Epidemiology* 32: 177–84.

Sledge WH, Tebes J & Rakfeldt J (1995) Acute crisis respite care. In: Phelan M, Strathdee G & Thornicroft G (eds) *Emergency Mental Health Services in the Community*. Cambridge: Cambridge University Press.

Stein LJ & Test MA (1980) Alternative to mental hospital treatment. 1. Conceptual model treateament program and clincial evaluation. *Archives of General Psychiatry* 37: 392–7.

Strathdee G (1990) The delivery of psychiatric care. *Journal of the Royal Society of Medicine* 83: 222–5.

Tyrer P, Turner R & Johnson A (1989) Integrated hospital and community psychiatric services and the use of psychiatric beds. *British Medical Journal* 299: 298–300.

World Health Organization (1973) *Psychiatry and Primary Medical Care*. Copenhagen: WHO regional Office for Europe.

Forensic psychiatry

Carine Minne and Oyedeji Oyebode

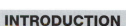

INTRODUCTION

Forensic psychiatry is a clinical sub-speciality concerned with all aspects of care and management of mentally disordered offenders. Other patients who pose considerable management difficulties, and who have not necessarily had conflicts with the law, can also be managed by forensic psychiatrists. Some general psychiatrists have a special interest in or responsibility for forensic psychiatry.

The term 'forensic' means pertaining to, connected with or used in courts of law – suitable or analogous to pleadings in court. Indeed, the Latin word 'forensis' was the forum or public place in ancient Rome where judicial processes were performed.

Forensic psychiatry was not an established sub-speciality until the 1970s. Prior to that, general psychiatrists cared for and became involved in court procedures dealing with mentally disordered offenders. The first textbook of forensic psychiatry was actually published in 1923 (Eastwood). Significant events over the years have, to some extent, been the drivers in improving the care and management provided to this patient population.

A review of services culminated in the Glancy Report (Department of Health and Social Security 1974), jointly produced with the then Department of Health and Social Services. It recommended that each regional health authority should develop secure hospital facilities for patients who could not be managed on open wards but did not require treatment in conditions of what was then termed special security. The suggestion was that 1000 beds in England and Wales should be provided.

In 1962, Graham Young, then aged 14, was committed to Broadmoor Hospital after conviction for the attempted poisoning of three people. He was conditionally discharged after 9 years and subsequently obtained a job in a photographic laboratory. He killed two colleagues by poisoning them within months of his discharge from hospital. This resulted in further public concern and the government appointed a committee, under the chairmanship of the late Lord Butler, to further review the services provided for mentally disordered offenders. This committee produced an important report (Home Office and Department of Health and Social Services 1975), which essentially changed the delivery of forensic psychiatric care. The main recommendation was for a regional secure unit (now termed medium secure unit) in each of the then regional health authorities.

In view of delays in these recommended developments, provisions for mentally disordered offenders were again reviewed resulting in the Reed Report (Department of Health and Home Office 1992). The final summary report specifically recommended that mentally disordered offenders should receive care and treatment from health and social services rather than custodial care. Essentially, the Reed Report recommended that mentally disordered offenders should be cared for

- by health and social services
- paying particular attention to the quality of care and the needs of the individual
- in the community rather than institutional settings, if possible
- under conditions of security appropriate to the patient's needs, bearing in mind their degree of dangerousness
- with a view to maximizing rehabilitation progressing to independent living
- as near as possible to their homes or families.

There were also recommendations for an increase in consultant and bed numbers.

In 1997 the Fallon Inquiry was established in response to a number of allegations about the working of the Personality Disorder Unit at Ashworth Special Hospital. This inquiry found many serious flaws and led to a number of recommendations being made when it was published in 1999. These recommendations addressed the current running of that Personality Disorder Unit as well as addressing future forensic psychiatry secure services, mental health legislation and policies.

The above inquiry report led to a review of security at the three English High Security Hospitals, Broadmoor,

Ashworth and Rampton. In 2000, the Tilt Report made several procedural and physical security recommendations, including security training needs for staff and the commission of annual prison service security audits, using standards specifically developed for high security hospitals. The focus of the recommendations was largely on physical security with many comparisons with provisions in prisons, without putting in context the complex clinical care provided by these hospitals.

Services where forensic psychiatry is practised

Forensic psychiatry is practised in a broad range of facilities as follows:

- high secure hospitals
- medium secure units
- forensic intensive care units
- general psychiatry in-patient services
- general psychiatry outpatient services
- community services, e.g.
  (a) bail hostels
  (b) probation services
- prisons

Forensic psychiatry patients, as other psychiatric patients, are looked after by multidisciplinary teams led by consultant psychiatrists, referred to as RMOs (Responsible Medical Officers). Forensic psychiatry teams in particular have embraced psychodynamic input by beginning to include psychodynamic psychotherapists, working directly with patients or by providing staff (or institutional) consultations. The offences committed by these patients can at times be perplexing or shocking with massive degrees of projection and splitting leading to mixed responses by different members of staff as well as demoralization or high risk of institutional ill-health. Providing direct and indirect psychodynamic input with individual patients and teams can offer better understanding of the nature of patients, interactions as well as improve relational security and the functioning of the institution.

MENTAL HEALTH ACT 1983 AND REFORM PROPOSALS

Definition of mental disorder

Mental disorder is currently defined by statute as 'mental illness, arrested or incomplete development of the mind, psychopathic disorder or any other disorder or disability of mind'. The four categories of mental disorder are as follows:

1 **Mental illness:** not defined in the 1983 Mental Health Act.

2 **Severe mental impairment:** means a state of arrested or incomplete development of mind, which includes severe impairment of intelligence and social functioning and is associated with abnormally aggressive or seriously irresponsible conduct on the part of the person concerned.

3 **Mental impairment:** means a state of arrested or incomplete development of mind (not amounting to severe mental impairment), which includes significant impairment of intelligence and social functioning and is associated with abnormally aggressive or seriously irresponsible conduct on the part of the person concerned.

4 **Psychopathic disorder:** defined as a persistent disorder or disability of mind (whether or not including significant impairment of intelligence), which results in abnormally aggressive or seriously irresponsible conduct.

Mental Health Act 1983 (England and Wales)

Civil Law

Part 2 of the 1983 Mental Health Act (MHA) provides for the detention of patients in hospitals or mental nursing homes for the medical treatment of mental disorder.

Medical treatment includes nursing care, habilitation and rehabilitation under medical supervision. There are various provisions under this part of the Act, which provide for detention of patients for a period of up to 28 days up to a maximum of six months in the first instance (see Chapter 40).

Criminal law

The 1983 Mental Health Act (England and Wales) consolidated the provisions within the 1959 Act and the Mental Health (open amendment) Act 1982. The provisions of the new Act were expected to have effect with respect to the reception, care and treatment of mentally disordered patients, the management of their property and other related matters. Part 3 of the MHA 1983 provides for the admission and detention in hospital of patients on the order of a court with medical recommendations. It is also concerned with guardianship orders and the transfer of patients to hospital or guardianship from penal institutions on the order of the Home Secretary. This part of the Act is related to remand in hospital for a report or treatment of an accused person. It also gives powers to courts to order hospital admission, guardianship or interim hospital orders. There is a provision in this section, which enables higher courts to restrict discharge from hospital. It also deals with transfer of sentenced and unsentenced prisoners from prison to hospital.

The Mental Health Act Commission set up in September 1983 is a Special Health Authority responsible to the

Secretary of State. The government hoped, in setting up the commission, that it would exercise a general protective function for detained patients, with a view to building up information over a period of time, which would help to provide a better understanding of mental health. The functions of the Commission are to:

- review how the powers and duties under the Act are carried out in respect of detained patients, including visiting and interviewing patients
- investigate complaints
- provide registered second opinion doctors where required by the Act and doctors to certify consent under section 57
- maintain the Code of Practice and advise ministers on amendments
- offer advice to Ministers on matters falling within the Commission's remit
- publish a biennial report.

Mental Health Review Tribunals were established under the Mental Health Act 1959 to provide an independent means to review the need for the continued compulsory detention of patients in psychiatric hospitals. Tribunal members (England and Wales) are appointed by the Lord Chancellor and each tribunal panel has three members: a lawyer as chairman, a medical member and a lay member. The legal member must be a judge for restricted patients.

The primary function of the Tribunal is to decide whether the patient should continue to be detained in hospital. The powers of the tribunal differ according to whether a patient is unrestricted, under Guardianship, restricted or transferred from prison.

The Mental Health Acts operational in Scotland (1984) and Northern Ireland (1986) are broadly speaking similar, but certain differences apply. In the Mental Health (Scotland) Act 1984, only mental illness and mental handicap come under the rubric of mental disorder and not psychopathic disorder. However, mental illness here is defined as also including a mental disorder that is persistent and manifested only by abnormally aggressive behaviour. Any detention lasting more than 28 days requires the approval of a sheriff, a legally qualified judge. Appeals against detention are heard by a sheriff and there are no Mental Health Review Tribunals. In the Mental Health (Northern Ireland) Act 1986, the situation is similar with mental illness and mental handicap, but in addition any other disorder or disability of mind. As with the Scottish Act, psychopathic disorder is not mentioned. In fact, here it is also specified that persons suffering from mental disorder by reason only of personality disorder are excluded from detention on these grounds alone.

Reform proposals of the MHA 1983

A White Paper published in December 2000 described the Government's proposals for legal reforms to reflect in particular the increase use of treatment in the community. The proposals are divided into two parts:

1. **The new legal framework:** provides a new broad definition of mental disorder: 'any disability or disorder of mind or brain, whether permanent or temporary, which results in an impairment or disturbance of mental functioning'. Unlike the Mental Health Act 1983, there would no longer be definitions of any particular categories of mental disorder or the concept of 'treatability'. An attempt to simplify the procedures of detention is outlined. There would also be a range of safeguards for patients' interests.

2. **High risk patients:** specific arrangements for people who are deemed to pose a significant risk of serious harm to others as a result of their mental disorder are also being proposed. In particular, the so-called 'dangerous severe personality disordered' who have not committed any offences but for whom the proposal includes some form of incarceration until they can be shown to be no longer dangerous, with inherent difficulties in quantifying and measuring risks. These have evoked strong views on ethical and moral grounds and, while writing this chapter, the debate continues.

CIVIL LAW. MENTAL DISORDER AND LEGAL IMPLICATIONS

Civil law involves one individual against another and relates to any matter defined by Parliament or the Courts as 'civil'. Essentially, civil law relates to laws concerning property, inheritance and contracts. The presence of mental disorder may have a legal effect on a person's civil rights, be they public (e.g. driving, jury service, standing for and voting in elections), personal (marriage, divorce and annulment and child care) or financial (entering into contracts and testamentary capacity). These issues are discussed in detail in Chapter 40.

OFFENDING AND MENTAL DISORDER

The relationship between offending and mental disorder is complex, involving many psychosocial aspects in general as well as risk factors specific to each offender. In order to begin to examine the complex relationship between different offences and mental disorder, one needs to be aware of the contribution of psychosocial aspects, which may be specific for any particular offender. These can be described under the headings of individual, family and social factors (Farrington 2000). Offending is one behavioural manifestation of antisocial behaviour arising in childhood that can persist into adulthood. There have been many studies indicating risk factors for offending and these need to be addressed in prevention programmes, focusing on the young, given the continuity that has been shown to exist between childhood antisocial behaviours and later adult antisocial behaviours.

All criminal acts are unique interactions between the perpetrator, the environment and sometimes the victim, and their interaction is unique on every occasion (Chiswick 1993). It is worth stating that the psychiatric services are only ever involved with a very limited number of offenders who are selected and not representative of the offender population as a whole. This further complicates any examination of links between particular offences and psychiatric disorders. Any links are also influenced by crime rates, prevalence of psychiatric disorders and application of the criminal justice system as well as how health and social policies are applied to mentally disordered offenders.

It can be helpful to look at the different kinds of offences that are committed before trying to link these with any particular mental disorder.

The crimes committed by mentally disordered offenders are essentially the same as those committed by the general population. They include:

- violent offences – from minor assault to homicide
- sexual offences – from indecent assault to rape
- property offences – acquisitive and destructive offences.

Violent crimes

Violent crimes include the following:

- *wounding*:
  (a) with intent to cause grievous bodily harm (Section 18, Offences Against the Person Act 1861)
  (b) with no intent to cause grievous bodily harm (Section 20 of the same act).
- *assault*:
  (a) occasioning actual bodily harm (Section 47 of the same Act)
  (b) common assault.

As with homicide, such offences can be associated with any form of mental disorder in the offender.

The contemporary terminology of 'child abuse and neglect' encompasses non-accidental injury, child neglect, non-organic failure to thrive and sexual and emotional abuse. Abuse varies from the most minor of assaults to the most life-endangering. Cordess (1995) provided a helpful illustration of the classification of child abuse and neglect, and child abduction.

Homicide is a general term for the killing of one human being by another. Legally, homicide is classified into lawful and unlawful homicide. Lawful homicide includes justifiable killings (e.g. on behalf of a state) and excusable homicide (e.g. an accident or reasonable mistake). Unlawful homicide is defined in common law as 'the unlawful killing of any reasonable creature or being and under the Queen's

peace, the death following within a year and a day of the deed'). This includes murder, manslaughter, killing of infants – which includes child destruction (a killing of a child before birth) and infanticide, and death by dangerous driving.

The psychiatric classification of homicides is divided into 'normal' and 'abnormal'. 'Normal' homicides occur:

- during the course of a crime
- for political reasons
- from 'normal' emotions such as anger, jealousy or revenge.

'Abnormal' homicides occur where the offender has a psychiatric disorder, which may include:

- psychosis – functional or organic
- neurosis – including affective disturbance
- personality disorder
- learning disability.

Sexual offences

The legal classifications of child sexual abuse are:

- incest
- unlawful sexual intercourse under 13 years (it is no defence for the minor to consent or for the adult to believe him/her to be over 16 years)
- unlawful sexual intercourse with a girl under 16 years but over 13 years
- indecency with children (inciting children to perform acts of gross indecency upon an adult or taking possessing or showing indecent photographs or films of a child)
- defilement of girls (encouraging them into prostitution)
- any other offence (e.g. buggery, indecent assault) where a child is the victim.

Glasser (1990) classifies paedophilia into two types, primary and secondary. Primary paedophilia is present when someone's sexual orientation is exclusively directed towards children and is often, if not always, associated with personality disorder. It has been shown that there is often a history of abuse in the perpetrator, although by no means do all those abused later become perpetrators. One psycho-analytic explanation for such behaviour is that there is an attempt on the part of the perpetrator to reverse an earlier actual or perceived trauma. Secondary paedophilia, on the other hand, is a consequence of some other pathology such as mental illness or other cerebral diseases or genetic disorders.

Violent sexual assault against adults include:

- rape (rape is seen predominantly as an act of violence expressed in sexual terms)
- buggery (this is anal intercourse with males or females, and anal or vaginal intercourse with animals, i.e. bestiality)

- indecent exposure (exhibitionism) (indecent exposure is an offence whereas exhibitionism is a paraphilia).

Property offences

Acquisitive property offences are:

- theft and handling stolen goods, including shop-lifting
- taking and driving away (motor vehicles)
- robbery
- blackmail
- burglary
- fraud and forgery.

Psychiatric illness is only rarely obviously associated with the above. Shop-lifting is predominantly carried out by 10- to 18-year-olds, but a small percentage of such offending is associated with affective disorder in middle-aged women in particular. Personality and developmental difficulties of adolescence are associated with the taking and driving away of motor vehicles.

There is no specific psychiatric condition associated with burglary but substance abuse and dependence is a common feature in such offenders. Domestic burglaries sometimes result in opportunistic acts resulting in crime not apparently planned, for example, in the sexual assault of a victim who happens to be at home during a burglary. In the assessment of such a case, one would have to take into consideration the nature of the psychopathology of the offender, whose disturbed internal world contained the ingredients for this opportunity to arise.

Destructive offences are:

- criminal damage
- arson (fire-setting).

Criminal damage is commonly part of a wider antisocial behaviour.

Lewis & Yarnell (1951) and Prins et al. (1985) have provided useful classifications of arson. There is no particular mental disorder associated with arson (fire-setting). The regular requests for psychiatric assessments of arsonists is most probably due to the public's concern about the dangerousness of the behaviour and the view that arsonists must surely be mentally disturbed. The majority of apprehended (most are not) fire-setters, however, are referred to the psychiatric services for assessment although no particular psychiatric diagnosis is associated with fire-setting. There are some interesting psychoanalytic speculations about the relationship between fire-setting and early disturbed sexual development, and attempts are being made to address this association more scientifically. Most arsonists are managed within the penal system although some do find their way to secure psychiatric hospitals. In terms of future dangerousness, studies show that about 30% repeat an arson offence but many will commit other types of offences.

SPECIFIC MENTAL DISORDERS AND OFFENDING

An estimate of the frequency of association between the various kinds of disorder and offending is of value in helping to determine the nature and extent of facilities required for appropriate treatment. Given what has been described in the previous section of this chapter about the complexity of any relationship, this is not easy to ascertain. However, that relationship between psychiatric disorder and violence attracts particular interest by virtue of public concern (which can be ignited unhelpfully through, for example, tabloid newspaper reports) and consequent concern by policy makers.

There have been a few attempts to quantify the ultimate risk posed by the person with a psychotic illness. Häfner and Böker (1973) jointly offered an estimate from a large offender sample in Germany. They were primarily interested in homicidal attacks. They calculated that the risk of a homicidal attack was 0.05% among people with schizophrenia and 10 times less among those with an affective psychosis. Mullen (1984) in reviewing various studies concluded that a risk of a homicidal attack by seriously mentally ill people is small and that the risk of suicide is about 100 times greater. For people with a psychotic illness, the illness itself is an important factor in precipitating some non-violent antisocial behaviour and probably most violence. There is beginning to be better recognition of the types of symptoms that render those prone the most vulnerable. It must be kept in mind that no person, psychotic or otherwise, ever acts entirely independently of his or her environment and, also, that special difficulties arise when there is a coexisting personality disorder.

Organic disorders

Lishman (1968) found that among head-injured people, post-traumatic antisocial behaviour was rare and almost exclusively confined to those with injuries of the frontal lobe. Subsequent studies have reconfirmed the importance of the frontal lobe or frontotemporal damage but also emphasized that premorbid personality traits may be as important as the location and extent of the injury in determining subsequent behavioural disturbances. A survey of sentenced prisoners in England and Wales (Gunn et al. 1991), evaluating a wide offender constituency, including non-violent offenders, found that only about 1% of them suffered from organic brain disorder.

Schizophrenia

There is still disagreement about the connection between schizophrenia and serious violence (Tidmarsh 1990). It is clearly a complex interaction and this applies to more minor offending as well as serious violence. There is no doubt that minor offences are more common than serious ones but that people with schizophrenia are over-represented among violent offenders when violence can occur during the acute or chronic phases of the illness. It is important to look at situational factors as well as the individual phenomenology. It is also important to keep in mind the contribution of alcohol or drug misuse in these cases as well as non-compliance with treatment.

Affective illness

The apparently low rate of affective illness in forensic psychiatry patient populations are likely to be underestimates as, for example, minor depressive episodes may not be noted or accepted by nonpsychiatric personnel and such cases therefore might not get referred to the psychiatric services. Even quite severe depression might be seen only as a reaction to having committed the offence and not also as a contributing factor. By far, the most common violent acts committed by depressed individuals are suicide and attempted suicide and one should always enquire about any homicidal ideation. The most widely known forensic psychiatry presentation of affective disorder is the killing of children by their depressed mothers and the killing of wives and sometimes also the children by depressed husbands. These are quite often followed by suicide. Suicide risk is greatest when the depressed individual's drive has returned, paradoxically, at the beginning of treatment. Rapid-cycling bipolar disorder in offender patients can be missed as they can be viewed by authorities as obstructive or nuisances. Some middle-aged women who shop-lift can present with an overt or more hidden depressive illness.

Personality disorders

It is known that personality disorders in psychiatry are usually mixed in type and a simple category does not offer much insight into an individual other than one dimension of his or her presentation. In order to provide the most appropriate management plan, the individual needs to have a thorough and preferably longitudinal assessment. Any of the mixed personality disorders may be associated with any kind of offending and substance misuse is a common associated finding. Female offenders are more often categorized as suffering from borderline personality disorder than are males who in turn, in relation to more serious crime, are categorized as suffering from antisocial personality disorder. The term psychopathic disorder should only be used in the legal context.

There is a strong association between the legal category of psychopathic disorder or, psychiatrically, antisocial personality disorder, and offending. Hare (1991) analysed the violent behaviours of 243 male prison inmates. Those suffering from antisocial personality disorder were found to be generally more violent than 'non-psychopaths'.

Specifically, 97% of them and 74% of the 'non-psychopaths' had received at least one conviction for a violent offence. In an earlier study (1983), Hare and Jutai showed that the mean number of charges per year free from violent offences was more than three times higher for those with antisocial personality disorder than the 'non-psychopaths'. There was also evidence to show that 'psychopaths' propensity for violence was not inhibited during incarcerations.

It should be stated that the relationship between personality disorder and offending is extremely complex and also controversial. There are various opinions on diagnoses, variations in assessing and differences in thoughts on treatability. There are also controversial mental health law proposals to introduce the preventive detention of certain people suffering from 'dangerous and severe' personality disorder, raising profound implications.

Mental impairment

Chiswick (1993) stated that among adult offenders in general, it is unlikely that the mentally impaired are over-represented although imprisonment for them seems to be a more likely outcome. This may be due to a greater chance of such people getting caught although it should be borne in mind that most people with such a handicap lead their lives unremarkably as part of the general population living in the community. Those more likely to be in such trouble are those who fall in the mild to moderate range of learning disability. Psychosocial factors such as social disadvantage and unstable home background are associated with offending in this population just as for the general population. Sex offences and arson are over-represented among offences committed by mentally impaired people (learning disabled) (Turk 1989). Mental impairment combined with antisocial traits does carry a high risk of offending. It is important to note that the use of hospital orders for the admission of mentally impaired offenders has fallen over the years which could be interpreted in two ways. Firstly, that these offenders are being dealt with through the community psychiatric services, perhaps jointly with the probation services, or, more worryingly, more are being imprisoned and not receiving appropriate help. Chiswick is of the view that the most vulnerable of this patient population are those that fall in the borderline IQ range who also have a superficial degree of social competence.

Neurosis

Many offenders fulfil the diagnostic criteria for one or more of the neurotic stress-related or somatoform disorders. Any causal connection, however, between the offence and a psychiatric diagnosis is more likely found with diagnoses of personality disorders. It is important to note that there is a close link between having a diagnosis of a personality disorder and suffering from neurotic symptoms whether or not these would amount to a separate diagnosis of neurotic disorder. It can be helpful to examine these neurotic conflicts and the symbolic meanings of particular offences for a given individual through offering psychodynamic psychotherapy.

Epilepsy

Chiswick (1993) stated that serious violence as an ictal phenomenon is exceedingly rare but, despite this, people with epilepsy were shown to be over-represented in the prisoner population compared with the general population (Gunn 1977) although this study has not been repeated. There is no evidence of a relationship between epilepsy and crimes of violence (Gunn & Taylor 1993) and the reason for this over-representation, if it is still the case, is unclear. It is possible that some degree of brain damage could be responsible for both the epilepsy and antisocial behaviour. Whitman et al. (1994) concluded that the important socio-economic correlate of epilepsy accounts for the association and some intrinsic link between epilepsy and violence. Similarly, violence in temporal lobe epilepsy is not simply an ictal phenomenon (Herzberg & Fenwick 1988).

THE MENTALLY DISORDERED OFFENDER AND THE CRIMINAL JUSTICE SYSTEM

Pre-trial stage issues

Patients can be referred for various reasons before a trial. A court may remand a defendant in custody and request a psychiatric report from there or a court may bail someone and ask for a psychiatric report to be prepared on them as an in-patient or as an outpatient. There are provisions in Part 3 of the 1983 MHA (Sections 35 and 36) that empower the court to remand a defendant to hospital for assessment or treatment. Requests for psychiatric assessment and reports can be from the court, the Crown Prosecution Service, the defence solicitor or the probation service. Generally, reports are requested as a routine for those persons charged with murder.

Court diversion

Court diversion schemes were introduced in England and Wales in 1989 on the background of the philosophy that the sick should be treated rather than punished. Further, people cannot be treated against their will in prisons because the provisions of the Mental Health Act do not apply in these institutions. James et al. (2002) stated that approximately 150 court diversion schemes are known to exist in England and Wales. The scheme is only one part of a comprehensive framework for diversion, together with psychiatric intervention at the police station and the remand prison. They also stated that the need for a range for such services is

evident from the levels of morbidity among those caught up in the criminal justice system. Various studies have shown a significant level of major mental health problems in these groups. Gunn et al. (1991) found 2% of the 5% sentenced prisoner population interviewed to be psychotic and 3% in need of transfer to an NHS hospital. The need for an early diversion to the health service from the criminal justice system is because unnecessary delays are encountered by these groups once in the system and they cannot be adequately and appropriately treated when in prison. The court diversion scheme is therefore an early process for identifying the mentally ill in the criminal justice system and for putting appropriate interventions in place when their mental health needs are properly identified. These schemes have effectively dealt with those charged with serious offences and minor offences. Further, many minor offenders are now filtered out at an early stage in the criminal justice system. The Revolving Doors Survey (1994) found that 'in those arrested who were thought to have a significant mental health problem, no further action was taken in 37%, 4% were cautioned and 9% bailed'.

There is a paucity of literature on the outcome of admission from court schemes. Joseph & Potter (1993) looked at 65 cases admitted to hospital through the court scheme. These were mostly admitted to open wards. Of these, 31% absconded and did not return, 22% received no benefit, 32% derived 'some benefit' from their admission and 45% 'benefited markedly'. A further study by Rowlands et al. (1996) reviewed the benefit of court diversion in 21 cases admitted to hospital in a 12-month period. They reported that those with psychosis benefited most from the intervention, with 'no benefit' in only 5.2% compared to 53% with alcohol/drug dependence.

Trial stage issues

Actus reus and mens rea

The term *actus reus* relates to the accused carrying out that particular unlawful act with which they have been charged.

The term *mens rea* relates to the accused person being capable of having a guilty mind at the time of commission of the unlawful act. It essentially amounts to intent. This is not a psychiatric concept but an abnormal mental state can influence the capacity to form intent or the qualitative nature of it. A psychiatrist can be required to give evidence in relation to capacity to form intent but not as to the fact of intent which is essentially a legal matter. In England and Wales at present, defendants less than 10 years old are not legally considered to be criminally responsible. Those aged between 10 to 14 years must have *mens rea* proven. They may be found not guilty because of insufficient *mens rea*.

Not all criminal offences require *mens rea*. In order to determine which do require *mens rea*, it is useful to distinguish between (1) offences that were developed by the judges at common law (e.g. murder, theft), and (2) newer offences created by statute and designed to deal with particular problems (e.g. pollution, factory safety).

Insanity defence

An accused may be found not guilty by reason of insanity under the MacNaughten Rules. Essentially, the rules apply when a person commits an offence because of a 'Defect of reason resulting from a disease of mind such that (s)he did not know the nature and quality of the act (s)he was doing or, if (s)he did know it, that (s)he did not know he was doing what was wrong'. This means that 'every man is to be presumed to be sane, and to possess a sufficient degree of reason to be responsible for his crimes, until the contrary be proved'. Medicolegal issues centre on the definition of 'disease of mind', which is not a medical concept. The 'mind' here refers to the mental faculties of reasoning, memory and understanding. 'Disease' here can be organic or functional, permanent or temporary, treatable or untreatable, internal or may manifest itself in violence and is prone to recur.

Diminished responsibility

This is a matter that can only be raised by the defence. Diminished responsibility has its roots in the common law of Scotland and was introduced into English law by the Homicide Act 1957 (Section 2(1)), which states that:

> Where a person kills or is a party to the killing of another, he shall not be convicted of murder if he was suffering from such abnormality of mind (whether arising from a condition of arrested or retarded development of mind, or any inherent cause or induced by disease or injury) as substantially impaired his mental responsibility for his acts and omissions in doing or being a party to a killing.

The burden of proof is on the defendant, on the balance of probabilities. It is accepted in about 80% of pleas for diminished responsibility.

Murder

The crime of murder is committed 'when a person of sound mind and discretion unlawfully kills any reasonable creature or being and under the Queen's peace with intent to kill or cause grievous bodily harm, the death following within a year and a day'.

This is subject to three exceptions. An offence that would otherwise be murder is reduced to voluntary manslaughter if the accused:

- was provoked
- suffers from diminished responsibility
- was acting in pursuance of a suicide pact.

Involuntary manslaughter, where the killing is not intended, can be either 'constructive' (where there was an intention to commit an unlawful or dangerous act) or 'gross negligence' (where there was disregard for the lives and safety of others).

Automatisms

Medical and legal concepts of automatism are not convergent and this is coupled with the fact that judgements on automatism have changed legal interpretation over the years. It is however important to stress that it remains an extremely rare condition. Automatism has defied a clear medical definition. Fenwick (1990) stated that an automatism is an involuntary piece of behaviour over which an individual has no control. The behaviour itself is usually inappropriate to the circumstances, and may be out of character. It may be complex, coordinated and, apparently, purposeful and directed, though lacking in judgement. Afterwards, the individual may have no recollection, or only partial and confused memory, for his actions. In organic automatisms, there must be some disturbance of brain function, sufficient to give rise to the above features. In psychogenic automatisms, the behaviour is complex, coordinated, and appropriate to some aspects of the patient's psychopathology. The sensorium is usually clear, but there will be severe or complete amnesia for the episode (see Chapter 26).

The legal definition of automatism was given by the Lord Chancellor, Viscount Kilmuir, in the case of Bratty v Attorney General for Northern Ireland (1963).

> The state of the person, though capable of action, is not conscious of what he is doing…it means unconsciousness, involuntary action and it is a defence because the mind does not go with what is being done … This is very like the words of a learned president of the Court of Appeal of New Zealand (Gresson P) in Regina v Cottle where he said; 'With respect, I would prefer myself to explain automatism as an action without any knowledge of action or action with no consciousness of what was being done'.

Fitness to plead

The issue of fitness to plead can be raised before a trial starts (Fig. 30.1). The rules to determine fitness to plead are determined by Section 1 of the Criminal Procedure (Insanity and Unfitness to Plead) Act 1991. To be fit to plead, a defendant should be able to:

- understand the charge and its implications
- enter a plea of guilty or not guilty
- challenge jurors
- instruct counsel
- follow the evidence in court.

Unfitness can be raised by the defence, prosecution or judge. The consequences of being found unfit to plead are determined by the 1991 Act above.

Prior to 1991, anyone found unfit to plead received a mandatory hospital disposal. Since the 1991 Act, if found

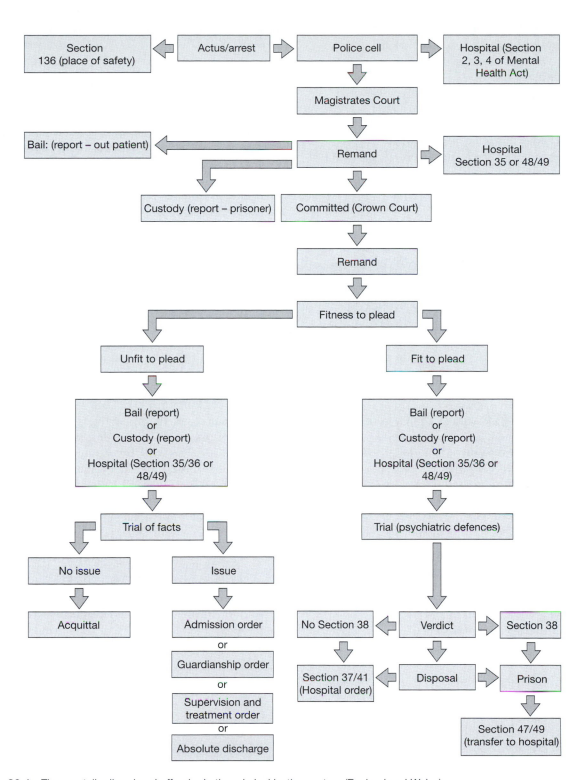

Figure 30.1 The mentally disordered offender in the criminal justice system (England and Wales).

unfit to plead, there is a trial of facts. If the defendant is found not to have committed the offence, he/she is released by the court. If hospital treatment is required following this and the person will not accept it voluntarily, admission would then be under civil section. If the defendant is found

to have committed the offence, the judge now has discretion as to disposal, and the following options are available:

- **Admission Order:** this is equivalent to a Hospital Order under Section 37, with or without a Restriction Order under Section 41 of the 1983 Mental Health Act. There is a mandatory Hospital Order with restriction without limit of time, where the offence is unlawful killing.

- **Guardianship Order:** also equivalent to section 37 of the 1983 Mental Health Act.
- **Supervision and Treatment Order:** this is equivalent to a probation order with a condition of psychiatric treatment. (Section 9(3), Criminal Justice Act 1991).
- **Absolute Discharge:** this is the disposal where the offence is a minor one and there are no indications for treatment and supervision in the community.

Multi-agency public protection arrangements (MAPPA)

Multi-agency public protection arrangements (MAPPA) were established by the Criminal Justice and Court Services Act (2000). The arrangements require police and probation to work together to manage the risk posed by dangerous offenders in the community. The MAPPA Guidance was issued in 2003 by legislation in a bid to achieve greater consistency of practice across different areas of the country. The plan was for the Prison Service to become part of the responsible authority with the police and the National Probation Service. Furthermore, there would be a statutory duty to cooperate by those agencies that, although not part of the Criminal Justice System, work with sex offenders. These agencies will include local health authorities and trusts, housing authorities and registered social landlords, social services departments, social security and employment service departments, youth offending teams, local education authorities, and electronic-monitoring providers. The responsible authority will be required to draw up and agree with each of the bodies concerned a memorandum setting out the ways in which they are to cooperate. Consistency is defined in the guidance as the MAPPA framework. It is stated that MAPPA is often understood as cooperation between police and probation locally, focused almost exclusively on the assessment and management of risk posed by offenders in the community. The vision is for MAPPA to be much broader and more complex than this. MAPPA will form the basis of public protection through a genuinely multi-agency partnership throughout England and Wales. The framework was developed from best practice in close consultation with practitioners. The framework strives to clarify what can be a complex set of arrangement for assessing and managing risk and provides the basis upon which more consistent public protection practice is established throughout England and Wales.

The four functions of the framework are:

- the identification of MAPPA offenders
- the sharing of relevant information amongst those agencies involved in the assessment of that risk
- the assessment of risk of serious harm, and
- the management of that risk.

PRISON PSYCHIATRY

Psychiatric health care in prisons has been a cause for concern over the years, particularly to do with the availability and quality of the care. The primary aim of prison is custody of its inmates; institutional practices are therefore of the utmost importance, and this places medical care in general in a less important role. Prisons usually have one or more full-time or part-time medical officers. A large number of these doctors do not have higher psychiatric training and psychiatric care is usually provided by visiting psychiatrists, generally employed on a sessional basis. Most of them have a main base in the National Health Service (NHS) and many are consultant psychiatrists or specialist registrars undergoing higher psychiatric training. There has, over recent years, been a trend for some prisons to contract out their health care service, which includes psychiatric care, but the success of this has been variable. There has been a review of health care provisions in the prisons with a view to prisoners receiving the same quality and level of care as pertains in the NHS. Formal partnership between prisons and the National Health Service was established in 1999 and commissioning responsibility was devolved to the Department of Health in 2003. There are plans to have 300 extra prison in-reach staff from April 2004 and the full integration of prison health care into the National Health Service in 2008. This will invariably lead to increased demands on the already stretched National Health Service.

Gunn et al. (1991) surveyed a prison population based on a 5% sample of men serving sentences. They looked at 406 young offenders and 1478 adult men, 404 and 1365 of whom agreed to be interviewed. Thirty-seven per cent of the men had psychiatric disorders diagnosed, of whom 0.8% had organic disorders, 2% psychosis, 6% neurosis, 10% personality disorder and 23% substance misuse. Thirty-five per cent were judged to require transfer to hospital for psychiatric treatment, 5% required treatment in a therapeutic community setting and a further 10% required further psychiatric assessment or treatment within the prison. By extrapolation, the sentenced prison population includes over 700 men with psychosis and around 1100 who would warrant transfer to hospital for psychiatric treatment.

RISK MANAGEMENT AND DANGEROUSNESS

Risk assessment and management has become an essential and prominent part of almost all mental health practice within the increasing 'culture of blame' and the wish for risk of untoward events happening being extinguished. It is of course impossible to practise psychiatry without some uncertainty although mental health professionals have a duty to provide the best treatment to and management of any given patient they have assessed. The Care Programme Approach (CPA) was implemented in 1991 after concerns about losing some severely mentally disordered individuals from mental health services after discharge, leaving them without the treatment they needed.

The essential elements of an effective care programme are:

- systematic assessment of health and social care needs(including accommodation) bearing in mind both immediate and longer term requirements
- a care plan agreed between the relevant professional staff, the patient, and his or her carers, and recorded in writing
- the allocation of a key worker whose job (with multi-disciplinary managerial and professional support) is to keep in close contact with the patient; to monitor that the agreed programme of care is delivered and take immediate action if it is not; and conduct a regular review of patient's progress and of his or her health and social care needs.

Following the implementation, there were still very rare homicide cases where patients known to the mental and social health services had killed while supposed to be receiving care in the community. The killing of a member of the public by Christopher Clunis, a man suffering from mental disorder and known to the different services, led to a public inquiry which set up a pattern for subsequent homicide inquiries.

In 1993, in order to further boost the application of the CPA, the then Health Secretary produced a 10-point plan for continuing to develop successful and safe community care. The emphasis here was on public protection first and the plan led to Supervised Discharge (implemented in 1996). This applied particularly to 'revolving door' patients who had shown a pattern of relapses after discharge from hospital. Also in 1993, the Supervision Register was introduced (implemented in 1994), with the stated intention being to ensure that the severely mentally ill received appropriate and effective care in the community. It was never clear how such a register would contribute to improving community care but many mental health professionals saw it as a cynical manoeuvre to deflect blame on to those asked to take responsibility for dangerous patients in what was still an inappropriately resourced and underfunded service. This register also raised particularly sensitive issues of confidentiality as it was to contain detailed information about the patient and list any history of violence or self-destructive behaviours and any current risk posed and the distribution of these details was widespread. The requirement for such registers has now been lifted.

Following the updating of the CPA with the National Service Framework in 1999, a further development ensued, that of Multi-Agency Public Protection Arrangements (MAPPAs). Since the year 2000 it has been a statutory duty for the police and probation to set up such panels, the cases of people who are considered a risk to the public and who are back in the community after hospitalization or imprisonment. Health and Social Services, as well as education and housing departments, are asked to be involved and their involvement may also eventually become statutory (see above). The primary intention of the CPA was stated as being the provision of a helpful way for the different professionals from various agencies to communicate better to ensure that each patient's needs were met as best as possible. A secondary intention for this new policy was to protect the public. With the introduction of the subsequent implementations, public protection is now felt to have become the primary focus, particularly with the increased emphasis on risk assessments and managements throughout mental health services, manifested by MAPPAs and DSPD (Dangerous and Severe Personality Disorder) pilot units.

Very few patients who have been violent are considered dangerous all the time. Most patients in high security are considered dangerous some of the time and only when certain ingredients, including a particular state of mind, come together. It is a task of the clinical team looking after these patients to continuously review these ingredients or factors and the totality of this is now called 'risk containment' (Monahan 1993). There are inherent difficulties in defining dangerousness and risk is a more helpful term to use. The term risk containment is used to describe the multifaceted approach required when considering a patient who has been dangerous. Snowden (1997) has provided a helpful way of considering risk containment under three broad headings.

The first heading is that of risk identification. In other words, what is the risk being considered? Is it a risk of harm towards the self or towards another? Is the risk one of relapse of a particular mental illness which is known to be associated with violent behaviour?

Secondly, once the risk is identified, one considers assessing that risk in terms of the frequency with which it might recur and the severity of any recurrence. As much information as possible should be obtained about the patient's background and past, previous and present behaviour as well as previous and present mental states. All possible sources of information should be sought by the different professionals in the clinical team, ranging from obtaining old school reports, to speaking with relatives or neighbours or examining police records or social work reports. This enables a thorough appraisal of as many facets as possible of a particular patient, leading to the best informed clinical judgement that can be made in assessing that risk. This is something which varies over time and therefore has to be constantly reappraised.

The third heading is that of clinical risk management and is about providing the patient with multidisciplinary treatment strategies that help reduce the frequency and severity of the identified and assessed risks.

Looking at it from the perspective of the whole institution(s), risk containment such as described above should be systematically reviewed and revised with regular clinical auditing and research. All these aspects of a patient's management also form part of the wider rubric of the Care Programme Approach, applied to all patients receiving treatment from mental health services, both in- and outpatients. Forensic psychiatry teams are particularly accustomed to looking after patients who have been dangerous but, essentially, apply the same basic skills of assessment that any psychiatric team uses, whether it is of harm to self or of harm to another.

Clinical risk assessment has begun to be replaced by actuarial approaches to risk (using instruments such as the Psychopathy Check List–Revised (Hare 1998)) which aims to apply empirically established associations between variables and the probability of future aggression. The actuarial approach should be integrated with a clinical approach although it should be remembered that, however good a risk assessment is, whether clinical, actuarial or combined, this will not make a significant impact on public safety (Petch 2001). Disasters can be prevented by offering high standards of care to avert the deterioration of a mental illness in a person known to be a risk but only a small proportion of those who are violent give any indication beforehand.

The shift of emphasis away from 'dangerousness' and towards a broader concept of risk assessment was summarized by Steadman et al. (1993), drawing on a report about violence from a public health perspective (US Department of Health and Human Services 1991) and a paper from the New York Academy of Medicine (1986):

- a move from a legal concept of dangerousness to a 'decision-making concept' of risk
- that prediction should be considered as being on a continuum rather than a 'yes/no' dichotomy
- that there should be a shift away from the notion that there can be single prediction of risk, to a recognition that there is a continuing process of risk assessment that must be incorporated into the day-to-day management of mentally disordered people.

Despite the current limitations in predicting violence, dangerousness continues to be a major consideration of mental health professionals when deciding whether to detain or release a mentally disordered patient. The NHS executive (1994) has published important guidelines on the discharge of mentally disordered people and their continued care in the community, which includes a section on assessing potentially violent patients. The Royal College of Psychiatrists (1996) has also published important guidelines on assessment and clinical management of risk of harm to other people.

In individual cases a past history of violence is regarded as one of the best predictors of future violence. Prins (1990) suggested nine questions, in no order of priority, which may help in the decision, summarized below:

1. Have past precipitants and stresses in the offender patient's background been removed or sufficiently alleviated?
2. What is this offender-patient's current capacity for dealing with provocation?
3. Have the clues to the offender-patient's self-image been explored in sufficient depth?
4. How vulnerable and fragile does the offender-patient seem to be? Were the circumstances of the original offence the last straw in a series of stressful events, although the individual sees everybody else as hostile?
5. Was the behaviour person-specific or aimed at society in general?
6. Has the offender-patient come to terms, in part if not in toto, with the offending act?
7. Have details about the original offence been examined?
8. Has the health care institution monitored the offender-patient's reaction to stress and temptation?
9. Has it been borne in mind that the offender-patient's denial of the original offence may reflect the truth?

FUTURE DEVELOPMENTS

The outcome of the Mental Health Act 1983 reform proposals referred to earlier in this chapter is awaited at the time of writing. The reforms within the Prison Medical Service are on-going and have been described under 'Prison psychiatry' in this chapter.

Forensic psychiatry secure services are currently being restructured nationally. There is a move towards scaling down the three large high security hospitals and providing smaller units. However, this will necessitate providing more long-term medium secure beds, which at present are often provided in conditions of high security. The provision of long-term medium security has been chronically inadequate within the NHS and it is hoped that this will start to improve. There are also moves towards shortening the average length of stay in high security but this will only work if long-term medium secure provisions are adequate. Many of these patients have chronic and enduring severe mental disorders that require long-term treatment in secure settings to enable them to engage with treatment and provide the necessary containment that has so often been absent in their lives beforehand.

The treatment of severe personality disorders remains controversial and a continued point of debate. We consider that the development of the speciality of forensic psychotherapy and other psychological treatments requires careful consideration. The understanding of personality disorders will otherwise always remain an enigma and people suffering from such disorders may otherwise never be in a position to receive help that they clearly require. Perhaps the inclusion of forensic psychotherapists in the clinical teams alongside further research in this area will improve what is currently known about this patient population and lead to an improvement in their management. Certainly, this was one of the strongest recommendations made in the Ashworth Report. There are many developments of services for those suffering from personality disorders, some, like the DSPD project, at the pilot stage. The document, 'Personality disorder, no longer a diagnosis of exclusion' is also an indication of how seriously the needs of those suffering from these disorders are being addressed. However, for these developments in services to work raises massive research and training implications. Highly trained and very experienced professionals from different disciplines will be needed to run such services or they will be doomed to fail. Given the particular kinds of psychopathology, the enactments possible, as well as the expectable dynamics, input from forensic psychotherapists, in such units will be essential if these facilities are to be adequately and safely provided.

Regarding the impact of the National Confidential Inquiry into Suicide and Homicide by People with Mental Illness, it is hoped that the learning process resulting from this will contribute to more robust risk management. A substantial number of patients cared for in forensic psychiatry settings are considered to be 'high risk' and it is hoped that any improvements in management can be adapted in a coordinated way and not simply end up as recommendations that cannot be implemented. It should also be remembered that risk is not something that can be extinguished but rather, is something that changes from moment to moment and can only be contained as best possible. One of the best ways to contain risk is to know your patient and his or her fluctuating mental state.

WRITING PSYCHIATRIC REPORTS AND APPEARING IN COURT

Preliminary matters

Medicolegal reports can be asked for by:

- probation officers
- defence solicitors
- crown Prosecution Service
- other mental health professionals
- social services.

Ensure that your instructions are adequate and that the request for such a report falls within your remit. Check exactly where the final destination of the report will be and ask for all available documents in relation to the case to be

made available to you by the referrer. Try to anticipate how many interviews you are likely to need, how much reading time and preparation time in order to make a realistic assessment of costs.

At the beginning of the first interview with the patient, ensure that the person is aware that the purpose of the assessment with you is to provide a report to the court and any matters arising during the course of the assessment could be mentioned in the report. It can be helpful to obtain that person's written consent for you to have access to any medical or other relevant files you may subsequently wish to request.

Planning the written report

1. State the name and date of birth of the person assessed.
2. Provide an introductory paragraph indicating who referred, why and the person's current situation (e.g. on bail, in prison) and any relevant Mental Health Act they may be under. If the person has been charged, then state what s/he has been charged with and how s/he is pleading. Refer to the dates and places of interviews held and all other information made available to you.
3. It is sensible to then proceed with a background history, including a picture of the family dynamics if this is possible from the material available. This can be followed by the personal history, including birth and development, schooling, any qualifications, employment record, drugs and alcohol history, forensic history, medical history, psychosexual history and psychiatric history.
4. The next section should be a detailed account of the index offence as reported by the person and contrasts if possible with information available such as witness statements. Any relevant psychological factors or aspects of the person's mental state at the time should be mentioned.
5. The person's mental state at the time of the assessment should now be described. It is helpful to describe not just the presence or absence of psychiatric symptoms but also, a reference to the psychodynamics apparent in the interaction between the assessor and the patient as this can give clues to treatability psychotherapeutically, for example, in cases of personality disorder.
6. The last section of the report should be headed conclusions and should begin with a very brief resume of the background and personal history. Give your opinion of any diagnosis/es and any implications within the Mental Health Act if this is relevant. Refer to the offence and your view on the importance or not of any psychological factors at that time. It can be helpful to a court to include a psychodynamic formulation

which contains current psychopathology, aetiological factors and any maintaining factors. The purpose of this would be to try to offer a picture of the offender's internal world to the court as a way of increasing everybody's understanding of the offence in relation to that particular individual and thereby improve the chances that the person will receive the most appropriate disposal. An opinion on suitability for treatment should be given if possible and if treatment is recommended, then it ought to be specified. The recommendations must be within the remit of the court and ought to be available. It is sensible to make any recommendations respectfully to the court and to mention any concerns you might have should those recommendations not be followed. A comment on prognosis is appreciated but not always possible.

[7] State your name and qualifications at the end and your current status within your profession. Date the report.

Appearing in court

[1] Preparation: read your report again to be familiar with its contents. It can be helpful to read any literature which can support your opinion and recommendations. If a long time has lapsed since the preparation of the report, you may need to consider a further interview with the person and provide an addendum to your report prior to the hearing.

[2] It is helpful to make yourself familiar with court procedures as this can help overcome feelings of anxiety induced by what may be perceived as a strange, threatening or even hostile atmosphere. Note which court you are appearing in, for example, Magistrates Court, Crown Court, High Court or Central Criminal Court.

[3] It is best to respect dress code and time. Generally, courts are very appreciative of professionals giving their time to assist.

[4] The following notes apply to all courts:

- announce your arrival to the clerk
- bow to the bench when you enter
- you will be shown where to sit
- be prepared for how you will want to be sworn in, as you will be asked
- when you say the oath, use this as an opportunity to gauge your voice projection
- check how to address the bench (e.g. the judge will be addressed as 'Your Honour' in Crown Court, or 'My Lord' or 'My Lady' in High Court)
- in the witness box, bring only your report and any notes you have prepared that you have checked can be disclosed, as this may be requested
- answer questions succinctly and do not attempt to answer questions beyond your remit especially when you are feeling pressed to do so

- when asked a question by a barrister or Queen's Counsel, turn towards the bench when replying. He/she is the person you are answering to
- remember that you are an impartial witness there to assist the court
- when you leave the court, bow again.

[5] It may be helpful to discuss your experience in court with colleagues afterwards, especially if you have had a difficult cross-examination.

FURTHER READING

Bluglass R & Bowden P (eds) (1990) *Principles and Practice of Forensic Psychiatry*. London: Churchill Livingstone.
Chiswick D & Cope R (eds) (1995) *Seminars in Practical Forensic Psychiatry*. London: Royal College of Psychiatrists.
Cordess C & Cox M (eds) (1998) *Forensic Psychotherapy: Crime, Psychodynamics and the Offender Patient*. Jessica Kingsley Publishers.
Doctor R (ed.) (2003) *Dangerous Patients: A Psychodynamic Approach to Risk Assessment and Management*. Karnac.

REFERENCES

Chiswick D (1993) Forensic psychiatry. In: Kendell RE & Zealley AK (eds) *Companion to Psychiatry Studies*. London: Churchill Livingstone.
Chiswick D (2000) Associations between psychiatric disorder and offending. In: Gelder MG, Lopez-Ibor Jr J & Andreason NC (eds) *New Oxford Textbook of Psychiatry*. Oxford: Oxford University Press.
Cordess C (1995) Crime and mental disorder: 1. criminal behaviour. In: Chiswick D & Cope R (eds) *Practical Forensic Psychiatry. Seminars in Practical Forensic Psychiatry*. Wiltshire: Redwood Press.
Department of Health and Home Office (1992) *Review of Health and Social Services for Mentally Disordered Offenders and Others Requiring Similar Services (Reed Report)*. London: Department of Health and Social Security.
Department of Health and Social Security (1974) *Revised Report on the Working Party on Security in NHS Psychiatric Hospitals (Glancy Report)*. London: Department of Health and Social Security.
Drivers and Vehicle Licensing Agency (1966) *For Medical Practitioners. At A Glance Guide to the Current Medical Standards of Fitness to Drive*. Swansea: DVLA.
Fenwick P (1990) Automatism. In: Bluglass R & Bowden P (eds) *Principles and Practice of Forensic Psychiatry*. London: Churchill Livingstone.
Glasser M (1990) Paedophilia. In: Bluglass R & Bowden P (eds) *Principles and Practice of Forensic Psychiatry*. London: Churchill Livingstone.
Gunn J (1977) *Epileptics in Prison*. London: Academic Press.
Gunn J, Maden A, Swinton M et al. (1991) Treatment needs of prisoners with psychiatric disorders. *British Medical Journal* **303**: 338–40.
Gunn J, Maden A & Swinton M (1991) *Mentally Disordered Prisoners*. London: Home Office.
Gunn J & Taylor PJ (eds) (1993) *Forensic Psychiatry Clinical, Legal and Ethical Issues*. Oxford: Butterworth-Heinemann.
Häfner H & Böker W (1973) *Crimes of Violence by Mentally Abnormal Offenders* (Transl. by H Marshall 1982). Cambridge: Cambridge University Press.
Hare RD (1983) Diagnosis of antisocial personality disorder in two prison populations. *American Journal of Psychiatry* **140**: 887–90.
Herzberg JL & Fenwick PBC (1998) The aetiology of aggression in temporal lobe epilepsy. *British Journal of Psychiatry* **153**: 50–5.
James D, Farnham F, Moorey H, Lloyd H, Hill K, Blizard R & Barnes TRE (2002) *Outcome Of Psychiatric Admission Through the Courts*. London: Home Office.

Joseph PL & Potter M (1993) Diversion from custody. I: psychiatric assessment at the magistrates' court II: effect on hospital and prison resources. *British Journal of Psychiatry* **162**: 325–34.

Lewis NDG & Yarnell H (1951) Pathological fire-setting. Nervous and Mental Disease Monographs No. 82. *Journal of Nervous and Mental Disease*. New York.

Lishman WA (1968) Brain damage in relation to psychiatric disability after head injury. *British Journal of Psychiatry* **114**: 373–410.

Mullen PE (1984) Mental disorders and dangerousness. *Australian and New Zealand Journal of Psychiatry* **18**: 8.

Prins H (1990) Some observations on the supervision of dangerous offender patients. *British Journal of Psychiatry* **156**: 157–62.

Prins H, Tennant G & Trick K (1985) Motives for arson (fire raising). *Medicine, Science and the Law* **25**: 257–78.

Revolving Doors (1994) *The Management of People with Mental Health Problems by the Paddington Police*. London: Revolving Doors Agency.

Rowlands R, Inch H, Rodger W & Soliman A (1996) Diverted to where? What happens to diverted mentally disordered offenders. *Journal of Forensic Psychiatry* **7**: 284–96.

Royal College of Psychiatrists (1996) *Assessment and Clinical Management of Risk of Harm to Other People*. Royal College of Psychiatrists Special Working Party on Clinical Assessment and Management of Risk. London: Royal College of Psychiatrists.

Smith R (1999) Prisoners: an end to second class health care? *British Medical Journal* **318**: 954–5.

Steadman HJ (1983) Predicting dangerousness among the mentally ill: art, magic and science. *International Journal of Law and Psychiatry* **6**: 381–90.

Tidmarsh D (1990) Schizophrenia. In: Bluglass R & Bowden P (eds) *Principles and Practice of Forensic Psychiatry*. London: Churchill Livingstone.

Turk J (1989) Forensic aspects of mental handicap. *British Journal of Psychiatry* **155**: 591–4.

Whitman S, Coleman T, Berg B, King L & Desai B (1980) Epidemiological insights into the socioeconomic correlates of epilepsy. In: Herman BP (ed.) *A Multidisciplinary Handbook of Epilepsy*, pp. 301–54. Springfield: Thomas.

Psychiatry of old age

Ajit Shah and Elizabeth Tovey

INTRODUCTION

The psychiatry of old age including demography, epidemiology, individual disorders and their management, suicide and attempted suicide and the principles of service delivery, are described in this chapter.

DEMOGRAPHY

Population projections throughout the world predict an increase in the elderly population over the next decade. In the UK there is a particular increase in the old old (over 80 years in age) compared to the young old (65 to 80 years in age). The prevalence of dementia doubles every 5.1 years after the age of 60. Thus, the absolute number of dementia cases will continue to increase. Although the prevalence of depression in the elderly is not age-related, the absolute number of cases will also increase.

EPIDEMIOLOGY

Dementia

The prevalence of dementia in the UK is up to 5.6% in the 10 million people who are over the age of 65 years (Copeland et al. 1987). There is broad agreement on the prevalence rates of severe dementia, but not of mild dementia. The prevalence of Alzheimer's disease, vascular dementia and mixed dementia are 46%, 20% and 10% respectively in those over 65 years, and 75%, 20% and 5% respectively in those over 75 years with dementia. Alzheimer's disease is more common in men and vascular dementia is more common in women.

The prevalence of dementia in nursing and residential home populations is 35–50% for mild/moderate dementia and around 30% for severe dementia. The prevalence of dementia among acutely ill and continuing care geriatric in-patients is 35–61% and up to 90% respectively.

Depression

The reported prevalence of depression in the elderly ranges from 11% to 16%. There is evidence that prevalence of depression increases with age in women (Copeland et al. 1987). The prevalence of depression in residential and nursing home populations is about 35%. The prevalence of depression in acutely ill and continuing care geriatric in-patients of up to 50% and 38% respectively has been reported.

Neurosis

The Liverpool study reported a prevalence of 2.4% for all neuroses (Copeland et al. 1987). The Guy's/Age Concern survey reported prevalence of 3.7% for generalized anxiety and 10% for phobias (7.8% agoraphobias, 1.3% social phobias and 2.1% specific phobias) (Lindesay et al. 1989). However, many of these individuals also had comorbid depression and thus the prevalence of pure neurosis is likely to be lower. Personality disorder has not been systematically studied in the elderly.

Schizophrenia and late paraphrenia

In the Liverpool study the prevalence of these disorders was 0.1% (Copeland et al. 1987).

DEMENTIA

Definition

The ICD-10 defines dementia as follows:

> Dementia is a syndrome due to disease of the brain, usually of chronic or progressive nature, in which there is impairment of multiple higher cortical functions, including memory, thinking, orientation, calculation, learning capacity, language and judgement. Consciousness is not clouded. The cognitive impairments are

481

commonly accompanied, and occasionally, preceded by deterioration in emotional control, social behaviour or motivation. This syndrome occurs in Alzheimer's disease, in cerebrovascular disease, and in other conditions primarily or secondarily affecting the brain.

Thus, dementia implies global intellectual deterioration. Moreover, functional impairment is a necessary prerequisite for the diagnosis of dementia (see Chapter 26).

Non-cognitive features

In addition to cognitive impairment, dementia encompasses several non-cognitive domains including disorders of behaviour, personality, mood, thought content and perception, and functional disability. These are nowadays referred to as behavioural and psychological signs and symptoms of dementia (BPSD).

Behaviour disturbances including agitation, aggression, wandering, pacing, restlessness, sleeplessness and sexual disinhibition are not uncommon and occur in over 50% of patients during the course of dementia (Burns et al. 1990a). Personality changes, including emergence of new personality features or an exaggeration of premorbid personality traits are common in dementia (Jacomb & Jorm 1996). Personality in this context includes the ability to express and experience emotions, however inappropriate.

The prevalence of depressive symptoms and depressive illness in Alzheimer's disease are 0–87% (median 41%) and 0–86% (median 19%) respectively (Wragg & Jeste 1989). The prevalence of depressive symptoms and syndrome is generally greater in vascular dementia than Alzheimer's disease.

Auditory, visual and olfactory hallucinations have been described (Burns et al. 1990b). A former classification of delusions (simple persecutory, complex persecutory, grandiose, and those associated with specific neurological deficits) has been modified into delusions of theft, delusions of suspicion and systematized delusions (Burns et al. 1990c). Four types of misidentification syndromes have been described (Burns et al. 1990b): people in the house, misidentification of mirror image, misidentification of television and misidentification of people. The prevalence of delusions, hallucinations and misidentification syndromes in Alzheimer's and vascular dementia varies: 20%–50%, 17–36% and 11–34% respectively (Burns et al. 1990b, 1990c).

Alzheimer's disease

Definition
The essential features for an ICD-10 diagnosis of dementia of Alzheimer's type are listed in Box 31.1. ICD-10 further classifies this dementia into four sub-groups: Dementia in Alzheimer's disease with (i) early onset, (ii) late-onset, (iii) atypical or mixed and (iv) unspecified. The DSM-IV definition of Alzheimer's disease is similar.

Pathology
Pathological changes include widening of sulci, narrowing of gyri and ventricular enlargement consistent with brain atrophy. Histological changes include senile plaques, neurofibrillary tangles, granulovacuolar degeneration and amyloid deposition in blood vessel walls in cortical and subcortical grey matter. Amyloid has been identified as the main ingredient of senile plaques. The severity of cognitive impairment and neurotransmitter changes are associated with the number of senile plaques (see Chapter 26).

Aetiology
First-degree relatives of Alzheimer's disease sufferers have a three-fold higher risk of developing the disorder, although most cases are sporadic. Three specific pathogenic loci and several risk-associated loci have been identified using linkage studies of family pedigrees. Autosomal dominant pattern of inheritance is observed in some families with early-onset disease. Patients with Down's syndrome, with trisomy 21 and variants, have a higher risk of developing Alzheimer's disease. Mutations in the amyloid precursor protein (APP) gene located on chromosome 21 have been identified as a cause of early-onset Alzheimer's disease. APP is a transmembrane glycoprotein and its derivative, beta-amyloid peptide, is found in amyloid plaques. APP gene mutations can cause the three secretase enzymes involved in the cellular processing of APP to produce more beta-amyloid. Mutations on presenilin-1 gene, located on chromosome 14, account for some early-onset familial Alzheimer's disease. A homologous gene, presenilin-2, on chromosome 1 has a similar effect. The precise function of the presenilin genes is unclear, but they may be involved in the transport and processing of APP within the nerve cell (see Chapter 3).

Apolipoprotein is found both in plaques and tangles. Moreover, Alzheimer's disease is associated with apolipoprotein E genes (ApoE) located on chromosome 19 (Saunders et al. 1993). ApoE exists in three forms in the

---

Box 31.1   Diagnostic guidelines for ICD-10 diagnosis of dementia in Alzheimer's disease

The following features are essential for a definite diagnosis:

Presence of dementia as described above

Insidious onset with slow deterioration. While the onset usually seems difficult to pin-point in time, realization by others that the defects exist may come suddenly. An apparent plateau may occur in progression

Absence of clinical evidence, or findings from special investigations to suggest that the mental state may be due to other systemic or brain disease which can induce a dementia (e.g. hypothyroidism, hypercalcemia, vitamin B_{12} deficiency, niacin deficiency, neurosyphilis, normal pressure hydrocephalus, or subdural)

Absence of a sudden, apoplectic onset, or of neurological signs of focal damage such as hemiparesis, sensory loss, visual field defects, and incoordination occurring early in the illness (although these phenomena may be superimposed later)

following order of frequency: ε3, ε4 and ε2. The various permutations individuals can have are ε3ε3, ε3ε2, ε3ε4, ε4ε4, ε4ε2 and ε2ε2. Having one ε4 allele increases the risk of having Alzheimer's disease four-fold and having two ε4 alleles increases the risk 16-fold. Presence of ε4 alleles can reduce the age of onset. However, about 40% of Alzheimer's disease patients do not possess an ε4 allele, so its presence is not necessary or sufficient for the development of Alzheimer's disease. Other risk modifying genes of possible importance include α1-antichymotrypsin gene and possible candidate genes on chromosome 12 (see Chapter 3).

Other risk factors include age, infections, autoimmune conditions, head injury, hypertension and hypotension, aluminium, previous history of depression, advanced maternal age at birth and thyroid disease. Diagnosis of rheumatoid arthritis, long term prescription of non-steroidal anti-inflammatory drugs, steroids and oestrogens are reported to be protective against the development of Alzheimer's disease.

Vascular dementia

Definition
The ICD diagnosis of vascular dementia assumes the general definition of dementia described earlier. ICD-10 vascular dementia is divided into several categories including acute onset, multi-infarct, subcortical vascular dementia, mixed cortical and subcortical dementia, other vascular dementia and unspecified. The DSM-IV criteria are similar. The probability of the diagnosis is increased by abrupt onset (possible index vascular event), stepwise decline (possible recurrent vascular events), presence of associated arteriosclerosis, focal neurological signs and symptoms, patchy cognitive deficits, relative preservation of personality, nocturnal confusion, hypertension and evidence of cardiovascular disease.

Pathology
In vascular dementia there may be gross or localized brain changes with atrophy and ventricular dilatation. There may be evidence of ischaemia and infarction in brain tissue, and arteriosclerosis in the major blood vessels. There are no characteristic neurochemical changes (see Chapter 26).

Aetiology
Risk factors for the development of vascular dementia include male sex, increasing age, oriental culture, hypertension, heart disease, strokes, diabetes, cigarette smoking and hyperlipidaemia.

Dementia with Lewy bodies

This dementia, also called cortical Lewy body disease and Lewy body dementia, is characterized by Lewy bodies in the cerebral cortex and the substantia nigra (see Chapter 26). It is also associated with reduction in acetylcholine transferase in the neocortex and reduced dopamine in the caudate nucleus. Variable prevalence of 6–15%, depending on sample types, has been reported.

Clinical features include fluctuating cognition with pronounced variations in attention and alertness, recurring visual hallucinations which are typically well formed and detailed, spontaneous motor features of parkinsonism and neuroleptic sensitivity (Consensus Guidelines for the Clinical Diagnosis of Dementia with Lewy Bodies (DLB) 1996). Repeated falls, transient disturbance of consciousness, systematized delusions and hallucinations in other modalities also occur. Mortality is increased in patients treated with neuroleptics. Severity of cognitive impairment is associated with the density of cortical Lewy bodies.

Other dementias

A number of other dementias occur in old age including those due to alcohol, fronto-temporal dementias, normal pressure hydrocephalus, neurosyphilis, and those due to vitamin deficiencies (see Chapter 26).

The management of dementias

Diagnosis
A detailed history, mental state examination, physical examination and special investigations are required for accurate diagnosis. A history from the patient and informants is essential, and should address previous medical history, current drug prescription, sensory impairment, physical symptoms and loss of function. A detailed cognitive assessment will allow accurate identification of the precise cognitive deficits and their functional consequences. This can be further supplemented by formal neuropsychometric assessment by a clinical psychologist, particularly when there are doubts about diagnosis. Physical examination will allow identification of the aetiology of dementia and any associated delirium, the severity of self-neglect due to dementia and sensory impairment. This should facilitate distinction between dementia, delirium superimposed on dementia, delirium alone and other mental illness. Table 31.1 illustrates some of the distinguishing features between delirium and dementia (see Chapter 26).

In general, the findings of the history and examination will guide as to which special investigations are needed. It may be necessary to perform some of the special investigations listed in Box 31.2 in order to further identify reversible causes of dementias and super-added delirium and identify the severity of self-neglect. Computerized axial tomography (CT) scans may allow identification of other structural pathologies like tumours and help in the differential diagnosis of dementias. They can help identify ischaemic changes and areas of infarction in vascular dementia and characteristic radiological features of normal

Table 31.1 Distinction between dementia and delirium

	Dementia	Delirium
Onset	Insidious	Acute
Decline	Relatively slow	Rapid
Level of conciousness	Alert	Clouding of conciousness
Sensory perceptions	No hypersensitivity	Hypersensitivity (e.g. hyperacusis)
Visual hallucinations	Less common	More common
Stability of mental state	Fairly stable	Fluctuating

Box 31.2 Special investigations in mental illness in the elderly

Commonly indicated
FBC
ESR
U & Es
Calcium
TFT
LFT
Glucose
B$_{12}$
Folate
Syphilis serology
MSU
Chest X-ray
CT brain
ECG

Sometimes indicated
EEG
Lumbar puncture
MRI scan

Box 31.3 Specific areas of information shared with carers

Diagnosis of dementia and its implications
Behaviour problems in dementia
Possible causes of the behaviour problem
How the problems are going to be managed
Results of any special investigations
Role of medication, if any
Need for day care
Need for respite care
Need, if appropriate, for admission into hospital
Need to refer to psychogeriatric services
What resources may be available to carers
Need for placement into a residential facility
Management of financial resources (Power of Attorney or Court of Protection)
Ability to drive a car

understand and cope with the behaviour disturbance. Both groups of carers may also require opportunities to ventilate their feelings. Relatives may be able to join support groups such as the Alzheimer's Disease Society in the UK, which provide information and peer group support.

Almost all drugs can cause delirium and many exacerbate the cognitive impairment of dementia. Thus, indications for their continued use should be reviewed. Any potentially reversible or partially reversible causes of dementia, hypothyroidism or neurosyphilis for example, should be treated. Common causes of delirium and behaviour disturbance such as constipation, urinary tract infection and chest infection should be rigorously sought and treated, and advice from specialist geriatric medicine services should be sought when appropriate. Optical, opthalmology or audiology opinion should be sought when sensory impairment is identified because their correction may improve cognitive deficits.

Early identification and intervention may avoid a full-blown crisis. Both professional and non-professional carers could be advised to use some simple calming strategies. Disturbed patients should be approached from the front, gently and calmly. Communication should be clear and unambiguous. Judicious use of touch and non-threatening postures may also be of value (see Chapter 35).

Pharmacological treatments

Acetylcholine deficit is common in Alzheimer's disease. Drugs designed to inactivate the acetylcholinesterase enzyme, which breaks down acetylcholine in the synaptic cleft, have been advocated to improve cognition. Three drugs in this group, donepezil (Gauthier et al. 2001), galantamine (Tariot et al. 2000) and rivastigmine (Rosler et al. 1998) are available in the UK and have modest efficacy for

pressure hydrocephalus. Magnetic resonance imaging (MRI), with better resolution, may also be of value. Functional MRI scanning, positive emission tomography (PET) and SPEC scanning are not normally used in routine clinical practice.

General treatment

After making a diagnosis of dementia, a simple explanation of the diagnosis, management plan and possible sequelae should be given to the patient and the professional or family carer. Box 31.3 illustrates some of the specific issues that should be addressed during such explanations. Professional carers and relatives often require considerable support to

improving cognitive impairment in mild to moderately severe Alzheimer's disease (see Chapter 38). There is increasing evidence that these drugs also improve Behaviour and Psychotic Symptoms of Dementia (BPSD) and function. Furthermore, rivastigmine has been shown to improve cognitive impairment and BPSD including apathy, anxiety, delusions and hallucinations in dementia with Lewy bodies (McKeith et al. 2000).

In the UK, the National Institute of Clinical Excellence (NICE) guidelines (see www.nice.org.uk) recommend that only those with a diagnosis of Alzheimer's disease and a Mini Mental State Examination score of 12 to 26 should be prescribed these drugs, usually in secondary care. Recently, another drug called memantine, which works by reducing overstimulation of the N-methyl-D-aspartate (NMDA) receptor by glutamate (memantine is NMDA antagonist), has been licensed in the UK for use in severe Alzheimer's disease (Reisberg et al. 2003). It improves cognition and also produces global improvement, although it is not covered by the existing NICE guidance.

The efficacy of other psychotropic drugs in the treatment of BPSD is unclear and probably modest. Research in this area is open to criticism because of poor methodology and it has been argued that psychotropics simply sedate the patient rather than modify target behaviour. A meta-analysis of 17 double-blind studies of older neuropleptics and placebo reported neuroleptics to be modestly effective in reducing behaviour disturbance (Schneider et al. 1990). However, neuroleptics can worsen confusion or cognitive impairment, so they should be used carefully and sparingly. Phenothiazines, for example, have potent anticholinergic properties which may worsen cognition and confusion and atypical neuroleptics, which have fewer extrapyramidal and anticholinergic side-effects may be more useful. Both risperidone (Katz et al. 1999) and olanzapine (Street et al. 2000) have been shown to have efficacy in the treatment of BPSD with a good side-effect profile. However, they increase risk for cerebrovascular events. Because of altered pharmacokinetics and pharmacodynamics in the elderly, small doses should be used with careful observations for side effects.

Short-acting benzodiazepines or chlormethiazole may be helpful in the management of acute disturbance in patients with dementia. However, tolerance, dependence and other side-effects mandate that they should be used briefly and avoided if at all possible. Carbamazepine and sodium valproate may have efficacy in the treatment of aggressive behaviour.

Antidepressants have proven efficacy for the treatment of depression in dementia. Ideally one of the newer antidepressants from the selective serotonin uptake inhibitor (SSRI) group or other newer antidepressants should be used because they have fewer anticholinergic side-effects. The SSRI, citalopam, has been shown to decrease agitation in double-blind studies and other drugs acting on the serotonin system have anecdotally been reported to reduce aggressive behaviour in dementia.

DEPRESSION

Clinical features

The clinical features of depression in the elderly are essentially similar to those in younger individuals. Agitation, retardation, hypochondriasis, cognitive impairment, and delusions of physical illhealth, persecution, poverty, self-blame, worthlessness and guilt are common; nihilistic delusions may occasionally occur. Hallucinations are unusual, but when they occur they are usually second person auditory hallucinations with a derogatory content (and are mood congruent). Cognitive impairment in depression may be mistaken for dementia, a phenomenon referred to as depressive pseudodementia. This can be discriminated from dementia by the clarity of onset, relatively rapid onset, its duration and speed of cognitive decline, the manner in which the patient answers the questions, presence or absence of higher cortical deficits and/or other depressive symptoms (Table 31.2).

Aetiology

The aetiology of depression can be divided into predisposing factors, precipitating factors and perpetuating factors. Predisposing factors can be classified into genetic factors, physical health, personality and social support. Up to 30% of late-onset depressions have a family history. Physical illness and its treatment may predispose to depression in up to 50% of medically ill elderly in-patients. Occult malignancies may present with depression and drugs like corticosteroids can produce depressive side-effects. Late-onset depression may be associated with anxiety-prone, avoidant and dependent personality. The association

Table 31.2 Significant clinical differences between depressive psuedodementia and dementia

	Pseudodementia	Dementia
Onset	Acute	Insidious
Course	Rapid	Insidious
Duration	Relatively brief	Permanent
Main complaint	Impaired memory	No complaints
Cognitive questioning	Cannot respond or does not know answer	Incorrect response
Higher cortical functioning	Intact	Impaired
Mood congruent delusions	Common	Uncommon

between depression and the presence of a confidant or an intimate relationship are unclear with some studies supporting and others refuting such a relationship.

Precipitating factors include independent adverse life events which are important in precipitating depression and are frequent in the preceding year. Bereavement is an important life event associated with depression in the elderly. However, not everyone with depression has experienced adverse life events and not everyone experiencing such events becomes depressed. Thus, other factors must operate. Personality traits, including an inability to form close relationships, a tendency to be helpless and hopeless, an inability to tolerate change and loss of control, and feelings of loneliness, despair and dependence on others may be vulnerability factors predisposing to depression. Both precipitating and predisposing factors may also act as perpetuating factors.

Management

An accurate diagnosis is essential in the treatment of depression and this can be achieved by satisfactory history from the patient and a collateral source, mental state examination and a thorough physical examination. This process will also allow exclusion of differential diagnosis. Table 31.2 summarizes the most significant differences between dementia and depressive pseudodementia. Physical examination and selected special investigations from the list in Box 31.2 will allow identification of self-neglect (dehydration or anaemia for example) and other physical illnesses (hypothyroidism or hypercalcaemia mimicking depression for example).

Treatment plans should be tailored to individual patients with regard to the severity of the depression and its aetiology. Treatment should be directed at predisposing factors, precipitating factors and perpetuating factors on the social, psychological and biological axis. Where possible, rectification or adjustment of correctable factors should be effected. Treatment should be divided into three phases: acute, aimed at remission of the index episode; continuation, aimed at preventing relapse of the index episode after treatment; and, maintenance, aimed at prevention of new episodes. First-line pharmacological treatment should be with newer antidepressants (selective serotonin reuptake inhibitors and related drugs, selective noradrenaline (norepinephrine) reuptake inhibitors and reversible monoamine oxidase inhibitors), which are as potent as older antidepressants but have fewer side-effects (see Chapter 38). In the elderly, due to altered pharmacokinetics and sensitivity, it is wise to start at small doses and increase doses slowly with close monitoring for side-effects. Efficacy may begin at three weeks but may not be observed for up to 10 weeks in some patients. After recovery antidepressant medication should continue for a longer period than in younger patients. The multicentre study from the Old Age Depression Research Interest Group (1993)

suggests a minimum maintenance period of two years, although a recent study did not show efficacy for sertraline in relapse prevention over a two-year follow-up period (Wilson et al. 2003).

Should an antidepressant appear ineffective the adequacy of dosage, compliance and treatment duration, improvement of perpetuating factors and the accuracy of the diagnosis should be examined before changing medication. If all these factors are satisfactory consideration should be given to changing the antidepressant to one from another chemical group. There are no hard and fast rules with regard to which treatment to adopt after first line antidepressants fail. It will be dictated by previous response, patient and carer preference and psychiatrist's preference.

ECT is well tolerated in the elderly (Benbow 1994). However, the recent NICE (www.nice.org.uk) guidelines recommend that ECT should only be used to achieve rapid and short-term improvement of severe symptoms, after an adequate trial of other treatments has proven ineffective or when the condition is thought to be potentially life threatening, in individuals with severe depression (catatonia, a prolonged, or a severe episode of mania). It controversially suggests caution in the use of ECT in the elderly. Depressive delusions, psychomotor retardation, agitation and other biological symptoms predict a good response (Benbow 1994). If exacerbation of confusion is an issue, unilateral ECT may be considered.

Most depressed elderly patients benefit from supportive psychotherapy and some may need more formal counselling. Cognitive–behavioural therapy and group psychotherapy are effective, while reminiscence therapy, problem-solving therapy, family therapy and more in-depth interpersonal psychotherapy may be of benefit but have not been systematically evaluated. Psychotherapeutic techniques must take account of factors associated with old age including memory, sensory deficits and articulation difficulties.

Prognosis

Over a 12-month follow-up period, between 35% and 68% of treated depressed patients remain well, between 14% and 29% remain continuously depressed, and between 12% and 19% relapsed (Baldwin & Jolly 1986). Over a 3-year follow-up period between 22% and 31% achieved lasting recovery, between 28% and 38% had a further episode with recovery, between 23% and 32% achieved partial recovery, and between 7% and 17% remained continuously ill (Baldwin & Jolly 1986). Mortality is also increased among depressed elderly patients.

MANIA

The prevalence of mania decreases with increasing age, but among patients with bipolar illness, mania may not infrequently present for the first time in old age. Up to 50% of first-degree relatives of such patients have affective disorders and such a family history is associated with early onset of illness. Two subtypes of mania have been described in elderly patients:

- affective disorder with depression in middle age and manic episodes late in life
- secondary mania in which the first affective episode is associated with coarse neurological disorder in an individual with low genetic loading.

The clinical presentation of mania in old age is similar to that seen in younger patients.

The pharmacological treatment of mania is essentially similar to that in younger patients, but should allow for the age-related altered pharmacokinetics and prolonged half-life of various drugs. Neuroleptics are of value in acute mania. Lithium and anticonvulsants, like carbamazepine and sodium valproate, can be of value in acute mania, but are also used for prophylaxis.

LATE PARAPHRENIA

In ICD-10 and DSM-IV late paraphrenia is subsumed under paranoid schizophrenia or persistent delusional disorder. Patients with late paraphrenia present for the first time in old age with persecutory delusions, auditory and/or visual hallucinations and Schneiderian first rank symptoms. Delusions of reference, hypochondriasis and grandeur, misidentification syndromes and hallucinations in other modalities may also occur. Affective symptoms are concurrently present in up to 60% of cases. Late paraphrenia patients do not show an obvious marked cognitive decline, but their performance on some cognitive test batteries is worse than normal ageing.

Late paraphrenia is commoner in women. They have sensory deficits including auditory and visual impairment. Personality features of suspiciousness, sensitivity, quarrelsomeness and unsociability are also associated with this disorder.

There are no controlled trials of neuroleptic usage in late paraphrenia, but anecdotally neuroleptics are accepted as the treatment of choice. Correction of sensory deficits may also help. All this should be coupled with social, psychological and occupational support.

SQUALOR SYNDROME

This syndrome is characterized by extreme self-neglect, domestic squalor, social withdrawal, apathy, tendency to hoard rubbish and lack of shame (Halliday et al. 2000). The annual incidence has been estimated as 0.5 per 1000 population over the age of 60 years. Sex ratio is unclear with conflicting reports. The vast majority of these individuals live alone and many are known to the community authorities, but they tend to decline offers of help. Financial hardship may be absent, many own properties and they come from all social classes. Physical illness and biochemical and haematological abnormalities commonly occur in these individuals. Deafness and visual impairment are common accompaniments.

Normal mental state is observed in up to 50% of cases. The remainder have the following diagnosis in order of decreasing frequency: dementia, paraphrenia or chronic schizophrenia, alcoholism and manic-depressive illness. Their subjectively measured personality characteristics are domineering, quarrelsome and independent.

Management should be along the lines of principles described for individual disorders earlier and consistent with general principles of management in old age psychiatry described below. Use of various legislations, including the Mental Health Act in the UK, in this syndrome has been described (Shah 1995).

SUICIDE AND ATTEMPTED SUICIDE

Suicide

A comprehensive recent review covering issues discussed in this section in greater detail is provided elsewhere (Shah & De 1998).

Epidemiology

There are large variations in elderly suicide rates across different countries. Generally, suicide rates in the elderly for both sexes are higher than the average rate in the general population. Suicide rates in the elderly for both sexes have declined over recent years in most countries.

Risk factors attributable to age, period and cohort membership will influence the suicide rate for any given age at a given time (Skegg & Cox 1991). Thus, individuals born in a particular cohort will have suicide rates peculiar to that cohort (cohort effect). Moreover, the individual's age at any given time within the cohort will further influence the suicide rate (age effect). Furthermore, environmental factors related to the period of study will further influence suicide rates (period effects). The period effect of the Second World War, detoxification of domestic gas and restricted barbiturate prescribing on reducing elderly suicide rates has been well demonstrated.

Correlates of suicide

Suicide rates in most countries are higher among elderly males than females. Male suicide rates continue to increase with age, whereas female suicide rates increase until about 60 years and decline thereafter. Elderly people who kill themselves often live alone, are lonely and are more likely to be widowed, single or divorced. Bereavement is an important precipitant and suicide rates are higher in the first few years after the death of spouse, particularly in men. Marital and family discord may be further precipitants.

Between 50% and 90% of elderly suicides have depressive illness at the time of their death. Severity of depression ranges from mild to severe and the duration from 6 to 12 months. A first episode of depression is a particularly vulnerable time with 20–35% of suicides occurring then. Symptoms of agitation, anergia, anhedonia, dysphoria, poor concentration, loss of weight, guilt, somatic preoccupations, hopelessness and insomnia are commonly associated with suicide in depressed elderly individuals.

Alcohol or substance abuse or dependence is present in up to 44% of elderly suicide victims. Alcohol may be the predominant intoxicating agent, may potentiate other poisonous agents like barbiturates or may be taken as 'Dutch courage' prior to suicide.

A smaller but significant proportion of elderly suicides have suffered from schizophrenia or paraphrenia with a prevalence of 6–17%. The relationship between elderly suicide and personality disorder has been less well examined. The prevalence of personality disorder in elderly suicide victims has been reported at 16% (with an odds ratio of 4) (Harwood et al. 2001). Personality trait accentuation of anankastic and anxious types were associated with suicide (Harwood et al. 2001).

Prevalence rates for dementia (prevalence of 4%) and delirium (prevalence of 7% for other organic disorders including delirium) are reported to be higher in elderly suicide victims than in the control group (Harwood et al. 2001). Up to 13% of elderly suicides may have been judged to have no formal mental illness.

Physical illness is present in up to 65% of elderly suicides and is often prolonged, sufficiently severe to cause acute discomfort or interfere with daily living. Up to 23% of elderly suicides receive in-patient investigation and treatment for their physical illness in the preceding year. Pain is a common accompaniment and present in up to 27% of cases and may be severe and associated with definite organic pathology such as ischaemic heart disease, post-herpetic neuralgia and chronic pain associated with the musculoskeletal system or hypochondriacal in nature. It has been speculated that both metastatic and non-metastatic effects of carcinoma can precipitate mental illness, which in turn can lead to suicide. A significant number of elderly suicides have an occult carcinoma; all these suicide victims also had depression and this concurs with the traditional observation that neoplasms may present with depression.

Medical contact

Up to 90% of elderly suicide victims are reported to have seen their general practitioner in the preceding three months and up to 50% in the week prior to suicide. Up to 20% had seen a psychiatrist in the preceding six months and about

50% of elderly suicide victims have a lifetime history of psychiatric contact.

Most studies report that a relatively small proportion of elderly suicide victims were being treated with antidepressants (12–53%), often utilizing subtherapeutic doses, while a significant proportion are treated with sedatives or hypnotics.

Methods

With increasing age, violent methods are used more frequently, particularly by men. Hanging, jumping from a height, drowning and suffocation are common means of suicide by the elderly in the UK, Japan, Finland, Singapore, New Zealand and Australia. In contrast to the US, Australia, Finland and New Zealand, shooting is uncommon in the UK, Singapore and Japan due to tighter firearms regulation. Suicide by inhalation of car exhaust fumes is increasing in the UK and New Zealand. Self-poisoning is generally more common in elderly women, but there has been a reduction in elderly suicides by self-poisoning in both sexes, largely due to a reduction in barbiturate poisoning. Suicides due to benzodiazepines and analgesics has increased in recent years, particularly in women. Analgesics are the commonest drugs taken in overdoses. Over 90% of such deaths are due to aspirin, paracetamol and dextropropoxiphene. Tricyclic antidepressants are now rarely used.

Suicide notes

Fewer elderly compared to their younger counterparts leave suicide notes because many are isolated and have no one to write to, while others have lost the ability to express themselves. When left, notes are often brief with a self-reproachful content. In one study only 43% of the victims left notes.

Attempted suicide

Elderly individuals account for up to 15% of all attempted suicides and most are unmarried, live alone, have relationship or financial difficulties or unresolved grief. Serious physical illness and pain are also associated with attempted suicides.

Depression may be present in over 90% of elderly individuals attempting suicide, and in some studies psychotic symptoms (including mood congruent depressive delusions), sleep disturbance and somatization were also common. Alcoholism and alcohol consumption before attempted suicide are common, and both lower and higher rates of organic brain syndrome have been reported. It has been suggested that many attempted suicides in late life are serious bids that have failed due to confusion from physical illness, overmedication and alcohol misuse.

Drug overdoses are the most common method (up to 90%) of attempted suicide in elderly patients, the drugs employed include minor tranquillizers, hypnotics, antidepressants and analgesics. Barbiturate self-poisoning has declined while non-opiate analgesic poisoning, particularly paracetamol and paracetamol-containing analgesics has increased. Self-poisoning is more common among women while wrist cutting, shooting, attempted drowning, jumping from heights and attempted asphyxiation are favoured by men.

PSYCHIATRY OF OLD AGE SERVICES

The management of individual disorders described above should be considered in tandem with the general provision of psychiatric services for elderly individuals. These services, in the UK, will now have to follow the standards set by the new National Service Framework for Older People

---

Box 31.4   The National Service Framework for Older People standards
Standard 1: Rooting out age discrimination
NHS & social services will be provided on the basis of clinical need regardless of age
Standard 2: Person-centred care
NHS and social care organizations treat older people as individuals and enable them to make choices about their own care through: (i) single assessment process; (ii) integrated commissioning arrangements; and (iii) integrated provision of services
Standard 3: Intermediate care
To promote independence and prevent unnecessary hospital admission by access to a range of services
To provide effective rehabilitation services to allow early discharge from hospital or avoid unnecessary admissions
Standard 4: General hospital care
Delivery of in-patient care through appropriate specialist care and by staff with appropriate skills
Standard 5: Strokes
The NHS in partnership with agencies will take action to prevent strokes
Those with a stroke will have access to specialist diagnostic services, be treated by specialist stroke service and they and their carers will be part of a multidisciplinary programme of secondary prevention and rehabilitation
Standard 6: Falls
The NHS working in partnership with councils will take action to prevent falls and their sequelae
Standard 7: Mental health in older people
Older people with mental health problems have access to mental health services, to ensure effective diagnosis, treatment and support, for them and their carers
Standard 8: Promoting an active healthy life in old age
The health and wellbeing of older people is promoted through a coordinated programme of action led by the NHS with support from councils

---

(NSF) (Department of Health 2001). There are eight specific standards as listed in Box 31.4.

Ideally the service should cater for a defined geographical area, and while a useful administrative cut-off age is 65 years, there must be some flexibility for patients with early onset dementia and graduates (patients who developed mental illness early in life and have grown old while receiving treatment in existing services for younger patients). Services should cater for all mental illnesses in old age, but some services do not receive graduates. The NSF, in Standards 1 and 7 (Box 31.4), recommends elimination of any age discrimination in service delivery for both early-onset dementia sufferers and graduates.

Sources and mode of referrals

Services may accept referrals either from other medical practitioners (closed referral) or from medical and non-medical staff (open referral). Referrals from general practitioners (GPs) has several advantages including avoidance of duplication of effort and substitution of the GP's role, the filtering of medically ill patients to geriatric medical services and continuation of management in the community (Shah & Ames 1994). In the open referral model the GP should be kept fully informed.

Site and nature of initial assessment

The initial assessment of a patient should ideally take place at the patient's home (Shah & Ames 1994). Home visits have no significant disadvantages. The advantages of home assessments include:

- consultation rate close to 100% (Benbow 1990)
- direct observation of the home environment (Benbow 1990)
- avoidance of unnecessary social work and occupational therapy assessment ordered from the outpatient clinic (Shah & Ames 1994)
- ready access to the patient's medication and attention to polypharmacy, poor compliance, drug interaction, dependence on benzodiazepines, and hoarding for overdose (Shah & Ames 1994)
- reduced stigma about attending a psychogeriatric clinic
- avoiding the irregularities in the timing and availability of the ambulance for transportation and avoiding the indignity of lengthy ambulance rides (Benbow 1990)
- personal costs of a trip to the clinic is avoided by the patient (Shah & Ames 1994).

Two appropriate members of the multidisciplinary team should assess the patient. This enables assessment from the perspective of two disciplines and provides safety from assaults and accusations. One member should be a doctor to facilitate mental state and physical examinations. Community psychiatric nurses have been involved in initial assessment, despite controversy over their use as filters between GPs and psychiatrists.

Multidisciplinary community meetings, similar to traditional ward rounds, are used to discuss new cases and their management, to facilitate liaison between team members, to cross-refer cases, to provide mutual support, and to discuss new plans, ideas and problems. Management should be based on the principle of case-management where the case-manager not only provides professional assistance from his/her discipline but also coordinates other management strategies. Standards 2 and 7 of the new NSF recommends development of close multidisciplinary working, integration between health and social services, development of a single assessment process across different disciplines and agencies, and agreed protocols between primary and secondary care for the assessment and management of dementia and depression.

Patients may require follow-up for further assessment, treatment, rehabilitation, monitoring of side-effects, monitoring of mental state, support for patient or carers and advocacy (Shah & Ames 1994). This may be at home, in the outpatient clinic or at a day-hospital.

OUTPATIENT CLINICS

Outpatient and specialist memory clinics can complement home visits with detailed neuropsychometry, and blood and radiological investigations (Shah & Ames 1994). Such clinics are being increasingly located in the general hospital because it allows access to a wide range of facilities. Memory clinics offer elective, detailed assessment of patients with dementia and related disorders, but due to the lengthy assessments such clinics are able to evaluate a relatively small number of patients. However, through Standard 7 of the NSF, the development of memory clinics is encouraged.

Day hospitals

Day hospitals are an important component of old age psychiatry services. They allow assessment, treatment, rehabilitation, long-term support, development of a social network and support for carers (Shah & Ames 1994). The UK Royal College of Psychiatrists recommend 90 day places for a population of 30,000 over 65-year-olds. Day hospitals cater both for functionally and organically ill patients, either in separate units or on separate days, and flexible day hospitals which are open at the weekend and during the evening are slowly emerging, with obvious advantages (Shah & Ames 1994). In rural areas travelling day hospitals have been developed.

In-patient care

There are three types of hospital admissions: assessment and/or treatment, respite and continuing care. The UK

Royal College of Psychiatrists recommends 45 acute beds and 90 continuing care beds for a population of 30 000 over the age of 65 years.

Factors that may contribute to an in-patient admission include severity of the illness, severity of the sequelae of the illness, insufficient social and community support at home, need for more detailed and intensive assessment, and implementation of certain treatments like ECT (Shah & Ames 1994). Respite admissions can be in stand-alone units, acute admissions wards or continuing care wards. They are usually intended to give carers a break. Some patients may require long-term (continuing care) admissions. In the UK, continuing care admissions are regulated by locally agreed criteria (between different agencies) following a department of health directive.

Role of the general practitioner

General practitioners play a vital role in the satisfactory functioning of psychogeriatric services. They see a significant amount of psychiatric morbidity and have good ability to recognize both depression and dementia, but adopt less good treatment strategies. The latter could be facilitated by the psychogeriatric service providing support and back-up with liaison clinics in general practice involving psychiatrists, community psychiatric nurses and social workers. Standard 7 of the NSF promotes close working between primary care and specialist old age psychiatry services through a range of models such as above and through development of agreed protocols for assessment and management of dementia and depression.

Liaison service

Psychiatry of old age services should provide a liaison service to departments of geriatric medicine and general hospitals, residential and nursing homes, social service and voluntary agency day facilities, voluntary organizations and other local government facilities. The liaison service should aim to share knowledge about psychiatry of old age with others and improve the ability of non-specialist professionals to detect and manage mental illness. This can be done on a case by case basis (consultation model) and by contributions to their meetings and open forum seminars (liaison model) or by both models.

Depressed medically ill elderly in-patients experience severe psychological distress, have more severe physical illnesses, have physical illnesses that are difficult to treat, are poorly compliant with treatment, have longer hospital admissions and have a higher mortality. Moreover, depression is poorly recognized and treated among geriatric in-patients and more than 80% of depressed elderly patients have no documented plans for the management of their depression following discharge. Furthermore, less than half of all elderly medically ill in-patients with depression are referred to psychiatrists and antidepressants are used infrequently and at inadequate doses.

The prevalence of mental illness in residential facilities including sheltered homes, hostels, residential homes, special accomodation homes and nursing homes is considerable. Residential facility staff and nursing home staff have limited psychiatric training, so psychiatric morbidity is often unrecognized in such facilities or, when recognized, poorly treated. There is considerable need for liaison service development in this area.

MENTAL HEALTH LEGISLATION AND ELDERLY PATIENTS

The application of mental health legislation to elderly patients is essentially the same as its application to younger patients in most jurisdictions. Thus, in England and Wales, for example, the various sections of the Mental Health Act 1983 apply equally to elderly and young patients. However, it is important to note that the mental health act does not allow for the treatment of medical illnesses in elderly individuals with mental illness. Recent case law has drawn attention to the issue of the established clinical practice of informally admitting patients unless they actively dissent even when they lack the capacity to consent to the admission ('the Bournewood case'); this is particularly common in subjects with dementia. The Court of Appeal ruled that an autistic patient who lacked capacity to consent to the admission and did not dissent was illegally detained. It was implied that all patients who lack the capacity to consent and do not dissent should be detained under the Mental Health Act. The House of Lords subsequently over-ruled this decision, thus providing a statutory basis for individual psychiatrists to admit patients who lack the capacity to consent, but do not dissent, without recourse to the Mental Health Act. This anomaly is likely to have safeguards in the proposed new Mental Health Act Bill. Although, such patients will still be admitted informally, they will have additional safeguards including a requirement to secure a second opinion, automatic hearing at the Mental Health Review Tribunal, access to a 'nominated' person and access to the specialist mental health advocacy service (all these are otherwise proposed to be reserved for detained patients).

REFERENCES

Baldwin RC & Jolley D (1986) The prognosis of depression in old age. *British Journal of Psychiatry* 149: 574–83.

Benbow SM (1990) The community clinic: its advantages and disadvantages. *International Journal of Geriatric Psychiatry* 5: 119–21.

Benbow SM (1994) Electro-convulsive therapy in later life. In Chiu E & Ames D (eds) *Functional Psychiatric Disorders of the Elderly*, pp 440–60. Cambridge: Cambridge University Press.

Burns A, Jacoby R & Levy R (1990a) Psychiatric phenomena in Alzheimer's disease IV: disorders of behaviour. *British Journal of Psychiatry* 157: 86–94.

Burns A, Jacoby R & Levy R (1990b) Psychiatric phenomena in Alzheimer's disease. II Disorders of perception. *British Journal of Psychiatry* 157: 76–81.

Burns A, Jacoby R & Levy R (1990c) Psychiatric phenomena in Alzheimer's disease. I: Disorders of thought content. *British Journal of Psychiatry* 15: 72–6.

Consensus Guidelines for the Clinical and Pathological Diagnosis of Dementia of Lewy Body Type (DLB) (1996) Report of the Consortium on DLB International Workshop held in Newcastle, UK 1996 for diagnosis. *Neurology* 47: 1124–34.

Copeland JRM, Dewey ME, Woods N et al. (1987) Range of mental illness among the elderly in the community. Prevalence in Liverpool using the GMS AGECAT package. *British Journal of Psychiatry* 150: 815–23.

Department of Health (2001) *National Service Framework for Older People.* London, Department of Health.

Gauthier S, Feldman H, Hecker J, Vellas B, Emir B et al. (2002) Functional, cognitive and behavioural effects of donepezil in patients with moderate Alzheimer's disease. *Current Medical Research Opinion* 18: 347–54.

Halliday G, Banerjee S, Philpot M & MacDonald A (2000) Community study of people who live in squalor. *Lancet* 355: 882–6.

Harwood D, Hawton K, Hope T & Jacoby R (2001) Psychiatric disorder and personality factors associated with suicide in older people: a descriptive and case-control study. *International Journal of Geriatric Psychiatry* 16: 155–65.

Jacomb P & Jorm A (1996) Personality change in dementia of Alzheimer's type. *International Journal of Geriatric Psychiatry* 11: 201–7.

Katz IR, Jeste DV, Mintzer JE, Clyde C, Napolitano J et al. (1999) Comparison of risperidone and placebo for psychosis and behaviour disturbance associated with dementia: a randomised, double blind trial. Risperidone Study Group. *Journal of Clinical Psychiatry* 60: 107–15.

Kivela SL, Pahkala K & Laippala P (1991) A one-year prognosis of dysthymic disorder and major depression in old age. *International Journal of Geriatric Psychiatry* 6: 81–7.

Lindesay J, Briggs K & Murphy E (1989) The Guy's/Age Concern survey. Prevalence rates of cognitive impairment, depression and anxiety in an urban community. *British Journal of Psychiatry* 154: 2317–29.

McKeith I, Del Ser T, Spano P, Emre M, Wesnes K, Anand R, Sain A, Ferrara R & Spiegel R (2000) Efficacy of rivastigmine in dementia with Lewy bodies: a randomised, double-blind, placebo-controlled international study. *Lancet* 356: 2031–6.

Old Age Depression Research Interest Group (1993) How long should the elderly take antidepressants? A double blind placebo controlled study of continuation/prophylaxix therapy with dotheipin. *British Journal of Psychiatry* 162: 175–82.

Reisberg B, Doody R, Stoffler A, Schmitt F, Ferris S, Mobius HJ and Memantine Study Group (2003) Memantidine in moderate to severe Alzheimer's disease. *New England Journal of Medicine* 348: 1333–41.

Rosler M, Retz W, Retz-Junginger P & Dennier HJ (1998) Effects of two-year treatment with cholinesterase inhibitor rivastigmine on behavioural symptoms in Alzheimer's disease. *Behavioral Neurology* 11: 211–16.

Saunders AM, Strittmater WJ, Schmechel D et al. (1993) Association of apolipoprotein E allele E4 with late-onset familial and sporadic Alzheimer's disease. *Neurology* 43: 1467–72.

Schneider LS, Pollock VE & Lyness SA (1990) A meta-analysis of controlled trials of neuroleptic treatment in dementia. *Journal of the American Geriatric Society* 38: 553–63.

Shah AK (1995) The use of legislation in cases of squalor. *Medicine, Science and the Law* 35: 43–4.

Shah AK & Ames D (1994) Planning and developing psychogeriatric services. *International Review of Psychiatry* 6: 15–27.

Shah AK & De T (1998) Suicide in the elderly. *International Journal of Psychiatry in Clinical Practice* 2: 3–17.

Skegg K & Cox B (1991) Suicide in New Zealand 1957–1986: the influence of age, period and birth-cohort. *Australia and New Zealand Journal of Psychiatry* 25: 181–90.

Street JS, Clark WS, Gannon KS, Cummings JL, Bymaster FP et al.

(2000) Olanzapine treatment of psychotic and behavioural symptoms in patients with Alzheimer's disease in nursing care facilities: a double-blind, randomised placebo controlled trial. The HGEU Study Group. *Archives of General Psychiatry* **57**: 968–76.

Tariot PN, Solomon PR, Morris JC, Kirshaw P, Lilienfeld S et al. (2001) A 5-month, randomised, placebo-controlled trial of galanthamine in AD. The Galanthamine USA-10 Study Group. *Neurology* **54**: 2269–76.

Wilson KCM, Mottram PG, Ashworth L & Abou-Saleh MT (2003) Older community residents with depression: long-term treatment with sertraline. *British Journal of Psychiatry* **182**: 492–7.

Wragg RE & Jeste D (1989) Overview of depression and psychosis in Alzheimer's disease. *American Journal of Psychiatry* **146**: 577–87.

PART 3

Diagnosis, investigation and treatment

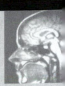

Clinical examination of psychiatric patients

Pádraig Wright, Julian Stern and Michael Phelan

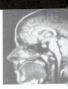

INTRODUCTION

The psychiatric interview is undertaken primarily in order to establish a diagnosis. It includes history-taking and the clinical examination of the mental state. However, the psychiatric interview is much more than a diagnostic process. It also helps to establish rapport between patient and doctor and to educate and motivate the patient.

Interviewing patients also serves an important therapeutic purpose. This is the goal for patients during psychotherapeutic consultations, but it also applies to all other patients for whom the opportunity to discuss problems with a sympathetic listener is often helpful. The many functions of the psychiatric interview are described in Box 32.1.

The diagnostic process in psychiatry differs from that in other medical disciplines in that:

- it relies almost exclusively on history-taking and clinical examination
- the account obtained from the patient must be corroborated by information from the patient's partner, children or other relatives, or from the family doctor, social worker or teacher, as appropriate.

Interviewing such third parties should only be undertaken with the patient's fully informed consent. However, such corroborative interviews should be the rule rather than the exception because psychiatric patients may, consciously or unwittingly, conceal important information. Verbal accounts from patients and third parties should be supplemented by written records from family doctors, hospitals or schools when appropriate. This is especially the case for events that occurred many years ago or for which the patient has only a second-hand account from parents or others.

Psychiatric interviews should be conducted in macroscopic settings that facilitate the patient's privacy and comfort and ensure the doctor's safety. These goals are relatively easy to achieve in psychiatric outpatient clinics but present challenges when patients are interviewed in their home (privacy and safety) or in general medical hospital departments (comfort, privacy and safety), and may be impossible to achieve in some settings, for example police stations or prisons.

The microscopic setting of the interview also warrants attention. Patients feel more at ease if seated at the same level as, and to one side of, rather than opposite, the doctor. One tried and trusted arrangement (Fig. 32.1) is for the doctor to sit at a fixed desk with the patient seated in a heavy or fixed chair to the doctor's left. The door should be to the doctor's right and should open outwards. This arrangement facilitates writing (for a right-handed doctor), eye contact between patient and doctor, and safety (the desk and patient's chair are virtually immobile, the door can be reached and opened quickly and, given that it opens outwards, cannot be barricaded from within the room). Safety is enhanced by ensuring that there are no potential weapons such as lamps, electrical cables or coat hangers in the interview room, and by telling a receptionist, nurse or other colleague that the interview is taking place.

The taking of a psychiatric history, assessment of a patient's personality, and performance of a mental state examination will now be described. Psychodynamic aspects of clinical examination and difficulties that may be encountered when interviewing psychiatric patients will also be discussed.

Box 32.1   The functions of the psychiatric interview

History-taking: undertaken in order to elicit the patient's account of problems and establish a differential diagnosis

Mental state examination: undertaken in order to establish the presence or absence of specific psychiatric symptoms and thus confirm a diagnosis on which treatment may be based

Establishing rapport

Education and motivation of the patient: undertaken in order to advise the patient about their illness or its treatment, about prognosis, and indeed about the processes of psychiatric evaluation and treatment

Treatment: may be the primary goal of the interview as in a formal psychotherapeutic interaction, or it may be an additional function as in the standard clinical interview

---

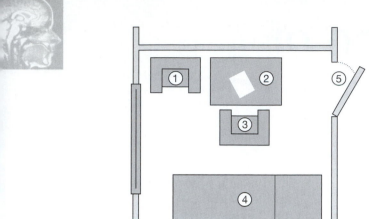

Figure 32.1 The layout of a room suitable for history-taking and clinical examination of psychiatric patients.

1. Patient's chair
2. Desk
3. Doctor's chair
4. Couch
5. Outward opening door

TAKING A PSYCHIATRIC HISTORY

Prior to the interview, care should be taken to ensure that patients and those accompanying them know the interviewing doctor's name and the location of coffee shops, toilets, etc. The interview should commence with introductions, a brief explanation of the purpose of the interview, and an estimate of the time available or required. Explain the need to take notes and reassure the patient about confidentiality. If the interview is medicolegal in nature, the doctor should explain who has requested and who may see any resulting report.

Establishing the reason for referral and the presenting complaint

Note-taking should commence with a brief record of the reason the patient was referred (depression not responding to antidepressant treatment, for example), the referring source (general practitioner, for example), and the expected outcome of the referral (confirmation of diagnosis or initiation of other treatment, for example).

History-taking proper should commence with the collection of demographic details. This is both necessary and, being emotionally neutral information as distinct from emotionally laden information, helps to establish rapport. Some patients may remain ill-at-ease at the end of this stage of the interview and it may be appropriate to continue eliciting relatively neutral information by proceeding with personal history and family history details, only returning to

the presenting complaint and history of the presenting complaint later in the interview. Otherwise, it is best to proceed as outlined in Box 32.2 and invite the patient to

---

Box 32.2 A scheme for eliciting and recording clinical information

The reason for referral

Brief demographic details

The reason the patient was referred (depression not responding to treatment)

The referring source (general practitioner, community nurse)

The expected outcome of the referral (confirmation of diagnosis, admission)

The presenting complaint

The presenting complaint (e.g. 'I feel miserable. Completely without hope')

The history of the presenting complaint

The duration of the presenting complaint

Potential precipitants

The mode of onset of symptoms

The severity of symptoms and their impact on the patient's life

Establishing the family history

Age, marital status, occupation, physical and mental health, and/or cause of death of first-degree relatives

The personality of each first-degree relative and the relationship each has with the patient

Family history of psychiatric illness (especially alcohol and drugs, psychiatric hospitalizations, and suicide)

Psychiatric illness in members of the extended family

Possible impact of events such as births, marriages and deaths upon the patient

Establishing the personal history

Gestation and birth, early development and ages at which milestones were attained

Childhood relationships with parents and siblings

Ages of starting and finishing school

Relationships with peers and teachers

Academic and sporting achievements

Employments (listed chronologically), reasons for changes in employment

Age at menarche and details of sexual relationships, sexual experiences, contraception and terminations of pregnancies

Age at marriage, duration of relationship before marriage, spouse's age, health and occupation, and sex and age of any children

The quality of the relationship between patient and spouse, and patient and offspring

Significant illness and surgical procedures

Psychiatric illnesses (durations of each, treatment received, doctor and/or hospital)

Previous episodes of unrecognized psychiatric illness

Current social situation (accommodation arrangements, income, make-up of household, domestic or financial difficulties)

Establishing the forensic history

Arrests, cautions, convictions, imprisonment or other punishment

Crimes admitted to but not detected

---

describe his/her problems. This is undertaken in order to establish the presenting complaint and to get a brief overview of the difficulties the patient is currently experiencing. A few words or a short phrase may be sufficient to describe the presenting complaint and it is usual to record the patient's own words. Thus it is preferable to write, for example, 'I feel utterly miserable – there is absolutely no hope for me,' rather than the word 'depression'.

Establishing the history of the presenting complaint

The duration of the patient's difficulties should next be established by asking, 'When did you last feel perfectly well?' or, 'When were you first troubled by these problems?'. Having established the nature and duration of the patient's problems, their history (potential precipitants, mode of onset of symptoms, severity of symptoms and treatment received to date) should next be established.

Potential precipitants should be identified when possible and may include psychosocial stresses (unemployment, domestic strife, poverty), physical illness (influenza, cancer) or its treatment, or non-adherence to maintainence therapy with antidepressants, antipsychotics or mood stabilizing drugs. An attempt should be made to differentiate between independent precipitants and those which may have arisen because of the patient's deteriorating mental health. Loss of employment because of poor performance consequent upon mental illness is but one example of the latter.

The mode of onset of symptoms is important in establishing a diagnosis and in determining a prognosis. Thus symptoms of sudden onset often suggest an identifiable and potentially treatable cause (head injury, psychosocial stress or illicit drugs) and a better outcome, whereas insidiously developing symptoms are more often associated with disorders with ill-defined aetiologies, symptomatic or no treatment, and poor outcomes. The severity of the patient's illness and the disability it causes must be evaluated by questions about changes in appetite, weight, sleep pattern and sexual behaviour, and by enquiries about how symptoms impact on the patient's personal, domestic, occupational and social functioning. Finally, the nature, duration and effect of any treatment received to date should be noted.

Establishing the family history

The age, martial status, occupation, physical and mental health, and cause of death of each of the patient's first-degree relatives (parents, siblings and offspring) should next be recorded. In addition, an attempt should be made to evaluate the personality of each first-degree relative, living or deceased, and to assess the relationship each has or had with the patient. A family history of psychiatric illness is often difficult to obtain because of stigma (see Chapter 11), because some mental illnesses are accepted as the norm within the family, or because alcohol or substance abuse is not regarded as mental illness. Specific questions must therefore be asked about alcohol and drugs, psychiatric hospitalizations, and suicide. In addition to information about first-degree relatives, information about psychiatric illness in members of the extended family should be sought. Finally, the possible impact of events such as births, marriages and deaths upon the patient and upon the atmosphere in the patient's home, both during childhood and currently, should be considered. The most important family history data may usefully be recorded in a genogram (see Fig. 32.2 for an example).

Establishing the personal history

A record of the patient's personal development, sexual development and relationships, past medical and psychiatric history, and current social circumstances is next obtained. Information is first collected about the patient's gestation and birth, early development and the ages at which milestones (sitting upright, standing upright, walking, talking and bladder and bowel control) were attained. The patient's childhood relationships with parents and siblings should also be evaluated, and the ages of starting and finishing school, relationships with peers and teachers, and academic and sporting achievements should be noted. Following this, employments should be listed chronologically and the reasons for changes in employment noted. It is especially important to note if new jobs represent advancement or decline in terms of responsibility and remuneration, because the latter may reflect progressive impairment consequent upon mental illness.

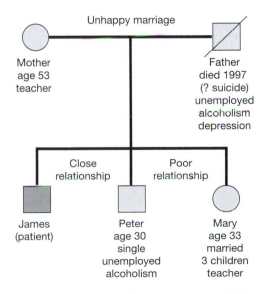

Figure 32.2 The use of a genogram for recording history information.

Following this, age at menarche and details of sexual relationships, sexual experiences, contraception and terminations of pregnancy are obtained as appropriate. Age at marriage, duration of relationship before marriage, spouse's age, health and occupation, and the sex and age of any children should also be recorded. The quality of the relationship between patient and spouse, and patient and offspring, should also be enquired into.

Details of all significant illness and surgical procedures are next recorded, followed by details of any psychiatric illnesses, including the durations of each, the treatment received, and the doctor and/or hospital attended. It is important to note that while patients may have no formal past psychiatric history, they may nonetheless have had previous episodes of psychiatric illness, recognized or unrecognized – such episodes must be enquired about.

The patient's current social situation refers to accommodation arrangements, income (from employment or from social welfare payments), make-up of household, and any domestic or financial difficulties. The suitability of accommodation and the patient's income and financial status are especially important as problems in these areas may impact upon psychiatric illness.

Establishing the forensic history

Forensic details may be elicited by asking the patient if they have ever been in trouble with the police (arrests, cautions, convictions, imprisonment or other punishment). Delinquency or crimes admitted to but not detected should also be noted and alcohol and/or substance abuse may also be enquired about at this time. It may be appropriate to corroborate the forensic history by reviewing police or court records in the case of some patients.

ASSESSING A PATIENT'S PERSONALITY

It is extremely difficult to evaluate a patient's premorbid personality during a psychiatric consultation and any opinion formed must be constantly reviewed in light of further contact with the patient and additional information from informants. Questions such as, 'If I had met you before you became ill, would I notice many differences between you then and you now?', 'How would your best friend (or spouse or work colleague) describe you?' or, 'How would you deal with a serious financial difficulty (unemployment, illness in your family)?' may allow some access to the patient's personality. Further information may be gained by enquiring about the patient's relationships (many or few friends, deep or superficial friendships), character (confident or self-deprecating, impulsive or cautious, independent or dependent, shy or gregarious) and usual mood (cheerful or despondent, optimistic or pessimistic, stable or emotional). Personal habits (tobacco, alcohol and substance use/abuse,

when first used/abused and current quantity used/abused per day, and expenditure on this) and attitudes (religious and moral, and also attitudes to psychiatry and psychiatric treatment) should also be enquired into. Finally, an individual's preferred leisure activities may reflect a preference for company or solitude, or intellectual, physical, competitive or creative pursuits. A brief enquiry into the patient's plans for the future may also be informative, although it is important to note that such plans may be heavily influenced by current symptoms, especially depression.

PERFORMING A MENTAL STATE EXAMINATION

The doctor will have become aware of many symptoms (and of the patient's cognitive ability) during the process of history-taking, but in performing a mental state examination, only those symptoms the patient is experiencing or exhibiting at the time of the examination should be recorded. History-taking will almost certainly indicate a probable diagnosis but it is nevertheless important to confirm this and to rule out other diagnoses by a systematic mental state examination, which carefully considers the patient's appearance, posture and movement, behaviour, speech, mood and affect, thought, perception, cognition and insight (see Box 32.3). The many clinical features that may be detected during the mental state examination are described in detail in Chapter 6 and are only referred to briefly, and in order to ensure continuity, below.

Appearance

Personal care may be impaired (schizophrenia, depression, dementia or alcohol or substance abuse), bizarre clothing or accessories may be worn (mania, depression, schizophrenia, dementia, anorexia nervosa, or organic psychiatric disorder) or stigmata suggestive of intravenous drug abuse or solvent abuse may be apparent.

Patients with dyspraxia may wear clothing backwards, may not wear underclothing, or may fasten buttons incorrectly. Facial appearance may reflect underlying mood, parkinsonism caused by antipsychotic medication, or organic disorder (thyroid disease, Parkinson's disease or supranuclear palsy), while tearfulness and crying are features of many psychiatric disorders, most noticeably depression.

Posture and movement

Patients may exhibit a slumped posture with slowed movements if depressed, while manic patients are usually overactive. Anxious patients may appear tense and hypervigilant and may sweat excessively. Patients with schizophrenia may exhibit mannerisms, stereotypes,

---

Box 32.3   A scheme for eliciting and recording the mental state examination

Appearance
Personal care and clothing
Stigmata suggestive of drug abuse
Facial appearance

Posture and movement
Posture
Movements
Tension, hypervigilance, excessive sweating
Mannerisms, stereotypies, echopraxia, flexibilitas cerea, negativism or excitement
Parkinsonism, akathisia, tardive dyskinesia, tics
Responding to auditory hallucinations

Behaviour
Irritability, distractibility and apathy
Overfamiliarity, importunateness, sexual inappropriateness
Social withdrawal, no eye contact, little conversation
Perplexity
Aggression and violence

Speech
Quantity of speech
Rate of speech
Volume of speech
Neologisms, thought disorders, punning, clang associations, flight of ideas, poverty of the content of speech
Perseveration, dysphasia or dysarthria

Mood and affect
Depression (enquire about suicide)
Elation
Anxiety
Depersonalization or derealization
Affect (appropriateness of mood, rate of change of mood)

Thought
Rate of thinking
Form of thought
Content of thought (delusions, over-valued ideas and obsessional thoughts)

Perception
Illusions
Hallucinations

Cognition
Orientation in time, place and person
Serial sevens, months of the year or days of the week backwards
Repeat and later recall the names of three unrelated objects (short-term memory)
Recount recent political or sporting news items (recent memory)
Dates of distant evens, birth dates of close relatives (remote memory)
Mini-mental state examination if appropriate

Insight
Illness
Nature of illness
Appropriate treatment

---

echopraxia, flexibilitas cerea, negativism or excitement, and parkinsonism, akathisia and tardive dyskinesia associated with antipsychotic treatment may also be evident. Schizophrenic patients may also be observed attending to or responding to auditory hallucinations. Patients with social phobia will appear extremely anxious in the presence of other people and the rituals undertaken by patients with obsessive-compulsive disorder may be evident. Tics may occur in isolation, in patients with anxiety disorders (especially obsessive-compulsive disorder) and in Gilles de la Tourette's syndrome.

Behaviour

In addition to the abnormalities of posture and movement described above, patients with psychiatric illness frequently exhibit abnormal general and social behaviour. This may be observed during the patient's interaction with relatives, other patients and hospital personnel, as well as during the formal psychiatric interview. Abnormalities of general behaviour include irritability (mania, agitated depression, alcohol withdrawal), distractibility (depression, mania, dementia) and apathy (depression, dementia).

Social behaviour is often severely compromised by psychiatric illness. Manic patients are overfamiliar and importunate, attempt to engage those around them in conversation, and may behave in a sexually inappropriate manner. Patients with schizophrenia or depression are often socially withdrawn, may not make eye contact, and do not easily engage in conversation, while demented patients may appear perplexed and may ignore social conventions. Aggression and violence is relatively uncommon but may be especially associated with mania, personality disorder, schizophrenia and alcohol or drug abuse.

Speech

The patient's speech is observed throughout the psychiatric interview and verbatim examples of speech should be recorded in order to illustrate the symptoms described below and in order to note the content of conversation which may reflect underlying psychopathology. Speech may be abnormal in quantity, rate, volume and/or tone.

The quantity of speech is typically reduced in depressed patients, who may not initiate conversation and may respond to questions with monosyllabic answers. Severely depressed patients may be mute. The rate of speech is also frequently reduced in depression, such that long pauses occur before an answer is made, as well as between words and sentences, and words are spoken more slowly than is usual. In contrast, manic patients speak spontaneously and rapidly, the quantity of speech is greatly increased, and jokes and puns are frequent. Patients with schizophrenia may exhibit an increased or reduced quantity and rate of speech, while anxious patients, especially those with obsessive-compulsive disorder, often answer with excessive detail.

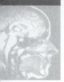

The volume of speech is increased in mania and reduced in depression, and sighing is also characteristic of depression. Normal speech is characterized by considerable variation in the tone of voice cadence, but this is reduced or lost in depressed patients who therefore speak monotonously.

In addition to the relatively measurable quantity, rate, volume and tone of the patient's speech, the doctor should also note neologisms (characteristic of schizophrenia), thought disorders such as derailment, word salad and verbigeration (which are also features of schizophrenia), and punning, clang associations and flight of ideas (mania). Poverty of the content of speech occurs in schizophrenia and is characterized by seemingly normal conversation that imparts very little information. Finally, perseveration, dysphasia and dysarthria may be apparent and are suggestive of organic pathology.

Mood and affect

The patient's mood may be apparent from the presenting complaint or from their appearance, motor activity, behaviour and/or speech. However, this information needs to be expanded upon by direct questions such as, 'What are your spirits like?' or, 'What is your mood like?' The most frequently detected abnormalities of mood are depression, elation, anxiety and depersonalization and/or derealization. The term euthymia is used to describe normal mood.

Depression is associated with tearfulness, guilt about the past, pessimism and unworthiness about the present, and hopelessness about the future. These emotions may reach delusional intensity and can lead to suicide. Thus, direct enquiry about suicide is a vital component of the mental state examination and should commence with questions such as, 'Have you ever been so miserable that you thought that life was not worth living?', proceeding if appropriate through questions such as, 'Have you thought of ways in which you might end your life?' and ending with detailed questions, about when, how and where suicide might occur and the steps that would be taken to conceal the attempt. There is no evidence that such questioning increases the risk of suicide and indeed many patients are relieved to have the opportunity to discuss their most distressing thoughts.

The elated mood of mania is readily apparent and may be transmitted to the interviewing doctor (infectious euphoria). In contrast to depressed patients, manic patients are often excessively self-confident and are extravagant in their claims about the past and their plans for the future. Close questioning about the reality of such claims and plans may cause the patient to become irritable.

Anxiety is often apparent from the patient's behaviour and its presence may be confirmed by questions such as, 'Do you feel more tense than usual?' or, 'Have you noticed yourself sweating (or your heart beating, etc.) more than usual?' Having established that symptoms of anxiety are present, further questioning is necessary in order to determine the precise anxiety disorder the patient is suffering from.

Comorbidity of anxiety disorders is such that it should be assumed that a patient with one anxiety disorder is also suffering from another anxiety disorder until proven otherwise.

Depersonalization and derealization are relatively common symptoms but are nonetheless difficult to enquire about and to confirm as present or absent. Depersonalization is often described as a feeling of detachment from reality or the sensation of being two-dimensional, or unable to experience emotions. Patients experiencing derealization may describe their surroundings as lacking depth, being like a film set, or as if constructed from cardboard.

Having evaluated the patient's mood, the patient's affect should also be noted. This refers to the appropriateness of mood, and the rate at which mood alters in response to a given situation. Patients whose mood varies rapidly are described as labile, while the terms bluntening or flattening of affect are used to describe those who exhibit a relatively unchanging neutral mood irrespective of circumstances. Finally, incongruity of affect, in which the patient's mood is the opposite of that expected in the circumstances (laughing when describing a recent bereavement, for example), may be evident.

Thought

Access to the thoughts of another is only possible through their speech or writings. Thoughts may be abnormal in rate, form (formal thought disorder) or content. Thus patients may complain that their thoughts are either excessively rapid or excessively slow, or may exhibit flight of ideas, thought retardation or poverty of thinking. Formal thought disorder is most common in schizophrenia and includes derailment, circumstantiality or loosening of associations, dribbling and thought-blocking.

Abnormalities of the content of thought include delusions, overvalued ideas and obsessional thoughts. Delusions may be primary and arise without precedent, or secondary and follow hallucinations, pathologically altered mood, or indeed other delusions. It is important to differentiate delusions from culturally or subculturally accepted beliefs, especially when exhibited by patients from different countries, religions or traditions to those of the interviewing doctor. Delusions of thought insertion, withdrawal or broadcast are commonly expressed by patients with schizophrenia (and are also passivity phenomena). Once identified, delusions should be classified as delusions of persecution, reference, infestation, nihilism, misidentification, infidelity, guilt, control or worthlessness, or as grandiose, religious, amorous or hypochondriacal delusions as appropriate.

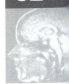

Overvalued ideas are strongly held and may influence the patient's behaviour, but they differ from delusions in that they usually exist in isolation and are also believed by at least a few other individuals in the patient's society.

Obsessional thoughts or images may be revealed by questions such as, 'Do some thoughts keep coming into your mind even though you do not want them to, and do you try to resist thinking them?' The content of obsessional thoughts may often be sexual or violent, and can be bizarre. However, patients recognize obsessional thoughts as their own, are distressed by them, find them embarrassing or senseless and usually, at least initially, try to resist them or to distract themselves from them.

Perception

Illusions and hallucinations are sometimes apparent from the behaviour of patients (brushing insects from the bedclothes or apparently attending to, or responding to, auditory hallucinations). More often, questions such as, 'Have you had any unusual experiences?' or, 'Have you ever heard sounds or voices when you were alone or that no one else could hear?', may be necessary. Hallucinations may be classified by the sensory modality they appear to involve (auditory, visual, olfactory, gustatory or tactile), as deep (often sexual) or superficial (formication), or as simple (noises or flashes of light) or complex (voices commenting about the patient) hallucinations. Hallucinations other than auditory hallucinations should always raise the suspicion of an organic psychiatric disorder.

Cognition

The cognitive ability of a patient may be examined by enquiring about orientation in time, place and person, and by simple tests of attention, concentration and memory (see Chapter 26). The ability or otherwise of a patient to cooperate with the interview and history-taking is often a good means of evaluating attention and concentration, but this should be supplemented by the serial sevens test, or by asking the patient to repeat the months of the year or days of the week backwards. Memory may be evaluated by asking the patient to:

- repeat and later recall the names of three unrelated objects such as an orange, a paper clip and a table (short-term memory)
- recount recent political or sporting news items (recent memory)
- provide dates of distant personal or newsworthy events, or birth dates of close relatives (remote memory).

If these simple tests suggest impairment, and in patients for whom a more detailed cognitive evaluation is appropriate, the mini mental state examination (Folstein et al. 1975)

should be completed. Formal neuropsychological evaluation may be appropriate in some patients.

Insight

Having taken a history and performed a mental state examination, the interviewing doctor should have a reasonably clear idea of a patient's interpretation of their experiences. However, it remains useful to formally ask the patient if anything is wrong, and if so, if this is due to illness or to some other cause. If illness is admitted to, it is important to determine if the patient believes it to be physical or psychological, and to warrant treatment and, if so, the nature of such treatment. Insight is often greatly impaired in psychotic patients, while patients with depression or anxiety disorders may have full insight into the nature of their problems and the appropriate treatments.

Having completed the mental state examination it is usual for the interviewing doctor to note their own subjective response to the patient, both because this may be informative in deciding upon diagnosis and because the doctor's attitude to the patient may influence treatment.

PSYCHODYNAMIC ASPECTS OF CLINICAL EXAMINATION

As made clear above, there is much more to the psychiatric interview than establishing a diagnosis. The psychiatrist must always be attuned to the psychodynamic issues inherent in any interaction with a patient, and must always consider the consequences of these issues.

Each interview with a patient involves a potentially intense emotional experience. The patient who is grieving for her dead child, the patient who accuses you of wanting to poison him, the pitifully thin woman who wants you to allow her to starve herself to death – each of these patients requires much from a psychiatrist, and each psychiatrist employs a variety of manoeuvres to cope with the waves of explicit and implicit demands, threats, and appeals made by the patient (and also by the patient's family and by other health professionals). These manoeuvres will sometimes be employed to safeguard the relationship between patient and doctor, and to allow the consultation to proceed in a productive way; but sometimes they will be used primarily for defensive purposes, to block out emotions which are too unsettling or disturbing for the psychiatrist. What is being alluded to is the presence of a state of emotional availability in the practitioner, which allows the patient to feel that his/her concerns, anxieties and conflicts are genuinely heard. If the patient feels pushed away or fobbed off, he or she may respond in a number of ways that may worsen the situation for both patient and psychiatrist. A suicidal patient may interpret the psychiatrist's apparent disinterest as another (perhaps final) rejection and make a suicidal gesture.

A depressed patient may feel that once again she is useless, and stop attending the clinic. A paranoid man may feel that the psychiatrist is only interested in the phenomenology of his delusions, and not in the associated despair, terror and confusion, and may then refuse to take his medication, which is now incorporated into his delusions as another agent that may poison him.

The temporal and spatial techniques described in the first part of this chapter, and the relatively structured mode of history-taking and mental state examination all serve a purpose. It is essential, for example, for patient and psychiatrist to have a safe physical environment. It is essential also that there is enough time for the interview, so that neither patient nor psychiatrist feels rushed. Sometimes it is useful to let the patient know how much time is available for the interview at the outset. One can then see how the patient makes use of such a time limit – whether he/she reacts to the announcement in a particular way (moaning, complaining, grateful or seemingly disinterested), and whether they make use of the time constructively or spend the session on seemingly trivial issues and then complain when the session ends that they have not been given the opportunity to talk about the real problem. This latter might occur in a patient with a paranoid and passive–dependent personality, for example.

Information gathering, in the formal sense described in the first part of this chapter, is important. However, there is much additional non-verbal and non-explicit information to be gleaned from the patient. Use is made of the stethoscope, the sphygmomanometer and of laboratory apparatus that measure arterial blood gas concentrations in cardiology. In psychiatry, the best instruments – metaphorical stethoscopes – are the psychiatrist's own emotions.

Transference, counter-transference, projective identification and acting out

The concepts of transference, counter-transference, projective identification and acting out are of crucial importance and are described in more detail in Chapter 36.

What are the expectations which both doctor and patient bring to the interview? They are partially socially determined, to do with the traditional power relationships and status of the doctor, hospital and patient (Mechanic 1968). But they are also personal, depending on the patient's earliest experiences with parents and carers, subsequent experiences with other figures of authority (teachers, grandparents, carers), and experiences with medical professionals. Thus the patient's (often unconscious) attitude, demeanour, and behaviour towards the doctor may reflect all sorts of past experiences and internalizations.

Similarly, the doctor brings his or her own set of attitudes, memories, and internal figures. One cannot expect to have the same underlying attitude towards both an elderly woman who reminds one of a dearly loved grandmother, as towards a young, arrogant man who reminds one, only too clearly, of an obnoxious younger sibling who might have displaced one from one's mother's breast when one was a mere toddler.

So each encounter involves the patient's transferences and the counter-transference of the practitioner. A traditional method for dealing with counter-transference in medicine in general, and in psychiatry in particular, is to pretend that it does not exist by employing a formulaic mode of history-taking and case management. However, Winnicott (1957) in his seminal paper, 'Hate in the counter-transference' described the psychiatrist caring for a psychotic or difficult patient as similar to a mother caring for a demanding baby – 'However much he loves his patients he cannot avoid hating them and fearing them, and the better he knows this the less will hate and fear be the motives determining what he does to his patients'.

Counter-transference, hate and malignant alienation

If counter-transference hatred is not recognized, the hateful feelings will be repressed and/or projected elsewhere. Watts & Morgan (1994) have described the defences used to avoid knowledge of counter-transference hate as including repression, reaction formation, projection and distortion/denial (see defence mechanisms in Chapter 36):

- Repression may seem safe as far as the psychiatrist is concerned, but the hatred may be conveyed by non-verbal messages such as inattentiveness, yawning, or watching the clock.
- With reaction formation (attempting to turn hate into its opposite, love) the psychiatrist becomes oversolicitous and may meddle, overprescribe or hospitalize the patient excessively.
- Projecting counter-transference hate, by thinking, 'I do not wish to harm that patient, it is he who wants to kill himself', for example, can lead the psychiatrist towards a nihilistic view of the patient as a 'hopeless case', to which the response may be either to do nothing or make a zealous attempt to control the patient.
- Distortion/denial implies that the psychiatrist selectively attends to clinical facts which support his views of the patient, and repudiates or devalues the patient's own experiences.

Watts & Morgan go on to describe a scenario of 'malignant alienation'. In this situation, patients, often with severe personality disorders, suicidal depression, long-standing violent tendencies, or those described as 'withdrawn psychotic' patients, have long-standing difficulties in communicating their needs effectively. They evoke counter-transference hate and this hatred is acted out by carers, rather than understood and made conscious. The 'difficult patient' is alienated and may finally be placed at high risk of suicide.

The concept of projective identification is of great importance (see Chapter 36). Steiner (1976) gives an example of a competent and experienced psychiatrist treating an anorexic woman. She came into the consulting room, 20 minutes late for her appointment, sullen, aggressive, and critical of the psychiatrist. He started off sympathetically, but found himself feeling increasingly inadequate. Eventually he commented, 'You do seem to find everything I say useless'. Later on he told her he was going to be leaving her in a couple of months and this evoked a furious outburst from her, with the patient accusing him of letting her down, and in particular of unreliability. The psychiatrist felt overwhelmed with guilt, and although he knew that in fact it was the patient who had been chronically unreliable over the period he had treated her, he was unable to recognize that her fury had to do with the fact that he had actually been helpful to her and how helpless she felt at the prospect of him abandoning her.

Through projective identification, this patient induced in her psychiatrist a state of mind in which he felt inadequate and unable to deal with her as he ought to. This was precisely the state of mind of the patient. Making him feel useless and helpless, and yet (later on) feeling that he could contain these feelings for her without being overwhelmed as she was, seemed to provide an important sense of relief for her. Thus projective identification, by producing such a state of mind in the doctor, can be seen as a primitive form of communication, 'through which a patient hopes that the doctor or therapist can experience something of what it is like to be in the patient's state of mind' (Steiner 1976).

The task of the psychiatrist is thus to respond to the patient's behaviour with firmness, understanding and empathy, to contain the projections, and not be provoked into inappropriate actions by them, and this requires external and internal stability.

External and internal stability

External stability can be facilitated by the provision of a stable setting – the same room, the avoidance of unnecessary interruptions during a consultation, informing the patient in advance of the duration of the session and so on. Psychiatrists in training may be obliged to be constantly available via pagers, but interruption of a session by pagers or telephones is antithetical to a good therapeutic alliance. It repeatedly indicates to the patient that time with the psychiatrist is not regarded by the psychiatrist as protected or precious in any way. The telephone on the desk, the pager in the pocket and even the writing of notes, may serve as a defensive armour (akin to a white coat and stethoscope) that prevents intimacy. If the phone is always about to ring, the pager about to go off, the door about to be knocked on, how deeply involved can the patient and the psychiatrist become?

Thus consultations should take place in a setting that is safe and not prone to unnecessary interruption. The psychiatrist should review the patient's notes before the session so that the first minutes of the session are not occupied with the psychiatrist reading letters of referral or previous notes, while the patient waits. If possible, the psychiatrist should avoid writing notes during the session and should focus fully on the patient's verbal and non-verbal communications, and on the psychiatrist's own affective responses towards the patient.

Support for this work is vital, and detailed, regular external supervision from a senior colleague (usually the consultant) is essential during the training phases of a psychiatrist's career. Thereafter, regular supervision remains desirable. Indeed, such supervision is a hallmark of the ideal practice of psychotherapy. Regrettably, most consultant psychiatrists receive no formal ongoing supervision of their work.

The work of a psychiatrist is often very different to that of a psychotherapist, but there are many areas of overlap and cross-fertilization. Thus the recommendations of the Royal College of Psychiatrists (1998) that each trainee psychiatrist in the UK have direct, supervised experience of treating patients using a number of psychotherapeutic modes, are significant. The concepts of transference, counter-transference, projective identification and acting out will only become meaningful when experienced in this way, and only then can they be harnessed throughout the rest of one's work in other fields within psychiatry. Other forms of support include staff support groups (optimally facilitated by an outside facilitator) and case discussion workshops during which 'difficult cases' may be considered. Personal psychotherapy or analysis will help one understand oneself, one's motivations, anxieties, blind-spots and prejudices, and will make one aware of one's own counter-transference and thus minimize the risk of inappropriate acting out with patients, colleagues and others.

DIFFICULTIES THAT MAY BE ENCOUNTERED WHEN INTERVIEWING PSYCHIATRIC PATIENTS

Psychiatrists need to elicit a great deal of information in a short time and ensure that patients are as comfortable as possible while doing so. They often fail to do this, and research has identified a number of common reasons. First, all doctors frequently fail to clarify exactly what a patient means, and will often accept the patient's jargon (for example, 'My nerves are driving me mad, doc'). A second common mistake is that of failing to respond to non-verbal cues. If a patient appears to be on the point of crying, for example, the doctor can usefully comment on the fact that the patient appears upset, rather than ignore it or move to another topic. A further common mistake that doctors may make is that of providing premature reassurance during interviews. By prematurely reassuring patients, a doctor effectively prevents them from fully explaining their concerns, and is more likely to cause upset than to reassure.

Psychiatrists need to be aware that there are many different ways to ask questions. At the beginning of an interview, it is appropriate to use open-ended questions ('Tell me about your problems' or, 'What is your sleep like?', for example) that are then followed up with closed questions to clarify certain points ('Did you first feel depressed or first feel anxious?' or, 'Do you have difficulty in falling asleep?', for example). Leading questions that imply an answer ('You don't sleep very well, do you?', for example) are generally best avoided, as are questions with multiple themes ('What're your sleep, appetite and energy like?'). Facilitating techniques should be used to encourage disclosure. These include silences that allow the patient time to think about a reply, brief empathic statements such as, 'That must have been extremely upsetting for you', the use of non-verbal cues such as nodding, and the maintenance of appropriate eye contact while the patient is speaking. It is very useful to present the patient with a brief summary of your understanding of their account of their problems, both in order to ensure an accurate record has been obtained and to impress upon patients that they have been listened to and their difficulties understood.

Certain types of patients and interview situations present particular difficulties to the psychiatrist. These are now discussed individually (see Chapter 35).

The stuporose patient

Stupor may be caused by schizophrenia (catatonic stupor), affective disorder (depressive or, very rarely, manic stupor) or hysteria (dissociative stupor), or by posterior diencephalic/upper mesencephalic lesions. Stuporose patients are mute, motionless and unresponsive to stimulation, but are otherwise completely conscious, aware and alert. They must be evaluated by observation of their behaviour, by physical examination, and by interviewing an informant. Catatonic stupor is suggested by negativism, waxy flexibility and other schizophrenic movement disorders (see Chapter 18), depressive stupor by tearfulness and a sad expression, and dissociative stupor by closed eyes and resistance to passive eye-opening. Evidence of diencephalic/mesencephalic lesions includes abnormally reacting, unequal pupils. Both stuporose patients and patients who exhibit mutism may sometimes communicate by reading and writing.

The elderly patient

The assessment of elderly patients differs from that of other patients in that sensory impairment may present difficulties and cognition and physical health must be thoroughly evaluated. Impaired hearing and vision may be overcome by conducting the interview in a quiet, well-lit room, by speaking slowly and clearly (not loudly) and by using written material and functioning hearing aids. It is often invaluable to have the help of a relative or friend who can communicate readily with the patient.

The mentally handicapped patient

Short, clear questions should be used when interviewing mentally handicapped individuals and any account obtained should be supplemented with an account from an informant. Particular attention must be paid to changes in behaviour and to biological features of psychiatric illness. Thus a mentally handicapped patient may be unable to complain of feeling depressed but may exhibit increased irritability, loss of appetite and weight, sleep disturbance and tearfulness. A definitive assessment and diagnosis may be impossible in the case of some severely mentally handicapped individuals, and it may be necessary to undertake a trial of treatment with, for example, antidepressants if depression is suspected.

The agitated patient

Interviewing agitated patients is difficult and may be dangerous (see Chapter 35). The doctor may have to confine questions to those that are immediately important, only completing the evaluation when the patient has improved following treatment. Agitated patients respond best to a quiet calm manner of questioning, and are most appropriately interviewed in open areas where they do not feel restrained. Help must always be readily available in the event that the patient becomes violent.

Interviewing patients via an interpreter

The ability to conduct an interview via an interpreter is an essential skill for any psychiatrist. Although it may often be necessary to utilize the interpreting skills of the patient's friends or relatives, a trained interpreter should always be used if available. This ensures privacy for the patient and precludes the risk of relatives allowing their own views of the situation to modify their translation. When working with an interpreter, three chairs should be arranged in a triangle and the doctor should speak directly to the patient, addressing them in the second person. The doctor can help the patient feel at ease and feel understood by paying attention while the patient answers and by responding to the patient's non-verbal cues. Summarizing and asking the patient to repeat important points will help ensure that the patient understands all questions and that the doctor has obtained an accurate account. Similar principles apply when interviewing a deaf person via a sign interpreter. However, it is best if the signing interpreter sits slightly behind and to one side of the doctor, and it is important that good lighting is provided, in order that signing can be seen clearly and interpreted accurately.

Emergency consultations

Emergency consultations often take place in less than ideal settings (in patients' homes, in police stations or with several other individuals present, for example) and sufficient time for a thorough assessment is rarely available. Nonetheless, the doctor should attempt to obtain an outline personal history and a clear account of the presenting complaint, its duration, and the mode of onset and severity of symptoms. This should suggest a probable diagnosis and the mental state examination should then concentrate on the symptoms associated with this diagnosis. Alcohol and drugs should be enquired about and a brief targeted physical examination undertaken if appropriate. A corroborating history from a relative or friend may be especially helpful during emergency consultations. In exceptional circumstances, this may be obtained without the patient's consent (see Chapter 35).

REFERENCES

Folstein MF, Folstein SE & McHugh PR (1975) 'Mini mental state' – a practical method for grading the cognitive state of patients for the clinician. *Journal of Psychiatric Research* **12**: 189–98.

Mechanic D (1968) Medical Sociology. New York: The Free Press.

Royal College of Psychiatrists (1998) *Higher Specialist Training Handbook*, 8th edn. London: Royal College of Psychiatrists.

Steiner J (1976) Some aspects of the interviewing technique and their relationship to the transference. *British Journal of Medical Psychology* **49**: 65–72.

Watts D & Morgan G (1994) Malignant alienation: dangers for patients who are difficult to like. *British Journal of Psychiatry* **164**: 11–15.

Winnicott DW (1957) *The Child, the Family and the Outside World*, pp. 49–78. London: Penguin.

Diagnosis and classification in psychiatry

David J Castle and Assen V Jablensky

INTRODUCTION

Classification in psychiatry has a long history, a story eloquently told by Berrios (1999), who makes the point that most reviews of classification systems in psychiatry have been 'written in terms of a "received view"', and that 'this contains two assumptions, that: (i) the activity of classifying is inherent to the human mind; and (ii) psychiatric "phenomena" are stable natural objects' (Berrios 1999, p.145). He articulates instead a 'conceptual history', assuming that all psychiatric classification systems are 'cultural products', and concludes, *inter alia*, that classifications are only valuable if they 'can release new information about the object classified'.

The history of the evolution of our major modern psychiatric diagnostic and classification systems, namely the American Psychiatric Association's *Diagnostic and Statistical Manual* (DSM) (American Psychiatric Association 1980, 1987, 1994) and the World Health Organization's *International Classification of Diseases* (ICD) (World Health Organization 1992) is rather more dry, and how much these systems really 'release new information' is debateable. But diagnostic criteria and classification systems in psychiatry are useful for a number of other reasons, as outlined by Jablensky (1999):

1 The enhancement of diagnostic agreement among clinicians, allowing improved reporting.
2 Improving reliability of diagnosis in research, such that comparisons can be made across studies.
3 Provision of an international reference system that ensures less 'idiosyncrasy' in teaching.
4 A 'demystification and transparency' in reporting and communication about psychiatric disorders and enhancing communication with non-professionals.

Also, as Kendell & Jablensky (2003) articulate, even if we do not accept many putative diagnostic entities in psychiatry as valid (i.e. as 'real'), it does not mean that they do not have utility. Indeed, Kendell & Jablensky (2003, p.4) conclude that 'Although most diagnostic concepts have not been shown to

be valid [in the sense of having demonstrable natural boundaries], many possess high utility by virtue of the information about outcome, treatment response, and aetiology that they convey. They are therefore invaluable working concepts for clinicians'.

Thus, this chapter provides a broad overview of diagnosis and classification in psychiatry. Some detail is given on our two predominant world systems, DSM and ICD, before a consideration of more generic issues such as how one determines whether a particular set of symptoms constitute a 'disorder' and how one goes about deciding whether disparate putative disorders relate to each other. We then consider alternative approaches to psychiatric classification, and close with a glimpse of what future psychiatric classifications might look like.

TYPES OF CLASSIFICATION SYSTEMS IN PSYCHIATRY

Broadly, psychiatry has embraced classification systems that fall into three main types, namely:

1 **Symptom-based:** this approach is commonly used in psychiatry. There is a long tradition to this approach, notably formulated comprehensively by Kraepelin, whose multi-edition 'textbook' became the basis of modern psychiatric classification systems. Kraepelin (1893) not only took account of cross-sectional psychopathology, but also included consideration of longitudinal course of illness, for example in his delineation of dementia praecox (with a poor longitudinal outcome) from manic depressive psychosis (with essentially an episodic course).
2 **Treatment-driven:** in pragmatic terms, a treatment-informed approach to psychiatric classification has intuitive appeal. However, the problem in psychiatry is that treatments are not entity-specific, but rather target (more or less) specific symptoms (e.g. antipsychotic medication for psychosis), behaviours (e.g. exposure/response prevention for compulsions), or

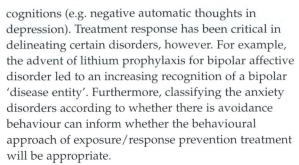

cognitions (e.g. negative automatic thoughts in depression). Treatment response has been critical in delineating certain disorders, however. For example, the advent of lithium prophylaxis for bipolar affective disorder led to an increasing recognition of a bipolar 'disease entity'. Furthermore, classifying the anxiety disorders according to whether there is avoidance behaviour can inform whether the behavioural approach of exposure/response prevention treatment will be appropriate.

3 **Aetiological:** ultimately, the 'true' classification of psychiatric disorders will be informed by an understanding of cause. Thus, Huntington's disease has been shown to be a true autosomal dominant condition localized to chromosome 4 (Huntington Disease Collaborative Group 1993). Alzheimer's disease has also been shown to have a genetic basis, but here subtypes have been revealed, with different genes coding for different types: for example, the amyloid precursor protein gene on chromosome 21 (autosomal dominant form) and other loci on chromosomes 19 and 14 (early onset form) (Masters & Beyreuther 1994). Furthermore, it is clear that there are important other influences in terms of susceptibility to Alzheimer's disease, leaving a 'pure' genetic classificatory system difficult to uphold (e.g. urban residence, cardiovascular risk factors: see Prince et al. 1994). It is also clear that the vast majority of psychiatric disorders are aetiologically multifactorial, and it is likely that such heterogeneity of cause will make aetiological classification problematic.

OUR CURRENT CLASSIFICATION SYSTEMS: DSM AND ICD

From the third edition of DSM in 1980 (American Psychiatric Association 1980), the notion has been to adopt essentially an 'atheoretical' approach, concentrating on clinical description, and not making any assumptions about aetiology. Thus, observed phenomena, along with longitudinal course, are the main factors determining definition of disorders and the grouping or otherwise of different disorders. Sets of specific 'operational' criteria are presented, in an attempt to enhance reliability.

Another feature of all editions of DSM since DSM-III has been the requirement for individuals to be assessed on a number of axes (see Table 33.1). This allows concurrent yet discrete assessment of various aspects of the functioning of the individual. Axes I and II encompass all the mental disorders, with personality disorders and mental retardation being on axis II and all other mental disorders being on axis I. Axis III is used for coding comorbid physical disorders, and axis IV is used to record the nature and severity of psychosocial stressors. Finally, axis V records the clinicians' assessment of the individual's overall level of functioning: this is performed using the Global Assessment of Functioning (GAF) scale, which ranges from 1-100 (higher score being better function) and which provides a number of anchors to enhance reliability.

The overall structure of DSM-IV-text revision (TR) (American Psychiatric Association 2000) axis I is:

- disorders usually first diagnosed in infancy, childhood, or adolescence
- delirium, dementia, and amnestic and other cognitive disorders
- mental disorders due to a general medical condition not elsewhere classified
- substance-related disorders
- schizophrenia and other psychotic disorders
- mood disorders
- anxiety disorders
- somatoform disorders
- factitious disorders
- dissociative disorders

Table 33.1 Comparison of DSM-IV and ICD-10	
DSM-IV	*ICD-10*
US-based, from American Psychiatric Association, but has wide acceptance around the world	World Health Organization; international, and includes diversity of opinions, including Third World
Not part of a general medical classification system	Part of a general medical classification system
Closed system	Open system
One version only	Clinical and research versions
Atheoretical	Groupings based on presumed shared aetiologies ('blocks')
Multiaxial, with personality disorders on a separate axis (Axis II)	Personality disorders and mental retardation included on Axis I
'Global functioning' assessed using Global Assessment of Functioning Scale (GAF)	'Disability' assessed using the Disability Assessment Schedule (WHO-DAS)

- sexual and gender identity disorders
- eating disorders
- sleep disorders
- impulse-control disorders not elsewhere classified
- adjustment disorders
- personality disorders.

There is an additional category, 'Other conditions that may be a focus of clinical attention', for coding such problems as medication-induced movement disorders and relational problems.

On axis II, the personality disorders are clustered into groups, as follows:

- Cluster A (odd, eccentric): paranoid, schizoid, and schizotypal personality disorders
- Cluster B (dramatic, emotional, erratic): borderline, histrionic, narcissistic, and antisocial personality disorders
- Cluster C (anxious, fearful): avoidant, dependent, and obsessive-compulsive personality disorders.

There is also a residual category 'personality disorder not otherwise specified', and a mooting of two further potential categories, namely 'depressive' and 'passive-aggressive (negativistic)' personality disorders. The clusters outlined above have some clinical utility, but are not supported robustly by research attempts at various forms of cluster analysis of personality disorders. Also, many people with personality disorders can meet criteria for a number of different DSM-IV-defined personality disorders.

ICD-10 has a rather different heritage, being a consensus system that needed to accommodate the views of clinicians and researchers in countries with sometimes rather disparate views about mental disorders (see Table 33.1). It grew out of ICD-9, which essentially presented a number of textual 'vignettes' to guide clinicians. ICD-10 comes in different versions, one for clinicians, and another (with more specific criteria) for researchers; the research version has many similarities to DSM-IV.

ICD-10 groups the psychiatric disorders in ten 'blocks' reflecting disorders with supposedly common aetiologies. The block of 'Organic' disorders includes disorders where the symptoms can be explained in terms of cerebral (e.g. Alzheimer's dementia) or systemic (e.g. delirium in the context of fever) pathology. Non-organic psychotic disorders (schizophrenia and related disorders) form another block, as do the mood disorders (which includes depression, bipolar affective disorder, cyclothymia, and dysthymia).

Disorders of personality are considered as a separate block, rather than being on a discrete axis as in DSM-IV. This block also includes 'enduring personality changes' considered not secondary to brain damage; examples include personality change in the context of catastrophic personal experiences such as prolonged captivity or torture.

The overall structure of ICD-10 (World Health Organization 1992) is as follows:

- organic, including symptomatic, mental disorders
- mental and behavioural disorders due to psychoactive substance use
- schizophrenia, schizotypal and delusional disorders
- mood (affective) disorders
- neurotic, stress-related and somatoform disorders
- behavioural syndromes associated with physiological disturbances and physical factors
- disorders of adult personality and behaviour
- mental retardation
- disorders of psychological development
- behavioural and emotional disorders with onset usually occurring during childhood and adolescence
- unspecified mental disorder.

HOW TO DETERMINE WHETHER SOMETHING IS AN ENTITY

An important issue when considering nosology and classification is how one determines whether something is a diagnostic entity. In their classic paper, Robins & Guze (1970) suggest the following as useful in determining whether a putative entity has validity (see Kendell and Jablensky 2003):

1. clinical profile, including symptoms and demography
2. aetiological parameters, notably family studies
3. laboratory tests, including radiology, psychological profiles and biochemical parameters
4. longitudinal course, including stability of diagnosis over time
5. ability to delimit the putative disorder from other disorders, by application of certain exclusion criteria.

In psychiatry it is the exception rather than the rule that our 'disorders' meet these criteria. Even our 'sacred symbol' (Szaz 1976), schizophrenia, does not perform well against these standards. Thus, the positive symptoms of schizophrenia (delusions and hallucinations) are germane to any psychotic state, being seen in bipolar affective disorder (Wing & Nixon 1975); intoxication with substances such as cannabis (Castle & Ames 1996) and amphetamines; prolonged alcohol use (Glass 1989); epilepsy (Toone 1991); and delirious states. Schneider (1959) attempted to delineate certain 'first rank' symptoms that are potentially pathognomonic for schizophrenia, but it is well recognized that these symptoms are also seen in other disorders, notably bipolar affective disorder (Wing & Nixon 1975). Also, attempts to find a 'point of rarity' between the symptoms of schizophrenia and affective disorders have largely failed (Kendell & Gourlay 1970, Kendell & Brockington 1980).

Kraepelin's conceptualization of dementia praecox was of a disorder with a poor longitudinal trajectory, as opposed to manic depression with essentially an episodic course but good interepisode functioning. This again has not been borne out in longitudinal studies. Indeed, many people with schizophrenia have a very good outcome, while a substantial proportion of those with manic depression do badly in the long term (see Murray et al. 1992).

Attempts at delimitation of schizophrenia from other disorders by application of exclusion criteria also run into difficulties. In particular, the insistence on the absence of organic brain disease is undermined by increasingly consistent findings of structural brain abnormalities in schizophrenia (McCarley et al. 1999), and is bedevilled by a particular propensity for the manifestation of positive psychotic symptoms to occur in the setting of substance use, in individuals who have a vulnerability to psychosis (see Castle & Ames 1996). Also, the affective disorder exclusion criterion belies the fact that many people with schizophrenia also exhibit depressive symptoms at some stage of their illness course (Siris 1991) and the lack of any consistent delineation of so-called schizoaffective disorder.

One of the other problems associated with attempting to define a core entity that really is schizophrenia, is that sets of criteria tend to be rather arbitrary and this may have profound implications for research as they force a circularity into the consideration of these putative disorders. For example, defining schizophrenia as a disorder with at least six months' illness duration, as in DSM-IV (American Psychiatric Association 1994), necessarily biases samples towards a poor outcome group; Research Diagnostic Criteria (RDC; Spitzer et al. 1978) have only two-week illness stipulation, with the inclusion of more patients with a relatively benign outcome. DSM-III (American Psychiatric Association 1980) arbitrarily imposed an age-at-onset cut-off for schizophrenia at 45 years, biasing samples towards younger ages. The Feighner criteria (Feighner et al. 1972) give loadings for a family history of schizophrenia, a long illness duration, and an early onset. The implications of such restrictions are evidenced strikingly in the male:female ratios for the different sets of diagnostic criteria. Thus, in a register-based first episode sample (Castle et al. 1993), more lenient RDC produced a male:female ratio of 1.2:1; for DSM-IIIR (American Psychiatric Association 1987) the ratio was 1.3:1, and for DSM-III (American Psychiatric Association 1980), 2.2:1. The stringent criteria of Feighner et al. (1972) excluded many more females than males, with resultant gender ratio of 2.5:1.

THE PROBLEM OF COMORBIDITY

Another problem with many psychiatric classification systems is the implicit attempt to pigeon-hole individuals and apply diagnostic labels to them. Regrettably this denies the fact that many people have more than one psychiatric disorder. Indeed, having one psychiatric disorder increases the risk of having another one. For example, in the National Comorbidity Survey in the US (Kessler 1995), if a respondent had one psychiatric disorder, they had a 56% chance of having another one as well. For example, it appears that people with schizophrenia have a particular predilection to depression, and certain anxiety disorders, notably obsessive-compulsive disorder (see Castle & Wykes 2003); whether the latter association indicates similar pathogenic factors remains a point of conjecture (see Gross-Isseroff et al. 2003).

Psychiatrists tend to be taught, and to think, in a very hierarchical way, such that certain diagnoses over-ride others (Foulds 1976). This can result in patients not being assessed or treated adequately in terms of the extent of their psychopathology. For example, it is well recognized that negative symptoms of schizophrenia can be secondary to, for example, depression, and the implicit belief by the clinician that such symptoms as social withdrawal and apathy are part and parcel of the schizophrenia process, may leave depression undiagnosed and untreated.

There is also the problem that as we cleave more and more putatively discrete disorders from the core, the core becomes the rag-bag deficit diagnosis. This is evidenced by the anxiety disorders, where panic disorder, the phobic disorders, and obsessive compulsive disorder have been reified, leaving generalized anxiety disorder as something of a default diagnosis (Tyrer 1984). The problem with this is that it may be seen as a general diagnostic dustbin, with a residue of a number of disorders that happen not to fit within the current nosology.

THE PROBLEM OF THE AXES

Both ICD-10 and all editions of the DSM since 1980 encompass the notion that psychiatric disorders can be conceptualized on a number of different axes. The multiaxial approach was foreshadowed by Rutter and colleagues (1969) in their classification of childhood psychiatric disorders, where developmental stage and intellectual functioning are classified on axes separate from the primary clinical diagnosis. DSM-III took the bold step of classifying personality disorders on a separate axis (axis II); this was not the case in ICD-10. While the DSM approach to personality disorders has been praised in that it raised the profile of the personality disorders, and enhanced the consideration of personality pathology, the downsides have been considerable. Perhaps most concerning is the implicit belief that disorders on axis II are untreatable. Indeed, when the axis II disorder 'depressive personality disorder' was found to respond to antidepressants, it was elevated to axis I (as dysthymia) (Akiskal et al. 1977); a similar tale can be told of cyclothymic personality disorder and cyclothymia (Akiskal 1983).

The obverse problem arises for schizotypal personality disorder, which can increasingly be considered a *forme fruste* of schizophrenia (see Battaglia & Torgerson 1996), in that it aggregates in families of probands with schizophrenia, shows similar eye tracking abnormalities as people with schizophrenia, and responds to antipsychotic medication.

Another problem is that of the labelling, usually pejorative, of people with 'personality disorders' (Lewis & Appleby 1988). What is too often the case is that the behaviours of such individuals are considered a manifestation of their Axis II pathology, whereas they are just as vulnerable (if not more so) to a number of Axis I disorders. Thus, people with so-called borderline personality disorder share many psychosocial risk factors with people with post-traumatic stress disorder (e.g. early sexual abuse) and depression (lack of supporting relationships, unemployment).

HOW TO DETERMINE WHETHER A PUTATIVE DIAGNOSTIC ENTITY BELONGS WITH OTHERS

A further consideration is how to determine whether one disease entity should be grouped with others. An example of such groupings of disorders is the so-called obsessive-compulsive (OC) spectrum of disorders, in which disorders are grouped because they share certain symptoms. In its broad conceptualization, the OC spectrum encompasses (see Hollander 1993):

- disorders associated with *bodily preoccupation*, including body dysmorphic disorder (BDD), anorexia nervosa, and hypochondriasis
- *neurological disorders*, including Tourette's syndrome and autism
- *impulse control disorders*, including pathological gambling, kleptomania, and trichotillomania.

Decisions about inclusion in the OC spectrum have been based on similarities with obsessive-compulsive disorder (OCD) in a variety of domains, such as symptoms, demographic features, course of illness, comorbidity, treatment response, joint familial loading, and presumed aetiology (reviewed by Castle & Phillips, 2004). The symptom domain (i.e. the presence of obsessions and/or repetitive behaviours) is the usual initial reason for considering a given disorder to be a potential spectrum candidate. However, it is clear that disorders should not be grouped together and considered related to one another on the basis of shared symptomatology alone. Indeed, the brain has a fairly limited repertoire in terms of the symptoms it produces. The fact that positive psychotic symptoms, for example, occur in schizophrenia, temporal lobe epilepsy, cannabis intoxication, borderline personality disorder and Huntington's disease does not imply that these disorders should be grouped together or considered related disorders (see Castle & Phillips, 2004).

A powerful potential 'grouping' variable for psychiatric disorders is shared aetiological factors. In terms of the OC spectrum, our knowledge of aetiology is limited, and the extent of 'sharing' of such parameters amongst putative members of the spectrum is variable. For example, BDD shows some familial aggregation with OCD, but other psychiatric disorders such as depression show much higher rates of aggregation in families of people with BDD. In a controlled family study, Bienvenue et al. (2000) found increased rates of BDD alone or BDD with hypochondriasis in relatives of probands with OCD, but hypochondriasis alone and impulse control disorders did not show any excess. In a separate study, somatization disorder, but not OCD, aggregated in family members of probands with hypochondriasis (Noyes et al. 1997). Thus, overall family studies of the OCD spectrum give only mixed support for aetiological links amongst some putative members.

Longitudinal course is also very variable amongst members of the putative OC spectrum. Thus, BDD tends to onset in adolescence and is fairly stable throughout life, if untreated (this is very similar to social anxiety disorder, not a member of the 'spectrum'), while the onset-age and longitudinal course of trichotillomania, for example, is far more variable. Demographic parameters also differ between members of the spectrum. Whilst OCD shows a roughly equal gender representation (males have a mean onset earlier than females), as does BDD (but no clear difference between the genders in onset-age), anorexia nervosa is essentially a disorder of girls.

Treatment response has been put forward as one of the most compelling justifications for grouping disorders in the OC spectrum. Again, the degree of support is variable across conditions. Thus, whilst OCD and BDD tend to respond to the serotonergic antidepressants (SRIs) and cognitive–behaviour therapy (CBT), trichotillomania does not (Van Minnen et al. 2003). And in any event, other disorders also appear to respond selectively to SRIs, notably premenstrual dysphoric disorder (PMDD; see Grady-Weliky 2003). A further twist is that some people with OCD do not respond to SRIs, suggesting to some observers that subtypes of OCD might have different biological underpinnings. For example, the findings that OCD in conjunction with tics tends to require the use of a dopamine-D_2 receptor blocker suggests dopaminergic involvement in what might be a relatively distinct subtype (see Lochner & Stein 2003).

Thus, the attempt to group a number of psychiatric disorders under the OC umbrella, while heuristically of potential utility, is defensible to a reasonable degree for only some members of the proposed spectrum, while the claim for other of the disorders is far more tenuous. Furthermore, if one was to accept for membership of the OC spectrum all of the potential candidate disorders, one would encompass a large slice of the entire DSM, raising further questions about the usefulness of such an exercise.

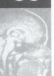

CLASSIFYING BEHAVIOURS

Another matter worthy of consideration is those psychiatric classification systems that have attempted to classify certain behaviours, rather than disorders as such. A good example is Pilowsky's (1978) classification of 'abnormal illness behaviours'. This is a brave attempt to make some meaning out of how people manifest illness behaviours, and the motivations behind the behaviours. This approach implicitly encompasses the sociological notions of 'illness behaviour' ('the ways in which given symptoms may be differentially perceived, evaluated and acted (or not acted) upon by different kinds of person' (Mechanic & Volkart 1960)) and 'sick role' (a 'partially and conditionally legitimated state' whereby the ill individual is granted certain societal privileges, but is expected to desire wellness, and act in a way compatible with professional advice, in getting better (Parsons 1964)).

Thus, Pilowsky (1978) considers 'abnormal illness behaviour' as those forms of illness behaviour that are 'either deemed ill suited to the most effective and parsimonious way of maximizing health, or judged to deviate markedly from the usual range of particular organismic states, or both'. To incorporate all manifestations of abnormal illness behaviour, Pilowsky's (1978) classification encompasses both 'somatically focused' as well as 'psychologically focused' behaviours, which may be either 'illness affirming' or 'illness denying'. There is a further subdivision, such that the motivation may be predominantly conscious or predominantly unconscious (see Box 33.1 for full exposition).

This scheme has an admirable comprehensiveness to it, but is compromised by the fact that individuals may adopt a number of different 'illness behaviours' either in parallel or in different settings at different times. An example is so-called 'accident neurosis', which Miller (1961) famously and polemically dismissed as essentially malingering, but which increasingly is recognized as a complex set of reactions to an accident, compounded to various degrees by legal processes and the potential for monetary 'reward'. Mayou (1996) has warned against the potential reification of post-traumatic stress disorder in this context, as a legally 'legitimized' disorder, the criteria for which the individual must meet in order to obtain legal redress and compensation.

ARE DIMENSIONAL APPROACHES BETTER?

Dimensional approaches to psychiatric classification have mostly been championed by psychologists rather than psychiatrists. Perhaps the best known is Eysenck's (1970) dimensional approach to personality. Thus, people are considered in terms of their behaviours and attitudes, to 'rate' along three dimensions, namely introversion–

Box 33.1   Pilowsky's classification of abnormal illness behaviour (see Pilowsky 1978)

Somatically focused abnormal illness behaviour

I.   Illness affirming
  A. Motivation predominantly conscious:
     1. malingering
     2. Munchausen's syndrome
  B. Motivation predominantly unconscious:
     1. neurotic:
        ● conversion reaction
        ● hypochondriacal reaction
     2. psychotic:
        ● hypochondriacal delusions associated with:
           (a) psychotic depression
           (b) schizophrenia
           (c) monsymptomatic hypochondriacal psychosis

II.   Illness denying
  A. Motivation predominantly conscious:
     1. illness denial in order to obtain insurance cover, employment
     2. denial to avoid feared therapies
  B. Motivation predominantly unconscious:
     1. neurotic:
        ● 'flight into health', e.g. non-compliance with therapy after myocardial infarct
        ● counterphobic behaviour, e.g. risk-taking associated with haemophilia
     2. psychotic:
        ● psychotic denial of somatic symptoms, e.g. as part of a hypomanic reaction
     3. neuropsychiatric:
        ● anosognosia, e.g. denial of hemiparesis

Psychologically focused abnormal illness behaviour

III.   Illness affirming
  A. Motivation predominantly conscious:
     1. 'pseudopatients' (simulation for research purposes)
     2. compensation seeking
     3. Ganser syndrome ('hysterical pseudodementia')
  B. Motivation predominantly unconscious:
     1. neurotic:
        ● 'psychic hypochondriasis'
        ● dissociative reactions
        ● psychogenic amnesia
     2. psychotic:
        ● delusions of memory loss

IV.   Illness denying
  A. Motivation predominantly conscious:
     1. denial of psychotic symptoms to avoid stigma, hospitalization, or gain discharge from care
     2. denial of psychotic illness to avoid perceived discrimination by, e.g. employers
  B. Motivation predominantly unconscious:
     1. neurotic:
        ● refusal to accept 'psychological' diagnosis or treatment in the presence of neurotic illness, personality disorder of dependency syndromes
     2. psychotic:
        ● denial of illness ('lack of insight') in psychotic depression, mania, schizophrenia
     3. neuropsychiatric:
        ● confabulatory reactions in, e.g. Korsakoff's psychosis

---

extroversion, neuroticism and psychoticism. Whilst useful enough in considering the personal makeup of individuals, and being to some extent predictive of psychiatric disorders *per se*, the approach does not help very much in deciding diagnosis or treatment. Thus, whilst dimensional approaches overall might be a closer reflection of 'truth', their utility in terms of whether they actually enhance our ability to treat people effectively and reliably, is questionable.

ALTERNATIVE APPROACHES TO PSYCHIATRIC CLASSIFICATION

There is little doubt that DSM-IV and ICD-10 are major achievements in that they bring clarity, explicit rules and reference points to the field of clinical investigation which has been beset with problems of low reliability and with scepticism about the value of diagnosis to the extent of perceiving it as an obstacle to the management of patients. In this sense, DSM-III and its successors, and ICD-10, have performed a therapeutic role. However, with many therapies, the initial enthusiasm about efficacy and novelty is followed by an increasing number of observations on complications, unexpected interactions, and adverse side effects that have to be judiciously taken into account if the real benefits of the therapy are to be sustained. It would be unfortunate if the acceptance of the present diagnostic systems stifles further discussion of their limitations, shortcomings and potential for misuse. Also, the need must be recognized for renewed research leading to alternative or complementary solutions for the classification problems in psychiatry.

One recent trend is in restoring to psychiatric research the syndromes and symptoms as basic units of observation by adopting a primarily syndromological approach to the clinical study of psychiatric conditions. The proposed rationale for this is that with the use of present-day research technologies it is more likely that significant associations between dynamic cerebral processes and psychopathology will eventually be found at the level of symptoms and syndromes rather than at the level of disorders as defined in the current diagnostic systems. Systematic studies of this kind have been proposed, and Van Praag (1993) coined the term 'functional psychopathology' for this reorientation of psychiatric research, in the expectation that 'functional psychopathology would be to psychiatry what physiology is to medicine'.

Similarly, the study of selected neurophysiological, cognitive and neurochemical markers, assessed as dimensions across the conventional diagnostic groups and in the general population, may reveal unexpected patterns of association with clinically significant symptoms, behaviour, or personality traits that might result in refined definitions of clinical entities and in better validated phenotypes for genetic research.

A third trend is the application of new statistical models to the analysis of the validity of existing systems and the generation of novel and, sometimes, radically different approaches to classification. One such approach focuses on the concept of prototype (Cantor et al. 1980) as an alternative to the classic category as the basic unit of classification. The difference here is that while a category must be defined in terms of necessary and sufficient characteristics, a prototype only requires a correlation with its defining features. The difficulty of fitting psychopathology and behaviour into tightly defined disease categories, which explains some of the shortcomings of the current diagnostic systems, is eliminated in a prototype-based classification by fiat, if we decide to forgo the objective that a psychiatric classification should mirror all the features of a biological classification. An extension of the prototype approach, using mathematical set theory and a generalized form of latent class analysis as a computational method, proceeds on the assumption that the concept of a discrete, 'crisp' disease entity may not be applicable to psychiatric disorders which could be better represented by 'fuzzy' sets, allowing for considerable variation and heterogeneity. Some early results of the application of this model to large psychiatric data sets on psychoses (Manton et al.. 1994) suggest that it may be possible to develop a classification based on a series of empirically derived 'ideal' or 'pure' types of disorders; that individuals may show quantifiable degrees of membership in more than one such 'pure' type; and that the classification has clinical relevance, including a high prognostic validity.

FUTURE PROSPECTS: CLINICAL OR BIOLOGICAL CLASSIFICATION IN PSYCHIATRY?

A point of view that is sometimes expressed – mainly by researchers with a biological orientation – is that clinical neuroscience will eventually replace psychopathology in the diagnosis of mental disorders, and that the phenomeno-logical study of subjective experience of people with psychiatric illnesses will be relegated to the domain of applied anthropology. For example, increases in knowledge about the biological causes and processes in schizophrenia would gradually lead to a model of clinical practice that regards psychopathology as an epiphenomenon of secondary importance for the diagnosis and treatment. This belated transformation of clinical psychiatry would simply reproduce developments in other medical disciplines where biochemical, electronic and imaging tools have replaced ancient, finely honed clinical skills such as the ability to elicit by palpation over 50 characteristics of the arterial pulse wave. Once the genes causing, or predisposing to, psychiatric disorders are mapped and cloned, diagnostic applications may become feasible in at least some disorders, as recent advances in familial Alzheimer's disease suggest.

In time, such developments would result in a completely redesigned classification of mental disorders, based on genetic aetiology. The categories of such a classification and their hierarchical ordering may recombine the present clinical diagnostic entities in many unexpected ways. Such a classification, the argument goes, would for the first time approximate a 'natural' classification in psychiatry.

This, indeed, is already happening in general medicine where molecular biology and genetics are transforming dramatically medical classifications. New organizing principles are producing new classes of disorders, such as mitochondrial diseases (Johns 1995). Large chapters of neurology are being rewritten to reflect novel taxonomic groupings like diseases due to nucleotide triplet repeat expansion (Rosenberg 1996; see Chapter 3). The potential of molecular genetic diagnosis in various medical disorders is increasing by leaps and bounds and it looks unlikely to bypass psychiatric disorders (Farmer & Owen 1996).

Although the majority of psychiatric disorders now appear to be much more complex from a genetic point of view than until recently assumed, there can be little doubt that molecular genetics and neuroscience will eventually have a major impact on our understanding of the aetiology and pathogenesis of psychiatric disorders. This is also likely to include a better understanding of the role of environmental and behavioural factors and of gene–environment interactions at different stages of individual development. However, the exact nature and extent of the impact of such advances on the diagnostic process in psychiatry and on the classification of psychiatric disorders is extremely difficult to predict. The outcome will ultimately depend not so much on the knowledge base of psychiatry per se, as on the social, cultural and economic forces that shape the societal perception of mental illness and thereby determine the nature of the clinical practice of psychiatry.

One possible outcome is, of course, what Eisenberg (1986) called 'mindless psychiatry' – a psychiatric practice guided by biological models of mental disorders, in which the subjective experience of psychopathology is an epiphenomenon. It corresponds exactly to what Karl Jaspers called 'the somatic prejudice' – one of the six fallacies that Jaspers identified in psychiatry – namely the belief 'that all psychological interest in schizophrenia will vanish when once the morbid somatic process that underlies it is discovered' (Jaspers 1963).

Another possible outcome is that clinical psychiatry will retain psychopathology at the core of its identity as a medical discipline uniquely dealing with the abnormal representations of reality in everyday consciousness. And, since classification is not only an abstract system representing the natural order of things, but also a tool of communication servicing practical needs, it must retain a relationship to the subjective world and to behaviour. Therefore, the speculation is that in the future psychiatry will evolve towards a dual classification – one grounded entirely within the realm of biological and medical classifications, with molecular genetic and neuroscience concepts as organizing principles, and another, dimensional or prototype-based, which would be unapologetically naturalistic in its design and isomorphic to the reality of clinical phenomenology. To prevent or redress the cognitive impoverishment of the discipline that might result from an uncritical adoption of a classification system as its *one* language, it behoves clinicians, researchers and teachers to reflect on the two realities and two cultures that meet on the common ground in psychiatry and ensure its vitality and relevance.

REFERENCES

Akiskal HG (1983) Dysthymic disorder: psychopathology of proposed depressive subtypes. *American Journal of Psychiatry* **140**: 11–20.

Akiskal HG, Djenderedjian AH, Rosenthal RH & Khani MK (1977) Cyclothymic disorder: validating criteria for inclusion in the bipolar affective group. *American Journal of Psychiatry* **134**: 1227–33.

American Psychiatric Association (1980) Diagnostic and Statistical Manual of Mental Disorders, 3rd edn. Washington, DC: APA.

American Psychiatric Association (1987) Diagnostic and Statistical Manual of Mental Disorders 3rd edn, revised. Washington, DC: APA.

American Psychiatric Association (1994) *Diagnostic and Statistical Manual of Mental Disorders*, 4th edn. Washington, DC: APA.

Battaglia M & Torgersen S (1996) Schizotypal disorder: at the crossroads of genetics and nosology. *Acta Psychiatrica Scandinavica* **94**, 303–10.

Berrios GE (1999) Classifications in psychiatry: a conceptual history. *Australian and New Zealand Journal of Psychiatry* **33**: 145–60.

Bienvenue OJ, Samuels JF, Riddle MA, Hoehn-Saric R, Liang KY, Cullen BAM, Grados MA & Nestadt G (2000) The relationship of obsessive-compulsive disorder to possible spectrum mechanisms: results from a family study. *Biological Psychiatry* **48**: 287–93.

Cantor N, Smith EE, French RS & Mezzich J (1980) Psychiatric diagnosis as prototype classification. *Journal of Abnormal Psychology* **89**: 181–93.

Castle DJ & Ames FR (1996) Cannabis and the brain. *Australian and New Zealand Journal of Psychiatry* **30**: 179–83.

Castle DJ & Phillips KA (2004) The OCD spectrum of disorders: a defensible construct? *Trends in Evidence-Based Neuroscience*. (In press)

Castle DJ, Wessely S & Murray RM (1993) Sex and schizophrenia: effects of diagnostic stringency, and associations with premorbid variables. *British Journal of Psychiatry* **162**, 658–64.

Castle DJ & Wykes T (2003) Depression and anxiety in schizophrenia. In: Castle DJ, Copolov D & Wykes T (eds) *Pharmacological and Psychosocial Treatments in Schizophrenia*, pp. 63–74. Martin Dunitz: London.

Cloninger CR (1999) A new conceptual paradigm from genetics and psychobiology for the science of mental health. *Australian and New Zealand Journal of Psychiatry* **33**: 174–86.

Eisenberg L (1986) Mindlessness and brainlessness in psychiatry. *British Journal of Psychiatry* **148**: 497–508.

Eysenck HJ (1970) A dimensional system of psycho-diagnosis. In: Mahrer AR (ed.) *New Approaches to Personality Classification*, pp. 169–207. New York: Columbia University Press.

Farmer A & Owen MJ (1996) Genomics: the next psychiatric revolution? *British Journal of Psychiatry* **169**: 135–8.

Feighner JP, Robins E, Guze SB, et al. (1972) Diagnostic criteria for use in psychiatric research. *Archives of General Psychiatry* **26**: 57–63.

Foulds GA (1976) *Hierarchical Nature of Personal Illness*. London: Academic Press.

Glass IB (1989) Alcoholic hallucinosis: a psychiatric enigma. *British Journal of Addiction* **84**: 29–41.

Grady-Weliky TA (2003) Premenstrual dysphoric disorder. *New England Journal of Medicine* **348**: 433–8.

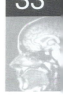

Gross-Isseroff R, Hermesh H, Zohar J & Weizman A (2003) Neuroimaging communality between schizophrenia and obsessive-compulsive disorder: a putative basis for schizo-obsessive disorder? *World Journal of Biological Psychiatry* **4**: 129–34.

Hollander E (1993). Obsessive-compulsive spectrum disorders: an overview. *Psychiatric Annals* **23**: 355–8.

Huntington's Disease Collaborative Group (1993) A novel gene containing a trinucleotide repeat that is expanded and unstable in Huntington's Disease chromosomes. *Cell* **72**: 971–83.

Jablensky A (1999) The nature of psychiatric classification: issues beyond ICD-10 and DSM-IV. *Australian and New Zealand Journal of Psychiatry* **33**: 137–44.

Jaspers K (1963) *General Psychopathology*. Transl. by J Hoenig and MW Hamilton. Manchester: Manchester University Press.

Johns DR (1955) Mitichondrial DNA and disease. *New England Journal of Medicine* **333**: 638–44.

Kendell RE & Gourlay J (1970) The clinical distinction between the affective psychoses and schizophrenia. *British Journal of Psychiatry* **117**: 261–6.

Kendell RE & Brockington IF (1980) The identification of disease entities and the relationship between schizophrenic and affective psychoses. *British Journal of Psychiatry* **137**: 324–31.

Kendell R & Jablensky A (2003) Distinguishing between validity and utility of psychiatric diagnoses. *American Journal of Psychiatry* **160**: 4–12.

Kessler RC (1995) The epidemiology of psychiatric comorbidity. In: Tsuang M, Tohen M & Zahner G (eds) *Textbook of Psychiatric Epidemiology*, pp. 179–98. New York: Wiley.

Kraepelin E (1893) *Psychiatrie*, 4th edn. Leipzig: Barth.

Lochner C & Stein DJ (2003) Heterogeneity of obsessive-compulsive disorder: a literature review. *Harvard Review of Psychiatry* **11**: 113–32.

Lewis G & Appleby L (1988) Personality disorder: the patients psychiatrists dislike. *British Journal of Psychiatry* **153**: 44–9.

Manton KG, Korten A, Woodbury MA, Anker M & Jablensky A (1994) Symptom profiles of psychiatric disorders based on graded disease classes: an illustration using data from the WHO International Pilot Study of Schizophrenia. *Psychological Medicine* **24**: 133–44.

Masters CL & Beyreuther K (1994). Alzheimer's disease: a clearer definition of the genetic components. *Medical Journal of Australia* **160**: 243–4.

Mayou R (1996) Accident neurosis revisited. *British Journal of Psychiatry* **165**: 399–403.

McCarley RW, Wible CG, Frumin M, et al. (1999) MRI anatomy of schizophrenia. *Biological Psychiatry* **45**: 1099–119.

Mechanic D & Volkert EH (1960) Illness behaviour and medical diagnosis. *Journal of Health and Human Behaviour* **1**: 51–8.

Miller H (1961) Accident neurosis. *British Medical Journal*, 919–98.

Murray RM, O'Callaghan E, Castle DJ, Lewis SW (1992) A neurodevelopmental approach to the classification of schizophrenia. *Schizophrenia Bulletin* **18**: 319–32.

Noyes R Jr, Holt CS, Happel RL, Kathol RG & Yagla SJ (1997) A family study of hypochondriasis. *Journal of Nervous and Mental Disease* **185**: 223–32.

Parsons T (1964) *Social Structure and Personality*. London: Collier-MacMillen.

Pilowsky I (1978) A general classification of abnormal illness behaviours. *British Journal of Medical Psychology* **51**: 131–7.

Prince M, Cullen M & Mann A (1994) Risk factors for Alzheimer's disease and dementia: a case-control study based on the MRC elderly hypertension trial. *Neurology* **44**: 97–104.

Robins L & Guze SB (1970) Establishment of diagnostic validity in psychiatric illness: its application to schizophrenia. *American Journal of Psychiatry* **126**: 983–7.

Rosenberg RN (1996) DNA-triplet repeats and neurologic disease [Editorial]. *New England Journal of Medicine* **335**: 1222–4.

Rutter M, Lebovici L, Eisenberg L, et al. (1969) A tri-axial classification of mental disorders in childhood. *Journal of Child Psychology and Psychiatry* **10**: 41–61.

Schneider K (1959) *Clinical Psychopathology*. Transl. by MW Hamilton. London: Grune & Stratton.

Siris SG (1991) Diagnosis of secondary depression in schizophrenia: implications for DSM-IV. *Schizophrenia Bulletin* **17**: 75–98.

Spitzer RL, Endicott J & Robins E (1978) Research Diagnostic Criteria (RDC): rationale and reliability. *Archives of General Psychiatry* **35**: 773–82.

Szaz TS (1976) Schizophrenia: the sacred symbol of psychiatry. *British Journal of Psychiatry* **129**: 308–16.

Toone BK (1991) The psychoses of epilepsy. *Journal of the Royal Society of Medicine* **84**: 457–9.

Tyrer P (1984) Classification of anxiety. *British Journal of Psychiatry* **144**: 78–83.

Van Minnen A, Hoogduin KAL, Keijsers GPJ, Hellenbrand I & Hendriks G-J (2003) Treatment of trichotillomania with behavioural therapy or fluoxetine: a randomised, waiting-list controlled study. *Archives of General Psychiatry* **60**: 517–22.

Van Praag HM (1992) *Make-Believes in Psychiatry or the Perils of Progress*. New York, Brunner Mazel.

Wing J & Nixon J (1975) Discriminating symptoms in schizophrenia. *Archives of General Psychiatry* **32**: 853–9.

World Health Organization (1992) *The ICD-10 Classification of Mental and Behavioural Disorders: Clinical Descriptions and Diagnostic Guidelines*. Geneva: World Health Organization.

Electroencephalography and neuroimaging

Pádraig Wright, Thordur Sigmundsson and James V Lucey

INTRODUCTION

Psychiatrists often bemoan the absence of biological markers for the diseases they study and treat, and critics of psychiatry frequently cite this absence as evidence that psychiatric illness does not exist. Electroencephalography has been used to investigate psychiatric illness for more than half a century but it has contributed little to our understanding of such illness. However, the use of increasingly sophisticated structural and functional neuroimaging, and indeed electrophysiological, techniques offers hope that we will soon more fully understand the neurophysiological correlates of psychiatric illness. Current and potential future applications to psychiatry of electroencephalography and of structural and functional neuroimaging will be discussed in this chapter.

ELECTROENCEPHALOGRAPHY IN PSYCHIATRY

The normal electroencephalogram

An electroencephalogram (EEG) is a recording of the electrical potential of the brain made at the scalp surface. The EEG α rhythm was first recorded with an Einthoven string galvanometer by Austrian psychiatrist Hans Berger in 1929, and until recently the EEG was the only non-invasive means of assessing brain function (Berger 1931).

An EEG is a recording of the electrical potential produced by inhibitory and excitatory post-synaptic electrical discharges from neuronal dendrites at the cortical surface. Such neurons constitute less than 5% of all neurons in the brain. The voltage recorded on an EEG is only 10% of that recorded on an electrocardiograph because the electrical resistance of the skull is high. An individual's EEG is largely genetically determined and several investigations have reported that EEGs recorded from monozygotic twins were almost identical (Dummermuth 1968). The EEG records changes in the electrical potential of the brain, which are detected as variations in voltage (10 to 100 microvolts) and frequency (0.5 to 40 Hz).

When recording an EEG, electrodes (usually 21) are placed on the scalp in a standard (or international) 10/20 arrangement, in which the electrodes are placed at points either 10% or 20% of the total distance along an imaginary line between two anatomical landmarks, for example the nasion and inion. Negative potentials cause an upward deflection on the EEG record, and either bipolar (between two electrodes) or common (between any single electrode and a fixed electrically neutral site such as the nose or ear lobe) reference potentials may be recorded. The arrangement of recording electrodes in use at a given time is referred to as a montage.

EEG recordings may be made with the patient either lying still or ambulatory, and nasopharyngeal (inserted via the nares) or sphenoidal (inserted inferior to the zygomatic arch) electrodes may be used to allow recordings from the inferior temporal lobe, especially prior to temporal lobe surgery. Depth electrodes are occasionally placed in the brain via burr holes, and electrocorticography may be undertaken by placing electrodes directly on the brain intra-operatively. More recent technological advances allow continuous portable EEG recording for 24 hours or more, simultaneous videotape display and recording of a subject's behaviour and EEG and thus their potential correlation, and the rapid computerized analysis of digitized EEG data. This latter facilitates brain mapping, in which EEG voltages or amplitudes are plotted on a map representing the brain and for which extensive comparative data from both healthy and psychiatric subjects are available (Fenwick 1992).

Normal EEG frequencies

The normal EEG frequencies are as follows:

- δ rhythm = 0.1–3.9 Hz
- θ rhythm = 4.0–7.9 Hz
- α rhythm = 8.0–13.0 Hz
- β rhythm = 13.0–40.0 Hz

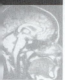

The α rhythm (30–50 microvolts) is the normal rhythm seen in a subject who is awake with his eyes closed. It is maximal over the occipital and, to a lesser extent, the parietal regions, and is often less evident over the dominant hemisphere. The β rhythm is present over the remaining frontocentral areas of the scalp. If the subject opens his eyes or undertakes mental activity, the α rhythm blocks or attenuates and is replaced by β rhythm all over the scalp. The β waves from different sites are out of phase and are said to be desynchronized. The δ and θ frequencies occur during sleep but are not present during wakefulness in adults, while τ and μ waves occur over the occipital and motor cortices respectively, and are caused by minimal ocular (scanning) and limb movements. A hypnotized subject exhibits the same EEG as one who is awake and alert, and minor abnormalities are common in EEGs recorded from healthy individuals.

Age and the EEG

Although EEG activity is evident from at least the second trimester of gestation (Eeg-Olofsson 1970), the EEG of a normal neonate reveals relatively little rhythmic electrical activity. Desynchronized δ and θ waves are evident in recordings from alert older infants. With increasing age, these are replaced by α rhythm from frontal, through temporal and parietal, and thence to occipital regions. In general, the EEG is dominated by δ rhythm until about the age of two years, by θ until about the age of five years, and by α activity thereafter until the adult EEG emerges.

The adult pattern of dominant α rhythm described above becomes evident in late adolescence and is referred to as the mature EEG. Frontal θ and posterior temporal δ waves may persist in some young adults (referred to as a maturational EEG) and there is some evidence that these rhythms are associated with personality disorder when they are present in later adulthood (referred to as an immature EEG).

From the seventh decade of life onwards, α waves are of lower voltage and frequency, and low-frequency rhythms such as δ waves may reappear. These changes are more evident in men than in women and may be accompanied by clinically insignificant temporal slow-wave foci (Obrist & Busse 1965).

Activation of the EEG

Suspected EEG abnormalities may not be evident during a standard recording. These may be revealed if the brain is stressed or otherwise activated in some way. The techniques used to unmask abnormalities hidden in the resting EEG record include:

- hyperventilation, which induces cortical hypocapnia, cerebral vasoconstriction and hypoxia, and may allow epileptic foci to become evident
- photic stimulation, in which a strobe light flashing at 8–15 Hz is used to capture the occipital α frequency, that is the α frequency adjusts to match that of the strobe

light (photic driving). This may allow epileptic foci to be seen and may even induce epileptic seizures, as may a flickering television screen
- barbiturates and neuroleptics, which may both be used to unmask epileptic foci.

The EEG and sleep

Sleep is similar to coma, in that it consists of inactivity and loss of awareness and responsivity. In contrast to the comatose individual, however, the sleeping individual either awakens spontaneously or can be roused. The EEG has been used extensively in the investigation of both the physiology of sleep and sleep disorders. Indeed physiological sleep is divided into five stages purely on the basis of changes observed in EEG recordings taken from sleeping subjects.

During sleep, the rhythm recorded on an EEG changes from the β rhythm of wakefulness, through occipital α rhythm when the eyes are closed, to the sleep EEG. Stages I (transitional sleep), II, III and IV of the sleep EEG are referred to as non-rapid eye movement (non-REM) or orthodox sleep, during which parasympathetic tone is increased, while Stage V is referred to as rapid eye movement (REM) or desynchronized sleep, during which sympathetic tone is increased. Stages III and IV are characterized by slow waves and are therefore sometimes referred to as slow wave sleep (SWS), or as synchronized sleep. The principal EEG features of sleep stages I through IV are summarized in Box 34.1.

Stage V or REM sleep is also called paradoxical sleep because while deep unconsciousness and marked atonia occur, paradoxically the EEG resembles that recorded during

Box 34.1   EEG features of sleep
Stage I
The α rhythm gradually disappears
Low-voltage desynchronized slow waves (δ and θ) appear
High-voltage sharp waves occur at the vertex
Stage II
Low voltages and δ and slower frequencies dominate the recording
Sleep spindles occur (sinusoidal 12–14 Hz of 0.5 sec)
K complexes occur (high-amplitude sharp positive/negative deflections)
Stage III
High-voltage slow waves all over the scalp
δ waves account for <50% of rhythm
Sleep spindles and K complexes diminish
Stage IV
High-voltage slow (δ) waves dominate the EEG
δ waves account for >50% of rhythm
Sleep spindles and K complexes are absent

Stage I (transitional) sleep, or when a subject is awake with his eyes closed. Thus low voltage, variable frequency waves and occasional α rhythm are recorded. The eyes exhibit rapid conjugate movements and physiological arousal is evident as tachycardia, tachypnoea, systolic hypertension, increased oxygen consumption, dilated pupils, penile tumescence or vaginal lubrication, increased cerebral perfusion and occasional myoclonic jerks. Dreaming is reported (and is vividly recalled) by 60–80% of individuals awakened from REM sleep, as compared to about 20% of subjects awakened from non-REM sleep. REM accounts for over 50% of sleep in childhood, for 25% in adulthood and for 10% of sleep in old age. REM changes on an EEG recorded during the daytime suggest either sleep deprivation, withdrawal from alcohol or from drugs that suppress REM (barbiturates, benzodiazepines), or narcolepsy.

The cycle from Stage I to V takes about 1.5 hours and is repeated 4 or 5 times per night (Fig. 34.1). Thus, sleep during the early part of the night is largely SWS, sleep during the later of the night is largely REM sleep, and overall most time is spent in Stage II sleep. The normal sleep/wake cycle is of 25 hours' duration (not 24 hours) and if deprived of sleep (or selectively of REM sleep) extra REM sleep, called REM-rebound, occurs when normal sleep is again possible. However, the function of sleep in general, and of REM sleep in particular, is unknown. Both total sleep deprivation and selective REM deprivation have real but relatively modest effects on formal tests of cognitive function, which can largely be compensated for by increased effort, at least in the short term. This cognitive deficit has been quantified as equivalent to that caused by a blood alcohol level of 0.05% (Falleti et al. 2003). However, performance on formal tests of cognitive function are not good indicators of occupational or other performance and there is growing evidence that sleep deprivation significantly impairs the working ability of, for example, doctors (Samkoff & Jacques 1991). It is important to note that sleep requirements vary greatly both between individuals and within individuals at different times and that 5 or 6 hours' sleep is sufficient for many people. In particular, sleep requirements diminish with age.

The circadian rhythm of secretion that hormones such as cortisol, prolactin, growth hormone and insulin exhibit is well known and some hormones exhibit a similar secretory pattern (which may be superimposed on the circadian pattern) during the sleep cycle. Thus growth hormone levels are maximal during SWS, prolactin levels peak during early Stage I and later Stage IV sleep, and testosterone levels increase continuously during sleep. There is also increasing evidence that seasonal and circadian patterns of hormone levels and behaviour may be controlled by rhythmic secretion of melatonin from the pineal gland. Melatonin levels are low during REM sleep and may be controlled by a putative biological clock in the suprachiasmatic nucleus of the hypothalamus which responds to light falling on the retina. Melatonin is effective in alleviating jet lag (during which the normal diurnal variation in body temperature and in cortisol and catecholamine secretion is disrupted) but there is no evidence that phototherapy for seasonal affective disorder acts by increasing melatonin levels.

The effects of psychotropic drugs on the EEG

Almost all psychotropic drugs affect the EEG and recordings from patients taking such drugs are effectively useless. The specific effects of the most frequently prescribed psychotropic drugs are presented in Box 34.2. It should also be remembered that barbiturates, benzodiazepines and antipsychotics all aggravate epileptic discharges.

The EEG and electroconvulsive therapy (ECT)

The EEG during an application of ECT is similar to that seen during a tonic/clonic seizure. Between applications of ECT, irregular slow waves (θ and δ) occur. These are most evident

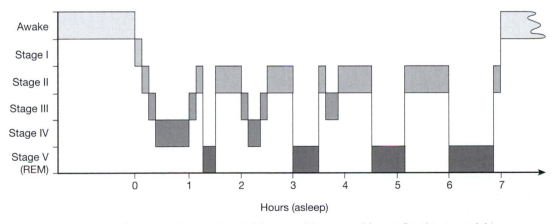

Figure 34.1 The cycle from sleep Stage I to V takes about 1.5 hours and is repeated four or five times per night.

Box 34.2   Effects of psychotropic drugs on EEG recordings
Barbiturates
Increased β and θ rhythms
Reduced α rhythm
Occasional δ waves
Benzodiazepines
Increased β and θ rhythms
Reduced α rhythm
Tricyclic antidepressants
Increased δ, θ and β rhythms
Antipsychotics
Increased β (low to moderate dosage)
Increased δ and/or θ (high dosage)
Lithium carbonate
No or minimal effects (therapeutic levels)
Increased δ and/or θ (high and toxic levels)

over the dominant hemisphere, especially the frontal lobe, and they persist for increasingly longer periods of time after each successive administration of ECT. Very high voltage slow waves appear towards the end of a course of ECT, and the α rhythm may disappear completely. The effects of ECT on the EEG gradually diminish following a course of treatment and they are no longer evident after between one and three months; prior to that, the EEG is impossible to interpret.

The EEG and psychiatric illness

The EEG is helpful in the diagnosis and monitoring of epilepsy and many other neuropsychiatric disorders, but is of more limited use when applied to psychotic, affective and anxiety disorders.

Epilepsy
The EEG is abnormal in about 15% of healthy subjects and normal in about 20% of patients with epilepsy, although activation procedures may reveal spikes (waveforms which rise and fall rapidly) in many of the latter. Epilepsy is therefore a clinical diagnosis which may be supported by the EEG. Spikes and waves (waveforms which rise rapidly and fall slowly) occurring in the α, θ and δ ranges in the inter-ictal EEG record are the hallmark of epilepsy. These may be focal (for example, over the temporal recording leads in temporal lobe epilepsy), unilateral or bilateral, and may be synchronized or desynchronized. Spikes and waves may combine to produce spike and wave complexes. These exhibit a high frequency in tonic/clonic epilepsy and a frequency of 3 Hz in classic absence epilepsy. Epilepsy is discussed in more detail in Chapter 26.

Acute organic psychosis and encephalitis
Metabolic disorders such as hypoxia, hepatic encephalopathy, vitamin B_{12} deficiency and hypoglycaemia cause diffuse slowing of the background rhythm and the occurrence of triphasic waves (which must be differentiated from triphasic sharp waves – see Creutzfeldt–Jakob disease below). The exception is withdrawal from alcohol or delirium tremens, in which the EEG may be normal and exhibit fast rhythms. Focal intracranial pathology, whether tumour, haemorrhage, abscess or infarct, may cause slow waves and perhaps epileptiform rhythms to arise in the leads over the lesion. The degree of change on the EEG depends on the site (cortical lesions are more easily detected than deeper lesions), size (a lesion <2 cm in diameter may cause no EEG changes) and rate of growth (a rapidly enlarging lesion is more likely to cause EEG changes) of the lesion. EEGs from patients with encephalitis may exhibit diffuse irregular slow waves and seizure patterns.

Dementia
There is a marked reduction in α waves and very low amplitude background rhythm (referred to as a flattened EEG) in Huntington's disease. In Alzheimer's dementia, there is accentuation of the normal changes that occur with ageing, so α rhythm is reduced and a disorganized θ rhythm evolves. The EEG in vascular dementia is similar to that of Alzheimer's dementia but with the addition of focal features over infarcts or haemorrhages. In Creutzfeldt–Jakob disease (CJD) a reduced background rhythm with characteristic triphasic sharp wave complexes with a frequency of 1–2 Hz occurs in up to 90% of patients. This may not be present initially and repeat recordings are necessary. These EEG changes have not been reported in new variant CJD in which neuropsychiatric symptoms, ataxia, myoclonus and dementia occur, nor in Gerstmann–Straussler–Scheinker (familial CJD) syndrome or iatrogenic CJD. The EEG is often normal in Pick's disease.

Personality, affective and anxiety disorders
An immature EEG (see above) is present in about 50% of patients with personality disorder (and in 70% of prisoners convicted of motiveless homicide) while EEGs from patients with affective disorders reveal an excess of non-specific abnormalities. Excess generalized low-amplitude θ and β rhythms occur in a significant proportion of patients with anxiety disorders.

Schizophrenia
Over 40% of schizophrenic patients have an abnormal EEG, the most frequent abnormality being the presence of low-amplitude epileptiform activity (especially with activation procedures). This proportion is highest in catatonic schizophrenia, with low-amplitude slow waves (δ and θ) and a reduced α rhythm occurring in catatonic stupor.

Schizophreniform psychosis associated with temporal lobe epilepsy is discussed in Chapter 18.

Evoked potentials

It has long been known that stimulation of peripheral sense organs alters the EEG, and that a sound or light may evoke a wave over the auditory or visual cortex respectively. Evoked waves are usually hidden by background EEG activity but they may be revealed by averaging, a computerized mathematical technique which greatly reduces background EEG 'noise'. A positive evoked wave occurring 300 milliseconds after a stimulus is conventionally referred to as the P300. P300 abnormalities have been reported in patients with dementia (delayed response and reduced amplitude) and in both schizophrenic patients (Muller et al. 2001) and their first-degree relatives (reduced amplitude) (Blackwood & Muir 1990).

Magnetoencephalography

Magnetoencephalography (MEG) utilizes modern super-conductor technology to record the minute magnetic fields generated by neuronal electrical activity. MEG thus has the same range of applications in psychiatry as the EEG but contrasts with electroencephalography in that it allows the detection of electrical activity throughout the brain without the need for intracerebral electrodes and it has greater resolution. The science of magnetoencephalography and its application to psychiatry is in its infancy and further developments are awaited.

STRUCTURAL NEUROIMAGING IN PSYCHIATRY

Neuroimaging is conveniently divided into structural and functional neuroimaging. The two most commonly used structural imaging techniques are computed X-ray tomography (CT) and magnetic resonance (MR) imaging. These have largely replaced the skull X-ray which will be briefly described. Technical aspects of CT and MR neuroimaging will then be reviewed and the clinical and research applications of these imaging techniques to psychiatry will be discussed.

Skull X-ray

The skull X-ray is of very limited use in modern psychiatric practice. Nonetheless, it allows detection of intracranial calcifications, especially hypophyseal calcification which, if present, enables radiologists to see any shift of midline structures caused by space-occupying lesions. Erosion of bone, for example of the sella turcica by pituitary tumours or the cranial vault by other brain tumours, can also be visualized on skull X-ray, as can thickening of the skull in Paget's disease. However, psychiatrists had recognized the limitations of skull X-ray even prior to the introduction of modern neuroimaging techniques. One study found no abnormality in 53 'routine' skull X-ray examinations and only one abnormality – a skull fracture – in 30 clinically indicated skull X-ray examinations (Larkin et al. 1985). It is of interest to note that Jakobi and Winkler in 1927 described ventricular enlargement in patients with schizophrenia examined with pneumoencephalography, a technique dependent on X-ray and the introduction of (radiolucent) air into the subarachnoid space via lumbar puncture.

Computed X-ray tomography (CT)

Like conventional X-ray, CT depends on measuring the amount of energy absorbed by tissues placed in front of an X-ray tube emitting high-energy photons, in order to produce an image. X-ray photons are attenuated by atoms in tissue, leading to the emission of an electron. X-rays are therefore a form of ionizing radiation. The degree to which tissues attenuate X-rays depends on their density, and attenuation values (CT values or Hounsfield units) have been calculated for various tissues relative to the attenuation value of water, arbitrarily set at 0 (Table 34.1). Photons passing through tissue sensitize photographic film in conventional X-ray, but are detected by photon detectors in CT.

In cranial CT, the X-ray tube and photon detectors rotate around the head in a transverse plane (usually the orbitomeatal plane through the orbits and the external auditory meatus, in order to minimize radiation to the eyes). The signal from the photon detectors is then transformed (using Fourier transformation) by computer in order to build a two-dimensional picture of a slice of healthy or abnormal brain (Fig. 34.2A) within a grid or matrix. Each square, or pixel (picture element) in this grid has a particular shade of grey determined by the attenuation value of the tissue. The advantages and disadvantages of CT and MR neuroimaging are presented in Box 34.3.

Table 34.1 CT or Hounsfield values for a range of human tissues	
Tissue	*CT/Hounsfield value*
Cerebrospinal fluid	+8
White matter	+15
Grey matter	+18
Bone	+200–500
Air	–500
Water	0

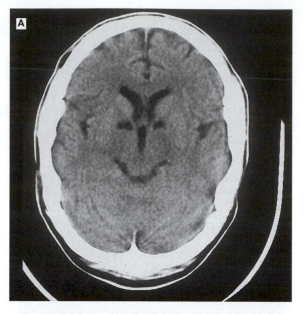

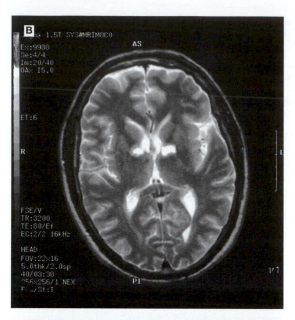

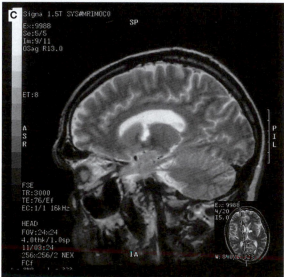

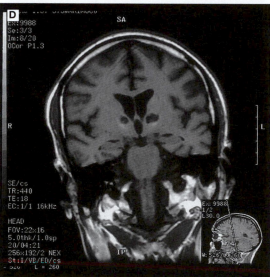

Figure 34.2 (**A**) CT of the head of a patient showing a bilateral white matter lesion involving the anterior limb of the internal capsule. (**B**), (**C**) and (**D**) are axial, sagittal and coronal MR images, respectively, of the same patient and are shown for comparison. Clinically, this lesion was associated with a behavioural syndrome identical to frontal lobe syndrome, indicating that most of the afferent fibres from the frontal lobe to the striatum were severed by the lesion.

(Images courtesy of Neuroimaging Department, Maudsley Hospital, London.)

Magnetic resonance imaging (MRI)

MR (or nuclear magnetic resonance, NMR) imaging depends on the detection of electromagnetic energy derived from interactions between atoms and an external magnetic field, in order to produce an image. Protium (^{1}H), the isotope accounting for 99.9% of hydrogen atoms, and the most abundant element in most living tissues, is effectively an unpaired proton that behaves like a moving charge, spinning and generating a magnetic field along its axis of

spin. Protons may be thought of as bar magnets or magnetic dipoles with a definite magnitude or vector and direction to their axis of rotation. Individual protons in living tissue are arranged randomly and their net magnetization is 0. When placed in an external magnetic field, protons align in the direction of the field (the B0 axis) and their net magnetization is no longer 0. They also 'wobble' like spinning tops along the axis of the magnetic field, a phenomenon called precession. The frequency of precession, or Lamour frequency, is measurable and is unique for each

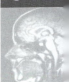

Box 34.3   Advantages and disadvantages of CT and MR neuroimaging

Advantages of CT

Widely available and relatively inexpensive

Examinations are rapid

Relatively safe

Can readily distinguish cerebrospinal fluid (CSF) from grey matter

Resolution may be enhanced by use of contrast agents

Superior to MRI in evaluating bony abnormalities and cerebral calcifications

Invaluable when MRI is contraindicated (patients on life-support systems, for example)

Disadvantages of CT

Does not effectively differentiate between white and grey matter

Poor resolution

Allergies to contrast agents

Exposure to ionizing radiation

Advantages of MR

Safe

More sensitive than CT in distinguishing between grey and white matter

Can identify ectopic grey matter

Can evaluate deep grey matter nuclei in the basal ganglia

Can evaluate white matter lesions (plaques in multiple sclerosis, infarcts)

Invaluable when examining brain regions near bone (temporal lobe, basal forebrain, cerebellum)

Allows imaging in three planes and reconstruction in any plane

Allows measurement of volumes

Disadvantages of MR

Relatively unavailable and expensive

Several absolute contraindications (aneurysm clips, pacemakers, paramagnetic metallic objects)

Some relative contraindications (pregnancy, claustrophobia)

---

element. In MRI, short radio-frequency pulses are applied to precessing tissue protons (at the precessing frequency and perpendicular to the external magnetic field) by a transmitter coil. This additional energy tips the protons through 90° or 180° causing protons that were precessing at random to precess in unison. Such protons absorb energy from the radio-frequency pulses, recover slowly (relax) and then release this energy such that it may be detected by a receiver coil. The strength of the signal detected by a receiver coil depends on the density of protons in the tissue being examined. Thus tissue differentiation is possible on MR images because hydrogen in living tissue is mostly in the form of water, the concentration of which differs in different tissues.

The relaxation time of protons is described by two different, but simultaneous, processes. The T1 (longitudinal or spin-lattice) relaxation time reflects the return of the net magnetization to the B0 axis, while the T2 (transverse or spin-spin) relaxation time reflects the return of random precession (dephasing of the spin coherence). T1 and T2 relaxation times differ by tissue, and radio-frequency pulses may be applied so that the differing T1 or T2 properties of the tissue are accentuated (T1 or T2 weighting). The spatial information required for an image is obtained by applying gradients to the static external magnetic field, such that protons will precess at slightly different frequencies along the gradient. The application of three such gradients at right angles to each other generates three 'slices' of tissue and allows for the construction of a three-dimensional image of the brain (Figs 34.2A, C and D; 34.3A and B; and Chapter 20, Fig 20.2). The thickness of each slice of tissue determines the size of each volume element (voxel) sampled (which is slightly less than 1 cubic millimetre in modern MRI scanners). The image is then reconstructed by computer in a similar manner to that described for CT, but with the important difference that images may be reconstructed in any plane.

Unlike ionizing radiation, there are no known biological hazards associated with magnetic fields or radiofrequency waves. MRI therefore offers a uniquely safe opportunity to study the brain. MRI is also superior to CT in differentiating between grey and white matter and, because images can be obtained in different planes and information sampled at different relaxation times, in investigating tissue characteristics. This intrinsic property of MRI not only provides structural information but also allows the collection of information about brain function (see below).

The role of CT and MR structural neuroimaging in psychiatry

Structural scans of the brain are undertaken for two reasons by psychiatrists: clinical investigation and research. The commonest clinical indications for neuroimaging are the exclusion or confirmation of suspected pathology responsible for focal neurological signs or symptoms and the investigation of suspected dementia (cortical atrophy supports the diagnosis, and the site and nature of brain abnormalities can help distinguish between the dementias). The intial scarcity of neuroimaging facilities meant that strict criteria (the presence of a focal neurological sign or atypical psychosis, for example) had to be met before imaging was undertaken. CT and MRI are now more widely available and clinical neuroimaging is increasingly recognized as an essential component of the clinical investigation of many psychiatric disorders (Box 34.4). However, it remains important to undertake a neurological examination prior to imaging, in order to facilitate interpretation of the CT or MR scan. In particular, the clinical question must be clearly formulated prior to MR because the image protocol and radio-frequency pulse sequences utilized by the radiologist are determined by the patient's symptoms and the implied brain region under investigation.

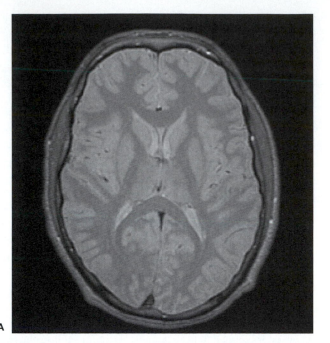
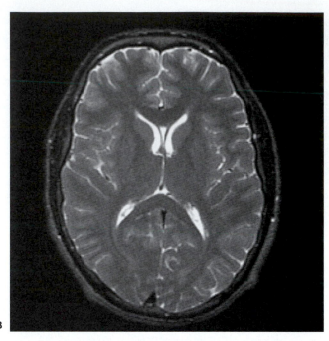

A   B

Figure 34.3 (A) and (B) are proton density and T2-weighted axial MRI images respectively taken from the same anatomical location in the head of a patient at the level of the basal ganglia.
(Images courtesy of Neuroimaging Department, Maudsley Hospital, London.)

Box 34.4   Clinical indications for structural brain scans
Dementia
Delirium
Catatonia
Movement disorder
Acute change in personality
First onset of psychosis
History of head trauma
History of seizures
Eating disorder
Electroencephalographic abnormalities
Focal neurological abnormalities
First onset of psychiatric symptoms after age 50 years
Atypical symptoms or course of illness

Structural neuroimaging has been used extensively in psychiatric research, especially in the psychoses and dementias, since Johnstone et al. (1976) first reported ventricular dilatation in patients with schizophrenia, using CT. Increasingly sophisticated neuroimaging techniques have been focused on identifying brain regions that differ between patients and comparison populations. Early work depended on manual measurement of the area of relatively large brain structures (ventricles) in cross-sections on CT scans. MRI subsequently provided the opportunity to examine both smaller structures poorly visible on CT (temporal lobe, cerebellum) and images of the brain in different planes. MRI also provided excellent separation between white and grey matter, which allowed segmentation of the brain into three components – white and grey matter, and cerebrospinal fluid (CSF). It is usual to refer to specific brain regions being investigated with CT or MRI as regions of interest (ROI), the volumes of ROIs being compared between groups either manually (by tracing them on a computer monitor and multiplying the area by the slice thickness to get the volume for each slice, the cumulative volume of ROIs on all slices providing an estimate of the volume of the structures being examined) or automatically (by using computer programs capable of segmenting the brain into grey and white matter and CSF and of calculating the volume of each component separately). More recently, it has become possible to analyse structural imaging data using methods first developed for analysing functional neuroimaging data (the recording of images with a template image in stereotactic space and the analysis of differences in grey or white matter intensities on a voxel (volume element) by voxel basis). In addition to the search for brain abnormalities specific to individual neuropsychiatric disorders, structural neuroimaging has also been used to monitor disease progress in patients with degenerative brain disorders (Fox et al. 1996), examine the effects of pharmacological treatments such as increased basal ganglia volume in patients treated with antipsychotic drugs (Chakos et al. 1995), and to co-register structural and functional neuroimaging data, for example PET with MRI.

FUNCTIONAL NEUROIMAGING IN PSYCHIATRY

Four functional neuroimaging techniques have established themselves in psychiatric research and their clinical applications are becoming increasingly important. Single photon emission tomography (SPET) and positron emission tomography (PET) depend on the administration of radioactive isotopes and the subsequent detection of gamma photons and positrons respectively. Functional MRI (fMRI) and MR spectroscopy (MRS) utilize MRI technology as described above.

Positron emission tomography (PET)

PET is the benchmark technique for functional imaging of metabolic processes such as regional cerebral blood flow (rCBF) or regional cerebral metabolism of glucose (rCMG). It involves the combination of two technologies, tracer kinetic assay (TKA) and CT. TKA involves the use of a radio-labelled, biologically active compound (the radionuclide tracer) and a mathematical model of its kinetics as it participates in a biological process. The PET scanner measures the tissue concentration of the tracer and produces a three-dimensional image of the anatomical distribution of the biological process being investigated.

The radionuclide tracers used during PET imaging are natural substrates or their analogues, combined with radioactive forms of natural elements (labels) such as ^{11}C, ^{13}N, ^{15}O and ^{18}F. These radiolabels emit radiation in the form of positrons that pass through the body and are detected externally, but that do not alter the biological process being investigated. Positrons are positively charged electrons that are emitted from the nucleus of some radioisotopes because they have an excess of protons and a positive charge, and are thus unstable. An emitted positron collides with electrons until it comes to rest and then combines with an electron to become a positronium. Since the positron is an anti-electron, the positron and electron annihilate each other and their masses are converted into electromagnetic energy. The mass of the electron and positron are equal, and equivalent to 511 kiloelectronvolts (keV) of energy. In a collision referred to as a true coincidence, the annihilation produces two 511 keV photons 180° apart. The scanner detects this energy. This is annihilation coincidence detection (ACD). Only true coincidences produce valid spatial information, so scanner designs try to maximize true coincidences and minimize scatter coincidences that produce 'noise'.

PET imaging (Fig. 34.4) requires a charged particle accelerator or cyclotron to produce positron-emitting isotopes and over 500 such isotopes have been produced by labelling with ^{15}O, ^{13}N, ^{11}C or ^{18}F. Compounds used with PET include H_2O^{15} for rCBF measurement and ^{18}F deoxyglucose (DG) for rCMG. PET imaging benefits from a low radiation exposure time:imaging time ratio, because PET radionuclides have short half-lives (^{15}O = 2 minutes, ^{18}F = 110 minutes). Dosimetry (here, used to ascertain the relationship between the radiation dose administered to the subject and the quality of the image detected) is determined by effects on organs throughout the body and not only by effects on the organ under investigation. In ^{18}F-DG PET imaging, 77% of the radiation dose is accounted for by photons of emitted ionization and only 23% by annihilation of positrons.

The CT technique in PET uses rigorous mathematical algorithms to produce tomographic images of projections from an object. PET scintillation detectors produce light when struck by radiation and image resolution depends on both detector resolution and the radiation cut-off frequency used. The signal to noise ratio is high and the tomographic planes are usually perpendicular to the long axis of the body. Early tomographic systems used ROI (regions of interest) analysis relying on manual placement of templates upon reconstructed images (see above). These were prone to inter-rater and intra-rater variability because anatomical localization was relatively unreliable. Modern PET imaging depends on computerized and automated systems for PET data analysis such as the Statistical Parametric Mapping or SPM system. Moreover, simultaneous anatomical localization of PET data using MRI – a process known as MRI co-registration – is increasingly available.

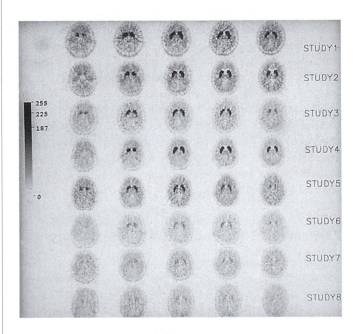

Figure 34.4 PET images of ^{11}C raclopride, a dopamine D_2 receptor ligand. The images are darkest in the striatum where the highest levels of ^{11}C raclopride occurs. Subject study 4 had placebo, and subject studies 1-3 and 5-8 had increasing doses of ziprasidone (2, 5, 10, 15, 20, 40 and 60 mg). The images show decreasing binding of ^{11}C raclopride due to ziprasidone's increasing occupancy of the dopamine D_2 receptor.
(Image courtesy of Dr C. Bench, MRC Cyclotron Unit, Hammersmith Hospital, London.)

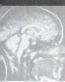

Single photon emission tomography (SPET)

SPET refers to a computerized emission tomographic system that depends on isotopes that emit single photons (as distinct from positrons in PET). Single photons are detected singly rather than in coincident pairs (as in PET). Collimation – the trapping of emitted photons and their direction towards the detector – is required because single photons are scattered randomly, and this means that most photons are absorbed by collimators and thus go undetected. Thus only a fraction of emitted photons are counted by SPET detector systems and SPET resolution is achieved at the expense of SPET sensitivity. The sensitivity of SPET is the degree to which the system responds to an incoming signal measured as counts per second (CPS) per slice (megaBequerel per litre or MBq/L). The most frequently used detector systems in clinical practice are rotating gamma cameras.

Once acquired, SPET data are organized as slices, and reconstructed separately from projections spaced over a 360° arc of rotation about the subject. The SPET detector system behind the collimator is made of sodium iodide crystals with photomultiplier tubes (PMTs) and SPET detector systems may have one large detector covered with many PMTs, or multiple detectors capable of higher count-rate detection and suitable for dynamic studies. Brain-dedicated SPET detector systems view the head from several angles simultaneously with separate scintillation detectors, while converging collimators increase the crystal surface area utilized for a given slice and thus maximize sensitivity. Reconstruction in transverse, coronal and sagittal planes is possible (Fig. 34.5). SPET images are collected over a much longer period of time and depend on many fewer photons than standard CT. Thus SPET images have more noise and less resolution than CT images. As with PET, ROI data analysis is still commonly used in SPET. However, SPM (see above) has recently been adapted for SPET. Ideal anatomical localization with SPET would require MRI co-registration as with PET, but in contrast to PET, this is difficult to achieve with SPET.

The role of PET and SPET in psychiatry

PET imaging techniques may be adapted to study metabolic processes such as the cerebral metabolic rate for glucose (with ^{18}F-DG) or cerebral protein synthesis (with ^{11}C-L-leucine). PET may also be utilized to investigate both presynaptic and post-synaptic receptor systems via different ligands, e.g. ^{18}F-fluoroethylspiperone for dopamine D_2 receptors. Multiple PET images may be overlapped in order to investigate simultaneous disease processes such as Parkinson's disease with or without Alzheimer's dementia.

SPET uses in neuropsychiatry include the examination of rCBF using ^{133}xenon (inhalation technique) or technetium 99m HMPAO, in the study of dementia, cerebral vascular disease and epilepsy. SPET receptor ligands include ^{123}iodine epidepride (which has been used extensively to investigate the dopaminergic system in schizophrenia), the substituted benzamide IBZM (which has also been used to investigate the dopaminergic system in schizophrenia) and ^{123}iodine Iomazenil (which has been used to examine the GABA receptor system in schizophrenia, alcoholism and anxiety)

For rCBF imaging, SPET represents a technique that is readily available and relatively inexpensive when compared to PET. Resolution similar to that achieved with second-generation PET is possible and, in contrast to PET, there is no need for an on-site cyclotron, and no need for arterial cannulation (essential with PET in order to achieve absolute levels of quantification). The disadvantages of SPET are nonetheless considerable. SPET techniques require collimation, the tissue volume sampled in each scan is substantially reduced, and SPET scans are generated by far fewer photons and must be collected over much greater periods of time than with PET scans. SPET ligands must therefore have a much longer half-life than PET ligands, so the capacity of SPET for repeated examinations is limited (this represents perhaps the greatest limitation of SPET). In contrast, PET may be used to repeatedly study serial brain states in the same individual. Regional CMG studies are not possible with SPET, nor is absolute quantification.

However, and despite the above, SPET presents real advantages to psychiatrists over and above those of cost and availability. These depend on technetium Tc 99m HMPAO, the ubiquitous SPET rCBF radionuclide, which has largely replaced ^{133}xenon inhalation in SPET rCBF studies. Xenon studies provided poor resolution and little information about deep cerebral structures. However, Tc 99m HMPAO is lipophilic and its uptake is proportional to blood flow for about five minutes after administration, following which it becomes hydrophilic and is no longer taken up by tissues. Thus a patient may receive an injection of the ligand some time prior to scanning, and SPET imaging at a later time (allowing for loss due to radiation decay) will reflect the rCBF during the five minutes following injection. This facilitates the study of patients with psychiatric disorders because the ligand may be injected in a calm environment, thus minimizing the influence of anxiety or hyperventilation on rCBF. Moreover, the specific anxiogenic potential of the SPET scanner is now much less of a problem.

Functional MRI (fMRI)

Increased neuronal activity raises the demand for metabolic energy and leads to an increase in regional cerebral blood flow. Local oxygen utilization changes the ratio of oxygenated to deoxygenated haemoglobin in blood. This in turn alters the MR signal from nearby hydrogen nuclei because deoxygenated haemoglobin is paramagnetic. This

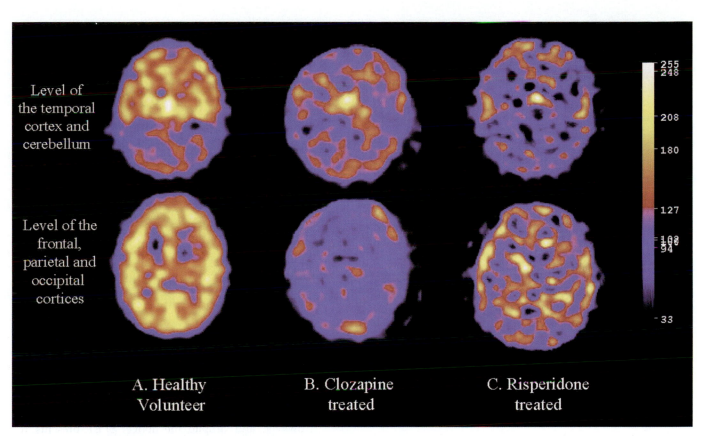

Figure 34.5 Single photon emission tomograms (SPET) of the brain using 123I-5-I-R91150, a ligand that binds selectively and reversibly with serotonin 5HT2A receptors. Binding of the ligand to the receptor (yellow and orange areas) is demonstrated in (**A**) a healthy volunteer at the level of the temporal cortex and cerebellum (upper image) and at the level of the frontal, parietal and occipital cortices (lower image). (**B**) displays binding at the same levels in the brain of a patient with schizophrenia treated with clozapine 450 mg per day while (**C**) displays binding at these levels in the brain of a patient with schizophrenia treated with risperidone 6 mg per day. These SPET scans indicate that both clozapine and risperidone bind to the 5HT2A receptor in vivo.

(Image courtesy of Dr. M. J. Travis, Institute of Psychiatry, London.)

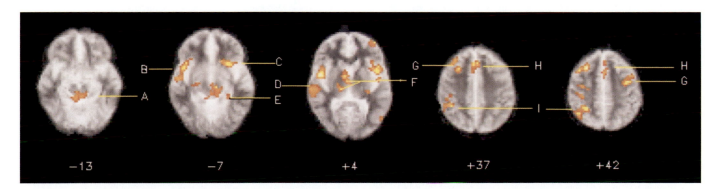

Figure 34.6 Functional MR imaging of brain activation during sampling of auditory hallucinations in schizophrenia. The five transverse sections are relative to the AC–PC plane, the numbers below the sections indicating their level with respect to this plane. The right side of the patient's brain is represented on the left side of each image and vice versa. The red to yellow colour scale illustrates regions active in phase with auditory hallucinations with the areas of greatest significance in yellow. The grey scale template was calculated by voxel-by-voxel averaging of the individual EPI images of 6 patients, following transformation into Talairach space. The main activations are in the right inferior colliculus (A), the right and left insulae (B and C), the right superior temporal gyrus (D), the left paraphippocampal gyrus (E) and the right thalamus (F). Similar activations are present in the middle frontal (G) and the anterior cingulate (H) gyri bilaterally, and in the right inferior parietal lobule extending into the superior lobule (I).

(Image courtesy of Dr S. Shergill, Institute of Psychiatry, London.)

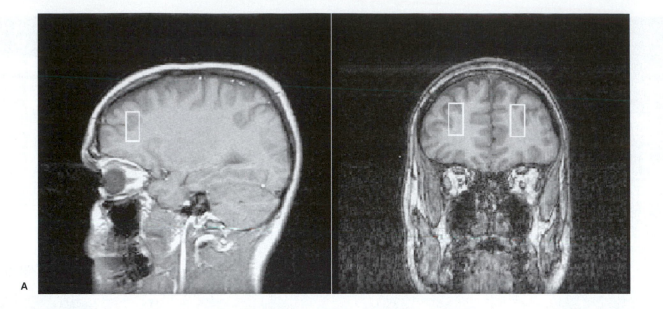

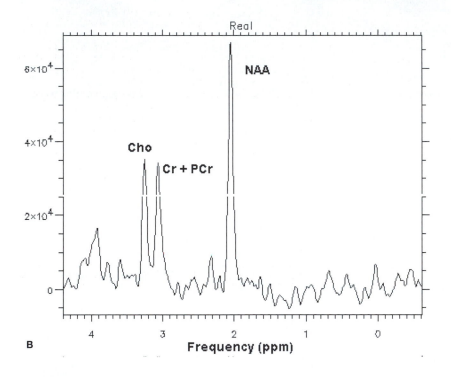

Figure 34.7 Magnetic resonance spectroscopy (MRS). (**A**) shows the location within the brain using coronal and sagittal magnetic resonance images of spectroscopic voxels from which a processed proton MRS spectrum may be derived. (**B**) displays a typical processed proton MRS spectrum from the frontal lobe in a healthy volunteer. The major metabolite peaks, N-acetyl aspartate (NAA) - an amino acid found only in neurons and therefore used as a neuronal marker, choline (Cho) and creatine and phosphocreatine (Cr1PCr), are indicated.

(Images courtesy of Neuroimaging Department, Maudsley Hospital, London.)

change in signal intensity is referred to as the blood oxygenation level dependent (BOLD) effect. Using recently developed techniques that allow the rapid acquisition of MR images (such as echoplanar imaging) data from numerous slices through the brain may be collected from an individual at rest or performing control or test procedures. The resulting fMR images may then be compared, areas of altered signal intensity identified and the underlying regional brain structures involved in a particular task determined (Fig. 34.6).

The excellent temporal and spatial resolution of the MR technology, its lack of ionizing radiation and its ease of use is revolutionizing neuroimaging and our understanding of the brain. It appears likely that this functional imaging technique will soon take its place in clinical psychiatric practice.

MR spectroscopy (MRS)

MRS is an MR dependent neuroimaging technique that allows quantification of brain neurochemistry. Radio-frequency pulses applied at the Lamour frequency cause protons to absorb, and later emit, energy (see above). However, the Lamour frequency of protons is modified by the electrons of nearby atoms which shield the protons from an external magnetic field. The extent of shielding depends on the atoms in the molecule in which the protons are incorporated. Thus protons in water molecules have a different Lamour frequency to protons in creatinine. This phenomenon, or chemical shift, may be presented graphically as points on the x-axis, each point representing the Lamour frequency of protons in different molecules. If quantitative data about the concentration of protons in specific voxels is then presented on the y-axis, an MR spectrum may be generated (Fig. 34.7).

The three metabolites detected most easily by MRS are N-acetyl aspartate (NAA), creatine1phosphocreatine (Cr1PCr) and choline (Cho). NAA is one of the most abundant amino acids in the brain. Its role is not yet fully understood but it is found only in neurons and may therefore be used as a neuronal marker (Maier 1995). MRS depended initially on detecting proton signals from relatively large single voxels (single voxel imaging). More recently, it has become possible to simultaneously detect signals from multiple voxels and thus to generate metabolite maps of the brain (chemical shift imaging) (Lim et al. 1998). In addition to protium (^{1}H), other isotopes that possess nuclear spin include fluorine (^{19}F), sodium (^{23}Na), phosphorus (^{31}P) and lithium (^{7}Li). This allows MRS detection in the brain of molecules that incorporate these isotopes, and phosphorus and proton MRS have been used extensively to investigate brain energy metabolism. Furthermore, the preliminary use of MRS in the evaluation of psychopharmacological compounds has already been reported (Maier 1995). It therefore appears likely that MRS, like fMRI, will soon have a place in clinical psychiatric practice (Malhi et al. 2002).

REFERENCES

Berger H (1931) Uber das electroenkephalogramm des Menschen III. *Archiv fur Psychiatrie und Nervenkrankheiten* **94**: 16–22.

Blackwood DHR & Muir WJ (1990) Cognitive brain potentials and their application. *British Journal of Psychiatry* **157**(suppl 9): 96–101.

Chakos MH, Lieberman JA & Alvir J (1995) Caudate nucleii volumes in schizophrenic patients treated with typical antipsychotics and clozapine. *Lancet* **345**: 456–7.

Dummermuth G (1968) Variance spectra of EEGs in twins. In: Kellaway P & Peterssen I (eds) *Clinical Electroencephalography of Children*. New York: Grune and Stratton.

Eeg-Olofsson O (1970) The development of the EEG in normal children and adolescents from the age of 1 through 21 years. *Acta Paediatrica Scandinavica* **208**(Suppl.).

Falleti MG, Maruff P, Collie A, Darby DG & McStephen M (2003) Qualitative similarities in cognitive impairment associated with 24 h of sustained wakefulness and a blood alcohol concentration of 0.05%. *Journal of Sleep Research* **12**(4): 265–74.

Fenwick PBC (1992) Use of the EEG in psychiatry. In: Weller M & Eysenck M (eds) *The Scientific Basis of Psychiatry*. London: WB Saunders.

Fox NC, Freeborough PA & Rossor MN (1996) Visualisation and quantification of rates of atrophy in Alzheimer's disease. *Lancet* **348**: 94–7.

Jakobi W & Winkler H (1927) Encephalographische studien auf chronisch schizophrenen. *Archiv fur Psychiatrie und Nervenkrankheiten* **81**: 299–332.

Johnstone EC, Crow TJ, Frith CD et al. (1976) Cerebral ventricular size and cognitive impairment in chronic schizophrenia. *Lancet* **ii**: 924–86.

Larkin EP et al. (1985) The X-ray department and psychiatry. *British Journal of Psychiatry* **146**: 62–5.

Lim KO, Adalsteinsson E, Spielman D et al. (1998) Proton magnetic resonance spectroscopic imaging with spiral-based k-space trajectories. *Archives of General Psychiatry* **55**: 346–52.

Maier M (1995) In vivo magnetic resonance spectroscopy: applications in clinical psychiatry. *British Journal of Psychiatry* **167**: 299–306.

Malhi GS, Valenzuela M, Wen W & Sachdev P (2002) Magnetic resonance spectroscopy and its applications in psychiatry. *Australia and New Zealand Journal of Psychiatry* **36**(1): 31–43.

Muller TJ, Kalus P & Strik WK (2001).The neurophysiological meaning of auditory P300 in subtypes of schizophrenia. *World Journal of Biological Psychiatry* **2**(1): 9–17.

Obrist WD & Busse EW (1965) In: Wilson WP (ed.) *Applications of Electroencephalography in Psychiatry*. Durham, NC: Duke University Press.

Samkoff JS & Jacques CH (1991) A review of studies concerning effects of sleep deprivation and fatigue on residents' performance. *Academic Medicine* **66**(11): 687–93.

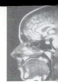

Emergency psychiatry

John M Cooney

INTRODUCTION

Emergency psychiatry encompasses that clinical practice which is directed towards the treatment of distressed patients with acute psychiatric disorders. Such treatment may involve reassurance, direction to other medical or non-medical resources, the prescribing of medication or admission to hospital. Whatever intervention is indicated, a psychiatric emergency demands that it be provided immediately. Thus, the role of the psychiatrist or mental health professional is primarily to make a decision on the further management of the patient. It follows therefore, that adequate information about the patient's presenting problem, and assessment of the individual and their circumstances in an objective manner, is critical. At all times consideration must be given to the safety of patients, professional colleagues and third parties.

Emergency psychiatry has considerable overlap with general psychiatry but it warrants consideration as a specialist topic for several reasons. The trend towards de-institutionalization means that vulnerable patients are exposed to rigors of daily life that are demanding and may be overwhelming. Psychiatric patients are more conspicuous in the community and in the media through the reporting of episodes of violence and this leads to subsequent public disquiet. This makes patients more likely to attend an emergency service either at their own request or at that of a third party. Debate continues as to the true prevalence of violent incidents committed by psychiatric patients and as to whether community care has resulted in their increase. There is no debate that one consequence of community care for psychiatrists and their colleagues is that risk has assumed primacy when dealing with patients. This is nowhere more evident than in emergency psychiatry – safe, coherent and rapid decision-making is paramount.

Clinicians working in an emergency situation must deal primarily with symptoms rather than with diagnoses. The environment in which emergency psychiatry is practised is often less controlled than a ward setting or a community base and patients or their relatives or friends may be unable or unwilling to provide collateral information. The clinical approach is therefore necessarily pragmatic and directed towards finding the best-fit solution within the constraints of the patient's symptoms and available services, effectively implementing this solution, and most importantly, documenting the process and decision. This calls for considerable common sense and judgement on the part of the clinician, as well as knowledge of psychiatry and of the applicable ethical and medicolegal environment.

This chapter will consider the general clinical approach to patients in the emergency context. Special consideration will be given to clinical presentations that are common, that cross diagnostic boundaries, and that are associated with the greatest degree of risk, especially the risk of violence and suicide. As patients present with symptoms it is more appropriate to address these rather than to address diagnoses. This approach also allows for consideration of the frequently changing elements of the emergency psychiatry consultation.

The assessments of emergencies occurs within the legal framework of common law. Thus, if there is an immediate threat to the integrity or safety of any individual, action may be taken to the extent that is necessary to neutralize the threat. Between this common law duty and the powers of compulsory detention and treatment most jurisdictions provide, lies the duty to care for and protect the individual civil rights of patients incumbent upon all psychiatrists. Thus, the provision of valid consent to treatment requires that the patient understands the likely nature and purpose of the proposed treatment and the consequences of not agreeing to it. A critical element in obtaining consent is consideration of how much information to make available. This is dictated by the Bolam Test, which directs disclosure only of the risks and consequences that a responsible body of medical opinion would disclose in identical circumstances. To proceed with treatment in the absence of valid consent constitutes battery. The responsibilities of duty of care require that a practitioner assesses and treats patients with a competence commensurate with their professional experience. This necessitates consulting with, or referring to, more experienced colleagues when appropriate. A wrong decision or a decision that leads to an untoward incident is not in itself negligent; a wrong decision made without following usual clinical procedures such as reading case notes, gathering available information and examining the patient may well represent negligence. However, the reality of emergency practice is that conditions are often less than ideal and usual sources of information may not be available. For example it may be necessary to assess a hostile patient, relatives may not be available, or clinical records may be missing. In the absence of adequate information, it is essential to briefly document this absence and the reasons for it.

The environment in which emergency psychiatry is practised often makes the protection of confidentiality a major issue. In order for patients to disclose intimate details about themselves and their illness, they must be confident that their privacy will be respected. Conflict arises with the threat of violence. If a clinician discovers that a patient constitutes a threat to another individual, under the Tarasoff Doctrine not only is it permissible to warn that person but there is an obligation to do so. However, in general, a psychiatrist is bound by the same ethical obligations in the emergency context as in standard clinical practice.

A GENERAL CLINICAL APPROACH TO PSYCHIATRIC EMERGENCIES

Behaviour that is considered abnormal, bizarre or uncharacteristic may be construed as evidence of mental illness. The role of the emergency psychiatrist is to establish if in fact the disturbance represents mental illness. Emergency evaluations typically take place in accident and emergency departments and there are often significant pressures on psychiatrists, and often relatively in-experienced psychiatrists, to satisfy the demands of other parties such as accident and emergency personnel, the police force or patients' relatives. Time may be more limited than is desirable. However, it is extremely uncommon for there not to be sufficient time available for adequate consideration of the patient and their problem. The major exception to this is when there is an immediate threat to the safety of an individual because of imminent or ongoing violence directed at self or at others. In contrast, potential damage to property represents only a relative reason for deferring a considered objective evaluation. Violence will be considered in more detail later.

The request for an emergency consultation

The request for an emergency consultation represents an important opportunity to influence outcome. For example,

while discussing the referral with the referrer, it may be possible to determine if the patient has attended another hospital or is a current patient there, in which case referral to that hospital should be advised unless there are specific contraindications. Otherwise, details of the patient and the referral source should be noted, and the names and contact details of relatives, carers and keyworkers recorded. Information as to the nature of the presenting complaint and the reason it represents an acute problem should be sought, in addition to relevant past history. It is often very useful to ask that a reliable informant accompany the patient and the availability or otherwise of such an informant may help in deciding where to evaluate the patient and whether to do so alone, with the collateral informant, or with a professional colleague.

Subjective emergency assessment of a patient

Psychiatry is above all else a clinical speciality and the interview with the patient forms the cornerstone of the assessment. Thus how it is conducted is crucial to the resolution of the presenting problem. A methodical approach ensures that vital information is not neglected. Dealing with acutely disturbed or frightened people is challenging and the need for a calm approach is paramount in order to ensure that the patient remains at ease during the interview. A calm approach is facilitated by a safe setting for the interview. The interview room should be readily accessible to other staff so that help is available if necessary, neither patient nor practitioner should feel trapped (but if there is only one exit it is best if the interviewer sits nearest to it), the room should be clean and suitably furnished and a panic alarm should be available in the event of the need to summon help quickly. It is unwise to interview a patient alone if threatening or violent behaviour has occurred recently or there is a past history of such behaviour. It may be useful to have a relative present to reassure and calm a patient, but it may be the patient's relatives who are threatening and they should not be interviewed alone in this case. It is essential to ensure that individuals who can provide collateral information remain available or contactable and their names, addresses and telephone numbers should be sought before the patient is interviewed.

It is rarely possible to obtain a full psychiatric history on every patient referred as an emergency. However, it is essential to obtain sufficient information to allow a full understanding of the presenting problem and permit the development of an acceptable course of action. As a minimum, and even in the most constrained circumstances, there should be sufficient information available for risk assessment. This topic has become a central issue in clinical practice and will be dealt with in more detail later.

Patients referred as emergencies are likely to be distressed, so it is very important to provide an adequate explanation of the evaluation process. Colleagues should be introduced and reassurance provided that advice or treatment is usually possible once an understanding of the problem is reached. It may occasionally be necessary to administer medication prior to the interview and careful clinical judgement should be exercised. Patients attending emergency services may be doing so for the first time, or may have a recurrence of chronic problems. The amount of time spent reassuring and orientating the patient should be tailored accordingly. Of necessity the emergency interview will focus on the presenting problem rather than on other areas of standard enquiry such as family or developmental history. Such information should be collected only if it is crucial to the onset of the presenting problem or points towards potential solutions, and seeking precipitants, predisposing and perpetuating factors is certainly a useful way of understanding the problem. It is also useful to estimate the patient's expectations and those of their carers because potential solutions will require their cooperation and help. Furthermore, a knowledge of expectations helps in framing explanations and recommendations.

Objective emergency assessment of a patient

The objective examination or mental state examination should occur in parallel with history taking. Observations of appearance and behaviour, and in particular of the patient's attitude to the evaluation and their emotional response to it are vital. Movement and speech may provide vital evidence of the patient's emotional state. Mood must always be assessed. **Specific enquiry must always be made about suicide**. The form and content of thought should be examined by direct questioning about perceptual abnormalities, passivity phenomena and delusions. Cognitive examination is crucial in determining whether the presentation has an organic basis or not. Thus orientation should be checked as a minimum and a more extended examination conducted if indicated. The Folstein mini mental state examination is a valid and reliable screening instrument for use in such situations. Assessment of insight is particularly important in determining further management (see elsewhere in this volume).

There is no situation in psychiatry in which physical examination is of more importance than in the emergency context. Commonly, patients are referred from the community by non-medical staff, general practitioners may only see a patient for a brief period and the referral circumstances may dictate postponement of physical examination. It is rarely possible or necessary to perform a complete physical examination on all patients referred as emergencies. Clinical judgement should therefore be exercised but as a minimum, vital signs should always be recorded and any abnormality pursued by appropriate examination and investigation. And on a practical note, it is

clearly easier to obtain a general medical or surgical opinion from a colleague in an accident and emergency department while a patient is there than after transfer to a psychiatric ward.

The collateral history is an extremely important source of information and may indicate potential solutions for the patient. Securing contact details for informants prior to the interview with the patient and then making time to discuss the patient with them is important. It is crucial to establish the nature of an informant's relationship with the patient and the patient's consent should be sought prior to speaking with any third party. Whether collateral information should be sought in the presence of the patient or separately is a matter of clinical judgement.

Completing the emergency assessment

It is imperative that attempts are made to obtain further relevant information from medical records or elsewhere when this exists and to note its absence if it does not exist or is not available. The complete emergency assessment of a patient will be based on the subjective and objective examinations and the evaluation of this additional material. A psychiatric diagnosis should be specified if there is one to be made, and if not, a thorough explanation of the problem is required.

THE PLAN OF TREATMENT

The plan of treatment follows from the assessment and the key issue concerns safety and risk. Thus the location at which help or treatment will be provided must be decided upon. A decision needs to be made as to whether admission is indicated, for example. This may be mandatory if there is significant risk of harm to the patient or others and an alternative solution is not possible in the wider community. Admission is also indicated for further assessment of a patient with a first psychotic episode. In general, such patients warrant admission for a period of observation to define their symptomatology further, and in order to rapidly conduct a battery of physical investigations. The availability of safe alternatives to admission always needs to be evaluated carefully, particularly where there is significant risk. It is rarely necessary to act directly contrary to the wishes of patients' relatives and it must be borne in mind that many psychiatric disorders are long-term conditions that the relatives of patients have been and will be involved with for much longer than individual members of medical teams. If a patient is admitted, the specific reasons for this and concerns about risk should always be made explicit to nursing colleagues. General practitioners and key workers in the community should be made aware of the names of emergency personnel and their contact details, prior to the patient being discharged from hospital.

Assessment and management of risk

The assessment of risk is inherent in good clinical practice and does not impose any further burden on psychiatrists. Risk is the probability that harm will occur and in contrast to dangerousness, it is a dynamic concept that varies over time and whose accuracy for short-term prediction is useful (Ferris et al. 1997). Emergency consultations have always been about risk, and Box 35.1 outlines the areas of specific enquiry that must be considered and documented because they inform the assessment and management of risk. It is clear that not all of this information will be available in the emergency setting but efforts to gather it subsequently must be made. Psychopathology has a small independent effect on risk and it has been estimated that if schizophrenia were preventable, crime in the community would only decrease

by 3% (Wessley 1997). It is important to note that, despite popular belief, there is evidence that patients act upon their delusions and are more likely to do so if these are affectively charged (Buchanan 1997). The most powerful predictors of risk operate in both patients and non-patients (Bonta et al. 1998) and include:

- criminal history/previous high risk behaviour
- antisocial personality
- substance abuse
- family dysfunction.

If risk assessment is concerned with establishing the likelihood of risk, risk management is about modifying outcome. When a risk is identified, there is a responsibility to act to ensure reduction of the risk. This entails the development of a management plan agreed upon by all involved in the patient's care. This should include contingency plans if problems arise, and contact details – personnel and location – for patients and their carers. The management plan should also include warning signs of incipient increase in risk and specify a date for review. In most psychiatric settings, the development of a risk management plan involves multidisciplinary team meetings, but this is not possible in the emergency situation. Pragmatic decisions therefore need to be made in the knowledge of the appropriate standards of clinical care under ideal circumstances.

Box 35.1 The assessment of risk (Royal College of Psychiatrists 1996)

History

Previous violence and/or suicidal behaviour

Evidence of rootlessness or 'social restlessness', for example few relationships, frequent changes of address or employment

Evidence of poor compliance with treatment or disengagement from psychiatric aftercare

Presence of substance misuse or other potential disinhibiting factors, for example a social background promoting violence

Identification of any precipitants and any changes in mental state or behaviour that have occurred prior to violence and/or relapse

Are these risk factors stable or have any of them changed recently?

Evidence of recent severe stress, particularly of loss events or the threat of loss

Evidence of recent discontinuation of medication

Environment

Does the patient have access to potential victims, particularly individuals identified in mental state abnormalities?

Mental state

Evidence of any threat/control override symptoms: firmly held beliefs of persecution by others (persecutory delusions), or of mind or body being controlled or interfered with by external forces (delusions of passivity)

Emotions related to violence, for example irritability, anger, hostility, suspiciousness

Specific threats made by the patient

Conclusion

A formulation should be made based on these and all other items of history and mental state. The formulation should, so far as possible, specify factors likely to increase the risk of dangerous behaviour and those likely to decrease it. The formulation should aim to answer the following questions:

How serious is the risk?

Is the risk specific or general?

How immediate is the risk?

How volatile is the risk?

What specific treatment, and which management plan, can bes reduce the risk?

AGGRESSION AND VIOLENCE IN THE EMERGENCY SETTING

Most aggression and violence in society is not due to mental illness. When violence occurs the issues of importance for the emergency psychiatrist are safety, recognition of the role of psychopathology and the initiation of measures to reduce the possibility of recurrence. Thus the psychiatrist must be able to:

- recognize signs of incipient violence and prevent it from occurring
- deal with violent incidents
- prevent recurrence of violence.

Therefore, the psychiatrist in such situations should avail him- or herself of known strategies for verbal diffusion of the threat of violence while assessing the underlying cause of the violence.

Threatened violence

The general principles outlined above should always be applied. When a request for an emergency consultation is made there will usually be some indication of the potential for violence. The details of this must be pursued before the

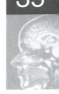

patient is assessed. This is critical because while non-psychiatrists can physically restrain the patient only a psychiatrist can apply the knowledge base required to examine for psychopathology and subsequently determine and implement an appropriate course of action. The emergency psychiatrist should therefore gather the available information and resist the urge to 'do something'. Clinical judgement is important and dealing with a patient you know well and who has previously been violent when psychotic requires a different approach from that applied to a patient presenting for the first time. Safety requires adequate consideration of the site of interview and the personnel who should be present, care should be taken with clothing, and potential weapons such as jewellery or scarves should be avoided.

The threatening patient should be approached from the front in a calm and confident manner. The personal space that should not be intruded on is four times larger than normal in violent persons and greater to the rear and sides than the front (Parks 1990) so the interviewer should be at least two metres from a threatening individual. Facial expression should be attentive and the patient should be addressed at a slight angle rather than face to face, which could be interpreted as confrontational. Prolonged direct eye contact should be avoided because patients in such situations will often stare intently. Hands should be kept in the midline because folded arms or hands on the hips can be construed as evidence of disrespect, hostility or confrontation in a person already aroused. The interviewer should not turn away from the patient to present the back. It is safer to turn to one side and move back if required for safety reasons.

When speaking to a threatening patient it is important to make a clear introduction and address the patient with respect, using their title (Mr, Mrs, etc.). Ask the patient what is troubling them and focus on the emotional content of their response. It is important to convey to the patient that their point of view will be listened to and empathized with, even if not agreed with. Contrary views to those of the patient should be expressed later, if at all. From time to time it is helpful to remind the patient of who you are and it can be helpful to induce an atmosphere of cooperativeness by discussing the elements of the patient's problem that can be agreed upon and resolved. It is not helpful to make unrealistic promises about further help. It is important to avoid making the patient lose face and to promote a sense of autonomy if possible, for example by offering medication if appropriate. It does not help to be confrontational or aggressive but equally, it must be professionally and dispassionately conveyed that violence is unacceptable. Acknowledging the person's capacity to harm others and offering the alternative solution of dialogue is one means of achieving this.

Clues to incipient violence will come from observation of the patient's appearance and behaviours – glaring, muscular tension, restlessness, and movements that are more rapid or deliberate are all warning signs, while speech that is louder, more strident and more profane reflects a patient's arousal and irritability.

Actual violence

Safety is paramount when violence occurs, and attempts to restrain a patient should not be undertaken when alone or in the absence of adequate numbers of personnel who have received training in restraint techniques. This implies at least five people – one per limb and one to control/protect the patient's head. It is preferable that one trained person be team leader and coordinate the response, and for the interviewing doctor to withdraw and allow the emergency team to act. Published guidelines address this topic and make suggestions for clinical standards in the management of situations involving violence, and psychiatrists should be familiar with these and with the procedures of the institution in which patients are assessed. Guidelines on the management of disturbed behaviour in inpatient psychiatric settings are being developed by NICE, the National Institute for Clinical Excellence, but are not yet available. However, considerable advice is contained within the publication entitled *Schizophrenia: Core Interventions in the Treatment and Management of Schizophrenia in Primary and Secondary Care* (NICE 2002).

When violence occurs, the emergency psychiatrist must consider three principal differential diagnoses:

1. Violence of organic origin:
   - drugs (iatrogenic and of abuse) and alcohol
   - brain trauma, tumours, infections, infarctions, inflammation, demyelination, degeneration and epilepsy. Systemic disorders including metabolic disturbances such as porphyrias, hypoglycaemia, electrolyte imbalances, uraemia, hepatic encephalopathy, and hypoxia. Endocrine dysfunction as in Cushing's and Addison's, thyroid disease (hyper- and hypo-), vitamin deficiency, infections and poisoning.
2. Violence of psychotic origin:
   - affective disorder and schizophrenia.
3. Violence of non-organic, non-psychotic (behavioural disturbance) origin:
   - where there is no acute or gross abnormality of brain or mind but when there may be abnormality of emotional development or maturation.

The management of violence will depend on which category the disturbed behaviour falls into. The general measures available to manage violence include:

1. Physical:
   - restraint
   - isolation or seclusion
   - medication.

2 Psychological:
- establish relationship
- provide alternatives to violence, such as taking medication or discussion.

3 Social:
- practical problem-solving about precipitants, e.g. advising about access to benefits.

More specific measures for managing violence depend upon which of the three causes is involved:

1 **Violence of organic origin:** safety and containment of violence have primacy, following which the underlying cause should be sought and treated. Verbal diffusion may be appropriate initially and frequent orientation of the patient is often helpful. Psychotropic agents should be used sparingly and titrated carefully against changes in mental state examinations. An intensive level of nursing care and observation should always be provided.

2 **Violence of psychotic origin:** safety and containment of violence have primacy. Consideration should be given to an organic cause in a patient known to suffer with a chronic psychotic disorder in the presence of new or uncharacteristic behaviour. Verbal diffusion should be attempted as a first option. If necessary, psychotropic agents should be administered initially for their psychomotor effects and should be titrated against arousal and agitation. Patients should subsequently be maintained on antipsychotic medication necessary to resolve psychotic symptoms. An intensive level of nursing care is necessary.

3 **Violence of nonorganic, nonpsychotic (behavioural disturbance) origin:** safety and containment of the patient are the first priorities. An organic or psychotic origin should be excluded in the course of the assessment. It is important to establish the basis for the incident in an empathetic and nonjudgemental manner. Verbal diffusion may be possible, for example by outlining options including medication (taking care that this was not the goal of the outburst in the first place). It may be useful to apportion responsibility for the disturbance as this clarifies the situation and is educational for perpetrator, psychiatrist and colleagues.

Seclusion

The maintenance of safety and/or the containment of violence may require the use of seclusion or pharmacotherapy. Indications for seclusion include:

- to prevent imminent harm to others, namely staff and other patients, if other means are inappropriate or ineffective
- to prevent imminent harm to the patient if other means are inappropriate or ineffective

- to prevent serious disruption of the treatment programme or significant damage to the environment
- to decrease the stimulation the patient receives
- at the patient's request.

Patients have expressed a preference for medication rather than prolonged restraint or seclusion in situations where they have behaved violently (Royal College of Psychiatrists 1998). This report confirms previous work by Harris et al. (1989) in which the following hierarchy of preferred treatments was conceived by patients and nursing staff:

- manual restraint and oral medication
- removal of clothing and intramuscular medication
- seclusion and restraint with constant observation.

There is very little comparative data examining the effects of seclusion compared with the effects of medication as required/requested, behavioural intervention or physical restraint. It is noteworthy that patients not only experience seclusion as traumatic but up to 50% are unaware of the reason for seclusion, while a similar proportion experience no benefit and 90% are unaware of being monitored while in seclusion (Harris et al. 1989).

Such findings have led to the formulation of clear guidelines for the use of seclusion. The emergency psychiatrist must be aware of the standards of good practice when seclusion is used, such as those produced by the Royal College of Psychiatrists (1998), which are as follows.

- Particular care is needed in heavily medicated, physically unwell or intoxicated patients.
- An observation schedule must be specified.
- A doctor must be present within the first few minutes of seclusion.
- A nurse must be in sight or sound throughout (present if the patient is sedated).
- There must be a nursing review every 15 minutes and a medical review every 4 hours.
- The patient must not be deprived of clothing and must be able to call for assistance.
- A full record of the seclusion incident must be made according to a specified format.

Nursing staff should receive training in the use of seclusion, and there is evidence that such training produces a reduction in violent incidents and thus a reduction in the need for seclusion and restraint.

Pharmacotherapy

Rapid tranquilization is the term used to describe the acute treatment of aggression or violence by pharmacological means. Despite the many concerns over the safety of agents used, it is striking how little clear objective data there is in this area. The trend in recent years has been for the use of lower doses of neuroleptics because of their cardiotoxicity in patients who may be dehydrated, nutritionally depleted, intoxicated or otherwise physically compromised. Benzodiazepines are used increasingly in parallel with antipsychotics in emergencies. In general, oral administration of medication is preferable, although clearly not always practicable. The emerging evidence base for parenteral administration of atypical antipsychotics is useful in focusing attention on this sometimes difficult to manage and difficult to study population. It should be borne in mind that the efficacy of newer agents has been established in patients who have been able to give consent and by definition, are not the most severely disturbed. Clinical practice will help the further evaluation of these agents in this more severely ill population. There is little difference in terms of time to onset of action between orally and intramuscularly administered medication (Dubin et al. 1985). Faced with a violent patient, these differences may seem relevant, however, and of course patients who refuse orally administered medication may require parenteral treatment.

Guidance on rapid tranquillization is available from NICE within the publication entitled *Schizophrenia: Core Interventions in the Treatment and Management of Schizophrenia in Primary and Secondary Care* (NICE 2002). The most important pharmacological recommendations made by NICE are as follows:

- Oral administration of medication is preferred to parenteral administration from the perspective of patients' dignity.
- When parenteral administration of medication is required, intramuscular administration is preferred to intravenous administration from the perspective of patients' safety.
- The intramuscular drugs recommended for rapid tranquillisation are haloperidol, lorazepam and olanzapine.
- A single drug is preferred to a combination of drugs whenever possible.
- If haloperidol (or another typical antipsychotic drug) is administered intramuscularly, an anticholinergic drug should also be administered in order to reduce the risk of acute dystonia and other extrapyramidal side-effects.
- Diazepam and chlorpromazine are not recommended for intramuscular administration.

The three drugs recommended by NICE for intramuscular use during rapid tranquillization will now be described and there will follow a description of other drugs that may also be used.

Haloperidol

This is probably the most widely used drug at present. It is a high-potency agent with low cholinergic, adrenergic, serotonergic and histaminergic binding, but it frequently causes extrapyramidal symptoms (see NICE recommendations above). Should haloperidol be administered by the intravenous (IV) or intramuscular (IM) route? The IV route is not recommended by NICE, while IV haloperidol produces a slightly more rapid onset of action, mean aggression scores fall only slightly more rapidly than following IM administration, and IV administration is associated with a higher risk of adverse effects. The usual dose is 5–10 mg, which may be repeated within one hour and continued up to a maximal dose of 60 mg in 24 hours. However, experimental evidence indicates that doses above 10–15 mg do not produce added benefit (Baldessarini et al. 1988).

Lorazepam

This short-acting (half-life 10–18 hours) benzodiazepine has inactive glucuronide metabolites and is well absorbed following intramuscular administration (in contrast to diazepam whose absorption is impaired by the acidic environment of active muscles). Effects are evident within one hour and persist for up to six hours. Acute dosage is 2–4 mg, which may be repeated after two hours.

Olanzapine

This is the only atypical antipsychotic available in the UK for intramuscular in the acutely disturbed patient. Reduction in agitation and disturbed behaviour is evident within 15 minutes (T_{MAX} is 30-40 minutes) and increases to a maximum at two hours (Wright et al. 2001). The initial dosage is 10 mg and further injections may be administered to a maximum cumulative dose of 20 mg in 24 hours. Acute dystonia was not observed during clinical trials. In addition to olanzapine, intramuscular formulations of ziprasidone are available in some countries. It is hoped that parenteral olanzapine and ziprasidone will allow tranquillization and early initiation of atypical antipsychotic therapy and thus an improved safety profile and smoother transition to atypical antipsychotic maintenance therapy.

Zuclopenthixol acetate

This oil-based preparation of the sedative thioxanthine zuclopenthixol is of proven efficacy in the rapid tranquillization of psychotically disturbed patients (Chakravarti et al. 1990). Its effects are prolonged – at least 72 hours – and it must never be administered as the first agent to neuroleptic-naive patients. Peak effects are seen 24–40 hours after administration. Single doses are from 50 to 150 mg and a single additional dose may be administered 1-2 days following the first or, more commonly, 2-3 days after the first, up to a maximum of 400 mg in two weeks. Maintenance medication should be commenced 2–3 days after the last injection. Chouinard et al. (1994) reported no difference in scores on the Brief Psychiatric Rating Scale (BPRS) between acutely psychotic schizophrenic patients treated with zuclopenthixol acetate 50–150 mg IM every 2–3 days when compared to patients receiving oral haloperidol 10–30 mg three times daily, while patients treated with haloperidol achieved benefit in terms of reduced hostility and fewer side-effects.

Chlorpromazine

This is used infrequently because of concerns about excess mortality, the potent α_1 adrenergic blockade and marked postural hypotension. It is not recommended by NICE and should be avoided in the elderly because of the risk of falls and subsequent fractures. Doses of 25–50 mg may be administered every 6–8 hours to a maximal dose of 1000 mg in 24 hours, although doses in excess of this have been used widely. Current caution is predominantly related to the indiscriminate nature of its antagonism of adrenergic, cholinergic, histaminergic and serotonergic receptors in addition to its high first-pass metabolism which means that parenteral doses are effectively 2–4 times that of oral doses.

Droperidol

This was widely used as an alternative to haloperidol, and for many was the drug of choice because it demonstrated superior efficacy in violent crises when compared to haloperidol (Resnick & Burton 1984; Thomas et al. 1992). However, droperidol was found to prolong the QTc interval on the electrocardiogram and was removed from clinical use. It was more sedative than haloperidol but it had a higher affinity for α_1 receptors and therefore increased liability to postural hypotension.

Diazepam

This may be administered by slow IV injection in doses of 5–10 mg and has a very rapid onset of action. There is danger of respiratory depression and tachyphylaxis may occur. The half-life of between 50 and 150 hours is relevant to chronic dosing, time to steady state and elimination kinetics.

Amylobarbitone sodium

Very rarely used in modern psychiatric practice, amylobarbitone may be given in a dose of 500 mg IM or IV, which may be repeated after 10 minutes (IV) or 30 minutes (IM). Dose-related central nervous system depression occurs and may be potentiated by other sedative drugs. Barbiturates induce hepatic microsomal enzymes with prolonged usage and are extensively metabolized by the liver. If administering this agent IV, it should be administered at a rate of 50 mg/min or less, because hypotension, laryngospasm and shock have been reported with more rapid rates.

Paraldehyde

Now very rarely used, paraldehyde should be stored in well-filled airtight bottles in complete darkness because of solvent action on rubber and polystyrene which leads to oxidation and the formation of acetic acid. It may cause toxic hepatitis (80% is metabolized in the liver) and up to 20% is excreted unchanged through the lungs. Given in doses of 5–10 mg paraldehyde induces sedation in about 15 minutes. This lasts for approximately eight hours. Paraldehyde causes considerable pain at the injection site.

Nadolol

This non-selective beta-blocker is not recommended for general use. It has a long half-life (14–24 hours), is not lipophilic and therefore does not cross the blood–brain barrier. It may be administered IM once daily in a dosage of 120 mg, as an adjunct to antipsychotic medication in aggressive patients with schizophrenia, and is significantly more effective than placebo (Allan et al. 1996). Contraindications to beta-blockade include asthma and peripheral vascular disease.

SUICIDE IN THE EMERGENCY SETTING

The assessment of suicide risk is one of the most fundamental tasks in psychiatry. Psychiatrists are taught that to enquire about suicide is a mandatory part of evaluation and that such enquiry does not of itself increase the likelihood of a person attempting suicide. Questioning should proceed from the more general to the specific and a standard schema (see Box 35.2) is useful to ensure a methodical approach.

Traditionally, the topics of suicide are dealt with by considering it in terms of suicide per se (or completed suicide) and of parasuicide (or deliberate self-harm). This division is based on differences between these phenomena in terms of demographics, prevalence and outcome. However, for the psychiatrist faced with self-destructive ideation or behaviour, such a division will not always be so apparent. A person's actions or behaviour can arise from many factors including but not necessarily limited to mental illness, so the task of assessing suicidal ideation or acts is to establish why it happened and determine the risk of it happening again. The clinical implication of this is that all patients expressing or carrying out acts of self-harm must be treated with extreme care.

Patients vary enormously in the amount of information that they will disclose about their motivation, the circumstances of the act and other important details. This may be because they are psychomotor retarded by depression and feel worthless and unable to trust anyone, or because they are embarrassed, or angry at not succeeding or at not being taken seriously. There are many reasons for reticence and it is essential for the evaluating psychiatrist to

---

Box 35.2 An example of a standardized scheme of questioning about suicide

How do you see the future?

Is life worthwhile?

Have you thought of harming yourself?

What have you thought of doing?

Have you done this? or How would you go about doing this?

What stops you? or What has stopped you from doing this?

gain sufficient information despite this. Generalizations about patients are dangerous (the clinical adage that the more readily patients disclose their suicidality, the less likely they are to be suicidal is almost certainly incorrect!) and counter-transference can distort clinical judgement, leading to over-identification and inappropriate reassurance that all will be well. The opposite reaction may also occur and it is not uncommon for psychiatrists and colleagues to feel hostility towards patients they perceive as manipulating them. Such feelings can distort the information-gathering process and must be recognized and used as clues to the objective clinical state of the patient (see Chapters 32 and 36).

The assessment of suicide risk may be informed by epidemiological data but must be firmly based on assessment of the individual patient, including evaluation of both risk factors and protective factors. The risk of suicide is not static and an attempt to gain a longitudinal view of its course from both patient and collateral sources is very useful. Box 35.3 provides a summary of risk factors for suicide. It should be noted that the factors listed in Box 35.3 that point to a lower risk of suicide do not imply that there is no risk. It should also be noted that the 75% increase in the suicide rate for young men since 1982, means that suicide is now the second commonest cause of death in this age group after road accidents.

In assessing the suicidal patient it is vital to enquire about:

- intent
- whether there is a psychiatric illness present or not
- the reasons for the act
- the likelihood of repetition or completion.

Intent is best estimated by considering sequentially the patient's preparation (planning, and so-called terminal events such as writing a note or letter, or making a will), the circumstances of the attempt (alone, precautions taken against discovery, belief that planned act was lethal), and the aftermath (not seeking help, stated wish to die, regret of failure). A first attempt that occurred impulsively, with rescue inevitable and using a method of low lethal potential may suggest an attempt by the patient to effect change, a degree of ambivalence, and a lower risk of completion.

Mental illness is a major risk factor for suicide and 90% of those completing suicide have a mental disorder. On the other hand, the majority of psychiatric patients do not kill themselves despite the high prevalence of suicidal ideation. This is not a cause for complacency but an attempt to put mental illness and suicide in perspective.

Of those with mental illness completing suicide, approximately 45% suffer with an affective disorder. In relation to depression, the single most important risk factor in the mental state is hopelessness, while patients with psychotic depression have a five-fold increase in risk relative to patients with major depression without psychotic features. Comorbid alcohol or drug abuse or dependence significantly escalates the risk. The lifetime suicide risk for patients with an affective disorder is generally quoted as 15%, although recent reappraisal of data with sophisticated statistics yields a lower estimate of 6% (Inskip et al. 1998). From a clinical perspective, however, the presence of affective disorder significantly increases the risk of suicide for an individual patient, particularly in the period immediately following diagnosis.

The lifetime risk of suicide for patients with schizophrenia is 10% and is greatest soon after the diagnosis and during any post-psychotic depressive phase, particularly if associated with demoralization and hopelessness. The post-discharge period also represents a time of great risk, requiring particular vigilance.

Alcohol dependence is associated with a lifetime risk of 15% for completed suicide and this risk does not diminish with the passage of time from diagnosis, while about 3–8% of patients with borderline personality disorder kill themselves (McGlashan & Heinssen 1988; Stone et al. 1987). These latter are at risk because of the instability of interpersonal relations, self-image and affect, and the impulsivity, that characterize the disorder. Thus while chronic self-harm may be a way of coping with life for such patients, it is important to recognize comorbid disorders such as depression and clearly evaluate such patients in a systematic manner when they present following self-harm (Kernberg 1984).

Not all patients presenting following self-harm have a diagnosable psychiatric illness. The suicide rate in the UK is 11/100 000, whereas the parasuicide rate for a city such as Oxford is 300/100 000 for women and 400/100 000 for men (National Task Force on Suicide 1996). About 1% of patients presenting with deliberate self-harm will go on to complete suicide during the following year (the majority during the following next six months) (Hawton & Fagg 1988). The rate of psychiatric disorder among this latter group is approximately 20% and thus the majority of patients presenting with deliberate self-harm do not suffer from a mental illness but have other problems that led them to act in this manner. Identification of the pertinent issues and definition of these problems is required as is explanation so that alternatives may be considered by the patient. Thus it is vital to establish the level of domestic and social support available to the patient and to gauge their own personal

Box 35.3   Risk factors for suicide
High-risk factors
Age >45, male, divorced or widowed, unemployed, conflictual interpersonal relationships, chaotic or conflictual family background, depression, alcohol/drug dependence, psychosis, personality disorder, chronic illness, chronic pain, neurological disorders
Low-risk factors
Age <45, female, married, employed, stable interpersonal relations, stable family background

resources as indicated by their capacity to form relationships, maintain employment, deal with adversity and have insight into, and some control over, their emotional state. This approach will facilitate the generation of a problem list (which may include a psychiatric diagnosis) and the clarification of risks and possible alternatives. Management of the patient will depend on this process and upon the personal, domestic, social and statutory supports available.

CONCLUSIONS

Emergency psychiatry cuts across all areas of psychiatric specialization and expertise. What distinguishes it as a speciality is the requirement to make a rapid and effective decision to resolve some need that has provoked presentation by the patient. To do this, the clinician simultaneously operates in two related but distinct clinical dimensions. The first dimension is represented by the need to assess the patient in a logical and methodical manner while all the time attending to safety. This process of assessment and attention to safety requires objectivity at a time and in a situation where there may be immense pressure to act immediately to resolve the problem. This is where the second dimension – the expertise and experience of the psychiatrist - can provide the comprehensive approach that is necessary for the safe and effective resolution of emergencies (see also Chapter 32).

REFERENCES

Allan ER, Alpert M, Sison CE et al. (1996) Adjunctive nadolol in the treatment of acutely aggressive schizophrenic patients. *Journal of Clinical Psychiatry* **57**: 455–9.

Baldessarini RJ, Cohen BM & Teicher MH (1988) Significance of neuroleptic dose and plasma level in the pharmacologic treatment of psychoses. *Archives of General Psychiatry* **45**: 79–91.

Bonta J, Hanson K & Law M (1998) The prediction of criminal and violent recidivism among mentally disordered offenders: a meta-analysis. *Psychological Bulletin* **123**: 123–42.

Buchanan A (1997) The investigation of acting on delusions as a tool for risk assessment in the mentally disordered. *British Journal of Psychiatry* **170**(suppl. 32): 12–16.

Chakravarti SK, Muthu A, Muthu PK, Naik P & Pinto RT (1990) Zuclopenthixol acetate: single dose treatment for acutely disturbed psychotic patients. *Current Medical Opinion Research* **12**: 58–65.

Chouinard G, Safadi G & Beauclair L (1994) A double blind controlled study of zuclopenthixol acetate and liquid oral haloperidol in the treatment of schizophrenic patients with acute exacerbation. *Clinical Psychopharmacology* **38**(suppl. 4): 5114–20.

Dubin WR (1985) Rapid tranquillization, the efficacy of oral concentrate. *Journal of Clinical Psychiatry* **46**: 475–8.

Ferris LE, Sandercock J, Hoffman B et al. (1997) Risk assessment for acute violence to third parties: a review of the literature. *Canadian Journal of Psychiatry* **42**: 1051–60.

Harris GT, Rice ME & Preseon DL (1989) Staff and patients' perceptions of the least restrictive alternatives for the short-term control of disturbed behaviour. *Journal of Psychiatry and Law* **17**: 239–63.

Hawton K & Fagg J (1988) Suicide and other causes of death following attempted suicide. *British Journal of Psychiatry* **159**: 359–66.

Inskip HM, Harris EC & Barraclough B (1998) Lifetime risk of suicide for affective disorder, alcoholism and schizophrenia. *British Journal of Psychiatry* **172**: 35–7.

Kernberg OF (1984) *Severe Personality Disorders: Psychotherapeutic Strategies*. New Haven, CT: Yale University Press.

McGlashan TH & Heinssen RK (1988) Hospital discharge status and long-term outcome for patients with schizophrenia, schizoaffective disorders, borderline personality disorder and unipolar affective disorder. *Archives of General Psychiatry* **45**: 363–8.

National Institute for Clinical Excellence (2002). Schizophrenia: Core Interventions in the Treatment and Management of Schizophrenia in Primary and Secondary Care. Online. Available at: www.nice.org.uk [accessed 26 May 2004].

National Task Force on Suicide (1996) Interim Report. Dublin: Government Publications.

Parks J (1990) Violence. In: Hillard JR (ed.) *Manual of Clinical Emergency Psychiatry*, pp. 147–60. Washington, DC: American Psychiatric Press.

Resnick MP & Burton BT(1984) Droperidol versus haloperidol in the initial management of acutely agitated patients. *Journal of Clinical Psychiatry* **45**: 298–9.

Royal College of Psychiatrists (1996) Special Working Party on Clinical Assessment and Management of Risk. Council Report CR 53. London: Royal College of Psychiatrists.

Royal College of Psychiatrists (1998) *Management of Imminent Violence*. College Research Unit.

Stone MH, Stone DK & Hurt SW (1987) Natural history of borderline patients treated by intensive hospitalization. *Psychiatric Clinics of North America* **10**: 185–207.

Thomas HJ, Schwartz E & Petrilli R (1992) Droperidol versus haloperidol for chemical restraint of agitated and combative patients. *Annals of Emergency Medicine* **21**: 407–13.

Wessley S (1997) The epidemiology of crime, violence and schizophrenia. *British Journal of Psychiatry* **170**(suppl. 32): 8–11.

Wright P, Birkett M, David S, Meehan K, Ferchland I et al. (2001) Double blind, placebo controlled comparison of intramuscular olanzapine and intramuscular haloperidol in the treatment of acute agitation in schizophrenia. *American Journal of Psychiatry* **158**: 1149–51.

Psychotherapy – individual, family and group

Julian Stern

INTRODUCTION

In this chapter, some of the features of the psychotherapies essentially derived from or related to the psychodynamic model, i.e. individual, group and family therapies, are described. Cognitive and behavioural models will be described in Chapter 37.

Psychotherapy is, according to Bateman et al. (2000), 'essentially a conversation which involves listening to and talking with those in trouble, with the aim of helping them understand and resolve their predicament'. It is a broad term used to describe many modes of treatment ranging from psychodynamic therapies to more focused (behavioural and cognitive) therapies, and may involve individual patients, families, couples or groups of otherwise unconnected patients. Therapists may work alone or in couples, supervised 'live' (as in some models of family therapy) or retrospectively.

The psychotherapeutic model also informs much of the work performed in other psychiatric settings, and psychotherapists are often called upon within psychiatry to perform functions other than the treatment of patients, for example consultations to staff groups or the offering of an opinion on a complicated patient or situation on a ward. Thus Gabbard (2000) describes a model of psychodynamic psychiatry that is 'an approach to diagnosis and treatment characterized by a way of thinking about both patient and clinician that includes unconscious conflict, deficits, and distortions of intrapsychic structures and internal object relations, and that integrates these elements with contemporary findings from the neurosciences' (p. 4).

JEROME FRANK'S 'COMMON FEATURES'

Jerome Frank (1961) identified a number of features that are common to all of the psychotherapies. These include:

- an intense emotionally-charged relationship with a person or group

- a rationale or myth explaining the distress and methods for dealing with it
- the provision of new information about the future, the source of the problem and possible alternatives that hold a hope of relief
- non-specific methods of boosting self-esteem
- provision of success experiences
- facilitation of emotional arousal
- the therapy takes place in a locale designated as a place of healing.

While all these factors might describe some of what occurs in psychotherapy, it is difficult to give a real 'flavour' or 'feel' for what goes on within a therapeutic relationship until one takes on a patient for psychotherapy under supervision. Then the full complexity, intrigue and interest of the relationship, of the patient's life, of terms such as transference or counter-transference, come alive. Psychotherapy can then begin to make sense, both as an explanatory model and as a method of treatment. It is in recognition of this, that the Royal College of Psychiatrists (1993) has made the psychotherapeutic treatment of patients a mandatory part of the training of each junior psychiatrist in the UK.

PSYCHODYNAMIC/PSYCHOANALYTIC PSYCHOTHERAPY

This mode of therapy, often termed 'psychotherapy' derives from the work of Sigmund Freud. 'The technique of psychodynamic therapy is a focus on the provision of conscious understanding, primarily through the use of interpretation of the patient's verbalizations and behaviour during the (psychotherapy) session' (Roth & Fonagy 1996, p. 5).

'The best way of understanding psychoanalysis is still by tracing its origin and development', wrote Freud in 1923, and it remains enlightening and enjoyable to read Freud's original works.

Box 36.1 presents an extremely condensed summary of Sigmund Freud's life and writings.

Freud's models of the mind

As Bateman & Holmes (1995) write, Freud's theories of the mind progressed through three main phases: the 'affect trauma' model; the topographical model; and the structural model.

The earliest model is the *affect trauma model*, where Freud was influenced by casualties of the Franco-Prussian war (where such casualties included cases of hysterical paralysis). The idea was of an accumulation of 'dammed up' affects inside the patient which, if released, would threaten psychic equilibrium, and potentially lead to symptoms.

A treatment gradually developed, initially involving hypnosis and subsequently the 'ventilation' of these affects and memories, leading to an emotional 'catharsis' via the fundamental rule of 'free association' with particular reference to repressed childhood memories of physical or sexual trauma. 'Free association' is a key technique in psychoanalysis, in which the patient is invited to talk about anything that comes into his/her mind as completely as possible, no matter how trivial, irrelevant or 'irrational' it may seem.

Why did Freud abandon hypnosis, having been so impressed by Charcot's work with hysterics in Paris, and Janet's descriptions of the successful use of hypnosis in the treatment of hysterics? First, Freud found it difficult to hypnotize some patients, and was also concerned about the possible role of suggestion in such treatments. Furthermore, in the case of Anna O, whom his colleague Breuer had treated (Freud & Breuer 1895) the importance of (sometimes erotic) transference had become manifest.

As Freud's biographer, Ernest Jones (1961, p. 148), wrote:

> (Breuer) decided to bring the treatment to an end...and bade her (Anna O) goodbye. But that evening he was fetched back to find her in a greatly excited state, apparently as ill as ever. The patient, who according to him had appeared to be an asexual being and had never made any allusions to such a forbidden topic throughout the treatment, was now in the throes of an hysterical childbirth, the logical termination of a phantom pregnancy that had been invisibly developing in response to Breuer's ministrations. Though profoundly shocked, he managed to calm her down by hypnotising her, and then fled the house in a cold sweat.

Freud recognized the importance of transference (see below), and over the next decade (1897–1908) abandoned hypnosis in favour of free association.

The *topographical model* implies a spatial model, in which different psychological functions are located in different places. The division of the mind into the unconscious, preconscious and conscious (see below) systems (Freud 1900) ushered in the second phase of Freud's work, still containing echoes of cerebral localization.

A fundamental idea derived from this phase is the contrast between the two principles of mental functioning, i.e. primary process and secondary process. Primary process

---

Box 36.1   Sigmund Freud (1856–1939)

1856 – born in Freiburg (Moravia)

1860 – family moves to Vienna

1873 – Freud enters medical school in Vienna

As a medical student he made original contributions to neurohistology

As a neurologist he made original contributions in the fields of aphasia and cerebral palsy

1885 – visits Charcot in Paris

1886 – returns to Vienna and marries Martha Bernays

1895 – publishes, with Breuer, *Studies in Hysteria*

1896 – publishes *Heredity and the Aetiology of Neuroses* in French. The word 'psychoanalysis' appears for the first time

For the next four decades he was extremely prolific, and his works are collected in the 24-volume 'Standard edition'.

Among his most famous cases were:
- Anna O (with Breuer): *Studies on Hysteria* (Freud & Breuer 1895)
- Dora: 'Fragment of an analysis of a case of hysteria' (1905a)
- Little Hans, a boy with a phobia of horses, whose father Freud saw: 'Analysis of a phobia in a five year old boy' (1909a)
- Rat Man: 'Notes upon a case of obsessional neurosis' (1909b)
- Schreber, a case of paranoia whom Freud wrote about but never saw as a patient: 'Psychoanalytic notes on an autobiographical account of a case of paranoia (Dementia paranoides)' (1911a)
- Wolf Man: 'From the history of an infantile neurosis' (1919)

1923 – first operation on his jaw and palate for what was incorrectly diagnosed as leukoplakia, but was cancer. He eventually undergoes more than 20 operations.

4th June 1938 – after the Nazis march into Austria, and Anna Freud is questioned by the Gestapo (in March 1938), Freud and his family leave Vienna for Paris, and arrive in London two days later.

September 1938 – the Freuds move to 20 Maresfield Gardens in Hampstead, London, Freud's last home and now home of the Freud museum.

23rd September 1939 – Freud dies.

thinking occurs in dreaming, fantasy, and infantile life; here the distinctions between opposites need not apply, nor do the differences between past, present and future. Secondary process thinking is rational and follows the principles of logic, time and space.

Freud differentiated between unconscious and preconscious phenomena. Unconscious phenomena are not available to the conscious mind, and have been actively repressed because of their unthinkable nature – a memory, feeling or thought that conflicts with our view of ourselves and of what is acceptable, and which would cause too much guilt, anxiety or psychic pain if it were acknowledged. These are to be distinguished from phenomena that are unconscious in a descriptive sense, but which are easily brought to mind, and therefore are neither subject to repression nor operating under the sway of primary process thinking, i.e. the system preconscious. The preconscious in the topographical model has a role both as a reservoir of accessible thoughts and memories, and as a censor capable of modifying instinctual wishes of the system unconscious, to render them acceptable to the conscious system.

In his book *The Interpretation of Dreams* (1900), Freud called dreams, 'The Royal Road to the Unconscious'. Other routes to the unconscious include the unravelling of 'parapraxes' (so-called Freudian slips), and interpretation in analysis, especially transference interpretations (see below).

Structural theory was described in 1923 by Freud, and remains firmly embedded in instinct theory. It does not replace the above models, although there is now more emphasis on three structural components of the personality, i.e. the id, super-ego and ego.

The 'id' operates under the sway of the pleasure principle, and is the part of the personality concerned with basic inborn drives, and sexual and aggressive impulses. The id is the 'dark, inaccessible part of our personality; what little we know of it we have learnt from our study of dream-work and the construction of neurotic symptoms, and most of that is of a negative character, and can be described only as a contrast to the ego...we call it a chaos, a cauldron full of seething excitations' (Freud 1933, p. 105-6). It is filled with energy reaching it from the instincts but it has no organization, and strives to satisfy instinctual needs subject to the observance of the pleasure principle – the achievement of pleasure and the avoidance of unpleasure or tension.

'Super-ego' subsumed a previous concept of the term, 'ego-ideal', an internal model to which the individual aspires or attempts to conform. The term 'super-ego' is used to describe conscience and ideals.

The 'ego' is a term used to describe the more rational, reality oriented and executive aspects of the personality, and like the super-ego is partly conscious and partly unconscious.

In Freud's structural theory, the ego has to mediate between internal and external pressures. It serves three masters – 'the external world, the super-ego and the id' (Freud 1933, p. 110).

When the attempt to mediate breaks down, neurosis is a common outcome. Neurosis occurs when 'people turn away from reality because they find it unbearable either the whole or parts of it ' (Freud 1911b, p. 35).

Freud believed various aspects of culture helped in the task of replacing the id-driven pleasure principle with the reality principle – including religion, science, education, and especially art.

Freud once described the aim of analysis as 'Where id was, there ego shall be', i.e. making more of one's actions, affects and impulses conscious and under volitional control.

Ego defence mechanisms

> The ego makes use of various procedures for fulfilling its task, which, to put it in general terms, is to avoid danger, anxiety and unpleasure. We call these procedures 'mechanisms of defence'.
>
> S. Freud (1937, p. 235)

Although Sigmund Freud first introduced the term 'defence', it was his daughter Anna Freud who in 1936 systematically listed nine defence mechanisms, and later added a tenth healthy mechanism (sublimation) and two others (Table 36.1). More have subsequently been added. Ego defence mechanisms are habitual, unconscious and sometimes pathological mental processes which are employed to resolve conflict between instinctive needs (id), internalized prohibitions (super-ego) and external reality.

The main features of defences, as summarized by Bateman & Holmes (1995), are:

- They may be normal and adaptive as well as pathological.
- They are a function of the ego.
- They are usually unconscious.
- They are dynamic and ever-changing, but may coalesce into rigid fixed systems in pathological states and personality disorders.
- Different defences are associated with different psychological states.
- Some defence mechanisms are seen as more mature, while others are seen as more primitive, e.g. splitting, projective identification.

The word 'primitive' is applied to defence mechanisms in three different contexts – developmental, motivational and diagnostic (Akhtar 1995). The developmental context proposes that certain defences are used very early on in life, while others do not appear until a certain degree of ego organization is evident. The motivational context refers to the type of 'psychic danger' which necessitates the use of particular defences.

Table 36.1 Mechanisms of defence (adapted from Bateman & Holmes 1995)

Primitive/Immature	Neurotic	Mature
Autistic fantasy	Condensation	Humour
Devaluation/denigration	Denial	Sublimation
Idealization	Displacement	
Introjection	Dissociation	
Splitting (the two components of which are idealization	Externalization	
and denigration, above)	Identification with the aggressor	
Projection	Intellectualization	
Projective identification	*Isolation*	
Passive aggression	Rationalization	
Turning against the self	*Reaction formation*	
	Regression	
	Repression	
	Reversal	
	Somatization	
	Undoing (magic undoing)	

Note: those in italics (regression, repression, reaction formation, isolation, undoing, projection, introjection, turning against the self, and reversal) were the nine mechanisms listed by Anna Freud, to which she later added sublimation, identification with the aggressor, and idealization.

The expression 'primitive defences' also has a diagnostic connotation. Kernberg (1970) argues that individuals with a lower level of character organization (which includes all the severe personality disorders) use defences which are different from those with a higher level of character organization (e.g. obsessional or hysterical characters). See Box 36.2 for associated mental states.

Repression

This is the most basic defence mechanism, and other defence mechanisms come into play when repression begins to fail. Thoughts or feelings which the conscious mind finds unacceptable are repressed from consciousness.

Denial

Denial is the refusal to recognize external reality. Thus, for example, a patient may have been clearly told of an unpleasant prognosis to his illness, but denies any memory of that conversation at a later date. This is not the same as conscious dishonesty or lying.

Projection

Projection involves the attribution of one's own unacknowledged or disowned feelings onto others. It may

---

Box 36.2 Defence mechanisms and associated mental states

Paranoia – projection, projective identification, splitting

Depression – turning against the self (Freud's classic paper, 'Mourning and Melancholia', 1917)

Phobias – displacement of affect

Obsessions – isolation, magic undoing, reaction formation

Hysteria – denial, projection, identification

---

be of delusional intensity, and is associated with paranoia. Thus, for example, a husband with powerful sexual fantasies towards other women may attribute his impulses and desires to his wife, and become extremely jealous and possessive towards her. As Rycroft (1972) writes, projection of aspects of oneself is preceded by denial, i.e. one denies that one feels such and such an emotion, or has a particular wish, but asserts that someone else has.

Identification

Identification refers to the process whereby self-representations are built up and modified during development, as opposed to the conscious copying of imitation.

Projective identification

A term coined by Klein (1946), this complicated concept combines features of projection with those of identification. She described projective identification as a process that begins in early infancy and consists of parts of the rudimentary self being split off and projected into an external object, often the mother. The latter then becomes identified with the split-off part, as well as possessed and internally controlled by it.

An example from psychiatric practice would be of a young woman patient who denies all aggression or sexuality in herself, but comes into a casualty department having cut her wrists and looking unkempt. The male psychiatrist finds himself having increasingly sadistic and sexualized thoughts while attending to her. At least some of these thoughts may be explained by her denial of her aggression and sexuality, the subsequent projection thereof onto the psychiatrist who identifies with the role ascribed to him of an aggressive, sexually abusive male (see 'Acting out', below). Kernberg (1992) describes how the individual using projective identification, 'projects an intolerable intrapsychic experience onto an object ... tries to control the object in a continuing effort to defend against the intolerable experience, and unconsciously in actual interaction with the object, leads the object to *experience what has been projected onto him*' (p. 159).

Reaction formation

Reaction formation refers to behaving or feeling in a way directly opposite to unacceptable (hostile) instinctual impulses. Thus someone who is (secretly) fascinated with faeces may disavow and deny all interest therein, and develop an obsessional need for cleaning the hands and/or perineum. The showing of excessive deference to a person in authority whom one actually resents or despises is another example of reaction formation.

Identification with the aggressor

This process, described by Anna Freud, has links with both reaction formation (in that there is a reversal of affects), and with identification. One way of seeking refuge from the pain of being badly treated is to identify with the aggressor and to treat another person in a similar way, thereby inducing in the other the unwanted pain of the experience. An example would be a man who was bullied and abused in childhood 'identifying with the aggressor' and becoming a sadistic tormentor of children himself.

Turning against the self

In this context, unacceptable aggression to others is turned indirectly onto oneself, for example, in hypochondriasis.

Displacement

When we are too afraid to express our feelings or affects directly towards the person who provoked them, we may redirect them towards another person or object ('kicking the dog'). Turning against the self is an example of displacement, and may involve deliberate self-harm or even suicide.

Regression

Regression involves the abandonment of one's adult functioning and reverting to more childlike modes of acting, feeling and behaving. This occurs (healthily) on holiday, when grown men and women build sand castles or wear fancy dress. In the face of disasters (personal, such as a sudden death, or societal, such as warfare or earthquake), we may also regress to a more childlike state, a more dependent way of behaving, and we then turn to adults or leaders in whom we can repose our trust.

Isolation and undoing

These mechanisms are part of the conceptualization of obsessional disorders. Freud initially described isolation as the feature that helped separate obsessional neurosis from hysterical conversion. If the individual did not 'convert' painful affects through repression into bodily symptoms (as in hysterical conversion), then the affect was 'neutralized' by 'isolation'. In isolation, a traumatic memory is denuded of any feeling.

> When something unpleasant has happened to the subject, or when he has done something which has a significance for his neurosis, he interpolates an interval during which nothing further must happen...the experience is not forgotten, but instead it is deprived of its affect, and its associative connections are suppressed or interrupted so that it remains as though isolated, and is not reproduced in the ordinary processes of thought.
>
> S. Freud (1926)

Undoing is also referred to as 'magical undoing' or 'doing and undoing'. Undoing allows the person to reverse hostile wishes which he believes he has already perpetrated in the 'doing'. This is seen most frequently in patients with obsessional symptoms.

> In obsessional neurosis the technique ... is first met with in the 'diphasic' symptoms, in which one action is cancelled out by the second, so it is as though neither action had taken place, whereas in reality, both have.
>
> S. Freud (1926)

The attempt to undo has a magical quality, aiming to reverse time, to attack the reality of the original hostile wish or thought, and recreate the past as though such intentions had never existed in the first place.

Splitting

This term refers to a splitting or division of an object into good and bad, 'idealized' and 'denigrated'. The child, according to Kleinian theory, will keep the mother split into two separate persons – the good, nurturant provider (idealized) and the mother who is unavailable, depriving, frustrating (denigrated). This 'split' characterizes the 'paranoid-schizoid' position (see below) and is gradually diminished with the acquisition of the 'depressive position', where there is a recognition of good and bad in the same person, and the development of 'ambivalence'.

A patient may tell his (female) psychiatrist that she is the only person who has ever understood him; she is destined for great things, and has remarkable empathy (idealization). After she disappoints him by being unavailable one day, he describes her as useless, incompetent and irrelevant (denigration). Splitting can also occur within a team, for example the same patient may describe some team members as hopeless and others as excellent. Splitting is seen as a primitive defence mechanism.

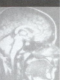

Acting out

Acting out is the direct expression of an unconscious impulse in order to avoid the awareness of the accompanying affect. This concept was initially described by Freud, in his paper 'Remembering, repeating, and working through'. In this important paper he describes how we all have a tendency towards unconsciously repeating relationships with important figures (primarily our parents), and this links closely with the concept of transference. Freud (1914) wrote about a 'repetition compulsion' and a tendency towards 'acting out' in the transference, i.e. acting towards one's therapist as if he/she were one's father, mother, etc. One of the aims of psychoanalysis or psychotherapy is to allow the patient to see his/her tendency towards such acting out, and to 'work through' this compulsion rather than repeatedly 'acting it out'.

Subsequent writers have distinguished between acting out within a psychotherapy session and outside a session, and some have suggested that the term 'acting out' should be reserved for events outside the session and 'acting in' for events inside the session. There is further confusion in that 'acting out' is a term now adopted within general psychiatry, usually with pejorative connotations, towards a patient who is 'misbehaving'. In addition, psychotherapists are now aware of the concept of 'acting out in the counter-transference', for example, a tendency to behave sadistically with a patient who might, by a process of projective identification (see above), project his/her disowned violence onto the therapist or psychiatrist. The therapist or psychiatrist then 'identifies' with this, and instead of being able to make sense of what is going on, an enactment occurs with the patient.

Intellectualization

This refers to thinking and speaking in jargon, rather than feeling.

Sublimation

Sublimation is seen as a healthy defence mechanism – the indirect expression of instincts without adverse consequences, e.g. great works of art, or hostility channelled into sport.

Psychosexual stages

Central to much of Freud's work was an explicit focus on sexuality and sexual fantasies. His stages of sexual development are summarized in Table 36.2.

Freud viewed adult sexuality as the outcome of a libidinal drive present from birth, and progressing through a number of 'pre-genital' phases, with pleasure bring derived from particular erotogenic zones associated with particular stages. Thus, initially he proposed an 'oral ' phase (before the age of one), where the infant derives satisfaction via the mouth, from sucking for example the nipple, or thumb ('auto-erotic'). This satisfaction appears to be independent of any nutritional/hunger needs in the infant.

Second, he described the 'anal' phase (ages 1–3), where immense gratification and pride is derived from gaining control over defecation, or the retention of faeces. This is followed by the 'phallic' phase, when the child develops more awareness and curiosity of his/her genitalia, with concomitant curiosity and anxiety about sexual differences. Freud also described the Oedipus complex and subsequent castration anxiety (see below) as pertaining to this phase. Following the phallic phase is 'latency' (6–12), a period of relative quiescence of sexual interest, perhaps even prudishness, with the child's interests turning towards the outside world, and to intellectual pursuits at school. Latency ends with puberty, when hormonal changes re-ignite the sexual drive and the 'genital' phase starts

The 'Oedipus complex'

For Freud, the ' Oedipus complex' was the nuclear complex from its discovery in 1897 to the end of his life. Derived from the Greek tragedy in which Oedipus unknowingly kills his father and has an incestuous relationship with his mother, the Oedipus complex is central to much of Freud's theorizing on psychosexual development, and has its female equivalent in the 'Electra complex'.

Modern analytic authors, especially those following Klein (see below) describe the 'Oedipus situation', which includes not only the sexual relation between the parents (the primal scene), but also focuses on the disappointment, sense of

Table 36.2	Freud's stages of sexual development	
Age	Stage	Features
0-1 year	Oral	Gratification by oral means from the breast in particular
1-3 years	Anal	Gratification via control over defaecation, a sense of self develops
3-5 years	Phallic	Further elaboration of Oedipal configuration and fantasies, with castration complex fears
5-12	Latent	The infantile stage of sexuality ends with the repression of the Oedipus complex, ideas from previous stages are repressed and denied expression
12-20	Puberty	Sexual drives are reawoken under the influence of hormonal changes

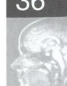

unfairness and wish for revenge evoked, when the young child is forced to confront that his or her (assumed) exclusive two-person relationship with the mother is actually not so exclusive, that there is a third person involved (father), and that in many circumstances (especially sexual) it is the child who is excluded by the mother–father dyad. 'Castration anxiety' is another term of Freud's, referring to the young boy's fear of castration as punishment for his Oedipal longings towards his mother.

Freud has been accused of writing from a masculine-biased point of view, especially pertaining to female sexuality. Beginning with the work of pioneering analysts such as Karen Horney, his work is seen as ignoring many important socio-economic and cultural dimensions, of being 'patriarchal' or 'phallocentric'. These critiques are beyond the scope of this chapter, but influence much of current psychoanalytic therapy as practised today.

Dreams

Freud considered *The Interpretation of Dreams* (1900) as his finest and most personal work, laying the foundations for the entire edifice of psychoanalysis. Insight such as this, he wrote 'falls to one's lot but once in a lifetime'. By analysing his own dreams, he came to the conclusion that 'a dream is the fulfillment of a wish'. Freed from the constraints of reality, under the sway of the pleasure principle, and in response to the day residue, i.e. recent events or preoccupations, the dreamer's deepest feelings and impulses are activated. The wishes, often of an infantile sexual nature are cleverly disguised by 'dream work', and the latent (underlying) content is disguised, censored, condensed, and displaced, emerging as the manifest content. Freud described four fundamental rules of dream work: condensation, displacement, conditions of representability and secondary revision.

In *condensation*, different elements are fused or combined into a single overdetermined image, which then requires unpacking. This is the means by which thoughts that are mutually contradictory make no attempt to do away with one another, but persist side by side.

Displacement resembles the work of a magician, the censor's attention being distracted by a shift of emphasis away from the area of maximal conflict or interest. Displacement allows an apparently insignificant idea or object to become invested with great intensity, which originally belonged elsewhere. This displacement takes place because consciousness finds the original object of these intense feelings (e.g. hatred or sexual longing towards a parent) unacceptable. The thoughts therefore undergo repression and appear in a disguised and displaced form.

A further aspect of dream work is what Freud describes as '*conditions of representability*', whereby dreams represent words in figurative form, in images. Freud saw this as the most interesting form of dream-work. An example (quoted in Perelberg 2000) is the representation of an important person by someone who is 'high up', at the top of a tower in a dream.

All dreams are subject to '*secondary revision*', an attempt by the dreamer to organize, revise and establish connections in the dream to make its account intelligible.

Freud's distinction between the latent and manifest content of dreams is important. The work that transforms latent thoughts into manifest dream content is called 'dream work', while the work in the opposite direction is the work of interpretation. The process of interpretation allows access to the wish expressed in the dream.

Freud's works

Amongst Freud's most important works are the case histories in Box 36.1, and also:

- 'Studies on Hysteria' (with Breuer) (Freud & Brewer 1895)
- 'The Interpretation of Dreams' (Freud 1900)
- 'Three Essays on the Theory of Sexuality' (Freud 1905b)
- 'Totem and Taboo' (Freud 1913)
- 'Remembering, Repeating and Working Through' (Freud 1914)
- 'Mourning and Melancholia' (Freud 1917)
- 'Beyond the Pleasure Principle' (Freud 1920)
- 'Group Psychology and the Analysis of the Ego' (Freud 1921)
- 'The Ego and the Id' (Freud 1923)
- 'New Introductory Lectures on Psychoanalysis' (Freud 1933).

DEVELOPMENTS FOLLOWING FREUD

All forms of dynamic psychotherapy stem from the work of Freud and psychoanalysis. C.G. Jung and Alfred Adler broke away before the First World War to form, respectively, the Schools of Analytic Psychology (Jung) and Individual Psychology (Adler).

While the neo-Freudians (Adler, Horney, Stack-Sullivan, Fromm) shifted the emphasis from biological to social processes, Jung developed his own school of analytical psychology which moved away from man's biological roots to a study of the manifestation of his psychological nature in myths, dreams and culture.

Alfred Adler (1870–1937)

Adler split from Freud in 1910, and is an important member of the group of neo-Freudians. Adler emphasized social factors in development. He gave more importance to aggressive strivings and the drive to power. Acutely aware

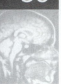

of sibling rivalry, he argued that neurosis originated in attempts to deal with feelings of inferiority, sometimes based on relative physical handicaps (organ inferiority), and this gave rise to a compensatory drive to power.

Similarly, he saw masculine protest in women as a reaction to their inferior position in society. He postulated an aggressive drive before Freud himself did, and although not mainstream, many of his ideas have been incorporated, e.g. inferiority complex, and the recognition that striving for power may reveal itself by its apparent opposite, i.e. retreat into manipulative weakness. He played a part in founding social and preventive psychiatry, and in the development of day hospitals, therapeutic clubs and group therapies.

Carl Gustav Jung (1885–1961)

Along with Adler, Jung was one of the first important figures to split away from Freud. He founded the School of Analytic Psychology. A basic organizing assumption running through his work is that the mind consists of far more than can be gained by experience, and this additional part is termed the collective unconscious.

Thus, there are three levels of the psyche – the conscious/unconscious (including the psyche), the personal unconscious and the collective unconscious (racial and universal features). He thus moved in an opposite direction from Adler and the neo-Freudians. For Jung, Freud's 'personal unconscious' and its complexes were 'banal and uninteresting'.

The persona is the outer crust of the personality, which is the opposite of the personal unconscious on a variety of dimensions, e.g. thinking versus feeling, sensuousness versus intuition, extrovert versus introvert (related to the direction of flow of mental energy).

For Jung, there was a deeper, transpersonal unconscious, something that reflects the history of the human species and indeed the cosmic order, and that arises prior to an individual's experience. Within this collective unconscious are the so-called archetypes, which may roughly be defined as universal nuclear mythic themes (The Hero, The Great Mother, etc.). The manifestations of the archetypes appear in a profusion of symbols that appear in dreams, disturbed states of mind and certain cultural products – for example, he claimed to have objective evidence of archetypes in the form of spontaneous production of symbolism that could not have been known to the subject by ordinary means, e.g. a schizophrenic patient has a vision of the sun as a wheel, which matches a similar vision reported in an ancient and forgotten text. His deep rejection of the primacy of ordinary experience and causality led Jung to seek manifestations of the collective unconscious in realms that are by and large today regarded as occult and mystical for example, alchemy, flying saucers and so on.

Archetypes can be defined as generalized symbols and images within the collective unconscious, and include:

- *animus* – the unconscious masculine side of the woman's female persona
- *anima* – the unconscious female side of the man's persona
- *complex* – a group of interconnected ideas that arouse associated feelings and effect behaviour.

Jungian analysis in Britain is organizationally separate from Freudian psychoanalysis, Jungian analysis being located mainly in the Society of Analytic Psychology (SAP), while Freudian psychoanalysis is under the auspices of the Institute of Psychoanalysis.

Object relations theorists (Fairbairn, Guntrip, Balint, Winnicott)

The early psychoanalytic view of sexuality as a pleasure-seeking drive, present from birth, appeared for some theorists to be too centred on the individual and his gratifications. Object relations theorists have suggested that the primary motivational drive in man is to seek a relationship with others. Rather than the individual deriving satisfaction through different means at different stages, starting with the oral phase, he seeks relationships with others, starting with the mother. In psychoanalysis, the term 'object' refers to that (usually a person) which is used to gratify a need. The original 'object' in Freud's theories was a maternal breast. A 'bad object' is an object whom the subject fears or hates, who is experienced as malevolent. An 'internal object' is derived from an external object by the process of introjection, and is located in internal reality. Object relations theory is thus the psychoanalytic theory in which the subject's need to relate to objects occupies the central position, in contrast to instinct theory, which centres on the individual's need to reduce instinctual tension.

Object relations theory was underpinned by experimental work, including the work of Harlow, whose work on infant primates illustrates the drive for attachment to 'objects', and Bowlby, whose work on maternal deprivation and the effects of separation of mother from infant is described below.

Object relations theory has been the dominant school in British analytic thinking, with key figures including Ronald Fairbairn in Scotland, Harry Guntrip in Leeds, Michael Balint and Donald Winnicott (see below); it plays a major or dominant role in the three traditions within the British Psychoanalytical Society.

The three traditions or groupings that have emerged within the British Psychoanalytical Society are:

- contemporary Freudians – Anna Freud, Joseph Sandler
- middle/independent group – Donald Winnicott, Michael Balint
- Kleinians – Melanie Klein, Wilfred Bion, Herbert Rosenfeld, Hanna Segal.

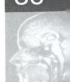

Donald Winnicott (1896–1971)

Winnicott trained initially as a paediatrician. It is to him that we owe the terms:

- primary maternal preoccupation
- good enough mother
- false self
- transitional objects.

Winnicott noticed that a change in the mental state of the mother towards the end of pregnancy seemed to attune her particularly towards the needs of her new baby. He argued that, initially, the mother's attention to the baby's needs protects the infant from impingements that disturb his 'going-on-being', which is a prerequisite for integration. Any impingement, be it external or internal in origin, produces catastrophic disintegration.

In the first months, he argued 'there is no such thing as a baby', i.e. there is only a mother–baby dyad. Slowly, by a process of gradual disillusionment, separation occurs. Initially the baby makes use of 'transitional objects', i.e. blankets, pieces of mother's clothing, etc. A 'transitional object' is treated by the subject as being halfway between himself and another person, typically a doll or piece of mother's clothing, which does not have to be treated with the consideration appropriate to that person. Such objects help children to make the transition from infantile narcissism to object-love, and from dependence to self-reliance.

The baby develops an ability to play, and an ability to 'be alone in the presence of the mother'. Play is an important concept in Winnicottian theory, and the ability to play is seen as similar to the ability to make use of therapy.

In his later writings he makes use of the concepts 'true self' and 'false self'. Winnicott believed that the drive-driven child conjured up in his mind an object suited to his needs, especially when excited. If at this precise moment the 'good enough mother', i.e. a mother attuned to his needs, presents him with just such a suitable object, a moment of illusion is created in the baby, who feels (omnipotently) that he has 'made' the object himself. The repetition of these 'hallucinatory' wishes and their realization by the mother leads the infant to believe he has created his own world. This omnipotence is healthy, leading to the development of a creative and healthy self. Only once this 'true self' has been established, can omnipotence be abrogated and the reality of pain and loss be faced. A child who grows up with a mother who is unable to facilitate this and the subsequent gradual 'disillusionment', will develop a compliant 'false self' that conceals frustrated instinctual drives.

Another extremely influential paper was Winnicott's 'Hate in the countertransference', written in 1947 (see paragraphs on 'Transference' and 'Counter-transference' below).

John Bowlby and attachment theory

John Bowlby (1907-1990) was an eminent British researcher and psychoanalyst who is associated with the concepts of 'attachment' and 'separation'. The main features of 'attachment theory' have been summarized as follows (Holmes 1993):

- Lorenz's work with birds and Harlow's work with monkeys suggests that the mother–infant relationship is not necessarily mediated by feeding. Bowlby postulated a 'primary attachment relationship' developing in the human infant at around 7 months, the main evolutionary function of which was to protect the subject from predation.
- This attachment relationship is characterized by 'proximity seeking', activated in young children by separation from an attachment figure, and in later life by threat, illness and fatigue.
- Attachment results in the 'secure base phenomenon'. When an individual is securely attached, he or she can engage in 'exploratory behaviour'.
- Separation leads to 'separation protest', in which efforts are made, often angry or violent, towards reunion. Permanent separation, i.e. loss, impairs the capacity of the individual to feel secure and to explore his/her environment.
- The individual carries inside him/her an 'internal working model' of the world, in which are represented the whereabouts and likely interactive patterns between self and his/her attachment figures.
- The 'attachment dynamic' is not confined to infancy and childhood, but continues throughout life. Development is a movement from immature to mature dependence, or 'emotional autonomy'.

Bowlby found himself increasingly marginalized within UK psychoanalytic circles (Holmes 1993), but his work remains important for both its clinical and research implications.

Mary Ainsworth, who worked with Bowlby at the Tavistock Clinic, subsequently developed the Strange Situation Test (SST) (Ainsworth et al. 1978), a reliable instrument for rating the attachment and security of a one-year-old infant to his/her parent, usually the mother. Three typical reactions to separation, reuniting with the mother and response to a stranger in the room were first described:

- the secure child – protests when mother disappears, but is easily pacified on her return and returns to exploratory play
- the insecure–avoidant child – does not protest much on separation, and on the mother's return hovers warily nearby, unable to play freely
- the insecure–ambivalent child – does protest, but cannot be pacified by the returning adult, pushing away toys and/or burying his/her head in the mother's lap.

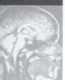

Subsequently, a fourth category has been recognized:

- the insecure–disorganized child – freezes on separation and seems unable to sustain any organized pattern of behaviour.

Longitudinal studies have followed the progress of infants rated on the SST, and a striking finding is the stability of the attachment patterns over time (Holmes 1993).

Subsequently, Main (1990) developed the adult attachment interview (AAI), for studying attachment phenomena in adults. Adults are interviewed in a semi-structured interview, in which they are asked to describe early memories, feelings and thoughts about their own parents. The interview is supposed to 'surprise the unconscious', and reveal feelings about current and past attachments and separations, and to tap into emotional responses to loss and difficulty. The interviews are then rated, according to the coherence of discourse rather than the memories per se. Once again, three main patterns emerge.

Current research involves administering the AAI to pregnant women, and then assessing the extent to which the offspring of securely attached mothers (as assessed by the AAI) are rated as having secure attachments on the SST a year later (see Fonagy et al. 2000).

Through the use of such instruments, and the studies mentioned above, it is now possible to trace lines of attachment reaching from a mother's sense of security in pregnancy through her child's infancy and early childhood and into pre-teen years.

Melanie Klein (1882–1960)

Melanie Klein developed a play technique in the psychoanalysis of children, and wrote extensively, about child and adult psychoanalysis. She came to the UK from Berlin in 1926, and took psychoanalysis, and the death instinct in particular, in a new direction, to account for destructive forces within the personality deriving from 'primary envy'.

She proposed two modes of functioning, which she described as the 'paranoid–schizoid' and the 'depressive' positions. The paranoid–schizoid position is characterized by the predominance of primitive defence mechanisms, i.e. denial, splitting and primitive projective identification. In the more mature depressive position, there is integration of the good and bad aspects of self and others ('objects'), with the realization that the person you hate is also the one you love, i.e. ambivalence. Most people oscillate, but some, e.g. those with borderline personalities, operate more in the paranoid–schizoid than the depressive position more of the time.

Kleinians understand the 'flux' between the two positions in their analysands (analytic patients) as the analysand being confronted in his/her internal world between two painful possibilities, the persecutory anxiety that is outstanding in the paranoid–schizoid position, and the guilt and feelings of devastation in the depressive position. In the paranoid–schizoid position, the focus is very much on aggression, or self- or other-directed destructiveness, much of it in the form of envy and fear of envy, and grandiosity; while in the depressive position the focus is on love, reparation and various other forms of regard for the object as well as destructiveness and guilt

Projective identification, initially described by Klein in 1946, is a more complex notion than Freud's 'projection'. In projective identification, the subject disowns or disavows an unwanted aspect of him/herself, and projects it into/onto the recipient who then introjects it, identifying with the role he/she has been placed in, and fulfils the role requirements of the projecting subject. This all occurs at an unconscious level, and represents a primitive mode of communication.

Thus, for instance, a patient suffering from 'borderline personality disorder', who in her childhood was repeatedly beaten and abused, may almost 'invite' a stressed psychiatrist to treat her harshly when she cuts her wrists again, evoking not only a sense of helplessness in the psychiatrist (i.e. she communicates her sense of helplessness), but also then provoking that he re-enact, unconsciously to him, early patterns to which she is so accustomed. Kleinian analysts, in particular, have advanced our understanding of counter-transference, projective identification, and the pressure placed by patients on their therapists, analysts or psychiatrists, to 'act out' within the therapeutic alliance

Wilfred Bion (1897–1974)

Bion was a prominent follower of Klein. He worked at the Tavistock Clinic, and contributed to Kleinian theory and the theory of Group Analysis. His concepts of 'container' and 'contained' are important in Kleinian theory. He derived this notion from his clinical work especially with borderline and psychotic patients. In his book *Learning from Experience* (1962), Bion writes:

> Melanie Klein has described an aspect of projective identification concerned with the modification of infantile fears: the infant projects a part of its psyche, namely its bad feelings into a good breast. Thence in due course they are removed and reintrojected. During their sojourn in the good breast they are felt to have been modified in such a way that the object that is reintrojected has become tolerable to the infant's psyche. From the above theory I shall abstract for use as a model the idea of a container into which an object is projected and the object that can be projected into the container; the latter I shall designate by the term contained (p. 90).

Thus the mother, if receptive to the infant's state of mind and capable of allowing it to be evoked in herself, could process it in such a way that, in an identifiable form, she could attend to it in the infant. In this way, something that in the infant is 'near-sensory' and somatic is transformed into something more mental, which could be used for thought or stored as memory. If the process badly backfires, severe problems in thinking, mentalizing and in emotional development occur.

Bion gave a name to these 'near-sensory' elements, calling them 'beta elements'. If they can be transformed into something more understandable, more within the realms of emotions, they are then termed 'alpha elements'. If the beta elements remain unprocessed, they might go out of the mind into three spheres-into the body (psychosomatic or hypochondriacal symptoms); into the perceptual sphere (perceptual hallucinations); or into action (Britton 1992, p.106).

Bion also described the concept of 'basic assumptions' or primitive states of mind, which are generated automatically when people come together in a group. He described the basic assumptions as:

- dependence, i.e. expecting solutions to be bestowed by the group leader
- fight/flight, i.e. fleeing from, or engaging in battle with enemies/adversaries, especially outside the group
- pairing, i.e. encouraging or hoping that individuals in the group would form a procreative couple, thus leading to the birth of a person or idea which would then provide salvation.

These basic assumptions may dominate the group, and interfere with its explicit 'work task', and so prevent creative change and development. 'Basic assumption groups' thus interfere with the exploration by the 'work group' of the feelings and the problems of the individuals in it.

Otto Kernberg (1928–) and Heinz Kohut (1913–1981)

These two prominent American analysts both had a particular interest in narcissistic personalities. Otto Kernberg, closer in perspective to the British Object Relations and Kleinian schools, emphasizes the paranoid substrate of the syndrome, and hence regards mistrust, rage and guilt about this rage to be the basic cause of the self-inflation in narcissism. He gives a special place to envy, underlying the narcissist's scorn for others, and considers chronic defences against such envy, especially devaluation, omnipotent control and narcissistic withdrawal, as a major aspect of the clinical picture of narcissistic personality disorder.

Kernberg has also written extensively on 'borderline personality organization'. He describes how for a coherent structuring of the self and for the internalization of object relationships, the early ego has to accomplish two tasks: the first involves the differentiation of self-images from object images that form part of early introjections and identifications; the second task involves the integration of

'all-good' images with their devalued 'all-bad' images (similar to the task of Klein's depressive position). As a result of this synthesis, somewhat ambivalent, albeit deeper and richer views of the self and of objects emerge. The failure of the second task characterize 'borderline personality organization'. The lack of synthesis results in the persistence of splitting as the main defensive operation of the ego. Primitive, unrealistic and contradictory self-representations continue to exist and are readily activated by environmental cues. The world appears to be populated by 'gods' and 'devils', but no true, integrated human beings.

Heinz Kohut, a leading proponent of 'self-psychology', would see the aetiology of narcissistic personality disorder in terms of parental empathic failure, and would emphasize the reparative function of the analyst, emphasizing empathy as a therapeutic tool. Kohut's self-psychology emphasizes deficit rather than conflict as the core of many modern ills, regards healthy narcissism as the foundation for good object relations, and highlights empathy and 'attunement' rather than interpretation as the curative factors in psychoanalysis.

Margaret Mahler (1897–1985)

Margaret Mahler was a prominent and influential analyst in the USA. In her theory of symbiosis and individuation–separation (derived from direct observations of children) she proposed that the psychological birth of the infant, i.e. the beginning in the child of a coherent sense of personhood, is distinct from the biological birth.

She postulated a sequence of maturational and developmental events through which a child must pass before becoming sufficiently separate enough from the mother, to permit the attainment of a fairly stable sense of being a unique individual. These phases are described as:

1. The 'autistic phase' in which the neonate is self-contained and encased as if by a psychophysiological barrier.
2. The 'symbiotic phase', in which a dual unity exists between mother and infant, the basic core of the infant's self awakens in a state of enmeshment with the mother's self.
3. The 'separation-individuation phase', consisting of four subphases:
   (a) differentiation subphase (4 or 5 to 8 or 9 months)
   (b) practising subphase (9–16 to 18 months)
   (c) rapprochement subphase (16–24 months) which, if overcome, is followed by a period designated
   (d) 'on the road to object constancy'.

In 'object constancy', a deeper, more ambivalent, but more sustained object representation is internalized: temporary frustrations can be withstood; this is accompanied by a more realistic, and less shifting view of the self. The attainment of object constancy assures the mother's lasting presence in the mental structure of the child (Akhtar 1995). Some similarities with Winnicott's notion of the acquisition of the 'true self' and the 'false self' can be noted.

Mahler (1971, p. 181) noted that a failure to achieve 'object constancy' is associated with clinical signs that indicate:

That the blending and synthesis of 'good' and 'bad' self and object image have not been achieved; that ego-filtered affects have become inundated by surplus unneutralized aggression; that delusions of omnipotence alternate with utter dependency and self-denigration; that the body image has become and remains suffused with unneutralized id-related erogeneity and aggressive, pent-up body feeling, and so on.

Akhtar (1995) has described six clinical manifestations of impaired object constancy:

- disturbances of optimal distance
- splitting and intensification of affects
- paranoid tendencies
- inordinate optimism and the 'someday' fantasy
- malignant erotic transference
- inability to mourn, nostalgia and the 'if only' fantasy.

Mahler's work has had a substantial influence on the theory and practice of psychoanalysis, more so in the USA than in the UK and Europe, as well as on the field of academic developmental psychology (Akhtar & Parens 1991, Nachman 1991).

Jacques Lacan (1901–1981)

The French analyst Jacques Lacan combined linguistics with psychoanalysis. He is particularly influential in France, but his influence on the practice of psychotherapy and psychoanalysis in the UK and USA is limited (although he is widely referred to among academics in the fields of linguistics, art history and philosophy). He did not stick rigidly to the 50-minute hour (see below), and his writings are complex.

In Lacan's view, the oedipal child enters into the world of 'signs', which convey to him the meanings of self, gender and the body, just as he is similarly confronted by language and grammar that he must assimilate in order to become part of the linguistic community.

Lacan described three developmental stages:

- a primordial period of unconscious infantile 'desire'
- a world of the 'imaginary' emerging from the 'mirror stage' in which the child first confronts his image and narcissistically (therefore incorrectly) assumes this to be his true self
- finally, the 'symbolic order' arising through the contact with language, the 'no(m) du pere', a linguistic expression of Freud's picture of the father's combined role as the necessary separator of child and mother, ego ideal and potential castrator.

At around the age of two years the child begins to acquire self-awareness and language. A crisis of development occurs then, as the primitive pre-oedipal unity of mother and child is shattered by the advent of the no(m) du pere – the name of the father and also the 'no' of the father, 'the prohibition placed like the archangel's sword at the gates of paradise by the jealous father' (Bateman & Holmes 1995).

THE PRACTICE OF PSYCHOTHERAPY AND PSYCHOANALYSIS

Psychotherapy is practised in a quiet, private room, with the therapist and patient either facing each other (sometimes at an angle) or with the patient lying on a couch, with the therapist sitting behind the patient's head. Sessions usually last 50 minutes (the so-called 'therapeutic hour') and direct questioning, reassurance and polite chatter are usually avoided. Sessions are at the same time every week, and may be as frequent as five times a week, or as infrequent as once a week, with the frequency fixed at the beginning of treatment (though subject to revision during the course of treatment). Treatment lasts many months, and often many years.

The boundaries and rules are strict, and therefore any 'boundary violation' or 'acting out' e.g. the patient arriving late, or storming out of the session, can be interpreted by the therapist at that time or at a later date. The deeper unconscious meanings of the patient's communications are of prime importance, and are brought to the surface, akin to an archaeologist's work, through the process of interpretation rather than didactic teaching or coaching.

Psychoanalysis as a treatment

Psychoanalysis involves daily (four to five times per week) sessions (of 50 minutes), with the patient lying on a couch, and the analyst sitting behind the patient. The duration of treatment can be for many years, and psychoanalysis is thus both time- and resource-consuming. The practice of psychoanalysis is thus restricted in the UK, almost exclusively, to the private sector, although many patients are treated at training institutions for a reduced fee.

The theoretical underpinnings of many of the briefer treatments (so-called brief dynamic therapy (see below)), derive from psychoanalysis, and many practitioners, whether analysts, therapists or other mental health professionals, have undergone their own analytic therapy.

Key concepts

Transference and counter-transference

Freud first made use of the term 'transference' in 1895, and initially regarded it as an obstacle to treatment. The patient is 'frightened at finding that she is transferring onto the figure of the physician the distressing ideas that arise from the content of the analysis'. Freud saw this as a 'false connection' between a person who was the object of earlier – often sexual or erotic – wishes, and the doctor.

By 1909 he was beginning to see that it could be an agent for therapeutic change. Positive and negative transference was described, and transference interpretations became central to the practice of psychoanalysis, especially Kleinian analysis.

However, not all interpretations are transference interpretations, and there is debate in analytic circles as to whether everything should be interpreted with reference to transference or not.

A good definition is provided by Greenson, (quoted in Bateman et al. 2000, p. 52):

> Transference is the experiencing of feelings, drives, attitudes, fantasies and defences toward a person in the present, which do not befit the person but are a repetition of reactions originating in regard to significant persons of early childhood, unconsciously displaced onto figures in the present. The two outstanding characteristics of a transference reaction are: it is a repetition, and it is inappropriate.

Transference occurs in many situations, including other doctor–patient relationships. One might treat a consultant, or a headmaster, or a priest in an inappropriate way, e.g. with anxiety, cheekiness, temerity, etc., unconsciously transferring one's basic attitude to one's father or another early authority figure, onto the figure in the present.

Psychotherapy requires that a therapeutic or working alliance be set up between the adult part of the therapist and the adult part of the patient, in order that one can investigate the relationship between the child part of the patient, and the therapist.

'Counter-transference' refers to the therapist's attitudes towards the patient. It was also initially regarded as a hindrance by Freud, and was one of the reasons why analysts were and are expected to undergo their own personal analyses. Any strong emotions the therapist felt towards the patient were initially seen to have originated from the therapist's own past, his/her own conflicts or unresolved problems, and thus inappropriately transferred onto the patient.

However, the concept was expanded to include not only the therapist's own personal 'baggage', but also particular affects and emotions which the patient evokes in his/her therapist, which had more to do with the patient than the therapist. Thus, a patient who is very 'passive–dependent' might project all of his/her unacknowledged hostility onto the therapist who then feels like getting rid of the patient. (The concepts of projection and projective identification as defence mechanisms are particularly relevant here.)

In an important paper Winnicott (1949) (see above) described 'Hate in the countertransference'. He described

patients' capacity to evoke feelings of hatred in their helpers, which are in some way appropriate. He relates this to the various ways in which a mother may, on occasions, hate her own infants. Like transference, counter-transference is ubiquitous, and it is essential that psychiatrists and mental health professionals learn to recognize it, and not act out their countertransference wishes, for instance by prematurely discharging an irritating patient. A constant monitoring of one's own affective state is necessary, and at all times it is important to try to ascertain whether a strong emotion – sadness, a rescue fantasy, boredom, sadism, etc. – is primarily emanating from the practitioner (fatigue due to a late night), or from the patient (sudden boredom, which may indicate the patient avoiding something, or the patient being subtly hostile to you).

Interpretations

Greenson (1967) has described three types of verbal communication contributing to therapeutic understanding, and all are used to a lesser or greater extent in therapy/analysis:

- clarification
- confrontation
- interpretation.

Clarification involves rephrasing and questioning. Confrontation draws attention to what the patient is doing, often repeatedly and sometimes unawares, e.g. arriving late, forgetting to pay the bill, etc. Interpretation offers new formulations of unconscious meaning and motivation.

Rycroft (1972) describes various types of interpretations. These include:

- dream interpretations – here the analyst discovers the latent (underlying) content of the dream by analysing its manifest content
- transference interpretations – often held to be the most powerful, i.e. interpreting the patient's behaviour/attitude in the consulting room towards the analyst, e.g. 'I think you are feeling pushed away by me in much the same way you felt pushed out by your younger sibling whom you are now complaining about'.
- correct interpretations – those that both adequately explain the material being interpreted, and are formulated in such a way and communicated at such a time as to make sense to the patient.
- premature interpretations – 'true' interpretations, but presented to the patient at a time when he/she is not yet ready to 'receive' or make sense of them.

Thus, just because a patient agrees with an interpretation, it does not follow that it is correct - the patient may just be very compliant. Conversely, if a patient disagrees with or dismisses an interpretation, it may be 'correct', but the patient may habitually reject the unpleasant truth about him/herself.

Therapeutic alliance

The therapeutic alliance or treatment alliance refers to 'the non-neurotic, rational, reasonable rapport which the patient has with his analyst and which enables him to work purposefully in the analytic situation' (Greenson & Wexler, 1969). Thus the therapeutic alliance refers to the ordinary, adult-to-adult relationship that the patient and therapist need to have in order to cooperate over their joint task. It involves the patient's willingness to abide by some of the basic rules (such as attendance, timekeeping, payment (in private sector psychotherapy)), and to be able to keep more primitive hostile impulses at bay (e.g. impulses towards acting out in a violent manner). In psychotherapy, the therapist thus sets up a therapeutic alliance between the adult part of the patient and the adult part of the analyst, in order to explore the way in which this relationship is distorted and coloured by the child part of the patient.

Psychotherapy can thus only be conducted satisfactorily if there is enough adult capacity or 'ego strength' in the patient to recognize, tolerate and sustain the paradox that, although he may have intense feelings towards the therapist 'as if' the latter were a parental figure, in reality this is not the case (see below).

Cawley's levels of psychotherapy

Cawley (1977) has usefully described 'levels of psychotherapy' ranging from Level 1 (informal, between friends) to Level 2 (formal therapy, primarily supportive and non-interpretative) to Level 3 (formal therapy dynamic/analytic, interpretative) (Table 36.3).

While almost any person with difficulties may benefit from Level 1 psychotherapy (supportive), a number of questions arise when considering patients for dynamic/analytic psychotherapy (Level 3).

Selection of patients for dynamic psychotherapy

Bateman et al. (2000, p. 190) list four selection criteria when considering who should be offered formal psychodynamic psychotherapy (Level 3):

1. That the person's difficulties are understandable in psychological terms.
2. That there is sufficient motivation for insight and change.
3. That the patient has the requisite ego strength.
4. That the person has the capacity to form and maintain relationships.

During the initial assessment interview, it should be possible to make a tentative psychodynamic formulation, which will take into account both the patient's past and his/her current difficulties. The patient's preparedness to think about problems is a parallel requirement. The patient's response to a trial interpretation can help in assessing this.

How does the patient respond to the therapist? Does he/she use excessive denial and/or projection as habitual defence mechanisms, disavowing all responsibility for all his/her difficulties, only blaming others. Does he/she 'really' want to change, or just moan at the therapist, using the therapist as a metaphorical dustbin?

What about 'ego strength'? The patient must be able to evaluate his/her experiences and integrate the competing demands of the motivational drives (id), conscience (super-ego) and external reality, while coping with the tensions they create. He/she needs to cope with emotions evoked without decompensating, acting too destructively, or becoming overwhelmed with anxiety. He/she also must keep in touch with the adult part of the self, i.e. maintain the working alliance with the therapist at the same time as getting into contact with the disturbed, needy, messy child within.

Therefore, one needs to know, will the patient cope with the end of each session, and with the therapist's absences? Hence there are a number of contraindications to psychodynamic psychotherapy (see below).

An alternative set of criteria is provided by Gabbard (1990), who suggests that the presence of the following 11 features indicates an expressive exploratory emphasis in psychotherapy:

- strong motivation to understand
- significant suffering
- ability to regress in the service of the ego
- tolerance of frustration

Table 36.3 Cawley's levels of psychotherapy	
Level	*Activity/process*
1. Outer (support and counselling)	1. Unburdening of problems to a sympathetic listener 2. Ventilation of feelings within a supportive relationship 3. Discussion of current problems with helper
2. Intermediate	4. Clarification of problems, their nature and origins 5. Confrontation of the defences 6. Interpretation of the transference and unconscious motives
3. Deeper (exploration and analysis)	7. Repetition, remembering and reconstruction of the past 8. Regression to less adult and more primitive levels 9. Resolution of conflicts by 'working through' them

- capacity for insight (psychological mindedness)
- intact reality testing
- meaningful object relations
- good impulse control
- ability to sustain work
- capacity to think in terms of metaphor and analogy
- reflective responses to trial interpretations.

Contraindications to psychoanalytic psychotherapy include:

- A patient who is actively *suicidal* (unless also being cared for by a psychiatric team).
- Repeated suicide attempts.
- A history of gross deliberate self-harm and/or violence towards others.
- A current drug or alcohol *addiction*.
- Serious *psychosomatic* conditions (with very concrete thinking and no wish to view the illness in another light). In general, patients with a fixed and long-standing tendency towards somatization are not regarded as good candidates for psychodynamic therapy. They are seen to deal with psychic conflict by somatizing. Somatization is seen as a defence against coming into contact with very primitive, disturbing fears, fantasies and memories. Some analytic authors (e.g. McDougall 1989) argue that somatization is a defence against psychosis. However, Guthrie & Creed (Guthrie et al. 1991) have written of encouraging results in treating patients suffering from irritable bowel disorder with dynamic therapy. In general, the prognosis with such patients depends on the fixity and chronicity of the 'psychic solution'.
- Patients suffering from a *psychotic* illness such as schizophrenia. In such patients, the impaired ego boundaries make dynamic therapy unviable. Unable to distinguish fantasy from reality, they are unable to distinguish between their own thoughts and those of others, and a psychotic transference may occur. Furthermore, engaging in therapy requires an 'as if' quality from the patient. For example: an elderly male therapist is not really your father, it is 'as if' he were your father. This 'as-if' quality is lacking in the patient suffering from an acute psychotic episode. There are some patients with psychotic illnesses, especially bipolar affective disorder, who can benefit from dynamic therapy while in remission (preferably in a unit attached to a psychiatric hospital).
- No evidence of the capacity to *form and sustain relationships* (relative contraindication). The capacity to form and sustain relationships is important as a prognostic indicator, and this may sound cruel: the very people who find this difficult may be deemed 'not suitable' for therapy using this criterion. Nonetheless, if the patient has never sustained a close relationship, it is likely that he/she will flee from therapy, either finding it useless or finding the therapist's absences too difficult to bear. This is not an absolute contraindication, and many schizoid patients are seen in therapy.

Brief dynamic psychotherapy

Holmes (1994) has defined brief dynamic psychotherapy (BDP) as a 'time-limited form of psychoanalytically-based therapy, usually lasting 6–40 sessions, characterized by a high level of therapist activity, and the attempt to work with a psychodynamic "focus" which links presenting problem, past conflict or trauma and the relationship with the therapist'.

Indications for BDP usually include motivation for change, a circumscribed problem, evidence of at least one good relationship in the past, and the capacity for 'psychological mindedness' (see below). Malan (1963) listed contraindications for BDP, including:

- chronic addiction
- serious suicide attempts
- chronically incapacitating phobic or obsessional symptoms
- evidence of grossly destructive or self-destructive acting out.

The patient needs to have the 'ego strength' to cope with the psychological turmoil following an emotionally charged session, without drowning his/her sorrows in alcohol or drugs. He/she also must be able to resist hitting a partner/spouse/therapist/shopkeeper following such a session, and must also resist self-harm.

The defence mechanisms in many patients with severe phobias and chronic obsessive-compulsive disorder tend to respond poorly to dynamic therapy and are generally better treated, in the first instance at least, by focused therapies (cognitive–behavioural), even though dynamic therapists may contribute to an understanding of their aetiology.

The patient, once accepted for BDP, will be informed of the number of sessions, the length of the sessions, whether homework is required (e.g. in cognitive analytic therapy), arrangements for holidays, and a post-therapy follow-up.

A focus is found, which brings together the patient's presenting problem, a past difficulty (often relating to a past loss or trauma), and the current transferential relationship to the therapist. Various authors describe different models and metaphors; for instance, Malan uses two triangles – the triangle of person and the triangle of defence. The triangle of person links the relationship with the significant other with the therapist and the parental figure; the triangle of defence links a hidden impulse for forgotten feeling, a defence, and the resulting anxiety.

Other key names in the field of BDP include Malan, Davanloo, Michael and Enid Balint, Luborsky and Mann.

One of the key features in brief or focused therapy is the active therapist; another feature is the focus right from the start on the termination, which will inevitably re-evoke feelings of loss, so central to many patients' problems. Thus,

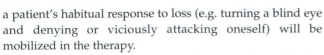

a patient's habitual response to loss (e.g. turning a blind eye and denying or viciously attacking oneself) will be mobilized in the therapy.

In brief dynamic therapy, constant supervision for the therapist is necessary, and personal therapy for the therapist highly desirable.

Cognitive analytic therapy

This is a relatively new therapy, devised by Anthony Ryle at St Thomas' Hospital, London, specifically for use in the UK National Health Service. It is a time-limited therapy, lasting 16 or sometimes 24 sessions. Ryle himself was influenced by the Russian cognitive scientist Vygotsky (Ryle et al. 1992).

In the therapy there are three R's, i.e. *reformulation* (the reshaping of the history and description of the present), therapy then being occupied with the patient being helped to *recognize* the recurrences of these unrevised patterns, so they can become open to *revision*.

The patient is given reading material from 'The Psychotherapy File', which describes a number of patterns of unrevisable, maladaptive procedures termed traps, dilemmas and snags. The patient then identifies which ones apply to him/her.

- Traps – negative assumptions generate acts which produce consequences which reinforce the assumptions.
- Dilemmas – the person acts as though available action or possible roles were limited to polarized alternatives (false dichotomies), usually unaware that this is the case.
- Snags – appropriate roles or goals are abandoned either because the individual makes an assumption that others would oppose them, or because they are perceived as forbidden or dangerous.

At the fourth session, the therapist provides a summary of his or her understanding of the history and its meaning, and describes how the strategies, used historically as a way of surviving, may now be maladaptive.

A diagram (sequential diagrammatic representation) may be used, and the patient will keep this. The patient feels understood and 'held' and becomes less defensive. Dreams, memories and feelings become accessible. Sessions thereafter are usually unstructured although homework is given. At the end, a goodbye letter is given to the patient, and patients are also asked to write their own evaluation.

> The emphasis of this therapy is upon the formation and use of accurate descriptions and the aim is that patients may learn to recognize automatic procedures in time to consider alternatives.
>
> Ryle et al. (1992, p. 402)

Interpersonal psychotherapy

This is a psychotherapy based on the ideas of the interpersonal school. Key figures include Stack-Sullivan,

Klerman and Weissman. Sullivan taught that psychiatry includes the scientific study of people and interpersonal processes, rather than an almost exclusive focus on the mind, society or the brain, and therefore the unit of study is the patient's interpersonal relations at any one time.

Initially, interpersonal therapy (IPT) was formulated as a time-limited weekly therapy for depressed patients. It makes no assumptions about aetiology, but uses the connections between the onset of the depressive symptoms and current interpersonal problems as a focus for treatment. It thus focuses more on current relationships than on enduring aspects of the personality, and the therapists take an active and supportive stance.

The therapy starts with a diagnostic phase, in which the patient's disorder is identified and explained. The therapist links the depressive symptoms to one of four interpersonal areas:

- grief
- interpersonal role disputes
- role transitions
- interpersonal deficits.

The therapist will then pursue strategies specific to one of these problem areas. In the final phase of treatment, the patient is helped to focus on the therapeutic gains and to develop ways of identifying and countering depressive symptoms should they recur in the future.

IPT has been described as an effective treatment both for depression and bulimia nervosa (Klerman et al. 1994).

Psychodynamic interpersonal therapy

This model, developed by RF Hobson in Manchester and more recently Guthrie and colleagues, is theoretically derived from psychodynamic principles, but also draws on humanistic and interpersonal concepts. Originally called the conversational model of therapy, the main task of the therapist is to develop with the patient a 'mutual feeling language' and a relationship of 'aloneness-togetherness'. There are seven different but interlinking components to the model:

- exploratory rationale
- shared understanding
- staying with feelings
- focus on difficult feelings
- gaining insight
- sequencing interventions
- making changes

Psychodynamic interpersonal therapy (PIT) can be used for either brief or long-term work. Guthrie (1999) describes the treatment in detail, and also provides evidence for the efficacy of PIT in depression, and the treatment of somatization

Family therapy

Family therapy can be defined as the psychotherapeutic treatment of a natural social system, the family, using as its basic medium conjoint family interviews.

Walrond-Skinner (1977)

Origins of family therapy

Family therapy has many origins. Freud recognized the importance of the family in the development of symptoms, and indeed his case of Little Hans (see above) was based on material supplied to him by the patient's father. However, Freud himself did not see families for therapy per se. Bowlby in 1940 and subsequently therapists from both sides of the Atlantic (including Dr John Bell from the Mental Research Institute, Palo Alto, California) described early experimental work with family group therapy, and this in turn influenced other clinicians in the development of a practice. Various clinical and philosophical influences provide the background to family therapy, including:

- General systems theory (Von Bertalanffy) – used particularly in family therapy with the concepts of concentric and overlapping systems and subsystems of interacting individuals. Within the system there is:
  (a) maintenance of homeostasis wherever possible, but there may be
  (b) crisis due to an external challenge, which may lead to
  (c) exploration of the problems and
  (d) reorganization and a new family homeostasis
- Cybernetics – the theory of control and communication between the individual and machine.

The three main schools of family therapy are structural, systemic and strategic (see Box 36.3).

Box 36.3   The main schools in family therapy

Structural (Minuchin): stressing dysfunction, hierarchies, redesigning the family system so that it approximates a normative model of clear but open boundaries between generational subsystems

Systemic (Milan school): using circularity, hypothesizing, neutrality, paradox and counterparadox

Strategic (Haley): using active interventions to fit the specific problem and the detail of how and when it occurs; has some similarities to a behavioural approach (looking at antecedents, behaviour and consequences – 'ABC')

Social constructionist approach, based on the awareness that the 'reality' therapists observe is 'invented', with perceptions being shaped by the therapists' own cultures and their implicit assumptions and beliefs, influenced by Foucault

Brief solution-focused therapy – this emphasizes the competencies of families and individuals

Psycho-educational approach (e.g. the work of Leff et al. (1985) in families with a schizophrenic member)

Psychoanalytic family and couple therapy

Salvador Minuchin is associated with the structural school of thought. He pioneered studies on urban slum families and researched 'psychosomatic families' and families with a member with an eating disorder. Minuchin also developed the use of a one-way screen for the training of therapists. This approach postulates that families tend to function well when certain family structures prevail, such as 'hierarchies' between generations within a family, with semi-permeable boundaries permitting a sufficient flow of information up and down, for example between parents and their children. The structural therapist would intervene with the aim of making the family structure approximate a 'normative model'. Techniques include challenging absent or rigid boundaries, 'unbalancing' the family equilibrium by temporarily joining with one member of the family against the others, or setting 'homework' tasks to restore hierarchies. This is a very active approach, challenging 'dysfunctional' alliances and coalitions within families, often deliberately inducing therapeutic crises, in order that the family discovers new resources and solutions to old problems and dilemnas.

In 1967, the Institute of Family Studies was founded in Milan, Italy, and between 1972 and 1974 they developed their notions of 'paradox' and 'counter-paradox'. In 1975, they entered into a different phase, rejecting notions of hierarchy and examining how different levels of meaning were related to one another in a circular pattern. They focused on pattern and information, rather than structural form, and this group became known as the Systemic/Milan School, whose approach began to be adopted in many developing centres throughout the world. They are also associated with the use of 'paradoxical injunctions', i.e. a technique where instead of the prescription being for change, the prescription is for the status quo to be maintained or even exaggerated.

The Milan systemic approach focuses on multi-generational family patterns, describing the interactions and struggles of family members over several generations. There is considerable emphasis on the making of (sometimes elaborate) hypotheses, both by the observing team behind the one-way mirror, and within the consulting room, within the therapist's mind and shared between therapist and family members. Other key principles include therapist 'neutrality', 'circularity' and 'reflexive questioning'. Systemic therapists become curious inquirers, who solicit information about various family members, and their beliefs and perceptions regarding relationships and interactions (Asen 2002).

The Palo Alto group (Bateson, Weakland, Jackson and Haley) conducted research at the Palo Alto (California) Mental Research Institute on the communications patterns in families with members showing schizophrenic symptoms. Adopting ideas from general systems theory and cybernetics to study family systems, they looked at communication processes and, in 1959, Jackson established the world's first family therapy centre for training, research and therapy. The core concept of communication theory has been extended to the notion that communication is part of a struggle for power within relationships. This group's work is referred to as strategic therapy or, alternatively, brief therapy. Initially, it was problem-focused and developed crisis intervention techniques.

Strategic family therapy aims to deliver interventions or 'strategies' to fit the presenting problem. The underlying assumption is that the symptom is being maintained by the apparent solution, i.e. the very behaviours that seek to suppress the presenting symptom. 'Reframing' is used as a major technique – the family's or patient's perceived problem is put into a different meaning-frame, thus providing new perspectives and therefore potentially making new behaviours possible.

More recently, De Shazer (1984) has developed 'solution focused therapy'. In Australia and New Zealand, Michael White and David Epston have developed similar solution-focused ideas, incorporating unique outcomes and the theory of narrative texts, whereby clients are encouraged through future time questions, or are asked to rewrite their own life stories.

Foundations of family therapy

Family therapy has broadened the focus of treatment from the individual to the family and social context, contending that individuals live not in isolation but within a social context, and are best understood by examining their relationships to others and the environment in which they interact. The notion of holism underlines the central concept. The whole is made up of more than a group of individuals, as it also includes the relationships between its members. A central concept, therefore, is of circular causality. Circularity implies that every member in a system influences the others and is influenced by them. When such an assumption is applied to a family in therapy, blame for the problem is not attributed to individuals, and problems are viewed with respect to relationships between people, or other systems, and may be an inevitable result of change across time.

The family is seen as a dynamic system that co-evolves with its environment. The family experiences continual fluctuation as it moves through its own family life-cycle and time. Carter & McGoldrick (1984) have presented a framework which details the six stages of the family life-cycle and the changes required from the family in order for it to proceed developmentally.

The symptom is believed to have occurred when the family has not appropriately adjusted to disruptions or transition points in the family life-cycle. Such transition points may include changes in the composition of the family (e.g. births, deaths or divorces), particular developments by individual members (e.g. change in residence, school or workplace) and unexpected changes (e.g. illness or retrenchment). Such changes may require negotiation of new rules or family structures. It is believed that the family is self-

regulating and thus will attempt to maintain stability or homeostasis. In response to fluctuations brought about by changes in the developmental life-cycle, or stresses from outside the family system, change in one family member may be counterbalanced by complementary changes in another member, in a process known as negative feedback.

Positive feedback has the opposite effect. A small deviation within the system may be exaggerated or amplified by other members. This process may explain how some problems develop and become out of control and how the same unhelpful solution is repeated.

A universal goal of family therapists is to remove the symptom and alleviate family distress, while other aims involve clarifying communication, solving problems and promoting individual autonomy. In most family therapies, there is the tendency to de-emphasize insight and promote action, and to concentrate on the present rather than the past (in contrast to individual psychodynamic psychotherapy). The therapist's role is as a change agent and is thus generally active and directive. The three main schools of thought in family therapy share these foundations. However, they differ in their levels of focus, methodology, and techniques.

Systemic therapy, like psychodynamic psychotherapy influences psychiatric practice way beyond the confines of particular patients being treated in specific psychotherapy settings. The systemic approach is well integrated especially in the field of child and adolescent psychiatry, less so within general adult psychiatry (Asen 2002).

Group psychotherapy and analysis

Group therapy and group analysis are popular and well-established modes of psychotherapy, practised, like individual and family therapy both in the private and public sectors. Many of the founding figures in group therapy and analysis were also trained in individual psychoanalysis (e.g. Wilfred Bion and Malcolm Pines). However, the theory and practice of group analysis is now a distinct discipline influenced not only by psychoanalysis but also by sociology, social psychology and organizational theory (Roberts 1995).

At least three models of group analytic practice can be discerned:

- analysis in the group – where an individual may be treated within a group context
- analysis of the group – where the leader/'conductor'/ therapist interprets the transference of the group to him/herself
- analysis through and of the group – especially associated with the work of Foulkes and the Institute of Group Analysis.

Wolf and Schwarz are associated with analysis in the group, similar to individual therapy in a group setting. Bion and Ezriel are associated with analysis of the group. Henry Ezriel proposed that in every meeting of a group it is possible to identify a common group tension. His method was for the 'conductor' (therapist) to identify three types of object relationship emerging from the common group tension:

- the 'required' relationship – a socially acceptable, safe, defensive mode of functioning, for example 'I will miss the group during the summer break'
- the 'avoided' relationship – which might include feelings of murderous rage about the therapist's long indulgent summer break
- the 'calamitous' relationship – which is the feared outcome of the avoided relationship being consciously acknowledged, for example murderous wishes could destroy therapist and group, incestuous wishes would lead to dire punishment.

Foulkes is associated with analysis through the group, i.e. the awareness of transpersonal phenomena and multiple levels of group functioning, including:

- level of current adult relationships
- level of individual transference
- level of shared feelings and fantasies (the level of archetypal universal images, similar to Jung's archetypes of the collective unconscious).

Yalom (1985) published *The Theory and Practice of Group Psychotherapy* having worked both in the USA and at the Tavistock Clinic in London. He describes a number of therapeutic factors specific to groups:

- universality
- altruism
- corrective recapitulation of the family group, i.e. what went wrong in the early family group can be repeated and recognized in the group, where in a more open and experiential atmosphere less maladaptive ways can be worked out
- imitative behaviour
- interpersonal learning
- cohesiveness
- existential factors, which include the recognition of responsibility in the face of our basic aloneness and mortality
- catharsis
- insight
- development of socializing techniques
- guidance
- instillation of hope.

Pairing and subgrouping can be destructive, as can inappropriate idealization of the therapist. In general, the maintenance of boundaries, including starting and finishing on time and preparation of the room, is part of the therapist's function.

While not all patients in the mental health setting will formally be involved in group therapy, all patients and staff are wittingly and unwittingly caught up in group processes.

Hobbs (in Holmes 1991) usefully describes a number of group processes within psychiatry. It is in order to better understand these processes that some wards or psychiatric teams make use of an outside facilitator in a staff support group, or a case discussion seminar. Even within these groups, there are further group dynamics of which to be aware (see Stern 1996).

Therapeutic communities

The term 'therapeutic community' (TC) is usually used in the UK to describe small, cohesive communities where patients (sometimes referred to as 'residents') have a significant involvement in decision making and the practicalities of running the unit. Key principles include collective responsibility, citizenship and empowerment, and TCs are structured in a way that deliberately encourages personal responsibility and discourages unhelpful dependency on professionals. Patients are seen as bringing strengths and creative energy into the therapeutic setting, and the peer group is seen as all-important in the establishment of a strong therapeutic alliance. The belief in flattening of hierarchies and delegated decision-making may be seen by outsiders as facilitating something anarchic, but in reality there is a deep awareness of the need for strong leadership and a safe therapeutic frame (Campling 2001).

The power of groups was demonstrated in the UK in the Second World War by the Northfield experiments, named after the Northfield Hospital in Birmingham. Here, an Army psychiatric unit was run along group lines, and some well-known figures, including Bion, Foulkes and Main, were involved. Bion went on to write about groups and became a prominent Kleinian theoretician. Foulkes is one of the founding fathers of group analysis, and Main described the therapeutic community, an institution where 'the setting itself is designed to restore morale and promote the psychological treatment of mental and emotional disturbance'. Main went on to create the influential example of the Cassel Hospital in Surrey.

Maxwell Jones founded the Belmont in the 1950s, later called the Henderson Hospital, in Sutton, Surrey. Here, the community is the main focus, and careful procedures for admission, discipline and discharge have been established over the years. Patients with severe personality disorders are often admitted, and the regime is characterized by what the anthropologist Rapoport (1960) termed 'permissiveness, reality-confrontation, democracy and communalism'.

Permissiveness encourages the expression and enactment of disturbed feelings and relationships, so that they can be examined by patients and staff alike. Differences between patients and staff are minimized, and decisions are made with residents having a majority vote (and often being harsher than staff members themselves). Permissiveness is usually limited to the verbal expression of feelings, and would be strongly confronted if it led to other members of the TC being emotionally hurt or damaged, or feeling marginalized or excluded. Racist comments, for example, would not go unchallenged in modern TCs (Campling 2001).

A further important observation form Rapoport's study was the repeated cycle of *oscillations*: times of healthy functioning, when residents were well able to manage responsibility and a level of therapeutic permissiveness; and other times when high levels of disturbed behaviour have meant that staff had to take a more active role. A further observation was the conflict between those whose main objective was preparing residents for the outside world, and those whose main objective was helping residents to better understand their inner worlds – a tension between 'rehabilitation' and 'psychotherapy' that still persists in many modern TCs. The Henderson is in many ways the prototypical therapeutic community.

Clark (1977) has described three important terms:

- *therapeutic community* or *therapeutic community proper* refers to the specific type of therapeutic milieu set up by Maxwell Jones and followers, e.g. Henderson, 'a small face-to-face residential community using social analysis as its main tool'
- *therapeutic milieu* is a social setting designed to produce a beneficial effect on those being helped in it, e.g. a sheltered workshop, hospital ward, hostel
- *social therapy* is the least specific term, employing the idea that the milieu or social environment can be used as a mode of treatment.

TCs have a long history of involvement in research. Much of this has been from a social science perspective and qualitative in nature. Some of it is of importance to other areas of psychiatry, for example methodological approaches to develop, describe and measure the therapeutic milieu, of which the Ward Atmosphere Scale developed by Moos is the best example. Over the past decade, researchers based at both the Henderson and the Cassel hospitals have produced methodologically sound research demonstrating the cost-effectiveness of their treatments (Dolan et al. 1996; Hinshelwood & Skogstad 1998; Norton 1996).

TCs are seen to have a valuable role to play within the future of mental health services. Within the NHS in the UK, they have established a niche for those suffering from severe emotionally unstable personality disorder, a group of high risk patients who become heavy users of services if they do not receive the intensive long term psychosocial therapy they require.

The application of TC ideas, like ideas from psychodynamic, systemic and group therapy, has had an important impact on the general practice of psychiatry.

RESEARCH IN PSYCHOTHERAPY

This is a vast topic, outside the realms of this chapter. The interested reader is referred to the publication by Roth &

Fonagy (1996), in which they systematically and critically review the literature on:

- which psychotherapeutic interventions are of demonstrable benefit to particular patient groups
- research evidence that would help funders of health care decide on the appropriate mix of therapies for their population and
- the extent to which one can draw on evidence of demonstrated efficacy in controlled research conditions and clinical effectiveness in services as delivered.

Two recent examples of sound research in psychotherapy are the work of Guthrie, Creed and colleagues in Manchester working with patients from a gastroenterology clinic, and the work by Leff et al. in London, researching systemic couple therapy for depression.

In their earlier study, Guthrie and colleagues (1991) studied the effects of psychodynamic interpersonal therapy on patients with irritable bowel syndrome (IBS). The treatment group received seven sessions of exploratory psychotherapy, while the control group received a similar number of sessions of supportive listening. At the end of the study a significantly greater improvement was found in the treatment group, rated by a gastroenterologist who was blind to the treatment groups. The study includes a placebo attention control and clearly showed that the improvement resulting from the psychotherapy was the result of the specific effect of the therapy, rather than as a result of spending time with an empathic and supportive therapist. In addition, only the most difficult patients, i.e. those with chronic, unresponsive symptoms, were included in the study. A more recent study by the same group (Creed et al. 2003) has looked at the cost-effectiveness of psychodynamic interpersonal therapy and paroxetine in patients with severe IBS. The results showed that both treatments were superior to treatment as usual in improving the physical aspects of health related quality of life measures, but there was no difference in the psychological component. During the follow-up year, the psychotherapy but not paroxetine was associated with a significant reduction in health care costs compared with treatment as usual. (A recent study by Drossman and colleagues (2003) highlights the efficacy of cognitive–behavioural therapy (CBT), and to a lesser extent desipramine, in a similar population.)

In the study by Leff et al. (2000) the relative efficacy and cost of couple therapy, antidepressant therapy and CBT were compared, for the treatment and maintenance of people with depression living with a critical partner or spouse. Patients in a long-term heterosexual relationship, who met defined criteria for depression were randomly allocated to the three treatments mentioned above. (The CBT drop-out rate was so high that this treatment option was soon deleted from the trial). The results were striking: over half (56%) of those allocated to drug treatment dropped out of the treatment compared with 15% of those offered couple therapy.

Subjects' depression improved in both groups, but couple therapy showed a significant advantage according to the Beck depression inventory, both at the end of treatment and after a second year off treatment. Overall, there was no difference in the total costs (adding the costs of psycho- or pharmaco-therapy to the costs of other services used). The authors conclude 'For this group, couple therapy is much more acceptable than antidepressant drugs and is at least as efficacious, if not more so, both in the treatment and maintenance phases' (p. 95).

These studies are methodologically very different from the traditional intensive, highly personal case study/research work carried out over months or years in psychoanalytic or psychotherapy practice. The tradition within most psychodynamic work remains that of detailed case histories, originating with Freud's own cases. Both are valuable sources of information about patients and psychological processes. Single case studies have a number of attractive features – they can be carried out in routine clinical practice, they do not necessarily require the facilities associated with more complex research, and can sometimes be completed fairly quickly. However, precisely because they are single case studies, the results cannot necessarily be generalized. The task of psychotherapy research in the future is to proceed with both modes of enquiry, and permit as much cross-fertilization between the two modes of research and practice as possible.

THE ROLE OF PSYCHOTHERAPY AND THE PSYCHOTHERAPIST WITHIN PSYCHIATRY

The relationship between psychiatry and psychotherapy is a complicated one. Hook (2001) has described some of the tensions, prejudices and anxieties which characterize this relationship.

Within psychiatric practice in Britain, and perhaps throughout the world, psychotherapy occupies a unique role. Not only is it a mode of treatment for some patients, it is also an explanatory model; not only is the psychotherapist called upon to fulfil numerous overt functions within the institution, there are also all sorts of other functions which a psychotherapist may be called upon or expected to fulfil, some more appropriate than others.

Overt roles of the psychotherapist

The 'overt roles' are the explicit functions for which the organization employs the practitioner. They are what might be included in a job description, and include:

- assessment of patients referred for psychotherapy
- treatment of such patients if appropriate – individual, groups, family, cognitive behavioural therapy, etc.

- consultations to various teams in the hospital – for instance, old age team, mother and baby unit, forensic or general adult psychiatry, etc.
- supervision of junior staff who are treating patients
- formal teaching for junior psychiatrists, and medical students, including those preparing for examinations
- the running of staff support groups for junior doctors and/or other teams on wards/community
- attending the weekly 'grand round'
- research
- informal (as required) consultations.

Over and above the many varied overt roles mentioned above, much more is provided.

Covert roles

Firstly, through intensive contact with supervisees, much psychological support is provided for psychotherapists as they struggle to cope with what it takes to work with mental disturbance. The model is of long-term focused care on an individual, and tries to make sense of symptoms and behaviour that would otherwise be described as unintelligible.

There is also the presence in the hospital of someone who, while functioning (hopefully) effectively and creatively, also states implicitly or explicitly that he/she has had or is having his/her own psychotherapeutic or analytic treatment. This generally facilitates others to ask for it themselves, so that the psychotherapist is often called upon by colleagues to help find a suitable therapist for themselves or their family members.

An allied role is to provide 'meaning' to the work publicly. Constantly at weekly academic meetings or 'grand rounds', fascinating cases are presented – of pathologically jealous men, of depressed mothers, of lonely migrants who have lost everything and evoke sadness in their carers; but within some minutes of these presentations beginning, these people are transformed into 'cases of', 'treatment-resistant depression', 'psychosis', 'post-traumatic stress disorder (PTSD)', and the patient is lost to the discussion. In fact, it is not only the patients who are transformed – sensitive, creative psychiatrists start trying to trump each other with regards to diagnosis, special investigations, reading the latest scan, discussing the latest research on the latest drugs. The patient and what he or she is, or means, or wishes, or fears, is lost. This is where the psychotherapist may try and come in, with notions of the unconscious, or family dynamics, of conflict or of countertransference, to try help make sense of what is going on internally, and between the patient and carer, and perhaps why some of the drugs are not being taken or are not 'doing the job properly'. On occasions, this is reassuring and helpful to the group and to the patient in the long run. On other occasions, when the anxiety in the group is too high, these comments are brushed

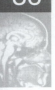
aside, and the discussion continues, seemingly untouched; this occurs sometimes when the patient is so anxiety-provoking that action takes precedence over thought; and sometimes when the person presenting the case, or the group as whole, is highly anxious (or perhaps sometimes when the point made by the therapist is just not useful!).

A third covert function is to provide a place where impossible patients can be disposed of. Three particular groups come to mind:

- So-called borderline women: attractive, seductive, self-destructive, who just refuse to improve on antidepressants and who make the young psychiatry trainee (or not so young consultant) distinctly uneasy.
- Slightly older patients, again predominantly women, who somatize, re-enacting their sadomasochistic object relations through contact with the medical profession, as well as their social network, and once again frustrating psychiatrists by refusing to get better.
- Thirdly, there are men who are not quite violent or perverse enough to be referred to forensic services, but who are uncomfortable to treat in general outpatient psychiatry, and who once again tend not to improve on antidepressant therapy.

These patients are the ambivalently charged gifts from psychiatric colleagues. The most intelligent and sympathetic of psychiatrists want these special patients to be got rid of, and dealt with even if they are totally unsuitable for therapy.

A final covert role, perhaps increasingly obvious now, is that there are many unconscious projections flying around the hospital and the psychotherapy department, and particular people within the department, carry those projections (often disavowed or undesirable attributes) 'perverse, greedy, interested in sex, lazy, feminine, effeminate', and so on. When these projections are too massive, and the splits between psychotherapy and psychiatry too wide, it becomes very difficult to function. The opposite is true too: when there is a denial of any difference, when psychotherapists deny their very different discipline and mode of thinking, then there is also likely to be a breakdown of effective and creative functioning.

The psychotherapist within the general psychiatry context has to function with the same capacity to think about the task at hand, and the greater social context, and his/her own contribution and feelings and prejudices, as when he/she is doing intensive individual therapy or analysis.

ADDITIONAL TOPICS

There are many other topics in psychotherapy that have not been covered in this chapter. These include areas such as child and adolescent psychotherapy (e.g. Anastosopolous et al. 1999), forensic psychotherapy (Welldon & Van Velsen 1997), psychotherapy across cultures (Kareem & Littlewood

1992), psychotherapeutic work with trauma victims (Garland 1998), work with the elderly (Porter 1991) and with addicts (Edwards & Dare 1996), psychodynamic work with patients with functional bowel disorders (Stern 1999) and patients with special needs or learning disabilities (Sinason 1992).

REFERENCES

Ainsworth MDS, Blehar MC, Walters E & Wall S (1978) *Patterns of Attachment: A Psychological Study of the Strange Situation*. Hillsdale, NJ: Erlbaum.

Akhtar S (1992) *Broken Structures: Severe Personality Disorders and Their Treatment*. New York: Jason Aronson.

Akhtar S (1995) *Quest for answers: A Primer of Understanding and Treating Severe Personality Disorders*. New York: Jason Aronson.

Akhtar S & Parens H (1991) *Beyond the Symbiotic Orbit. Advances in Separation-individuation Theory*. Hillsdale, NJ: The Analytic Press.

Anastasopolous D, Laylou-Linos E & Waddell M (1999) *Psychoanalytic Psychotherapy of the Severely Disturbed Adolescent*. London: Karnac Books.

Asen E. (2002) Integrative therapy from a systemic perspective. In: Holmes J & Bateman A (eds) *Integration in Psychotherapy: Models and Methods*. Oxford: Oxford University Press.

Bateman A, Brown D & Pedder J (2000) *Introduction to Psychotherapy*. London: Routledge.

Bateman A & Holmes J (1995) *Introduction to Psychoanalysis: Contemporary Theory and Practice*. London: Routledge.

Bion WR (1962) *Learning from Experience*. London: Heinemann.

Britton R (1992) Keeping things in mind. In: Anderson R (ed.) *Clinical Lectures on Klein and Bion*. London: Routledge.

Campling P (2001) Therapeutic communities. *Advances in Psychiatric Treatment* **7**: 365–72.

Carter E & McGoldrick M (1984) *The Family Lifecycle*. New York: Gardner Press.

Cawley RH (1977) The teaching of psychotherapy. *Association of University Teachers of Psychiatry Newsletter* **19**: 36.

Clark DH (1977) The therapeutic community. *British Journal of Psychiatry* **131**: 553–64.

Creed F, Fernandes L, Guthrie E et al. (2003) The cost-effectiveness of psychotherapy and paroxetine for severe irritable bowel syndrome. *Gastroenterology* **124**: 303–17.

Dare C, Eisler I, Russell G & Szmukler G (1990) Family therapy for anorexia nervosa; implications from the results of a controlled trial of family and individual therapy. *Journal of Marital and Family Therapy* **16**: 1–26.

De Shazer S (1984) The death of resistance. *Family Process* **23**: 11–17.

Dolan B, Warren F, Menzies D et al. (1996) Cost-offset following specialist treatment of severe personality disorders. *Psychiatric Bulletin* **20**: 413–17.

Drossman D, Toner B, Whitehead W et al. (2003) Cognitive behavioural therapy versus education and desipramine versus placebo for moderate to severe functional bowel disorders. *Gastroenterology* **125**: 19–31.

Edwards G & Dare C (1996) *Psychotherapy, Psychological Treatments and the Addictions*. Cambridge: Cambridge University Press.

Fonagy P, Steele M, Steele H et al. (2000) The predictive specificity of Mary Main's Adult Attachment Interview. In: Goldberg S, Muir R & Kerr J (eds) *John Bowlby's Attachment Theory: Historical, Social and Clinical Significance*. Hilldale, NJ: Analytic Press.

Frank J (1961) *Persuasion and Healing*. Baltimore, MD: Johns Hopkins Press.

Freud S (1900) *The Interpretation of Dreams*. Standard edition IV–V. London: Hogarth Press.

Freud S (1905a) *Fragment of an Analysis of a Case of Hysteria*. Penguin Freud Library, vol. 8.

Freud S (1905b) *Three Essays on the Theory of Sexuality*. Penguin Freud Library, vol. 7.

Freud S (1909a) Analysis of a phobia in a five year old boy ('Little Hans'). In: *The Wolfman and Other Cases*. 2002 edition. Penguin Freud Library, vol. 9.

Freud S (1909b) Notes upon a case of obsessional neurosis. In: *The Complete Psychological Works of Sigmund Freud*. Standard edition, vol. 10. London: Hogath Press.

Freud S (1911a) *Psychoanalytical Notes on Autobiographical Account of a case of Paranoia (Dementia Paranoides)*. Standard edition, vol. 11. London: Hogarth Press.

Freud S (1911b) *Formulations on the Two Principles of Mental Functioning*. Penguin Freud Library, vol. 11.

Freud S (1913) *Totem and Taboo*. Penguin Freud Library, vol. 13.

Freud S (1914) *Remembering, Repeating and Working Through*. Standard edition II. London: Hogarth Press.

Freud S (1917) 'Mourning and melancholia'. In: *The Complete Psychological Works of Sigmund Freud*. Standard edition, pp. 237–60. London: Hogarth Press.

Freud S (1919) From the history of an infantile neurosis (the 'Wolfman'). In: *The Wolfman and Other Cases*. 2002 edition. Penguin Freud Library, vol. 9.

Freud S (1920) *Beyond the Pleasure Principle*. Penguin Freud Library, vol. 11.

Freud S (1921) *Group Psychology and the Analysis of the Ego*. Penguin Freud Library, vol. 12.

Freud S (1923) *The Ego and the Id*. Penguin Freud Library, vol. 11.

Freud S (1926) *Inhibitions, Symptoms and Anxiety*. Standard edition, vol. 22. London: Hogarth Press.

Freud S (1933) *New Introductory Lectures on Psychoanalysis*. Penguin Freud Library, vol. 2.

Freud S (1937) *Analysis Terminable and Interminable*. Standard edition, vol. 23. London: Hogarth Press.

Freud S & Breuer J (1895) *Studies on Hysteria*. Standard edition II. London: Hogarth Press.

Gabbard G (2000) *Psychodynamic Psychotherapy in Clinical Practice*. Arlington, VA: American Psychiatric Press.

Garland C (ed.) (1998) *Understanding Trauma: A Psychoanalytical Approach*. London: Duckworth and Co.

Gay P (1995) *The Freud Reader*. London: Vintage Press.

Greenson R (1967) *The Technique and Practice of Psychoanalysis*. London: Hogarth Press.

Greenson R & Wexler R (1969) The non-transference relationship in the psycho-analytic situation. *International Journal of Psycho-Analysis* **50**: 27–39.

Guthrie E (1996) Psychotherapy for somatization disorders. *Current Opinion in Psychiatry* 9: 182–7.

Guthrie E, Creed FH, Dawson D et al. (1991) A controlled trial of psychological treatment for irritable bowel syndrome. *Gastroenterology* 100: 450–7.

Guthrie E (1999) Psychodynamic Interpersonal therapy. *Advances in Psychiatric Treatment* 5(2):135–45.

Hinshelwood R & Skogstad W (1998) The hospital in mind: in-patient psychotherapy at the Cassel Hospital. In: Pestalozzi J (ed.) *Psychoanalytic Psychotherapy in Institutional Settings*. London: Karnac.

Holmes J (1991) *Textbook of Psychotherapy in Psychiatric Practice*. London: Churchill Livingstone.

Holmes J (1993) Attachment theory: a biological basis for psychotherapy. *British Journal of Psychiatry* 163: 430–8.

Holmes J (1994) Brief dynamic psychotherapy. *Advances in Psychiatric Treatment* 1(1): 9–15.

Hook J (2001) The role of psychodynamic psychotherapy in a modern general psychiatry service. *Advances in Psychiatric Treatment* 7(6): 461–8.

Jones E (1961) *The Life and Work of Sigmund Freud*. New York: Basic Books.

Kareem J & Littlewood R (1992) *Intercultural Therapy: Themes, Interpretations and Practice*. Oxford: Blackwell Scientific Publications.

Kernberg O (1970) Apsychoanalytic classification of character pathology. *Journal of the American Psychoanalytic Association* **15**: 641–85.

Kernberg O (1992) *Aggression in Personality Disorders and Perversions*. New Haven, CT: Yale University Press.

King P & Steiner R (1992) *The Freud–Klein Controversies 1941–45*. London: Routledge.

Klein M (1946) Notes on some schizoid mechanisms. In: Klein M *Envy and Gratitude, and Other Works*, vol 3, pp. 1–24. London: Hogarth Press.

Klerman GL & Weissman MM (1994) *New Applications of Interpersonal Psychotherapy*. Washington, DC: American Psychiatric Press.

Klerman GL, Weissman MM, Rounsaville BJ & Chevron ES (1994) *Interpersonal Psychotherapy of Depression*. New York: Basic Books.

Leff JP, Kuipers E, Berkowitz R & Sturgeon D (1985) A controlled trial of interventions in the families of schizophrenic patients:two year follow-up. *British Journal of Psychiatry* **146**: 594–600.

Leff J, Vearnals S, Brewin C et al. (2000) The London Depression Intervention Trial. *British Journal of Psychiatry* **177**: 95–100.

Mahler MS (1971) A study of the separation-individuation process and its possible application to borderline phenomena in the psychoanalytic situation. *Psychoanalytic Study of the Child* 26: 402–24.

Main M (1990) *A Typology of Human Attachment Organisation with Discourse, Drawings and Interviews*. New York: Cambridge University Press.

Malan D (1963) *A Study of Brief Psychotherapy*. London: Tavistock Publications.

McDougall J (1989) *Theatres of the Body: A Psychoanalytic Approach to Psychosomatic Illness*. London: Free Association Books.

Nachman PA (1991) Contemporary infant research and the separation-individuation theory of Margaret S Mahler. In: Akhtar S & Parens H (eds) *Beyond the Symbiotic Orbit. Advances in Separation-Individuation Theory*. Hillsdale, NJ: The Analytic Press.

Norton K (1996) Management of difficult personality disorder patients. *Advances in Psychiatric Treatment* 2(5): 202–10.

Perelberg RJ (2000) *Dreaming and Thinking*. London: Karnac Books.

Porter R (1991) Working with the elderly. In: Holmes J (ed.) *Textbook of Psychotherapy in Psychiatric Practice*. London: Churchill Livingstone.

Rapoport RN (1960). *Community as Doctor: New Perspectives on a Therapeutic Community*. London: Tavistock Publications.

Roberts J (1995) Reading about group psychotherapy. *British Journal of Psychiatry* **166**: 124–9.

Roth A & Fonagy P (1996) What works for whom? *A Critical Review of Psychotherapy Research*. New York: Guilford Press.

Royal College of Psychiatrists (1993) Guidelines for psychotherapy training as part of general professional psychiatric training. *Psychiatric Bulletin* **17**: 695–8.

Rycroft C (1972) *A Critical Dictionary of Psychoanalysis*. London: Penguin Books.

Ryle A, Spencer J & Yawetz C (1992) When less is more or at least enough. Two cases of 16-session cognitive analytic therapy. *British Journal of Psychotherapy* 8(4): 401–12.

Sharpe M, Hawton K, Simkin SS, et al. (1996) CBT for chronic fatigue syndrome. A randomized controlled trial. *British Medical Journal* **312**: 22–6.

Sinason V (1992) *Mental Handicap and the Human Condition: New Approaches from The Tavistock*. London: Free Association Books.

Stern JM (1996) Group processes in a case discussion workshop for community psychiatric nurses. *Journal of Psychiatric and Mental Health Nursing* 3(6): 355–60.

Stern JM (1999) Psychoanalytical psychotherapy with patients in a medical setting. *Psychoanalytic Psychotherapy* 13: 51–68.

Walrond-Skinner S (1977) *Family Therapy. The Treatment of Natural Systems*. London: Routledge and Kegan Paul Ltd.

Welldon E & Van Velsen C (1997) *A Practical Guide to Forensic Psychotherapy*. London: Jessica Kingsley Publishers.

Whale J (1992) The use of brief focal psychotherapy in the treatment of chronic pain. *Psychoanalytic Psychotherapy* 6: 61–72.

Winnicott DW (1947) Fear of breakdown. *International Review of Psycho-Analysis* 1: 103–7.

Winnicott DW (1949) Hate in the counter-transference. *International Journal of Psycho-Analysis* 30: 69–74.

Yalom ID (1985) *The Theory and Practice of Group Psychotherapy*, 3rd edn. New York: Basic Books.

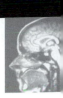

Behavioural and cognitive psychotherapies

Stirling Moorey

INTRODUCTION

Over the last 30 years, cognitive–behavioural therapies (CBTs) have established a central place in the psychological treatment of many disorders. Evidence for their effectiveness is substantial. CBT has consistently been shown to be superior to waiting list and 'treatment as usual' conditions, and is usually at least as effective as drug treatment, though its superiority over other active forms of psychotherapy is more controversial (see Roth & Fonagy 1996). The relative simplicity of its theory and practice, together with the empirical evidence makes this approach increasingly appealing to clinicians and managers alike. Cognitive–behavioural therapy covers a broad spectrum from simple, technical, theory-free behavioural techniques at one end to complex treatment packages based on cognitive theories at the other (Box 37.1). Most practice occupies a middle ground. This chapter will cover behavioural approaches first, since they are of historical significance and still highly effective treatments in their own right, and will then consider cognitive therapy, focusing mainly on the contribution of A.T. Beck.

BEHAVIOUR THERAPY

Learning theory

In the first half of the 20th century, John Watson championed the cause of psychology as 'a purely objective branch of natural science'. His *behaviourism* viewed all our actions as the products of conditioning: thoughts, feelings and motives are mere epiphenomena. In 1920 he described how he was able to condition a fear response in an 11-month-old child named Little Albert by pairing the appearance of a furry white rat with a loud noise (Watson & Rayner 1920). Every time the child touched the rat a loud noise was made. The infant developed a fear of the rat which generalized to other stimuli such as cotton wool and even gentlemen with white beards! Watson's pupils developed a method for

deconditioning anxiety in children which was probably the first example of behaviour therapy. Two types of conditioning exist: classical and operant.

Classical conditioning

Watson was strongly influenced by the work of the Russian physiologist, Pavlov. His work on conditioning salivation in dogs is well known. In a typical Pavlovian experiment, a physiological response such as salivating to the sight of food is studied. The food is termed the *unconditional* stimulus (UCS) and salivation is termed the *unconditional response* or *reflex* (UCR). Presentation of the food is repeatedly paired with a *conditional stimulus* (CS), for instance a bell. When the bell is then rung without the food the dog salivates. This salivation to the bell is the *conditional response* or *reflex*.

Pavlov found that the strength of conditioning is increased by a number of factors:

- if the unconditional stimulus (food) follows the conditional one (bell)
- if there is a short delay between the unconditional stimulus and the conditional stimulus
- the intensity of UCS and CS: bigger pieces of food or a louder bell.

Behaviour therapists have been particularly interested in the application of classical conditioning theory to anxiety. Phobias in particular can be seen as forms of conditioned

---

Box 37.1 Definitions

Behaviour therapy is a treatment approach originally derived from learning theory, which seeks to solve problems and relieve symptoms by changing behaviour and the environmental contingencies that control behaviour

Behaviour modification is an approach to change behaviour in clinical and non-clinical settings based on operant conditioning

Cognitive therapy is a treatment approach derived from cognitive theories which seeks to solve problems and relieve symptoms by changing thoughts and beliefs

Cognitive behaviour therapy (behavioural–cognitive therapy) refers to the pragmatic combination of concepts and techniques from these therapies in clinical practice

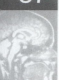

fear responses to given stimuli. This model has been applied to simple phobias, agoraphobia, social phobia and obsessive-compulsive disorder. As an explanation of the development of most phobias, the conditioned fear model is inadequate (e.g. only 23% of animal phobias are associated with a prior traumatic experience with the animal; McNally & Steketee 1985). This has led to the idea that we may be *prepared* to acquire certain fears on evolutionary grounds (Seligman 1971). The classical conditioning model has been very influential in the development of exposure therapy, because of the evidence from animal studies of how fears can be deconditioned. Joseph Wolpe was the first person to apply these principles in a significant way to psychiatric patients. His method was based on the premise that one physiological state (relaxation) was incompatible with another (anxiety), a concept termed reciprocal inhibition. Thus, if a phobic patient could relax in the presence of a phobic stimulus, the anxiety response could be deconditioned. His *systematic desensitization* is a technique in which phobic patients are taught deep muscle relaxation, and then imagine feared stimuli in an increasing hierarchy of anxiety (Wolpe 1958). Exposure therapy for anxiety disorders depends on the process of *habituation*. This process, which is still incompletely understood, is one in which repeated exposure to a stimulus leads to a decrement in orienting responses and arousal within an exposure session.

Operant conditioning

Classical conditioning describes how an organism responds to its environment. Operant conditioning (Skinner) is more concerned with the way that behaviour acts or operates on the environment to produce consequences. Behaviour which gets the environment to react in a rewarding manner is more likely to be repeated. A *reinforcer* is any environmental response which increases the frequency of a behaviour. For animals this is often food, but for human beings more subtle things like money or social acceptance may be reinforcing. Animals and humans will be able to detect situations where they are more likely to receive a reward. These situations then *cue* a behavioural response which elicits reinforcement. For instance, if a mother gives a child a sweet to keep it quiet in a supermarket when it starts to shout, it will soon learn to have a tantrum every time it is taken there. The supermarket acts as a cue, the tantrum is the behavioural response and the sweet the reinforcement.

Modern developments of conditioning theories

Although conditioning theories are out of fashion at the moment, they have progressed a long way since the days of Pavlov and Skinner. It has been established that this form of learning does not depend on the organism being a mere passive responder to the environment or just acting in a random way. Modern theories of conditioning emphasize how the process involves the acquisition of knowledge about the relationship between an action and the occurrence of a

reinforcer, rather than a simple stimulus–response reflex (Adams & Dickinson 1981). If an animal is trained to perform an action to obtain food, and then the food is separately paired with an aversive stimulus, the simple conditioning model would predict that there would be no change in the trained behaviour: the behaviour would be reflexly conditioned, and so the animal would not predict that the result of the behaviour would be aversive. Of course, the animal is much less likely to perform the behaviour. The organism is therefore making predictions about the consequences of behaviour. These new ideas have some similarities with cognitive theories of learning and there is a rapprochement between the two approaches (Rapee 1991).

Characteristics of behaviour therapy

In contrast to psychoanalytic approaches to therapy, behavioural therapy is far more structured and directive. The emphasis is on here-and-now problems that can generate goals that are specific, measurable, and attainable. This allows desired outcomes to be defined and assessed. A patient with agoraphobia might set a goal of being able to travel by herself 10 stops on a tube train at rush hour. It is easy to decide if a goal as operationally defined as this has been met by the end of therapy. Therapists routinely measure outcome with each patient and change therapy techniques on the basis of research evidence. The therapeutic relationship is collaborative, but the therapist is in control. Usually the rationale for treatment is discussed with the patient and the patient is set clear tasks within and between sessions. Because of this clear focus behaviour therapists are usually able to set criteria for the sort of patients they can treat. If a patient cannot identify clear problems and goals, or if a patient is not willing to accept and comply with the treatment plan they will not be taken on for therapy.

Exposure therapy

Exposure is a simple and easily learned treatment for anxiety disorders that has been shown to be effective in numerous clinical trials. Despite the attraction of more sophisticated cognitive models, 60–80% of patients with anxiety are likely to respond to straightforward behaviour therapy. Therapy for phobias (simple phobia, agoraphobia, social phobia) lasts for 8–15 sessions. Sessions involving therapist-aided exposure may last two hours, but other sessions, where homework is reviewed and new homework set may only need 30 minutes. As with many cognitive and behavioural techniques, active participation of the client is necessary for the therapy to be effective. Since this involves confronting the situation which the patient is avoiding, whether it be social gatherings, tube trains or dirt, the therapist needs to be skilled in persuading the patient to comply. The first step in therapy therefore involves the explanation of the rationale of exposure. Patients are taught about the nature and function of anxiety and told

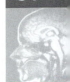

that symptoms although unpleasant are not dangerous. They are told that with exposure the anxiety symptoms will reduce within the session (*habituation*), and that with each successive session the initial anxiety response will become less. While a single very prolonged exposure session (*flooding*) may be sufficient to eliminate some phobias, most patients prefer to approach the problem in a more gradual way (*graded exposure*). The patient and therapist then construct a hierarchy of feared situations, and the patient is encouraged to enter these feared situations in a graded way. The hierarchy is constructed so that there is a gradual increase in the feared characteristics of the stimuli at each stage. Initial sessions may require therapist-aided exposure, but most patients can then go on to carry out homework assignments on their own (Marks 1987). Modelling has also been employed as an aid to exposure (Bandura 1971): if a patient is too frightened to approach a feared stimulus themselves the therapist can model a coping response, e.g. by approaching and handling a spider. Recent work has shown that many patients can carry out self-exposure effectively with only minimal intervention from the therapist. See Box 37.2 for the characteristics of effective exposure therapy.

Case example

Jim was a 50-year-old manager of a betting shop who had been seriously assaulted during a robbery. On his way back from depositing the day's takings he was attacked by two men who thought he still had the money. His front teeth had been knocked out and he suffered severe bruising. At the time he feared for his life. A year later, when he was referred by his GP, he had still not been able to return to work. He had symptoms of post traumatic stress disorder, including high levels of anxiety, hypervigilance, nightmares and avoidance of travelling alone in parts of the East End of London where he lived. Jim understood that he was overreacting to many situations, but still found himself irrationally afraid of any young men. He was able to draw up a hierarchy of feared situations and set about exposing himself to these systematically. Progress was not always smooth. Early on in the therapy, a local man with mental health problems threatened him with a gun in the street! He understandably needed encouragement to continue the programme. With perseverance he was able to spend longer periods helping out in the shop, and was very pleased to find that he could strike up mutually agreeable conversations without seeing the customers as potential attackers. At the end of 12 sessions of therapy he was at the top of the hierarchy except for being able to carry large sums of money. He decided that it was not a reasonable

expectation of his firm that he should do this alone and he eventually left his job.

In obsessive–compulsive disorder (OCD), exposure is combined with response prevention. In this disorder, obsessional fears are usually neutralized by rituals, such as checking, hand washing, etc. The therapist helps the patient construct a hierarchy of stimuli which trigger intrusive thoughts, and then supports the patient in exposure to these cues without engaging in the neutralizing behaviour. For instance, a patient with a fear of contamination by dog faeces might scrub their hands many times a day, and avoid walking in places where they have seen dog faeces. Exposure could begin with the patient touching dusty surfaces and resisting the urge to wash their hands. As he or she progresses up the hierarchy he or she could move on to touching carpets, shoes, etc. It would also be important to overcome avoidance by deliberately walking in the park or down a street where the patient has seen dogs defaecating. At home they might have elaborate rituals to prevent supposed contamination from getting into the house, e.g. taking off shoes with gloves and leaving them in a 'dirty' area of the house, having a shower. The behavioural programme would expect the patient to walk into the house without removing shoes and to live with the anxiety until it reduces.

There is strong evidence supporting the contention that if the patient is able to engage in the behavioural programme the therapy will be effective. For specific phobias 70–80% of patients are successfully treated. For agoraphobia exposure has been shown to be more effective than waiting list and attention controls and as effective as medication (see De Rubeis & Crits Cristoph 1998 for a recent review). The effects of exposure seem to persist over time whereas relapse rates are higher for drug treatments (Marks et al. 1975). The combination of exposure and high dose benzodiazepines is less effective than exposure alone (Marks et al. 1993). In the short term antidepressants plus exposure is the most effective treatment for panic and agoraphobia (see review by Van Balkom et al. 1997) but in the longer term these effects may be lost (Mavissakalian 1993). Despite the consistent findings of efficacy of behaviour therapy in agoraphobia, many patients are left with residual symptoms. Only one-third of subjects meet strict criteria for full recovery. Meta-analytic studies have shown exposure to be an effective treatment for social phobia (Chambless & Gillis 1993). Exposure produces an improvement in 80% of OCD patients who engage (Marks & O'Sullivan 1988) and this persists over two years (Kasvikis & Marks 1988). As with agoraphobia a significant proportion of patients, while improved, still have symptoms after therapy.

Behaviour modification and social skills training

Behaviour modification is the name given to techniques based on the principles of operant or Skinnerian

Box 37.2	Characteristics of effective exposure
Real life, rather than imagination (Emmelkamp & Wessels 1975)
Prolonged rather than brief (Stern & Marks 1973)
Makes use of regular self-exposure tasks (McDonald et al. 1978)

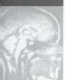

conditioning: behaviour that is followed by pleasant consequences will increase in frequency, while behaviour that is followed by unpleasant consequences will be less likely to be repeated. Through a careful *behavioural analysis* the links between the circumstances in which a particular behaviour occurs and the consequences of the behaviour are established. The therapist establishes the setting conditions for the behaviour (e.g. an alcoholic walking past a pub), the nature of the behaviour itself, and the reinforcing consequences (pleasant sense of inebriation, escape from painful feelings). This behavioural analysis is often referred to by the mnemonic *ABC: Antecedents Behaviour Consequences*.

Behaviour modification addresses both antecedents and consequences. The behavioural analysis will show how unwanted behaviour is being reinforced or how desirable behaviour is not receiving reinforcement. What is aversive or rewarding will vary between individuals and cannot be assumed. In the past behaviour modification has relied too much on tangible rewards like food or cigarettes, where in fact human behaviour is reinforced by more subtle factors like social contact and praise. *Aversive techniques* can be effective but often elicit aversive emotional reactions which complicate the process of relearning. They are also contentious ethically. In practice they are confined to cases where the behaviour to be punished is life threatening or has dire social consequences, e.g. substance misuse and some sexual deviations. More commonly undesirable behaviour is reduced by replacing it with a more socially acceptable behaviour which is reinforced, e.g. orgasmic reconditioning in sexual problems. Wherever possible therapists look for ways to reinforce prosocial behaviour by pairing it with a reward. The target behaviour is not always present at the beginning of therapy, and initially it may be necessary to reward an approximation to the desired goal and then to *shape* the response by rewarding successively closer approximations.

Operant conditioning techniques lend themselves well to single-case study designs. A behaviour that is to be increased is measured at baseline and a change observed with the intervention. When the intervention is stopped the behaviour is seen to decrease in frequency. A direct causal relationship can be established, but the strength of this method is also its weakness, because in many situations the clinician wants the behavioural change to persist when therapy has stopped. There are various ways in which generalization of behavioural change can be encouraged. One method is to degrade the relationship between stimulus and response by giving only intermittent reinforcement. Theorists have argued that by giving the patient more responsibility for regulating and rewarding their own behaviour, improvements can be maintained after therapy (Kanfer & Karoly 1972).

Another important component of any cognitive–behavioural work is skills training. This approach is not based on a single model of learning, and in fact often uses operant techniques to help reinforce and maintain gains in skills. The skills training approach usually involves a cognitive–behavioural analysis of the skills deficits, followed by teaching the skill and a period of practice with feedback within the session as well as practice outside the session. This method has been applied to a variety of skills. *Problem-solving* was originally introduced by D'Zurilla & Goldfried (1971). There is evidence that some patients who experience repeated life-crises and resort to parasuicide have problem-solving deficits (Hawton & Catalan 1987). Problem-solving training has been used with suicidal patients (Hawton & Catalan 1987). Difficulties in interpersonal skills are found in people with chronic mental illness, marital problems and in the parents of children with behavioural problems. *Social skills training* has been used in depression (Bellack et al. 1983), social phobia (Trower et al. 1978) and schizophrenia (Falloon 1988). A skills training approach is also used in assertiveness training and anxiety management training. See Box 37.3 for features common to the behavioural/ cognitive therapies.

> **Box 37.3 Common features of behavioural/cognitive therapies**
>
> Broad social learning theory assumptions: maladaptive thoughts and behaviours are learned and can be unlearned
>
> Primary interest in here-and-now, observable problems
>
> Focus on measurable, operationally defined problems and goals
>
> Structured, directive therapy sessions
>
> Collaborative therapeutic relationship
>
> Use of self-monitoring and self-help assignments between sessions
>
> Evaluation of treatment efficacy
>
> Use of empirical research evidence in applying treatment

COGNITIVE THERAPY

Cognitive theories

The 1970s saw a critique of the more simplistic forms of behaviourism (Mahoney 1974). Brewer (1974) reviewed studies of human conditioning and found that subjects were always *consciously* aware of the association between stimulus and response that was being conditioned. Conscious mental processes became a legitimate area of study. Meichenbaum began to look at the self-verbalizations of children with attention deficit disorder (Meichenbaum & Goodman 1971) and schizophrenics (Meichenbaum & Cameron 1973). He developed self-instructional methods to help people guide their own behaviour. Meichenbaum coined the term 'cognitive behaviour modification' for this integration of cognition into behaviour therapy (Meichenbaum 1977). Even more radical mentalism was present in the ideas of Albert

Ellis and A.T. Beck. Both had trained as psychoanalysts but had become more interested in conscious than unconscious processes. Ellis' Rational Emotive Behaviour Therapy (REBT) (Ellis 1962) and Beck's cognitive therapy (Beck 1976) see emotional disorder and behavioural problems as secondary to irrational beliefs or faulty information processing. Beck's systematic approach to identifying the cognitive disorder associated with diagnoses such as depression (Beck et al. 1979) and anxiety (Beck et al. 1985), as well as his efforts to test the efficacy of his therapy, have led to a widening acceptance of the cognitive model among behaviourists. Cognitive behaviour therapy spans the whole spectrum from behavioural techniques to cognitive therapy.

The essence of all cognitive theories is that we are not controlled by events, but by the meanings we give to events. The way in which we interpret, evaluate and encode information about the world influences our emotions and behaviour. Several people can experience the same event, yet have very different perceptions of it. In the cognitive model, this even applies to apparently aversive life events like cancer (Moorey 1996, Moorey & Greer 2002). Two women with breast cancer may have exactly the same stage of disease and prognosis. One might see the illness as a challenge, and adopt an optimistic attitude to the future, while the other might assume that her life is over and develop a helpless/hopeless attitude. Different types of cognitive therapy adopt different emphases. Beck's cognitive therapy focuses on errors in information processing, while Ellis' REBT attends less to faulty inferences and more to the fundamental evaluations we make about the world, as shown in irrational beliefs. These two approaches could be termed rationalist, since they assume an objective reality about which we can make objective judgements (Mahoney 1995a). More recently social constructionism has influenced some writers, who see reality as exclusively socially derived. *Constructivist cognitive therapy* (Mahoney 1995b) again attends to the personal meaning we give to events, but is less empirical. The task of this form of therapy is to help people to expand their options and choose a new more individually helpful way of seeing the world, not necessarily a more realistic or logical one.

Beck's cognitive model

Beck's cognitive therapy is the most studied and most widely practised. It is also appealing to psychiatrists since Beck has developed specific cognitive models for different diagnostic categories, and is firmly wedded to empiricism. According to Beck, patients with psychiatric disorders process information in a biased way, and the nature of the bias differs for different conditions. In depression there is a pervasive negative view of the self, the world and the future. In anxiety, there is a shift in attention leading to exaggerated awareness of physical or social danger. In paranoid states, the person is primed to find injustice or prejudice against

themselves in the actions of others. There is evidence that normal individuals have a self-serving bias in thinking, but there is usually sufficient reality testing available to allow people to change their beliefs on the basis of new information. In psychiatric disorders biases in thinking and behaviour trap the patient in a particular mind set. Beck has identified *cognitive distortions* or thinking errors which lead the patient to attend selectively to information consistent with faulty beliefs and filter out information that does not fit (see Box 37.4).

Once a particular way of seeing the world is established, the patient will act in accordance with his or her beliefs. Behaviours consistent with maladaptive beliefs then create a vicious cycle and help to maintain the distorted cognitions.

The cognitive model of depression

In depression there is a negative view of the self, the world and the future (the *negative cognitive triad*). Events which confirm this negative view (e.g. failures and mistakes) are remembered, while events which contradict it (e.g. successes) are forgotten or ignored. The content of consciousness reflects this underlying shift in perception, and the depressed person has *negative automatic thoughts* which seem to them realistic, but are usually spontaneous, distorted thoughts. Negative thinking also contributes to the behavioural deficits in depression. If the future seems hopeless, there is little point in doing anything, or if you believe that you are inadequate it is better to avoid people in case you get rejected. Reduced activity and social withdrawal means less opportunities for finding pleasure or

---

Box 37.4 Thinking errors

All or nothing thinking

You see things in black and white, missing all the shades of grey in between. If you are depressed you may think 'If I can't do *everything* I used to do, then there's no point in doing *anything*'. If you do less well than usual you may think, 'If I don't succeed, I must be a *total* failure'.

Overgeneralization

From a single event, you predict a never ending pattern of loss or defeat which may be exaggerated and not based on fact.

Magnification and selective attention

You focus on the negative aspects of the problem and selectively attend to them. You tend to filter out or disqualify more positive information. If you face an operation you remember all the possible side-effects, but fail to hear that they are extremely rare.

Arbitrary inference

Instead of looking at the evidence available you jump to conclusions. For instance, if a loved one is late coming home you might conclude, 'He's had an accident!'

Labelling

Here the distortion leads to a global, overgeneralized negative view of yourself. You label yourself as hopeless, incompetent, and invalid or a victim.

achievement, and so a vicious spiral of increasing depression is created (Williams 1995). There is substantial evidence for the presence of negative thinking in depression , and for a bias in autobiographical memory which leads to the retrieval of negative memories in preference to positive ones (Williams 1995).

The cognitive model of anxiety

In anxiety the self is seen as *vulnerable,* the world *dangerous,* and the future *uncertain.* Schemas associated with vulnerability are seen to be of evolutionary usefulness in energizing the organism and preparing for fight or flight from danger (Beck et al. 1985, Beck & Clark 1997). The problem in anxiety disorders is that these danger schemas are activated inappropriately in non-threatening situations. Once anxiety is present the cognitive apparatus selectively attends to threat (e.g. a grandparent suddenly becomes aware of all the dangers in a children's playground), overestimates the chance of disaster (the grandparent becomes convinced that their grandchild will inevitably fall off the climbing frame) and underestimates the opportunities for rescue or coping (the grandparent frets about what she will do if the child falls and fears she won't be able to cope). Once this selective attention is operating, danger signals in the internal or external environment become predominant and this reinforces the anxiety. Again avoidance and various safety behaviours are seen as maintaining factors in anxiety disorders. As in depression, there are underlying assumptions (this time about the world being a dangerous place, about the individual being vulnerable, etc.), which may be dormant until triggered by a life event.

Cognitive models of specific anxiety disorders

Cognitive therapists have taken this basic model of anxiety and modified it for panic (Clark, Barlow), generalized anxiety disorder (Wells, Borkovec), hypochondriasis (Warwick) and social phobia (Clark & Wells) (see Wells 1997 for a discussion of these different models). Much of this work has been carried out at Oxford, where the approach has been to identify the particular beliefs and behaviours that maintain the disorders. These models (Table 37.1) have in common a description of:

- bias in information processing
- selective attention
- maladaptive behaviours – avoidance and safety behaviours.

In panic disorder, there is a catastrophic misinterpretation of bodily sensations. The patient selectively attends to bodily sensations of autonomic nervous system activity and mistakes them for signs of impending disaster. The misinterpretations are specific to the sensation: breathlessness – suffocation, chest pain – heart attack, etc. Agoraphobic symptoms may arise out of avoidance of situations where panics have occurred. More subtle avoidance is seen when the person acts to prevent the feared catastrophe taking place, by avoiding exercise if they fear a heart attack. This prevents them from testing the negative belief and helps to maintain the disorder. A similar process takes place in hypochondriasis but the mis- interpretations are not of impending disaster. The person with health anxiety will see bodily symptoms as signs of disease which might be life threatening but which are not imminently life threatening. Safety behaviours include reassurance seeking from family and medical professionals and obsessional checking for signs of disease. In panic and health anxiety the focus of attention is usually on bodily symptoms, but in generalized anxiety disorder it is worry which is the cause of distress. According to Wells, any negative events can set off worry (e.g. unpleasant news material, intrusive thoughts). Worry is then chosen as a coping strategy (often because of beliefs that it helps problem solving or prevents bad things happening), but once this happens negative beliefs about worry (e.g. that worry can cause stress or that the person will lose control of their thinking) set in and a vicious cycle is set up, perpetuating the anxiety. Clark (1996) has carried out a number of compelling experiments specifically designed to test his model of panic. More limited evidence is available so far for the other anxiety models (Wells 1997).

A similar approach has been taken by Salkovskis (1985) to obsessive-compulsive disorder. Here the source of the problem is not the intrusive thoughts themselves but the interpretation the person makes of them. Intrusive thoughts are actually quite common in the general population,

Table 37.1	Cognitive models of anxiety disorders			
	Panic disorder	*Hypochondriasis*	*Generalized anxiety disorder*	*Social phobia*
Bias in information processing	Catastrophic misinterpretation	Non-catastrophic misinterpretation	Misinterpretation of any situation as threatening	Misinterpretation of social threat
Selective attention	Bodily sensations of autonomic nervous system activity	Any bodily sensations	Worrying thoughts	Image of self as a social object
Safety behaviours	Avoidance of exercise, controlling breathing	Reassurance seeking, checking for symptoms	Thought control, avoidance	Avoiding eye contact, monitoring of speech

occurring in 80% of individuals, and the content of normal and abnormal obsessions is similar (Rachman & de Silva 1978, Salkovskis & Harrison 1984), but in obsessive–compulsive disorder these thoughts are seen as threatening. They usually imply that the person has some responsibility for the content of their thoughts. A man who had intrusive thoughts of jumping in front of a tube train, or swerving in the face of oncoming traffic, saw these as indications that he might be schizophrenic, and that he might actually lose control and do what he feared. Another patient experienced intrusive thoughts of friends and family being attacked. He believed that this meant that he was an evil person, otherwise why would he have these images? This overdeveloped sense of responsibility for intrusions leads the obsessional patient to try to suppress them. But these attempts at thought control paradoxically make the intrusions stronger and more frequent. Rituals are seen as strategies for neutralizing intrusive thoughts. So, the person who feared his images of violence meant he was bad would say to himself 'I'm not bad' and would make gestures with his arms to ward off the images. Someone with intrusive thoughts that he might forget to turn off the gas and so be responsible for the death of everyone in his house will obsessionally check the taps are turned off many times before he can leave the house.

Vulnerability to emotional disorder

So far, we have looked at the way in which cognitive theory explains different emotional disorders. In Beck's model, vulnerability to a disorder comes from the existence of underlying dysfunctional assumptions or schemas. We all need to have assumptions about the world in order to make sense of the 'blooming, buzzing confusion' of reality. Schemas help us to select and organize experience and predict what is going to happen next. If we have a stable, supportive family upbringing, we develop positive schemas. We see ourselves as basically worthwhile and competent. We see others as potentially supportive and well inclined. We see the world as generally a positive place. If on the other hand we have aversive experiences in childhood, we may see ourselves as worthless or incompetent, others as critical or abusive, and the world as dangerous or hostile. We all have some positive and some negative core beliefs. Often the negative beliefs remain dormant if we have positive life experiences in childhood and adulthood. Sometimes we avoid them by developing conditional assumptions about the world. These 'if-then' beliefs predicate self-worth on the world being a certain way. They are global, absolute and rigid, and predispose to emotional problems. Examples of dysfunctional assumptions predisposing to depression would be:

- I must always be nice to people.
- It is terrible to be rejected.
- I can only be happy if I have a successful life.

- If I make a mistake, it means I am a failure.
- If I do not have someone to love me, I must be worthless.

Critical incidents may lead to the activation of these beliefs and the core beliefs associated with them. Not all negative life events will lead to depression. The key is the personal meaning of the event, and whether or not it fits with a person's underlying assumption. Thus someone with a belief that he can only be happy if he is loved may cope with the loss of a job but not the loss of a relationship. Beck suggests that themes of success or perfection are associated with autonomous personality styles, while themes of loss and rejection are associated with sociotropic personality style. Autonomous individuals will be sensitive to failure experiences, while sociotropic individuals will be sensitive to interpersonal loss or rejection. There is some evidence to support the idea that interpersonal life events trigger depression in sociotropes, but less evidence as yet for the autonomy-failure connection (Blackburn 1996).

Cognitive model of personality disorders

In DSM-IV Axis I disorders, there are positive core beliefs which allow the person to function reasonably well between episodes. In Axis II disorders, the negative core beliefs are near the surface most of the time, and the associated maladaptive assumptions and interpersonal strategies give rise to what we term personality disorders (Fig. 37.1). For example, a woman had developed epilepsy in childhood and had been 'wrapped in cotton wool' by her parents. She

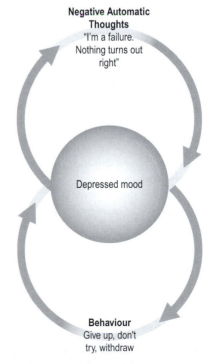

Figure 37.1 The cognitive model.

571

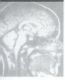

believed that she was basically weak and unable to cope alone, but that if she had someone to rely on she could survive in life. She saw herself as incompetent, the world as a difficult place, and others as a source of support and rescue (*core beliefs*). Her *conditional assumption* was: If I have someone to look after me, I will be alright. And the interpersonal strategy that flowed naturally from this was to attach herself to people stronger than herself (*compensatory strategy*). In psychiatric terms she had a dependent personality disorder. Beck et al. (1990) have defined the relevant core beliefs and compensatory strategies for all the DSM personality disorders. A similar approach has been taken by Young who describes Early Maladaptive Schemas, which are the equivalent of Beck's core beliefs. Young's Schema-focused Therapy (Young et al. 2003) employs cognitive, behavioural, interpersonal and affective strategies to activate and restructure the schemas laid down in early childhood experience.

Characteristics of cognitive therapy

Cognitive therapy, like other behavioural and cognitive-behavioural approaches is a time-limited, structured therapy aimed at helping individuals cope with emotional problems and achieve symptom relief as well as reducing the chances of relapse. Like behaviour therapy it is structured, problem-focussed and outcome oriented, placing great importance on the empirical testing of its theoretical and practical applications. In contrast to some forms of behaviour therapy, it always embeds its therapeutic techniques within a case conceptualization based on cognitive theory. The therapy takes place in weekly 50 minutes sessions (12-20 sessions in total) spaced over 3-6 months. Because cognitive therapy seeks to change patients' longstanding beliefs about themselves and the world, it is necessary to establish a sound therapeutic alliance. Rather than tell patients their beliefs are unfounded, the therapist uses questioning and guided discovery to demonstrate that the beliefs are illogical or unhelpful. Beck coined the term 'collaborative empiricism' to describe the special nature of the relationship in cognitive therapy where patient and therapist test out the hypotheses of the cognitive model as applied to the patient's problems. The therapy teaches a sceptical approach to cognitive events, encourages achieving distance from thoughts as a prelude to learning to modify them and thereby gain control over powerful negative feelings. While still requiring patients to engage actively in therapy, it has a set of techniques to work with patients who are sceptical, and so may be applicable to a wider range of less 'motivated' patients.

Conceptualization

Therapy is embedded in the cognitive model, and a conceptualization is developed for each patient to guide the treatment. For patients with clear diagnoses, the cognitive model for that particular disorder allows the therapist to plan a course of treatment and predict pitfalls. The assessment of the patient will therefore start with a cross-sectional problem-focused analysis of behaviour, cognition, emotion and physiological reactions. If a patient is depressed, the therapist will look at how the negative view of the self, the world and the future is operating in his or her life. He will assess the behavioural deficits which might be preventing the patient from engaging in activities to promote a sense of achievement, pleasure or control, and how negative automatic thoughts led to these behavioural deficits. He would also be interested in the somatic symptoms of depression (e.g. is insomnia a problem? What are the patient's negative thoughts about their sleep disturbance?). Early experiences are important in shaping cognitive schemata (core beliefs and assumptions) and so developmental factors are also significant in a CBT assessment. How have early experiences led to certain core beliefs? What assumptions and compensatory strategies have arisen out of them? Have their been any critical incidents which have triggered the current episode? At the beginning of therapy various observer and self-report measures are used to establish a baseline so that the effectiveness of therapy can be assessed (e.g. Beck Depression Inventory, Beck Anxiety Inventory, Fear Questionnaire, Young's Schema Questionnaire). These instruments also give information about symptoms and cognitions which are of use in conceptualizing the case.

Case example

Philippa was a 35-year-old clerical worker with an 8-year history of panic and agoraphobia. She was unable to use public transport or to walk any distance alone. Her coping strategy was to ride everywhere on her bike, but she could only do this during daylight. She had 2–3 panics a week and felt pessimistic about the effectiveness of therapy: she had been treated for five years in analytic psychotherapy, and reported little or no improvement with her symptoms of panic and avoidance. Philippa was the daughter of an alcoholic. She had witnessed her father acting in an uncontrolled and sometimes aggressive fashion. She felt that the family pretended that her father did not have a problem, and kept it secret from the world. She was brought up in a strict religious family but was no longer religious.

By asking questions about her symptoms and inducing some of the panic feelings in the session through imagery, the therapist was able to map the interactions between her thoughts, feelings and behaviours. During a panic, she started to feel out of control as she became more and more anxious. She feared that she would suddenly start crying in public, resulting in people rejecting her, or, even worse, taking pity and trying to help. At the height of the panic she would have an image of herself as a madwoman lying on the floor flailing about and moaning. As therapy progressed, she

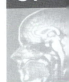

revealed that her sister had a bipolar affective disorder, and she feared that she too might be mad. She had not told her previous therapist this for fear of what they would think. She had been living with her sister some years before, when she had her first manic episode. Having seen her sister lose control and be admitted to hospital involuntarily she thought the same might happen to her. Whenever she got panic symptoms she interpreted the anxiety as impending loss of control and catastrophized that she would go mad and be forceibly detained. The full conceptualization could not be developed until the 7th session, which illustrates how assessment in CBT is an ongoing process throughout treatment.

Initial phase of cognitive therapy

The initial phase of therapy concentrates on listening to the patient's account of their problems and forming a conceptualization as described above. At the same time, the patient is introduced to the ideas and structure of the therapy including the use of homework assignments. Self-help reading material can be used to aid the process of explanation (e.g. Fennell 1989). The conceptualization is shared with the patient as it is developed. This is helpful in building up an alternative picture of the problems. For instance, the depressive may attribute inactivity to laziness, while the cognitive conceptualization might reframe this inactivity as a symptom of depression associated with hopelessness. The basic idea to get across at this stage is that thoughts are not reality. Therapy is about clearing a space to examine thoughts and beliefs to see if they are realistic or helpful. In the first sessions problems are defined and the patient's goals for therapy established. Behavioural techniques are used to test out negative thoughts with a view to initial symptom management. In depression behavioural techniques include scheduling activities which give patients a sense of mastery or pleasure, graded tasks to help patients achieve success step by step, and specific experiments to test negative predictions. In anxiety, relaxation or distraction strategies might be taught to help the patient establish a sense of control. The aim in cognitive terms is to decrease the frequency of negative thinking and thus to improve symptoms. At all times these interventions are used in sessions to furnish evidence for the cognitive model, to point out where predictions are erroneous, where positive experiences are dismissed or minimized, where self-expectations are unrealistic and how these negative interpretations contribute to emotional responses and behavioural and environmental consequences.

Middle phase of therapy

Thought monitoring and challenging

As symptoms improve, the treatment becomes more cognitive. The patient is likely to need help in sessions to identify initially specific thoughts and in the use of a structured monitoring sheet. Techniques such as mental action replay are used to bring an incident vividly back to mind in session with a view to identifying negative automatic thoughts. Other techniques include role-play of interpersonal scenarios and exposure to specific cues or bodily sensations that are subject to misinterpretation. The patient is taught to recognize and record automatic thoughts as they occur. This involves noticing the situation where the emotional reaction occurred (What was happening? What were you thinking?), the emotion experienced (depression, anxiety, anger, shame, etc.), and the cognition (thought, image or meaning associated with the situation). Patients may need some practice in keeping this diary and distinguishing thoughts and emotions. Once automatic thoughts can be recognized, the patient is helped to challenge them, that is, scrutinize them to assess their accuracy and usefulness. It is important that the therapist does not take on a lecturing or bullying stance in this work. Beck emphasizes the use of *Socratic questioning* in challenging thoughts, that is using questions that lead the patient in coming to his/her own conclusions. Persuading or arguing with the patient is likely to be counterproductive. In many cases the patients thoughts may well be true in which case the therapist needs to help the patient find the underlying meaning that makes the thought so arousing of emotion.

Patients can be taught questions to ask themselves when they identify an automatic thought:

- What is the evidence for and against the thought? The patient is taught to weigh the thought against the balance of evidence. The evidence against is often initially overlooked as a result of selective memory bias. Often the evidence may be insufficient and a behavioural experiment may be devised to gather relevant evidence, e.g. expressing feelings or revealing weakness to test out other people's reactions.
- Is there an alternative way of looking at this? The patient is taught to open up the range of their perspective and to frame the event/thought in a different way. Looking at the event through someone else's eyes may aid this process (How would a friend look at this? What would I say to a friend if he or she said this?).
- What is the effect of thinking this way? The patient can remind him/herself of the dysfunctionality of the negative interpretation and how it may lead to self-defeating consequences including confirmation of the negative thought.
- What thinking error am I making? The patient can look for overgeneralizations, black-and-white thinking, etc., as an aid to answering the negative thought (Box 37.4).
- Supposing the thought is true, what does it mean about you, the world, the future? The patient can then

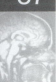

challenge both the validity of the underlying thought and the reasoning by which he/she reaches it.

As a result of these challenges the patient can produce answers to their original thought which may affect their emotions. Often a patient will need several sessions to work on and finally deal with key disturbing thoughts that have troubled them for some time. Sometimes there is a dramatic reduction in the degree to which the patient believes the thought, but usually the strength of the belief reduces by increments.

Behavioural experiments

When a patient completes a thought record, it is helpful for them to develop an action plan from it (Greenberger & Padesky 1995). This often involves setting up a behavioural experiment to confirm or test the conclusions of the examination of the thoughts. For instance, Philippa (see above) feared that she would become manic depressive like her sister. In the session she was able to identify many similarities with her sister, but only a few differences. Through guided discovery the therapist helped her to see that she was assuming that her likeness to her sister was based on their both sharing a vulnerability to mental illness, but there could be other reasons for similarities such as inherited characteristics, etc. She decided that as homework she would ask *all* her siblings about their similarities and differences. Behavioural experiments can be the most powerful way of disproving negative thoughts.

Sometimes it is necessary to do the experiments in the session. With anxiety disorders this usually involves an exercise to induce the symptoms (through imagery, role play or hyperventilation), followed by asking the patient to drop their safety behaviours. The effect is that the symptoms are less marked when the patient gives up the strategy they think is actually saving them. Thus, a panic patient who fears he is going to have a heart attack exercises during the panic and proves his heart copes perfectly well, or an obsessional patient exposes himself to the intrusive thought without trying to suppress it and discovers that it becomes less troublesome.

Final phase of therapy

The final stages of therapy deal with the identification and challenging of dysfunctional assumptions and preparation for future problems as a means of relapse prevention. Challenging dysfunctional assumptions can involve the same questioning as in dealing with automatic thoughts. However, their more abstract nature makes them less susceptible to challenges with reference to the evidence. More use is made of pointing to their dysfunctionality, to the consequences of holding such beliefs with regard to negative emotional states, goal attainment and other people's welfare. Final challenging involves further behavioural change and experiment in acting contrary to these beliefs and testing out

the consequences. One of the implications of this work later in therapy is that it involves placing the patient up against his/her vulnerability and acts to strengthen their ability to deal with negative events. Working with core beliefs may take even longer. Techniques include reviewing evidence over the lifecycle for the core belief, dispelling the 'all-or-nothingness' of the belief using a continuum technique and keeping a log of evidence for more positive beliefs (Padesky 1994). The final stages in therapy include the recapitulation of what has been learned in therapy and the formulation of a plan to deal with future problems. This is often written down as an action plan for coping with setbacks.

Efficacy of cognitive therapy

Cognitive therapy has been most intensively investigated in depression (see De Rubeis & Crits Cristoph (1998) and Deckersbach et al. (2000) for recent reviews). It has been shown to be more effective than waiting list controls and unstructured therapies for outpatients with depression. In the majority of studies CT is as effective as antidepressant medication. There is evidence to suggest that cognitive therapy may reduce relapse rates when compared to antidepressant medication when both are withdrawn after three months (26% relapse in the CT condition, 64% relapse in the medication condition). Paykel et al. (1999) compared maintenance antidepressants with and without 20 weeks cognitive therapy, in patients who had made a partial response to drug treatment. The relapse rate in the medication plus cognitive therapy condition was 29% compared with 47% in the medication only condition. In recurrent depression maintenance, CBT can be as effective as maintenance medication (Blackburn & Moore 1997). Most trials that investigated the combination of CT with antidepressants have not found the combination to be any more effective than the two treatments alone. Stuart & Bowers (1995) reviewed eight studies of cognitive therapy with depressed inpatients (203 patients altogether). They found that the combination of cognitive therapy and medication was more effective than medication alone in the treatment of this more severely depressed group. Mindfulness-based cognitive therapy is a promising new development which teaches patients with recurrent depression to observe nonjudgementally their negative thoughts rather than ruminate about them. There is evidence that this can reduce relapse rates (Teasdale et al. 2000).

There is evidence for the effectiveness of cognitive therapy in a range of anxiety disorders (see De Rubeis & Crits Cristoph 1998) including panic (where 85% patients become panic-free), panic with agoraphobia, generalized anxiety disorder, social phobia and obsessive-compulsive disorder (Table 37.2). The effects of therapy persist at follow-up. While studies show its superiority over waiting list and treatment as usual controls, it is more difficult to demonstrate superiority over other treatments. Gould et al.

Table 37.2   Evidence of effectiveness of cognitive–behavioural therapy

Strongest evidence for efficacy (large number of RCTs)	Good evidence for efficacy (several RCTs)	Some evidence for efficacy (more trials needed)
Depression	Hypochondriasis	Borderline, antisocial and avoidant personality disorders
Agoraphobia	Post-traumatic stress disorder	Self-harm behaviours
Panic disorder	Schizophrenia	Bipolar affective disorder
Social phobia		Substance misuse
Specific phobia		
Obsessive-compulsive disorder		
Bulimia nervosa		
Sexual dysfunction		
Chronic fatigue syndrome		

RCT = Randomized controlled trial

Box 37.5   CBT and medication

Depression

CBT is as effective as antidepressant medication in outpatients with depression

The combination of CBT and antidepressants may be more effective than either alone in severe (inpatient) depression

Combination of CBT and medication in mild–moderate (outpatient) depression is not more effective than either alone

After ending treatment, relapse rates are lower with CBT than antidepressants

Anxiety

Drug treatments have a higher relapse rate than CBT on discontinuation

Antidepressants plus exposure are the most effective treatment for panic and agoraphobia in the short term, but are not superior to CBT at long-term follow-up

Combining exposure and medication (particularly high dose benzodiazepines) may decrease long term efficacy

---

(1995) found that studies of panic with or without agoraphobia generally reported that treatments combining exposure and cognitive restructuring were most effective. There is some suggestion that cognitive treatments are more effective for panic treatments, while exposure is more effective for avoidance in agoraphobia. Both cognitive therapy and behaviour therapy are effective for generalized anxiety disorder (Box 37.5); CBT is as effective as antidepressant medication, but at follow up the gains from medication tend to be lost (Gould et al. 1995).

CBT has been found to be effective for bulimia nervosa (Fairburn & Cooper 1989, Fairburn et al. 1991), but insufficient evidence is available regarding anorexia. In bulimia CBT is superior to antidepressants, waiting list controls and other psychotherapies, particularly for symptoms of the eating disorder and affective symptoms. There have been few trials of CBT for personality disorders. A form of therapy called dialectical behaviour therapy has been found to reduce parasuicidal behaviour in borderline personality disorder (Linehan et al. 1991, Verheul et al. 2003).

Cognitive–behavioural therapy in psychosis

One of the most exciting developments in CBT in the last 10 years has been its application to psychosis. Three approaches have been demonstrated to be of benefit in schizophrenia.

Family interventions in schizophrenia

Following on from work which showed that high expressed emotion (EE), in a family with a schizophrenic member, was associated with higher relapse rates, Leff et al. (1982) developed a family intervention to reduce high EE. Other behavioural interventions (e.g. Falloon 1988) do not focus purely on high EE. The various approaches share in common a focus on positive areas of family functioning and increasing family structure and stability (through problem-solving, goal-setting, cognitive restructuring, etc.). Randolph et al. (1994) reported a comparison of behavioural family therapy with routine care over one year in a clinical setting. At the end of the year 15% of the therapy group relapsed compared with 55% of the control group.

Coping enhancement, compliance, and relapse prevention

Cognitive–behavioural interventions have also been used to teach patients how to recognize their particular relapse profile and to enhance coping strategies (see for instance Birchwood & Tarrier 1992).

CBT for hallucinations and delusions

Following the pioneering work of Kingdon & Turkington (1994), there has been a growing interest in the application of cognitive techniques in psychosis as an adjunct to antipsychotic medication. The therapy needs to be more flexible than standard cognitive therapy, and a great deal of emphasis is placed on establishing a good therapeutic relationship before any challenging of beliefs takes place. Kuipers et al. (1997) describe the more flexible approach that was needed in their controlled trial:

When necessary, treatment was arranged in locations convenient to the client, including home visits and proactive outreach following non-attendance. Within sessions the therapist was highly sensitive to changes in mental state and in particular the occurrence of paranoia. Active attempts were made to manage such problems so as to ensure that clients did not feel unduly pressured and to prevent treatment from becoming aversive. If necessary sessions were cut short or rearranged. Difficult topics were discussed only when clients felt able to do so.

As in all cognitive therapy, it is important to develop a shared model of the problems, gradually building up alternative explanations for symptoms the patient assumes are based on reality. The story of how the symptoms first appeared and what they meant to the patient is elaborated, and it is often possible to see that the first psychotic experiences occurred in states of altered consciousness through the impact of stress, sleep disturbance or drugs (Kingdon & Turkington 1994). If symptoms can be reconceptualized as stress reactions, the patient is then more willing to consider examining them and testing the validity of their beliefs. Delusional beliefs and beliefs about hallucinations are gently challenged and behavioural experiments devised. In addition, most of these treatment packages also teach coping strategies, challenge negative self-concepts and work on social disability and relapse. Evidence is beginning to emerge of the effectiveness of this therapy in improving symptoms. For instance, compared with treatment as usual, CBT showed a significant reduction in overall symptomatology (Kuipers et al. 1997): 50% of the CBT group were treatment responders, compared to 31% of the control group. Comparisons with befriending or supportive therapy tend to show similar effects in the short term, but more benefit from CBT at follow up. A recent meta-analysis (Pilling et al. 2002) concluded CBT produced higher rates of 'important improvement' in mental state and demonstrated positive effects on continuous measures of mental state at follow-up. CBT also seems to be associated with low drop-out rates. Current research is focusing on the impact of CBT in first episode psychosis to find out if early intervention can prevent relapse and long term disability.

CBT for bipolar disorder is in its infancy, but techniques now exist to help patients detect and attenuate hypomanic episodes. Lam et al. (2003) have demonstrated that CBT reduces bipolar episodes and admissions.

CONCLUSIONS

Cognitive–behaviour therapy is a broad church that embraces a variety of behavioural and cognitive theories and techniques. Its flexibility allows it to be applied to a wide range of conditions and there is increasing evidence for its effectiveness (see Table 37.2). Despite this empirical backing,

CBT should not be considered a panacea. While statistical superiority over controls is well established the *clinical significance* of results is sometimes less dramatic, with many patients improved but still symptomatic. Like all therapies CBT requires participation from the patient, and it may be less helpful with people who are unable or unwilling to engage in the self-help strategies required of them. Finally, the very convincing evidence for CBT still lies in the realm of research studies, often with single diagnosis groups. Demonstrating its usefulness in the clinical world with patients with mixed diagnoses and multiple problems is the challenge for cognitive behaviour–therapy in the 21st century.

FURTHER READING

Beck JS (1995) *Cognitive Therapy: Basics and Beyond*. Guilford Press.
Hawton K, Salkovskis PM, Kirk J & Clark DM (eds) (1989) *Cognitive Behaviour Therapy for Psychiatric Problems*. Oxford: Oxford Medical Publications.
Stern R & Drummond L (1991) *The Practice of Behavioural and Cognitive Psychotherapy*. Cambridge University Press.
Wells A (1997) *Cognitive Therapy of Anxiety Disorders*. Chichester: Wiley.

REFERENCES

Adams CD & Dickinson A (1981) Instrumental responding following reinforcer devaluation. *Quarterly Journal of Experimental Psychology* **33B**: 109–21.
Bandura A (1971) *Principles of Behavior Modification*. New York: Holt, Rhinehart & Winston.
Beck AT (1976) *Cognitive Therapy and the Emotional Disorders*. New York: International Universities Press.
Beck AT & Clark DA (1997) An information processing model of anxiety: automatic and strategic processes. *Behaviour Research and Therapy* **35**(1): 49–58.
Beck AT, Rush AJ, Shaw BF & Emery G (1979) *Cognitive Therapy of Depression*. New York, Guilford Press.
Beck AT, Emery G & Greenberg RL (1985) *Anxiety Disorders and Phobias: A Cognitive Perspective*. New York: Basic Books.
Beck AT, Freeman A & Associates (1990) *Cognitive Therapy of Personality Disorders*. New York: Guildford Press.
Bellack AS, Hersen M & Himmelhoch JM (1983) A comparison of social skills training, pharmacotherapy and psychotherapy for depression. *Behaviour Research and Therapy* **21**: 101–7.
Blackburn IM (1996) Cognitive vulnerability to depression. In: Salkovskis P (ed.) *Frontiers of Cognitive Therapy*, pp. 250–65. New York: Guilford Press.
Blackburn IM & Moore RG (1997) Controlled acute and follow-up trial of cognitive therapy and pharmacotherapy in out-patients with recurrent depression *British Journal of Psychiatry* **171**: 328–34.
Birchwood M & Tarrier N (1992) *Innovations in the Psychological Management of Schizophrenia: Assessment, Treatment and Services*. Chichester: Wiley.
Brewer W (1974) There is no convincing evidence for operant or classical conditioning in adult humans. In: W Weimer & D Palermo (eds) *Cognition and the Symbolic Processes*, vol. 1, pp. 1–42. Hillsdale, NJ: Erlbaum.
Chambless DL & Gillis MM (1993) Cognitive therapy of anxiety disorders. *Journal of Consulting and Clinical Psychology* **61**: 248–60.
Clark DM (1996) Panic disorder: from theory to therapy In: Salkovskis P (ed.) *Frontiers of Cognitive Therapy*, pp. 318–44. Guilford Press.
Deckersbach T, Gershuny BS & Otto MW (2000) Cognitive behavioural therapy for depression: applications and outcome. *Psychiatric Clinics of North America* **23**: 795–809.

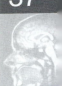

De Rubeis RJ & Crits Cristoph P (1998) Empirically supported individual and group treatments for adult mental disorders. *Journal of Consulting and Clinical Psychology* **66**(1): 37–52.

D'Zurilla TJ & Goldfried MR (1971) Problem solving and behaviour modification. *Journal of Abnormal Psychology* **78**: 107–26.

Ellis A (1962) *Reason and Emotion in Psychotherapy*. New York: Lyle Stuart.

Emmelkamp PMG & Wessels H (1975) Flooding in imagination versus flooding in vivo for agoraphobics. *Behaviour Research and Therapy* **13**: 7–15.

Fairburn CG & Cooper PJ (1989) Eating disorders. In: Hawton K, Salkovskis PM, Kirk J & Clark DM (eds) *Cognitive Behaviour Therapy for Psychiatric Problems*, pp. 277–314. Oxford: Oxford Medical Publications.

Fairburn CG, Jones R, Peveler RC, Carr SJ, Solomon RA, O'Connor ME, Burton J & Hope RA (1991) Three psychological treatments for bulimia nervosa. *Archives of General Psychiatry* **48**: 453–69.

Falloon IRH (ed.) (1988) *Handbook of Behavioural Family Therapy*. London: Unwin Hyman.

Fennell MJV (1989) Depression. In: Hawton K, Salkovskis PM, Kirk J & Clark DM (eds) *Cognitive Behaviour Therapy for Psychiatric Problems*, pp. 169–234. Oxford: Oxford Medical Publications.

Gould RA, Otto MW & Pollack MH (1995) A meta-analysis of treatment outcome for panic disorders. *Clinical Psychology Review* **15**(8): 819–44.

Greenberger D & Padesky CA (1995) *Mind Over Mood: A Cognitive Therapy Treatment Manual*. New York: Guilford Press.

Hawton K & Catalan J (1987) *Attempted Suicide: A Practical Guide to its Nature and Management*, 2nd edn. Oxford: Oxford University Press.

Kanfer FH & Karoly P (1972) Self control: a behaviouristic excursion into the lion's den. *Behavior Therapy* **3**: 398–416.

Kasvikis Y & Marks IM (1988) Clomipramine, self-exposure and therapist accompanied exposure in obsessive-compulsive ritualisers: two-year follow up. *Journal of Anxiety Disorders* **2**: 291–8.

Kingdon DG & Turkington D (1994) *Cognitive Behaviour Therapy of Schizophrenia*. Hove: Lawrence Erlbaum.

Kuipers E, Garety P, Fowler D, Dunn G, Bebbington P, Freeman D & Hadley C (1997) London–East Anglia randomised controlled trial of cognitive–behavioural therapy for psychosis. I: effects of the treatment phase. *British Journal of Psychiatry* **171**: 319–27.

Lam DH, Watkins ER, Hayward P, Bright J, Wright K, Kerr N, Parr-Davis G & Sham P (2003) A randomized controlled study of cognitive therapy for relapse prevention for bipolar affective disorder: outcome of the first year. *Archives of General Psychiatry* **60**: 145–52.

Leff J, Kuipers L, Berkopwitz R, Eberlein-Fries R & Sturgeon D (1982) A controlled trial of intervention in the families of schizophrenic patients. *British Journal of Psychiatry* **141**: 121–34.

Linehan MM, Armstrong HE, Suarez A, Allmon D & Heard H (1991) Cognitve–behavioral treatment of chronically parasuicidal borderline patients. *Archives of General Psychiatry* **48**: 1060–4.

McNally RJ & Steketee GS (1985) Etiology and maintenance of severe animal phobias. *Behaviour Research and Therapy* **23**: 431–5.

Mahoney MJ (1974) *Cognition and Behavior Modification*. Cambridge, MA: Ballinger.

Mahoney MJ (1995a) Theoretical developments in the cognitive psychotherapies. In: Mahoney MJ (ed.) *Cognitive and Constructive Psychotherapies: Theory, Research and Practice*, pp. 3–19. New York: Springer.

Mahoney MJ (ed.) (1995b) *Cognitive and Constructive Psychotherapies: Theory, Research and Practice*. New York: Springer.

Marks IM (1987) *Fears, Phobias and Rituals: Panic Anxiety and their Disorders*. New York: Oxford University Press.

Marks IM, Hodgson R & Rachman S (1975) Treatment of chronic OCD 2 years after in vivo exposure. *British Journal of Psychiatry* **127**: 349–64.

Marks IM & O'Sullivan G (1988) Drugs and psychological treatments for agoraphobia/panic and obsessive-compulsive disorders: a review. *British Journal of Psychiatry* **153**: 650–8.

Marks IM, Swinson RP, Basoglu M, Kuch K et al. (1993) Alprazolam and exposure alone and combined in panic disorder with agoraphobia. *Journal of Psychiatry* **162**: 776–87.

Mavissakalian M (1993) Combined behavioral therapy and pharmacotherapy of agoraphobia. *Journal of Psychiatric Research* **27**(Suppl 1): 179–91.

McDonald R, Sartory G, Grey SJ, Cobb J, Stern R & Marks IM (1978) Effects of self-exposure instructions on agoraphobic patients. *Behaviour Research and Therapy* **17**: 83–5.

Meichenbaum D (1977) *Cognitive Behaviour Modification: An Integrative Approach*. New York: Plenum Press.

Meichenbaum D & Cameron R (1973) Training schizophrenics to talk to themselves: a means of developing attentional controls. *Behavior Therapy* **4**: 515–34.

Meichenbaum D & Goodman J (1971) Training impulsive children to talk to themselves: a means of developing self-control. *Journal of Abnormal Psychology* **77**: 115–26.

Moorey S (1996) When bad things happen to rational people: cognitive therapy in adverse life situations. In: Salkovskis P (ed.) *Frontiers of Cognitive Therapy*, pp. 450–70. Guilford Press.

Moorey S & Greer S (2002) *Cognitive Behaviour therapy for People with Cancer*. Oxford: Oxford University Press.

Padesky CA (1994) Schema change processes in cognitive therapy. *Clinical Psychology and Psychotherapy* **1**(5): 267–78.

Paykel ES, Scott J, Teasdale JD et al. (1999) Prevention of relapse in residual depression by cognitive therapy: a controlled trial. *Archives of General Psychiatry* **56**: 829–35.

Pilling S, Bebbington P, Kuipers E et al. (2002) Psychological treatments in schizophrenia: I. Meta-analysis of family intervention and cognitive behaviour therapy. *Psychological Medicine* **32**: 763–82.

Rachman SJ & de Silva P (1978) Normal and abnormal obsessions. *Behaviour Research and Therapy* **16**: 233–8.

Randolph ET, Eth S, Glynn SM, Paz GG, Leong GB, Shaner AL, Strachan A, Van Vort W, Escobar JI & Liberman RP (1994) Behavioural family management in schizophrenia. Outcome of a clinic-based intervention. *British Journal of Psychiatry* **164**: 501–6.

Rapee RM (1991) The conceptual overlap between cognition and conditioning in clinical psychology. *Clinical Psychology Review* **11**: 193–203.

Roth A & Fonagy P (1996) *What Works for Whom? A Critical Review of Psychotherapy Research*. London: Guilford Press.

Salkovskis PM (1985) Obsessive-compulsive problems: a cognitive–behavioural analysis. *Behaviour Research and Therapy* **23**: 571–83.

Salkovskis PM & Harrison J (1984) Abnormal and normal obsessions: a replication. *Behaviour Research and Therapy* **27**: 549–52.

Seligman MEP (1971) Phobias and preparedness. *Behavior Therapy* **2**: 307–20.

Stern R & Marks IM (1973) Brief and prolonged flooding: a comparison in agoraphobic patients. *Archives of General Psychiatry* **28**: 270–6.

Stuart S & Bowers WA (1995). Cognitive therapy with inpatients: review and meta-analysis. *Journal of Cognitive Psychotherapy* **9**(2): 85–92.

Teasdale JD, Segal ZV, Williams JMG, Ridgeway V, Soulsby J & Lau M (2000) Prevention of relapse/recurrence in major depression by mindfulness-based cognitive therapy. *Journal of Consulting and Clinical Psychology* **68**: 615–23.

Trower P, Bryant B & Argyle M (1978) *Social Skills and Mental Health*. London: Methuen.

Van Balkom AJLM, Bakker A, Spinhoven P, Blaauw BMJW et al. (1997) A meta-analysis of the treatment of panic disorder with or without agoraphobia: A comparison of antidepressants, behavior, and cognitive therapy. *Journal of Nervous and Mental Diseases* **185**(8): 510–16.

Verheul R, Van Den Bosch LM, Koeter MW, De Ridder MA, Stijnen T & Van Den Brink W (2003) Dialectical behaviour therapy for women with borderline personality disorder: 12-month, randomised clinical trial in the Netherlands. *British Journal of Psychiatry* **182**: 135–40.

Watson JB & Rayner R (1920) Conditioned emotional reactions. *Journal of experimental psychology* **3**: 1–14.

Wells A (1997) *Cognitive Therapy of Anxiety Disorders*. Chichester: Wiley.

Williams JMG (1995) *The Psychological Treatment of Depression*, 2nd edn. London: Routledge.

Wolpe J (1958) *Psychotherapy by Reciprocal Inhibition*. Stanford, CA: Stanford University Press.

Young JE, Klosko JS & Weishaar ME (2003) *Schema Therapy: A Practitioner's Guide*. New York: Guilford Press.

Psychopharmacology

Pádraig Wright and David Perahia

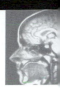

INTRODUCTION

This chapter provides an account of basic and clinical psychopharmacology, the former describing neurotransmitters and neuroreceptors and the latter including a discussion of pharmacokinetics and psychotropic drug development. The chapter concludes with a discussion of the main classes of psychotropic drugs.

BASIC PSYCHOPHARMACOLOGY

The human brain accounts for 2% of our bodyweight but utilizes 10% of the energy and 20% of the oxygen that we consume. Glucose is metabolized in the brain as in all other tissues by oxidative phosphorylation with the production of adenosine triphosphate. In addition, glucose is converted to glutamate, gamma-amino butyric acid (GABA) and aspartate in the brain via the GABA shunt in which the enzyme glutamate decarboxylase catalyses the conversion of glutamate to GABA.

Every substance that enters the brain must cross the blood–brain barrier (BBB). The BBB maintains brain glucose levels at the expense of general blood glucose levels via a sodium-linked active transport system, and prevents the passage of immunoglobulins, viruses and bacteria into the brain. Lipid-soluble substances, including lipid-soluble drugs, readily cross the BBB. Lipid-insoluble drugs can only pass into the brain very slowly.

Neurotransmitters

Neurotransmitters are substances that transfer signals across synapses between presynaptic and postsynaptic neurons. Postsynaptic neurons are subsequently either activated or inhibited. Neurotransmitters (Figure 38.1) may be defined as substances that:

- are synthesized in the presynaptic neuron

- are stored inactively in the presynaptic terminal
- are released from the presynaptic terminal when the presynaptic neuron depolarizes
- bind to a receptor at, and cause an effect (opening or closing of ion channels) in, the postsynaptic neuron, and
- have a presynaptic reuptake mechanism and/or degrading enzymes in the synapse that inactivate them.

Dopamine (DA), noradrenaline (norepinephrine) (NA), serotonin (5HT), acetylcholine (Ach), GABA, glutamate and glycine are the most important neurotransmitters and these will now be discussed in some detail. Other neurotransmitters include neuropeptides (endorphins, somatostatin, cholecystokinin, vasoactive intestinal peptide, angiotensin, neurotensin and substance P), neurohormones (corticotrophin and thyrotrophin release hormones) and the neuronally synthesized gases, nitric oxide (see phosphodiesterase type 5 inhibitors below) and carbon monoxide.

Dopamine

The three dopaminergic systems of most importance to psychiatry originate in the midbrain and diencephalon and are depicted in Figure 38.2.

The mesocorticolimbic system

Dopaminergic neurons project from the ventral tegmental nucleus to the limbic, septal and frontocortical areas. The psychopharmacology of the mesocorticolimbic system may be summarized as follows:

- Drugs of abuse such as alcohol, cocaine and amphetamine release DA at the nucleus accumbens. It is therefore believed that this system is involved with reward and pleasure.
- All effective antipsychotic (AP) drugs are D_2 receptor antagonists. It is therefore believed that excess mesocorticolimbic dopaminergic function may underpin schizophrenia, especially its positive symptoms.
- Frontal D_1 receptors appear to play an important role in normal cognitive function, and deficient

579

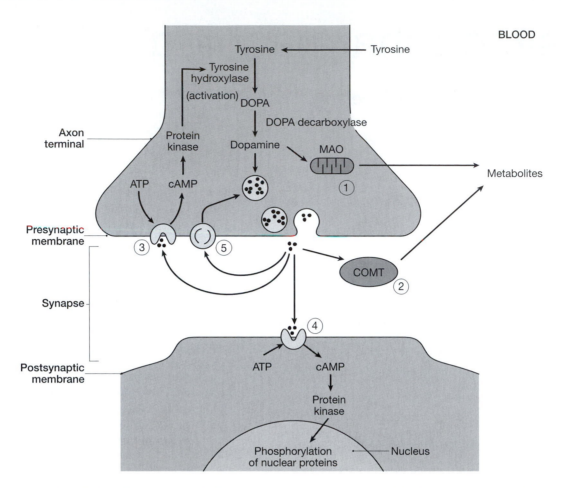

Figure 38.1 Dopamine (and serotonin and noradrenaline) is (1) degraded by monoamine oxidase (MAO) in presynaptic mitochondria, and (2) by synaptic catechol-o-methyltransferase (COMT) in the synapse. Dopamine binds to (3) presynaptic, as well as (4) postsynaptic membrane receptors, and is (5) actively transported back into the axon terminal. (From original drawing by Pádraig Wright.)

mesocorticolimbic dopaminergic function in the prefrontal and cingulate cortex has been implicated in the negative symptoms of schizophrenia.

- Mesocorticolimbic dopaminergic dysfunction has been implicated in mood disorders, particularly depression (prefrontal cortex/cingulate gyrus, nucleus accumbens), and in psychomotor retardation (dorsolateral prefrontal cortex, caudate nucleus).

The nigrostriatal system

Dopaminergic neurons project from the substantia nigra to the striatum. Degeneration of this system causes Parkinson's disease while blockade of D_2 receptors here by AP drugs causes extrapyramidal syndromes such as dystonia, akathisia and Parkinsonism.

The tuberoinfundibular system

Dopaminergic neurons project from the arcuate nucleus of the hypothalamus to the pituitary gland. DA inhibits the release of prolactin and blockade of D_2 receptors here by AP drugs causes hyperprolactinaemia.

Biochemistry

DA is synthesized from phenylalanine via L-tyrosine and degraded by monoamine oxidase (MAO) and catechol-o-methyltransferase (COMT) to homovanillic acid (HVA) (Figure 38.3). DA receptors are subdivided into the D_1-like GS coupled (D_1 and D_5) and the D_2-like G1 coupled (D_2, D_3 and D_4) classes (see below).

Clinical aspects

All AP drugs are potent D_2 receptor antagonists and many are also potent $5HT_{2A}$ receptor antagonists. Improvements in positive and negative symptoms are thought to result from altered dopaminergic function in the limbic and prefrontal cortex respectively.

Tricyclic (TCA) antidepressant (AD) drugs inhibit the reuptake of DA to the presynaptic neuron by the DA transporter while monoamine Type A oxidase inhibitor (MAOI) AD drugs increase synaptic DA by inhibiting MAO, its catalytic enzyme.

Amphetamines increase synaptic DA by causing its release into the synapse and both amphetamines and cocaine potently inhibit the DA reuptake transporter.

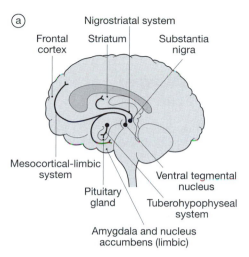

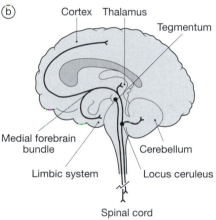

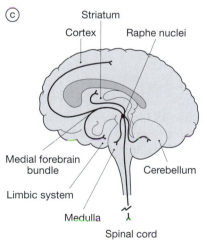

Figure 38.2 Schematic representation. (a) The mesocortico-limbic and nigrostriatal dopaminergic systems originate in the midbrain and project to the frontal cortex and limbic system, and to the striatum, respectively. The tuberohypophyseal dopaminergic system originates in the diencephalon and projects to the pituitary gland. (b) Noradrenergic neurons originating in the locus ceruleus project to the cortex, limbic system, thalamus, cerebellum and spinal cord. Tegmental noradrenergic neurons project to the brainstem and spinal cord. (c) Serotonergic neurons arise in the raphe nuclei and project to the cortex, limbic system, striatum, cerebellum, medulla and spinal cord. (From original drawing by Pádraig Wright.)

Noradrenaline (norepinephrine)

Noradrenergic neurons originate in the locus ceruleus in the floor of the fourth ventricle (Fig. 38.2). They project especially to the medulla and spinal cord, the cerebellum, the limbic system and thalamus, and the cortex. Noradrenergic systems are believed to be critical to arousal, attention, mood and pain because:

- activity in noradrenergic neurons in the locus ceruleus increases in response to novel or aversive stimuli
- α_1 and α_2 receptor antagonists cause sedation
- many antidepressant (AD) drugs increase noradrenergic neurotransmission and
- some AD drugs effectively alleviate pain.

Biochemistry

Noradrenaline (norepinephrine) is synthesized from phenylalanine (via dopamine) and degraded by MAO and COMT to 3-methoxy-4-hydroxy phenylglycol and 3-methoxy-4-hydroxymandelic acid respectively (Figure 38.3). Noradrenergic receptor subtypes include α_1 and α_2 and $ß_{1-3}$ (see below).

Clinical aspects

Abnormalities of noradrenergic function are believed to play a role in depression and bipolar disorder. TCA AD drugs increase synaptic NA by inhibiting its reuptake to the presynaptic neuron by the NA transporter.

MAOI AD drugs increase synaptic NA by inhibiting MAO, its catalytic enzyme. There are two types of MAO, MAO-A and MAO-B. MAO-A is the most efficient in degrading NA (and 5HT) and its irreversible inhibition by MAOIs (especially phenelzine) may impair the metabolism of both dietary tyramine and sympathomimetic drugs such as phenylpropanolamine and cause severe hypertension. Moclobemide, a reversible inhibitor of MAO-A, may pose less of a risk in this regard.

Amphetamines increase synaptic NA by promoting its rapid release into the synapse and both amphetamines and cocaine potently inhibit the NA reuptake transporter.

Serotonin

Serotonergic neurons originate in the dorsal and median raphe nucleii in the brainstem (Fig. 38.2). They project to the medulla and spinal cord, the cerebellum, the limbic system and striatum, and the cortex. Serotonergic systems are believed to be critical to sleep, appetite and mood because:

- reduced serotonergic function may cause insomnia and depression
- enhanced serotonergic function may cause appetite reduction and weight loss
- most AD drugs increase serotonergic neurotransmission.

Biochemistry

Serotonin (5HT) is synthesized from tryptophan and degraded by MAO to 5-hydroxyindolacetic acid (Fig. 38.3).

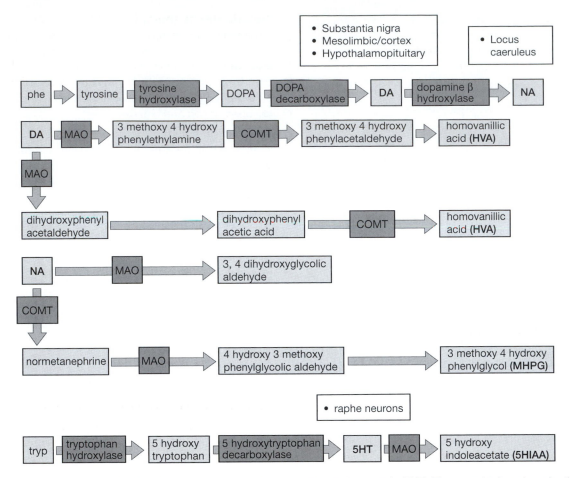

Figure 38.3 Synthetic and metabolic pathways of: noradrenaline, dopamine and serotonin (5HT). These are broken down by the monoamine oxidase enzymes located in presynaptic mitochondria. Noradrenaline and dopamine are also broken down by the synaptic enzyme catechol-O-methyltransferase (COMT). Monoamines are all actively transported back into the neuron from the synaptic cleft by specific transporters. (From original drawing by Pádraig Wright.)

Serotonergic receptor subtypes include $5HT_{1A-1F}$, $5HT_{2A-2C}$, $5HT_3$, $5HT_4$, $5HT_{5A-5C}$, $5HT_6$ and $5HT_7$.

Clinical aspects

Abnormalities of serotonergic function are believed to be important in depression, anxiety, psychosis (many AP drugs are potent $5HT_{2A}$ receptor antagonists) and nausea (5HT reuptake inhibitor ADs cause nausea while ondansetron, a potent $5HT_3$ receptor antagonist, is an effective antiemetic). Selective 5HT reuptake inhibitor (SSRI) AD drugs such as fluoxetine and paroxetine increase synaptic 5HT by inhibiting its reuptake to the presynaptic neuron by the 5HT transporter. TCAs such as amitriptyline and impiramine (tertiary amines) have a similar effect while most TCAs cause the release of 5HT into the synapse. MAOIs increase synaptic 5HT by inhibiting MAO, its catalytic enzyme.

Amphetamines increase synaptic 5HT by causing its release into the synapse while lysergic acid diethylamine (LSD) and psilocybin are $5HT_{1A}$ and $5HT_{2A}$ and HT_{2C} partial agonists.

Acetylcholine

Acetylcholine (Ach) plays a critical role in the central nervous system where cholinergic neurons project from the septal nucleii and nucleus basalis of Meynert in the ventromedial globus pallidus, to the hippocampus, amygdala and thalamus, and cortex. Cholinergic neurons appear to be critical to memory because they degenerate in dementia. Cholinergic neurons projecting from the brainstem to the basal ganglia play a role in the modulation of movement.

Biochemistry

Ach is synthesized from acetyl-CoA and choline by the enzyme choline acetyl transferase and degraded by acetylcholinesterase to acetic acid and choline. Cholinergic receptors may be either:

- nicotinic (rapidly acting and excitatory) and found at the neuromuscular junction and some sites in the brain, or
- muscarinic (slowly acting and excitatory), of which there are 5 subtypes, M_{1-5}, found in the brain and in cardiac and smooth muscle.

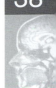

Clinical aspects

Many drugs used in psychiatry have potent anticholinergic or atropine-like effects and may cause dry mouth, increased sweating, blurred vision, constipation and urinary retention. Anticholinergic/antimuscarinic drugs are administered to overcome the rigidity and bradykinesia of both idiopathic and iatrogenic Parkinsonism. Dysfunction of M_1 receptors has been implicated in dementia while dysfunction of M_2 receptors has been implicated in mania. Acetylcholinesterase inhibitors such as donepezil may slow cognitive decline in dementia (see below).

Gamma-amino butyric acid

Gamma-amino butyric acid (GABA), the main inhibitory neurotransmitter in the brain, is found in the substantia nigra, striatum (caudate, putamen and globus pallidus) and hypothalamus as well as in the cerebellum (Purkinje cells) and spinal cord.

Biochemistry

GABA is synthesized from glutamate via the GABA shunt and degraded to succinic acid. GABA receptors are subdivided into $GABA_A$ (ion channel receptors) and $GABA_B$ (G-protein coupled receptors) classes.

Clinical aspects

Loss of GABA neurons in the striatum occurs in Huntington's chorea and GABA dysfunction has been implicated in both anxiety and epilepsy because benzodiazepine (BZD) drugs, potent postsynaptic $GABA_A$ receptor agonists, are very effective anxiolytic and antiepileptic drugs.

Glycine

Glycine is second only to GABA as the most important inhibitory neurotransmitter in the brain. It is synthesized from serine.

Glutamate

Glutamate and aspartate are the major excitatory neurotransmitters in the brain. Glutamate binds to either ion channel or ionotropic receptors such as N-methyl, D-aspartate or NMDA receptors, or to G-protein coupled metabotropic receptors (of which there are six subtypes).

Clinical aspects

Glutamate plays a critical physiological role but is also a potent neurotoxin implicated in the pathophysiology of stroke, head injury and epilepsy. NMDA antagonists such as lamotrigine and memantine have therefore been developed. Phencyclidine and ketamine are antagonists of the NMDA receptor and are psychotomimetic.

Opioid peptides

Opioid peptides include the endorphins and enkephalins and their β-endorphin, ACTH, dynorphin/neo-endorphin and enkephalin precursors. Opioid peptides are largely involved in mediating stress reactions and pain.

Substance P

Substance P is the neurotransmitter within the substantia gelatinosa of the spinal cord where it plays a role in the transmission of pain. This peptide also appears to play a role in depression.

Neuroreceptors

Neurotransmitters bind to neuroreceptors which are classified into 'superfamilies', of which the two most important are the ligand gated ion channel receptors and the G-protein coupled receptors.

Ligand gated ion channel receptors

Neuronal depolarization depends on the opening of ion channels in the neuronal membrane and the subsequent influx of sodium ions (Na^+) and efflux of potassium ions (K^+). The response of a neuron to ion channel receptor activation by either the natural ligand/neurotransmitter or a drug is rapid and brief. Examples of this mechanism include the action of Ach at the cholinergic nicotinic receptors of the neuromuscular junction, and GABA at $GABA_A$ receptors in the brain

The ion channel of the cholinergic nicotinic receptor opens when Ach binds to it, allowing the influx of Na^+ ions and resulting in an excitatory postsynaptic potential. Glutamate receptors behave similarly.

$GABA_A$ receptors in the brain differ from nicotinic and glutamate receptors in that they open in response to GABA and allow the influx of both K^+ and chloride ions (Cl^-). This results in an inhibitory postsynaptic potential. BZD drugs such as diazepam have high affinity for, and are agonists at, the $GABA_A$ receptor. Binding of a BZD drug to the $GABA_A$ receptor enhances the effect of GABA and causes a greater influx of K^+ and Cl^- than binding of GABA alone.

G-protein coupled receptors

Some receptors are linked to ion channels and enzymes by guanine triphosphate binding, or G, proteins. The G-protein is embedded in the intracellular surface of the cell membrane and it is activated when a ligand binds to the receptor. The activated G-protein then either stimulates or inhibits adenylate cyclase or other second messengers.

Examples of G-protein coupled receptors include adrenergic receptors that bind catecholamines (α_1 and α_2, β_{1-3}), serotonergic receptors ($5HT_{1A-1F}$, $5HT_2$), and dopaminergic receptors (D_1-like G_S coupled and D_2-like G_I coupled).

It will be noted from the above that all of the receptors important to psychiatry, with the exception of the ion channel glutamate and $GABA_A$ receptors, are G-protein coupled.

CLINICAL PSYCHOPHARMACOLOGY

Clinical psychopharmacology encompasses the sciences of pharmacokinetics and psychotropic drug development.

Pharmacokinetics

The fate of any drug ingested by an individual may be described by its pharmacokinetics – i.e. how it is absorbed, distributed within the body, metabolized and eliminated.

Absorption

Psychotropic drugs may be administered orally, intramuscularly (IM) or intravenously (IV). Orally administered drugs are absorbed in the stomach and proximal small intestine, the rate of absorption depending on the lipid solubility of the drug, whether the stomach is empty or full and concomitant treatment with other drugs that delay gastric emptying.

Orally administered drugs are initially absorbed more rapidly than they are eliminated and plasma level gradually increases. The peak plasma level or C_{MAX} is reached when the rates of absorption and elimination are equal (Fig. 38.4). The time taken to reach this point is referred to as T_{MAX}. The plasma level of the drug falls following C_{MAX} because the rate of elimination increasingly exceeds that of absorption. The time taken for the plasma level to fall to half of any given value is referred to as its half life or $t_{1/2}$.

It will be appreciated that second and subsequent doses of a drug add to the plasma level already achieved by a first dose. With continued dosing the rate at which drug enters the body eventually comes to equal the rate at which it is removed from the body and a relatively constant plasma level is achieved. This is referred to as steady state and the time taken to achieve it with continued dosing is equal to four or five half-lives ($4–5 \times t_{1/2}$).

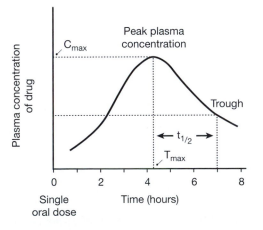

Figure 38.4 A diagram of peak plasma concentration (C_{max}), the time taken to reach peak plasma concentration (T_{max}) and the half-life ($t_{1/2}$) of a drug (single oral dose of drug administered at time 0).

Distribution

Bioavailability refers to the proportion of a drug administered by any route that may be recovered from the systemic circulation. Bioavailability is 100% for IV administered drugs. It is always <100% for orally administered drugs because absorption is rarely 100% and/or because some proportion of absorbed drug is metabolized while passing through the liver (first pass metabolism). The effect of incomplete absorption and/or first pass metabolism may range from insignificant to marked.

The distribution of absorbed drugs throughout the body depends on the extent to which they bind to plasma proteins and their lipid solubility. Most psychotropic drugs bind extensively to plasma proteins and are highly lipid soluble. Only unbound or free drug is able to cross the BBB and exert an effect.

Metabolism

Most psychotropic drugs undergo oxidative metabolism by the cytochrome P450 or CYP system of enzymes. The ingestion of alcohol or other drugs (notably antiepileptic drugs) may increase or decrease hepatic metabolism by competing for enzymatic sites or by the induction of metabolic enzymes. This can have clinically significant effects on the plasma concentration of some drugs.

Most psychotropic drugs have active metabolites and some of these are as active as the parent compound. Thus norfluoxetine and nortriptyline have AD activity equivalent to their parent compounds, fluoxetine and amitriptyline. It is obvious, but nonetheless worth stating, that lithium, an element, cannot be metabolized!

There are generally few restrictions on the use of psychotropic drugs in patients with mild to moderate liver disease. Lithium, disulfiram and donepezil are safe but the following should be noted:

- phenothiazines are particularly hepatotoxic and should be avoided
- lofepramine and monoamine oxidase inhibitor AD drugs should be avoided
- sodium valproate is hepatotoxic and should be avoided
- BZD drugs with long $t_{1/2}$ should be avoided because their metabolism is impaired.

Elimination

Psychotropic drugs are generally eliminated from the body by renal excretion of water soluble metabolites. The rate of elimination of a drug is usually proportional to its plasma concentration, a phenomenon referred to as first-order elimination kinetics. Some drugs (alcohol when its plasma concentration reaches 10 mg per 100 ml, for example) are subject to zero-order elimination kinetics in which elimination mechanisms become saturated and elimination proceeds thereafter at a constant rate and is not proportional to the drug's plasma concentration.

Despite the fact that psychotropic drugs are generally eliminated by renal excretion, there are generally no restrictions on the use of such drugs in patients with mild to moderate renal impairment. However, chloral hydrate, lithium and acamprosate should be avoided in patients with moderate renal impairment, and clozapine is contra-indicated in severe renal impairment.

Psychotropic drug development

Pharmaceutical companies wishing to licence a new prescription psychotropic drug for clinical use must satisfy the requirements of regulatory authorities such as the European Medicines Evaluation Agency in Europe as to the drug's quality, safety and efficacy. All drugs therefore undergo stringent preclinical and clinical evaluations before they are licensed for clinical use.

Preclinical evaluations include:

- quality testing to ensure each tablet or parenteral formulation contains exactly the ingredients, and is stable under the storage conditions and for the period of time or shelf-life, stated in its license
- in vitro toxicological and pharmacodynamic testing in cultured cells and tissues and
- in vivo toxicological, pharmacodynamic and behavioural testing in a range of animals (rodents, non-rodents and primates).

Clinical evaluations include:

- Phase I open-label, single, escalating and multiple-dose clinical studies in small numbers of healthy volunteers, the majority of whom are male because teratogenicity of the compound has not yet been excluded. These studies are designed to determine the safety and pharma-cokinetics of the new drug, to evaluate drug–drug interactions and, when possible, to determine dose.
- Phase II open-label and double-blind, single, escalating and multiple-dose clinical trials in relatively small numbers of patients suffering with the disease the new drug is designed to treat. These trials are designed to further evaluate safety, pharmacokinetics and pharmacodynamics, and to determine appropriate dosages and dosing regimens.
- Phase III clinical trials designed to provide statistical evidence that the drug being developed is more effective than placebo and at least as effective and safe as a comparator drug (a drug that has already been licensed to treat the disease being investigated). Phase III trials usually involve large numbers (thousands) of patients treated double-blind with various doses of the drug being developed, a comparator and/or placebo.
- At the time of writing the preclinical and clinical studies required before a psychotropic drug may be licensed may take as long as 10 years to perform and may cost up to $1 billion.

THE MAIN CLASSES OF PSYCHOTROPIC DRUGS

There now follows an account of the pharmacokinetics and pharmacodynamics of the main classes of psychotropic drugs, and of their efficacy and safety. Our knowledge of drugs is changing constantly and the most up to date sources of information available should be consulted regularly. In the UK these include:

- the *Summary of Product Characteristics* or SPC, available from the manufacturers of a drug
- the *British National Formulary* (BNF), available online (www.bnf.org)
- the guidance available from the National Institute of Clinical Excellence (NICE), available online (www.nice.org.uk)
- the guidance available from the Committee on Safety of Medicines (CSM), available online (www.mca.gov.uk/aboutagency/regframework/csm/csmhome.htm).

The main groups of psychotropic drugs are now discussed in the following order:

- antipsychotic drugs
- antidepressant drugs
- antimanic drugs
- lithium and other mood-stabilizing drugs
- drugs used in the treatment of anxiety disorders including sedative and hypnotic drugs
- drugs used in the treatment of psychiatric disorders in children
- antiepileptic drugs
- drugs used in the treatment of erectile impotence, premature ejaculation and antisocial sexual behaviour
- drugs used in the treatment of dementia
- drugs used in the treatment of Parkinsonism and related disorders
- drugs used in the treatment of alcohol and drug dependency.

Antipsychotic drugs

Antipsychotic (AP) drugs are conventionally divided into the newer atypical and older typical groups. The atypical AP drugs include three dibenzazepines (clozapine, the archetypal atypical AP drug, olanzapine and quetiapine), and several drugs with diverse structures (amisulpride, aripiprazole, risperidone, sertindole, ziprasidone and zotepine).

The typical AP drugs include the phenothiazines such as chlorpromazine, the thioxanthines such as flupenthixol and the butyrophenones such as haloperidol. Haloperidol may be regarded as the archetypal typical AP drug.

Pharmacokinetics and pharmacodynamics

The AP drugs have relatively similar pharmacokinetics and pharmacodynamics. Thus:

- they are rapidly and completely absorbed at the proximal small intestine, reaching C_{MAX} in 1-4 hours
- they are subject to extensive first pass metabolism
- their $t_{1/2}$ is generally of several days' duration (although the $t_{1/2}$ of depot preparations many extend over many weeks)
- their plasma protein binding is in excess of 90%
- they are metabolized almost exclusively, and very extensively, in the liver, almost no parent drug being excreted.

Mechanism of action

Without exception, all effective AP drugs have a relatively high (and largely dose-dependent) affinity for mesolimbic (A10) postsynaptic D_2 receptors at which they are potent antagonists. Occupancy of at least 65% of D_2 receptors appears to be both necessary and sufficient for their antipsychotic efficacy.

The affinity of AP drugs for nigrostriatal (A9) postsynaptic D_2 receptors appears to determine their extrapyramidal safety. Atypical AP drugs differ from typical AP drugs in that they have relatively low affinity for nigrostriatal D_2 receptors. They also have relatively high $5HT_{2A}$ to D_2 receptor binding ratios. These properties, possibly combined with interactions with other receptor types, may be responsible for the extrapyramidal safety profile of atypical APs.

More recently, a fast dissociation hypothesis of AP efficacy and safety has been proposed (Kapur & Seeman 2001). This suggests that D_2 receptor occupancy produces the antipsychotic effect but that rapid dissociation from the D_2 receptor (rather than occupancy of $5HT_{2A}$ or other receptors), accounts for extrapyramidal safety.

Efficacy

AP drugs are effective in treating acute episodes of schizophrenia, mania and other psychoses, in preventing relapse in patients with schizophrenia and other psychoses, and in preventing relapse in patients with bipolar disease when mood-stabilizing drugs are ineffective or are not tolerated.

Schizophrenia

It is generally accepted that AP drugs are all equally effective in alleviating both the positive symptoms of schizophrenia and in treating other acute psychoses. There is some evidence that atypical AP drugs are more effective than typical AP drugs in alleviating negative symptoms and in reducing depressive symptoms, suicidal behaviour and completed suicide (Meltzer et al. 2003, Wright & O'Flaherty

2003). More recent evidence suggests that atypical AP drugs such as olanzapine and possibly risperidone may improve cognitive function in patients with schizophrenia (Bilder et al. 2002).

Atypical AP drugs have been recommended as the first-line treatment for almost all patients with schizophrenia by NICE in the UK (2002a) and other similar authorities. It seems reasonable to extrapolate this recommendation to other patients who require AP drugs, for example those with acute mania (Box 38.1).

Treatment should commence with an adequate dose of a single atypical AP drug. If this is ineffective after 2–3 weeks the dose should be increased and treatment continued for a further 2–3 weeks. If treatment remains ineffective this drug should be discontinued, a second atypical AP drug should be prescribed and the same two-stage process should be repeated. If the second atypical AP drug proves ineffective, treatment with clozapine should be commenced. If the first atypical AP drug is not tolerated the patient should be switched to treatment with the second atypical AP drug. If this is not tolerated the patient should be switched to treatment with clozapine.

Clozapine is used as a second-line AP drug in patients with treatment resistant schizophrenia (inadequate efficacy of two different AP drugs prescribed in adequate doses for an adequate duration of time) and/or extrapyramidal side-effects caused by other AP drugs. Patients treated with clozapine require haematological monitoring because of the risk of agranulocytosis (see below).

Patients who refuse oral AP therapy or who are agitated may require a parenterally administered AP drug. Parenteral formulations of atypical AP drugs have recently become available and IM olanzapine is reported to reduce agitation as effectively as, but more rapidly than, IM haloperidol (Wright et al. 2001).

Box 38.1   National Institute of Clinical Excellence guidelines on atypical antipsychotics for schizophrenia

The atypical antipsychotics (amisulpride, olanzapine, quetiapine, risperidone and zotepine) should be considered when choosing first-line treatment of newly diagnosed schizophrenia

An atypical antipsychotic is considered the treatment option of choice for managing an acute schizophrenic episode when discussion with the individual is not possible

An atypical antipsychotic should be considered for an individual who is suffering unacceptable side-effects from a conventional antipsychotic

An atypical antipsychotic should be considered for an individual in relapse whose symptoms were previously inadequately controlled

Changing to an atypical antipsychotic is not necessary if a conventional antipsychotic controls symptoms adequately and the individual does not suffer unacceptable side-effects

Clozapine should be introduced if schizophrenia is inadequately controlled despite the sequential use of two or more antipsychotics (one of which should be an atypical antipsychotic) each for at least 6–8 weeks

The starting dose, dose range and available formulations of the atypical AP drugs that are currently licensed in the UK are presented in Table 38.1.

The relapse rate in untreated schizophrenia reaches almost 100% after two years. Long term maintenance AP drug therapy is therefore essential for the majority of patients and should be continued indefinitely.

The majority of patients with schizophrenia do not realise that they are ill and they are therefore understandably reluctant to take AP drugs. This, and the adverse effects associated with these drugs, mean that adherence to maintenance AP drug treatment is problematic. Injectable depot formulations of AP drugs reduce this problem to some extent in that patients may be more wiling to accept an IM injection every few weeks than tablets every day. A depot formulation of risperidone has recently become available in the UK. The pharmacokinetics of depot AP drugs differ significantly from those of orally administered AP drugs in that $t_{1/2}$ may be of several weeks and steady state may not be reached for several months.

Bipolar disorder

The relapse rate in untreated bipolar disorder is as high or higher than that in untreated schizophrenia. Bipolar patients are frequently treated with AP drugs when mood stabilizing drugs are ineffective or are not tolerated. Maintenance therapy should also be continued indefinitely in these patients because the risk of relapse never diminishes. Of the atypical AP drugs, olanzapine, quetiapine and risperidone have recently been approved for the treatment of acute mania (see below) and olanzapine has been approved for the

prevention of manic and depressive relapse in patients with bipolar disease (Tohen et al. 2003).

Safety

All effective AP drugs have a high affinity for, and are potent antagonists at, D_2 receptors but AP drugs also exert an effect at many other neuroreceptors. Antagonism at the $5HT_{2A}$ receptor may confer enhanced efficacy against negative symptoms but activity at other central receptors is, in the main, regarded as being responsible for adverse effects (Table 38.2).

The adverse effects listed in Table 38.2 occur to a great extent with all typical AP drugs. Atypical AP drugs also cause anticholinergic, antiserotonergic and antiadrenergic adverse effects but they are much less likely to cause antidopaminergic adverse effects such as extrapyramidal syndromes and, in some cases, hyperprolactinaemia.

AP drugs may also cause impaired temperature regulation, insomnia, dizziness, headache, confusion, gastrointestinal disturbance, blurred vision, contact sensitization, rashes, (cholestatic) jaundice and blood dyscrasias including leucopenia and agranulocytosis.

The *British National Formulary* (2003) lists the most significant adverse effects associated with atypical AP drugs as weight gain, dizziness, postural hypotension (which may be associated with syncope or reflex tachycardia in some patients) and extrapyramidal symptoms occasionally including tardive dyskinesia on long-term administration. Hyperglycaemia and sometimes diabetes mellitus may also occur and neuroleptic malignant syndrome has been reported. More recently, it has been recognized that AP

Table 38.1 The initial daily dose, daily dose range and available formulations of the atypical AP drugs that are currently licensed in the UK

	AP drug	Initial dose	Dose range	Available formulations
First-line AP drugs	Aripiprazole	10 mg	10–30 mg	Tablets
	Amisulpride	400–800 mg	400–1200 mg	Tablets Liquid
	Olanzapine	10 mg	5–20 mg	Tablets Orodispersible tablets Intramuscular injection
	Quetiapine	50 mg	300–750 mg	Tablets
	Risperidone	2 mg	4–16 mg	Tablets Orodispersible tablets Liquid Depot injection
	Zotepine	75 mg	75–300 mg	Tablets
	Sertindole[2]	4 mg	12–24 mg	Tablets
Second-line AP drugs	Clozapine[1]	12.5–25 mg	200–900 mg	Tablets

Notes:

[1] In order to use clozapine, both prescribers and patients must be registered with CPMS, the Clozaril Patient Monitoring Service

[2] Sertindole has been reintroduced following an earlier suspension because of concerns about arrhythmias (QTc prolongation); its use is restricted to patients who are intolerant of at least one other AP drug and are enrolled in a clinical study

Table 38.2 Adverse effects attributable to the antagonism of AP drugs at different types of neuroreceptors	
Neuroreceptor effect	Adverse effect
Anticholinergic	Dry mouth, constipation (occasionally, paralytic ileus in older patients), dry eyes, blurred vision, closed angle glaucoma, urinary hesitancy, urinary retention (especially in males with prostatic hypertrophy), sexual dysfunction, mild tachycardia (because of reduced vagal tone), impaired memory and confusion
Antiserotonergic	Weight gain (antihistaminergic mechanisms also proposed)
Antiadrenergic	Dizziness, postural hypotension (may lead to falls and hip fractures in older patients), sexual dysfunction
Antidopaminergic	Extrapyramidal syndromes, hyperprolactinaemia

drugs increase the risk of cerebrovascular events and mortality in elderly patients with dementia.

Clozapine is associated with an increased risk of agranulocytosis and patients being treated with it require haematological monitoring. Reversible neutropenia occurs in 3% of clozapine treated patients while 0.8% of patients developed agranulocytosis prior to the introduction of haematological monitoring.

Their safety profile means that AP drugs should be prescribed cautiously in patients with hepatic and renal impairment, epilepsy, Parkinson's disease, prostatism, blood dyscrasias and closed angle glaucoma. Some AP drugs cause photosensitivity. AP drugs are relatively contraindicated in patients with impaired consciousness and phaeochromocytoma.

Extrapyramidal adverse effects

Acute dystonia, Parkinsonism, akathisia and tardive dyskinesia were described in patients with schizophrenia before the advent of AP drugs but typical AP drugs greatly increase the risk of these disorders. Acute dystonia occurs immediately or within a few days of treatment with an AP drug, especially in young male patients. Parkinsonism may only develop after many weeks of treatment and is commonest in older female patients. Akathisia occurs equally in both sexes and usually develops during the first few days or weeks of treatment.

Tardive dyskinesia is commonest in older female patients. Its incidence in patients treated with typical AP drugs is about 5% per year and the cumulative prevalence is between 20% and 25%. The incidence and cumulative prevalence in patients treated with atypical AP drugs is significantly lower.

Neuroleptic malignant syndrome

The neuroleptic malignant syndrome (NMS) consists of extrapyramidal symptoms (rigidity), fluctuating consciousness (delirium, stupor) and autonomic lability (hyperthermia, tachycardia, hypo- or hypertension, sweating, pallor, salivation and urinary incontinence). Marked elevation of creatinine phosphokinase occurs and thromboembolism and renal failure caused by myoglobinuria secondary to muscle necrosis are common. Untreated, death occurs in 10% to 20% of affected patients.

Neuroleptic malignant syndrome is a medical emergency that is best treated in an intensive care unit. Antipsychotic therapy must be discontinued, the patient's temperature normalized, fluid and electrolyte balance maintained and secondary infection treated. Diazepam, dantrolene or bromocriptine may be useful, as may amantadine and L-dopa. Recovered patients usually have no sequelae. Further antipsychotic treatment should be with a drug from a different chemical group and dosage should be increased extremely slowly and with careful monitoring.

Hyperprolactinaemia

Hyperprolactinaemia, a side-effect of all typical AP drugs, causes hypo-oestrogenaemia, and is associated with a number of different adverse effects in men and women:

- Men: gynaecomastia, impotence, loss of libido and impaired spermatogenesis.
- Women: galactorrhoea, amenorrhoea, altered ovarian function, loss of libido and an increased long-term risk for osteoporosis.

Aripiprazole, olanzapine, quetiapine and clozapine do not appear to be associated with significant hyperprolactinaemia, in contrast to both amisulpride and risperidone and to the typical AP drugs. Reducing risk for hyperprolactinemia is highly desirable given that impotence in men and loss of libido in both sexes may impair the quality of patients' lives and their adherence to treatment, while osteoporosis may present a longer term personal and public health risk (Naidoo et al. 2003).

Cardiovascular adverse effects

Sudden cardiac death has long been reported in otherwise healthy young people, especially men, treated with AP drugs. The causes of such deaths may include:

- Prolongation of the QTc interval on the electrocardiogram, which may lead to ventricular tachyarrhythmias and death. This is more likely to occur in patients who are hypokalaemic or have high

sympathetic tone, both of which situations may prevail in agitated, overactive patients. The atypical AP drug sertindole has been reintroduced for use in the UK following an earlier suspension because of concerns about arrhythmias (see Table 38.1). Amisulpride, olanzapine, quetiapine, risperidone and zotepine appear to have no clinically significant effect on the QTc interval. Of the typical AP drugs, droperidol is no longer available in the UK and thioridazine is restricted to second-line treatment of schizophrenia in adults under specialist supervision because of QTc prolongation.

- NA α_1 blockade – some AP drugs, especially in high dosage, may cause marked NA α_1 blockade and lead to profound hypotension.
- Concomitant treatment with drugs that act synergistically to cause cardiorespiratory collapse, for example BZD drugs.

Antidepressant drugs

The efficacy of AD drugs appears to depend on their ability to increase synaptic concentrations of some or all of the biogenic amines NA, 5HT and DA, which in turn enhances neurotransmission across the synapse. The mechanisms by which AD drugs increase synaptic concentrations of biogenic amines include:

- inhibition of the transporter molecules responsible for the reuptake of NA, 5HT and DA from the synapse to the presynaptic neuron
- inhibition of MAO, the catalytic enzyme for NA, 5HT and DA
- blockade of presynaptic NA and 5HT neuroreceptors which prevents negative feedback by NA and 5HT at these receptors and thus permits the presynaptic neuron to continue secreting NA and 5HT.

The AD drugs may be pragmatically classified into the newer and older groups. The newer AD drugs include the following:

- selective 5HT reuptake inhibitors (SSRI) including citalopram and its isomer escitalopram, fluoxetine, fluvoxamine, paroxetine and sertraline
- 5HT/NA reuptake inhibitors (SNRI) venlafaxine and duloxetine
- reversible MAO Type A inhibitor moclobemide (sometimes referred to as a RIMA, a reversible inhibitor of MAO-A drug)
- a miscellaneous group that includes mirtazapine (a presynaptic NA α_2 and $5HT_{2A, 2C \& 3}$ antagonist), reboxetine (a selective NA reuptake inhibitor) and tryptophan (the essential amino acid precursor of 5HT).

Buproprion (a DA reuptake inhibitor) is licensed as an adjuvant to cigarette smoking cessation in the UK but not as an antidepressant (see below).

The older AD drugs include the following:

- tricyclic (TCA) AD drugs amitriptyline, amoxapine, clomipramine, dothiepin, doxepin, imipramine, lofepramine, nortriptyline and trimipramine (NA and 5HT reuptake inhibitors)
- TCA-related AD drugs maprotiline (a tetracyclic selective NA reuptake inhibitor), mianserin (a tetracyclic and largely selective NA reuptake inhibitor) and trazadone (a tetracyclic 5HT reuptake inhibitor and α_1 noradrenergic antagonist)
- the MAO-A inhibitor (MAOI) AD drugs including isocarboxazid, phenelzine and tranylcypromine.

Pharmacokinetics and pharmacodynamics
Newer antidepressant drugs
Selective serotonin reuptake inhibitors The SSRIs are slowly but completely absorbed from the proximal small intestine and reach C_{MAX} in 4–8 hours. First pass metabolism is extensive. The $t_{1/2}$ of SSRIs ranges from 10 hours (paroxetine, fluvoxamine) to 72 hours (fluoxetine). Protein binding exceeds 90% for most SSRIs but is approximately 75% for citalopram and fluvoxamine.

SSRIs selectively inhibit the reuptake of 5HT via the 5HT transporter molecule from the synapse to the presynaptic neuron. They also weakly inhibit the reuptake of NA from the synapse to the presynaptic neuron.

Experimental tryptophan depletion: Tryptophan (see below) is an essential amino acid precursor of 5HT that raises synaptic 5HT concentrations simply by providing more substrate for conversion to 5HT. Experimental tryptophan depletion (excess intake of neutral amino acids will saturate the brain's amino acid transporter and prevent tryptophan uptake) causes rapid and marked lowering of mood in depressed patients who have been successfully treated with AD drugs acting on 5HT systems. This effect is not evident in similar patients successfully treated with AD drugs acting on NA systems.

Serotonin/noradrenergic reuptake inhibitors The SNRI venlafaxine is readily absorbed from the proximal small intestine and reaches C_{MAX} in two hours. It is subject to extensive first pass metabolism and has a $t_{1/2}$ of approximately five hours. Its plasma protein binding is approximately 25%. Venlafaxine inhibits the reuptake of 5HT at lower doses and of both 5HT and NA at higher doses via their transporter molecules.

Duloxetine has a $t_{1/2}$ of approximately 12 hours while its plasma protein binding is approximately 95%. It has no active metabolites. Duloxetine is an even more potent inhibitor than venlafaxine of 5HT and NA reuptake from the synapse.

Moclobemide The RIMA moclobemide is readily absorbed from the proximal small intestine and reaches C_{MAX} in one hour. It is subject to extensive first pass metabolism and has a $t_{1/2}$ of approximately two hours. Its

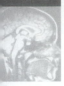

plasma protein binding is approximately 50%. Moclobemide increases synaptic concentrations of NA, 5HT and, to a lesser extent, DA by reversibly inhibiting their catalytic enzyme, MAO-A.

Mirtazapine   Mirtazapine is readily absorbed from the proximal small intestine and reaches C_{MAX} in two hours. It has a $t_{1/2}$ of approximately 30 hours. Mirtazapine increases synaptic concentrations of both 5HT and NA by means of antagonism at presynaptic α_2 noradrenergic and $5HT_{2A, 2C \& 3}$ receptors.

Reboxetine   Reboxetine is readily absorbed and reaches C_{MAX} in two hours. Plasma protein binding is extensive. It is a selective NA reuptake inhibitor with no appreciable effect on 5HT or MAO systems.

Tryptophan   Tryptophan is available for use in combination with other AD drugs in patients who have been depressed for at least two years and who have not responded to AD monotherapy.

Older antidepressant drugs

Tricyclic and tricyclic related antidepressant drugs   The TCA AD drugs have relatively similar pharmacokinetics and pharmacodynamics. Thus

- absorption is rapid and almost complete at the proximal small intestine and C_{MAX} is reached in 2–6 hours
- they are subject to extensive first pass metabolism and only 50% of absorbed drug appears in the systemic circulation. Many TCA AD drugs have active metabolites
- their $t_{1/2}$ is approximately 24 hours
- their plasma protein binding is up to 95%
- they are eliminated via the kidney.

TCA AD drugs increase synaptic concentrations of both NA and 5HT (and DA to a much lesser extent) by inhibiting their reuptake to the presynaptic neuron. The secondary amines desipramine and nortriptyline inhibit NA reuptake to a much greater extent than 5HT reuptake while clomipramine has the opposite effect.

Experimental noradrenaline (norepinephrine) depletion: Experimental NA depletion (accomplished by treatment with α methyl paratyrosine which inhibits tyrosine hydroxylase, the enzyme that catalyses the conversion of tyrosine to DOPA and thence to DA and NA) causes marked lowering of mood in depressed patients who have been successfully treated with AD drugs acting on NA systems. This effect is not evident in similar patients successfully treated with AD drugs acting on 5HT systems.

Monoamine oxidase inhibitor drugs   The MAOIs are readily absorbed from the proximal small intestine and reach C_{MAX} in 1–2 hours. They are subject to extensive first pass metabolism and have a $t_{1/2}$ of approximately 2–4 hours. MAOIs are transformed by MAO into products that irreversibly inactivate MAO. The effect of an MAOI therefore persists long after the MAOI itself is no longer detectable and is only reversed by synthesis of new enzyme. MAOIs increase synaptic concentrations of NA, 5HT and DA by inhibiting MAO-A and B.

Efficacy

AD drugs are effective in:

- treating major depressive disorder and similar syndromes
- preventing new episodes of depression in patients who have been successfully treated for major depressive disorder and similar syndromes
- treating depressive relapse in patients with bipolar disorder (bipolar depression)
- treating anxiety disorders including obsessive-compulsive disorder, panic disorder, post-traumatic stress disorder, generalized anxiety disorder and social phobia (see below)
- treating bulimia nervosa (see below)
- treating chronic pain syndromes including diabetic neuropathy and postherpetic neuralgia (TCAs and SNRIs but not SSRIs)
- treating nocturnal enuresis in children
- treating premature ejaculation (SSRIs only).

Major depressive disorder

Newer AD drugs are no more effective than older ones in treating depression but they are safer in overdose and generally have fewer side-effects. Furthermore, treatment with most newer antidepressant drugs may be initiated at the therapeutic dose. This precludes subtherapeutic dosing and shortens time to recovery. Newer AD drugs are therefore recommended as the first-line treatment for the vast majority of patients and especially for:

- patients with histories of overdosing, intolerance to older AD drugs or poor adherence to treatment
- patients with general medical disorders, particularly cardiovascular disorders
- patients taking concomitant medications.

Older AD drugs may be appropriate for some patients, for example lofepramine might be prescribed for an individual who responded to it previously. MAOIs should be reserved for second-line treatment of depression and atypical depression by a psychiatrist familiar with their effects.

Treatment should commence with an adequate dose of a single newer AD drug. If this is ineffective after 2–3 weeks the dose should be increased and treatment continued for a further 2–3 weeks. If treatment remains ineffective this drug should be discontinued, a second newer AD drug should be prescribed and the same two-stage process should be repeated. If the second drug proves ineffective the treatment strategies described below for treatment-resistant depression should be considered. The importance of treatment with an adequate dose of AD drug for an adequate duration of time cannot be overemphasized.

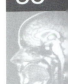

If the first newer AD drug prescribed is not tolerated the patient should be switched to treatment with a second newer AD drug. If this is not tolerated a third AD may be prescribed or the treatment strategies described below for treatment-resistant depression should be considered.

When switching patients from one class of AD to another, the following rules should be observed:

- an interval of two weeks should elapse between discontinuing treatment with an MAOI and commencing treatment with either an SSRI, a TCA or another MAOI
- an interval of two weeks should elapse between discontinuing treatment with an TCA and commencing treatment with an MAOI
- an interval of one week (five weeks in the case of fluoxetine) should elapse between discontinuing treatment with an SSRI and commencing treatment with an MAOI.

The starting dose, dose range and available formulations of the AD drugs currently licensed in the UK are presented in Table 38.3.

Patients who respond to AD drug therapy and then discontinue treatment have a high risk of relapse, especially during the first 12 months following recovery (Geddes et al. 2003). The majority of such patients should continue to take the same AD drug they responded to at the same dosage for at least six and ideally 12 months after recovery. Such prophylactic therapy may need to be continued indefinitely in some patients. The eventual discontinuation of prophylactic AD drug therapy should be tapered over several weeks in order to prevent the occurrence of discontinuation syndrome (see below).

Major depressive disorder in children and adolescents

In December 2003 the CSM advised that the benefit/risk balance was unfavourable for sertraline, citalopram and escitalopram (and unassessable for fluvoxamine) in the treatment of individuals under the age of 18 years for major depressive disorder, and that only fluoxetine has been shown in clinical trials to have a favourable benefit/risk balance for such individuals.

Bipolar depression

It is generally accepted that AD monotherapy should be avoided in the management of depressive relapse in patients with bipolar disorder because of the risk of inducing acute mania (SSRIs are probably safer than TCAs in this regard). Such patients should therefore be treated with an AD drug and a concomitantly administered mood-stabilizing drug such as lithium, valproate or olanzapine (see below).

Treatment-resistant depression

The following strategies may be useful in the management of treatment resistant depression:

- consider misdiagnosis and/or comorbidity
- consider non-compliance, inadequate dosage or inadequate duration of treatment
- prescribe a drug from a different AD class (including MAOI) or prescribe venlafaxine if not already tried
- consider dual drug therapy with either an AD drug and an atypical AP drug, an AD drug and lithium, an AD drug and tryptophan or two AD drugs from two different classes (TCA with SSRI or TCA with MAOI)
- consider triple drug therapy with an AD drug, lithium and tryptophan
- consider the addition of thyroxine (as liothyronine) to one of the above strategies.

Safety

AD drugs primarily modify NA- and 5HT-mediated neurotransmission but they also exert an effect at many other central and peripheral receptors. These latter effects are, in the main, regarded as being responsible for the adverse effects of ADs.

Newer antidepressant drugs

SSRIs commonly cause nausea, dyspepsia, crampy abdominal pain and diarrhoea and all patients should be warned of this likelihood. These adverse effects will disappear in most patients after 7–10 days of treatment. In contrast, if headache occurs, it is likely to persist. Sexual dysfunction (diminished libido, erectile and ejaculatory impotence and anorgasmia) is much more common with SSRIs than TCAs and may affect as many as 1 in 3 patients. This is a major cause of treatment discontinuation in the later stages of recovery and during prophylaxis. Less common adverse effects associated with SSRIs include:

- psychomotor arousal (which may be an advantage to some patients)
- extrapyramidal syndromes
- hyponatraemia (especially in older patients)
- serotonin syndrome, characterized by confusion, fever, myoclonus, chorea, seizures and coma. This also occurs with venlafaxine. It is more likely to occur if SSRIs or SNRIs are administered with MAOIs.

Seizures may also occur. SSRIs have no effect on cardiac function and are therefore safe in overdosage (see below). They may cause mild anorexia and weight loss, although paroxetine may be associated with weight gain.

A discontinuation syndrome occurs in 1 in 3 patients within 24 hours of abruptly discontinuing treatment with SSRIs. The symptoms may be moderate or severe and include anxiety, mood disturbance, gastrointestinal disturbance, dizziness, paraesthesia, sleep disturbance and an influenza-like syndrome. SSRI discontinuation syndrome is most common with paroxetine which has a short $t_{1/2}$ and very uncommon with fluoxetine which has a long $t_{1/2}$ and an active major metabolite with a long $t_{1/2}$. SSRI

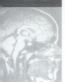

Table 38.3   The initial daily dose, daily dose range and available formulations of the AD drugs that are currently licensed in the UK

	AD drug	Initial dose	Dose range	Available formulations
Newer AD drugs	Citalopram	10–20 mg	20–60 mg	Tablets Liquid
	Duloxetine	60 mg	60 mg	Capsules
	Escitalopram	10 mg	10–20 mg	Tablets
	Fluoxetine	20 mg	20 mg	Capsules Liquid
	Fluvoxamine	50–100 mg	100–300 mg	Tablets
	Mirtazapine	15 mg	15–45 mg	Tablets
	Moclobemide	300 mg	150–600 mg	Tablets
	Paroxetine[1]	20 mg	20 mg	Tablets Liquid
	Reboxetine	8 mg	8–12 mg	Tablets
	Sertraline	50 mg	50–200 mg	Tablets
	Tryptophan[2]	3 grams	3–6 grams	Tablets
	Venlafaxine	75 mg	75–375 mg	Tablets Capsules
Older AD drugs	Amitriptyline	75 mg	150–200 mg	Tablets Liquid
	Amoxapine	100–150 mg	150–300 mg	Tablets
	Clomipramine	10 mg	30–250 mg	Tablets Capsules
	Dothiepin	75 mg	150–225 mg	Tablets Capsules
	Doxepin	75 mg	75–300 mg	Capsules
	Imipramine	75 mg	150–20 mg	Tablets
	Isocarboxazid	30 mg	30–60 mg	Tablets
	Lofepramine	140–210 mg	140–210 mg	Tablets Liquid
	Maprotiline	25–75 mg	75–150 mg	Tablets
	Mianserin	30–40 mg	30–90 mg	Tablets
	Nortriptyline	75–10 mg	75–150 mg	Tablets
	Phenelzine	45 mg	45–90 mg	Tablets
	Tranylcypromine	20 mg	20–30 mg	Tablets
	Trazadone	100–150 mg	100–600 mg	Tablets Capsules Liquid
	Trimipramine	50–75 mg	150–300 mg	Tablets Capsules

Notes:
The above dosing recommendations refer only to the treatment of depressive disorder and dosing recommendations may differ when the AD drugs listed are used in the treatment of anxiety or eating disorders (see below)
[1] In order to use tryptophan both prescribers and patients must be registered with OPTICS, the Optimax Information and Clinical Support unit
[2] The CSM recently recommended 20 mg as the daily dose of paroxetine in the treatment of depression and several anxiety disorders (see below)

discontinuation syndrome may be avoided by gradual discontinuation of SSRIs over several weeks.

Older antidepressant drugs
TCAs are potent Ach, α_2 noradrenergic and H_1 neuroreceptor antagonists and some are also D_2 antagonists. These properties and as yet undefined central mecanisms are responsible for the adverse effects presented in Table 38.4. It is thought that the general increase in noradrenergic tone associated with TCAs is responsible for the anxiety, agitation, tremor and increased sweating experienced by some patients. TCAs also have Class I or membrane stabilizing antiarrhythmic properties and may cause heart

block in healthy individuals. TCAs are highly cardiotoxic in overdosage because:

- a reservoir of potentially absorbable drug remains available in the proximal small intestine for a prolonged period following ingestion because their anticholinergic effects delay gastrointestinal motility
- their Class I antiarrhythmic properties slow ventricular conduction and promote ventricular tachyarrhythmias
- they impair alveolar gas exchange and cause hypoxia, hypercapnia and acidosis. Acidosis in turn reduces protein binding and increases available free drug.

In contrast to TCAs (with the exception of lofepramine), SSRIs have no appreciable effect on cardiac function and are relatively safe in overdosage. As is the case with many drugs, TCAs may cause rashes, hypersensitivity reactions, leucopenia, agranulocytosis, eosinophilia, thrombocytopenia and hyponatraemia (especially in older patients and possibly due to inappropriate secretion of antidiuretic hormone). NMS occurs rarely. Mianserin and trazadone are associated with increased risks of white cell dyscrasias and priapism respectively.

MAOIs may cause a potentially fatal hypertensive crisis because they inactivate MAO in the gut and prevent the neutralization of ingested sympathomimetic substances (dietary tyramine and histamine and drugs such as phenylpropanolamine and ephedrine). Patients being treated with MAOIs must be warned against eating certain foods (meat, soya or yeast etracts, mature cheeses, pickled herring, broad bean pods), drinking full bodied red wines or taking cough remedies containing phenylpropanolamine and ephedrine. These restrictions do not apply to patients treated with moclobemide.

The adverse effects associated with MAOIs include hypotension, insomnia and psychomotor arousal. MAOIs have no effect on cardiac function but they may cause dry mouth, constipation, urinary hesitancy and retention, sexual dysfunction and confusion. Phenelzine is a rare cause of peripheral neuropathy.

Antimanic drugs

The antimanic drugs include AP and BZD drugs along with lithium, carbamazepine and valproate (Keck 2003). These are all discussed in more detail elsewhere in this chapter.

Patients with acute mania (manic episode) almost always require hospitalization and treatment with antimanic drugs in order to rapidly control their behaviour and reduce risk, reduce their agitation and distress, alleviate their psychotic symptoms and prevent further episodes of mania. In general, AP drugs reduce manic symptoms in 1–2 days, lithium takes 1–2 weeks to be effective and carbamazepine and valproate have an intermediate onset of action.

Olanzapine, quetiapine and risperidone are approved for the treatment of acute mania and the vast majority of patients should be treated with one of these atypical AP drugs, either alone or in combination with BZD drugs (Goodwin & Young 2003). Parenteral administration of such drugs may be required, either because patients refuse oral therapy or in order to reduce risk. Patients with less severe mania may be treated with either lithium or carbamazepine alone, or with modest doses of atypical AP drugs.

Approximately half of all manic patients will not respond adequately to the treatments described above. Such patients will require combination therapy with an atypical AP drug and either lithium or carbamazepine. Clozapine has also been used successfully to treat patients with treatment resistant mania.

Lithium and other mood stabilizing drugs

Prophylactic mood-stabilizing drugs are recommended for patients who have experienced one of the following:

Table 38.4 Adverse effects attributable to the antagonism of TCA AD drugs at different types of neuroreceptors	
Neuroreceptor effect	Adverse effect
Anticholinergic	Dry mouth, constipation (occasionally, paralytic ileus in older patients), dry eyes, blurred vision, closed angle glaucoma, urinary hesitancy, urinary retention (especially in males with prostatic hypertrophy), sexual dysfunction, mild tachycardia (because of reduced vagal tone), impaired memory and confusion
Antiadrenergic (primarily α_1 antagonism)	Dizziness, postural hypotension (may lead to falls and hip fractures in older patients), sexual dysfunction, dry mouth, constipation
Antihistaminergic (primarily H_1 antagonism)	Sedation (impairs occupational and driving ability but may be a benefit for some patients), weight gain (antiserotonergic mechanisms also proposed)
Antidopaminergic	Extrapyramidal syndromes, hyperprolactinaemia (especially likely with amoxapine and clomipramine)
Complex central mechanisms	Lowered seizure threshold with increased risk of epileptic seizures, induction of manic episode (more likely in patients with recognized or unrecognized bipolar disorder)

- two manic episodes
- an episode of mania and an episode of depression, or
- a single manic episode that caused very significant personal, domestic or occupational impact.

Some patients with recurrent depressive illness also benefit from mood-stabilizing drugs.

The mood-stabilizing drugs that are currently available include lithium salts, the antiepileptic drugs valproate, carbamazepine and lamotrigine and the atypical AP olanzapine (Goodwin & Young 2003). Lithium salts represent first-line prophylactic monotherapy but approximately 1 in 3 patients relapse while taking them. Such patients may benefit from second-line prophylactic treatment with carbamazepine or valproate, either alone or in combination with lithium salts. Typical AP drugs (including depot formulations) represent the third line prophylactic treatment in patients with bipolar disorder. The atypical AP drugs carry a low risk for tardive dyskinesia and olanzapine has recently been approved for the prevention of manic and depressive relapse in patients with bipolar disease. It remains to be seen if the atypical APs become established as first-line mood-stabilizing drugs.

Lithium

Lithium salts will now be discussed (the antiepileptic and AP drugs are discussed elsewhere in this chapter).

Pharmacokinetics and pharmacodynamics

Lithium is an alkali metal that may be administered as either its lithium carbonate or lithium citrate salt. The active component of both is the lithium cation (Li^+). Lithium:

- is rapidly and completely absorbed at the proximal small intestine and, to a lesser extent, the stomach
- reaches C_{MAX} in 1–2 hours and has a $t_{1/2}$ of approximately 24 hours (currently available tablets are coated so as to delay absorption and produce a non-toxic C_{MAX} approximately four hours after administration and effective blood levels throughout the day)
- has a narrow therapeutic window, being largely ineffective at serum levels below 0.4 mmol/l and toxic at levels above 1.5 mmol/l
- is not bound to plasma proteins and is eliminated unchanged via the kidney.

Mechanism of action   The mechanism of action of lithium is unknown. It may modify neuronal second messenger systems or stabilize neuronal membranes.

Efficacy

Lithium is indicated for the treatment of manic episode and the prevention of relapse in bipolar disorder. It is a second-line (after continuation of treatment with a newer type of AD drug) or adjuvant treatment (in combination with a newer

type of AD) for the prevention of new depressive episodes in unipolar depressive disorder. Lithium may also be used to control aggressive or self-mutilating behaviour.

The daily dosage should be increased gradually until serum lithium measured 12 hours after administration is maintained in the range 0.4–1.0 mmol/l (it was previously recommended to maintain serum lithium measured 12 hours after administration in the range 0.6–1.2 mmol/l but this is now regarded as excessive for most patients). It is usual to measure serum lithium weekly while the dose is being titrated to the therapeutic range and every three months thereafter. Patients taking lithium require baseline and regular laboratory investigations in addition to serum lithium assays (see below).

Approximately 50% of patients in whom treatment with lithium is abruptly discontinued will develop mania within 1–2 weeks (Verdoux & Bourgeois 1993). Rebound mania may be avoided by gradual discontinuation of lithium over 6–8 weeks if treatment must cease.

Safety

The majority of patients taking lithium experience adverse effects even when their serum lithium levels are maintained within the therapeutic range. The body systems affected by these adverse effects include:

- central nervous system – dysphoria, emotional and cognitive dulling (especially memory impairment) and tremor (this becomes more evident as serum lithium increases and may predict toxicity)
- endocrine and reproductive systems – asymptomatic goitre, hypothyroidism (thyroid function should be evaluated every 6–12 months) and teratogenicity (there is an increased risk of cardiac malformations, especially Ebstein's anomaly, if lithium is taken in the months before conception and/or during the first trimester. Lithium is secreted in breast milk and may cause neonatal hypothyroidism in breastfed babies
- genitourinary system – polyuria, increased urinary output, diabetes insipidus and, very rarely, renal failure
- gastrointestinal system – increased or decreased salivation, metallic taste (caused by secretion of lithium in saliva), polydipsia, nausea, vomiting, mild diarrhoea and weight gain
- skin – rash, exacerbation of existing or development of de novo psoriasis and hair loss
- cardiovascular system – clinically insignificant flattening or inverting of T waves on ECG and, rarely, symptomatic conduction defects.

Lithium toxicity is evident in some patients with serum lithium levels of 1.5 mmol/l and in almost all with levels greater than 2.0 mmol/l. It usually develops over 1–2 days and may be precipitated by dehydration, impaired renal function, concomitant infection, treatment with diuretics or deliberate overdose. The adverse effects that may be present in the non-toxic state worsen during the initial stages of toxicity and patients experience severe vomiting and diarrhoea, marked thirst, polydipsia and polyuria and develop a coarse tremor. With increasing toxicity, the clinical picture progresses through hypertonicity, choreoathetoid movements, ataxia and dysarthria to delirium, seizures, renal failure and impaired consciousness. Untreated, cardiovascular collapse, coma and death soon follow.

Toxicity may be prevented by advising patients of the importance of hydration and by temporarily discontinuing lithium and encouraging hydration at the first signs of toxicity.

Drugs used in the treatment of anxiety disorders including sedative and hypnotic drugs

The use of antidepressant, benzodiazepine and non-benzodiazepine drugs in the treatment of anxiety will now be discussed, as will sedative and hypnotic drugs.

Antidepressant drugs as anxiolytics

Older ADs are effective in treating anxiety disorders but their adverse effects militate against patients taking them. Newer ADs appear to be as effective in treating anxiety disorders as older ADs but cause fewer adverse effects and are therefore better tolerated by patients. The main difference between using newer ADs to treat anxiety and using them to treat depression is that somewhat different dosages are required (see Table 38.5).

Benzodiazepine drugs

The risk of dependence is high with benzodiazepine (BZD) drugs and the last two decades have seen attempts to curb widespread prescribing. Nonetheless, the BZDs remain the most widely used anxiolytic and hypnotic drugs.

The BZDs available in the UK include alprazolam, chlordiazepoxide, clobazam, clonazepam, clorazepate, diazepam, flunitrazepam, flurazepam, loprazolam, lorazepam, lormetazepam, midazolam, nitrazepam, oxazepam and temazepam.

Pharmacokinetics and pharmacodynamics

Individual BZDs differ in the rate at which they are absorbed from the gastrointestinal tract. Diazepam is rapidly absorbed, for example, and reaches C_{MAX} in approximately one hour. In contrast, temazepam is absorbed slowly and has a C_{MAX} of three hours. Absorption of BZDs following IM administration is erratic. However, while the IM route has no therapeutic advantage over the oral route, it may be necessary to administer BZDs IM if it not possible to do so by the oral or IV route. Liquid formulations of BZDs are absorbed rapidly if administered rectally, C_{MAX} being reached in 15–30 minutes.

Protein binding of BZDS is generally >90% but it is 75% for alprazolam.

Table 38.5 The disorder, initial daily dose and daily dose range of the newer AD drugs that are currently licensed for the treatment of anxiety disorders in the UK (dosing for the treatment of bulimia nervosa is also included)

AD drug	Anxiety disorder(s)	Initial dose	Dose range
Citalopram	Panic disorder	10 mg	20–60 mg
Escitalopram	Panic disorder	5 mg	10–20 mg
Fluoxetine	Obsessive-compulsive disorder	20 mg	20–60 mg
	Bulimia nervosa	60 mg	60 mg
Fluvoxamine	Obsessive-compulsive disorder	50 mg	100–300 mg
Paroxetine[1]	Panic disorder	10 mg	20–50 mg
	Obsessive-compulsive disorder	20 mg	20–60 mg
	Social phobia	20 mg	20–50 mg
	Post-traumatic stress disorder	20 mg	20–50 mg
	Generalized anxiety disorder	20 mg	20 mg
Sertraline	Obsessive-compulsive disorder	50 mg	50–200 mg
	Post-traumatic stress disorder (women)	25 mg	50–200 mg
Venlafaxine	Generalized anxiety disorder	75 mg	75 mg
Moclobemide	Social phobia	300 mg	600 mg

[1] The CSM recently recommended 20 mg as the daily dose of paroxetine for the treatment of social anxiety disorder, generalized anxiety disorder and post-traumatic stress disorder (and depression – see above) while 40 mg is the recommended daily dose for the treatment of obsessive-compulsive disorder and panic disorder

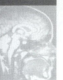

Individual BZDs differ significantly in their lipid solubility. This is lowest for lorazepam and temazepam and highest for midazolam (which therefore rapidly crosses the BBB).

The $t_{1/2}$ of individual BZDs differ dramatically and this and the fact that many have active metabolites with long $t_{1/2}$ of their own complicates their clinical use. Flurazepam, for example, has a $t_{1/2}$ of 1-2 hours but its active metabolite desalkylflurazepam has a $t_{1/2}$ of 75 hours. Flurazepam therefore has a longer effective $t_{1/2}$ than the $t_{1/2}$ of the parent compound would suggest. Taking into account the $t_{1/2}$ of parent drug and the $t_{1/2}$ of any active metabolites, it is possible to divide BZDs into those with very short, short, medium and long durations of action (Table 38.6). In general, BZDs with (i) very short and short durations of action are useful hypnotics that cause little daytime sedation but that carry a risk of dependence; while (ii) those with medium and long durations of action are useful anxiolytics with a reduced risk of dependence but a tendency to cause daytime sedation. BZDs are metabolized in the liver by simple conjugation with glucuronic acid to produce water soluble glucuronides that are excreted by the kidney or by complex pathways with several steps, for example demethylation or dealkylation followed by glucuronidation.

Mechanism of action   BZDs are potent postsynaptic GABA$_A$ receptor agonists. Physiologically, GABA binds to the β subunit of the GABA$_A$ receptor following which Cl⁻ ions enter the neuron and generate an excess negative charge (hyperpolarization) that prevents the neuron from reaching action potential. BZDs bind to the α subunit of the GABA$_A$ receptor. This alters the β subunit, facilitates its ability to bind GABA and causes the ion channel to open. It is thought that BZDs exert their anxiolytic and anticonvulsant effects by facilitating GABA induced neuronal inhibition at specific neuroanatomical locations.

Efficacy

BZDs are indicated at the lowest effective dose and for the shortest possible time for the treatment of severe anxiety disorders and severe insomnia. They should not be prescribed for mild anxiety or mild insomnia.

BZDs are also useful in psychiatric emergencies and in epilepsy (see Chapter 26) and have many uses as sedatives in general medicine and dentistry.

Anxiety disorders   Long-acting BZDs may be used to prevent severe anxiety occurring in response to a discrete stimulus. Fear of air travel, for example, may be prevented by 2–5 mg of diazepam or 10–15 mg chlordiazepoxide administered a few hours before the flight. This represents a reasonable use of BZDs because air travel is a relatively infrequent undertaking for most people, dependence is therefore unlikely and a BZD may permit a business trip or holiday. In contrast, the use of BZDs to alleviate distress in bereaved individuals is probably best avoided because they are likely to impair the adjustments of the normal grieving process.

Chronic anxiety disorders such as panic disorder and generalized anxiety disorder respond to long acting BZDs. Long term treatment with BZDs carries with it the risk of dependence and tolerance but short term treatment (2–4 weeks) is appropriate while awaiting the effects of a safer long term treatment such as an SSRI or cognitive therapy.

Insomnia   Very short-acting BZDs may be useful in the short term (1–3 weeks) treatment of insomnia when initial insomnia is present. Thus:

- patients in whom insomnia has no apparent cause may benefit while awaiting the effects of behavioural treatments and education in sleep hygiene, while
- patients in whom insomnia is caused by depression may benefit from such treatment while awaiting the effects of AD drugs.

Very short acting BZDs may cause withdrawal symptoms but generally do not cause 'hangover' the next day.

Short-acting BZDs may be useful in the short term (1–3 weeks or less) treatment of insomnia when interrupted sleep occurs. They are unlikely to cause withdrawal symptoms but frequently cause 'hangover' the next day.

Equivalent doses   It is often helpful to know the equivalent doses of different BZDs, for example when converting the daily dose of a BZD that a patient is dependent upon to the equivalent daily dose of diazepam in

Table 38.6 BZD drugs with very short, short, medium and long durations of action			
Hypnotics		Anxiolytics	
Very short	*Short*	*Medium*	*Long*
Loprazolam	Flunitrazepam	Alprazolam	Clorazepate
Lormetazepam	Flurazepam[1]	Lorazepam	Chlordiazepoxide
Temazepam	Nitrazepam	Midazolam[2]	Clobazam
		Oxazepam[2]	Clonazepam
			Diazepam
Notes: 1 See commentary on t1/2 of flurazepam above 2 Midazolam is used to induce anaesthesia and is not widely used in psychiatric practice			

order to facilitate gradual withdrawal of BZDs. The *British National Formulary* gives approximate equivalent doses for diazepam 5 mg as chlordiazepoxide 15 mg, loprazolam 0.5-1.0 mg, lorazepam 0.5 mg, lormetazepam 0.5-1.0 mg, nitrazepam 5 mg, oxazepam 15 mg and temazepam 10 mg.

Safety

BZDs are effectively free of the adverse effects that may be regarded as common to all drugs such as headache and gastrointestinal disturbance, appear to have no cardiac or autonomic effects and even in significant overdose are generally only fatal if taken in combination with other drugs with synergistic effects or with alcohol.

The adverse effects commonly associated with BZDs include drowsiness, sedation, dizziness and ataxia, especially in older patients in whom falls may occur. Psychomotor performance is impaired and reaction time increased, adverse effects that may affect drivers and those who operate machinery and that are potentiated by alcohol. High doses of BZD administered IV and/or to BZD naïve patients may cause respiratory depression. Flumazenil, a BZD antagonist, may be used to reverse this.

Paradoxical disinhibition Patients treated with BZDs may appear 'drunk' and this can progress to verbal and physical hostility. It is thought that this syndrome occurs because the dose of BZD prescibed is not sufficient to cause tranquillization but is sufficient to cause disinhibition and 'drunkeness'. An increase in the dose will usually resolve the problem.

Tolerance, dependence and withdrawal syndrome It was recognized soon after BZDs became available that tolerance (the need for increasingly higher doses to achieve the same clinical effect) to their sedative effects occurs rapidly. It was also observed that delirium and seizures may occur if high doses of BZDs are abruptly withdrawn. These findings led to attempts to reduce the use of BZDs and the number of prescriptions issued has declined in the last decade.

The BZD withdrawal syndrome consisting of anxiety, insomnia, weight loss, drowsiness, headache, sweating, myalgia, arthralgia, derealization, depersonalization, visual illusions, hyperacusis, tinnitus and paraesthesia was described by Petursson & Lader (1981). This may occur within hours or days in patients abruptly withdrawn from BZDs with very short or short durations of action and within days or weeks in patients abruptly withdrawn from BZDs with medium or long durations of action. It resolves within 2–4 weeks. The symptoms of the BZD withdrawal syndrome are similar to those for which BZDs are often prescribed and this may led to further inappropriate prescribing of BZDs.

Dependence seems to occur more readily with prolonged use of BZDs, which have very short or short durations of action. The treatment of BZD dependence relies upon:

- prevention – local or national prescribing guidelines or those of the Committee on Safety of Medicines or CSM (Box 38.2) should be adhered to

- gradual withdrawal – convert the daily dose of the BZD the patient is dependent upon to the equivalent daily dose of diazepam and reduce this dosage at a guide rate of 1 mg per week or 5 mg per month. A dose should be maintained at any given level if withdrawal syndrome recurs and only reduced further when it resolves.

Box 38.2   Committee on Safety of Medicines prescribing guidelines for BZD drugs

Benzodiazepines are indicated for the short-term relief (2-4 weeks only) of anxiety that is severe, disabling or subjecting the individual to unacceptable distress, occurring alone or in association with insomnia or short-term psychosomatic, organic or psychotic illness

The use of benzodiazepines to treat short-term 'mild' anxiety is inappropriate and unsuitable

Benzodiazepines should be used to treat insomnia only when it is severe, disabling, or subjecting the individual to extreme distress

---

Non-benzodiazepine drugs

A number of non-BZD GABA$_A$ receptor agonists have become available in the last decade. These include the imidazopyridine zolpidem, the cyclopyrrolone zopiclone and the pyrazolopyrimidine zalepon. These have very short (zalepon) or short (zolpidem and zopiclone) durations of action and are licensed for the short term treatment of insomnia. Their efficacy and safety is similar to that of BZDs. Tolerance and a withdrawal syndrome may occur and adherence to the prescribing guidelines applicable to BZDs may be wise.

Sedative and hypnotic drugs

Chloral hydrate and triclofos sodium are safe, short acting hypnotics with few adverse effects. They rarely cause hangover and are frequently used to treat insomnia in older patients. The prescribing guidelines applicable to BZDs should be followed when they are prescribed.

Barbiturates and paraldehyde are occasionally used to tranquillize patients who have not responded to other treatments or are in status epilepticus.

Antihistamines, and low doses of older AP drugs are also widely used for their sedative or hypnotic properties.

Drugs used in the treatment of psychiatric disorders in children

Children differ from adults in their ability to absorb (usually faster), metabolize (usually faster) and eliminate drugs and psychotropic drugs are not tested extensively in children during clinical development. Great care is therefore required when treating children with such drugs and the manufacturer of the drug or the *British National Formulary* should always be consulted.

The disorders for which psychotropic drugs are widely prescribed during childhood include nocturnal enuresis, attention deficit hyperactivity disorder (ADHD), autism, sleep disorders, tic disorders and conduct disorder in children with learning disability. Children with anxiety disorders, depression and psychosis may also require medication.

Nocturnal enuresis

The first-line treatment of nocturnal enuresis is behavioural because this is generally effective. Drug therapy is appropriate after seven years of age if behavioural treatment is ineffective or not possible and may be used alone or in combination with behavioural treatment. Short term drug therapy in children under seven years of age to cover periods away from home may be appropriate.

Imipramine (0.5–1.0 mg/kg) before going to bed is usually effective within 1–2 weeks. Amitriptyline is also used. The mechanism of action may involve direct anticholinergic effects on the bladder. Desmopressin (20–40 micrograms orally or by intranasal spray) before going to bed is also useful. Its adverse effects include fluid retention, hyponatraemia (which may cause seizures), headache, nausea, vomiting, nasal congestion and rhinitis. Treatment with imipramine or desmopressin should be reviewed every three months before a further three months of treatment is commenced. Treatment may need to continue for some years.

Oxybutynin is an anticholinergic drug that may be effective in children with treatment-resistant nocturnal enuresis caused by detrusor instability. Such treatment should only be initiated by a specialist following urodynamic studies.

Attention deficit hyperactivity disorder

The frequency with which attention deficit hyperactivity disorder (ADHD) is diagnosed and with which stimulant medication is prescribed to treat it is increasing. Concern that medication is being used to modify extreme but appropriate childhood behaviour is probably unfounded and the response of children with ADHD to effective medication is among the most rapid and most dramatic in psychopharmacology.

The stimulant drugs licensed for the treatment of ADHD in the UK are methylphenidate, which is widely prescribed, and dexamphetamine, which is prescribed less frequently. Both are controlled drugs and subject to the prescription requirements of the Misuse of Drugs Regulations, 2001. Atomoxetine, a non-stimulant drug that has recently become available, is not a controlled drug (and is licenced to treat ADHD in both children and adults).

Methylphenidate

Pharmacokinetics and pharmacodynamics Methylphenidate is rapidly absorbed and protein binding is low. Hepatic metabolism and elimination are rapid, providing a $t_{1/2}$ of approximately three hours and clinical effects of approximately five hours duration. The drug must be administered 3–4 times per day (see below).

Methylphenidate causes the release of NA, DA and 5HT from, and blocks the reuptake of DA and NA to, presynaptic neurons, especially in the striatum.

Efficacy Methylphenidate is administered in a dosage of 0.3–0.7 mg per kg per day. It is usually commenced at a dose of 5 mg twice daily and increased every 3–4 days until a beneficial effect is obtained or adverse effects prevent further dose increase. It is rarely necessary to dose above 60 mg per day. A long acting formulation that is administered once daily in a dose range of 18–54 mg is available.

Most children with ADHD respond rapidly and significantly to methylphenidate or similar drugs. For example, Elia et al. reported in 1991 that 96% of children showed behavioural improvement, while a recent review of clinical trials by Greenhill et al. (1999) concluded that stimulants such as methylphenidate 'show robust short-term efficacy and a good safety profile'. Methylphenidate also remains effective in the long term. However, the effect of treating ADHD during childhood and adolescence with methylphenidate and other stimulants on eventual adult function is unclear.

Methylphenidate is recommended by the National Institute for Clinical Excellence (2000) '…for use as part of a comprehensive treatment programme for children with a diagnosis of severe attention deficit hyperactivity disorder…'. However, clinical trials do not, in fact, provide evidence that educational or behavioural treatment programmes provide additional benefits over and above medications alone (MTA Cooperative Group 1999). Indeed Taylor (1999) has stated that behavioural treatment alone is unlikely to be effective and that medication should always be considered.

Children whose ADHD has responded to methylphenidate will require prolonged treatment and may benefit from so called drug-holidays during which treatment is suspended, partly as a means of assessing the need for continuing medication.

Safety The adverse effects commonly associated with methylphenidate include nervousness, insomnia, urticaria, fever, rash (which may progress to exfoliative dermatitis and erythema multiforme), anorexia, nausea, dizziness, palpitations, headache, dyskinesia, drowsiness, hypertension, tachycardia, angina, abdominal pain and weight loss. Organic psychosis may occur and abuse and diversion for recreational use are recognized. Greenhill et al. (1999), on the basis of a literature review, reported no evidence of harmful effects from prolonged treatment.

Dexamphetamine

Pharmacokinetics and pharmacodynamics The mechanism of action of dexamphetamine is similar to that of methylphenidate.

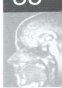

Efficacy The efficacy of dexamphetamine is similar to that of methylphenidate. However, it should be regarded as a second-line treatment for children who do not respond to methylphenidate because of the risk of dependence and organic psychosis. Dexamphetamine is administered in a dosage of 5–20 mg per day with a maximum dosage of 40 mg per day in older children and adolescents.

Safety The adverse effects commonly associated with dexamphetamine include insomnia, irritability, euphoria, tremor, headache, seizures, anorexia, growth retardation (height should be monitored), hypertension, dry mouth, tachycardia and sweating. Tics have been reported, organic psychosis may occur and dependence, tolerance and diversion for recreational use are recognized.

Atomoxetine

Pharmacokinetics and pharmacodynamics Atomoxetine is rapidly absorbed and is 98% protein-bound. Hepatic metabolism is via the cytochrome P450 2D6 pathway and the $t_{1/2}$ of five hours in extensive metabolizers is increased to 24 hours in poor metabolizers.

Atomoxetine is a highly selective inhibitor of the NA reuptake transporter. It increases synaptic concentrations of NA in the prefrontal cortex but has no effect on 5HT levels.

Efficacy Atomoxetine may be administered to children and adolescents under 70 kg in bodyweight in an initial dose of 0.5 mg per kg per day. This may be increased after three days to 1.2 mg per kg per day. The total daily dose may be administered as a single dose or as two equal doses. Most children with ADHD respond significantly over 4–6 weeks to atomoxetine and its efficacy has also been established in adults with ADHD.

Atomoxetine may be administered to children and adolescents over 70 kg in bodyweight, and to adults, in an initial dose of 40 mg per day. This may be increased after three days to 80 mg per day and, if necessary, after two weeks to 100 mg per day.

Individuals whose ADHD has responded to atomoxetine will require prolonged treatment.

Safety The adverse effects commonly associated with atomoxetine include dry mouth, insomnia, nausea, decreased appetite, constipation, dizziness, headache, sweating, sexual problems and palpitations. Modest increases in heart rate and blood pressure may occur. Atomoxetine was not associated with QT interval prolongation, with abuse or with diversion for recreational use during clinical trials.

Other treatments

The AD drugs imipramine and desipramine may represent a useful alternative to methylphenidate for some patients.

Autism

Psychotropic drugs play a modest but useful role in the alleviation of symptoms associated with autism:

- atypical AP drugs, usually in low dosage, may help in the short term treatment of agitation or aggression
- stimulants and atomoxetine may help when ADHD symptoms are present, although they may worsen tic disorders
- AEDs should be prescribed for the control of seizures
- SSRIs may help in the management of anxiety, agitation and stereotypic behaviours.

Sleep disorders

Reassurance, education and behavioural treatment rather than psychotropic drugs are the mainstay of the management of sleep disorders in children. Sedating antihistamines such as alimemazine (trimeprazine) 2 mg per kg daily, chloral hydrate 30–50 mg per kg daily or diazepam 0.1–0.3 mg per kg daily are occasionally prescribed for brief periods.

Diazepam 0.1–0.3 mg per kg daily or paroxetine 20–40 mg daily are very occasionally prescribed for night terrors.

Tic disorders

The motor and vocal tics of Gilles de la Tourette syndrome are commoner in children with autism, obsessive-compulsive disorder and ADHD than in otherwise healthy children. Clonidine (titrated to a maximum dose of 10 micrograms per kg per day), haloperidol (0.5–1.0 mg three times daily and slowly increased to a maximum of 10 mg daily or until a response is obtained) and pimozide are recognized treatments and atypical AP drugs and SSRIs are also used.

Conduct disorder

The use of psychotropic drugs for the primary purpose of controlling behaviour in children with learning disability is inappropriate because their adverse effects cause distress, impair cognition and may worsen the behaviour for which they were originally prescribed. Environmental management and psychological therapies are therefore the preferred treatments for such individuals. Psychotropic drugs should be prescribed for children with learning disability when the primary purpose is the short term control of a crisis or the long term treatment of a psychiatric disorder such as schizophrenia or depression.

AP drugs are widely prescribed for the control of agitation, self harming and aggression in children with learning disability. Such individuals have brain damage by definition and are therefore at great risk of developing extrapyramidal adverse effects (which may exacerbate rather than reduce agitation and aggression) if treated with typical AP drugs. Atypical AP drugs in the lowest effective dose for the shortest duration of time necessary should therefore be the first choice if it is necessary to prescribe AP drugs for children with learning disability. Children with learning disability who have a psychotic disorder (at least

2% of such individuals have schizophrenia, for example) may benefit from prolonged treatment.

Like AP drugs, antiepileptic drugs (AEDs) are also widely prescribed in children with learning disability, both in the treatment of epilepsy and recurrent mood disorders and in an attempt to reduce episodes of disturbed behaviour. Their use in the latter situation should only be commenced with recording of the target behaviour before and during treatment and with great attention to adverse effects. AEDs should be discontinued if the balance of benefits and risks proves unfavourable.

Newer AD drugs may help children with learning disability who have depression and may also reduce the frequency and severity of self harming in some such individuals. Stimulant medications and atomoxetine may be beneficial if ADHD is present.

Anxiety disorders
SSRIs may be useful in the treatment of anxiety disorders, including obsessive-compulsive disorder, in childhood (see CSM advice, p. 591). Psychotropic medication has no place in the management of school refusal unless there is an underlying psychiatric disorder.

Depression
The efficacy and safety of fluoxetine has been established in the treatment of depression in childhood (see CSM advice p. 591). Older AD drugs should be avoided.

Psychosis
Psychotic disorders are rare in childhood. Their treatment is with atypical AP drugs prescribed at low dosage, the dose being slowly titrated upwards until a response is obtained.

Antiepileptic drugs

Antiepileptic drugs (AEDs) are widely prescribed for the treatment of both epilepsy and bipolar disorder. The general pharmacological treatment of epilepsy will now be considered briefly. Following this, the AEDs available in the UK for the treatment of bipolar disorder – valproate, lamotrigine and carbmazepine – will be discussed.

General pharmacological treatment of epilepsy
New AEDs have been introduced in the last decade and the use of AEDs in combination is now better understood. Nonetheless, two or more AEDs should only be prescribed in combination when monotherapy with several alternative AEDs has proved ineffective because of the increased risk of toxicity and drug interactions.

The plasma levels of some AEDs should be monitored (especially when prescribed in combination because of the risk of AED–AED interactions such as the induction of enzymes by carbamazepine) but the rule is that the patient, not the laboratory value, should be treated. Thus if seizures are controlled and the patient is not experiencing adverse effects, AED levels above the advised range may be acceptable. Conversely, if levels are within the advised range but seizures continue, dosage may be increased until efficacy is achieved or until adverse effects occur. Equally, the dosage should not be increased if it is effective, despite AED levels being below the advised range. Regular full blood counts and evaluations of thyroid, renal and hepatic function are advised with some AEDs.

The clinician is most often faced with the treatment of patients with either partial or focal epilepsy (which may or may not generalize) or with generalized epilepsy.

Partial or focal epilepsy
The recommended first-line monotherapy drugs for partial or focal epilepsy are carbamazepine, lamotrigine, phenytoin and valproate. If none of these drugs are effective two of them may be prescribed in combination. Alternatively, a drug such as acetazolamide, clobazam, clonazepam, gabapentin, tiagabine, topiramate or vigabatrin may be added to the most effective monotherapy identified. Barbiturates have little place in the contemporary treatment of partial or focal epilepsy.

Generalized epilepsy
First-line monotherapy for generalized epilepsy depends on the type of seizure, as follows:

- tonic/clonic seizures – carbamazepine, lamotrigine, phenytoin or valproate. Barbiturates have little place in the treatment of tonic/clonic epilepsy
- absence seizures – ethosuximide or valproate, the latter also being effective in patients who experience both tonic/clonic and absence seizures
- myoclonic seizures – clonazepam, ethosuximide, lamotrigine or valproate. Some patients gain further benefit from the addition of piracetam to one or other of these AEDs.

Status epilepticus
Status epilepticus consists of recurrent seizures without recovery of consciousness between them. Treatment requires immediate intravenous lorazepam. Intravenous diazepam, midazolam and clonazepam may also be used. Paraldehyde or anaesthesia may occasionally be required.

If seizures are not controlled within 30 minutes, or if they recur, an intravenous loading dose of phenytoin and a subsequent phenytoin infusion should be administered. Patients with status epilepticus are best treated in an intensive care unit.

Contraception and reproduction
AEDs such as carbamazepine induce the metabolism of ethinyloestradiol and either an alternative method of contraception or a contraceptive pill (or combination of pills)

containing a dosage of 50 micrograms ethinyloestradiol daily is necessary.

Women with epilepsy should plan their pregnancies and should consider withdrawing AEDs before conception and during pregnancy. However, it is almost certainly safer to take AEDs while pregnant than to have seizures. Carbamazepine is probably the least teratogenic AED. Folate supplements are advised for women taking AEDs (and are now advised for all women) before and during pregnancy and vitamin K supplements are advised for pregnant women taking carbamazepine or phenytoin.

Discontinuation of antiepileptic drugs

Patients who have not had seizures for a prolonged period may wish to discontinue their AEDs. Any decision to do so must be based upon:

- the length of time the patient has been free of seizures (a two-year minimum is recommended)
- the normality of the electroencephlogram (EEG) with current AED treatment (it would be unwise to withdraw treatment from a patient whose EEG exhibits significant epileptic activity despite treatment with AEDs)
- the side-effects of current AEDs
- social factors (occupation, need for a driving licence and hobbies).

A careful record of seizure type and frequency must be made and an EEG recorded before reducing dosage, when dosage is reduced to half the initial dosage and when AEDs are stopped. Any increase in seizure frequency or severity, or deterioration in the EEG, should lead to the planned withdrawal being reconsidered.

Alternative psychosis or forced normalization

Some epileptic patients who are being effectively treated with AEDs may experience depression, mania and/or psychotic symptoms in association with a reduction in seizures and normalization of their EEG. This alternative psychosis or forced normalization may be alleviated by a slight reduction in AED dosage such that the EEG exhibits epileptic activity and/or occasional seizures occur.

Valproate

Pharmacokinetics and pharmacodynamics

Valproate is a branched chain fatty acid that is absorbed and metabolized (by oxidative enzymes) rapidly. Plasma protein binding is 10% while $t_{1/2}$ is 10–16 hours. Valproate does not induce metabolic enzymes but it inhibits enzymes that metabolize carbamazepine, ethosuxamide, lamotrigine and phenytoin and causes their plasma levels to increase. Semisodium valproate (or divalproex) is a dimer composed of two valproate molecules.

Mechanism of action Valproate causes upregulation of $GABA_B$ receptors and also enhances 5HT neurotransmission.

Efficacy

In addition to use in patients with epilepsy, valproate may also be prescribed as an antimanic drug in the treatment of acute mania, or as a mood-stabilizer in the prophylaxis of bipolar disorder in patients unresponsive to or intolerant of lithium. In this case it may be prescribed alone or in combination with lithium.

Treatment with valproate should be commenced at 200 mg twice daily (250 mg twice daily for semisodium valproate) and increased by 200 mg per day (250 mg per day for semisodium valproate) every 2–3 days. Patients with mania may require doses of up to 2000 mg daily (2250 mg daily for semisodium valproate) while 1000 to 2000 mg daily (1250–2250 mg daily for semisodium valproate) are usually adequate for prophylaxis. Plasma valproate levels of 50–150 mg/l are recommended. However, clinical status is the best determinant of a patient's optimal dose.

Safety

Nausea, ataxia, tremor, weight gain and reversible hair loss (although regrown hair may be curly) are the commonest adverse effects of valproate. Less common but more serious adverse effects include:

- hepatotoxicity, which may be fatal in children and in patients taking other AEDs in addition to valproate. Liver function should be evaluated before commencing and during the first six months of treatment with valproate
- Stevens–Johnson syndrome
- pancreatitis, hyperammonaemia with confusion and asterixis (clinical chemistry parameters should be monitored)
- blood dyscrasias including leucopenia and pancytopenia (haematological parameters should be monitored).

Valproate is teratogenic and may cause congenital cardiac defects and neonatal seizures if taken during pregnancy.

Lamotrigine

Pharmacokinetics and pharmacodynamics

Lamotrigine is absorbed and metabolized (oxidative enzymes) rapidly. Plasma protein binding is 50% while $t_{1/2}$ is 24 hours. Lamotrigine neither induces nor inhibits metabolic enzymes.

Mechanism of action Lamotrigine blocks fast Na^+ channels in neurons and reduces the neuroexcitatory effect of glutamate.

Efficacy

In addition to use in patients with epilepsy, lamotrigine may also be prescribed as an AD drug in the treatment of major depressive disorder, an AD drug in the treatment of bipolar depressive disorder, or a mood-stabilizer in the prophylaxis of bipolar disorder in patients who experience predominantly depressive relapses and are unresponsive to or intolerant of lithium (Cookson et al, 2002).

Lamotrigine does not seem to be an effective antimanic drug and is probably not an effective mood-stabilizer in the prophylaxis of bipolar disorder in patients who experience predominantly manic or mixed relapses.

Treatment with lamotrigine should be commenced at 25 mg daily for two weeks and increased slowly (by 25–50 mg per day) every 2–3 weeks. The usual maximum dose is 100–200 mg daily. The dose of lamotrigine should be reduced in patients who are also taking valproate. Clinical status is the best determinant of a patient's optimal dose.

Safety
Vomiting, dizziness, drowsiness, headache, diplopia, ataxia and confusion are the most common adverse effects. About 10% of patients develop a rash and slow titration of dose helps to minimize this risk. Any rash must be monitored extremely carefully because it may progress to Stevens–Johnson syndrome and toxic epidermal necrolysis. Patients should be advised to seek medical attention immediately if a rash or influenza-like syndrome develops.

Carbamazepine
Pharmacokinetics and pharmacodynamics
Carbamazepine is a dibenzazepine derivative that is absorbed and metabolized (by cytochrome 3A4 enzymes) rapidly. Plasma protein binding is 85% while $t_{1/2}$ varies from 50 hours when initially administered to five hours during chronic administration because carbamazepine induces its own metabolic enzymes. These induced enzymes also reduce blood levels of lamotrigine, valproate, AP drugs, barbiturates, clobazam, clonazepam, ethinyloestradiol (see advice on contraception above), ethosuximide, phenytoin, TCAs, tiagabine, topiramate and warfarin. Carbamazepine does not inhibit metabolic enzymes.

Mechanism of action Carbamazepine blocks NMDA receptors and this reduces the neuroexcitatory effect of glutamate. Carbamazepine also inhibits 5HT neuro-transmission.

Efficacy
In addition to use in patients with epilepsy, carbamazepine may also be prescribed as an antimanic drug in the treatment of acute mania, and as a mood-stabilizer in the prophylaxis of bipolar disorder in patients unresponsive to or intolerant of lithium. In this case it may be prescribed alone or, more often, in combination with lithium.

Evidence for the efficacy of carbamazepine as an antimanic or mood-stabilising drug is much less convincing than that for lithium, valproate, olanzapine and lamotrigine and its use appears to be declining.

Treatment with carbamazepine should be commenced at 200 mg twice daily and increased by 200 mg per day every 2–3 weeks. Patients with mania may require doses of up to 1600 mg daily while 500 mg daily is usually adequate for prophylaxis. Plasma carbamazepine levels of 4–12 mg/l are

recommended but these are of limited value. Clinical status is the best determinant of a patient's optimal dose.

Safety
Nausea, headache, dizziness, ataxia, diplopia and confusion are the commonest adverse effects of carbamazepine. Less common but more serious adverse effects include:

- an itchy erythematous rash in at least 1 in 10 patients. The risk of this may be reduced by slow titration of dose. Carbamazepine must be withdrawn if this rash is significant or if it occurs in association with fever and/or haematological abnormalities (leucopenia, thrombocytopenia). Clinical chemistry and haematological parameters should be evaluated before and during the first month of treatment
- Stevens–Johnson syndrome, agranulocytosis, aplastic anaemia
- cholestatic jaundice, hepatitis, acute renal failure, hyponatraemia, oedema, osteomalacia
- lymphadenopathy
- gynaecomastia, galactorrhoea, impotence
- dyskinesia, psychosis, depression, aggression.

Carbamazepine is probably the least teratogenic AED available but may cause neural tube defects if taken during pregnancy. Women should ideally discontinue treatment with it three months prior to conception and should not take it during pregnancy. They should take folate supplements both pre-conceptually and during pregnancy, especially if carbamazepine must be continued during pregnancy.

Drugs used in the treatment of erectile impotence, premature ejaculation and antisocial sexual behaviour

Drugs used in the treatment of erectile dysfunction (ED) may be divided into the newer phosphodiesterase type 5 (PDE5) inhibitors, which are administered orally, and the older drugs, which are usually administered by intracavernosal injection.

Phosphodiesterase type 5 inhibitors
Sildenafil, tadalafil and vardenafil are all potent and highly selective inhibitors of phosphodiesterase type 5 (PDE5) when administered orally (see Table 38.7). PDE5 inhibitors

Table 38.7 The initial daily dose, daily dose range and available formulations of the PDE5 inhibitors currently licensed in the UK

PDE5 inhibitor	Initial dose	Dose range	Available formulations
Sildenafil	50 mg	25–100 mg	Tablets
Tadalafil	10 mg	10–20 mg	Tablets
Vardenafil	10 mg	10–20 mg	Tablets

enhance erection by preventing the degradation of cyclic guanosine monophosphate (cGMP) by PDE5, thus facilitating nitric oxide-cGMP-mediated smooth muscle relaxation in the corpus cavernosum. This permits erection in response to sexual stimulation but does not cause erection in the absence of such stimulation. These three drugs are effective in approximately 70% of patients. Tadalafil may be taken 0.5–12 hours before anticipated sexual activity and remains effective for 36 hours or more. Sildenafil and vardenefil must be taken no more than one hour before anticipated sexual activity and have a shorter duration of effect. The PDE5 inhibitors have been used in the treatment of sexual dysfunction associated with SSRI AD drugs.

Adverse effects include headache, dyspepsia, flushing, rhinitis, and sinusitis. Abnormal colour vision has been reported with sildenafil. Priapism may occur, especially in patients with sickle-cell anaemia, multiple myeloma or leukaemia. PDE5 inhibitors should be used cautiously if the penis is anatomically deformed and are contraindicated in patients taking nitrates.

Older drugs

Older drugs for the treatment of erectile impotence are administered by intracavernosal injection and include papaverine, a smooth muscle relaxant, which may be effective alone or in combination with phentolamine, a short-acting α_1 noradrenergic antagonist, which is usually administered in combination with papaverine, and alprostadil or prostaglandin E_1, which may also be administered intraurethrally.

The use of these drugs is limited by the need for intracavernosal injections, which produce erections when administered as a direct response to the drug and independently of sexual stimulation, and the need to complete sexual activity within approximately one hour of injecting. The most troublesome adverse effect is priapism which may require urgent aspiration of the corpus cavernosum, intracavernosal injection of phenylephrine or adrenaline, or surgery.

Premature ejaculation

SSRIs cause delayed ejaculation, an adverse effect that may be used to advantage in the treatment of premature ejaculation.

Antisocial sexual behaviour

Cyproterone acetate, medroxyprogesterone, the luteinizing hormone analogue goserelin and the butyrophenone benperidol are occasionally used to reduce libido and control antisocial sexual behaviour in men.

Drugs used in the treatment of dementia

Four drugs are currently licensed in the UK for the symptomatic treatment of dementia in Alzheimer's disease.

A number of other drugs that are not specifically licensed for this purpose are also occasionally used including anti-inflammatory (based on Schneider's 1996 report that Alzheimer's disease is less common in patients with rheumatoid arthritis) and antioxidant drugs, oestrogens and neuroprotective drugs or nootropics (such as piracetam and co-dergocrine).

Acetylcholinesterase inhibitors

The most obvious neuronal and neurotransmitter loss in Alzheimer's disease is of cholinergic neurons and Ach. Acetylcholinesterase degrades Ach and acetylcholinesterase inhibitors have been developed in the hope that they would increase Ach levels in the brain and reduce the symptoms of Alzheimer's disease. Donepezil, rivastigmine and galantamine are the three acetylcholinesterase inhibitors that are currently available in the UK. NICE guidance should be followed when they are prescribed (Box 38.3).

Donepezil

This reversible non-competitive inhibitor of central acetylcholinesterase is licensed for the treatment of mild to moderate dementia in Alzheimer's disease (usually defined as a Mini-Mental State Examination score of >12). It has little effect on peripheral acetylcholinesterase.

Donepezil is almost completely absorbed in the upper gastrointestinal tract, has a C_{MAX} of three hours and $t_{1/2}$ of three days. Protein binding is >90%. Donepezil is administered once daily in a dose of 5–10 mg.

Donepezil may cause gastrointestinal (nausea, vomiting, anorexia, diarrhoea), central nervous system (fatigue, headache, insomnia, dizziness, convulsions, NMS) and

---

Box 38.3 National Institute of Clinical Excellence guidelines on Alzheimer's disease

NICE has recommended (January 2001) that, for the adjunctive treatment of mild and moderate Alzheimer's disease in those whose mini mental-state examination (MMSE) score is above 12 points, donepezil, galantamine and rivastigmine should be available under the following conditions:

- Alzheimer's disease must be diagnosed in a specialist clinic; the clinic should also assess cognitive, global and behavioural functioning, activities of daily living, and the likelihood of compliance with treatment
- Treatment should be initiated by specialists but may be continued by general practitioners under a shared-care protocol
- The carers' views of the condition should be sought before and during drug treatment
- The patient should be assessed 2–4 months after maintenance dose is established; drug treatment should continue only if MMSE score has improved or has not deteriorated and if behavioural or functional assessment shows improvement
- The patient should be assessed every six months and drug treatment should normally continue only if MMSE score remains above 12 points and if treatment is considered to have a worthwhile effect on the global, functional and behavioural condition

cardiovascular (syncope, bradycardia, atrioventricular block) adverse effects. It may also cause rash and urinary retention.

Galantamine
This reversible competetive inhibitor of acetylcholinesterase has benefits in mild to moderate dementia in Alzheimer's disease, and adverse effects, similar to those of donepezil.

Rivastigmine
This pseudo-irreversible non-competitive inhibitor of acetylcholinesterase has benefits in mild to moderate dementia in Alzheimer's disease, and adverse effects, similar to those of donepezil. It is rapidly absorbed and C_{MAX} is reached in one hour. Protein binding is <50%. Rivastigmine is initially administered in 1.5 mg doses twice daily and its maximum dose is 6 mg twice daily.

N-methyl-D-aspartate antagonists
Memantine is the only NMDA receptor antagonist available in the UK for the symptomatic treatment of dementia in Alzheimer's disease.

Memantine
Memantine modifies glutamate transmission and is licensed for the symptomatic treatment of moderate to severe dementia in Alzheimer's disease. Its daily dose is 5-10 mg. Its adverse effects include headache, tiredness, dizziness, confusion and hallucinations. Increased libido may also occur.

Vascular dementia
Cerebrovascular disease can both exacerbate Alzheimer's disease and cause a discrete vascular dementia in the absence of other pathology. Measures aimed at preventing cerebrovascular disease (or at preventing its progression if it is already evident) will therefore prevent (or prevent the progression of) vascular dementia. Such measures include:

- cessation of cigarette smoking
- management of obesity
- prophylactic use of drugs that reduce platelet adhesiveness (aspirin, dipyridamole) and
- identification and treatment of hypertension, diabetes mellitus and hyperlipidaemia.

Drugs used in the treatment of parkinsonism and related disorders

A significant proportion of patients treated with typical AP drugs and a much smaller proportion treated with atypical AP drugs, TCA or SSRI AD drugs or with lithium develop acute dystonia, parkinsonism, akathisia or tardive dyskinesia. These extrapyramidal system (EPS) adverse effects cause personal distress, functional disability and militate against future compliance with prophylactic AP treatment, thereby increasing patients' risk of relapse. EPS adverse effects are also stigmatizing – patients suffering with them look and behave abnormally and this impacts upon social acceptance and rehabilitation. It is probable therefore that the single most important advantage of atypical over typical AP drugs is their greatly reduced propensity for causing EPS adverse effects.

Parkinson's disease is caused by a deficiency of DA and a relative excess of cholinergic neurotransmission at muscarinic neuroreceptors in the basal ganglia. It has long been treated with anticholinergic (or more correctly antimuscarinic) drugs. These have almost no activity at the nicotinic receptor. Drugs that enhance dopaminergic neurotransmission in the basal ganglia are also used but these are not effective in alleviating the EPS adverse effects associated with AP drugs and may exacerbate psychotic symptoms. They will not be discussed further.

Pharmacokinetics and pharmacodynamics
The anticholinergic drugs currently available in the UK include benzatropine, benzhexol (or trihexyphenidyl hydrochloride), biperiden, orphenadrine and procyclidine.

Anticholinergic drugs are generally well absorbed from the gastrointestinal tract, have T_{MAX} of 1–2 hours and $t_{1/2}$ of approximately 10–16 hours. Procyclidine is slowly absorbed and has a T_{MAX} of 6–8 hours. Benzatropine has a longer duration of action than the other anticholinergic drugs.

Mechanism of action
The normal inhibition of cholinergic neurotransmission in the caudate and putamen by DA is blocked by AP drugs. This leads to a relative excess of cholinergic neurotransmission and may cause acute dystonia and parkinsonism. Anticholinergic drugs prevent this cholinergic excess by blocking muscarinic M_1 neuroreceptors.

Efficacy
Anticholinergic drugs are not required by the majority of patients treated with atypical AP drugs and should not be prescribed prophylactically for patients taking typical AP drugs because:

- while a significant proportion of such individuals will develop EPS adverse effects, not all will
- anticholinergic drugs modify the therapeutic effect of AP drugs
- anticholinergic drugs may cause psychosis, confusion (especially in high dosage and/or in elderly patients) and acute organic reaction
- anticholinergic drugs have euphoriant and stimulant properties and may cause dependence and
- anticholinergic drugs may increase the risk of developing tardive dyskinesia.

The anticholinergic drugs appear to be equally effective in alleviating EPS adverse effects. Therefore when treatment with an anticholinergic drug is required, the choice of drug should be based on safety and tolerability considerations. Anticholinergic drugs are effective in treating:

- acute dystonia: they work rapidly and may be administered IM or IV if a more rapid effect is desired or if swallowing is difficult because of muscle spasm. Once acute dystonia has been successfully treated either the dose of AP drug should be reduced, the patient should be switched from a typical AP drug to an atypical AP drug or prophylactic anticholinergic medication should be prescribed

- parkinsonism: once parkinsonism has been successfully treated either the dose of AP drug should be reduced, the patient should be switched from a typical AP drug to an atypical AP drug or prophylactic anticholinergic medication should be prescribed.

Akathisia occurs in up to 50% of patients treated with typical AP drugs. It responds variably to anticholinergic drugs and management strategies include reducing the dose of AP drug, switching a patient being treated with a typical AP drug to an atypical AP drug, beta-blocking medication or benzodiazepines.

There are no satisfactory treatments for tardive dyskinesia. Anticholinergic drugs should be avoided because they are not effective and probably worsen it (this is also why they should not be prescribed prophylactically for every patient treated with AP drugs). Prevention by use of atypical AP drugs is therefore critically important. Otherwise, very slowly reducing the dose of AP drug or switching a patient being treated with a typical AP drug to an atypical AP drug, including clozapine, may help.

Safety

The adverse effects of anticholinergic drugs include nausea, constipation, drowsiness, dry mouth, blurred vision, dilated pupils, confusion, hallucinations, worsening of narrow angle glaucoma and acute urinary retention in patients with prostatic hypertrophy.

Orphenadrine has marked membrane stabilizing effects and a $t_{1/2}$ of up to 20 hours. A lethal dose may therefore be no more than 10 times the therapeutic dose. Therefore it probably has no place in psychiatric practice.

Anticholinergic drugs cause euphoria and are widely abused by patients for whom they are prescribed and by other individuals. This euphoriant effect is most evident with benzhexol and procyclidine. Sudden discontinuation of treatment with anticholinergic drugs can cause cholinergic rebound characterised by restlessness, insomnia, diarrhoea, abdominal pain, movement disorder and salivation. Anticholinergic drugs should therefore be discontinued gradually.

Drugs used in the treatment of alcohol and drug dependence and cigarette smoking

Drugs to help individuals withdraw from and maintain abstinence in opiate and alcohol misuse and in cigarette smoking should only be prescribed as part of a programme of treatment that also includes education and counselling (see Chapters 27 and 28). Rapid and ultra rapid opiate detoxification are not recommended by the UK Advisory Council on the Misuse of Drugs and will not be described.

Opiate misuse

Methadone, buprenorphine and lofexidine are useful in withdrawal from opiates while naltrexone may help in maintaining abstinence.

Methadone

Methadone is a long acting opioid μ receptor agonist that may be substituted for diamorphine and that will prevent withdrawal symptoms. It is less sedating and has a longer $t_{1/2}$ (24 hours) than morphine. It is usually administered as a once daily oral solution in a concentration of 1 mg per ml but an injectable formulation is available. It is intrinsically addictive and should only be prescribed for individuals who are dependent upon opiates. The initial daily dose is 10–20 mg and this is increased by 10–20 mg per day until withdrawal symptoms have been controlled. The usual daily dose is then 40-60 mg (see Chapter 28). Withdrawal is accomplished by gradually reducing the daily dosage at a rate that is agreed between the patient and the psychiatrist.

The adverse effects of methadone include nausea, vomiting, constipation and drowsiness. Sweating, arrhythmias, hypothermia, hallucinations, dysphoria and rash may also occur. Respiratory depression and hypotension may occur at relatively high doses.

Buprenorphine

Buprenorphine is a partial antagonist at the opioid μ receptor that will prevent withdrawal symptoms if substituted for diamorphine. However, it may precipitate withdrawal symptoms in patients dependent upon higher doses of opiates because of its partial antagonist properties.

Buprenorphine is subject to extensive first pass metabolism and must be administered sublingually. It is therefore important to instruct patients appropriately. Buprenorphine is initially prescribed at a dose of 0.8–4.0 mg daily. This may be gradually increased to a maximum of 32 mg daily. Withdrawal is accomplished by gradually reducing the daily dosage at a rate that is agreed between the patient and the psychiatrist.

The adverse effects of buprenorphine are similar to those of methadone.

Lofexidine

Lofexidine is an α_2 adrenergic agonist like clonidine (which is occasionally used for a similar purpose). It acts centrally to reduce NA secretion and thus reduce sympathetic tone. It will effectively prevent withdrawal symptoms in patients who are opiate dependent.

Lofexidine is usually prescribed in a dosage of 0.2 mg daily. This is gradually increased by 0.2–0.4 mg daily to a maximum dose of 2.4 mg daily.

The adverse effects of lofexidine include dry mouth, throat and nose, drowsiness, bradycardia and hypotension (it should not be administered if the pulse rate is below 50 beats per minute and/or if systolic blood pressure is less than 90 mm Hg). Sedation and coma may occur.

Naltrexone

Naltrexone is an orally administered opioid antagonist that neutralizes the euphoriant effects of opiates and alcohol. It may therefore trigger withdrawal symptoms in opiate dependent individuals. It my help formerly opiate dependent individuals maintain abstinence. Naltrexone may also be used for opiate withdrawal in hospitalized patients.

It is prescribed at a dose of 25–50 mg daily. Once an appropriate daily dose has been determined the drug is usually administered on three days per week. Its adverse effects include nausea, vomiting, anorexia, diarrhoea, abdominal pain, anxiety, headache, insomnia, fatigue, sweating, lacrimation, hypothermia, rash and sexual dysfunction.

Alcohol misuse

BZDs with a long duration of action will prevent or greatly diminish alcohol withdrawal symptoms (see Chapter 27). Chlordiazepoxide is widely used for this purpose and is commonly prescribed at an initial dose of 40–200 mg daily in divided doses. This dose is then gradually reduced over 7–14 days. Chlormethiazole may be used in a similar manner to chlordiazepoxide but it is now only recommended for hospitalized patients.

Alcohol dependent individuals are frequently vitamin deficient and thiamine deficiency causes damage to the periaqueductal structures which leads to Wernicke's encephalopathy and Korsakoff's psychosis (see Chapters 26 and 27). Patients withdrawing from alcohol should be treated with thiamine or multivitamin preparations.

Disulfiram

Disulfiram irreversibly inhibits acetaldehyde dehydrogenase and causes acetaldehyde to accumulate following ingestion of alcohol. Elevated blood acetaldehyde causes facial flushing, severe headache, palpitations, tachycardia, hypertension, respiratory distress, nausea and vomiting. These symptoms commence within 15–30 minutes of ingesting alcohol and persist for several hours. Tachyarrhythmias, hypotension, collapse and occasional deaths occur if large quantities of alcohol are consumed. Alcohol challenge in which the effects of disulfiram are demonstrated to a patient taking disulfiram by administering a small quantity of alcohol is strongly discouraged.

Patients must be alcohol-free for at least 24 hours before disulfiram is administered (and for at least seven days after it is discontinued). It is usually prescribed in an initial dose of 800 mg daily. This is gradually reduced over 5–7 days to a maintenance dose of 100–200 mg daily. Patients must be warned that a disulfirm/alcohol interaction may be triggered by alcohol in some foods, in cough remedies and in toiletries such as aftershave lotions. They should also be encouraged to carry a card advising that they are being treated with disulfiram.

The adverse effects of disulfiram in the absence of alcohol include nausea, vomiting, drowsiness, halitosis, metallic taste and reduced libido. Dermatitis, hepatitis, peripheral neuritis and encephalopathy may also rarely occur. Disulfiram inhibits dopamine β hydroxylase and elevates brain concentrations of DA. This may exacerbate schizophrenia and may rarely cause psychosis in otherwise healthy individuals.

Acamprosate

Acamprosate is thought to be both a GABA receptor agonist and a glutamate receptor antagonist (Whitworth et al. 1996). It seems to reduce craving for alcohol and may help formerly dependent individuals maintain abstinence.

Treatment should be commenced as soon as possible after alcohol withdrawal. It should be continued for at least one year and should be maintained during relapse. Dosage is 666 mg three times daily for individuals weighing more than 60 kg and 666 mg in the morning and 333 mg in the afternoon and evening for those weighing less than 60 kg. Its adverse effects include gastrointestinal disturbance and rash. Alterations in libido may also occur.

Cigarette smoking

Individuals who wish to discontinue cigarette smoking may benefit from nicotine replacement therapy or buproprion. These should be prescribed in accordance with NICE guidelines (National Insititute for Clinical Excellence 2000b) (Box 38.4).

Nicotine replacement therapy

Products are available that allow the administration of nicotine by sublingual (gum, lozenges), transdermal (patches) or transmucosal (nasal spray, inhaler) routes. The daily dosage of any product should be titrated to the quantity of cigarettes smoked daily, maintained at this dosage for three months and then gradually reduced over a further period of three months.

Nicotine products may cause nausea, hiccups, dyspepsia, headache, palpitations, insomnia, abnormal dreams, myalgia, anxiety and somnolence.

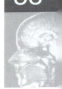

Buproprion

Buproprion is a NA and DA reuptake inhibitor that has almost no antagonist effect at neuroreceptors. Most of its effects are mediated by its metabolite, hydroxybuproprion.

Buproprion should be commenced two weeks before an agreed smoking cessation date at an initial dose of 150 mg daily. This dose is increased to 150 mg twice daily after one week and maintained at this for a further nine weeks. Buproprion should then be gradually discontinued.

The adverse effects of buproprion include gastrointestinal disturbance, impaired concentration, anxiety and alterations in taste. Rarely, psoriasis may be exacerbated and Stevens–Johnson syndrome and psychosis may occur. The CSM has advised that buproprion is contra-indicated in patients with a history of seizures or eating disoders, a CNS tumour or who are experiencing acute symptoms of alcohol or benzodiazepine withdrawal.

Special populations of patients

The treatment of children, women and elderly patients with psychoactive drugs merits special attention. Care must also be exercised when prescribing psychoactive drugs for motorists or individuals who operate machinery.

Children

Great care is required when treating children with psychoactive drugs because:

- they generally absorb, metabolize and eliminate drugs more rapidly than adults
- drugs are not extensively tested in children during clinical development, and
- formulations may not be available to allow precise dosing based upon body weight.

Most psychotropic drugs used to treat children are prescribed off label in that they are not specifically licensed for use in children. There are no psychoactive drugs that are specifically contraindicated in children (see p. 591 for CSM advice on the use of SSRIs for the treatment of major depressive disorder in individuals under 18 years of age) but the manufacturer of the drug or a reference such as the *British National Formulary* should be consulted for dosing information (see Chapter 13 also).

Women

Women receive twice as many prescriptions for psychoactive drugs as men but are largely excluded from clinical trials of new drugs because of the unknown potential for teratogenesis. The treatment of female patients with psychoactive drugs during their reproductive years therefore requires particular care (see Chapter 23).

Oral contraceptive pill

Psychotropic drugs that induce hepatic enzymes and increase the metabolism of both the combined and progesterone-only oral contraceptives include carbamazepine (see above), phenytoin, modafinil, phenobarbital and primidone. Women taking such drugs should either use an alternative method of contraception or take an oral contraceptive that provides 50 micrograms of ethinyloestradiol per day.

Reproductive function

Psychoactive drugs should be avoided in women who are planning to become pregnant or who are already pregnant. However, this is not always possible and when a decision is taken to commence or continue a psychoactive drug during pregnancy because the potential benefit outweighs the potential risk, the following guidelines should be applied:

- avoid treatment during the first trimester when the risk of teratogenicity is greatest if at all possible
- use the lowest effective dose possible
- ensure women taking antiepileptic drugs as mood-stabilizers or for epilepsy take appropriate doses of folate supplements before conception and during pregnancy in order to reduce the risk of neural tube defects (such advice is now applicable to all women contemplating pregnancy)
- use established rather than recently introduced drugs because more information on their use during pregnancy is available
- consult the manufacturer of a drug for up to date information on its use in pregnancy.

Drugs of choice during pregnancy include carbmazepine and fluoxetine. Acamprosate, antiepileptic drugs other than carbamazepine, benzodiazepines, tricyclic ADs, lithium (see above) and quetiapine should be avoided.

Most psychoactive drugs are secreted in breast milk and although concentrations may be low, breastfeeding infants are at risk of the same adverse effects as adults taking such drugs. Guidelines similar to those applied to pregnant women should therefore be applied to women who are breastfeeding. Breastfeeding women may take AD drugs but should avoid acamprosate, lithium, risperidone (risk of dystonia), quetiapine and clozapine (risk of agranulocytosis).

Hyperprolactinaemia
Typical AP drugs frequently cause hyperprolactinaemia which in turn causes hypo-oestrogenaemia, anovulation and amenorrhoea. Sexually active women taking such drugs are therefore relatively unlikely to become pregnant. Women switched from typical AP drugs to atypical AP drugs that do not cause hyperprolactinaemia should be advised about the return of menstruation and the risk of pregnancy.

Hyperprolactinaemia caused by typical AP drugs may cause hypo-oestrogenaemia and increase the risk of osteoporosis (see above). Prolactin sparing atypical AP drugs may therefore be particularly appropriate when treating female patients (see above and Chapter 18).

Elderly patients
Older patients experience twice as many adverse effects as younger patients because drug absorption, metabolism and elimination decreases with age, and drug interactions are more likely because such patients may require simultaneous treatment with several drugs.

Psychoactive drug therapy should be commenced at the lowest possible dose in older patients, the dose being increased slowly thereafter while vigilance is maintained for adverse effects ('start low and go slow'). Confusion is a frequent adverse effect of psychotropic drug therapy in older patients and drug-induced postural hypotension or sedation may lead to falls that result in hip fractures and subsequent morbidity and mortality.

Motorists
Many psychoactive drugs cause impaired attention, drowsiness and sedation, particularly when treatment is initially commenced or dosage increased. Patients who drive or operate machinery should be warned of these effects and advised of the synergistic effects of such drugs with each other and with alcohol. They should be specifically warned that it is illegal to drive while driving ability is impaired by drugs.

REFERENCES

Bazire S (2002) *Psychotropic Drug Directory 2001*. Dinton: Quay Books.
Bilder RM, Goldman RS, Volavka J, Czobor P, Hoptman M, Sheitman B, et al. (2002) Neurocognitive effects of clozapine, olanzapine, risperidone, and haloperidol in patients with chronic schizophrenia or schizoaffective disorder. *American Journal of Psychiatry* **159**:1018–28.
British National Formulary (2004) London: British Medical Association and Royal Pharmaceutical Society of Great Britain. Online. Available at: www.bnf.org [Accessed April 2004].
Committee on Safety of Medicines. Online. Available at: www.mca.gov.uk/aboutagency/regframework/csm/csmhome.htm [Accessed August 2004].
Cookson J, Taylor D, Katona C (2002) *Use of Drugs in Psychiatry*. London: Gaskell.
Elia J, Borcherding BG, Rapoport JL & Keysor CS (1991) Methylphenidate and dextroamphetamine treatments of hyperactivity: are there true nonresponders? *Psychiatry Research* **36**(2):141–55.
Geddes JR, Carney SM, Davies C, Furukawa TA, Kupfer DJ, Frank E & Goodwin GM (2003) Relapse prevention with antidepressant drug treatment in depressive disorders: a systematic review. *Lancet* **361**(9358): 653–61.
Goodwin GM & Young AH (2003) The British Association for Psychopharmacology guidelines for treatment of bipolar disorder: a summary. *Journal of Psychopharmacology* **17**(4 Supl. 3–6).
Greenhill LL, Halperin JM & Abikoff H (1999) Stimulant medications. *Journal of the American Academy of Child and Adolescent Psychiatry* **38**(5): 503–12.
Henry J (1997) Fatal toxicity index. *Drug Safety* **16**: 374–90.
Jacobson SJ, Jones K, Johnson K, Ceolin L, Kaur P, Sahn D, Donnenfeld AE, Rieder M, Santelli R, Smythe J et al. (1992) Prospective multicentre study of pregnancy outcome after lithium exposure during first trimester. *Lancet* **339**(8792): 530–3.
Kapur S & Seeman P (2001) Does fast dissociation from the dopamine D_2 receptor explain the action of atypical antipsychotics?: A new hypothesis. *American Journal of Psychiatry* **158**(3): 360–9.
Keck PE (2003) The management of acute mania. *British Medical Journal* **327**: 1002–3.
Meltzer HY, Alphs L, Green AI, Altamura AC, Anand R, Bertoldi A, Bourgeois M, Chouinard G, Islam MZ, Kane J, Krishnan R, Lindenmayer JP & Potkin S; International Suicide Prevention Trial Study Group (2003) Clozapine treatment for suicidality in schizophrenia: International Suicide Prevention Trial (InterSePT). *Archives of General Psychiatry* **60**: 82–91.
MTA Cooperative Group (1999) A 14-month randomized clinical trial of treatment strategies for attention-deficit/hyperactivity disorder. Multimodal Treatment Study of Children with ADHD. *Archives of General Psychiatry* **56**(12): 1073–86.
Naidoo U, Goff DC & Klibanski A (2003) Hyperprolactinemia and bone mineral density: the potential impact of AP agents. *Psychoneuroendocrinology* **Suppl. 2**: 97–108.
National Institute for Clinical Excellence (2000) *Guidance on the Use of Methylphenidate for ADHD*. London: NICE. Online. Available at: www.nice.org.uk [Accessed August 2004].
National Institute for Clinical Excellence (2001) *Donepezil, Rivastigmine and Galantamine for the Treatment of Alzheimer's Disease*. London: NICE. Online. Available at: www.nice.org.uk [Accessed August 2004].
National Institute for Clinical Excellence (2002a) *Schizophrenia: Core Interventions in the Treatment and Management of Schizophrenia in Primary and Secondary Care*. London: NICE. Online. Available at: www.nice.org.uk [Accessed August 2004].
National Institute for Clinical Excellence (2002b) *Guidance on the use of Nicotine Replacement Therapy (NRT) and Bupropion for Smoking Cessation*. London: NICE. Online. Available at: www.nice.org.uk [Accessed August 2004].
Petursson H & Lader MH (1981) Withdrawal from long term benzodiazepine treatment. *British Medical Journal* **283**: 643–5.
Schneider LS (1996) New therapeutic approaches to Alzheimer's disease. *Journal of Clinical Psychiatry* **57**(Suppl. 14): 30–6.
Taylor E (1999) Development of clinical services for attention-deficit/hyperactivity disorder. *Archives of General Psychiatry* **56**(12): 1097–9.
Tohen M, Goldberg JF, Gonzalez-Pinto Arrillaga AM, Azorin JM, Vieta E, Hardy-Bayle MC, et al. (2003) A 12-week, double-blind comparison of olanzapine vs haloperidol in the treatment of acute mania. *Archives of General Psychiatry* **60**(12): 1218–26.

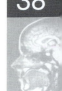

Verdoux H & Bourgeois M (1993) Short-term sequelae of lithium discontinuation. *Encephale* **19**(6): 645–50.

Whitworth AB, Fischer F, Lesch OM, Nimmerrichter A, Oberbauer H, Platz T, Potgieter A, Walter H & Fleischhacker WW (1996) Comparison of acamprosate and placebo in long-term treatment of alcohol dependence. *Lancet* **347**(9013): 1438–42.

Wright P, Birkett M, David S, Meehan K, Ferchland I, Alaka K, et al. (2001). Double blind, placebo controlled comparison of IM olanzapine and IM haloperidol in the treatment of acute agitation in schizophrenia. *American Journal Psychiatry* **158**: 1149–51.

Wright P & O'Flaherty L (2003) AP drugs: atypical advantages and typical disadvantages. *Irish Journal of Psychological Medicine* **20**: 24–7.

Psychosurgery and ECT

John M Cooney

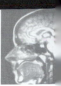

INTRODUCTION

The treatments described in this chapter have aroused considerable interest because they are perceived as inhumane, punitive and open to abuse by the medical/ psychiatric establishment. Both were introduced in the 1930s, before the advent of modern pharmacotherapy, and they developed in a somewhat haphazard way. However, increasing interest in the nature of consciousness and the role of the brain has been accompanied by further examination of these procedures and of their place in the treatment of mental disorders.

PSYCHOSURGERY

History

Trephination, boring holes in the skull for the relief of mental distress, has been practised in a wide array of cultures such as New Guinea, Tahiti and, particularly, in Peru and Bolivia, while reports of this practice date back some 4000 years in Europe. Psychosurgery in the modern era commenced with work by Burckhardt in Switzerland, in 1891. He removed areas of cortex from frontal and parietal regions in six patients, one of whom died, and two of whom developed epilepsy. Subsequently, the Russian neurosurgeon, Puseep, ablated the frontoparietal tracts of three patients with manic depression in 1910. He did not report his work until the 1930s.

In 1949, Egas Moniz was awarded the Nobel Prize for Medicine in recognition of his role in the development and introduction of psychosurgical techniques for the treatment of mental disorders. This remains the only Nobel Prize in psychiatry. The award reflected the importance of developing an intervention that had a relatively reliable effect in attenuating severe symptoms in patients at a time when there were no effective therapeutic alternatives. World War II saw an enormous expansion in the numbers of psychiatric admissions, such that 25% of beds in the USA were occupied by psychiatric patients. Up to 20% of patients with manic depression were hospitalized for 15 years and there was a 25% mortality in patients with schizophrenia (Swayze 1995). Effective treatments were urgently required.

Moniz, a Portuguese neurologist who had undertaken research on cerebral angiography, attended the 2nd International Congress of Neurology in London in 1935. There he heard of the experimental psychosurgery of Jacobsen and Fulton that caused profound behavioural change in primates. Later that year, his neurosurgical colleague Lima performed frontal leucotomies on psychotic patients. Moniz hypothesized that what we now refer to as neural plasticity was lost in psychiatric patients who then developed fixed neuronal connections. His report (Moniz 1936) of the first 20 patients indicated a good outcome from the procedure. Following this, other groups developed similar procedures, most notably the neurosurgeons Freeman and Watts in the USA. This era was one in which Papez described the 'circuit' in the limbic system in 1937, and Kluver and the neurosurgeon Bucy identified the dramatic effects of temporal lobectomy on aggression. These reports provided strength for the theoretical basis on which psychosurgery was predicated. By the early 1950s, Freeman and colleagues believed that psychosurgery was a first-line treatment for mental illness and were advocating early surgery in an attempt to improve prognosis.

The first era of psychosurgery ended in the 1950s for the following reasons:

- There was concern at the deleterious effect of psychosurgery on personality noted in about 60% of cases (with approximately 4% developing the so-called 'cabbage' personality in addition to other forms of morbidity and, indeed, mortality).
- Delay & Deniker (1952) first administered chlorpromazine in the 1950s.
- Janssen synthesized haloperidol in the 1950s.
- There was concern about the outcome of psychosurgery in terms of the impact on the course of the illnesses treated.

Swayze (1995) comprehensively reviews this period and reports follow-up data on 9284 patients in England and Wales who had a single leucotomy between 1942 and 1954. Of these, 41% were recovered or greatly improved, 28% minimally improved, 25% unchanged and 2% worse. There was a 4% mortality. Improvement was more likely in those with an affective illness with 63% recovered or greatly improved, while among patients with schizophrenia, only 30% fell into this best-outcome category. It is important to note that these patients were operated on for symptoms rather than specific diagnoses. Furthermore, postsurgical outcome figures do not differ greatly from those following the natural history of the illnesses. Sexual deviation and aggression were also treated via posteromedial hypothalamotomy or by the creation of unilateral non-dominant hypothalamic lesions. Reports are limited by small numbers of patients, but reduction of target symptoms with preservation of endocrine function was usual.

The second era of psychosurgery commenced with the introduction of stereotactic techniques in the 1950s. This coincided with a reduction in the number of patients undergoing psychosurgery, and a refinement of the procedures with increased localization of lesions and rigorous attempts to limit collateral damage. But even as technological breakthroughs allowed these improvements, the tide of public and professional opinion was swinging against psychosurgical interventions except in the most resistant of cases.

Psychosurgical techniques

The most commonly employed psychosurgical techniques in the treatment of mental illness are listed in Box 39.1.

Cingulotomy

This technique was introduced in 1962 at the Massachusetts General Hospital. It remains one of the most commonly performed procedures and is used for the treatment of intractable anxiety, pain, depression and, notably, obsessive-compulsive disorder (OCD). The technique involves stereotactically introducing electrodes into the cingulate bundles bilaterally and briefly heating their tips to 80–85°C. Ballantine et al. (1977) have described the evolution and

---

Box 39.1 The most commonly employed psychosurgical techniques in the treatment of mental illness

1. Cingulotomy (bilateral lesions in cingulate bundles)
2. Capsulotomy (bilateral lesions in the anterior limb of the internal capsule)
3. Stereotactic subcaudate tractotomy (bilateral lesions inferior to the head of the caudate nucleus and superior to the orbital cortex)
4. Limbic leucotomy (combined stereotactic subcaudate tractotomy and cingulotomy)

---

refinement of the placement of electrodes in this procedure, with progression towards deeper placement in the cingulum involving the superficial layers of the corpus callosum.

The original rationale for this intervention was the interruption of the main connection between frontal lobe and hippocampus, and a large part of the thalamic radiation. However, magnetic resonance (MR) evaluation of a series of patients who had a cingulotomy has demonstrated that the distribution of lesions frequently included the anterior internal capsule and did not always involve the cingulum itself (Sachdev & Hay 1996).

Approximately 30–70% of patients with OCD who have a cingulotomy have a good outcome. Clearly, these figures do not tell of the complexity of outcome. Most series are reported as personal (or single institution) figures and therefore are not directly comparable across centres. Most reports categorize outcome into four or five groups ranging from best outcome to poorest. Allied to this is the evidence that procedures in a single institution do not produce consistent anatomic lesions. The safety of cingulotomy is not in doubt. In three series reported in the literature, involving over 400 patients, there was no surgical mortality and only three cases of postoperative epilepsy, all controlled with medication. In terms of neuropsychological functioning, there is no decrement in IQ or memory using the Weschler Adult Intelligence Scales (WAIS). However, poorer performance on the Wisconsin Card Sorting Test (WCST) has been documented, indicating impairment of the formation and shifting of response sets, a function of the frontal lobes (Cummings 1995). There is no significant personality change following cingulotomy for OCD.

The modest efficacy of cingulotomy is more impressive in light of the low morbidity and mortality of the procedure, and considering the relatively intractable nature of symptomatology preoperatively. Cingulotomy has also been used in the treatment of aggression per se, but the results obtained have been inconsistent with remission rates of approximately 45%.

Capsulotomy

The anterior limb of the internal capsule relays fibres from the frontal cortex to the thalamus and thereafter to other sites in the limbic system. In capsulotomy bilateral lesions are produced in the region under local anaesthesia and light sedation. It is indicated in the treatment of depression and OCD. Electroencephalography (EEG) show that there is immediate slowing of the EEG over frontal areas, indicating interruption of frontothalamic loops, and this pattern is predictive of outcome even though the changes in electrical activity persist in only 20% of cases. Using ^{133}Xe inhalation, Kullberg & Risberg (1978) showed a reduction in frontal blood flow following this procedure. Position emission tomography (PET) scanning shows a reduction in ^{11}C glucose utilization in the medial frontal cortex following treatment of patients with OCD. This is of interest as it represents a decrement from relatively high glucose utilization, a finding at variance with the bulk of the literature in relation to OCD. It has been suggested that this finding may be accounted for by the severity of illness in patients presenting with treatment-resistance as one of the eligibility criteria for surgery. The neuropsychological effects of capsulotomy have been studied extensively. General measures of intelligence using the WAIS indicate preservation of IQ. However, there are subtle alterations in specific tests of frontal lobe function. There is a reduction in the scores obtained using the WCST and in particular an increase in perseverative errors in some subjects. It should be noted that follow-up at seven years did not identify any further deterioration in performance of these tasks, and indeed there was an improvement in some.

Blood flow changes with cingulotomy are not as extensive as those seen with capsulotomy and are largely confined to the upper frontoparietal region. In terms of clinical efficacy, two studies have compared capsulotomy with cingulotomy and demonstrated superior, more enduring results with capsulotomy (Fodstad et al. 1982; Kullberg 1977). These studies highlight one of the problems with contemporary psychosurgery. Both reports are of small sample sizes, the former includes patients with anxiety disorders and OCD, and *ad hoc* outcome measures are used by each group.

Stereotactic subcaudate tractotomy (SST)

In this procedure, white matter is lesioned beneath the head of the caudate nucleus and above the orbital cortex by inserting yttrium-90 rods that have a half-life of 60 hours. Developed by Geoffrey Knight in the UK, the principal indication for this is depression but it is also used in the treatment of anxiety disorders and OCD. Postmortem data on subjects who previously underwent SST identify lesions in the white matter of the ventral orbital lobe. There are secondary degenerative changes seen in the dorsomedial nucleus of the thalamus (an area affected by anterior capsulotomy also).

Neuropsychologically, there is no change seen in general measures of IQ, as with the other techniques described. In the immediate postoperative period, there is considerable confusion and significant impairment on many neuropsychological measures. At six months, there is improvement in attentional and verbal recall scores, but a slight fall in visual recall and frontal lobe task performance. Slowing of the EEG in the frontal region within weeks of surgery is associated with a good prognosis, as with capsulotomy. In all patients EEG changes do not persist at six months. In keeping with the clinical course improving over months, there is oedema seen on structural imaging post-operatively, with some volume loss and ventricular enlargement visible at three months. These findings do not increase subsequently. Regional blood flow is decreased in the orbitofrontal area and anterior cingulate cortex, and this

is associated with a good prognosis. Increased blood flow in the parietal lobe is associated with a poorer outcome. Urinary metabolites of noradrenaline (norepinephrine) are reduced immediately and at one year postsurgery and this too correlates with clinical outcome. A good outcome is seen in approximately 50% of patients with affective disorders and a poor result in 20% of this patient group. With anxiety disorders, these figures are 45% and 25% respectively.

Limbic leucotomy

This procedure is essentially a subcaudate stereotactic tractotomy with a cingulotomy. The primary indications are depression, anxiety disorder and OCD though there is anecdotal evidence of efficacy in Gilles de la Tourette syndrome. The largest series of 66 patients (Mitchell-Heggs et al. 1976) reports clinical improvement in 76% of subjects undergoing the procedure.

Psychosurgical interventions are reserved for the most resistant of cases who have had adequate clinical trials of all possible therapeutic interventions. The treatment of choice for OCD is anterior capsulotomy whereas SST is the preferred option for depression. Rigorous preoperative and postoperative assessment of psychopathology and neuropsychological measures are crucial in patients undergoing these procedures. Furthermore, most patients will require pharmacotherapy and/or psychological treatments postoperatively.

ELECTROCONVULSIVE THERAPY (ECT)

History

Reports of the efficacy of seizures in treating psychiatric disturbances date back to the 16th century. Phillipus Paracelsus used camphor by mouth to induce seizures for the treatment of mania, as did Von Auenbrugger in the 17th century. Ladislas Von Meduna was not aware of this work when he introduced intramuscular camphor for the treatment of schizophrenia in 1934, having noted that epilepsy and schizophrenia rarely coexist and having observed the beneficial effects of epileptic seizures in catatonia. This observation has not been borne out by subsequent epidemiological data but it provided a rational basis for the therapeutic induction of seizures. At the time, Von Meduna's report of 10 out of 26 patients with schizophrenia recovered, with three more improved and 13 unchanged, was compelling. Von Meduna soon changed the induction agent to intravenous pentylenetetrazol, which was better tolerated and more reliable.

In 1938, Cerrletti and Bini successfully employed electrical stimulation in the treatment of a mute catatonic patient. The next major development was the introduction of neuromuscular blockade using curare, by AE Bennett in the UK. Prior to this, induced seizures were associated with a

50% incidence of vertebral compression fractures and of other fractures and dislocations. This problem was further resolved in 1951 when the synthetic neuromuscular blocker suxamethonium was introduced along with general anaesthesia for ECT. The development of ECT has seen efforts to refine the technique to maximize efficacy and minimize side-effects, to establish indications and outcomes and to understand the mode of action. As a consequence, landmark studies by Lancaster on unilateral ECT (Lancaster et al. 1958), Ottoson on the requirement for seizures (1960) and the Medical Research Council (1965) have established the clinical efficacy of ECT. Efficacy has been further confirmed by blinded trials against so-called sham-ECT (Potter & Rudorfer 1993).

Methodological issues

ECT involves the application of electrical current to the head, which represents a potential difference across which there is a given resistance. Ohm's law states that the potential difference (voltage) is equal to the product of current (measured in coulombs) and resistance (measured in ohms). Resistance in ECT comes from the impedance of scalp, skull and brain between the two electrodes, the skull contributing over 80% of this. Modern ECT machines deliver an alternating current, the magnitude of which is constant in brief pulses (1–2 milliseconds). This is more physiological and contrasts with the former practice using sine wave current which resulted in increased electrical current delivered, and cognitive deficits following, treatment (Scott 1994).

ECT 'dosage'

The seizure threshold is the minimum charge required to induce a seizure and can vary 40-fold between individuals. Work by Sackheim et al. (1993) demonstrated the importance of stimulus strength relative to seizure threshold. A weak stimulus does not cause a seizure; an excessive stimulus causes a seizure but is also likely to cause memory impairment and confusion. The seizure threshold may be accurately measured by the application of gradually increasing stimuli, but is more usually estimated as it increases with age and male sex. Advocates of estimating threshold point out that repeated electrical stimulation increases the possibility of adverse cardiac events (McCall 1996) but acknowledge that a higher dosage (of the order of 30%) may be administered (Petrides & Fink 1996). Current recommendations are that the charge should exceed the seizure threshold by 150–250% for unilateral non-dominant (ULND) ECT and by 50–100% for bilateral ECT (Weiner 1994). ECT has potent effects on this threshold such that it rises with continued treatment. During a course of ECT, seizures should be monitored to determine the impact of this. Ottoson (1960) suggested the seizure was the most

crucial determinant of efficacy, but more recent work indicates that a seizure in itself is not enough. Effective ULND ECT requires that the stimulus exceed the seizure threshold by a greater amount than for bilateral ECT, pointing to the involvement of other elecrophysiological considerations (Weiner 1994). Seizure duration should be greater than 25 seconds and may be measured by a single-lead EEG or by the cuff technique. This requires a cuff from a sphygmomanometer to be inflated above systolic pressure on one limb just before the muscle relaxant is administered, thus preventing paralysis of that limb and allowing the seizure to be visualized.

Electrode selection and placement

Electrode placement may be either bilateral or unilateral. The American Psychiatric Association (1990) suggested that, if treatment is needed urgently or there has been a failure of unilateral ECT, bilateral placement should be used. If it is imperative to minimize cognitive side-effects, then ULND ECT is advisable. In contrast, the Royal College of Psychiatrists (1995 – these guidelines are currently undergoing revision) advocates the use of bilateral treatment because of concerns about stimulus intensity, dosing, overall efficacy and reliability with unilateral ECT.

For bilateral ECT, electrodes should be placed frontotemporally 4 cm above the midpoint of an imaginary line between the tragus and the external canthus (Fig. 39.1a and b). When administering ULND ECT, one electrode is placed at the right frontotemporal position, the other 4 cm inferior to the midpoint of a line joining the right and left tragus in a coronal plane on the right side of the head (Fig. 39.1c).

ECT is usually administered to patients twice weekly in the UK and three times a week in the USA. More frequent applications are associated with a shorter time to remission but a higher incidence of cognitive problems. It is worth noting that the seizure threshold is higher with bilateral ECT than ULND for the first few treatments. This suggests that ULND ECT is more likely to be effective. However, one study showed an increased rate of missed seizures with ULND ECT (McAndrew et al. 1967). The McAndrew placement, which allows a shorter distance between electrodes than the d'Elia placement, was used in this study. The other factor with ULND ECT is the quality of electrode contact with the scalp, as there is frequently hair in the region of placement and this may be a source of resistance.

Consent

Preparation of patients for ECT requires informed consent, preoperative anaesthetic evaluation and consideration of the facilities required for the safe treatment of patients. The nature of such facilities is described by guidelines such as those produced by the Royal College of Psychiatrists (1995).

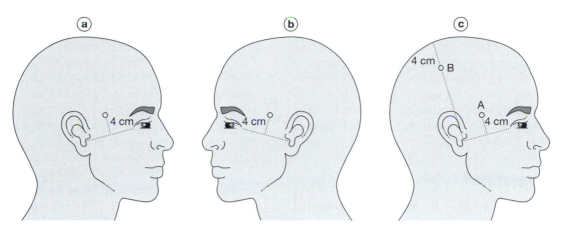

Figure 39.1 Placement of electrodes for bilateral administration of ECT: Electrodes are placed 4 cm above the midpoint of a line joining the tragus and the external canthus on the right (a) and left (b). (c) Unilateral non-dominant ECT: Electrode A is placed as for bilateral ECT; electrode B is 4 cm inferior to the midpoint of a coronal line from the right to the left tragus, on the right side. Electrodes A and B are approximately 10 cm apart. (From original drawings by Pádraig Wright.)

Similarly, the complex issue of informed consent and how to obtain it in a valid manner consistent with peer practice is described by, for example, the Royal College of Psychiatrists (1995) and the American Psychiatric Association (1990). The essential components of informed consent are explanations of the reasons for treatment, the nature of ECT and its side-effects, the use of a general anaesthetic, the nature of the desired outcome and the expected consequences of not having treatment.

Anaesthesia

Prior to ECT the medical history should be reviewed, the patient examined physically and appropriate investigations conducted. These will include a full blood count, urea and electrolytes and an ECG and chest X-ray if over 40 years old. Patients should also be evaluated by an anaesthetist prior to ECT.

Prior to administering ECT, equipment for ECG monitoring, blood pressure measurement and oxygen saturation is connected to the patient and intravenous access is established. The most commonly used anaesthetic is methohexitone sodium, a short-acting barbiturate administered in doses ranging from 0.75 to 1 mg/kg in a 1% solution. Thiopentone has been associated with arrhythmias, perhaps as a result of inadequate ventilation (Dubovsky 1994), propofol attenuates hypertension and tachycardia but may raise the seizure threshold and ketamine is associated with psychotic symptoms with repeated use in adults. Suxamethonium is the most commonly used muscle relaxant. The adequacy of muscle relaxation can be assessed by the disappearance of fasciculations. Pseudocholinesterase deficiency is so rare that routine screening is not warranted, but where it is detected (prolongation of muscle relaxation) other agents such as atracurium may be used. It is important

that the patient is oxygenated with 100% oxygen via the face mask prior to the ECT stimulus, as deoxygenation has potent anticonvulsant effects.

Some centres administer atropine or glycopyrrolate prior to treatment to dry secretions and block vagally mediated bradycardia, but this is not routinely used because it may prolong confusion and indeed predispose to arrhythmias. The beta-blockers esmolol and labetolol have been used to attenuate the sympathetic surge, and resulting increase in blood pressure, associated with ECT.

Medications and ECT

The American Psychiatric Association (1990) recommend that medication be discontinued prior to ECT because drugs influence seizure threshold. Benzodiazepines, carbamazepine and sodium valproate have anticonvulsant properties and increase the chance of treatment failure. Most antidepressants and neuroleptics lower the seizure threshold and thus increase the stimulus relative to the convulsive threshold and increase the likelihood of adverse cognitive problems. The Royal College of Psychiatrists (1995) highlights reports of increased seizure duration with continuation of selective serotonin reuptake inhibitors (SSRIs), particularly in young women. Where possible, drugs should be discontinued but if a full washout is not possible because of half-life (sertraline and paroxetine require two weeks and fluoxetine five weeks, for example) then drug treatment should be continued. In this case, the initial stimulus should be lower than usual, of the order of 50 millicoulombs, and the anaesthetist should be alerted so that intravenous diazepam can be administered if the seizure duration exceeds 90 seconds. Monoamine oxidase inhibitors need not be discontinued while moclobamide may have anticonvulsant properties and thus contribute to inadequate seizures. Lithium is the subject of conflicting reports with respect to toxicity with ECT, but it is pro-convulsant and therefore the recommendation for antidepressants should be observed. Caffeine acts as an antagonist at the adenosine type 1 receptor and may increase seizure duration. This can be of use where there is apparent resistance to seizure induction and caffeine sodium benzoate 500–2000 mg can be administered intravenously 10 minutes before ECT (Shapira et al. 1987).

Neurobiology of ECT

The principal clinical indication for ECT is the treatment of affective disorders, most commonly severe depression that is resistant to conventional antidepressants (Box 39.2). The theories that have been developed to explain the efficacy of ECT therefore focus on its effects in depression. Thus, the biological impact of ECT has been studied most intensively in neuronal systems implicated in depression and the effects of ECT have been compared to those of standard antidepressants. Definitive explanations are awaited, but progress emanates from both animal models and clinical studies, the latter of which are more feasible given the consensus on many of the methodological issues alluded to above.

The observation that ECT has marked anticonvulsant activity given that it raises seizure threshold led to the hypothesis that this was its mode of action. Evidence to support this derives from the kindling model of affective disturbances (Post & Weiss 1995). Anticonvulsants such as carbamazepine, sodium valproate and lamotrigine have well-defined mood-stabilizing properties and raising the seizure threshold is associated with the production of a peptide with anticonvulsant properties in the cerebrospinal fluid in animals (Tortella & Long 1985). ECT also causes disruption of the bloodbrain barrier with increased permeability and alterations in cerebral blood flow. It is generally accepted that mood disorders are associated with regional deficits in blood flow (Soares & Mann 1997). ECT

Box 39.2 Indications and contraindications for ECT

Indications
1. Severe depression, especially depression with biological (weight-loss, psychomotor retardation and/or early morning wakening) and/or psychotic (delusions) features
2. Treatment-resistant depression
3. Postpartum affective psychosis
4. Catatonic stupor
5. Treatment-resistant mania
6. Some neurological disorders (see text)

Contraindications
1. Contraindications to general anaesthesia
2. Raised intracranial pressure (see text)

---

studies have identified both decreases and increases in local blood flow with treatment (Bonne et al. 1996 and Rudorfer et al. 1997). However, methodological considerations in the rapidly developing field of neuroimaging make direct comparisons between studies difficult. There is a generalized slowing of the EEG following ECT and the persistence of δ and θ activity in the prefrontal region is a marker for therapeutic efficacy (Sackheim et al. 1996). Similarly, a good prognosis is associated with reduction in rapid eye movement density (Grunhaus et al. 1994).

Central systems mediating stress responses have an important role in the mediation of affective disorders. Overactivity of the hypothalamic-pituitary-adrenal (HPA) axis has been implicated in the biology of depression. Effective pharmacological antidepressant treatment reduces HPA activity, probably by down-regulation of central glucocorticoid and mineralocorticoid receptors. ECT also reduces HPA activity (Nemeroff et al. 1991). However, results using the dexamethasone suppression test (DST) are inconsistent. Recent reports have highlighted the role of the DST in identifying nonresponders to pharmacological interventions, but there is more limited evidence for this in relation to ECT (Ribiero et al. 1993). Prolactin, a stress-sensitive hormone that is elevated in response to seizure (and may distinguish between epileptic and nonepileptic seizures) is elevated in response to ECT and there is evidence that stimulus intensity is related to the magnitude of prolactin release (Zis et al. 1996). Thyroid release hormone is elevated following ECT (in animals) and thyroid stimulating hormone (TSH) is also elevated following ECT. Over the course of treatment, TSH concentration declines in parallel with the reduction in seizure length.

A variety of neurochemical changes have been described following ECT. Both antidepressants and ECT reduce the number of α_1 adrenoreceptors (Mann & Kapur 1994) but while pharmacological antidepressant agents cause a down-regulation of $5HT_2$ receptors, ECT increases $5HT_2$ receptor density (Cooper et al. 1995). There is an up-regulation of D_1 dopamine receptors and cAMP accumulation in the aftermath of electrically induced, but not chemically induced, seizures (Sackheim et al. 1995). Overactivity of cholinergic systems has been associated with depression and ECT causes reduced muscarinic receptor density in the cortex and hippocampus (Nutt & Glue 1993). What is most intriguing about ECT is the emerging evidence for differential regional effects, for example on the type 1 kainate receptor, which has increased density in the dentate but reduced density in the region of the CA_1 neurons of the hippocampus (Porter et al. 1996).

Safety

The mortality for ECT is 2 per 100 000 treatments, which is no higher than that expected with anaesthesia. The biggest risk is of cardiac mortality and this is particularly evident at the time of the procedure and in the following 15 minutes, owing to haemodynamic instability (see above). Identification of risk and evaluation of the risk/benefit ratio is required. The commonest side-effects of ECT are headache, drowsiness, confusion and memory impairment, the latter of which is perhaps the most significant. The principal memory defects are of short-term anterograde loss with spotty defects in retrograde memory. The mechanism of this is unclear, but phenomenologically the problem is primarily one of memory consolidation and may reflect disruption of protein synthesis in crucial temporal lobe structures (Devanand et al. 1994). There is no evidence that ECT causes structural damage, either from neuroimaging or from postmortem or preclinical studies (Devanand et al. 1994) (Box 39.2).

Indications

Guidance on the use of ECT has been provided by the National Institute for Clinical Excellence (2003), whose general recommendations are that:

- ECT should only be used in the management of patients with sever depression, prolonged or severe mania or catatonia
- ECT should not be used as a maintenance therapy in depression
- ECT should not be used in the treatment of schizophrenia other than when catatonia is present.

Depression

Depression is the primary indication for ECT and accounts for at least 85% of treatments (Box 39.2). Soon after the introduction of ECT for schizophrenia, it was clear from observation that it had considerable efficacy in the treatment of depression in schizophrenia. Direct confirmation of that hypothesis came in the 1960s with the publication of large-scale trials demonstrating its superior efficacy over antidepressants. In the 1970s and 1980s, evidence to support this efficacy accumulated from studies using sham-ECT. ECT is particularly useful in treating postpartum depression and treatment-resistant depression, and is safe and may be life-saving in depressed patients who refuse to eat. There is consensus that ECT is effective in 75–85% of cases of major depression.

The three factors that have been identified as predictors of a good response to ECT are:

- psychomotor retardation
- delusions
- a history of previous response to ECT, which is the most robust predictor of all.

Mania

ECT is an effective treatment for mania in 80% of patients. There are three prospective controlled trials in the literature and six retrospective studies; these have been reviewed by Mukherjee et al. (1994). The efficacy of ECT is especially impressive because in many studies patients were resistant to conventional antipsychotic/lithium combinations. It is clinical lore that patients with mania require more frequent administrations of ECT than depressed patients. Recent studies found no significant differences between twice or five times weekly treatment, however, and neither is there evidence that patients with mania require a more prolonged course of treatment than used in depression. The response rate among manic patients resistant to conventional pharmacological management is of the order of 60% but the relapse rate among this group is increased. There are no systematic data available on the efficacy of continuation or maintenance therapy with lithium or antipsychotic drugs.

Schizophrenia

The use of ECT in schizophrenia has fallen dramatically, so there is a limited data set from the modern era of comparative and sham-ECT studies. However, in patients with catatonia, ECT may be life-saving. The clinical differentiation of lethal catatonia, neuroleptic malignant syndrome and malignant hyperthermia may not be possible clinically and this is an indication for emergency ECT. Work by May & Tuma (1965) identified antipsychotics as the treatment of choice in schizophrenia with 95% of patients discharged within a year. The one-year discharge rate was 80% for those treated with ECT. Recently, there have been reports of success in treating clozapine-resistant schizophrenic patients with ECT and clozapine in combination as soon as possible (Rudorfer et al. 1997), the argument for this aggressive strategy being the finding that delay in instituting effective treatment in schizophrenia impairs prognosis.

Neurological disorders

There is clear evidence for a therapeutic benefit from ECT in patients with Parkinson's disease (Factor et al. 1995). Mood disorders occur in up to 60% of patients with multiple sclerosis and while ECT is an effective treatment, 20% of patients experience a neurological deterioration (Krystal & Coffey 1997). The risk for patients with raised intracranial pressure receiving ECT is of herniation of the brainstem. This has previously been considered an absolute contraindication but with clear delineation of the risk/benefit ratio and use of adjuvant supportive treatments such as corticosteroids and antihypertensives, successful treatment is possible. Patients suffering from chronic pain syndromes with affective symptoms have reportedly also benefited from ECT. Intractable epilepsy is a further occasional indication for ECT.

ECT is a safe, reliable treatment that has developed technologically to the point where the risks are clearly definable. There is undoubtedly a significant problem with the public and professional perception of ECT and the pendulum of opinion has swung from the widely perceived authoritarian prescription of ECT to the point where members of lower socioeconomic groups and ethnic minorities are seen as less likely to be treated with ECT because of the perceived imposition of a 'punitive or harsh' treatment on a doubly disadvantaged group. In contrast, insurers will insist on the most efficient form of treatment (Olfson et al. 1998) and ECT, although in use for over 60 years, remains the most effective treatment available for depression (McCall 2001). It is clearly unethical to neglect to offer a safe and potentially effective form of treatment to patients suffering from disorders that are, at best, only partially responsive to other contemporary interventions.

Brain stimulation techniques

Transcranial magnetic stimulation (TMS), vagal nerve stimulation (VNS) and deep brain stimulation (DBS) are all techniques that are being evaluated in the treatment of neuropsychiatric disorders. They have variously shown promise in affective disorders and trials are underway refining methodological issues. TMS, in common with ECT is non-invasive. High frequency repetitive TMS to the left prefrontal cortex to younger patients with depression in the absence of psychosis is suggested (Gershon et al. 2003).

REFERENCES

American Psychiatric Association (1990) *The Practice of ECT: Recommendations for Treatment, Training and Privileging.* Washington, DC: American Psychiatric Association Inc.

Ballantine HT, Levy BS, Dagi TF & Girius IB (1977) Cingulotomy for psychiatric illness; report of 13 years experience. In: Sweet WH, Obrador S & Martin-Rodriguez JG (eds) *Neurosurgical Treatment in Psychiatry, Pain and Epilepsy*, pp. 333–54. Baltimore: University Park Press.

Bonne O, Krausz Y, Shapira B et al. (1996) Increased cerebral blood flow in depressed patients responding to electroconvulsive therapy. *Journal of Nuclear Medicine* 37: 1075–80.

Cooper SJ, Kelly CB & McClelland RJ (1995) Affective disorders: 3. Electroconvulsive therapy. In: King DJ (ed.) *Seminars in Clinical Psychopharmacology*, pp. 224–58. London: Gaskell.

Cummings J (1995) Anatomic and behavioural aspects of frontal-subcortical circuits. *Annals of the New York Academy of Sciences* 769: 1–13.

Delay J & Deniker P (1952) Trente-huit cas de psychoses traitees par la cure longee et continue de 4560RP. Le congres des Al. de Langue Fr. In: *Compte Rendu de Congres*. Paris: Masson et Citie.

Devanand DP, Dwork AJ, Hutchinson ER, Bolwig TG & Sackheim HA (1994) Does ECT alter brain structure? *American Journal of Psychiatry* 152: 1403.

Dubovsky SL (1994) Electroconvulsive therapy. In: Kaplan HI & Saddock BJ (eds)
Clinical Psychiatry, pp. 2129–40. Baltimore: Williams & Wilkins.

Factor SA, Molho ES & Brown DL (1995) Combined clozapine and ECT for the treatment of drug-induced Parkinson's disease. *Journal of Neuropsychiatry and Clinical Neurosciences* 7: 304–7.

Fodstad H, Strandman E & West KA (1982) Treatment of chronic obsessive compulsive states with stereotactic anterior capsulotomy or cingulotomy. *Acta Neurochirurgica* (Wien) 62: 1–23.

Gershon AA, Dannon PN, Grunhaus L (2003). Transcranial magnetic stimulation in the treatment of depression. American Journal of Psychiatry 160: 835–45.

Grunhaus L, Shipley JE, Eiser A et al. (1994) Sleep electroencephalographic studies after ECT. *Archives of General Psychiatry* 2: 39–51.

Krystal AD & Coffey CE (1997) Neuropsychiatric considerations in the use of electroconvulsive therapy. *Journal of Neuropsychiatry and Clinical Neurosciences* 8: 283–92.

Kullberg G & Risberg J (1978) Changes in regional cerebral blood flow following stereotactic neurosurgery. *Applied Neurophysiology* 41: 79–85.

Kullberg G (1977) Differences in effect of cingulotomy and capsulotomy. In: Sweet WH, Obrador S & Martin Rodriguez JG (eds) *Neurosurgical Treatment in Psychiatry, Pain and Epilepsy*, pp. 301–8. Baltimore: University Park Press.

Lancaster NP, Steinert RR & Frost I (1958) Unilateral electroconvulsive therapy. *Journal of Mental Science* 104: 221–7.

Mann JJ & Kapur S (1994) Elucidation of the biochemical basis of the antidepressant action of electroconvulsive therapy by human studies. *Psychopharmacology Bulletin* 30: 133–40.

May PRA & Tuma AH (1965) Treatment of schizophrenia. An experimental study of five treatment methods. *British Journal of Psychiatry* 111: 503–10.

McAndrew J, Berkey B & Matthews C (1967) The effects of dominant and non-dominant unilateral ECT as compared to bilateral ECT. *American Journal of Psychiatry* 124: 483–90.

McCall WV (1996) Asystole in electroconvulsive therapy: report of four cases. *Journal of Clinical Psychiatry* 57: 199–203.

McCall WV (2001) Electroconvulsive therapy in the era of modern psychopharmacology. *International Journal of Neuropsychopharmacology* 4: 315–24.

Medical Research Council (1965) Clinical trial of the treatment of depressive illness. *British Medical Journal* i: 688–91.

Mitchell-Heggs N, Kelly D & Richardson AE (1976) A further review of sub-caudate limbic leucotomy. *British Journal of Psychiatry* 128: 226–40.

Moniz E (1936) Essai d'un traitement churgurical de certain psychoses. *Bulletin de l'Academie de Medecine* (Paris) 115: 385–92.

Mukherjee S, Sackheim HA & Schnur DB(1994) Electroconvulsive therapy of acute manic episodes: a review of 50 years experience. *American Journal of Psychiatry* 151: 169–76.

Nemeroff CB, Bissett G, Akil H et al. (1991) Neuropeptide concentrations in the cerebrospinal fluid of depressed patients treated with electroconvulsive therapy. *British Journal of Psychiatry* 158: 59–63.

National Instutute for Clinical Excellence (2003) *Guidance on the use of Electroconvulsive Therapy*. Online. Available at: www.nice.org.uk [accessed 26 May 2004].

Nutt DJ & Glue P (1993) The neurobiology of ECT: animal studies. In: Coffey CE (ed.) *The Clinical Science of Electroconvulsive Therapy*, pp. 213–34. Washington, DC: American Psychiatric Press.

Olfsen M, Marcus S, Sackheim HA, Thompson J & Pincus HA (1998) Use of ECT for the inpatient treatment of recurrent major depression. *American Journal of Psychiatry* 155: 22–9.

Ottoson JO (1960) Experimental studies of the mode of action of electroconvulsive therapy. *Acta Psychiatrica Neurologica Scandanavica* 145: 69–97.

Petrides G & Fink M (1996) The 'half-age' stimulation strategy for ECT dosing. *Convulsive Therapy* 12: 138–46.

Porter RHP, Burnet PWJ, Eastwood SL & Harrison PJ (1996) Contrasting effects of electroconvulsive shock on mRNAs encoding the high affinity kainate receptor subunits (KA_1 and KA_2) and cyclophilin in the rat. *Brain Research* 710: 97–102.

Post RM & Weiss RB (1995) The neurobiology of treatment resistant disorders. In: Bloom FE & Kupfer DJ (eds) *Psychopharmacology: The Fourth Generation of Progress*, pp. 1155–70. New York: Raven Press.

Potter WZ & Rudorfer MV (1993) Electroconvulsive therapy – a modern medical procedure. *New England Journal of Medicine* 328: 882–3.

Ribeiro SL, Tandon R, Grunhaus L & Greden JF (1993) The DST as a predictor of outcome in depression: a meta-analysis. *American Journal of Psychiatry* 150: 1618–29.

Royal College of Psychiatrists (1995) The second report of the Royal College of Psychiatrists special committee on ECT.

Rudorfer MV, Henry M & Sackheim HA (1997) Electroconvulsive

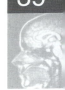

therapy. In: Tasman A, Kay J & Lieberman JA (eds) *Psychiatry*, pp. 1535–56. Philadelphia: WB Saunders.

Sachdev P & Hay P (1996) Site and size of lesion and psychosurgical outcome in obsessive-compulsive disorder: a magnetic resonance imaging study. *Biological Psychiatry* **39**: 739–42.

Sackheim HA, Prudic J, Devanand DP et al. (1993) Effects of stimulus intensity and electrode placement on the efficacy and cognitive effects of electroconvulsive therapy. *New England Journal of Medicine* **328**: 839–46.

Sackheim HA, Devanand DP & Nobler MS (1995) Electroconvulsive therapy. In: Bloom FE & Kupfer DJ (eds) *Psychopharmacology: The Fourth Generation of Progress*, pp. 1123–41. New York: Raven Press.

Sackheim HA, Luber B, Katzman GP et al. (1996) The effects of electroconvulsive therapy on quantitative electroencephalograms: relationship to clinical outcome. *Archives of General Psychiatry* **53**: 814–27.

Scott AI (1994) Contemporary practice of electroconvulsive therapy. *British Journal of Hospital Medicine* **51**: 334–8.

Shapira B, Lerer B, Gilboa D et al. (1987) Facilitation of ECT by caffeine pretreatment. *American Journal of Psychiatry* **144**: 9.

Soares JC & Mann JJ (1997) The functional neuroanatomy of mood disorders. *Journal of Psychiatric Research* **31**: 393–432.

Swayze VW (1995) Frontal leucotomy and related psychosurgical procedures in the era before antipsychotics (1935–1954): a historical overview. *American Journal of Psychiatry* **152**: 505–15.

Tortella FC & Long JB (1985) Endogenous anticonvulsant substance in rat cerebrospinal fluid after a generalised seizure. *Science* **228**: 1106–8.

Weiner RD (1994) Treatment optimisation with ECT. *Psychopharmacology Bulletin* **30**: 313–20.

Zis AP, Yatham LN, Lam RM, Clark CM, Srisurapanont M & McGarvey K (1996) Effects of stimulus intensity on prolactin and cortisol release induced by unilateral electroconvulsive therapy. *Neuropsychopharmacology* **15**: 263–70.

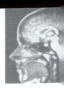

Psychiatry, ethics and the law

Séan Whyte

INTRODUCTION

This chapter is essentially about rules. To a greater extent than doctors in other specialties, psychiatrists operate within several complex, overlapping and occasionally contradictory sets of rules. At times these rules can seem supportive: for instance, giving a person treatment against their wishes is made much easier by knowing that this is widely accepted (in specific circumstances) as being in that person's best interests, and that you are following a proper legal procedure which is there to protect them and you. At other times, these same rules can seem restrictive, as for example when a patient's discharge from hospital is delayed until a full Care Programme Approach (CPA) meeting can be held. Some of the sources of the rules applicable to psychiatrists are shown in Box 40.1; these specific sets of rules, and others, are examined in the later sections of this chapter.

ETHICS IN PSYCHIATRY

Why are ethics – that is, personal or professional moral codes – relevant in psychiatry? Is not psychiatry, like the rest

---

of medicine, essentially one of the sciences, where an objective assessment is made of the patient's signs and symptoms, a diagnosis is reached, and treatment is prescribed by reference to a body of scientific knowledge about disease? Even if one regards science itself as being independent of moral and value judgments (and many scientists and philosophers do not – see, for instance, Fulford et al 1994) the processes of diagnosis and treatment in practice inevitably introduce moral questions. What is the 'norm' of speech or behaviour to which to compare this person's speech or behaviour? How do you decide whether a person's relationships count as 'unstable' (part of the definition of borderline personality disorder)? Which of the patients who might benefit from currently expensive or scarce treatments such as clozapine, rivastigmine or cognitive–analytic therapy will be given them? Add to this mix the fact that psychiatrists are expected to judge who is capable of making their own decisions and who is not, and that most psychiatrists are licensed to detain people in hospital against their will, and it becomes clear that many of the decisions psychiatrists make have a significant ethical component.

Ethical frameworks

The first, and perhaps most famous, statement of ethical principles relating to medicine was that of the ancient Greek physician Hippocrates. An abridged version of Hippocrates' Oath is shown in Box 40.2; many of the principles he formulated are still considered relevant today. The World Medical Association has produced more detailed and contemporary oaths, including the Declaration of Geneva for all doctors (World Medical Association 1968), the Declaration of Helsinki, which covers biomedical research (World Medical Association 2000), and the Declaration of Madrid, which applies specifically to psychiatrists (World Medical Association 1996). In the UK, the General Medical Council has produced its own list of doctors' duties, some of which are shown in Box 40.3; the Royal College of Psychiatrists has endorsed this and produced a companion

---

Box 40.1 Some of the sources of rules affecting psychiatrists
Legal sources
Mental Health Act 1983
Common Law
Quasi-legal sources
Care Programme Approach (CPA)
'Working Together' guidance
Ethical sources
Hippocratic Oath
Geneva, Helsinki and Madrid Declarations
General Medical Council
Royal College of Psychiatrists

manual applying these duties to psychiatric practice (Royal College of Psychiatrists 2000).

There are many such codes of professional ethics, mostly embodying the same general values, but differing in detail. With such a profusion of detailed guidance, it can be difficult to see the underlying ethical principles. A useful conventional way of summarizing these ethical codes is the Four Principles of Childress & Beauchamp (1967).

The four principles

These are four general principles that most philosophers accept underlie both the common morality and guidelines in professional ethics. They are independent of any particular moral system or theory (such as Kantianism, utilitarianism, virtue ethics or casuistry, all of which propose coherent sets of moral rules), but they provide a framework for looking at different sets of ethics. A discussion of these principles, and their relationship with moral systems and with codes of psychiatric ethics, can be found in Bloch et al. (1999). The four principles are:

- **Non-maleficence:** often stated as 'first do no harm,' this principle states that the doctor should avoid doing anything that would harm the patient.

Box 40.2   The Hippocratic Oath (abridged, after Temkin & Temkin 1967)

I swear by Apollo Physician and Asclepius and Hygieia and Panaceia and all the gods and goddesses...that I will fulfil according to my ability and judgment this oath and this covenant: ...I will apply dietetic measures for the benefit of the sick according to my ability and judgment; I will keep them from harm and injustice.

I will neither give a deadly drug to anybody if asked for it, nor will I make any suggestion to this effect...

Whatever houses I may visit, I will come for the benefit of the sick, remaining free of all intentional injustice, of all mischief and in particular of sexual relations with both female and male persons, be they free or slaves.

What I may see or hear in the course of the treatment...which on no account one must spread abroad, I will keep to myself ...

If I fulfil this oath and do not violate it, may it be granted to me to enjoy life...; if I transgress and swear falsely, may the opposite...be my lot.

Box 40.3   The duties of a doctor (General Medical Council 2001, abridged)

You must:
    Make the care of your patient your first concern
    Respect patients' dignity and privacy
    Listen to patients and respect their views
    Keep your professional knowledge and skills up to date
    Recognize the limits of your professional competence
    Be honest and trustworthy
    Respect and protect confidential information
    Avoid abusing your position as a doctor

- **Beneficence:** this principle states that the doctor should promote the welfare of patients. A balance should be sought which maximizes benefits to the patient (health, disease prevention, etc.) and minimizes harms (pain, disability, side-effects, etc.).
- **Autonomy:** doctors should respect the autonomy of patients, which means both respecting their right to make decisions for themselves (provided that they have the capacity to do so) and promoting their ability to make decisions, such as by providing useful information.
- **Justice:** doctors should treat patients according to what is fair, due or owed. Among other things, this implies that benefits (such as specific treatments) should be distributed fairly amongst all those in need of them. This is perhaps the most controversial principle, as there is so much room for disagreement over what is 'fair' and who is 'in need.'

HOW THE LAW APPLIES TO DOCTORS

The codes of ethics described above are not directly enforced: that is, they are intended to guide practice, rather than representing rules which must be followed to the letter. A different set of rules governs what powers doctors have, and determines when doctors should be punished for their actions. In this chapter, the focus is on the law in England and Wales, but in most cases broadly similar provisions apply in the rest of the UK and elsewhere.

The law of negligence

This is a very broad law, covering situations where a doctor, in their professional capacity, has done something they should not have done (negligence by commission) or has not done something they should have done (negligence by omission). Negligence is not a crime, and so doctors found to be negligent cannot be imprisoned or otherwise punished. Negligence is a civil wrong or 'tort,' and if the doctor (the defendant) is found to be negligent, he or she must pay damages to the person making the complaint (the plaintiff). The idea is that the damages restore the plaintiff to the financial position they would have been in had the negligence not occurred – for instance by replacing certain lost earnings from work while in hospital – and compensate the plaintiff for nonfinancial hardships, such as pain and suffering.

A plaintiff claiming that a doctor (or any other person) has been negligent must demonstrate three things: that the defendant owed them a *duty of care*; that the defendant has *breached* that duty; and that this breach led directly to the plaintiff suffering *damage*. These points are illustrated by the case vignettes in Box 40.4.

Mrs Anderson acquires pneumonia and goes to Dr Hooper for treatment. Dr Hooper prescribes amoxicillin without first checking her notes. Mrs Anderson returns a few days later with erythema multiforme; on reviewing her notes, Dr Hooper sees that sensitivity to penicillin has been reported in the past. Dr Hooper starts her on erythromycin instead, to which the infection responds. While Mrs Anderson is recovering in bed, she suffers minor injuries when a box falls off the wardrobe on top of her. After a total of three weeks, Mrs Anderson recovers and is able to return to work.

Case 1

Mrs Anderson's employer sues Dr Hooper for the loss of Mrs Anderson's labour for the three weeks. This case falls on the first hurdle: Dr Hooper does not owe the employer a duty of care.

Case 2

Mrs Anderson sues Dr Hooper for her injuries arising from the box falling on her, which she says would not have happened had she been prescribed erythromycin to start with and returned to work earlier, before the box fell. This case falls on the third hurdle: the damage is too remote from Dr Hooper's actions.

Case 3

Mrs Anderson sues Dr Hooper for the pain and suffering caused by the erythema multiforme, and the loss of earnings from the additional days she spent off work. This action succeeds: Dr Hooper owed her a duty of care; Dr Hooper breached that duty by prescribing her a drug to which he should have known she was sensitive; and the damages were a direct and reasonably foreseeable consequence of this.

In general, doctors owe a duty of care to all of their patients; they probably owe a duty of care to people they offer medical treatment to in 'good Samaritan' acts; and they may sometimes owe a duty of care to their patient's carers with whom they have had dealings. However, there is no duty of care to others with whom the doctor has no special or 'proximate' relationship, such as the patient's employer in Case 1.

Not all damage suffered by the plaintiff will be compensated for: the damage suffered must not be too remote from the breach of the duty of care. The usual test for remoteness applied by the courts is whether the damage was *reasonably foreseeable* (Wagon Mound 1961). Thus in Case 2 Dr Hooper cannot be liable for Mrs Anderson's injuries from the box falling on her, as this was not reasonably foreseeably a consequence of his actions.

A common area of disagreement in negligence actions is whether the doctor's actions or omissions amounted to a breach of the duty of care. In Case 3, this is reasonably straightforward: reactions to amoxicillin are common and Dr Hooper should know about them; it is also reasonable to expect Dr Hooper to check Mrs Anderson's notes before prescribing. The legal test used is whether the defendant did something which a 'prudent and reasonable' person would not do, or did not do something which a 'reasonable [person], guided [by ordinary] considerations' would do (Blyth 1856). In medical cases, the specific version of this test is known as the Bolam test: has the doctor 'acted in accordance with a

practice accepted as proper by a responsible body of [doctors] skilled in that particular art'? (Bolam 1957). For example, it is not negligent to use a new treatment that most doctors in the specialty might not use, provided that there is a responsible body of medical opinion in favour of the practice. The Bolam test has been reconsidered many times by the courts but has so far survived with only minor amendments (such as that the responsible body of medical opinion must have a 'logical basis': Bolitho 1997).

How the law of negligence applies to medical treatment has been controversial for many years, as it causes antagonism between patients and doctors, frequently leaves patients dissatisfied, and is expensively inefficient for both the NHS and doctors (or their defence associations). It is currently under review by the government and may be replaced with a no-fault administrative compensation system in the future.

Battery and other relevant laws

Two other areas of law are also relevant here. Firstly, if a doctor's treatment of a patient is grossly negligent and the patient dies (as, for example, was the case when an anaesthetist failed to recognize that a ventilator had been disconnected: R v Adomako 1994), the doctor can be prosecuted for manslaughter. Secondly, if a doctor examines a patient or gives a treatment which involves any form of physical contact and does not have the patient's informed consent to the procedure, the doctor may have committed battery, which is both a tort and a crime. Issues of consent are discussed in the next section.

CONSENT AND COMPETENCE

In order to carry out any procedure on a patient, a doctor must first ensure that the patient, if they are able to, has consented to the procedure. This applies to psychiatrists, although there are some complications related to the Mental Health Act, which are discussed in a later section. Imagine that a psychiatrist wishes to give a patient electroconvulsive therapy (ECT) for depression. Hearing the patient say 'yes' to the procedure, or signing a consent form (both of which are forms of *assent*) is not in itself consent – the psychiatrist must also be sure that the assent is valid before it becomes consent. The components of a valid consent are shown in Box 40.5; the criteria are identical for deciding whether a patient's refusal of consent is valid.

Box 40.5 Components of valid consent

For valid consent, the assent (or refusal) should be:
- un-coerced
- informed
- competent

Coercion and information

In this context, 'un-coerced' means that the person is free to make their decision without any undue influence or pressure from any other person (such as the patient's carer trying to bully the patient into refusing ECT because the carer has moral objections to it).

'Informed' means that the person has been given, or already has, all the information relevant to making a decision. This information must be given in a form appropriate to the person concerned: for instance, when giving information to a child or a learning-disabled patient, a doctor might have to use simpler and therefore less accurate language than when talking to an intelligent adult.

How much information to provide will depend on the nature and severity of the patient's condition, the complexity of the treatment, the risks of the treatment, and how much detail the patient wants to know – although the patient must be told enough to be able to make an informed decision, even if they say they do not want any detailed information. Some of the items that the General Medical Council recommends be covered are shown in Box 40.6.

Competence

As well as being provided with sufficient information, and being free to make their own decision, the patient must also be capable of making a decision – i.e. they must be competent. (In legal settings, competence is referred to as 'capacity'; the two terms are effectively interchangeable.) The components of competence are listed in Box 40.7; these are derived from a landmark High Court case (Re C 1994) and subsequent developments in the case law. However, the government has proposed a Mental Incapacity Bill, which if passed in the future would reform this area of law; the

---

Box 40.6 Types of information that will usually be required (General Medical Council 2001)

The purpose of the investigation or treatment

Details and uncertainties of the diagnosis

Options for treatment including the option not to treat

Explanation of the likely benefits and probabilities of success for each option

Known possible risks or side effects

The name of the doctor who will have overall responsibility

A reminder that the patient can change his or her mind at any time

---

Box 40.7 Components of competence

Comprehension and appreciation

Belief

Retention

Weighing in the balance

Expression

---

proposed definition of capacity is subtly different from the current definition. For more information, see the draft bill (Department for Constitutional Affairs 2003).

Comprehension and appreciation

Comprehension means that the patient must be able to understand, at an intellectual level, all the information that is relevant to making the decision. The depth of understanding does not have to be as great as the doctor's: a basic understanding of the key points is all that is required.

Appreciation refers to the ability to see the significance of the information, i.e. to relate it to one's own personal situation. In some situations, a certain amount of background knowledge or experience may be necessary in order to appreciate the information presented. For example, a young child or a person with a severe learning disability might comprehend 'death' and be able to explain that it means that a person 'isn't there any more', but might not have the maturity to be able to contemplate their own death as a possible consequence of a particular course of action.

Belief

This relates to an ability to use the information, and is most clearly illustrated by conditions in which this ability is impaired. For example, a patient with bipolar disorder might have the grandiose delusion that they were invincible and all-powerful. They might, therefore, disbelieve a doctor who told them that they had a heart condition that might kill them – and as a result refuse to accept treatment for it.

Retention

The information need only be retained for long enough to use it in making a decision. In relation to a decision to accept a cup of coffee, therefore, being able to remember the options available (e.g. white or black, with or without sugar) for a period of a few seconds will probably suffice. This would be possible, for instance, in a patient who had no anterograde memory because of hippocampal damage in Alzheimer's disease, but whose 'auditory loop' was intact. By contrast, a person wanting to make and complete the sale of a house might need to be able to hold a significant quantity of information in memory for several weeks or months.

Weighing in the balance

To do this, a person must be able to hold the arguments for and against a proposed course of action simultaneously in mind, and then aggregate them in some way in order to reach a decision. The *process* of aggregation has to be logical (in the sense that it cannot be based on schizophrenic magical reasoning, for instance), but the *outcome* (i.e. the decision reached) does not have to be one which others would regard as sensible or rational. It is well established that reaching an unwise decision does not, of itself, make a person incompetent.

Expression

This was not mentioned by the court in Re C, but is implicit in its decision (and was expressly noted as a requirement of capacity by the Law Commission in its 1997 report on mental incapacity). Any decision, no matter how carefully thought about, is of no use unless the person concerned can express it in some way to those around them. This communication might be verbal (oral or written), or nonverbal (such as a nod of the head), or implied by a person's actions (such as reaching for the sugar when offered an unsweetened cup of coffee).

Children

Unlike adults, children under the age of 16 are not presumed by the law to be competent; the default situation is that a parent must give or refuse consent on their behalf. However, children under 16 can be competent to give consent if they have 'sufficient understanding and intelligence to... understand fully what is proposed' (Gillick 1985). The courts have refused to clarify what this means, stating that it is up to the doctor to decide whether a child is Gillick-competent or not; it is suggested that the criteria for competence in Box 40.7 should be applied to make this decision. A Gillick-competent child can consent to treatment even if the parents refuse; however, a parent's consent can override a child's refusal of consent even if that child is Gillick-competent (Re W 1993); and even if both child and parents refuse, the doctor can still apply to the High Court for permission to proceed in the child's best interests (something which is not a possibility when the patient is an adult).

To complicate matters further, the situation is different for children aged 16 or 17. The Family Law Reform Act 1969 states that 16- and 17-year-olds are, like adults, presumed to be competent unless they are shown not to be, and allows them to consent to treatment in their own right. However, Re W explicitly applies to 16- and 17-year olds, so parents can override the child's refusal of consent as with children under 16.

This is the legal situation at the time of writing. However, the Human Rights Act 1998 has come into force since these judgments, and it is possible that the current right of parents to override a competent child's consent will be overturned in a future case brought under the Act. Furthermore, if the proposed Mental Incapacity Bill (Department for Constitutional Affairs 2003) is enacted, 16- and 17-year-olds will be treated as full adults for these purposes.

If the patient is incompetent

When an adult patient cannot consent for themselves, nobody has the right to consent on their behalf. Instead, the common law – that is, law that results from the decisions of higher courts, rather than from Acts of Parliament – governs what happens when a patient is found to be incompetent. In this situation, the doctrine of necessity applies. As described by Lord Goff in Re F (1990),

(1) there is 'a necessity to act when it is not practicable to communicate with the assisted person,' i.e. when they are incompetent; and

(2) 'the action taken must be such as a reasonable person would in all circumstances take, acting in the best interests of the assisted person'.

The House of Lords has gone on to make it clear that the common law doctrine of necessity covers all situations where a patient is incompetent (such as long-term nursing home care of a patient with Alzheimer's dementia), not just emergency situations (Bournewood 1998).

The General Medical Council (GMC) has suggested that a number of factors must be taken into account when deciding what is in the best interests of the 'assisted person.' These are listed in Box 40.8. Note that although the views of others may provide useful information, they are not binding: the decision is the doctor's.

If the proposed Mental Incapacity Bill (Department for Constitutional Affairs 2003) is made law, it will replace the doctrine of necessity for incompetent patients, and will require doctors to take account of factors such as those in the GMC's list.

Emergency situations

The law governing emergency situations is the same as that described in the sections above. If the patient is known to be competent, their consent must be sought for any care and treatment; if known to be incompetent, the common law doctrine of necessity applies. However, in an emergency it may not be possible to assess a patient's competence, or to give the information that would be required to make an informed decision. In such an emergency, a doctor can provide treatment 'limited to what is immediately necessary to save life or avoid significant deterioration in the patient's

---

Box 40.8 Factors to consider when deciding what is in a patient's best interests (General Medical Council 2001)

Options for treatment or investigation which are clinically indicated

Any evidence of the patient's previously expressed preferences, including an advance statement

Your own and the health care team's knowledge of the patient's background, such as cultural, religious, or employment considerations

Views about the patient's preferences given by a third party who may have other knowledge of the patient, for example the patient's partner, family or carer

Which option least restricts the patient's future choices, where more than one option (including nontreatment) seems reasonable in the patient's best interest

health' (General Medical Council 2001), unless that treatment conflicts with the terms of a valid advance directive. As soon as the patient is competent and there is time to give information, they must be told what has been done and their consent must be sought for any further treatment.

Fluctuating competence and advance directives

Competence is not static: a patient can be competent to make one sort of decision and not competent to make another, and even with respect to a single decision, they may be competent at one time and not at another (for instance, this is common in the early stages of Alzheimer's dementia where there are periods of lucidity). In these situations, it may be possible to increase the chance that a patient will be competent at any given time: in the case of the patient with Alzheimer's dementia, for example, this might mean interviewing them at a time of day when they are their most alert, conducting the interview in a comfortable, quiet and familiar environment, and ensuring a trusted relative or friend is present.

When a previously competent patient becomes in-competent, it is permissible to continue to rely on consent given when they were competent; it is preferable to have recorded the consent, and the fact of their competence at the time, in writing (General Medical Council 2001). When the patient becomes competent again, their consent should be reviewed with them before treatment continues.

When a competent patient anticipates future incompetence, they may make a formal record of their future wishes in an advance directive. Provided that the directive is sufficiently clearly worded and specifically covers the proposed treatment, doctors are probably legally bound to respect it, although this has not yet been tested in court in the UK. If the proposed Mental Incapacity Bill (Department for Constitutional Affairs 2003) comes into effect, advance directives will be made binding on doctors, and rules will be established for determining whether they are valid.

THE MENTAL HEALTH ACT 1983

This is the chief piece of legislation affecting psychiatrists in England and Wales. Independently of the common law powers described above, it empowers psychiatrists to detain certain patients for assessment and treatment, and to give them certain sorts of treatment without their consent. A breakdown of the parts and sections of the Act is shown in Box 40.9. A discussion of all sections of the Act is beyond the scope of this chapter; for full details, refer to Jones (2002), or to the Mental Health Act Online (Institute of Mental Health Act Practitioners 2003).

Box 40.9 Principal sections of the Mental Health Act

Part II – compulsory admission to hospital and guardianship

Section 2: admission for assessment

Section 3: admission for treatment

Section 4: emergency admission for assessment

Section 5: detention of an informal inpatient

Section 7: guardianship

Section 12: approval of doctors to use the Act

Section 17: leave of absence from hospital

Section 25a: supervised discharge from hospital

Part III – patients concerned with criminal proceedings

This part provides for patients to be sent to mental hospital from court and from prison (see Chapter 30)

Part IV – consent to treatment

Section 57: treatments requiring consent and a second opinion (e.g. psychosurgery)

Section 58: treatments requiring consent or a second opinion (e.g. ECT, long-term antipsychotic treatment)

Section 62: urgent treatment

Part V – Mental Health Review Tribunals

This part provides for a system to allow patients to appeal against their detention

Part X – miscellaneous

Section 135: warrant to search for and remove patients

Section 136: mentally disordered persons found in public places

---

Principles: the basis for detention

As explained above, the basis for authorizing treatment under the common law doctrine of necessity is that the patient is incompetent. However, the basis for detention under the Act largely ignores competence. The criteria for detention for treatment under Section 3 of the Act are shown in Box 40.10; the specific criteria vary slightly for other sections, but the principles are the same.

The basis for detention is an uneasy compromise between the patient's individual needs (as assessed by the professionals – not as seen by the patient themselves) and society's desire to stop patients harming themselves or others. It is also biased towards hospital treatment. The current Mental Health Act is being reviewed by the government; during the consultation process, some have suggested a Medical Incapacity Act (e.g. Zigmond 1998), which would merge the Mental Health Act with the proposed Mental Incapacity Act, to create a single regime based purely on competence (i.e. the patient's individual needs) that applies to all treatments with no distinction between mental and physical illness. However, the government has proposed moving the basis for detention in the opposite direction, in favour of public protection (Department of Health 2002): if the proposed Mental Health Bill is enacted, detention will be allowed solely in order to

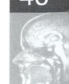

> **Box 40.10   Criteria for detention under Section 3 of the Mental Health Act**
>
> The patient must have a mental illness (or certain other disorders)
>
> The disorder must be severe enough ('of a nature or degree') to need treatment in hospital
>
> Voluntary treatment is not appropriate (usually because the patient is refusing admission)
>
> Detention in hospital is necessary in the interests of:
>
> - the patient's health, and/or
> - the patient's safety (for example, to stop them committing suicide), and/or
> - other people's safety (for example if the patient is violent)
>
> Two appropriate doctors (usually a psychiatrist approved under the Act and another doctor who knows the patient) and an approved social worker agree on using the Section

protect others, if the risk of harm is great enough; and compulsion will extend to treatment in the community. For a discussion of the issues raised, see the Mental Health Review website (Royal College of Psychiatrists 2003).

Key provisions

A few of the Sections of the Act listed in Box 40.9 will be commonly encountered, and you should be familiar with them.

- **Section 2:** allows a person meeting the criteria in Box 40.10 to be detained for up to 28 days for assessment of their condition. They may be suspected of having any mental disorder (including delirium or intoxication where there is diagnostic confusion, but not including substance misuse or sexual disorders in isolation).
- **Section 3:** allows a person meeting the criteria in Box 40.10 to be detained for up to six months for treatment. Unlike Section 2, it can be renewed. Only specified categories of mental disorder can be grounds for detention: mental illness, psychopathic disorder (roughly speaking, a legal term for personality disorder) and mental impairment (learning disability). If the patient falls into one of the latter categories, they can only be detained if their condition is treatable.
- **Section 4:** provides for an emergency procedure when only one doctor is available and the admission cannot be delayed. The patient must still meet the other criteria in Box 40.10. It only authorizes detention for up to 72 hours, but can be extended to 28 days if a second doctor later recommends this.
- **Section 5:** is a similar emergency procedure for use when the patient has already been admitted to hospital (i.e. is on a ward – being in A&E does not count as having been admitted). Section 5(4) allows a senior nurse to detain the patient for up to six hours to see a doctor; Section 5(2) allows a nominated doctor to detain the patient for up to 72 hours so that an assessment for Section 2 or 3 can take place.

- **Sections 7 and 25a:** these sections (guardianship and supervised discharge) are very similar: both allow for an outpatient to be monitored by a community supervisor (usually a community psychiatric nurse (CPN) or social worker). The supervisor has the power to require the patient to live in a particular place, to go to other places for medical treatment, education, or occupation, and to let the supervisor in to see them. Note that the supervisor does not have the power to make the patient accept treatment – just to take them to the place of treatment.
- **Sections 57, 58 and 62:** these sections deal with treatment. For up to three months, doctors can give patients treatments for mental disorder (not for other conditions) without consent; after three months, if the patient still refuses consent, treatment can only continue if an independent doctor agrees that the treatment is necessary. However, some treatments are exceptions to this, and from the start can only be given if the patient consents or if there is a second opinion in favour (e.g. ECT); other treatments require both consent and a second opinion (e.g. psychosurgery). However, Section 62 allows such treatments to begin immediately if they are urgently needed to save the patient's life or prevent serious deterioration.
- **Sections 135 and 136:** give the police powers to take people whom they suspect are mentally unwell to a place of safety (usually A&E or a psychiatric assessment unit, sometimes the police station). The latter covers people found in a public place; the former allows the police, acting with a doctor and a social worker who has obtained a magistrate's order, to break into private property to remove a person suspected of being mentally unwell.

Involuntary patients not covered by the Act

In recent years, the courts have become more aware that there is a group of patients who are not giving informed consent to treatment, but are not detained under the Act (see, most notably, Bournewood 1998). These involuntary informal patients are treated indefinitely under common law; none of the safeguards against abuse (such as appeals tribunals or managers' hearings) which exist for patients detained under the Act apply to them. It has been estimated that this applied to approximately 22 000 people in 1998. Part 5 of the Mental Health Bill (Department of Health 2003), if it becomes law, will provide basic safeguards for this group of patients without requiring them to be formally detained.

The Care Programme Approach (CPA)

This is a set of policies introduced by the Department of Health in 1991 and made more extensive and binding in 1999

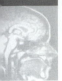
(Department of Health 1999a). The key features of the CPA are shown in Box 40.11 (see Chapter 29).

Box 40.11 The main element of the Care Programme Approach (CPA)

Systematic arrangements for assessing the health and social needs of people accepted into specialist mental health services

The formation of a care plan which identifies the health and social care required from a variety of providers

The appointment of a care coordinator to keep in close touch with the service user and to monitor and coordinate care

Regular review and, where necessary, agreed changes to the care plan

---

OTHER ACTS RELEVANT TO PSYCHIATRY

A number of other laws have particular application to mentally unwell patients. These are summarized in Box 40.12 and explained briefly below.

Box 40.12 Subjects of other laws relevant to psychiatry

Appointeeship
Powers of attorney
The Court of Protection
Driving
Marriage
Voting
Jury service
Making contracts
Child protection
Confidentiality and record-keeping

Protecting vulnerable patients

Three main systems exist for protecting the financial interests of patients who are unable to look after those interests themselves:

- **Appointeeship:** if it decides that a person claiming benefits is unable to act for themselves, the Benefits Agency has the power to appoint somebody who is in regular contact with the claimant and is acceptable to them, to manage their benefits on their behalf.
- **Powers of attorney:** a person who is at present competent, but who anticipates that they will become incompetent, can sign an Enduring Power of Attorney, which allows a nominated person to act for them in their financial affairs. It can come into effect immediately, or whenever the person becomes incompetent. If the Mental Incapacity Bill (Department for Constitutional Affairs 2003) is made law, these will be replaced with Lasting Powers of Attorney, which will allow the

nominated person to make decisions on welfare and health care matters as well as financial ones.

- **The Court of Protection:** when a person who has not previously signed a power of attorney becomes incompetent, the Court of Protection can appoint a receiver to manage their financial affairs – although this is only usually necessary if their affairs are complicated or no informal agreement can be reached on what is in the person's best interests under common law. The process is complicated and bureaucratic and the costs are deducted from the incompetent person's estate. If the Mental Incapacity Bill (Department for Constitutional Affairs 2003) becomes law, the Court's procedures will be simplified, and the new Court-appointed deputies will be able to make welfare and health care decisions as well as financial ones.

Social activities

Mentally unwell people are sometimes prevented from taking part in activities that affect the rest of society, or are made subject to special conditions. These activities include driving, marriage, voting, jury service and entering into contracts:

- **Driving:** the Driver and Vehicle Licensing Agency (DVLA) requires all drivers to inform it of any medical or related condition that might affect fitness to drive (or that the treatment for which might affect fitness to drive). The rules are complicated; they can be found on the DVLA website (Driver and Vehicle Licensing Agency 2003). As an example, a person who is currently psychotic cannot drive; a person with bipolar disorder who has had several episodes cannot drive until they have been well for more than six months and DVLA has given permission; and a person with an anxiety disorder can drive without DVLA needing to be informed. The duty to inform the DVLA rests with the patient concerned; patients are often understandably reluctant to reveal their illness or treatment to the DVLA, as they know (or fear) that they will be told they are not allowed to drive. This can put their GP or psychiatrist in a difficult position. Guidance from the General Medical Council (2001) states that, if the patient cannot be persuaded to inform the DVLA, and if the doctor reasonably believes that they are continuing to drive, the doctor must disclose the patient's condition to the medical advisor at the DVLA.
- **Marriage:** the Marriage Act 1983 only allows persons with 'sufficient mental capacity' to marry. However, the courts have held that the degree of competence required to marry is very low indeed – a basic understanding of marriage meaning that a man and a woman will stay together indefinitely will suffice. If a person is subsequently found to have had 'unsoundness of mind',

which meant that they lacked this capacity when they married, the marriage can be annulled.

- **Voting in elections:** under the common law, the returning officer must satisfy himself that a voter is competent to discriminate amongst the candidates, and to perform other tasks associated with voting, before he can allow them to vote. This capacity test is strict enough to exclude a number of severely mentally disordered people – but it is almost never enforced. In addition, patients who are detained in mental hospitals following conviction or certain other court orders are disbarred from voting. However, informal patients and those detained under part II of the Mental Health Act are now allowed to register to vote using the hospital as their address, provided they have been in hospital for a sufficient period.

- **Jury service:** the Juries Act 1974 contains very broad restrictions on jury service: any person who 'suffers or has suffered from... mental disorder... and on account of that condition either (a) is resident in a hospital or other similar institution; or (b) regularly attends for treatment by a medical practitioner OR is under guardianship OR [is] 'incapable' of managing his financial affairs, is prevented from serving on a jury. This includes, for example, a person who had a first episode of depression three months ago, has fully recovered, and is taking antidepressants for a further six months (a minimum recommendation to prevent a recurrence).

- **Entering into contracts:** in general, a person is bound by any contracts they make even if mentally unwell at the time. The only exception to this is that a person can be released from a contract by the court if they can demonstrate that it was not a contract for the 'necessaries' of life (a term defined by the Sale of Goods Act 1893), that they did not understand what they were doing or were otherwise incompetent to make the contract, and that the other party to the contract was unaware that they were incompetent.

Child protection

A full discussion of the law relating to child protection, which is relevant to psychiatrists working in the child and family field, is beyond the scope of this chapter. However, psychiatrists working with adult patients will often come into contact with their patients' children. In this situation, they have a duty to work in partnership with social services

Box 40.13 Characteristics of good records
Clear
Identifiable (i.e. patient's name, date of birth, your name, etc.)
Objective
Contemporary
Original and unaltered
Signed and dated

Box 40.14 Situations in which confidential information might be released (General Medical Council 2001)
Education
Research
Clinical audit
Public health monitoring
Administration and planning
Public interest disclosure

and other agencies to ensure that the children are properly assessed and have their needs met; and, if they suspect abuse, they have a duty to report this. Further information can be found in the publications *Working Together* (Department of Health 1999b) and *What to do if you're worried a child is being abused* (Department of Health 2003).

Confidentiality and record-keeping

All doctors have a duty, both ethically and under the law, to keep information they receive from patients confidential within the team of professionals caring for that patient. This includes keeping good records of that information (see Box 40.13). Patient information is regulated by the Data Protection Act 1998, and psychiatrists working within the NHS have to comply with policies produced by their local 'Caldicott guardian,' who is responsible for ensuring that confidential patient information is handled appropriately.

There are, however, situations where it may be permissible to release confidential information. These are listed in Box 40.14. The first five situations are rarely controversial. In these, patients' consent to the disclosure must be sought wherever practicable; if it is not practicable, disclosure may still be acceptable provided that the information is anonymized and its disclosure has no personal consequences for the patient, and occasionally in other situations.

Public interest disclosure is more problematic. This covers situations where there is a benefit to others or to society at large which outweighs the patient's interest in keeping the information confidential (and society's interest in being able to trust doctors to keep information confidential) – such as the prevention or detection of serious crime, the protection of vulnerable children, and protecting other road users from a dangerous driver. Full guidance on specific situations can be found in the General Medical Council's booklet *The Duties of a Doctor: Confidentiality* (General Medical Council 2001)

REFERENCES

Bloch S, Chodoff P & Green SA (eds) (1999) *Psychiatric Ethics*, 3rd edn. Oxford: Oxford University Press.
Bolam v Friern Hospital Management Committee [1957] 2 All ER 118.
Bolitho v City & Hackney Health Authority [1997] 4 All ER 771.

Bournewood (1998) In Re L (by his next friend GE). Online. Available at: www.publications.parliament.uk/pa/ld199798/ldjudgmt/jd980625/inrel01.htm [Accessed 20 September 2003].

Blyth v Birmingham Waterworks [1856] 156 ER 1047.

Childress J & Beauchamp TL (1994) Chapters 3–6 in *Principles of Biomedical Ethics*, 4th edn. New York: Oxford University Press.

Department for Constitutional Affairs (2003) Draft Mental Incapacity Bill. Cm 5859-i. Online. Available at: www.lcd.gov.uk/menincap/legis.htm [Accessed 20 September 2003].

Department of Health (1999a) *Effective Care Co-ordination in Mental Health Services: Modernising the Care Programme Approach: A Policy Booklet*. Online. Available at: www.doh.gov.uk/nsf/polbook.htm [Accessed 20 September 2003].

Department of Health (1999b) *Working Together to Safeguard Children: Government Guidance on Inter-agency Co-operation*. Online. Available at: www.doh.gov.uk/quality5.htm [Accessed 20 September 2003].

Department of Health (2002) *Draft Mental Health Bill*. Cm 5538-i. Online. Available at: www.doh.gov.uk/mentalhealth/draftbill2002/index.htm [Accessed 20 September 2003].

Department of Health (2003) *What to do if you're worried a child is being abused: Children's Services Guidance*. Online. Available at: www.doh.gov.uk/safeguardingchildren/index.htm [Accessed 20 September 2003].

Driver and Vehicle Licensing Agency (2003) *Medical Rules*. Online. Available at: www.dvla.gov.uk/at_a_glance/content.htm [Accessed 20 September 2003].

Fulford KWM, Gillett G & Soskice JM (eds) (1994) *Medicine and Moral Reasoning*. Cambridge: Cambridge University Press.

Gillick v West Norfolk and Wisbech Area Health Authority [1985] 3 All ER 403.

General Medical Council (2001) *Good Medical Practice: The Duties of a Doctor*. Online. Available at: www.gmc-uk.org/standards/guidance.htm [Accessed 20 September 2003].

Institute of Mental Health Act Practitioners (2003) *The Mental Health Act Online*. Online. Available at: www.markwalton.net/guidemha/index.asp [Accessed 20 September 2003].

Jones R (2002) *Mental Health Act Manual*, 8th edn. London: Sweet & Maxwell.

Law Commission (1997) *Who Decides? Making Decisions on Behalf of Mentally Incapacitated Adults*. Cm 3803. London: TSO.

Re C (Adult: Refusal of Treatment) [1994] 1 WLR 290.

Re F (Mental Patient: Sterilisation) [1990] 2 AC 1 at 75H.

Re W (A minor) (Wardship: Medical Treatment) [1993] Fam 64.

Royal College of Psychiatrists (2000) *Good Psychiatric Practice*. Council Report CR83. Online. Available at: www.rcpsych.ac.uk/publications/cr/cr83.htm [Accessed 20 September 2003].

Royal College of Psychiatrists (2003) *Reform of the Mental Health Act 1983*. Online. Available at: www.rcpsych.ac.uk/college/parliament/MHBill.htm [Accessed 20 September 2003].

R v Adomako [1994] 5 Med LR 277.

Temkin O & Temkin C (eds) (1967) *Ancient Medicine: Selected Papers of Ludwig Edelstein*. Baltimore, MD: Johns Hopkins University Press.

Wagon Mound No.1: Overseas Tankship (UK) Ltd v Morts Dock & Engineering Co [1961] AC 388.

World Medical Association (1968) *Declaration of Geneva: International Code of Medical Ethics*. Online. Available at: www.wma.net/e/policy/c8.htm [Accessed 20 September 2003].

World Medical Association (1983) *Declaration of Madrid: Ethical Guidelines for the Practice of Psychiatry*. Paris: World Medical Association.

World Medical Association (2000) *Declaration of Helsinki: Ethical Principles for Medical Research Involving Human Subjects*. Online. Available at: www.wma.net/e/policy/b3.htm [Accessed 20 September 2003].

Zigmond AS (1998) Medical incapacity act. *Psychiatric Bulletin* **22**: 657–8.

Index

N.B. page numbers in **bold** denote material in tables or boxes, and page numbers in *italic* denote material in figures, where there is no textual reference to the material on the same page.